Orthofix External Fixation
in Trauma and Orthopaedics

Springer

London
Berlin
Heidelberg
New York
Barcelona
Hong Kong
Milan
Paris
Singapore
Tokyo

Giovanni De Bastiani, A. Graham Apley and Anthony Goldberg (Eds)

Orthofix External Fixation

in Trauma and Orthopaedics

Springer

Anthony Goldberg MBBS, MPharm, FFPM
Group Medical Director, Orthofix® srl
Via delle Nazioni, 9
37012 Bussolengo (Verona), Italy

ISBN-13:978-1-4471-1178-8
British Library Cataloguing in Publication Data
Orthofix external fixation in trauma and orthopaedics
1. External skeletal fixation (Surgery)
I. De Bastiani, Giovanni II. Apley, A. Graham (Alan Graham)
III. Goldberg, Anthony
617.1'5
ISBN-13:978-1-4471-1178-8

Library of Congress Cataloging-in-Publication Data
Orthofix external fixation in trauma and orthopaedics / Giovanni De Bastiani, A. Graham Apley, and Anthony Goldberg, eds.
p. ; cm.
Includes bibliographical reference and index.
ISBN-13:978-1-4471-1178-8 e-ISBN-13:978-1-4471-0691-3
DOI: 10.1007/978-1-4471-0691-3

1. Fracture fixation. 2. Bone lengthening (Orthopedics) I. Title: Orthofix external fixation. II. De Bastiani, Giovanni, 1921– III. Apley, A. Graham (Alan Graham) IV. Goldberg, A. A. J. (Anthony Aaron Joseph)
[DNLM: 1. External Fixators. 2. Bone Lengthening—methods. 3. Fracture Fixation—methods. WE 185 O615 2000]
RD103.E88.O78 2000
617.1'5—dc21

00-020079

Softcover reprint of the hardcover 1st edition 2000

Project-managed, designed and typeset by Bookcraft Ltd, Stroud, UK

28/3830-543210 Printed on acid-free paper SPIN 10135784

Contents

Preface

The philosophy of external fixation has changed dramatically over the past few decades. Wide usage in the earlier part of the last century, often for inappropriate indications, coupled with a lack of appreciation of the biomechanics of fracture healing, served to highlight the problems which could be associated with the technique when transfixing pins and multibar structures conferring uncompromising rigidity were employed. With these early systems the results frequently compounded the conditions they were intended to treat; pin track infection, which could proceed to osteomyelitis, and worse still, to amputation in some instances, was seen as a major drawback and the incidence of non-union was high. This came to a head with use of the then available frames during World War II, and led the US Surgeon General to put an embargo on the use of external fixation devices in the United States.

All this was to change, however, due largely to the vision of one man, whose training and expertise spanned the disciplines of both physiology and orthopaedics. Giovanni De Bastiani knew instinctively, that designed intelligently and applied appropriately, external fixation could be used to complement the natural processes of fracture repair. He directed his energies to this end, and working with Giovanni Faccioli, a precision engineer, he produced, in the late 1970s, the first prototype Orthofix Dynamic Axial fixator. This was a lightweight, monolateral device with tapered, non-transfixing bone screws, which could introduce micromovement and loading at the fracture site at the correct points in the healing cycle, to encourage the development and maturation of bridging callus. The concept of "dynamization" was born. Fracture healing was expedited, and pin track infection appreciated as something that could be controlled, if not entirely eradicated.

Things did not stop here. If they had, there would have been no need for this book. De Bastiani and his team in Verona developed and tested a series of modular attachments to the standard range of fixators for the treatment of more complex fractures of the long bones and the pelvis. At the same time they realized that the monolateral fixator could, with minimal modification, be used to distract and manipulate the callus formed in response to a deliberately produced osteotomy. Suddenly it became possible to lengthen limbs with congenital or traumatic shortening and to correct deformity using material generated within the body itself in response to an applied stimulus. The influence of the Verona school spread rapidly, fostered by regular seminars held in Verona, and attended by surgeons from all parts of the world.

Wide usage brought with it an abundance of ideas from practising surgeons, many of which were tested and subsequently incorporated within the Orthofix range. These included fixators which could be used in association with fractures in and around the wrist, elbow, knee and ankle and which would permit early mobilization of the joints, and miniature fixators to treat fractures of the digits. Improvements to the original lengthening device with the introduction of a highly versatile modular rail construct has had a major impact on limb salvage and reconstruction, and the recently developed hybrid fixation system has combined the best features of both monolateral and circular fixation.

The present volume is intended as a tribute to Giovanni De Bastiani. It brings together, for the first time, the in-depth experience of scientists and surgeons throughout the world, whose practices in all areas of orthopaedic trauma and limb reconstruction have been influenced and enhanced by the devices he conceived and made available. They have themselves, in addition, been responsible in many instances, for major developments in devices and techniques based upon his original ideas.

Anthony Goldberg

Giovanni De Bastiani

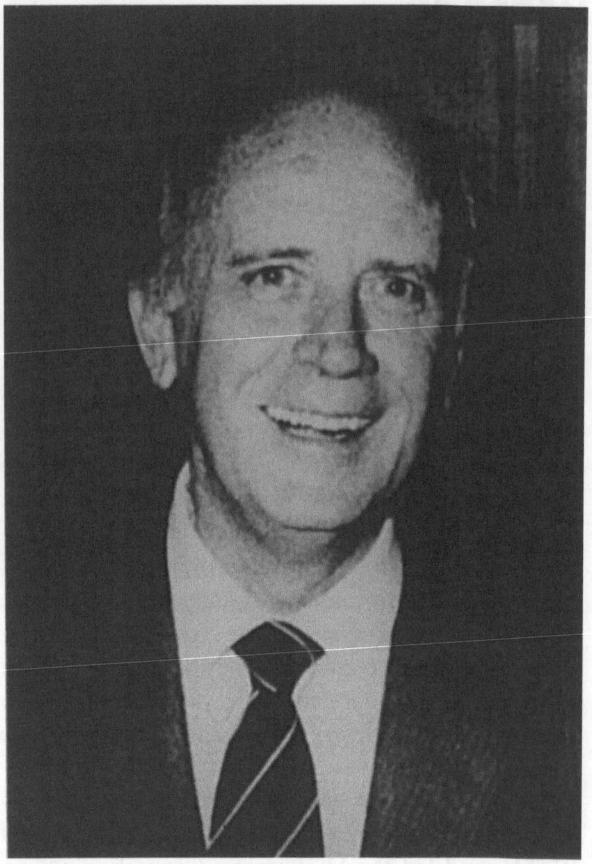

Giovanni De Bastiani was born in Bari, Italy on 24 May 1921. He qualified in medicine at the University of Padua in 1947 and in 1949 became an assistant in the department of Human Physiology. In 1954 he was appointed Professor of Human Physiology, and in the same year began a clinical appointment with Professor C. Pais in the Orthopaedic Clinic of the University of Genoa.

In 1957 he completed specialist training in trauma and orthopaedics, and started working with Professor Casuccio in the Orthopaedic Department of the University of Padua. In 1959 he was made Professor of Orthopaedics in the University and received a number of distinction awards over the succeeding years for his scientific and clinical work. In 1970 he became Head of the Department of Trauma and Orthopaedics in the newly-built hospital of Borgo Roma in Verona.

Possessed of an open and enquiring mind, he was always ready to explore and evaluate new methods of treatment spanning a wide range of conditions. His initial work in Verona centred on problems involving the hip in children and adults, and in the design of improved forms of prostheses for both idiopathic and acquired forms of hip disease. During this time he also developed a strong interest in the factors involved in fracture repair, bringing his formidable background in physiology to bear in an appreciation of the problems involved and the ways in which these might be addressed. His dissatisfaction with existing forms of osteosynthesis, coupled with his belief in the value of external fixation as a valid treatment modality, dictated the subsequent course of his research.

Between 1978 and 1979 he established a group with clinical and engineering expertise to study in depth the problems associated with external fixation which at this time was still regarded as a treatment of last resort. This was a direct result of the many problems experienced by other workers due to the biomechanical inadequacy of existing frames and problems at the pin–bone interface, which were associated with a high incidence of non-union and infection. This research led to the concept of "dynamization" to promote callus formation and consolidation, and culminated in the development of the first Dynamic Axial Fixator. This was designed specifically to answer many of the current criticisms of external fixation and was the forerunner of the Orthofix range of external fixators. De Bastiani and his group in Verona have subsequently published many papers on the safe use of external fixation in a range of trauma indications and have had a major influence in altering the perception of this method of treatment by the orthopaedic fraternity.

De Bastiani also established a firm place for external fixation in many other orthopaedic indications. Many of these are a direct result of his development of the technique of "callotasis", or callus distraction, which has had a major impact on the treatment of limb length inequality and bone loss.

Giovanni De Bastiani retired in 1991, but the work he initiated continues to be developed and refined in many parts of the world.

Lodovico Renzi Brivio
Director, Department of Orthopaedics and Traumatology
Carlo Poma Hospital, Mantua, Italy

Alan Graham Apley

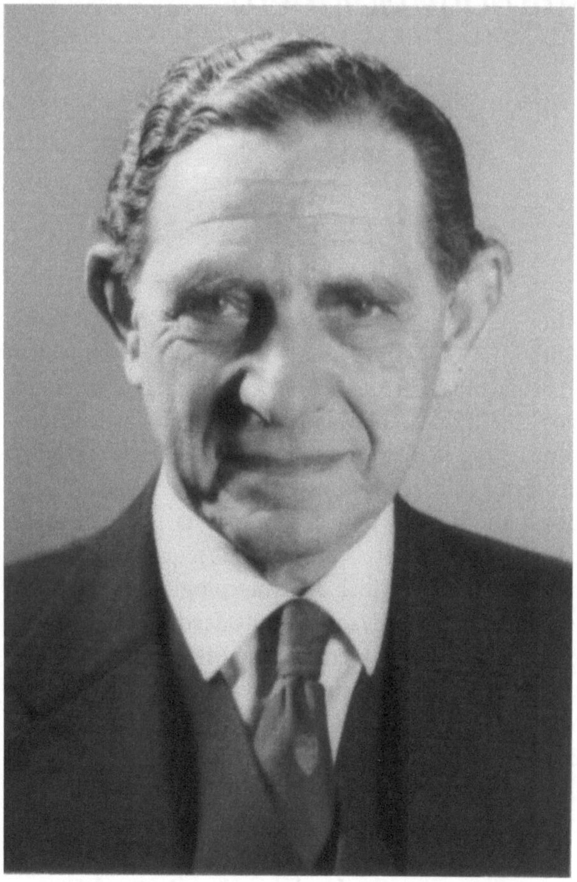

While those contributing to this book are presenting their wealth of experience in the treatment of fractures and their complications, it is impossible to think of fracture healing without acknowledging the influence of Alan Apley. He was, without doubt, one of the most charismatic figures in orthopaedics in the twentieth century. He left an indelible impression on the practice of orthopaedic surgery and on all those who read his works, met him on teaching courses, or heard him speak at meetings.

In his early professional life Alan Apley served with the Army, being invalided out in 1947. In that year he was appointed as a consultant at the Rowley Bristow Orthopaedic Hospital near London, and also at St Thomas' Hospital in London. In these early days he worked with George Perkins whose leitmotif was the functional treatment of fractures. This philosophy profoundly influenced Alan Apley, who throughout his life campaigned for treatment of "the whole patient" when confronted with any fracture. One of his major contributions was to emphasize the importance of physiological loading as an essential component of the early, as well as the later treatment of fractures; joints must be used as soon as possible after injury to a limb, and the bone and fracture loaded.

Alan Apley also recognised the need to be able to convey knowledge to others. He was a brilliant teacher. His lectures, chairmanships and communications by the written word gripped his audience or reader, and many have improved their teaching by listening to Alan Apley. As Editor of the *Journal of Bone and Joint Surgery* he was also able to help authors to transform dry scientific papers into concise, precise and readable form. Thousands of surgeons attended his courses held at weekends at Pyrford Hospital near London and his enthusiasm steered many of these embryonic surgeons towards orthopaedics.

In individual dicussions Alan Apley would give you all his attention. As a very junior registrar I visited his hospital on a Sunday morning with one other similarly trained registrar, and Alan Apley went round his patients teaching two junior visitors for two and a half hours.

Much of his teaching concerned the assessment of patients with fractures and the proper treatment of these. He had a special interest in external fixation. This form of treatment allows minimally invasive surgery to be carried out at the site of a wound, and enables limbs to function early after injury. His teaching would stress that skilful and meticulous care was needed in order for the treatment to fulfil its possibilities for the individual patient.

This book comprises articles which convey the subtle influences of both Alan Apley and Giovanni De Bastiani on all its authors and is a worthy tribute to their outstanding impact on orthopaedic surgery.

John Kenwright
Nuffield Professor of Orthopaedics,
Nuffield Orthopaedic Centre, Oxford

Anthony Goldberg

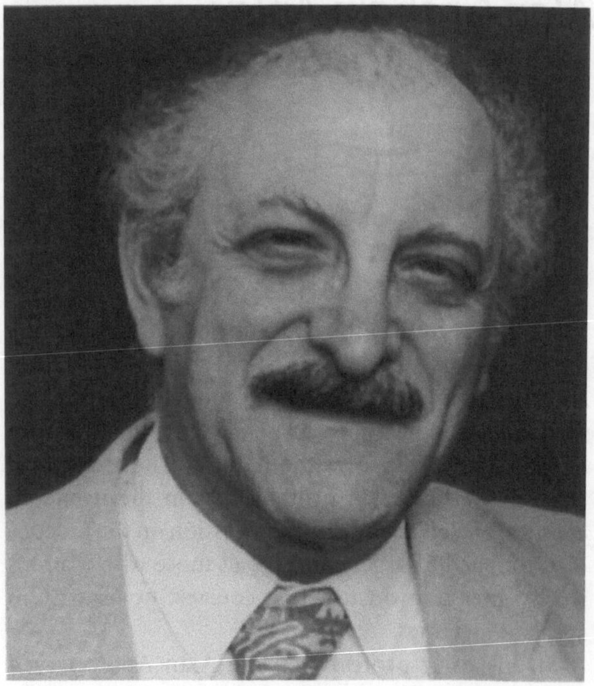

After graduating in Pharmacy at London University, Anthony Goldberg spent a year in the Department of Pharmacology, at the School of Pharmacy, where he carried out research into the properties of fast and slow contracting skeletal muscle under the supervision of Professor G. A. H. Buttle and Professor W. C. Bowman. He was awarded an MPharm for a thesis based on this research, and was subsequently elected a member of the British Pharmacological Society. He was then offered a place to study Medicine at University College Hospital, graduating MBBS in 1966.

He entered the Pharmaceutical Industry in 1968 as Medical Adviser to the Research Department of the Boots Company in Nottingham. Here he was involved in the design and implementation of some of the first clinical studies of ibuprofen in the rheumatic diseases. He additionally held honorary clinical posts in Rheumatology at the Hackney Hospital, and later at Chase Farm Hospital, the Prince of Wales Hospital and the North Middlesex Hospital and was elected to membership of the British Society for Rheumatology. He was also at that time visiting lecturer in the Department of Pharmacology at Strathclyde University in Glasgow, where he lectured on clinical trial methodology. A natural-born communicator, he also played a major role within the Boots Company in the training of sales personnel and lectured to Medical audiences on many occasions.

In 1972 he was appointed Head of Clinical Research, UK with the Boots Company, where, in addition to his clinical responsibilities, he worked closely with both the Marketing and Regulatory Affairs Departments.

He left the Boots Company in 1973 to become an Independent Medical Consultant to the Pharmaceutical and Healthcare Industries. During the succeeding years he controlled major projects for several companies, including Reckitt and Colman, Hydron Europe, Electrobiology Limited and Pharmax. He was elected to the Board of Pharmax in 1982 as a non-executive director and was acting Medical Director for fourteen years. In 1980 he was elected a member of the British Institute of Regulatory Affairs (BIRA).

In 1983, through his connections with Electrobiology, he was introduced to Orthofix External Fixation in Verona and met Professor De Bastiani for the first time. His relationship with the Italian Company developed over the ensuing period, and when the Company was acquired by an international consortium in 1987, he was appointed Medical Director. In 1989 he was elected a Founder Fellow of the Faculty of Pharmaceutical Medicine of the Royal Colleges of Physicians.

In addition to his responsibility for clinical research, he has been heavily involved in the creation of technical and promotional material. His ongoing commitment to surgeon training in external fixation techniques has enabled him to play a major role in the development of the basic and advanced seminars for surgeons which are held regularly in Verona, and he chaired these courses personally for a number of years. He was also responsible for coordinating the annual courses in external fixation in trauma and orthopaedics at the Royal College of Surgeons of England. As Group Medical Director of the expanding family of Orthofix companies, he maintains his interest in all these areas.

He has edited or co-edited the proceedings of many scientific congresses, meetings and seminars throughout his career in the industry.

James Richardson
Professor of Orthopaedics, Keele University, UK

Contributors

E. Alcivar A.
Director
Clinica Alcivar
Guayaquil, Equador

Roberto Aldegheri
Associate Professor
Institute of Clinical Orthopaedics and Traumatology
(Director: Prof. B. Bartolozzi)
University of Verona
Verona, Italy

F. Ali
Specialist Registrar in Orthopaedics
Northern General Hospital
Herries Road
Sheffield S5 7AU, UK

A. Graham Apley (deceased)
Professor, formerly Honorary Director
Department of Orthopaedics
St Thomas' Hospital
London, UK

Hannu T. Aro
Professor of Orthopaedic Surgery
Department of Surgery
University of Turku
20520 Turku, Finland

A. Atzei
First Assistant
Department of Hand Surgery
Policlinico G.B.Rossi
Verona, Italy

J. Bennek
Professor, and Head
Department of Paediatric Surgery
University of Leipzig
Leipzig, Germany

A.H. Broekhuizen (deceased)
Department of Surgery
Academic Medical Centre
Amsterdam, Holland

E. Brug
Professor
Klinic und Polyklinik fur Unfall- und Handchirurgie
Westfalische Wilhelms-University Munster
Münster, Germany

Edmund Y. S. Chao
Professor, Director
Orthopaedic Biomechanics Laboratory
Department of Orthopaedic Surgery
Johns Hopkins University School of Medicine
Baltimore, MD 21205-2196, USA

R. G. Checketts
Professor and Consultant Orthopaedic Surgeon
Sunderland Royal Hospital
Kayll Road
Sunderland SR4 7TP , UK

L. Cugola
Head
Department of Hand Surgery
Policlinico G.B.Rossi
Verona, Italy

Mark T. Dahl
Minnesota Limb Length Center
Minneapolis, Minnesota, USA

A. Donadelli
Institute of Clinical Orthopaedics and Traumatology
(Director: Prof. B. Bartolozzi)
University of Verona
Verona, Italy

L. Donnan
Senior Lecturer, Child Specialist Centre
Royal Children's Hospital
Parkville, Victoria 3052, Australia

M. El Shazley
Senior Lecturer
University of Sheffield
Orthopaedic and Traumatic Surgery Research Group
Clinical Sciences
Northern General Hospital
Sheffield S5 7AU, UK

J.J. Elting MD
Bassett Healthcare
One Associate Drive
Oneonta, New York, USA

Thomas Gausepohl
Senior Trauma Surgeon
Department of Trauma, Hand and Reconstructive Surgery
St. Vinzenz Hospital
Cologne, Germany

Gerfried Giebel
Professor
Klinik für Unfall- und Wiederherstellungs-Chirurgie
Krankenhäuser des Märkischen Kreises
Lüdenschied, Germany

C. Glorion
Department of Paediatric Orthopaedics
Paris-West Medical Faculty
Hôpital Raymond-Poincaré
Garches, France

J.R.W. Hardy
Consultant Senior Lecturer
Dept of Orthopaedic Surgery
University of Bristol
Winford Unit
Avon Orthopaedic Centre
Southmead General Hospital
Bristol BS10 5NB, UK

M. Hashmi
Clinical Fellow in Complex Trauma and Limb Reconstruction
University of Sheffield
Orthopaedic and Trauma Surgery Research Group
Clinical Sciences
Northern General Hospital
Sheffield S5 7AU, UK

J. Kenwright
Nuffield Professor of Orthopaedics
The Nuffield Department of Orthopaedic Surgery of Oxford University
Nuffield Orthopaedic Centre
Headington
Oxford, UK

W. Klein
Director of Trauma and Reconstructive Surgery
Stadtkrankenhaus Wolfsburg Klinik für Unfallchirurgie
38440 Wolfsburg, Germany

Haruo Kojimoto
Associate Professor
Osaka Medical Center and Research Institute for Maternal and Child Health
Izumi-shi
Osaka, Japan

J. Langlais
Department of Paediatric Orthopaedics
Paris-West Medical Faculty
Hôpital Raymond-Poincaré
Garches, France

F. Lavini
First Assistant
Institute of Clinical Orthopaedics and Traumatology
(Director: Prof. B. Bartolozzi)
University of Verona
Verona, Italy

A.G. MacEachern
Consultant Trauma and Orthopaedic Surgeon
Regional Specialty Adviser, South West Region
Torbay Hospital
South Devon Health Care Trust
Torbay
Devon, UK

Konrad Mader
Department of Trauma, Hand and Reconstructive Surgery
St. Vinzenz Hospital
Cologne, Germany

B. Magnan
First Assistant
Institute of Clinical Orthopaedics and Traumatology
(Director: Prof. B. Bartolozzi)
University of Verona
Verona, Italy

J.L. Marsh
Professor
Department of Orthopaedics
University of Iowa Hospitals and Clinics
Iowa City, USA

Steve Meletiou
Charlotte Orthopaedic Specialist
1915 Randolph Road
Charlotte, North Carolina 28207, USA

S. Nayagam
Consultant
Departments of Orthopaedic and Trauma Surgery
Royal Liverpool Children's Hospital and
Royal Liverpool University Hospitals
Liverpool, UK

L. Nogarin
Professor, and Director
Department of Orthopaedics and Traumatology
Vicenza Hospital
Vicenza, Italy

M. H. H. Noordeen
Consultant Orthopaedic Surgeon
The Royal National Orthopaedic Hospital Trust
The Middlesex and University College Hospitals Trust
The Great Ormond Street Childrens' Hospital Trust
London, UK

Monica Otterburn
Sister, Orthopaedic/Fracture Clinic
Sunderland Royal Hospital
Kayll Road
Sunderland SR4 7TP, UK

Dietmar Pennig
Professor and Director
Department of Trauma, Hand and Reconstructive Surgery
St. Vinzenz Hospital
Cologne, Germany

A. Pizzoli
Institute of Clinical Orthopaedics and Traumatology
(Director: Prof. B. Bartolozzi)
University of Verona
Verona, Italy

J.C. Pouliquen
Professor
Department of Paediatric Orthopaedics
Paris-West Medical Faculty
Hôpital Raymond-Poincaré
Garches, France

M. Püllen
Abteilung für Allgemeinchirurgie,
Marien-Hospital Gelsenkirchen,
Virchowstrasse 122
45886 Gelsenkirchen, Germany

A. Rebeccato
First Assistant
Department of Orthopaedics and Traumatology
Vicenza Hospital
Vicenza, Italy

Amanda Rees
Consultant Orthopaedic Surgeon
Rotherham District General Hospital
Moorgate Road
Rotherham S60 2UD, UK

L. Renzi Brivio
Director
Department of Orthopaedics and Traumatology
Carlo Poma Hospital
Mantua, Italy

J. B. Richardson
Professor of Orthopaedics
Keele University, UK
The Robert Jones and Agnes Hunt Orthopaedic and District Hospital NHS Trust Oswestry
Shropshire, UK

Mark Rickman
Specialist Registrar in Orthopaedics
The John Radcliffe Hospital
Headley Way
Headington
Oxford OX3 9DU, UK

Michael Saleh
Professor of Orthopaedic, Trauma and Reconstructive Surgery
University of Sheffield
Northern General Hospital
Sheffield, UK

S. Salvagno
Director, Scientific Affairs
Orthofix srl,
Via delle Nazioni 9
Bussolengo,
Verona, Italy

Brian W. Scott
Consultant Paediatric Orthopaedic Surgeon
St James University Hospital
Beckett Street
Leeds LS9 7TF, UK

John Scott
International Medical Adviser
Medical Department
Orthofix srl,
Via delle Nazioni 9
Bussolengo, Verona, Italy

R. B. Simonis
Consultant Orthopaedic Surgeon
St Peter's Hospital,
Chertsey
Surrey, UK

A.H.R.W. Simpson
Professor of Orthopaedics and Trauma
University of Edinburgh
Edinburgh, Scotland

S. Toksvig-Larsen
Department of Orthopaedics
Lund University Hospital
Lund, Sweden

Giampaolo Trivella
First Assistant
Civile Maggiore Hospital, Borgo Trento
Verona, Italy

A.E. Weale
Consultant Orthopaedic Surgeon
Bristol Royal Infirmary
Bristol, UK

S. Winckler
Professor
Direktor der Klinik für Unfallchirurgie,
Otto-von-Guericke-Universität
39120 Magdeburg, Germany

Natsuo Yasui
Associate Professor
Department of Orthopaedic Surgery
Osaka University Medical School
2–2, Yamada-oka, Suita,
Osaka 565-0871, Japan

Acknowledgements

The substance of several chapters first appeared in other publications, the publishers of which the editors and publisher thank for permission to reproduce copyright material.

Chapter 23 appeared in *Injury* (in press)
Chapter 28 appeared as 'The Sheffield Hybrid Fixator' in *Orthopaedic Product News* May/June 1998, p. 33–5
Chapter 32 appeared as Chapter 9 in *Tibia & Fibula* ed C Court-Brown and D Pennig, Butterworth-Heinemann, 1997
Chapter 46 appeared as 'Pitfalls and complications in leg lengthening: The Sheffield experience' in *Seminars in Orthopaedics* Vol. 7, No 3 (Sept) 1992: p. 207–22
Chapter 49 appeared as 'Non-union surgery. Part II. The Sheffield experience – one hundred consecutive cases. Results and lessons. in *International Journal of Orthopaedic Trauma* 1992; 2: p.19–24
Chapter 50 appeared as 'Bifocal surgery for deformity and bone loss after lower limb fractures' in *Journal of Bone and Joint Surgery* 77-B, No 3, p. 429–34
Chapter 55 appeared as 'Articulated distraction of the hip' in *Clinical Orthopaedics and Related Research* Vol 301, 1994 (April), p. 94–101, published by J B Lippincott

Part I The Scientific Basis of Orthofix External Fixation

A History of External Fixation

1

A.G. Apley and M.H. Noordeen

"History is bunk!" If you believe this remarkable statement with which, in 1919, Henry Ford stunned a courtroom, then you might as well turn to the next chapter. But if you agree with others who maintain that "those who neglect the mistakes of history are condemned to repeat them", then read on.

Very few ideas are truly "new" in surgery, although notable exceptions are gene manipulations and organ transplants. Most new ideas are merely revivals of old ones, long buried in the mists of time, lost in the whims of fashion and fad, or abandoned because technique lags behind imagination. These ideas may re-awaken when the time is ripe. External fixation is a typical example.[1] An early description is found in the writing of Hippocrates,[2] but even he is believed to have described methods of treatment used for centuries by his predecessors.[3] Hippocrates' account is worth quoting.

> One should sew two balls of Egyptian leather, such as are worn by persons confined for a length of time in large shackles, and the balls should have coats on each side, deeper toward the wound, but shorter towards the joints; and the balls should be well stuffed and soft, and fit well, the one above the ankle, and the other below the knee. Sideways it should have below two appendages, either of a single or double thong, and short, like loops, the one set being placed on either side of the ankles, and the other on the knee. And the upper ball should have others of the same kind in the same line. Then taking four rods, made of the cornel reed, of equal length, and of the thickness of a finger, and of such a length that when bent they will admit of being adjusted to the appendages, care should be taken that the extremities of the rods bear not upon the skin, but on the extremities of the balls. There should be three sets of rods, or more, one set a little longer than the other, and another a little shorter and small, so that they may produce greater or less distension, if required. Either of these sets of rods should be placed on this side and that of the ankles. If these things be properly contrived, they should occasion a proper and equable extension in a straight line, without giving any pain to the wound; for the pressure, if there is any, should be thrown at the foot and thigh. And the rods are commodiously arranged on either side of the ankles, so as not to interfere with the position of the limb; and the wound is easily examined and arranged.
>
> And, if thought proper, there is nothing to prevent the two upper rods from being fastened to one another; and if any light covering be thrown over the limb, it will thus be kept off from the wound. If then, the balls be well made, handsome, soft and newly stitched, and if the extension by the rods be properly managed as has been already described, this is an excellent contrivance; but if any of them do not fit properly, it does more harm than good.

It would be tedious to pursue the subject through the centuries, so let us skip a couple of millennia.

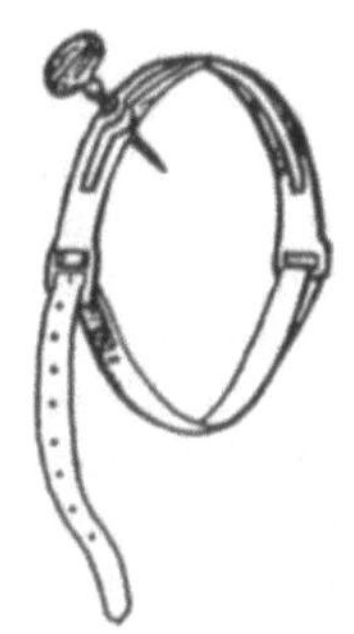

Fig. 1.1 Early fixators held the bone between at least two metal points, except Malgaigne's "point" (of 1840) in which one side is held firmly in a strap.

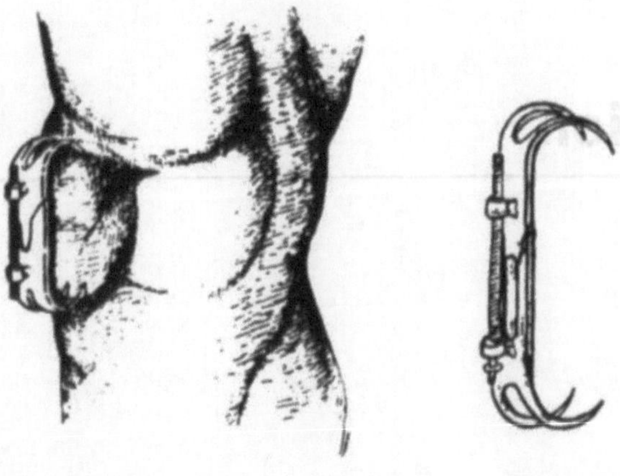

Fig. 1.2 Malgaigne's claw (1843) was used for fixation of patellar fractures.

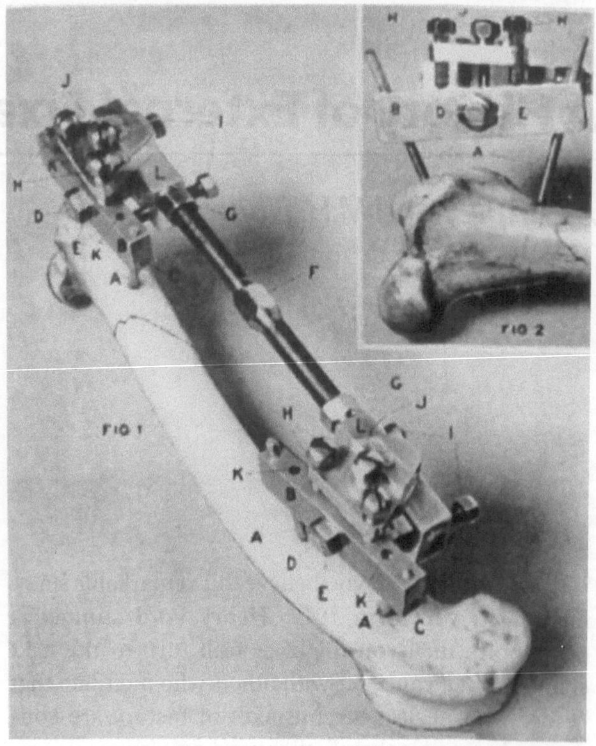

Fig. 1.3 The Stader splint

Malgaigne in the 1840s is credited with the first use of "pins" for attaching external devices to bone. These were the early rudimentary fixators (Fig. 1.1, Fig. 1.2). Shanz, Reidel and Anderson used nails and screws to control the bone, and also developed the concept of non-parallel pin insertion as a means of firmer control over the bone fragments. The pins were fixed in plaster, incorporated as a circular plaster encasement.

Stader, a veterinary surgeon, observing the poor tolerance of such devices in dogs, suggested a metal adjustable connecting bar (Fig. 1.3), and used this configuration successfully in dogs. Lewis, Breidenback and Stader[4] then further modified this for humans and used it on their first patient in 1937. They reported 20 patients, with 3 pin track infections (15 per cent), all of which healed on pin removal. Their description of the technique is immaculate; little has changed!

> Careful skin preparation is essential, and the same surgical aseptic safeguards should be observed as in any surgical procedure on bones. The splint should only be applied in the operating room, and careful sterilization is of course necessary.
>
> **Placement of pins** As a general rule the upper pin assembly is placed first. Place one of the pins into the pin handle or in a flexible shaft drill and tighten it firmly into place with the set screw. Introduce this pin through the desired hole in the pin bar and then hold this assembly in the right hand. With the left hand, accurately determine entrance point. Steadying the area with the skin stretched toward the fracture by the left hand, the right hand introduces the pin and by firm, steady pressure forces the pin through the skin and soft tissues in the outer cortex of the upper fragment of the bone.
>
> By firm pressure and rotation, the pin is firmly seated into the outer cortex. Then, by deep palpation upon the medial side of the limb the upper fragment is steadied while the pin bar is brought into parallel alignment with the long axis of the upper fragment by means of slightly altering, if necessary, the angle of introduction of the pin which up to this point has only been seated. After the upper fragment and pin bar have been brought into parallel alignment, continue pressure and rotation of the pin through the outer cortex, through the medullary canal, and then through the inner cortex.
>
> Care should be exercised so that the pin points definitely emerge through the inner cortex. This can be ascertained by a gradual release of resistance as the pin points start to emerge'.
>
> The insertion of the pins is difficult in some instances, especially so where the cortex of the bone is unusually thick. If this difficulty is met with, drilling a hole with a bone drill slightly less in diameter than the pins to be used, will overcome the problem. The pin is then introduced through the track of the drill, after the drill has been withdrawn.
>
> When using a drill it must be passed through the pin block in order that the hole being drilled will assume the proper angle. The drill should seat well into the distal cortex and when the pin is inserted it should be forced through the opposite cortex by pressure and rotation.
>
> An alternative method is to insert the pin into a motor-driven drill handle, adapted to receive the pin. No preliminary drilling is required, but care must be taken to see that the pin is not driven too far through the distal cortex.
>
> If, in the first Roentgenograms taken after the instrument has been applied, it is found that the pins

project through the distal cortex too far into the soft parts, they can be withdrawn to the proper depth.

As soon as the first pin has been inserted, the handle is unlocked from the pin and another pin fitted into the handle. The second pin is then introduced through the proper pin hole in the same pin bar while an assistant raises the pin bar about one-quarter of an inch above the surface of the skin. The second pin is then applied in a similar manner as the first, emerging through the inner cortex as above described.

The second pin assembly is then placed in position. When all four pins have been placed, they should be locked with the small hexagonal wrench by means of set screws in the end of each pin bar.

Applying the extension bar Adjusting screws should be unscrewed so they will not interfere with slipping the extension bar on to the pin bars. Lock nuts on extension bar should be loosened so as to facilitate extension or contraction as well as rotation.

From a strictly mechanical point of view there is no reason why, if one had two inches of overriding in a given fracture, the extension bar could not be so adjusted that it would slip onto the pin bars with this degree of overriding being present, with the idea of then proceeding to overcome shortening and then the other types of displacement. From experience however, it has been shown that much time can be saved if the operator will grasp the pin assembly in each hand and manually overcome as much of the overriding as possible, before applying the lateral extension bar. In this way fully 75 per cent of the reduction manoeuvres will be accomplished in 30 seconds time. While the operator maintains this position the assistant adjusts the extension bar to the right length and slips the stud bolts through the holes in the pin bar and then proceeds to screw on the nut. Before the operator lets go of the pin bar assemblies, the adjusting screws are snugly set with the fingers only. By properly manipulating extension bar nut the proper degree of extension can easily be secured. This can be checked in many instances by deep palpation.

Mediolateral alignment A mediolateral alignment of either segment is secured by proper manipulation of adjusting screws. Obviously, when this adjustment is being made, nut should be slightly loosened. After it has been secured, nut should be firmly tightened.

Anteroposterior alignment Each segment can be manipulated in this plane by set screws. The patient is then moved to the Radiologic Department, where final manipulations are accomplished either under fluoroscopic guidance or by taking several Roentgenograms.

The question has often been asked as to whether the pins should be put in place with the aid of the fluoroscope? The answer is definitely "No".

1. Too much Fluoroscopy would be necessary, which would endanger the patient and the operator.
2. By having an accurate knowledge of the anatomy involved, fluoroscope guidance is unnecessary.
3. Sterile surgery is impractical in the Radiologic Department.

A very important factor in the treatment of fractures is to see that firm impaction of the fragment is secured. As a final adjustment it is well to slightly impinge the fragmented ends upon each other. By firmly settling all adjusting screws, the entire instrument becomes locked and now acts as a splint.

Seepage does not indicate infection. It means that at the junction that the pins made with the skin there was a small amount of serous discharge, which usually formed a crust about the pin. When the pin was removed, healing occurred within a few weeks. Since the pin bar has been made of plastic instead of metal the seepage has decreased so that there are 10 cases in which no seepage took place.

This seepage is due to galvanic current set up by the use of two different metals, the pin being stainless steel and the pin bar duralumin. In other words the metal-to-metal contact gives a high dielectric value whereas with a material of high insulating value the electrical potential is nil.

There were three real infections, in two of which abscesses formed and had to be incised and drained. They healed quickly after incision, without any evidence of osteomyelitis. One infection, the femur case, resulted in a severe infection with osteomyelitis and death. In this patient, an old man aged 84, the dressings and the pins were continuously contaminated with urine and faeces, due to involuntary micturition and defecation. The patient was constantly picking at and removing the dressings, so that it was impossible to avoid secondary contamination of the pin wounds.

Lewis, Breidenback and Stader drew the following conclusions:

1. A new splint for reducing and immobilising fractures of the shafts of the long bones is presented.
2. Early transportation of the patient is possible, as contrasted to the impossibility of early transportation where traction suspension is used. This is of importance in bombed areas, either in civil or military surgery.
3. The splint is simple to apply and correction of malposition of the fragments is possible in all three planes of space even up to the time that fibrous union has occurred.
4. Early weight-bearing and continued use of the contiguous joints is permitted and urged, and this prevents muscle atrophy and stiffening of the joints from occurring.
5. After-treatment is reduced to a minimum as muscle strength is retained and joint function carried on.
6. Seepage around the pins is usually due to galvanism and not to infection. It is not an indication

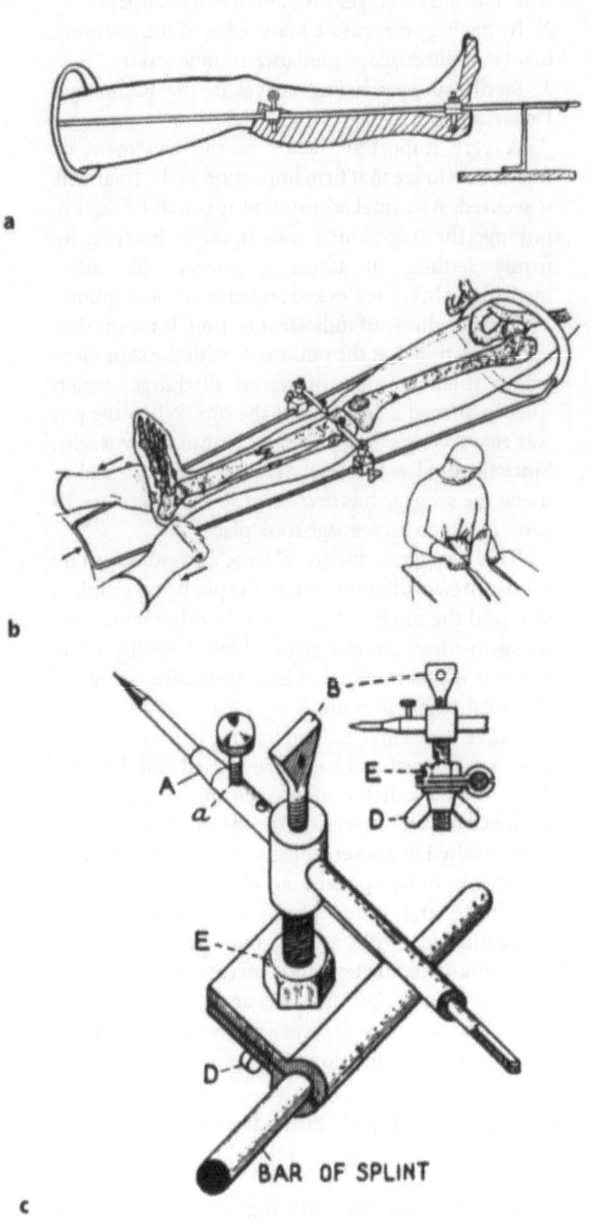

Fig. 1.4 **a** McKee clamps on a Thomas splint with plaster slab to reinforce fixation against movement in a sagittal plane. **b** Reduction of a fracture by traction. **c** McKee clamp for holding Steinmann nail to the side-bars of the Thomas splint.

for removing the pins unless accompanying signs of inflammation are present.

There were many variations on this theme including McKee's method[5] where a Thomas splint was used to connect Steinmann pins (Fig. 1.4).

External fixators, however, received a poor reputation after World War II and were feared as giving a consistently high complication rate.[6] Clearly this was not the universal view. Hey Groves, that brilliant innovator, was referring to his work on external fixation when, in

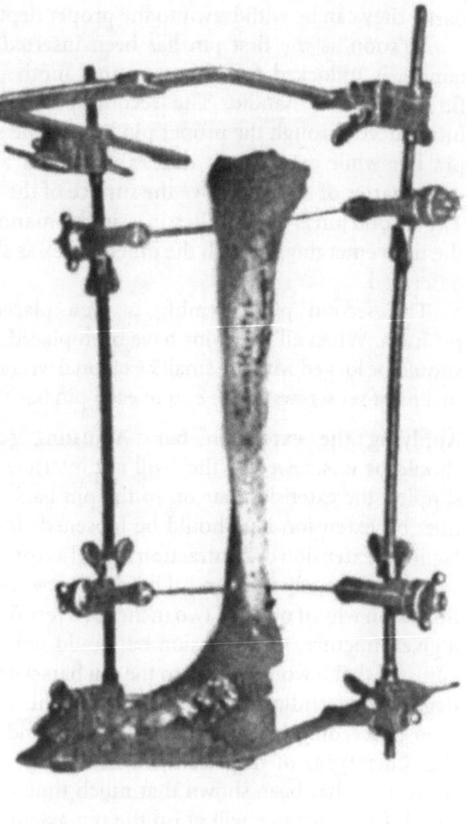

Fig. 1.5 Block's distraction unit (1923).

1921, he wrote[1] "there can be no doubt, as far as the evidence of these experiments goes, that this method of indirect fixation of fractures gives a more perfect union of the bones than any direct method that I have performed." (This quotation from his *Modern Methods of Treating Fractures* may be valid, but the adjective "modern" has a curiously hollow ring.)

Soft pin fixators were resurrected by the persistent efforts of Burny and Vidal.[7] Although the 1970s were dominated by bilateral frame constructs, De Bastiani and his colleagues popularised the uniaxial technique and introduced the important concept of "Dynamization".

The use of the wire frame for fractures was pioneered by Herzberg and Klapp[8] during the Balkan wars, and Martin Kirschner developed wire with a self drilling trocar tip. Although techniques for limb lengthening were already established, including the use of wire traction by Codovilla, Weber Block[9] developed the first distraction unit with threaded rods and tension wires (Fig. 1.5), in 1923. Several versions subsequently followed including that of Hempel, Goetze and finally the models popularised by Ilizarov,[10] which have been used for bone transport as well as lengthening.

The use of external fixators, therefore, has its origins deeply rooted in history; further refinements of technique were described by Abbot and Saunders (1939).[11]

Developments of external fixation, in terms of size of defect, tension across the defect, soft tissue injury, the timing of distraction, the stability of fixation and its effect on healing, as well as the rate and rhythm of healing are on the way.[12]

Clearly the art, principles and techniques of external fixation have blossomed; its science is still in bud.

References

1. Groves E.W. Hey, (1921) *Modern Methods of Treating Fractures* Wright: Bristol
2. Adams F, (trans) (1939) *The Work of Hippocrates* Williams and Wilkins: Baltimore
3. Peltier, L, 'An Abridged Report on External Skeletal Fixation: Hippocrates', *Clin Orthop* 1989; 241: 3–4.
4. Lewis K.M., Breidenback L., Stader (1942) 'The Stader Reduction Splint for Treating Fractures of the Shafts of Long Bones', *Ann Surg* 116: 623–36.
5. Charnley J, (1950) *The Closed Treatment of Common Fractures,* Churchill Livingstone
6. Belivens F, Editorial Comment *Clin Orthop* 1989; 241: 2.
7. Burny F, (1979) 'Elastic External Fixation of Tibial Fractures: study of 1421 cases' in Brooker A F and Edwards C C, (eds) *External Fixation: The Current State of the Art* Williams and Wilkins: Baltimore
8. Klapp F, 'Precursors of the Ilizarov technique' *Injury* 24 Supp 2: S24–S28
9. Klapp R, Block W (1930) *Die Knochenbruchbehandlung mit Drahtzügen* Urban and Schwarzenburg, Berlin, Vienna.
10. Ilizarov G, (1971) 'Basic Principles of Transosseal Osteosynthesis by Compression and Distraction' *Orthop Travmatol Protez* 7 (Russian)
11. Abbot LC, Saunders JB, (1939) 'The Operative Lengthening of the Tibia and Fibula, A preliminary report on the further development of principles and techniques' *Ann Surg* 110: 961–991.
12. Kenwright J, White SHA, 'A Historical Review of Limb Lengthening and Bone Transport' *Injury* 1993; 24 Suppl. 2: S9–S19.

SECTION 2 BIOLOGICAL CONSIDERATIONS

The Biology of Fracture Repair and the Role of Dynamization

2

J. Kenwright and J.B. Richardson

Introduction

External skeletal fixation is used widely and the indications for selecting this method of treatment are nearly always clear. There is, however, controversy regarding its place in the treatment of diaphyseal fractures, particularly in the leg. There is concern that healing may be inhibited, and that this may be associated with the treatment method itself; there is, however, no evidence in the literature that healing is delayed in groups of fractures where external fixation has been employed. When used by advocates of the method, very high rates of rapid fracture healing are recorded; both De Bastiani and his co-workers[1] and Checketts[2] have shown very low non-union rates when large groups of tibial diaphyseal fractures have been treated by external skeletal fixation. How can such high success rates be achieved?

Many factors affect the healing of fractures, not least the severity of the initial injury.[3] In this chapter the influence of mechanical factors will be discussed. The overall requirements for successful external fixation will first be presented. This will be followed by a description of the sequence of biological and mechanical changes seen during the healing of a fracture. The influence of mechanical conditions on fracture healing will then be reviewed. Finally, a treatment programme which embraces present experimental and clinical knowledge will be proposed.

Requirements for Successful Healing with External Fixation

There are certain prerequisites for successful fracture healing, and the following are particularly important when employing external skeletal fixation for the treatment of diaphyseal fractures.

1. As with all fractures there must be viable bone, and when using external fixation there must be no major bony defect if spontaneous bone healing is to occur. The soft tissue vascularity must also be adequate. No fractures will heal without these two features. In addition, there must be no serious infection.

2. Stability is needed to prevent loss of fracture position. In the early days after injury, sufficient stability can be difficult to achieve if comminution is severe.

3. Sound bone screw connections are needed and this interface must enable maintenance of effective fixation throughout the treatment, which may exceed six months.

4. Finally, the mechanical conditions must be appropriate for the different phases of fracture healing. The remainder of this chapter will address this last problem.

Fracture Healing, The Biological Process and the Mechanical Stages of Healing

Mechanical Influences on Fracture Healing

Intact Bone and its Responses

Bone is a dynamic tissue highly sensitive to changes in mechanical demands. The early observations of Wolff[4] led to his law on bone remodelling, which incorporates the concept that both the distribution and the mass of bone tissue are determined by the prevailing forces. More recent experimental work has shown that very short periods of appropriate dynamic mechanical stimulation induce adaptive remodelling in intact bone (Lanyon et al, 1982).[5] The continual remodelling process not only maintains an appropriate structural support of the body throughout normal function, but also replaces areas of microdamage resulting from everyday activity. In addition, bone is unique in its ability to restore near normal tissue architecture following gross fracture and subsequent repair. The pattern of this healing process is acutely sensitive to mechanical influences acting during the period of repair. Nearly all fractures need an artificial support system to stabilize the bone fragments and this fixation device plays a major role in determining the mechanical environment of the fracture site and thus subsequent bone healing.

Mechanical Influences and the Pattern of Healing

A considerable number of clinical and experimental investigations have attempted to define the mechanical conditions which will be ideal for the different stages of fracture healing. Different mechanical conditions are needed in the initial stages of granulation tissue formation, in the subsequent formation of external callus in secondary bone healing and in the remodelling phases. The timing of the development of these tissues will vary in patients who have sustained serious injuries to the soft tissues and to the blood supply of the healing bone (Fig. 2.1).

Both clinical and experimental studies have shown the acute sensitivity of fracture healing to mechanical influences, and the pattern of healing varies markedly with small changes in these. Aro and Chao[6] have recently defined the patterns of fracture healing that can be seen under different mechanical conditions and shown that these vary considerably according to the configuration of the fracture site. Simple formulae for the patterns of healing associated with different mechanical conditions can be found in the literature. In practice, these formulae are much too simple, but they form the basis for an understanding of fracture repair and its relationship to mechanical influences.

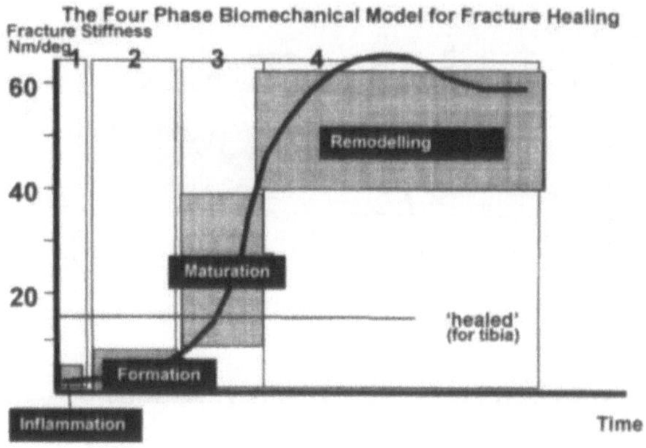

Fig. 2.1 The different phases of fracture healing can be mapped in relation to the rising stiffness of the healing fracture. Phases of inflammation, callus formation, maturation and remodelling are normal sequential phases of fracture healing.

Within the first few days of injury the fracture haematoma differentiates to granulation tissue and there is a primary callus response; this phenomenon is seen in both direct and indirect bone healing and is not thought to be susceptible to mechanical influences. Direct, or primary bone healing is seen after rigid stabilization associated with accurate reduction and minimal inter-fragmentary movement.[7] In this type of healing osteons cross the fracture line where the bone fragments are in direct contact. These conditions rarely occur, however, and if they do, they will almost certainly not exist uniformly throughout the fracture surfaces. Gaps exist which are initially filled with woven bone which is subsequently replaced by lamellar bone. In direct healing, external callus is not seen and normal bone strength is not restored for many months. Furthermore, any revitalized bone at the fracture site must be remodelled, and this will further prolong the healing process (Fig. 2.2).

Indirect, or secondary bone healing is seen in conditions of relative instability, when bridging external callus leads to progressive reduction of inter-fragmentary movements. This biological stabilization is then followed by a long-term remodelling phase in

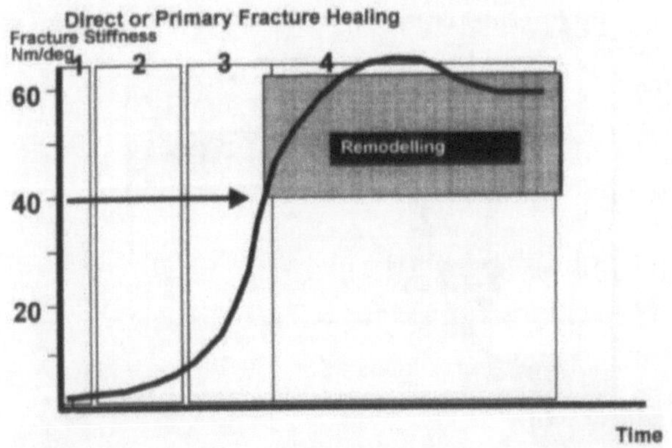

Fig. 2.2 The effect of providing a relatively stiff environment for the healing fracture. Reduced micromovements allow the survival of osteoblasts at the fracture site which form bone directly across the fracture gap without the need for callus. A rigid plate thus bypasses the first three phases of fracture healing and acts as "prosthetic callus". Healing proceeds slowly through the natural process of remodeling.

which woven bone is replaced with lamellar bone, and this restores the normal microscopic architecture. In this type of healing, restoration of mechanical integrity is rapid and the bone can withstand physiological forces within a short period. The cellular processes involved in the differentiation of tissues that form the bridging callus are acutely sensitive to the mechanical environment and may be inhibited if the characteristics of inter-fragmentary movement are not within defined boundaries.[8,9]

Recent development of a finite element analysis model of callus growth points to the timing of movement being more critical for the human patient than the size of the movement.[10] Measured movements of fractures managed in Orthofixation were transferred to a model in which each unit of tissue was determined by the forces acting on it, shear and strain, and the distance from the nearest blood supply. Patterns of granulation tissue and cartilage are seen to develop, and a critical moment is reached at the point of callus bridging.

Granulation tissue can survive in high strain environments, cartilage in intermediate ones and osteoblasts are active when strain rates are low. All three types of tissue will increase in quantity if the appropriate stimulus is maintained. The Kummerian principle of efficiency applies: no more tissue than is required will form, as the process is self-limiting. Tissue formation increases the polar moment of inertia at the fracture site and so movement is limited. This same principle applies in Wolff's law of bone remodelling, regulating the amount of bone at every point in the skeleton to only that required to keep stresses below a certain level.

The conundrum of tissue growth is the conflict inherent in a new tissue developing at a fracture site. Healing will occur in the tissues surrounding the fracture site, which become subjected to very high strain. Granulation tissue, however, is adapted to survive in areas of high strain, and cartilage can form under relatively high strain and also relatively low oxygen tension. The conundrum is the difficulty in moving from one type of tissue to another, as seen in fracture healing. Low strains are necessary for transformation to occur to a tissue adapted to low strains, such as osteoblasts. If the transformation does not occur across the whole field of healing tissue, then since the loads are shared in series, those tissues which have a low stiffness will continue to have high strains, and those areas which transform into stiffer tissues an increasingly lower strain.

Application of a uniform field of movement from day to day is therefore important. Increasing the load during the first 6 weeks following tibial fracture will be needed to maintain this movement in the face of an increasing volume and stiffness of healing tissue. If the movement is then continued, callus growth may continue, but maturation of cartilage to bone will not be possible.[11]

When a bridge of bone forms across the healing endochondral areas, dramatic changes in fracture site movement occur. The resulting reduction in movement allows the transformation of cartilage to bone.

Healing Pattern and External Skeletal Fixation: Which Type of Healing Is Best?

External skeletal fixation presents two special problems. First, there is nearly always a significant fracture gap despite attempts at reduction. Effective healing across such a gap has to be by external callus formation (Fig. 2.3), otherwise it will be many months before there is a significant return of mechanical strength. There are other patterns of bone healing that can occur to fill gaps, but the large gaps seen when using external skeletal fixation are associated with very delayed healing if external callus formation is inhibited. Healing can occur through intramedullary callus[7] but this is often associated with slow healing and a healing pattern which is at risk of refracture (Fig. 2.4).

External skeletal fixation is associated with a second problem; there is a race against the development of screw track infection which nearly always occurs if frames are left on long enough. The fracture needs to

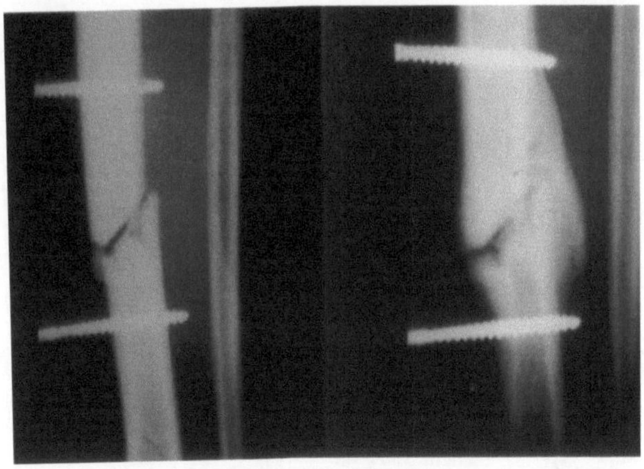

Fig. 2.3 These X-rays show the pattern of healing frequently seen when using external skeletal fixation. There was a small gap at the tibial fracture site even after careful reduction (left), and healing has occurred by external callus formation (right); without such callus, healing would have taken a very long time.

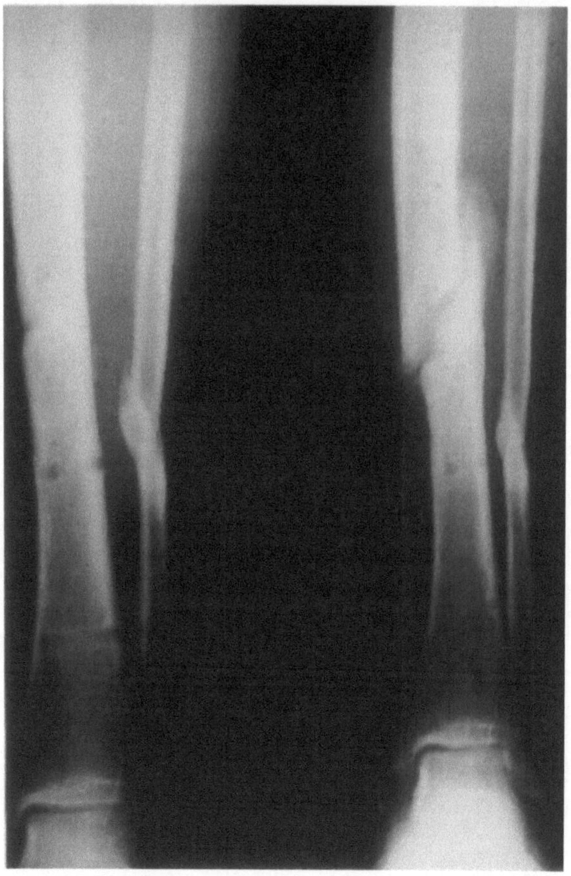

Fig. 2.4 The X-ray on the left shows healing of a tibial fracture which has occurred without the production of external callus, although intra-medullary callus has formed. The X-ray on the right shows the refracture which followed frame removal; this refracture healed rapidly.

become strong rapidly so that frames can be removed early. If intramedullary nail fixation is used these factors do not apply so strongly. It does appear, therefore, that ideally external callus is needed for healing when external skeletal fixation is employed for the treatment of fractures.

Optimal Mechanical Conditions for External Callus Formation: Clinical Evidence

There is no rigorous clinical evidence which enables definition of the "window" of mechanical conditions ideal for external callus formation, but there is considerable circumstantial evidence to suggest the existence of such a window. In femoral fractures treated by Apley and Perkins' method[12] (traction without a splint), macromovements with angulations of up to 5–10° can occur in the early days after injury; this is associated with massive external callus formation (Fig. 2.5). By contrast, if external fixation is combined with supplementary internal fixation, which suppresses interfragmentary movement, callus formation is inhibited (Fig. 2.6).

Clearly, there is clinical evidence that some degree of micromovement enhances callus formation; the importance of the timing of application of such micromovement, however, is not known. Fractures treated in casts are known to move considerably in the early days after injury;[13] for example, fractures of the tibia treated in plaster with early weightbearing often heal with extensive callus formation.[14,15] Furthermore, external callus forms most abundantly where there is early and continued cyclic micromovement at the fracture site, as seen in healing rib fractures. External fixation is often relatively rigid in order to have sufficient strength to maintain reduction of long bone fractures. This rigidity inhibits the natural stimulus for callus growth. External fixation does, however, allow for the application of controlled loads to the fracture.

Optimal Mechanical Conditions: Experimental Studies

Cyclic Micromovement

Many experimental studies have defined the broad limits of mechanical environment which result in the different patterns of healing. In most of these, it has not been possible to define the precise conditions operating at the fracture site.

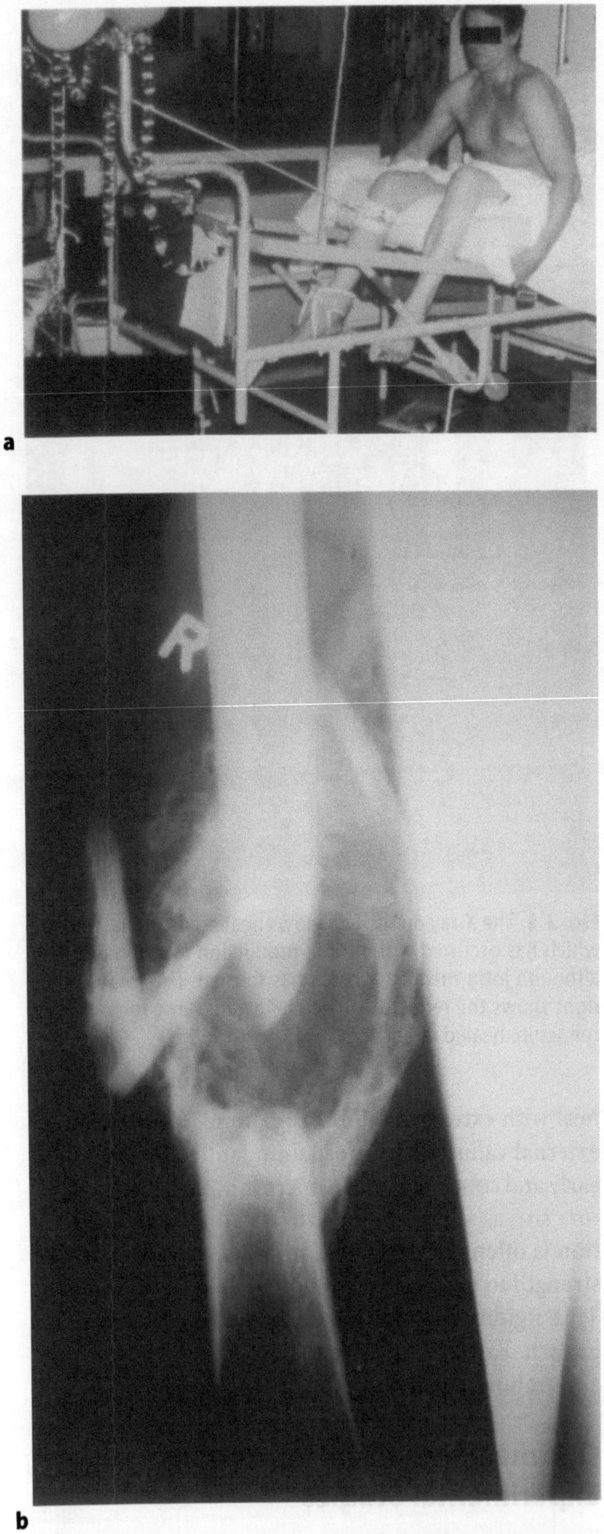

Fig. 2.5 **a** Apley and Perkins described the use of a split-bed, traction and early movement of the joints for the treatment of femoral diaphyseal fractures. Movement of up to 25° at the fracture site was common in the early stages of treatment. **b** Massive external callus formed with this functional treatment.

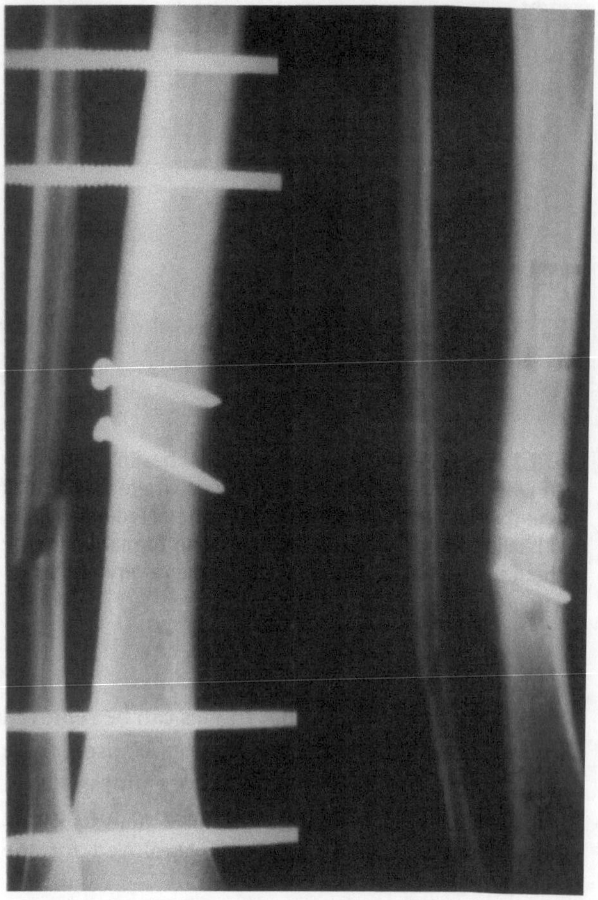

Fig. 2.6 This shows (left) the inhibited healing seen in a tibial fracture when external fixation was combined with internal fixation; the 2 screws have inhibited inter-fragmentary movement and hence external callus formation. Some healing might eventually have occurred at this fracture, but … (right) when the frame was removed 3 months from injury the fracture was unhealed; deformation occurred at the fracture site associated with this incomplete healing.

Defined micromovement regimes have been applied across experimental osteotomies. In sheep tibia small amounts of micro-strain applied at an early stage following osteotomy will enhance external callus formation.[9]

In these studies, very short periods (17 minutes per day) of 500 cycles of axial cyclical movement applied at a high strain (30 per cent) led to an enhanced healing response. These experimental studies support those of others in that it would appear important for there to be a small amount of applied strain every day within a few weeks of injury for external callus to be formed. There is a window of appropriate strain and too little or too much inhibited healing under these experimental conditions; 60 per cent of applied strain led to inhibited healing as also did 5 per cent.

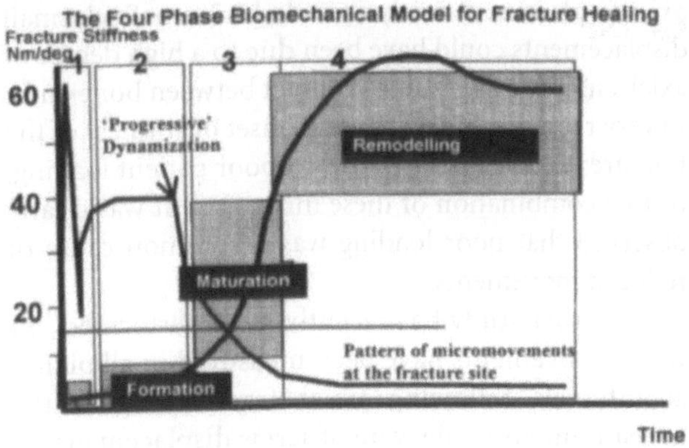

Fig. 2.7 Fracture site movements are seen to fall at the end of callus formation. This fall results from both the bulk and the beginnings of maturation of the callus. Calcification then proceeds across the callus and when this bridges the callus, micromovements are further reduced. Walking on a tibial fracture is the normal drive to the movements, and these occur in proportion to the stiffness of the fracture site. Unlocking the fixator column on an Orthofix fixator helps to reduce cyclic micromovement.

The timing of the application of the micromovement was crucial in these experiments. If such strain was not applied until 6 weeks after the osteotomy, healing was very markedly inhibited.[8] The direction of application of micro-strain may also be an important influence. It has been shown that fracture healing is very sensitive to shear deformation, an excess of which predisposes to the development of non-union of experimental osteotomies.[16,17] Cyclical loading has been compared with continuous compression and has been shown to enhance the later stages of fracture healing in rabbits.[18]

Progressive Dynamization

It also seems important for the resorption gap that usually occurs at the fracture healing site to decrease in its axial axis if rapid healing is to occur. It has been demonstrated that controlled collapse of the callus at the fracture site leads to a more rapid return of bone strength in groups of experimental fractures treated with external skeletal fixation, and Claes et al[19] have found that gaps inhibit healing.

The original Orthofix was designed by De Bastiani to allow a release of the axial forces in the external frame. He advised that this should occur after formation of the callus. His background in physiology gave him the understanding that natural forces would work to advantage once callus was forming. This technique entered the literature as "dynamization", but it is completely different from the application of controlled early cyclic micromovement, also termed "dynamization". Progressive dynamization actually reduces micromovement at the fracture site.[20] It is this reduction of micromovement which allows the survival of osteoblasts at the fracture site. Maturation of the external callus is thus aided by progressive dynamization. Closure of the fracture site is seen following unlocking of the fixator body, and once bridging of calcified callus is seen across the fracture site, there is a rapid fall in cyclic micromovement (Fig. 2.7). The scene is then set for full calcification of callus, and phase three of the healing process is well under way.

Little is known about the ideal mechanical conditions for remodelling, but some degree of loading and micro-strain is needed for the process to proceed effectively and so restore the normal mechanical properties of the bone. It has been suggested, however, that cyclic movements must be less than 20μm to allow remodelling across the fracture gap.[21]

Terminology and Summary of Ideal Mechanical Conditions

1. Fracture fixation must be *stable* enough to prevent gross loss of fracture position.
2. Experimental evidence suggests that there is an appropriate window for the level of micromovement needed at the fracture site in order for external callus to be formed. This micromovement is cyclical and needs to be applied within a short interval after the fracture, for only a small number of cycles per day.
3. There is clinical and experimental evidence that gap closure (what De Bastiani meant by "dynamization") instituted after an interval of several weeks of cyclic micromovement, enhances healing and does not lead to malposition or significant shortening.[1]
4. Some loading of the tissues is probably needed in the maturation phase of fracture healing. Too much loading at this stage could cause excessive strain in a fracture line through the healing callus. This is the most likely cause of hypertrophic non-union.

Should the Treatment Protocol be Adjusted to Control the Mechanical Environment?

At the time of initial stabilization of a severe diaphyseal fracture, factors designed to achieve stability override factors which relate to fracture healing. It may be difficult to obtain sufficient stability to maintain a reduced position. It is only after a short interval that the surgeon will need to consider factors which may enhance fracture healing and decide whether to make the constant adjustments needed to maintain the ideal mechanical conditions. Most fractures will heal even if no adjustments are made and this thought will pass through the surgeon's mind.

Will Bio-Feedback Lead to Self-regulation of the Mechanical Conditions?

It is theoretically possible that the patient will load the limb sufficiently to achieve ideal mechanical conditions at the fracture site through bio-feedback mechanisms. The patient may adjust the loading on the leg to make allowance for different stiffnesses of fixation and configurations of fracture sites and so adjust the fracture mechanics appropriately. Does such a self-adjustment of the mechanical conditions occur in practice?

In order to address this question a further series of experimental studies were performed by our research team.[22] Different frame stiffnesses were used to stabilize tibial osteotomies in two groups of sheep. In one group, in which the osteotomy was stabilized by a flexible frame, the loading increased steadily with time as did the healing. In this group, more effective healing was seen than in the second group in which a very stiff frame had been employed. During the first two weeks, the sheep with the stiffer fixators were able to place more weight on the leg but the mechanism which allowed this did not seem to be able to permit sufficient mechanical loading to enhance healing in this group. The bio-feedback mechanism had not been strong enough.

The movement occuring at the fracture site at different stages of fracture healing in patients has also been measured. Lippert[13] calculated fracture movements in several patients with tibial fractures from measurements of the displacement of pins inserted in the bone; movements were measured during different activities in patients treated with plaster casts. These studies in very small groups of patients, show large displacements of tibial fractures in the first 6 weeks after injury and axial displacements of up to 0.5cm are associated with normal healing patterns.

In a similar study in our department, a group of 45 patients who had sustained tibial fractures had axial movements monitored under dynamic loading conditions throughout their treatment.[23] The fractures were treated by external fixation and the relative displacement of the screws was again measured and fracture site movements calculated. Only very small displacements were seen in the first 6 weeks after injury. The displacements varied greatly between patients, but axial displacement rarely exceeded 0.2mm. Such small displacements could have been due to a high degree of axial stability as a result of contact between bone ends; to very rapid healing with early onset of stiffness of the fracture; to a very stiff frame; to poor patient loading, or to a combination of these influences. It was clearly observed that poor loading was a common cause of reduced movements.

A further study has recently been performed[24] in which movements have been measured in all planes at intervals following tibial fracture; again the measurements made were of screw displacement. In some patients there was hardly any movement in any plane. It is clear from these studies that there are certain patients whose fractures move by amounts which are outside the window of appropriate strain defined by previous studies as being needed for callus formation.

What Action Can Be Taken?

In order to approach the ideal mechanical environment, three types of action can be taken when treating patients.

I. Adjust frame mechanics
II. Control patient activity
III. Define duration of frame application

I. Frame mechanics

Frame mechanics can be adjusted, and many of the pioneers in the field of external skeletal fixation have advocated this.

i. Passive Cyclic Micromovement/Dynamization: Burny[25] advocates elasticity and initially applies a frame which, while very flexible, is sufficient to maintain fracture stability without loss of position; low non-union rates are seen in the published results.

ii. Applied Cyclic Micromovement/Dynamization: With externally applied loading of tibial fractures via external fixation frames, the fracture site is subjected to small amounts of cyclic micromovement, and this has been shown to enhance healing.

Eighty-four patients with fractures of the tibial diaphysis were randomly allocated to treatment by external skeletal fixation using an experimental unilateral frame employed either in fixed mode, or in a mode which allowed the application of a small amount of predominantly axial micromovement.[26] Statistically significant differences were observed between the two treatment groups; healing was significantly faster in those patients whose fractures had been subjected to micromovement (Fig. 2.8).

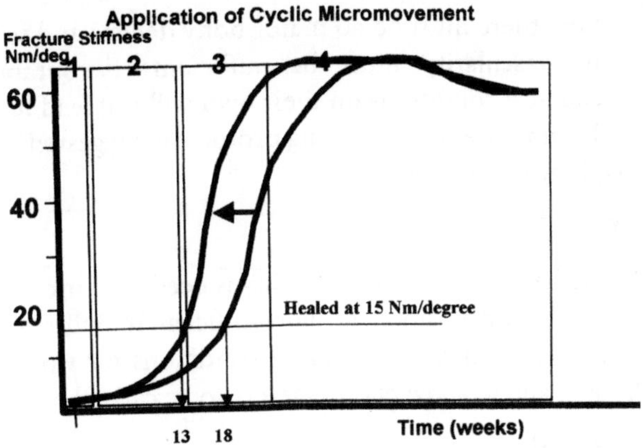

Fig. 2.8 In a prospective randomised trial of tibial fractures, the application of 1mm of cyclic micromovement in the first three weeks following fracture led to a significant increase in the rate of rise of fracture stiffness. Stiffness was not measured above 40Nm/degree, but it is probable that the subsequent pattern of stiffness is as shown.

iii. Progressive Dynamization: Behrens[27] has recommended that frames be dismantled progressively during healing to allow late loading of the fracture.

iv. Lazo-Zbikowski[28] has designed a bilateral telescoping frame to enhance progressive loading of the fracture.

v. Both Cyclic and Progressive Dynamization: The Dynamic Axial Fixator (Orthofix) has the facility to provide both types of dynamization to the healing fracture at appropriate times. Richardson et al[20] have shown that early loading of these frames allows cyclic micromovement to occur if the load is sufficient, and this occurs even in stable fractures. In the most recent model a mechanism has been incorporated to permit the application of cyclic micromovement before the patient can weightbear. This frame also allows closure of the fracture gap and transfer of the load to the fracture site when a central body locking nut is loosened; this releases a telescopic function within the body of the device. No loss of fracture position or significant shortening has been observed.

The balance of evidence in patients suggests that adjustment of the frame mechanics will allow differences in mechanical environment at the fracture site to be maintained, and thus enhance healing rates.

II. Fracture Loading

Whatever the frame mechanics, movements at the fracture will be minimal if patients do not allow the leg to function. They should therefore be encouraged to load the leg early, in order to allow cyclic micromovement at the fracture site soon after injury; loading is also needed to allow the fracture gap to collapse when frames are used in a telescopic dynamization mode. Richardson et al[20] have shown that patients can be encouraged to load their fractures at an early stage when using the Orthofix DAF fixator.

Groups of patients were monitored postoperatively and loading and fracture movements were measured in 6° of freedom via a transducer attached to the screws. Patients were kept under close supervision until they were able to weightbear effectively and it was seen that small amounts of cyclic micromovement could always be produced at the fracture site under these conditions.

Further studies of fracture movement measured in this way have shown that simple dorsiflexion and plantar flexion of the foot will also produce similar degrees of displacement at the fracture site.[29] These studies on the displacement of the fractured bone ends under treatment conditions for tibial fractures also showed that controlled axial collapse of the healing tissues occurs when the telescopic function is opened on the DAF; this axial displacement occurred within one hour of loosening the central body locking nut.

III. Frame Time

Great caution is needed in determining when a frame should be removed, in order to prevent refracture and to prevent non-union. Very early removal of frames and the application of functional casts, at, for example, 6 weeks from injury, and before sufficient callus has developed to reduce gross movements at the fracture site, may predispose to non-union. There is no rigorous evidence to support this impression, but many surgeons who use external skeletal fixation frames have noted that early removal of frames, as soon as the soft tissues have healed, may be associated with a high incidence of non-union; removal under these conditions probably allows too much movement at this stage of healing.

A Definition of Fracture Healing

Measuring the stiffness of the fracture provides a measure of the return of function. Radiographs, by contrast, provide anatomical information. Both are useful in the assessment of healing, as is clinical examination of the healing fracture. In a study of 124 tibial fractures where stiffness was measured (but removal of the frame was on clinical and radiological grounds) there were 8 cases of refracture. In all cases the stiffness was below 15 Nm/degree at the time of frame removal. In the subsequent 95 patients frames were removed and the patients allowed free weightbearing when the measured fracture stiffness had reached 15Nm/degree in the sagittal plane – there were no cases of refracture.[30]

This provided evidence for a stiffness of 15 Nm/degree to be considered a safe level of stiffness at which to remove a fixator from a healing tibial fracture. Similar evidence in leg lengthening supported a value of 15 Nm/degree for the tibia, but 20 Nm/degree for the femur. If there is malunion, an unduly heavy patient or the possibility of poor cooperation, a higher figure may be appropriate. Treatment in a plaster cast indicates that a lower level of stiffness may be possible for removal of the splint.[31] It is probable that a stiffness of 10 Nm/degree is applicable in arthrodesis.[32] In external fixation or callotasis of the radius we find that a stiffness of 2 Nm/degree is appropriate.

Summary: What Should Be Done?

Most fractures will heal eventually, but in some, healing will be delayed if the mechanical conditions are not appropriate for the various stages of fracture healing. If external skeletal fixation is employed, biological and mechanical conditions must be suitable for callus formation; there must be no major bony defects and soft tissue vascularity must be sufficient. Favourable mechanical conditions on their own will not lead to a healed fracture. The following protocol is suggested for diaphyseal fractures.

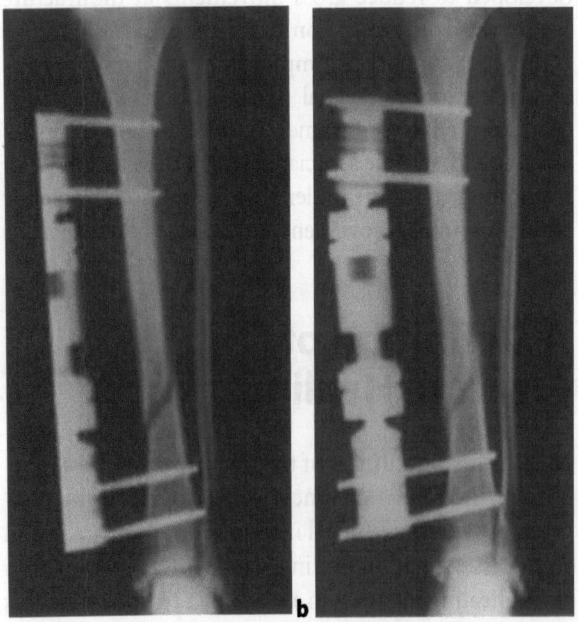

Fig. 2.9 Oblique diaphyseal fracture of the tibia. **a** Prior to the institution of dynamization, minimal evidence of callus, **b** good external callus formation following dynamization of the fracture.

Phase I

Immediately after injury, stability is needed to prevent loss of fracture position, to allow sufficient mobilization to prevent ARDS, to maximise conditions for wound healing and to allow plastic surgery to be carried out.

Phase II

Shortly after injury, and certainly within two weeks, some micromovement is needed at the fracture site; this can be achieved either by physiotherapy, by limb loading or by means of applied cyclic micromovement/dynamization (Fig. 2.9).

Phase III

After an interval of 4–6 weeks, progressive dynamization should be allowed. In this, the telescopic facility is released, allowing closure of minor fracture gaps. Further loading of the fracture is encouraged at this stage. Some degree of caution is needed in relation to the dynamization of fractures by this last manoeuvre, which assumes that there is no major risk of gross shortening of the limb. Shortening beyond that seen at the time of initial presentation is very rare in tibial diaphyseal fractures unless there is gross loss of longitudinal stability.

References

1. De Bastiani G, Aldegheri R and Renzi Brivio L, 'The treatment of fractures with a dynamic axial fixator' *J Bone Joint Surg* [Br] 1984; 66-B: 538–45
2. Checketts RG, Moran CG, Jennings AG, '134 Tibial shaft fractures managed with dynamic axial fixation' *Acta Orthop Scand* 1995; 66: 71–4
3. Nicoll EA, 'Fractures of the tibial shaft' *J Bone Joint Surg* [Br] 1964; 46B: 373–87
4. Wolff J, (1892) *Das Gesetz der Transformation der Knochen* A. Hirschwald: Berlin
5. Lanyon LE, Goodship AE, Pye CJ and MacFie JH, 'Mechanically adaptive bone remodelling' *J Biomech* 1982; 15: 141–54
6. Aro HT, Chao EYS, 'Bone-healing patterns affected by loading, fracture fragment stability, fracture type, and fracture site compression' *Clin Orthop* 1993; 293: 8–17
7. McKibbin B, 'The biology of fracture healing in long bones' *J Bone Joint Surg* [Br] 1978; 60B: 150–62
8. Goodship AE, Cunningham JL and Kenwright J, 'Strain rate and timing of stimulation in mechanical modulation of fracture healing' *Clin Orthop* 335 (Suppl) 1998; 105–15
9. Goodship AE, Kenwright J, The influence of induced micromovement upon the healing of experimental fractures. *J Bone Joint Surg* [Br] 1985; 67B: 650–5

10. Kenwright J, Gardner T, 'Mechanical influences on tibial fracture healing' *Clin Orthop* 1998; 335: 179–90
11. Lindholm RV, Lindholm TS, Toikkanen S and Leino R, 'The effect of forced inter-fragmentary movements on the healing of tibial fractures in rats' *Acta Orthop Scand* 1970; 40: 721–8
12. Apley AG, Solomon L *Apley's System of Orthopaedics and Fractures* 1990; Butterworths: London
13. Lippert FG, 'Three dimensional measurement of tibia fracture motion by photogrammetry' *Clin Orthop* 1974; 105: 130–43
14. Sarmiento A, Gersten LM and Sobol PA, 'Tibial shaft fractures treated with functional braces. Experience with 780 fractures' *J Bone Joint Surg* [Br] 1989; 71B: 602–9
15. Sarmiento A, Latta LL, *Functional Fracture Bracing* 1995; Springer: Heidelberg
16. Yamagishi M, Yoshimura Y, 'The biomechanics of fracture healing' *J Bone Joint Surg* [Am] 1955; 37A: 1035–68
17. Park S-Y, O'Connor K, McKellop H and Sarmiento A, The influence of active shear or compressive motion on fracture-healing. *J Bone Joint Surg* [Am] 1998; 80A: 868–78
18. Wolf JW, White AA, Punjabi MM and Southwick WO, 'Comparison of cyclic loading versus compression in the treatment of long bone fractures in rabbits' *J Bone Joint Surg* [Am] 1981; 63A: 805–10
19. Claes L, Wilke H-J, Rübenacker S, 'Interfragmentary strain and bone healing: an experimental study' *Trans Orthop Res Soc* 1989; 14: 568
20. Richardson JB, Gardner TN, Hardy JRW et al 'Dynamisation and tibial fractures' *J Bone Joint Surg* [Br] 1995; 77B: 412–6
21. Perren SM, 'Physical and biological aspects of fracture healing with special reference to internal fixation' *Clin Orthop* 1970; 136: 175–96
22. Goodship AE, Watkins PE, Rigby HS and Kenwright J, 'The role of fixator frame stiffness in the control of fracture healing: An experimental study' *J Biomech* 1993; 26: 1027–35
23. Kershaw CJ, Cunningham JL and Kenwright J, 'Tibial external fixation, weight bearing, and fracture movement' *Clin Orthop* 1993; 293: 28–36
24. Gardner TN, Evans M, Simpson AHRW, Turner-Smith A, '3-dimensional movement at externally-fixated tibial fractures and osteotomies during normal patient function' *J Clin Biochem* 1994; 9: 51–9
25. Burny FL, 'Elastic External Fixation of Tibial Fractures: Study of 1421 Cases' in Brooker Jr AF, Edwards C (eds), *External Fixation: The Current State of the Art. Proceedings of the Sixth International Conference on Hoffman External Fixation* 1979; Williams & Wilkins: Baltimore, p 55–73.
26. Kenwright J, Richardson JB, Cunningham JL, White SH, Goodship AE, Adams MA, Magnussen PA and Newman JH 'Axial movement and tibial fractures' *J Bone Joint Surg* 1991; [Br] 73B: 654–9
27. Behrens F, Searls K, 'External fixation of the tibia: basic concepts and prospective evaluation' *J Bone Joint Surg* [Br] 1986; 68B: 246–54
28. Lazo-Zbikowski J, Aguilar F, Mozo F, Gonzalez-Buendia R and Lazo JM, 'Biocompression external fixation' *Clin Orthop* 1986; 206: 169–84
29. Gardner TN, Evans M, Hardy J, Kenwright J, 'Dynamic interfragmentary motion in fractures during routine patient activity.' *Clin Orthop* 1997; 336: 216–25
30. Richardson JB, Cunningham JL, Goodship AE, O'Connor BT and Kenwright J, 'Measuring stiffness can define healing of tibial fractures' *J Bone Joint Surg* [Br] 1994; 76B: 389–94
31. Kay PR, Ross ERS and Powell ES, 'Development and clinical application of an external fixator monitoring system' *J Biomed Eng* 1989; 11: 240–4
32. Richardson JB, 'The mechanics of fracture healing' 1989; MD Thesis, University of Aberdeen

The Biology of Callus Distraction: Callotasis

3

N. Yasui and H. Kojimoto

Introduction

Callus distraction (callotasis) is a method of bone lengthening introduced into clinical practice by De Bastiani et al in the 1980s.[1] A long bone is sectioned at the diaphysis, stabilized for two weeks, and then subjected to gradual distraction using a rigid external fixation device. The distraction gap fills with growing callus that is destined to develop into solid bone. A slow rate of distraction does not break the bridging callus; it stimulates osteogenesis. The bone is thus lengthened without the need for bone grafting.

The fundamental principle of callus distraction was established by Ilizarov who had been engaged, since the 1950s, in basic and clinical research on the effect of tension-stress on tissue regeneration.[2,3] Ilizarov demonstrated how gradual traction of the bony callus stimulates not only osteogenesis but also growth and regeneration of the surrounding soft tissues, such as skin, muscles, nerves and blood vessels. The principle that governs the stimulation of tissue growth and regeneration during distraction, though poorly understood, is called the Law of Tension–Stress.[2,3]

Most current techniques of bone lengthening are based on the common principle of osteotomy and subsequent slow progressive distraction using an external fixation device. The type of osteotomy, timing, rate of distraction and the external fixation device to be used differs between different authors.[1-10] Ilizarov and his group, for example, performed a percutaneous corticotomy, attempting to preserve intramedullary circulation and to achieve progressive distraction at rates of 0.25 mm/6 hours using a circular fixator with a cross-tension wire system.[2,3,4] De Bastiani et al performed an open subperiosteal corticotomy and instituted a waiting period of 10–15 days before commencing distraction with a rigid monolateral fixator.[1,5]

In this chapter, the authors review their experimental studies on the basic histology of callus distraction and discuss the mechanism of tissue growth and regeneration during distraction. They also review the scientific background to the practical techniques of bone lengthening and evaluate the optimum conditions for osteotomy, the timing and rate of distraction, and the design of external fixation.

The Histology of Callus Distraction

Since 1986, we have been engaged in a series of animal experiments to demonstrate the histology and microangiography of callus distraction.[11-13] Over 100 rabbits were used in the course of these studies and details of the experimental conditions have been described elsewhere.[11] Briefly, a rigid monolateral external fixator (Orthofix M-100) was applied to the antero-medial aspect of tibia with four self-tapping screws and the bone was sectioned subperiosteally at the mid-diaphysis. Distraction usually began 10 days following operation and proceeded at a rate of 0.25mm every 12 hours.

a. The Waiting Period

Following osteotomy, a waiting period was observed before distraction began. The sequence of histological events in this period was essentially that of the fracture healing process. A haematoma forms and becomes organized. The necrotic tissue is then phagocytosed by inflammatory cells. Meanwhile, the cells within the deep layer of the periosteum proliferate and lift the fibrous layer of the periosteum away from the bone cortex. Radiographs showed that the external callus was first formed in an uncalcified state and subsequently became calcified (Fig. 3.1). By seven days, the callus around the osteotomy site contained hypertrophic cartilage, while the subperiosteal callus distant from the osteotomy site consisted of already calcified new bone trabeculae.

Various chemotactic factors, growth factors and cytokines are involved in the process of callus formation during this period. Bone morphogenetic protein (BMP), for example, may exude from broken bone matrix and stimulate mesenchymal cells to proliferate and differentiate into either chondrogenic or osteogenic cells.[14] The vascular nutrition and mechanical environment also affect the quality and quantity of callus formation.

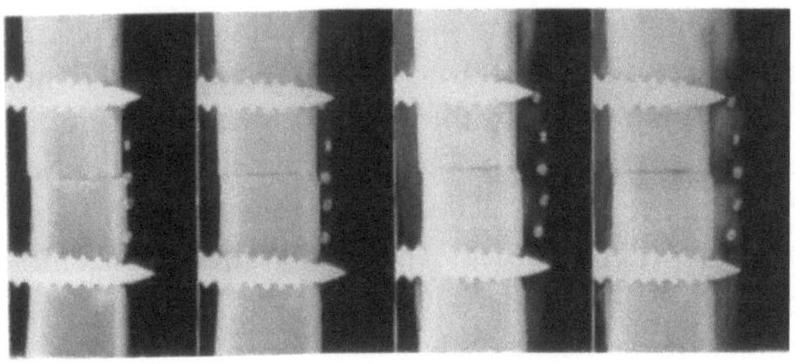

Fig. 3.1 The formation of external callus during the waiting period. The metal markers are sutured to the periosteum at the time of operation.

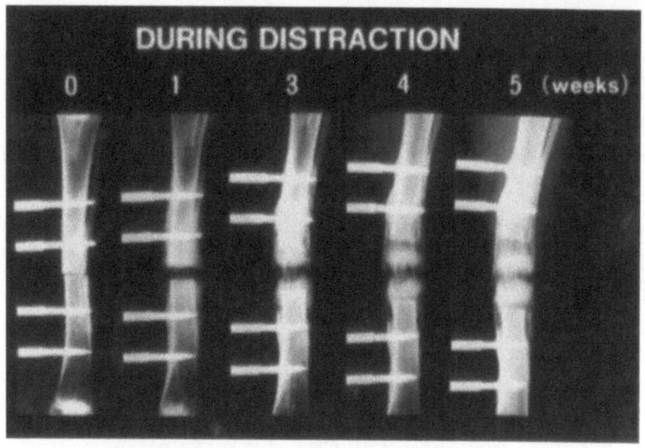

Fig. 3.2 The process of callus elongation and remodelling.

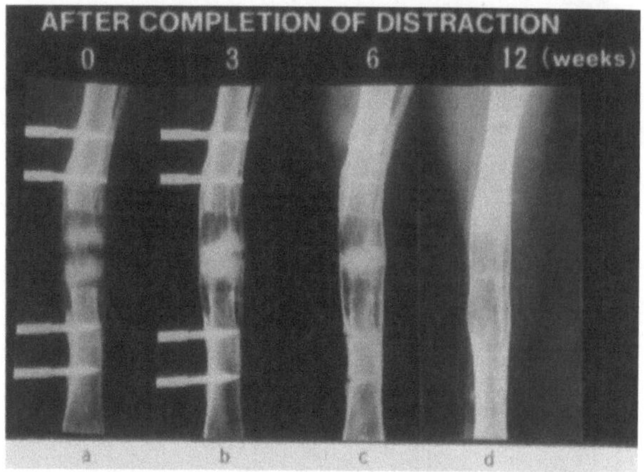

Fig. 3.3 The process of callus elongation and remodelling.

b. The Distraction Period

When slow progressive distraction was carried out, the callus filling the distraction gap showed three distinct zones radiographically (Fig. 3.2, 3.3). Elongation appeared to occur in a central radiolucent zone which was bounded by two sclerotic zones. Histologically, this central radiolucent zone consisted of longitudinally orientated fibrous tissue, while the sclerotic zones were formed by fine cancellous bone (Fig. 3.4). Some longitudinal fibres were seen to bridge the whole length of the distraction gap without interruption, while in other areas, the longitudinal fibres were interrupted by clusters of red blood cells. There were many fibroblast-like cells aligned along the longitudinal fibres (Fig. 3.5). Some of those cells were elongated parallel to the tension vector and had become hypertrophic. The origin of these cells was uncertain, but they appeared to retain the potential to respond to tension-stress and to differentiate into either osteogenic or chondrogenic cells.

The red blood cells between the longitudinal fibres were formerly considered to be extravasated haematocytes resulting from haemorrhage (Fig. 3.4). When a histological section was prepared following microangiography, however, many red blood cells between the longitudinal fibres were washed out and replaced by magnesium colloid (Fig. 3.5). These results indicated that the cells were intravascular circulating haematocytes existing within sinusoid-like structures developed between the elongated longitudinal fibres.

The proximal and distal ends of the longitudinal fibres merged with fibro- and hyaline cartilage, which contained hypertrophic chondrocytes arranged in columnar fashion (Fig. 3.6). The matrix of the hypertrophic chondrocytes had been invaded by cells derived from the bone-marrow. New bone had been formed on the surface of the eroded cartilage. Most of

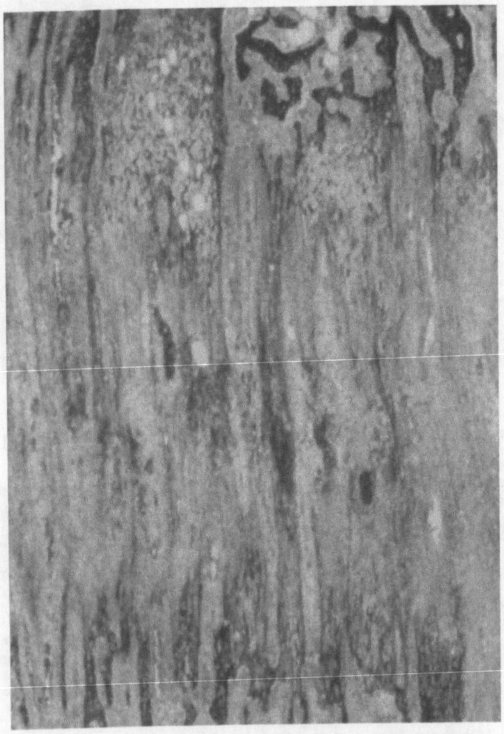

Fig. 3.4 Longitudinal section of the lengthened segment.

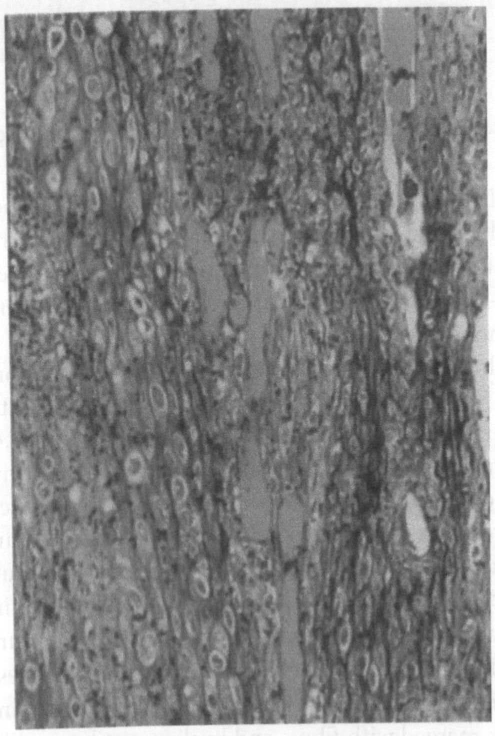

Fig. 3.5 Higher power magnification of the central growth zone. Round cells between the longitudinal fibres seem to be a response to tension-stress. Newly formed blood vessels are filled with magnesium colloid, a marker dye for micro-angiography.

the hypertrophic chondrocytes appeared to die when their pericellular matrix was penetrated, but some seemed to survive and change to osteoblastic cells (Fig. 3.7).

The columnar arrangement of the chondrocytes in the transitional region from cartilage to bone indicated that the mode of ossification was endochondral. Some longitudinal fibres, however, appeared to translate directly into new bone, suggesting the participation of another mechanism. Round hypertrophic cells between the longitudinal fibres morphologically resembled chondrocytes (Fig. 3.5), but did not necessarily produce cartilage matrix and seemed to change directly into osteogenic cells. As lengthening proceeded, the endochondral bone formation declined and the direct bone formation became more prominent.

Throughout the entire period of distraction, the cells controlling new bone formation must keep up a high level of osteogenic and proliferative activity. Although some growth factors and cytokines released after osteotomy may stimulate the initial callus formation,[14] the mechanism which maintains cell proliferation and differentiation during distraction is not understood. It is possible, however, that continuous tension-stress gives a signal to the cells to maintain proliferative activity without losing their differentiated phenotype. These cells may have some mechanoreceptors and affect each other through the autocrine/paracrine system.

c. Union and Remodelling Period

After the completion of distraction, the two sclerotic zones become fused, then shrink and are eventually absorbed (Fig. 3.3). At the end of the experiment there was tubular bone with a new cortex. Histology demonstrated that concurrently, the centre of the sclerotic zone was absorbed in a rate-limited manner from the bone marrow side. Bony trabeculae in the circumferential region remained to form a new cortex.

The Mode of Ossification

The histological findings presented here suggest that the mode of ossification during callus distraction, especially in the early stage of lengthening, is predominantly endochondral. Recently, however, opposing histological observations have been published by various authors.[2,3,8,15,16]

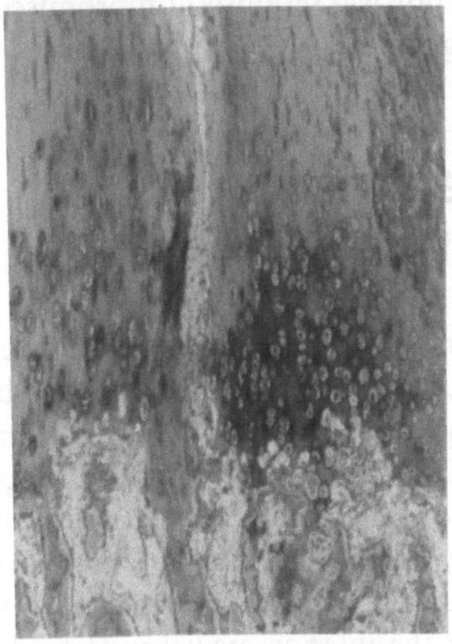

Fig. 3.6 Transitional region from cartilage to bone.

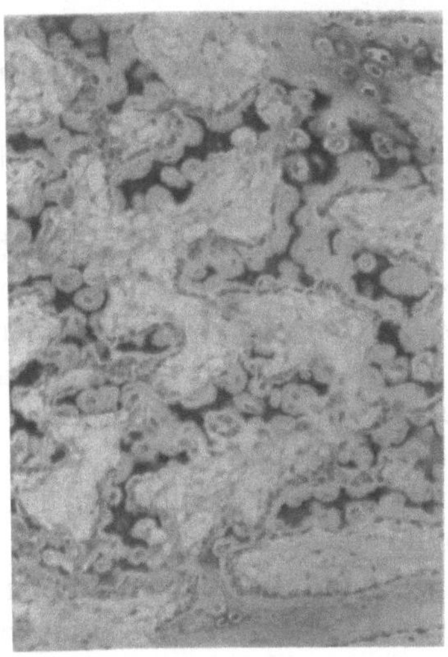

Fig. 3.7 New bone trabeculae containing cartilage remnants.

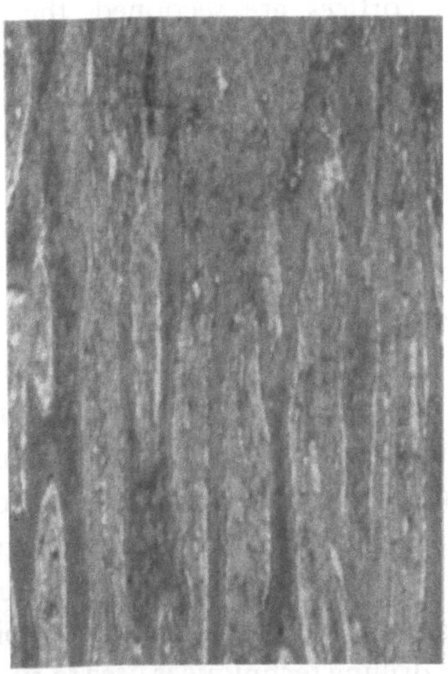

Fig. 3.8 Longitudinal section of canine specimen. New bone is formed predominantly by membranous ossification.

Delloye et al[15] performed canine forearm lengthening using the Ilizarov device and demonstrated that most of the new bone resulted from membranous ossification. They observed some atypical endochondral ossification during the initial stage of lengthening, but concluded that membranous ossification remained the main mechanism of bone formation during distraction.

Pablos and Canadell[8] presented an experimental study performed by Arrien, who compared an open and a percutaneous osteotomy in femoral lengthening in lambs. They concluded that the ossification of the lengthening zone was essentially desmal when the bone was sectioned by percutaneous osteotomy, whereas in the open osteotomy group, desmal ossification coexisted with endochondral ossification.

Ilizarov[2,3] reviewed a series of canine tibial lengthenings performed at his institution. He reported that when unstable frames were used for fixation, the distraction gap was filled with poorly differentiated connective tissue with large islands of cartilage. With stable fixation, more active and more direct osteogenesis proceeded in the distraction zone, bypassing the cartilaginous phase.

We also performed canine tibial lengthening to determine whether the histological discrepancy was due to the different experimental conditions or to the animal species. A larger Orthofix fixator was used for the canine experiment, but all the other experimental conditions were the same as those used in the rabbit experiment. Histology clearly showed more direct bone formation and much less cartilaginous tissue in the canine model (Fig. 3.8), suggesting that the ossification process differs, not qualitatively but quantitatively, according to the animal species. This is not surprising when one considers that the fracture repair process differs in subtle ways between different animal species. Moreover, one needs to consider the stage of lengthening when comparing the histology in different reports. It is true that in rabbit bone lengthening more endochondral bone is formed in the earlier stages of lengthening, and that direct bone formation becomes the main mechanism when new bone formation reaches a plateau at an advanced stage of lengthening.

The Role of the Periosteum and Endosteum

From a practical point of view, it is important to perform the osteotomy for bone lengthening with maximum care to preserve the surrounding soft tissues. It is also useful, however, to understand the role of the periosteum and endosteum in bone healing during lengthening. We designed the following experiment with rabbit tibial lengthening.[11] In one group, the periosteum was intentionally removed from the bone segments at the time of osteotomy, while in the other group, the bone marrow cavity was scraped out from both bone ends before the periosteum was sutured and the bone ends repositioned.

The results were remarkably consistent. When the periosteum had been removed at the operation, external callus formation was seriously compromised and the experiment was often interrupted by fracture. Although endosteal callus formed normally during the waiting period of 10 days, its amount was insufficient for it to be safe to begin distraction. When the bone marrow cavity had been scraped and the periosteum preserved, on the other hand, no obvious effects were observed on external callus formation. Despite the fact that endosteal callus formation was severely disturbed in this group of animals, bone lengthening was successful. These findings suggest that preservation of the periosteum is more important than careful corticotomy if bone lengthening by callotasis is to succeed.[11]

The Blood Supply and the Rate of Distraction

An osteotomy, no matter how carefully it is performed, must disturb the blood circulation. We have demonstrated the process of re-vascularization in rabbit tibial lengthening by microangiographic studies.[13] At various stages of lengthening, the animals were perfused with barium sulphate under general anaesthesia. The bone was then fixed, decalcified, sliced and examined radiographically.

Although the intramedullary blood vessels were, of necessity, sectioned by transverse osteotomy at the time of surgery, the blood circulation had recovered by the end of the waiting period. The formation of new blood vessels around the osteotomy site was detected by day 4, while the formation of periosteal callus was barely detectable in the radiographs. When distraction was carried out at rates of 0.35–0.7 mm/12 hours, some blood vessels maintained continuity across the osteotomy site, and bone lengthening was successful. When distraction was performed at a rate of 1.4mm/12 hours, however, the bridging vessels, which had formed across the osteotomy site during the waiting period, were completely disrupted. As a result, new bone formation was seriously compromised, and bone lengthening failed.[13]

The Technique of Osteotomy

Although most current techniques of bone lengthening are based on the principles developed by Ilizarov, the techniques of osteotomy differ between different authors. Ilizarov himself recommended performing either a compactotomy at the metaphysis or a corticotomy at the diaphysis, attempting to preserve the intramedullary circulation. In tibial lengthening, for example, the anterior, medial and lateral cortices of the proximal metaphysis are sectioned with a chisel through a small incision and the posterior cortex is divided by osteoclasis. Kawamura et al[7] and Monticelli and Spinelli[9] also performed percutaneous corticotomy.

De Bastiani et al[1] performed an open subperiosteal corticotomy using a pre-drilling technique. A series of holes 4.8mm in diameter drilled around the anterior two-thirds of the bone circumference was joined using a scalpel without damaging the bone marrow. The posterior cortex was broken manually but the integrity of the posterior periosteum was preserved.

We agree that both percutaneous corticotomy and compactotomy are theoretically valid because both periosteal and endosteal structures are important for bone healing. From the practical point of view, however, it is not easy to achieve genuine corticotomy with the preservation of intramedullary blood vessels. No matter how carefully the anterior and mediolateral bone cortices are sectioned, the process of manual fracture of the posterior bone cortex can easily damage the endosteal blood vessels.

Delloye et al[15] in experimental studies on dogs, reported that there were no differences in the amounts of newly formed bone and the patterns of bone healing after corticotomy and osteotomy.

Experimental studies, performed by ourselves and reviewed in this chapter, have clearly shown that preservation of the periosteum is more important than careful corticotomy. In our current clinical practice, therefore, we perform a percutaneous osteotomy without attempting to preserve the intramedullary circulation. The lateral approach is used for femoral osteotomy, and the anterior approach for tibial lengthening. A pre-drilling technique is used to avoid a crack extending to involve a pin hole. Through a small 1.5cm skin incision, a drill guide with a diameter of

2.5–3.2mm is applied to the bone cortex. Holes are then drilled passing through the bone marrow cavity, a stop on the drill preventing damage to the soft tissues beyond the opposite cortex. The drill holes are joined using a chisel and complete separation of the fragments confirmed with the image intensifier. The duration of the waiting period depends on the age of the patient, the quality of the bone to be lengthened, and the aetiological background. For tibial or femoral lengthening in achondroplastic patients, for example, five to seven days may be enough, while for small bones such as metatarsals, it may be better to wait three weeks before distraction.

The Stability of Fixation

It is now widely accepted that fixation which is too rigid causes stress shielding and delay in bone healing, and that some micromotion parallel to the bone axis stimulates osteogenesis. Very little is known, however, about the degree of micromotion desirable for new bone formation. Some confusion exists among orthopaedic surgeons as to whether elastic fixation is better than rigid fixation to promote faster bone healing.

Ilizarov demonstrated that the external fixation must be rigid enough to eliminate undesirable micromotion at an osteotomy. Bone healing is disturbed when an unstable frame configuration is used for distraction.[2,3]

Paley et al[17] evaluated the mechanical properties of different external fixators used in limb lengthening. They concluded that the Orthofix unilateral fixator with the thick half pin system was the most rigid and the Ilizarov circular fixator with a cross-wire tension system was the least rigid with respect to stiffness, shear, and axial motion. Recently, the Ilizarov system has been modified in western countries, and it is now possible to connect half pins to a circular frame.

We believe that, although some micromotion may stimulate callus formation during the distraction phase, it may delay bone union during the neutralization period. The authors prefer a rigid fixation period for at least a few weeks after the completion of distraction. Fixation with any kind of external fixator is not too rigid for this purpose. Once bony union has been obtained, the external fixator is shortened 1mm so that the union site is subjected to limited mechanical stress. Full dynamization is subsequently allowed to enhance the consolidation and to improve the bone atrophy caused by stress shielding. After consolidation is confirmed clinically and radiologically, the pins are removed in a step-wise manner, so that further mechanical stimulation is applied to the bone.[18]

Bone Remodelling

Most orthopaedic surgeons know from clinical experience that various mechanical stresses infuence the patterns of bone growth and remodelling. The principle which governs the adaptation of bone to mechanical stress is known as Wolff's law[19] which states that a bone, when bent by a mechanical load, adapts by depositing new bone on the concave side and resorbing the bone on the convex side. The compression force, rather than the tension stress, is generally considered to accelerate new bone formation.

Wolff's law does not explain the mechanism of new bone formation during progressive distraction, but it is applicable to the remodelling of the bone after union is complete. The lengthened segment should receive ordinary mechanical stresses after the external fixation device has been removed. The circumferential region of the lengthened segment strengthens to form new cortex, while the centre of the lengthened segment is absorbed and replaced by bone marrow. When bending occurs in the lengthened segment, accidentally or intentionally, new bone is deposited on the concave side and bone resorption occurs on the convex side.

The Distraction of Soft Tissues

Regardless of the type of osteotomy, bone lengthens only at the site of the osteotomy. The soft tissues around the osteotomy site, therefore, must be subjected to excessive local stretching during distraction. The muscles, especially those that have their origins or insertions across the osteotomy site, must be subjected to extreme local tensile stress. Do these muscles tear at the level of the osteotomy site, or is there a mechanism to relieve local stretching?

We performed an experimental study to examine the mode of elongation of muscle and periosteum during slow progressive distraction of the callus.[12] Using a rabbit tibial lengthening model, the periosteum and fascia of the triceps surae muscle were marked with small stainless steel wires at the time of operation. Changes in the anatomical relationship between the bone and the soft tissue markers were monitored radiographically. We found that the periosteum slid over the bone cortex during distraction, mitigating local stretching of the muscle around the osteotomy site. The elongation of muscle appeared to occur throughout the muscle substance and not simply at the site of the osteotomy.[12]

References

1. De Bastiani G., Aldegheri R., Renzi Brivio L. and Trivella G. 'Limb lengthening by callus distraction (callotasis)'. *J Pediatr Orthop* 1987; 7:129–34
2. Ilizarov G.A. 'The tension-stress effect on the genesis and growth of tissues. Part I. The influence of stability of fixation and soft-tissue preservation.' *Clin Orthop* 1989; 238:249–81
3. Ilizarov G.A. 'The tension-stress effect on the genesis and growth of tissues. Part II. The influence of the rate and frequency of distraction. '*Clin Orthop* 1989; 239:263–85
4. Paley D. 'Current techniques of limb lengthening.' *J Pediatr Orthop* 1988; 8:73–92
5. Aldegheri R., Trivella G., Renzi Brivio L., Tessari G., Agostini S. and Lavini F. 'Lengthening of the lower limbs in achondroplastic patients.' *J Bone Joint Surg* [Br] 1988; 70-B: 69–73
6. Dalmonte A. and Donzelli D. 'Comparison of different methods of leg lengthening.' *J Pediatr Orthop* 1988; 8:62–71
7. Kawamura B., Hosono S., Takahashi T., Yano T., Kobayashi Y., Shibata N. and Shinoda Y. 'Limb lengthening by means of subcutaneous osteotomy.' *J Bone Joint Surg* [Am] 1968; 50–A: 851–78
8. De Pablos J. and Canadell J. 'Methods of bone lengthening and their application.' *Serv Public Univ Navarra*, 1990
9. Monticelli G. and Spinelli R. 'Leg lengthening by closed metaphyseal corticotomy.' *Ital J Orthop Traumatol* 1983; 9:139–52
10. Wagner H. 'Operative lengthening of the femur.' *Clin Orthop* 1978; 136: 125–42
11. Kojimoto H., Yasui N., Goto T., Matsuda S. and Shimomura Y. 'Bone lengthening in rabbits by callus distraction.' *J Bone Joint Surg* [Br] 1988; 70-B: 543–9
12. Yasui N., Kojimoto H., Shimizu H. and Shimomura Y. 'The effect of distraction upon bone, muscle, and periosteum.' *Orthop Clin North Am* 1991; 22: 563–7
13. Yasui N., Kojimoto H., Sasaki K., Kitada A., Shimizu H. and Shimomura Y. 'Factors affecting callus distraction in limb lengthening.' *Clin Orthop* 1993; 293: 55–60
14. Wozney J.M. 'Bone morphogenetic protein and their gene expression' in *Cellular and Molecular Biology of Bone* (Noda M. ed) Academic Press, San Diego, 1993
15. Delloye C., Delefortrie G., Coutelier L and Vincent A. 'Bone regenerate formation in cortical bone during distraction lengthening. An experimental study.' *Clin Orthop* 1990; 250: 34–42
16. Aronson J. et al 'The histology of distraction osteogenesis using different external fixators.' *Clin Orthop* 1989; 241: 106–16
17. Paley D., Fleming B.S., Catagni M. Kristiansen T. and Pope M. 'Mechanical evaluation of external fixators used in limb lengthening.' *Clin Orthop* 1990; 250: 50–7
18. Yasui N., Kawabata H. and Nakanishi H. 'Bilateral and bifocal lengthening in the tibia and the femur using a segmental slide lengthener.' *Int J Orthop Trauma* 1993; 3: 87–8
19. Albright J.A. 'Bone: Physical properties.' in *The Scientific Basis of Orthopaedics* Appleton Century Croft, New York, 1979

The Biology of Soft Tissue Distraction

4

J. Kenwright and A.H.R.W. Simpson

Introduction

When undertaking leg lengthening, there are three aims:

i. To achieve significant increases of between 10 per cent or more of the original length; the limb may be smaller than the normal limb in all dimensions, and new tissue needs to be created in all the structures of the limb.
ii. To minimise temporary morbidity.
iii. To prevent permanent loss of function.

Where modern programmes of lengthening are employed, strong and proliferative new bone can usually be created. The programme must be adjusted to encourage this to form within the distraction gap, in order to shorten treatment times, but premature healing must be avoided. In patients with congenital abnormalities particularly, the soft tissues within the shortened leg are frequently contracted, and fixed deformities exist at joints. The programme must allow the tissues to grow and adapt to the new length, without worsening the underlying soft tissue abnormality.

While lengthening of bone and soft tissue may be easy in many instances, in association with certain pathologies it is difficult, and high complication rates have been described (Paley,[1] Dahl et al[2]). Dahl has shown that the incidence of complications is related closely to the severity of the underlying problem for which lengthening is needed. Five grades of severity are described, based upon the percentage shortening in the limb. The severity grading needs to be increased if there are additional risk factors for the development of complications, such as the presence of congenital abnormality. Dahl also reviewed the "learning curve" for surgery for different severity groups (see Ch. 45), and demonstrated that complication rates decreased dramatically as experience increased (in excess of 30 patients).

Lengthening programmes may therefore need to be adjusted, based upon a knowledge of the predicted responses of the bone and soft tissues in individual patients. Some of the knowledge we have gained in respect of these responses is reviewed below.

Loads Acting Upon the Tissues During Leg Lengthening

Load cells were attached to external skeletal fixation frames, and the axial load acting during leg lengthening, measured in patients (Leong et al,[3] Simpson et al)[4]; similar studies have been performed in experimental models (White and Kenwright,[5] Aronson et al,[6] Li et al).[7] Both the tissues in the distracted bony segment and the soft tissues of the lengthened limb contribute to these measured resistances to distraction. The relative contribution of each element varies from patient to patient and at different periods of distraction, but in many instances the measured axial force reflects primarily the resistance of the soft tissues (Simpson et al).[4] These studies showed that very low maximum axial force levels were reached during lengthening in patients suffering from post-traumatic shortening, whereas high peak levels of 1500 Newtons could be reached during the lengthening where shortening was associated with congenital abnormality (Fig. 4.1) These surprisingly high levels will cause deformation of simple external fixation frames and result in deformity at the osteotomy site; there will also be a risk of complications developing within the soft tissues due to the excess tension. The axis of the deforming force may lie well lateral or medial to the bone and needs to be

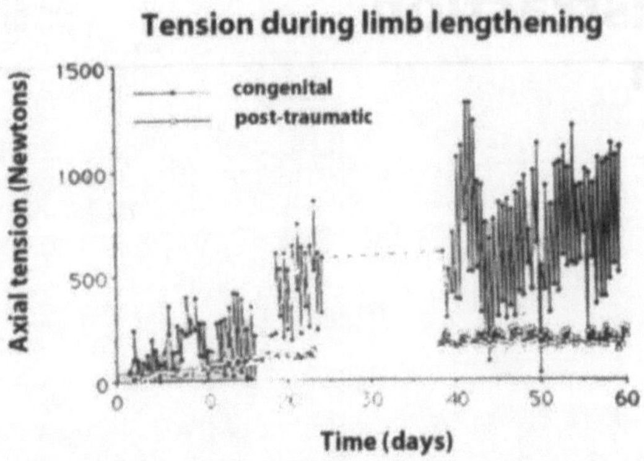

Fig. 4.1 Axial soft tissue tensions measured sequentially for 60 days following leg lengthening in patients with shortening due to congenital abnormality or previous femoral fracture.

resisted by the use of an appropriate frame configuration (Simpson et al).[8]

Responses of the Soft Tissues

1. Skin

This tissue tolerates lengthening very well. New skin is created readily under the influence of a distension force in plastic surgical skin expansion techniques, and skin rarely causes a problem during leg lengthening unless there is severe tethering of previous scars. The skin around external fixation screws does not respond so well to progressive distraction. Wherever possible, screws should be placed at a site where minimum excursion will occur around the screws during joint movement. Screws designed with a sharp leading edge will cut through the skin during distraction, or the use of thin tensioned wires may lessen the scarring caused by the migration of screws and wires which inevitably occurs during distraction. Unremitting pressure on the skin, caused by poor screw placement, will cause necrosis and should be avoided.

2. Muscle

There is scarcity of knowledge regarding the response of muscle to leg lengthening, yet the behaviour of the muscles often limits the ultimate gain in length that can be achieved. Temporary muscle dysfunction is commonly seen, but permanent disability can also occur, particularly in patients with congenital shortening or shortening associated with poliomyelitis, (Sofield et al).[9] The muscle may not adapt to the enforced lengthening and muscle weakness and stiffness of the adjacent joints may be permanent.

Kawamura et al[10] demonstrated that biochemical abnormalities may occur under experimental conditions in normal muscles after gradual distraction, with only a 10 per cent increase in limb length.

Ilizarov[11] suggested that regions of distracted muscles may develop the appearance of embryonic tissue. The morphology and function of muscle has been studied for different distraction rates in an experimental adult model of leg lengthening in our department (Kenwright and Simpson,[12] Simpson et al[13,14]) and these studies have shown that muscle response is acutely sensitive to the rate of lengthening. In groups of adult rabbits, the muscles in the leg were distracted by an external skeletal fixation device (Orthofix M100) applied to the medial surface of the tibia; an osteotomy was also created. Lengthening was performed twice daily at daily distraction rates of 0.4mm to 4.0mm and continued until a 20 per cent increase in the initial length of the tibia had been achieved.

No abnormalities were seen in any of the observations made in the contralateral limbs which had not been distracted, or in limbs subjected to a sham operation. The active force developed during twitch contractions was measured for each length (Gordon, Huxley and Julian)[15] and almost complete adaptation occurred at distraction rates of 1mm per day and less. Little adaptation was seen at high rates of distraction, and the sarcomere length was increased following distraction at rates which exceeded 1mm per day. Such increases in length reflect inefficiency in muscle function. Matano et al[16] have shown that sarcomere length can recover in experimental models. In our studies it was considered of importance that rapid rates of distraction caused prominent overstretching, and that there was loss of alignment of the contractile tissue with disruption of the sarcomere pattern as seen on electron microscopy.

Histological examination demonstrated evidence of cell damage at rates in excess of 1mm per day, with whorled muscle fibres and centralization of nuclei. Extensive necrosis was seen at even higher rates (Fig. 4.2). We also observed an increased perimyseal and endomyseal fibrosis in many specimens, but again, not in the sham group nor in contralateral limb muscles. The extent of fibrosis was related to the rate of distraction and was seen in all specimens distracted at rates of 1mm per day or above. Passive tension curves showed that there was a relative increase in muscle stiffness in all groups except those distracted at the very slowest rate (0.4mm/day). An increase in

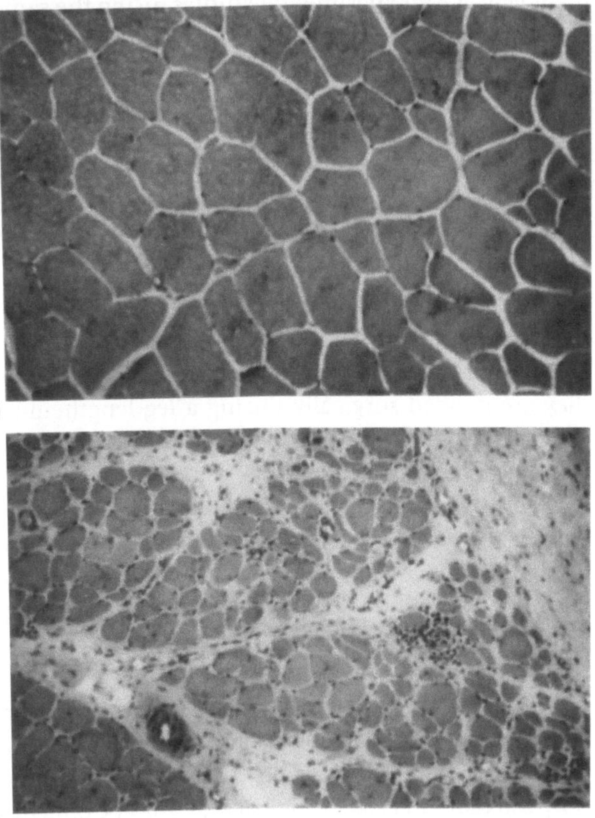

a

b

Fig. 4.2 **a** Cross-section of adult rabbit muscle following distraction at a rate of 0.3mm per day divided into increments; the muscle has remained normal. **b** Cross-section of adult rabbit muscle following distraction at a rate of 2mm per day in two increments; widespread fibrosis and abnormal muscle fibres are evident.

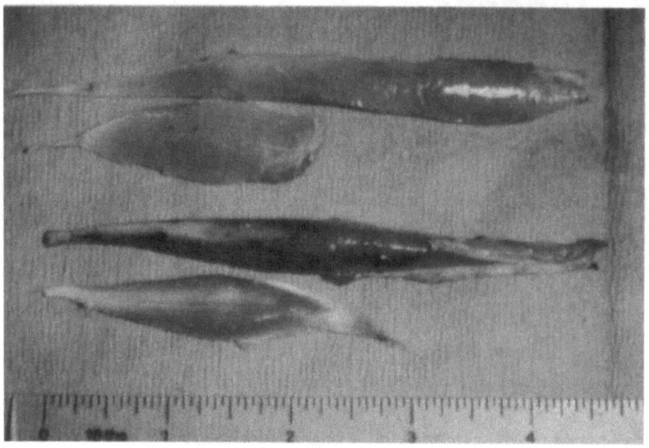

Fig. 4.3 Muscle specimens from the rabbit following experimental distraction: the upper two specimens are tibialis anterior and the lower two soleus. The upper specimen in each pair is the distracted muscle, which in each case is greater in length and in total volume than the corresponding muscle from the unoperated limb.

stiffness in a muscle will result in a need for the antagonist to exert more force to produce the same joint movement, and the system will therefore be less efficient. Increased stiffness may also cause a reduced speed of muscle response, and if this were to be permanent, it could lead to disability in conditions such as running and jumping. The cause of the fibrosis is not clear, but similar changes are seen in ischaemia.

A further basic question has remained unanswered until recently, namely, does lengthening promote growth of muscle tissue, or do the muscle fibres merely stretch? Ilizarov[11] demonstrated that "embryonic muscle" tissue may form within distracted muscle, and suggested that this indicated muscle growth. The observed histological response, however, could indicate either damage, or an overall growth response of the contractile tissues of the muscle. In our experimental studies, the muscles increased in length and in overall volume during lengthening (Fig. 4.3). At rates of less than 0.7mm per day (applied in two separate increments) the muscles became longer, and the cross-sectional area of the muscle fibres did not decrease, thus indicating an absolute increase in contractile tissue. There was a significant increase in the number of sarcomeres placed in a longitudinal manner within the muscle, and this also represents an increase in contractile tissue. Other recent experimental studies have labelled the cells which are dividing within distracted muscle and demonstrated that many newly dividing cells are seen during distraction (Szoke et al).[17] By means of other labelling techniques (detection of a muscle specific protein, Desmin), the cells were confirmed to be myoblasts or myotubes, and these authors conclude that lengthening leads to muscle proliferation.

Can these observations be applied to clinical practice in the treatment of patients? We simulated the leg-lengthening protocols used in clinical orthopaedics and showed that both muscle fibres and the ensheathing fibrous tissues are damaged at rates of distraction of 1.0mm per day and above, even when this is applied in two increments. The rate of 1mm per day has frequently been used in other experimental models, and is also commonly used for patients. It is not possible to compare absolute values between patients and experimental models, but it would appear that muscle and connective-tissue damage can be prevented by the use of very slow distraction. It may therefore be important to use slow rates of distraction which will allow effective myogenesis, particularly in patients with underlying loss of normal muscle compliance.

3. Tendons

Very little is known about the response of tendons to lengthening, though it is recognised that they do not adapt well, and that tendon tightening occurs after small percentage increases in the length of a limb segment (Fig. 4.4). Experimental studies, using the same model as that developed for muscle (Szoke et al),[18] have shown that tendons do adapt to distraction with a proliferative response and an increase in their length, but that 60 per cent of the total increase in length of the musculotendinous complex occurs within the muscular component. In skeletally immature animals, the percentage contribution to overall increase in length from the tendon is greater. Experience in the treatment of cerebral palsy has shown that tendon lengthening leads to weakness of the muscle, and this principle may also apply to tendons when they are divided surgically during a leg lengthening programme. The musculo- tendinous complex is best distracted progressively, unless there is initial major tendon contracture, when surgical lengthening of the tendon will have to be performed. Unfortunately, this latter situation frequently exists. Theoretically, it is best to stretch tendons, but marked early tightening leads to deformity, and this in turn places muscles at a mechanical disadvantage.

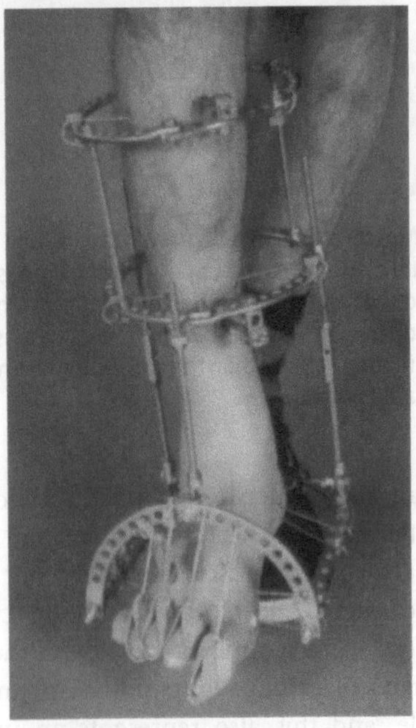

Fig. 4.4 Contracture of the long flexor tendons during leg lengthening; splintage may help to minimise this type of problem when using unilateral frames, or circular frames as demonstrated here.

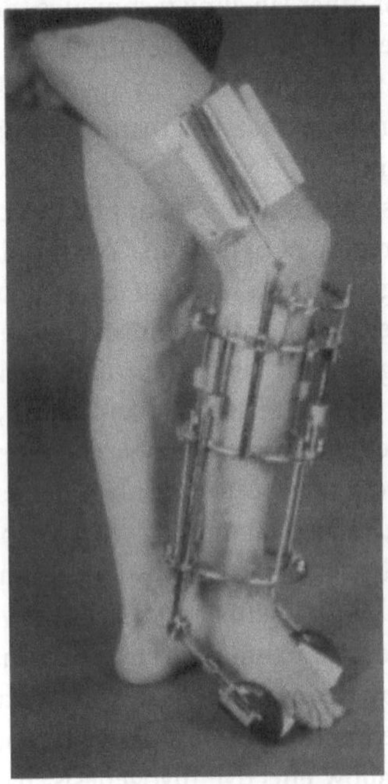

Fig. 4.5 Splints such as these help in the rehabilitation of joint and muscle function following lengthening.

Once muscles, and particularly those in the anterior compartment of the lower leg, have become weakened, the stronger calf muscles will predominate, and deformity will rapidly ensue. At this stage, it may be difficult with physiotherapy alone to produce the muscle strength necessary to prevent such contracture and tendon lengthening should be considered. Splints and rigorous rehabilitation must also be employed, to help prevent contracture of the musculotendinous complex (Fig. 4.5).

It is very important to stretch passively all muscle groups within the lengthened limb segment, on several occasions each day. The proliferation of epimyseal and perimyseal tissue was seen in experimental studies, and led to decreased compliance of the muscles. Fixed contracture will occur in these muscles. This process also occurs in patients under-

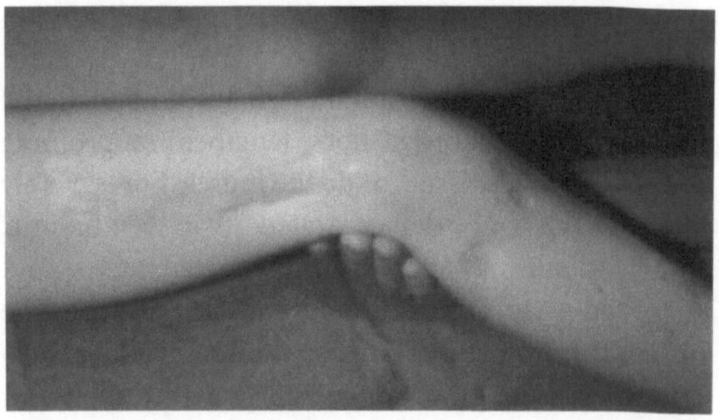

Fig. 4.6 Relative quadriceps shortening occurs frequently during leg lengthening in congenital shortening; if severe, quadricepsplasty should be performed.

going lengthening, and the risk can be reduced by concentrating upon passive stretch regimens during physiotherapy. The risk of contracture is considerable, however, even in those muscle groups in which less tension develops, due to the lengthening increments, e.g. the quadriceps muscle, and it is particularly important to stretch passively both the muscles in which there is great tension, and their antagonists (Fig. 4.6).

4. Joints

Great care must be taken of joints, both during the lengthening and the consolidation phases. Temporary loss of joint function is almost invariably seen in limb lengthening, but the incidence of permanent joint damage, or the risk of development of late degenerative joint disease, is not known. Three types of joint problem need to be considered.

(i) Loss of Range of Movement

This readily occurs during lengthening, for various reasons, which include (a) pain at the operation site, which inhibits the use of adjacent joints; (b) restricted movement associated with transmuscular screws or wires placed close to the joint; (c) low grade infection in screw tracks in the proximity of joints, which may worsen the problem by causing further discomfort or periarticular fibrosis; (d) the development of axial tension within muscles which act across the joint, so that the muscles are temporarily too short.

(ii) Function of the Articular Cartilage

The long-term effect of limb lengthening on the function of the articular cartilage within adjacent joints is not known. Experimental lengthening of 30 per cent has, however, been shown to lead to considerable fibrillation of the articular cartilage in the adjacent

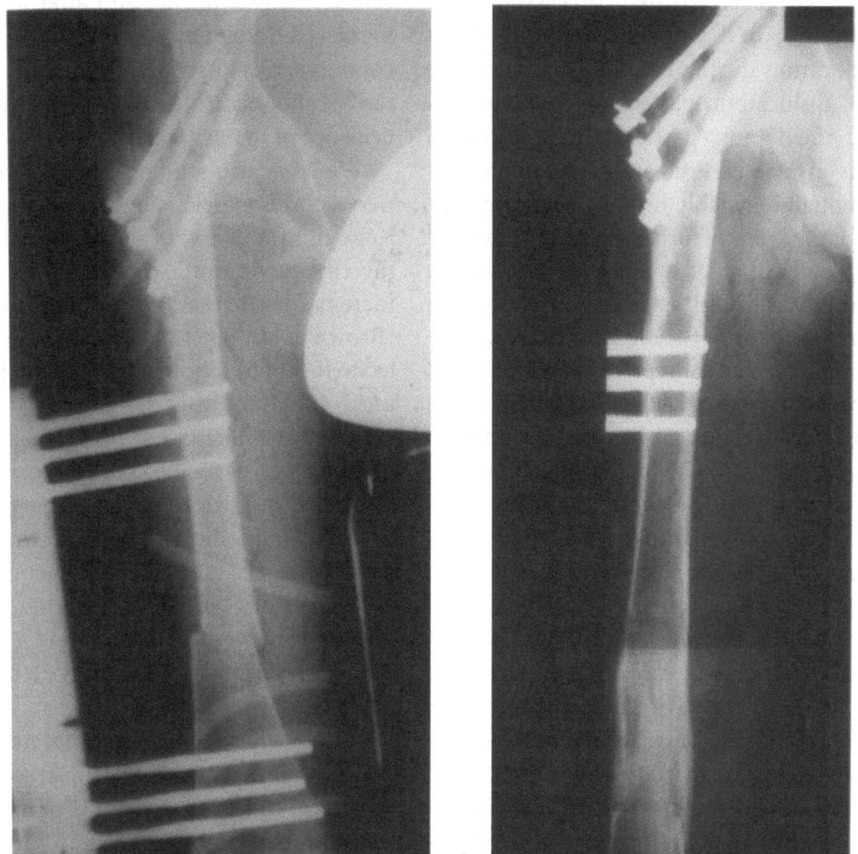

a b

Fig. 4.7 **a** Arthrodesis has been performed prior to leg lengthening in this patient with a pre-existing unstable hip joint, and the osteotomy for lengthening has been performed in the distal femur. **b** Leg lengthening has been successfully achieved without dislocation of the hip joint.

joint. This change was not seen in control, or in sham operated limbs (Stanitsky).[19]

Joint reaction forces have been measured directly from load cells placed both within the hip and the knee joints during simulated femoral lengthening in cadavers (Brad et al).[20] Continuous, moderately high joint forces were recorded within the hip joint particularly where the osteotomy was made through the proximal femur; 2.5cm of distraction led to measured loads of 14lbs acting across the articular surfaces of the hip joint. Much higher forces than these are probably exerted during lengthening in patients with congenital shortening of the limb (Simpson et al).[4] The level of these axial forces recorded from the external fixation frame in patients, correlated with the loss of range of joint movement. In practice, therefore, maintenance of an effective range of movement during lengthening probably means that no excessive forces are acting across the articular cartilage.

(iii) Prevention of Dislocation

Patients who have been treated successfully for dysplastic dislocation of the hip joint are often at risk of further dislocation during lengthening. The knee joint may also dislocate in patients with congenital shortening of the femur, particularly in those in whom there is associated cruciate ligament insufficiency. A potentially unstable hip or knee joint may well dislocate at the levels of force which act across the joint during lengthening. If a hip joint shows any signs of instability, surgical stabilization should be performed, preferably prior to lengthening (Fig. 4.7).

Ilizarov developed the concept of stabilization of joints by extension of the external fixation system across the joint. Such procedures may prevent joint subluxation and the occurrence of deformity, but large compressive forces can also develop. These can be reduced by designing the frame configuration so that the joint is isolated between two frames; distraction can then be applied across the joint with reduction of the axial compressive forces caused by the lengthening. The joint immobilization associated with any of these techniques may, however, lead to damage of cartilage. In practice, risks and advantages need to be balanced, and occasionally frames will need to be extended across joints.

In clinical practice, it would also seem very important to maintain joint function throughout the treatment period. Patients suffer discomfort, and will often be reluctant to move their joints during the first week following osteotomy. Intensive, but sympathetic rehabilitation is needed at this time. The use of epidural anaesthesia and CPM can be very helpful.

5. Nerves

Major nerve damage is uncommon with the distraction regimens used in clinical practice. Nerves can be damaged at the time of insertion of wires, when Ilizarov techniques are used. Paley[1] advises that any loss of nerve function seen immediately after operation should be treated by decompression of the nerve. This procedure increases the potential for excursion of the nerve, and allows subsequent lengthening to be undertaken. If nerve dysfunction develops during distraction, lengthening should be stopped and not recommenced until function has returned; it may then be recommenced at a very slow rate.

Most clinical studies record a very low incidence of permanent loss of nerve function. Galardi et al[21] noted that conduction velocity was nearly always reduced during leg lengthening. In our unit, a study was performed (Davies et al)[22] to examine the effects on nerve function of (a) the operation and (b) the subsequent lengthening. In 16 patients the conduction velocity before, during and after leg lengthening was measured. In patients with congenital shortening, the conduction velocity was frequently reduced temporarily, and occasionally patients developed clinical evidence of nerve damage.

We have also studied the effect of distraction on nerve under experimental conditions (Simpson and Kenwright).[23] Nerves can tolerate a 10 per cent acute increment without loss of function, but a 15 per cent incremental increase led to marked loss of function (Brown et al).[24] A 12 per cent increment in one stage led to loss of function which did not become apparent until 48 hours after lengthening; at this time the conduction velocity fell precipitously. The response of rabbit nerves to gradual distraction was also investigated. Radiologically opaque markers were attached to nerves and the response of the whole nerve to distraction was studied. Distraction increments in excess of 2 per cent per day in these adult rabbits led to loss of nerve function. Severe perineural fibrosis was also seen after gradual nerve lengthening of 2 per cent per day.

It does appear, therefore, that nerves will lengthen well, within the spectrum of distraction regimes used in clinical practice. In clinical practice, however, the common peroneal nerve seems particularly prone to damage. This may occur as a result of the pressure to which it is subjected at the level of the neck of the fibula rather than the axial tension occurring from the lengthening process.

Conclusions

Most writing on leg lengthening concentrates on the response of the bone, but it can be seen that the response of the soft tissues frequently limits the total length that can be achieved. In addition, the problems that develop within the soft tissues lead to most of the serious complications that can accompany limb lengthening. The clinical and experimental studies described here have shown that the soft tissues, like bone, are acutely sensitive to the distraction regime. Each soft tissue component will respond to the new length by an increase in total tissue, but each tissue is also acutely sensitive to damage. The risk of damage varies according to the pathology which has caused the leg length inequality. Each patient needs to be assessed for his or her individual response, and the programme may also need to be modified from a standard protocol at any stage, in accordance with the observed responses of the soft tissues. An inappropriate regimen of distraction applied to the osteogenesis gap will lead to poor quality of bone or premature union; situations which are retrievable. Inappropriate regimens of distraction applied to the soft tissues may result in permanent disability.

References

1. Paley D: 'Problems, obstacles, and complications of limb lengthening by the Ilizarov technique.' *Clin Orthop* 1990; *250: 81–104*
2. Dahl MT, Gulli B, Berg T. 'Complications of limb lengthening: A Learning Curve.' *Clin Orthop* 1994; 301: 10–18
3. Leong JCY, Ma RYP, Clark JA, Cornish LS, Yau ACMC. 'Viscoelastic behaviour of tissue in leg lengthening by distraction.' *Clin Orthop* 1979;139: 102–9
4. Simpson AHRW, Cunningham JL, Kenwright J. 'Forces in tissues during leg lengthening. A clinical investigation.' *J Bone Joint Surg* [Br] 1996; 78B: 979–83
5. White SH, Kenwright J. 'The importance of delay in distraction of osteotomies.' *Orthop Clin North Am* 1991; 22: 569–79
6. Aronson J, Harp JH, Hollis JM 'In vitro measurement of mechanical forces generated during distraction osteogenesis.' *Trans Orthop Res Soc* 1991; 37:440.
7. Li G, Simpson AHRW, Triffit JT. 'Rapid bone remodelling is accompanied by apoptosis during distraction osteogenesis.' ASAMI International Meeting in New Orleans, USA, March 1998
8. Simpson AHRW, Gardner T, Evans M, Herling G, Kenwright J. 'Prevention of deformity during leg lengthening.' *Clin Orthop* 1997; 341: 224–32
9. Sofield HA, Blair SJ, Millar EA 'Leg lengthening: a personal follow-up of forty patients some twenty years after the operation.' *J Bone Joint Surg* [Am] 1958; 40A: 311–22
10. Kawamura B, Hosono S, Takahashi T, Yano T, Kobayashi Y, Shibata N, Schinoda Y. 'Limb lengthening by means of subcutaneous osteotomy.' *J Bone Joint Surg* [Am] 1968; 50A: 851–77
11. Ilizarov GA 'The tension-stress effect on the genesis and growth of tissues: part I. The influence of stability of fixation and soft-tissue preservation.' *Clin Orthop* 1989; 238: 249–81
12. Kenwright J, Simpson AHRW. 'Soft tissue responses to leg lengthening.' *Journées Montpelliéraines de Chirugie Orthopédique*, Montpellier, June 1994
13. Simpson AHRW, Cunningham JL, Kenwright J. 'Compliance of tissues during leg lengthening – a clinical study.' European Orthopaedic Research Society, 1995 *J Bone Joint Surg* [Br] 1996; Suppl: 33
14. Simpson AHRW, Williams PE, Kyberd P, Kenwright J, Goldspink J. 'The response of muscle to limb lengthening.' *J Bone Joint Surg* [Br] 1995; 77B: 630–6
15. Gordon AM, Huxley AF, Julian FJ 'The variation in isometric tension with sarcomere length in vertebrate muscle fibres.' *J Physiol Lond* 1966; 184: 170–92
16. Matano T, Tamai K, Kurokawa T 'Adaptation of skeletal muscle in limb lengthening: a light diffraction study on the sarcomere length in situ.' *J Orthop Res* 1994; 122: 193–6
17. Szoke G, Lee SH, Bradley J, Kyberd PJ, Kenwright J, Simpson AHRW. 'Response of muscle to limb lengthening.' *J Bone Joint Surg* [Br] 1996; 78B (Suppl I): 40
18. Szoke G, Lee S, Kyberd P, Williams P, Simpson AHRW. 'The response of tendon to limb lengthening.' British Orthopaedic Research Society, Bristol, March 1995. *J Bone Joint Surg* [Br] 1995; 77B: 327
19. Stanitski DF, 'The effect of limb lengthening on articular cartilage: An experimental study.' *Clin Orthop* 1994; 301: 68–72
20. Brad W, Olney MD, Jayaraman G. 'Joint reaction forces during femoral lengthening.' *Clin Orthop* 1994; 301: 64–7
21. Galardi G, Comi G, Lozza L, Marchettini P, Novarina M, Facchini R, Paronzini A 'Peripheral nerve damage during limb lengthening.' *J Bone Joint Surg* [Br] 1990; 72B: 121–4
22. Davies PR, Simpson AHRW, Mills K. 'Nerve function during limb lengthening.' *J Bone Joint Surg* [Br] 1994; 76B (Suppl II and III): 143
23. Simpson AHRW, Kenwright J. 'The response of peripheral nerves to lengthening.' British Orthopaedic Research Society, 1992. *J Bone Joint Surg* [Br] 1992; Supplement II 74B: 326
24. Brown RA, Pedowitz RA, Kwan MK, Rydevik BL, Lee SV, Massie J, Woo SL-Y, Hargens AR, Garfin SR. 'The effect of acute stretch upon conduction properties of the rabbit tibial nerve.' *Orthopaedic Transactions* 1989; 13: 256

The Measurement of Fracture Healing

5

J.B. Richardson and J.R.W. Hardy

Interpreting the success of external fixation depends on the use of appropriate end-point measures. Not all end-points used in clinical studies are accurate or appropriate, however, and the wide variety of end-points used to assess fracture healing implies that there is no "gold standard" definition for it. Outcome measures for bone healing that have been investigated in the past include: (1) complications of treatment or injury, (2) time to clinical union (Ellis 1958a, Matthews et al 1974, Apley and Solomon 1982), (3) time to removal of plaster (Johnson and Pope 1977), (4) joint function (McMaster 1976), (5) direct fracture stiffness (Hammer et al 1984, Richards J and Mintowt-Czyz 1985, Richards 1987, Goodship and Lanyon 1988, Hente et al 1991, Richardson and O'Conner 1993, Richardson et al 1994), (6) indirect fracture stiffness (Jorgensen 1972, Burny 1968, Burny et al 1978, Burny et al 1984, Nishimura 1984, Cunningham et al 1987, Richardson et al 1992, Draper et al 1994, Nordeen et al 1995), (7) radiographs (Nicholls et al 1979), (8) the increasing area of callus (Lindholm et al 1970), (9) the size of the callus at clinical healing (Spencer 1987, Oni et al 1988a), (10) time to full weightbearing (Lawyer and Lubbers 1980), (11) Ultrasound (Floriani et al 1967, Abendschein and Hyatt 1972, Gerlanc et al 1975, Sekiguchi and Hirayama 1979, Christensen et al 1987, Benirschke et al 1993, Heckman et al 1994) and scintigraphy (Oni et al 1989).

Clinical Union

The commonest quoted end-point used to describe fracture healing is clinical union. Clinical union is determined by clinical impression. Time to clinical union depends on the reduction both of detectable symptoms and of the signs of abnormal movement at the site of a healing fracture. It is thus both inaccurate and subjective (Matthews et al 1974). The ability to weightbear through a new callus or the lack of tenderness at a fracture site can be transient. A patient, able to bear weight in the clinic on removal of his cast, may find that the new callus breaks following a relatively minor fall or undergoes fatigue failure with a long walk.

Time to full weightbearing is less often used as an end-point than independent weightbearing. A patient may be full weightbearing before independent weightbearing. Independent weightbearing is usually defined as the time at which all external support is no longer necessary. A patient treated by crutches and intramedullary nailing is independent when finally weightbearing without crutches, whereas a patient treated by crutches and external fixation is independent when finally weightbearing without crutches and without the external fixator. This clinical appearance of early healing following intramedullary nailing can lead to missed late atrophic non-union or hypertrophic non-union which may present as fatigue failure of the fixation device.

Radiographic Measures

Radiographs are used to measure deformity and assess fracture healing. Since X-rays were discovered by Röntgen in 1894, few radiographic measures of fracture healing have been proposed. The initial appearance of callus on radiographs has been observed to occur between 6 and 8 weeks, which is thought to coincide with a change in the levels of ionised calcium (Hardy et al 1993). Time to callus bridging has been proposed as a useful measure of fracture healing. This occurs in the second phase of fracture healing, at about 7 weeks from fracture. This may be some 9 weeks before clinical union and so cannot predict those patients who will, by enthusiastic weightbearing, develop a hypertrophic non-union. More often than not, papers describe the use of radiographs to demonstrate "complete union" without describing the method of making this diagnosis (Donald and Seligson 1983).

Radiographs are traditionally considered as poor measures of fracture healing. Spencer used the "fracture healing response" which was the ratio of the largest diameter of the healing mass measured from radiographs taken at 90° to each other, and the bone diameter at the fracture site on the same radiograph (Spencer 1987). With this method, good correlation was found between "fracture healing response" and time to clinical union.

Oni used Spencer's method, which he renamed the Callus Index, and also used equations to calculate callus as a volume of an ellipse and the bone volume as a perfect cylinder. He compared these with time to union and other end-points but found no correlation (Oni et al 1991).

Remodelling of cortical bone seems the best radiographic indicator of the strength of bony union (Panjabi et al 1985). Strength of bony union seems related to the number of trabeculae crossing the fracture gap (Claes et al 1985). Others have shown convincingly that a clinician's ability to determine effective osseous union using radiographs is poor (McKeown et al 1932, Eskelund and MunkPlum 1950, Nicholls et al 1979).

Tomograms, computerised axial tomography and magnetic resonance imaging have been used to assess fracture union but these cannot yet be used on a regular basis for end-point estimation because of cost.

Callus Growth

There have been rigorous studies on the histomorphometric and biomechanical properties of healing callus in animals (Koskinen 1959, Rokkanen and Slätis 1964, Lindholm and Törnkvist 1980, Lindholm and Törnkvist 1981, Sarmiento et al 1977, Markel et al 1991). There have also been studies that have used planimetery or radiographs to measure callus size in animals (Rokkanen and Slätis 1964, Mølster et al 1983). Urist and Johnson correlated the radiological and histological appearances of callus in man and explained that the "X-ray shows little more than a silhouette of the denser calcium deposits in the fracture site" (Urist and Johnson 1943).

Past authors, studying human fracture healing, have largely ignored the changes in the size of callus in animals demonstrated by six published studies (Lindsay and Howes 1931, McKeown et al 1932, Lindsay 1934, Falkenberg 1961, Lindholm et al 1970, Mølster et al 1982). Brighton and Krebs found a progressive increase in ultimate strength and stiffness in healing fibular fractures in rabbits as healing progressed. Lindsay and Howes studied fibular fractures in rats by subjecting the healing fractures to a simple bending test. They demonstrated a progressive increase in strength which correlated with increasing mineralization of the fracture and increasing callus area. After the twenty-first day, there was a decrease in strength and a decrease in callus area followed by a gradual increase in strength to normal levels despite a further decrease in callus size (Lindsay and Howes 1931). McKeown et al from the same group demonstrated in the rat that serial radiographs were of distinct value in determining the fracture strength only up to the formation of the largest diameter callus; thereafter their value diminished (McKeown et al 1932). Lindsay later found a direct correlation between the breaking strength of the healing fracture and the size and weight of the whole bone. He noted that breaking strength varied according to three phases of fracture healing: fibrosis, calcification, and structural reorganization (Lindsay 1934). Falkenberg noted, from observing healing osteotomies of the radius in rabbits, a peak in callus area between 20 and 30 days following fracture. From 20 to 60 days, the callus area decreased by 50 per cent, but the absolute tensile strength increased 100 per cent. He observed that an increase in mineral content correlated with the increase in callus strength in the late stages of fracture healing. Falkenberg concluded that the initial rapid increase in the ultimate tensile strength occurred with increasing callus area, and the quality of the callus improved more slowly in conjunction with fracture remodelling. A combination of increasing mineral content, reorientation of the hydroxyapatite crystals, and secondary osteon formation contributed to the late increase in strength of the healing fracture (Falkenberg 1961).

It is not only an increase in mineral content that is associated with an increasing stiffness. Sarmiento et al recognised the importance of the bulk of callus in the early stages of fracture repair (Sarmiento et al 1977) but failed to investigate the increasing diameter of fracture callus in man by measuring its extent on radiographs.

The size of callus was previously thought to be determined by the size of the fracture haematoma (Potts 1932, Hulth 1989). Proliferation of the

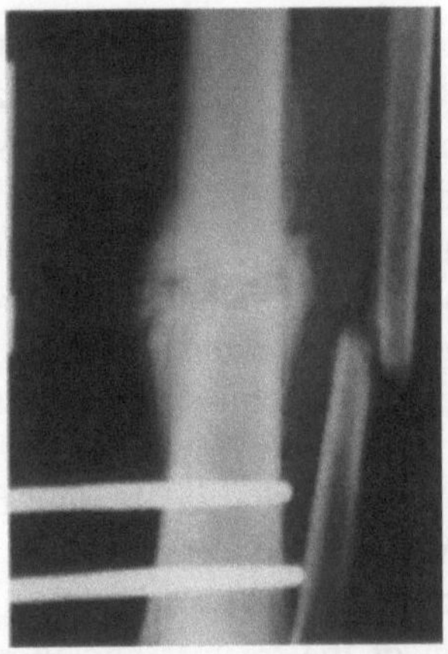

Fig. 5.1 Large callus which has built up over a 16 week period with full weightbearing from 2 weeks following fracture. Note the lamellation of callus adjacent to the pin which has been laid down by the cambial layer of the periosteum in response to fracture site movement.

periosteum must be responsible in part for the size of callus as we see radiographically the onion skin appearance associated with proliferation of periosteal callus (Fig. 5.1).

Aro et al demonstrated that the radiographic size of fracture callus correlated well with actual callus size measured by histomorphometry (Aro et al 1985). Therefore, radiographic measures in humans should be a good representation of the actual callus present. The comparison of changing callus diameter and fracture stiffness with time has recently been published (Hardy 1997).

If callus growth is a phenomenon stimulated by micromovement, then removal of an external fixator when a fracture has reached the desired stiffness that predicts the "healed" fracture (15 Nm/deg) (Richardson et al 1994) should be accompanied by evidence of continued remodelling. Clinical impression suggests that no refracture occurs when an external fixator is removed above a fracture stiffness of 15 Nm/deg but serial observations of callus growth and subsequent remodelling have provided an objective indication that even after removal of a fixator above 15Nm/deg a restimulation of callus growth occurs. This suggests that the patient's progress must continue to be monitored after fixator removal (Hardy 1997).

Refracture

Refracture seems to depend on the type of injury and the treatment used. The refracture rate following removal of plates used for treating tibial shaft fractures can be as low as 1.7 per cent to 2.4 per cent (Böstman 1983, Bilat et al 1994). This is probably because few plates are removed before 18 months, by which time bone has remodelled the cortical defect. Failure of bone in these circumstances is probably from a single load rather than fatigue loading. Fracture may occur at the original site or through one of the screw holes. Most refractures occur through a screw site after plating and are associated with sport (Pinder 1973).

Refracture is a common complication of external fixation following premature removal. It has been reported to occur in between 3 per cent and 13.8 per cent of patients following external fixation (Rommens et al 1986, Gershuni and Halma 1983) and is twice as common when supplementary lag screws are used (Krettek et al 1991). Some authors have blamed the rigidity of the fixator for this delay in healing and the high refracture rate without allowing for differences in the severity of the injury between the groups studied (Gershuni and Halma 1983). However, even if patients treated with relatively stiff frames, like the Hoffmann frame, are converted early to plaster cast or braces, the refracture rate can be as high as 4.1 per cent (Schröder et al 1986).

New methods of determining progression of fracture healing by the serial measurement of fracture stiffness have been reported to help to reduce this refracture rate (Richardson et al 1992). However, it is unlikely that measurement of fracture stiffness, which is the Young's modulus of fracture callus, can predict failure from overloading with a single load or through cyclic loading (fatigue). Callus, like bone, is probably highly susceptible to stress concentrations, and crack propagation through the bridge of peripheral callus from the fracture site requires a relatively small portion of the total failure energy. Pugh and Dee observed that for bone, as with any composite material, fatigue failure "often occurs within the apparent elastic limit of a material [below the yield stress]. The fracture typically begins at a stress concentration... and progresses along a microscopic amount with the application of each cycle of loading." (Pugh and Dee 1989).

Fracture Stiffness

The mechanical function of bone is to support and protect. To perform these functions bones need to be stiff. A break in the continuity of a bone reduces this stiffness. It seems obvious therefore, to measure fracture healing as a return to pre-fracture stiffness. Recent investigators have made use of the mechanical properties of healing callus to study the progress of fracture healing. The unscientific extrapolation of elasticity to ultimate strength (Mather 1967) has resulted in a common misuse of stiffness as a definition of the "healed" fracture.

White et al (1977) have described four stages of mechanical healing: (1) springy, rubbery callus low in stiffness, (2) resilient callus higher in stiffness, (3) hard callus with high stiffness and refracture through the original site, and (4) hard bone with high stiffness and fracture through a new site on ultimate testing.

To understand how the stiffness of a healing bone can be of use to the clinician one must have a grasp of the basic biomechanical properties of intact bone. Two types of stress may act on a bone, normal stress and shear stress. Normal stress is the force per unit area, perpendicular to the area on which it acts. Shear stress is the force per unit area acting parallel to the surface.

Strain is the change in dimension produced by a force. There are two types of strain: longitudinal and shear. Longitudinal strain is a change in length relative to the original length. Shear strain is an angular deformation measured as angular change at a right angle to the plane of interest. Strain can be measured. Stress exists within a material and can only be determined indirectly. Normal stress at a surface is considered as pressure which is measurable (Evans 1973).

The elasticity of a material is its capacity to return to its original shape following removal of a load. When strain is proportional to stress, a material is said to obey Hooke's Law, and when strain is plotted against stress, a straight line results. Stress divided by strain determines the modulus of elasticity of a material such as bone (Young's modulus = E).

The slope of stress over strain increases as the rigidity (stiffness) of a material increases, so a rigid material has a higher elastic modulus than an easily deformed material. As callus becomes calcified, and its structure changes, its modulus of elasticity changes. However, the stiffness of the whole healing bone is dependent on more than just the callus material that surrounds the fracture gap. The stiffness of a limb is not only dependent on the material properties of bone but also on its structure and geometry.

When unbroken bone is stressed beyond its elastic limit, it exhibits plastic behaviour and fails to return to its original dimensions once the load has been released (Burnstein et al 1972). The linear relationship between stress and strain no longer applies. In other words, a permanent deformation occurs. Progressive increase in load eventually results in a fracture. The strength of a bone refers to its resistance to fracture. Likewise, the definition of a healed bone should be one which has returned to its original strength. The yield strength refers to the stress at its elastic limit. The ultimate strength is the stress at the point of fracture. In a ductile material, the point of maximum stress appears to occur prior to fracture. This is because stress is a force per unit area, and a plastic material undergoes a local decrease in cross-sectional area during plastic yield (necking). The plastic property makes bone, and probably callus, twice as strong as it would be if it did not yield before ultimate failure (Burnstein et al 1972). Bone, and by inference callus, will fail at a lower stress if the load is cycled (fatigue failure). This property presents a problem for the surgeon who is often asked by patients, anxious to return to exercise or sport, whether their fracture has healed.

The toughness of a material is its resistance to fracture. Toughness signifies the strain energy (work) built up in a material as load is applied. It is dependent on strain, as well as on stress, and so two materials with the same breaking strength may absorb markedly different amounts of energy prior to fracture. When a bone is stressed to failure, and stress is plotted against strain, the area under the curve is equal to the work done (stored energy). When tested in tension, cortical bone can elongate by approximately 0.75 per cent of its original length before permanent deformation occurs.

Bone and callus are composite materials that exhibit viscoelastic properties. This means that their mechanical properties (the shape of the stress/strain curve) are dependent on the rate of stress application; the more rapid the rate of applied load, the greater the modulus and ultimate strength.

Thus stiffness is not the same as strength. To measure the return in ultimate strength of a broken bone necessitates testing to failure. This has been done on animals (Lindsay and Howes 1931) but cannot be done in man for obvious reasons.

The strength of a healing bone seems to correlate with the number of osteons that cross the fracture gap (Claes et al 1985). This suggests that the ultimate strength of a healed bone should be similar whether it is achieved by primary or secondary healing (Aro et al 1988). The advantage of secondary bone healing is that external callus forms rapidly and is mechanically sound enough to allow weightbearing in the early period before remodelling. Remodelling then imparts further stiffness and strength sufficient to resist the normal forces impacting upon the intact tibia.

A fracture in a long bone normally heals by the formation of a strong bridge of callus. The formation of a callus bridge sufficient to heal a tibial shaft fracture takes on average 16 weeks. After this, a patient can walk comfortably unaided. Once the callus bridge is able to prevent fracture site movement on weightbearing, below an unknown threshold level, then the fracture site is remodelled by the cutting osteons into stronger lamellar bone. At the stage in healing where clinically detectable fracture site movement is prevented, weightbearing becomes painless. This may be because the callus is large enough and strong enough to resist the bending that stretches the well-innervated periosteum around the maturing callus. Callus provides stiffness by virtue of its structure and composition, and the latter changes with time (Slätis and Rokkanen 1965).

Stiffness measurement in a healing fracture is not a simple measurement of Young's modulus of elasticity. Direct fracture stiffness is the stiffness of the healing limb unsupported by an immobilization device and it is a measure of the soft tissues as well as of the fibula and tibia. For example, a reduced, axially stable fracture with an intact periosteum will have a stiffness to bending by virtue of an intact fibrous periosteum (Hardy et al 1996).

The stiffness of a healing limb can be defined as:

$$stiffness = {}^{load}\!/_{displacement}$$

Fracture stiffness is calculated in units of Newton metres per degree (Nm/deg). The stiffness of intact bone is about 60 Nm/degree. The advantage of measuring stiffness, rather than strength, is that it causes no pain and does not harm the healing callus, provided failure does not occur.

Early stiffness measurements were called stability measurements, and were derived from the measured deflection on radiographs before and after loading the tibia in the sagittal plane (Jernberger et al 1970, Hammer et al 1984).

In 1984, Professor Bourgois compared theoretical and experimental results of strain gauge measurements from Hoffmann fixators applied to cadaveric tibiae. This is indirect stiffness measurement. He used cuts in a tibia with an intact fibula, and one with a divided fibula, to weaken the bone progressively. The calculated degree of weakening plotted against the bending moment showed a simple hyperbolic relationship (Bourgois and Burny 1984) which correlated well with his theoretical model (Bourgois and Burny 1972). Bourgois and Burny were cautious, suggesting that fracture stiffness measured in this way could not be used to diagnose the healed fracture. They wrote, "From theoretical studies, we conclude that when the curve becomes asymptotic, the callus stiffness is not that of normal bone but represents some 20–50 per cent of this value and not full healing" (Bourgois and Burny 1972). The models used in these studies are an over-simplification of the structure and constitution of callus surrounding a fracture gap. The variation in site, size, shape, and rate of callus production seen in the patients studied for this thesis and other series gives some insight into the variables on which stiffness must depend (Richards 1985).

One clear advantage of strain-gauging an external fixator is that measurements can be performed from the earliest time after fracture (Mintowt-Czyz and Richards 1986, Draper et al 1994). A disadvantage of indirect fracture stiffness measurements seems to be an unpredictable refracture rate (Richardson et al 1992). A further disadvantage is that the measurements become inaccurate when the pins loosen (Churches et al 1985).

Different frame types have an influence on the measured stiffness. It is obviously better, therefore, to perform stiffness measurements without the influence of a frame. This is only possible as fracture healing progresses into the second phase, characterised by calcification of the callus, which occurs between 6 and 8 weeks (Hardy et al 1993). With earlier removal there is a risk of pain and loss of reduction with most fractures.

Techniques for measuring a direct bending stiffness in one plane are becoming well-established as a measure of fracture healing (Goodship and Kenwright 1985, Cunningham et al 1987, Richardson and O'Connor 1993, Richardson et al 1994). The reproducibility and accuracy of direct fracture stiffness has recently been evaluated (Hardy et al 1994).

Both direct and indirect fracture stiffness measurements have been used to define the "healed" fracture. Different stiffnesses have been proposed as definitions, the latest recommendation being 15 Newton metres per degree (Richardson et al 1994). In this historical cohort study of patients with fracture stiffness measurements and clinical union measurements, two groups were compared. The first was a series of patients who had indirect fracture stiffness measurements. In this group the external fixation device was removed on clinical grounds and in many cases replaced with a cast brace. The second, a group of patients from various sources, had direct fracture stiffness measurements. The refracture rate was compared. Patients whose fixation was removed on clinical grounds had a 6.8 per cent refracture rate, as against no refractures when fixators were removed above a stiffness of 15 Nm/deg. This suggests that fracture stiffness is a more reliable outcome measure than clinical methods and complements clinical examination (Richardson et al 1994).

Fracture Stiffness

The Technique

A thorough investigation into the accuracy and reproducibility of fracture stiffness has identified variables that need to be taken into account when using this technique for monitoring the progress of healing (Hardy et al 1994, Hardy 1997). Fracture stiffness measurements seem to be both accurate and reproducible. Performing stiffness measurements predicts those patients not progressing to union. In patients with a healing fracture it allows removal of the fixator at the earliest opportunity. While the rate of clinical refracture is not as low as predicted by earlier investigations (Richardson et al 1994), it is low.

Stiffness measurements should be made after the first appearances of calcified callus on radiograph. By eight weeks most fracture sites can be gently manipulated without producing pain. Most patients fear removal of their fixator, anticipating that it will be painful. Measurements are best performed after the patient has first been reassured. The following is a description of the use of the Orthometer® (Orthofix srl, Verona, Italy).

A full explanation of the procedure is followed by placing the patient's leg over a support at the knee acting as a lever with the heel resting on the load cell (Fig. 5.2). The fixator is then carefully removed. Discomfort before or during the test should prompt replacement of the fixator with a repeated attempt at stiffness measurement two weeks later.

Removal of a fixator can be uncomfortable. Holding the fixator to counterbalance the torque of undoing the fixator clamps prevents discomfort. Patients are often reassured by clinical examination which shows that movement at the fracture site is not necessarily painful. Apart from reassuring the patient this manoeuvre also provides the clinician with a clinical impression of how fracture site stiffness is progressing.

Following removal of the fixator, the patient's pins should be cleaned using a swab soaked in 70 per cent isopropyl alcohol. This has the advantage of physically removing dried blood, reducing the risk of transmission of infective agents to health workers, and of transmission of staphylococcal organisms from one of the patient's pin sites to another.

Before the stiffness measurements are made it is important to ensure that the tibia and fibula are in the same plane, horizontal to the plane of the load cell at the heel and that the patient can line up the rotation of the foot against a distant object in order to begin each measurement with the same amount of rotation of the tibia. Rotation can affect the variability of the results (Hardy et al 1994). The goniometer is then attached to the fixator pins as directed by the manufacturer (Fig. 5.3).

For each patient, 5 measurements are performed. The patient's face should be watched for signs of discomfort during the procedure. A folded piece of elastic bandage or other suitable material may be used to comfortably apply pressure over the fracture site (Fig. 5.4).

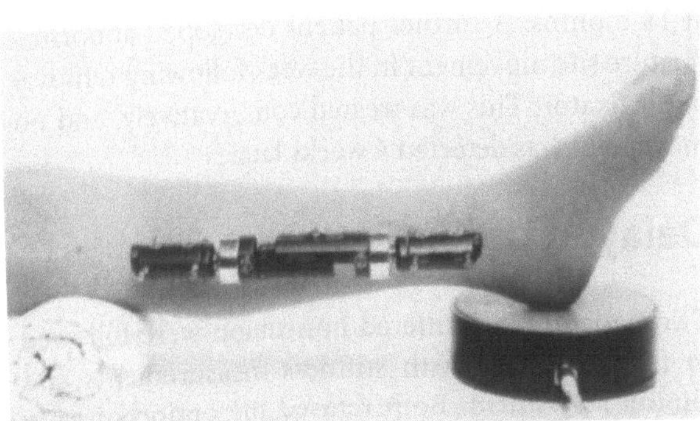

Fig. 5.2 The knee should be rested on a roll of towelling with the patient's heel on the centre of the load cell prior to taking the measurements that are required for the Orthometer® to calculate stiffness.

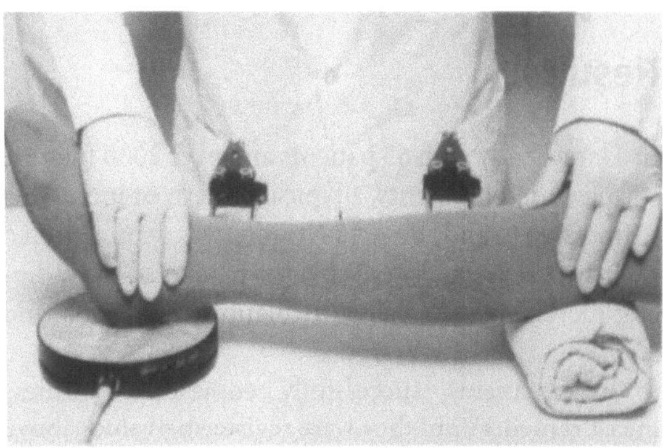

Fig. 5.3 Check that the malleoli are in the same horizontal plane and ask the patient to line up their big toe with a distant object so that the same rotation is maintained throughout the procedure.

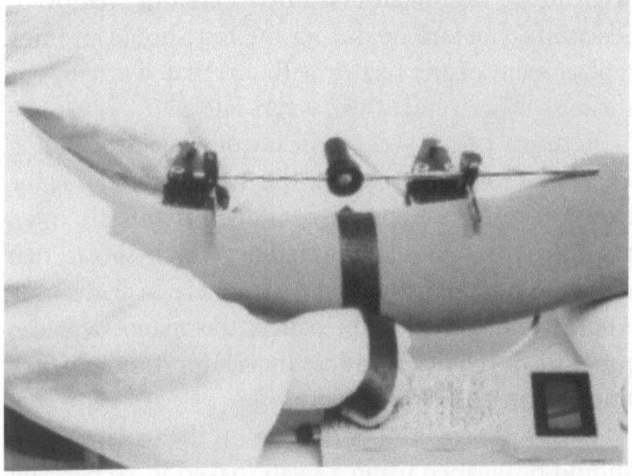

Fig. 5.4 While performing each measurement the clinician should look for signs of discomfort on the patient's face.

When a stiffness of 15 Newton meters per degree is reached and there is clinical and radiographic evidence of union, the fixator and pins can be removed. The clinician should not be afraid to persist with the treatment if there are any clinical doubts as to healing, particularly when healing is tested in the plane at right angles to the plane of stiffness measurement. The criteria for union should include: (1) radiographs confirming a healing fracture, (2) absence of fracture site movement or tenderness, (3) the ability to walk around the department comfortably without the fixator, and the ability to stand on the affected leg unsupported for more than 20 seconds.

If the measured fracture stiffness is below 15 Nm/deg, the fixator should be carefully replaced in its original position. This is made easier by using a fixator which maintains its position on loosening the pin clamps (Orthofix®) and by marking the position of the fixator on the pins before removal of the fixator.

Results

In a large study with 65 patients and over 2000 fracture stiffness measurements, a typical pattern of increasing stiffness up to and above 15 Nm/deg was demonstrated (Hardy et al 1994). These changes paralleled the radiographic changes in callus formation (Figs. 5.5a and 5.5b.).

Fifty patients successfully completed stiffness measurements until they were registering values above 15 Nm/deg. The mean stiffness at removal of the fixator for the 50 patients over 15 Nm/deg was 23.62 Nm/deg (range 15.11–44.38). The mean was skewed by the few patients referred towards the end of treatment rather than at the beginning. The number of patients successfully measured from a stiffness below 15 Nm/deg to above 15 Nm/deg was thirty-five. The mean stiffness at removal of the fixator for these 35 patients was 21.95 Nm/Deg (range 15.11–34.55).

No patient experienced pain and no complaints have been received to date as a result of the stiffness measurement. No patient lost reduction of the fracture position but particular care was taken to prevent too early removal of the fixator in patients with unstable fractures.

Discontinuity Pattern

Nearly all patients had a progressive increase in stiffness which could roughly be fitted to a hyperbolic graph as predicted by Bourgois. In 12 patients, however, the progressive increase in stiffness was interrupted by a sudden reduction in stiffness associated with a clinical loss of stability. This was always associated with an increase in the bearing of weight through the limb or an increase in the exercise taken by the patient. Two patients demonstrated a progressive decrease in stiffness from an initial stiffness well above 15 Nm/deg. These patients were young men who had fracture patterns in which, on reduction of the fragments, the fracture site was rigidly held in all planes.

Fatigue Refracture

Two patients refractured within two weeks of removal of their fixators and two suffered late refractures over the 12 months following fixator removal. One patient ignored advice against undertaking excessive activity on removal of the fixator and subsequently developed a hypertrophic non-union (Fig. 5.6). He reached a stiffness of 14.78 Nm/deg at 23 weeks and only healed at 18 months. A further patient developed abnormal fracture site movement in the week following removal of his fixator. This was treated conservatively, and no movement was detected 4 weeks later.

Delayed Union Pattern

Two patients who suffered non-union were followed to fracture union with stiffness measurements and clinical assessment. Both refused the option of early bone grafting when this was discussed from 24 weeks. Four patients showed no progression of fracture stiffness before 24 weeks and underwent a change of treatment with bone grafting.

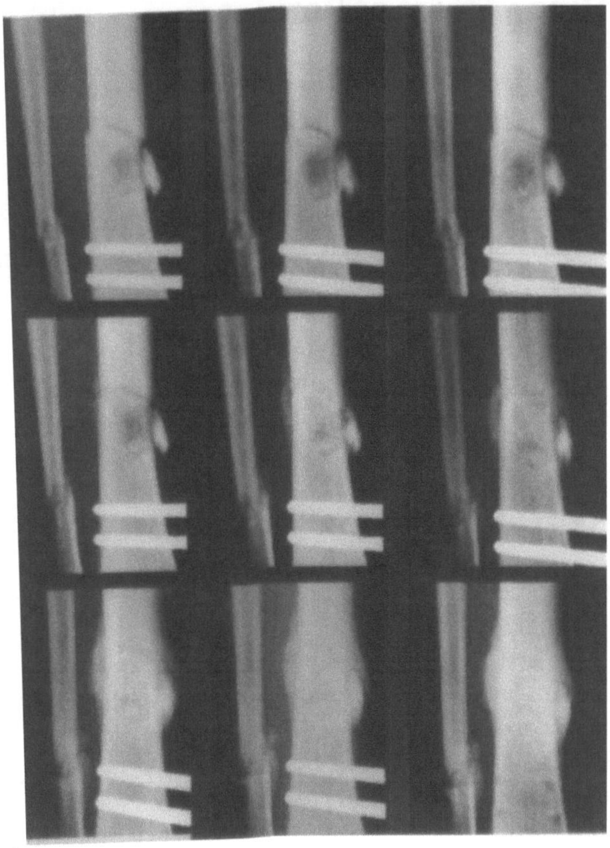

a

Asymmetrical Stiffness

In two patients rotation of the limb by 5° caused a 5–25 per cent change in the stiffness measurement. The change was either greater or less than the reading with the tibia and fibula in the same horizontal plane. This was probably due to the fibula, and to the irregular distribution of the callus.

The effect of rotating the limb by 90° to test stiffness in the sagittal plane was variable. In most patients at a stiffness of around 15 Nm/deg there was a lower stiffness in the plane 90° to the normal. This drop was demonstrated on 30 occasions while testing stiffness. It seemed to be due to the predominance of mature callus posteriorly and the state of healing of the fibula fracture if present. The bigger drops in stiffness were associated with the absence of fracture site movement in the antero-posterior plane but presence of sagittal movement at 90° to the normal plane. In these patients the fixator was left on until little movement could be detected at 90° to the normal plane. On twelve occasions, measuring fracture stiffness in two planes, patients had a higher stiffness 90° to the normal plane. This occurred in those with mature callus and/or an intact or healed fibula.

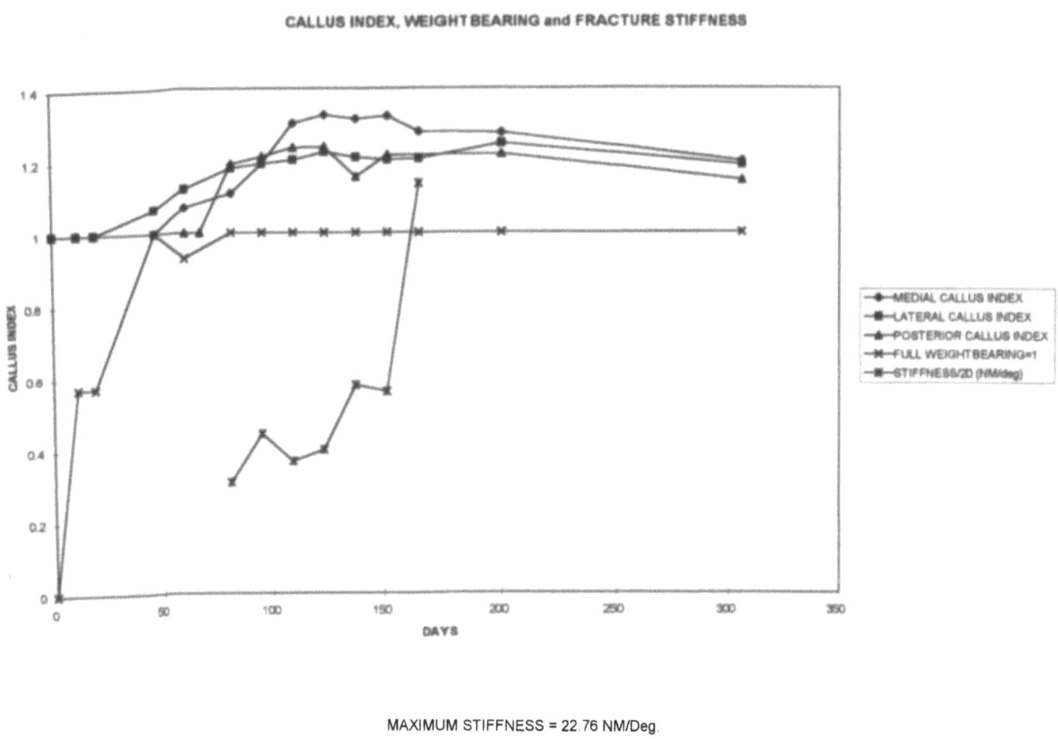

b

Fig. 5.5 The radiographs in **a** are represented in the changes in callus diameter as measured by callus index in **b** (Hardy 1997). The rising stiffness is associated with an increasing diameter of callus measured from the radiographs.

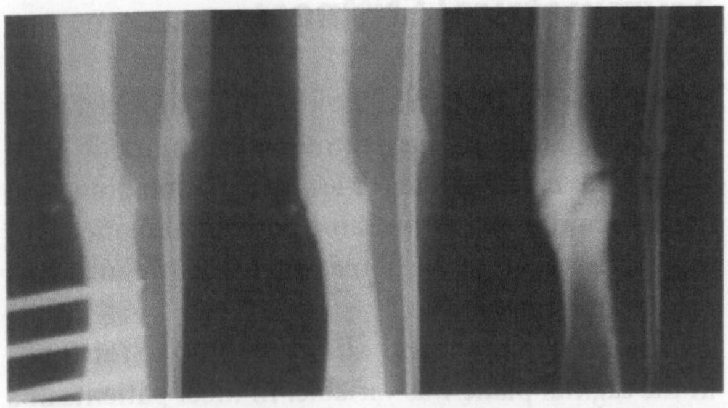

Fig. 5.6 Hypertrophic non-union developed after removal of the fixator at a value above 15Nm/deg in this heavy patient who refused operative treatment.

Loading Rate Effects

It was noticed, during the early part of this study, that the stiffness recordings were reduced if the duration of load was made shorter than the time between the start and end signals (Hardy et al 1994). This is probably due to the hysteresis effect of the complex material being tested. It is thus important to ensure that the load is applied for the entire period of time between the audible signals. A subjective change in the rate of application of the load did not alter the measured fracture stiffness.

Hinge Effect of Periosteum

During the course of the study it was discovered that if the limb was lifted before measurement, the measured stiffness would drop markedly in some patients. Lifting caused an increased angulation of above 2° in some patients, which significantly lowered the fracture stiffness measurement (Fig. 5.7). In 3 patients it caused a greater than 50 per cent drop in stiffness.

The drop seen with lifting reverses with progression of healing. One patient was followed up until this trend towards a drop in stiffness had reversed. The reversal occurred 2 weeks after he had reached a stiffness of 15 Nm/deg.

Reproducibility of Measurements

Overall accuracy of the prototype apparatus used in this study was estimated at ± 3 per cent.

To test the reproducibility of the prototype, the median and standard deviations of all five measurements on each patient at each sitting were used. Two hundred and thirty-two sessions of five stiffness measurements in the normal plane were sorted in ascending order of stiffness and ranked according to three ranges of stiffness. The median of five measure-

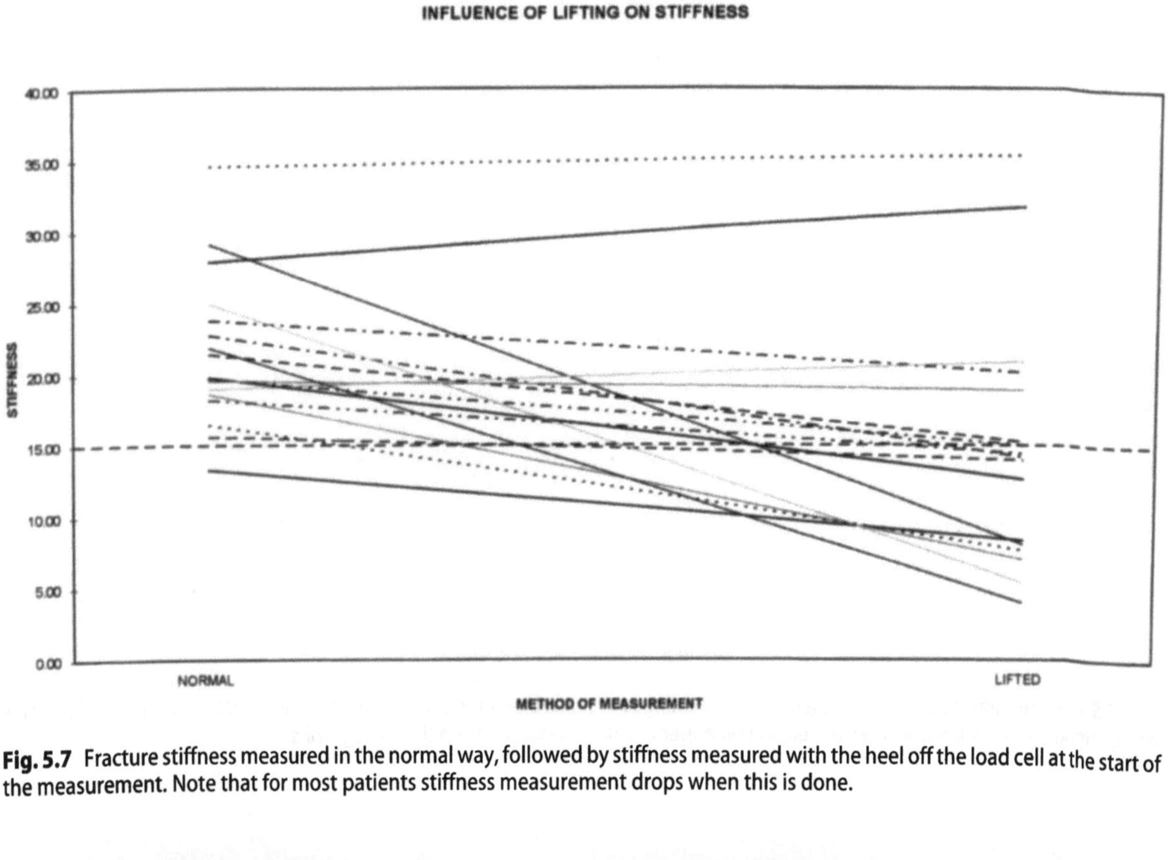

Fig. 5.7 Fracture stiffness measured in the normal way, followed by stiffness measured with the heel off the load cell at the start of the measurement. Note that for most patients stiffness measurement drops when this is done.

ments at each sitting was calculated as well as the standard deviations. Median values were close to mean values in all cases but the geometric mean was considered a more appropriate estimate of the average for five measures. The standard deviations were then expressed as a percentage of the median stiffness for 5 measures. All these percentages were then averaged in each range to give an idea of the reproducibility of the stiffness measurements (Table 5.1). This shows that in the range of stiffness from 7.29 Nm/deg to 39.0 Nm/dg the Coefficient of Variance is 10.7 per cent. Lower stiffness measurements seem less reproducible.

Stiffness Range Nm/Deg	Number of Patients Measured 5 times	Coefficient of Variance (%)
0.75 – 7.28	78	13.8
7.29 – 13.27	78	10.7
13.28 – 39.0	76	10.7

Table 5.1 Measurements ranked according to stiffness and divided into 3 groups to assess reproducibility of the measures in the stiffness ranges quoted.

Discussion

The advantage of serial measures of fracture stiffness is that they show the biomechanical progress of the callus and therefore complement the progress detected clinically. Radiographic determination of fracture healing has been demonstrated to be unpredictable (Nicholls et al 1979). Clinical examination is one method of assessing healing but it may leave patients in a fixation device for longer than would have been necessary. Refracture on removal of the device may occur in up to 6 per cent of patients unless a more objective measure of fracture healing is used. Initial studies, using the described method, suggested that the tibia is strong enough to be unsupported when the stiffness has reached 15 Nm/degree, and using this as a minimum level of stiffness before removal of the fixator reduces the refracture rate (Cunningham et al 1987, Richardson et al 1994). This figure may be too low in some circumstances, however.

One must be careful when interpreting the results of direct fracture stiffness in the light of the unusual cases demonstrated here. There are many obvious variables not previously considered in early reports of this measurement in the literature (Hammer et al 1984, Goodship and Lanyon 1988, Hente et al 1991, Richardson and O'Conner 1993). Sudden drops in stiffness of the order of magnitude of 3 per cent of previous recordings are likely to be due to measurement variation. Much larger reductions in stiffness are likely to be due to sudden fatigue failure of bridging callus. These reductions in stiffness may be managed by a period of 6 or more weeks of reduced weightbearing. Unusual patterns of changing stiffness may be due to the circumstances of reduction where a perfect, and unusually stiff, reduction probably loses its original stiffness due to the natural resorption of the necrotic bone ends with time (Charnley 1961). This is the first time this phenomenon has been demonstrated and suggests that resorption of the bone ends of a well reduced fracture takes place about the 5th to 9th week after fracture in man.

Fracture stiffness measurements have been shown to be a reproducible, and probably accurate measure of the progress of fracture healing. A standard deviation of 5 weeks for most sub-groups of tibial fractures allows a clinical trial to be performed with 42 patients to examine a treatment expected to improve healing by 5 weeks. This was recently used in a multi-centre study of BMP2. True accuracy could only be determined if there was a better independent measure of healing. In this series at least two patients had a symptomatic refracture despite a stiffness of 15 Nm/deg. Fracture stiffness at this level cannot predict the strength of the newly formed callus. It is therefore important to warn the patient that refracture can occur with an excessive single load or through fatigue.

Measurements are most repeatable when in the upper ranges of measurement. This is close to the point when a patient is reaching 15 Nm/deg (Cunningham et al 1987, Richardson et al 1992). An et al noted that calculated measurement of fracture stiffness using a strain gauge system on an external fixator bar was only sensitive until it reached 25 per cent of the stiffness of the intact bone (An et al 1988). This represents around 16 Nm/deg. This limitation was thought to be due to the stiffness of the fixator itself.

The plastic nature of early callus has been demonstrated. The clinical implication of this early plasticity is that if a fixator is to be removed to perform direct stiffness measurements then it is best to use a fixator in which the position of the pin holding clamps does not change. This will enable the original position to be duplicated on replacing the fixator until the next series of measurements is due. The Orthofix® fixator permitted this without complications for the patients. A marker should be used, before removal of the fixator, to indicate the position of the fixator on the pins so that it can be resited in exactly the same place.

Factors that reduce the reproducibility of the method, such as rotation of the limb, should be avoided. Caution should be exercised in patients who have reached 15 Nm/deg in the normal plane but who have a much reduced stiffness on lifting or who still have movement in the sagittal plane. These patients have obviously not yet healed and may go on to fatigue fracture.

Patients were advised to rest after fixator removal if the fracture site began to ache with excessive exercise. Patients were also instructed by showing them, on radiographs, the state of fracture callus at the time of removal of the fixator. The analogy of fatigue fracture of a coat hanger wire was used to warn them that excessive weightbearing in the early period after removal of the fixator could result in fatigue fracture of the newly formed callus.

Other obvious factors to consider include any malalignment of the limb, and excessive weight in a patient, since these will increase the bending moments applied to the healing fracture site.

Historically, the figure of 15 Nm/deg was calculated from indirect, as against direct, stiffness measurements (Richardson et al 1992). Until now no study has objectively investigated the variables to demonstrate that 15 Nm/deg is an insufficient level of stiffness for direct fracture stiffness measurements in some patients (Hardy et al 1994). It is clear from our understanding of biomechanical principles that stiffness is not the same as strength. This is as Bourgois and Burny suggested in 1972 and is borne out by the results of this study. Fracture stiffness should be used to measure the rate of healing in conjunction with clinical methods for optimal management of patients treated by external fixation.

Bibliography

Abendschein WF and Hyatt GW. 'Ultrasonics and physical properties of healing bone'. *J Trauma* 1972; **12**: 297–9.

An K-N, Kasman RA, Chao EYS. 'Theoretical analysis of fracture healing monitoring with external fixators.' *Eng Med* 1988; **17**: 11–5.

Apley AG and Solomon L. *Concise system of orthopaedics and fractures.* Butterworths: London 1982.

Aro HT, Eerola E, Aho AJ. 'Determination of callus quantity in 4-week-old fractures of the rat tibia.' *J Orthop Res* 1985; **3**: 101–8.

Aro HT, Kelly PJ, Lewallen DG, and Chao EYS. 'Comparison of the effects of dynamisation and constant rigid fixation on rate and quality of bone osteotomy union in external fixation.' Proc. 34th Ann. Meeting of the Orthopaedic Research Soc., Atlanta, Georgia. 1988.

Benirschke SK, Mirels H, Jones D, Tencer AF. 'The use of resonant frequency measurements for the non-invasive assessment of mechanical stiffness of the healing tibia.' *J Orthop Trauma* 1993; **7**: 64–71.

Bilat C, Leutenegger A, Ruedi T. 'Osteosynthesis of 245 tibial shaft fractures: early and late complications.' *Injury* 1994; **25(6)**: 349–58.

Böstman OM. 'Rotational refracture of the shaft of the adult tibia.' *Injury* 1983; **15(2)**: 93–8.

Bourgois R and Burny F. 'Measurement of the stiffness of fracture callus in vivo. A theoretical study.' *J Biomechanics* 1972; **5**: 85–91.

Bourgois R and Burny F. 'Feasibility of bone healing measurement with external fixation: Experimental Study.' *Orthopaedics* 1984; **7(4)**: 673–6.

Burny F. 'Etude par jagues de déformation de la consolidation des fractures en clinique.' *Acta Orthop Belgica* 1968; **34**: 917–27.

Burny F, Bourgois R, Dankerwolcke M, Moulart F. 'Utilisation clinique de jagues de constrainte-situation actuelle et perspectures d'avenir.' *Acta Orthop Belgica* 1978; **44**: 895–920.

Burny F, Dankerwolcke M, Bourgois R, Domb M, Saric O. 'Twenty years experience in fracture healing measurement with strain gauges.' *Orthopaedics* 1984; **7**: 1823–6.

Burnstein AH, Currey JD, Frankel VH, Reilly DT. 'The ultimate properties of bone tissue: The effects of yielding.' *J Biomechanics* 1972; **5**: 35–44.

Charnley J. *The Closed Treatment of Common Fractures* 3rd Ed. 1961. Churchill Livingstone: London.

Christensen AB, Tougaard L, Dyrbye C, Vibe-Hansen H. 'Resonance of the human tibia.' *Acta Orthop Scand* 1982; **53:** 867–74.

Churches AE, Tanner KE, Harris JD. 'The Oxford external fixator and the effects of bone pin loosening.' *Eng Med* 1985; **14:** 3–11.

Claes L, Burri C, Gerngross H, and Mutschler W. 'Bone healing stimulated by plasma factor XIII. Osteotomy experiments in sheep.' *Acta Orthop Scand* 1985; **56:** 57–62.

Cunningham JL, Evans M, Harris JD, Kenwright J. 'The measurement of stiffness of fractures treated with external fixation.' *Eng Med* 1987; **16**: 229–32.

Donald G and Seligson D. 'Treatment of tibial shaft fractures by percutaneous Küntscher Nailing.' *Clin Orthop* 1983; **178**: 64–73.

Draper ERC, Strachan RK, McCarthy ID, and Hughes SPF. 'Early biomechanical detection of delayed bone union in an animal model.' *J Bone Joint Surg* [Br] 1994; **76-B [Supp II and III]**: 88.

Ellis H. 'The speed of healing after fracture of the tibial shaft.' *J Bone Joint Surg* [Br] 1958; **40-B:** 42–6.

Eskelund V and MunkPlum C. 'Experimental Investigations into the healing of fractures.' *Acta Orthop Scand* 1950; **19**: 433–40.

Evans FG. *Mechanical properties of bone* 1973. Ed. Thomas: Springfield, Illinois

Falkenberg J. 'An experimental study of the rate of fracture healing.' *Acta Orthop Scand* Suppl. 1961; **50**: 1.

Floriani L, Debevoise H, Hyatt GW. 'Mechanical properties of healing bone by the use of ultrasound.' *Surg Forum* 1967; **18**: 468–70.

Gerlanc M, Haddad D, Hyatt GW, Langlon JT, Hilaire P. 'Ultrasonic study of normal and fractured bone.' *Clin Orthop* 1975; **111**: 175–8.

Gershuni DH and Halma G. 'The AO external skeletal fixator in the treatment of severe tibia fractures.' *J Trauma* 1983; **23(11)**: 986–90.

Goodship AE and Kenwright J. 'The influence of induced micromovement upon the healing of experimental tibial fractures.' *J Bone and Joint Surg* [Br] 1985; **67-B**: 650–5.

Goodship AE and Lanyon LE (eds). *European Biomechanics* 1988 Butterworth:London

Hammer R, Edholm P, Lindholm B. 'Stability of union after tibial shaft fracture.' *J Bone Joint Surg* [Br] 1984; **66-B**: 529–34.

Hardy JRW, Conlan D, Hay S, Gregg PJ. 'Serum ionised calcium and its relationship to parathyroid hormone after tibial fracture.' *J Bone Joint Surg* [Br] 1993; **75-B**: 645–9.

Hardy JRW, de Jonge EJ, Richardson JB. 'Fracture stiffness.' *J Orthop Techniques* 1994; 2: 177–89.

Hardy JRW. 'Tibial Diaphyseal Fracture Healing.' MD Thesis.

1997;University of Leicester, UK.

Heckman JD, Ryaby JP, McCabe J, Frey JJ, Kilcoyne RF. 'Acceleration of tibial fracture healing by non-invasive, low-intensity pulsed ultrasound.' *J Bone Joint Surg* [Am] 1994; **76-A**: 26–34.

Hente R, Cheal EJ, Hagerty T. 'Differentiation of repair tissue under controlled strain gradients.' 37th Ann. Meeting Orthop Res Soc Anaheim, California. 1991; **16(2)**: 479.

Hulth A. 'Current concepts of fracture healing'. *Clin Orthop* 1989; **249**: 265–84.

Jernberger A. 'Measurement of the stability of tibial fractures: a mechanical method.' *Acta Orthop Scand* 1970; **Suppl 139**.

Johnson RJ and Pope MH. 'Tibial shaft fractures in skiing.' *Am J Sports Med* 1977; **5(2)**: 49–61.

Jorgensen TE. 'Measurements of stability of crural fractures treated with Hoffman osteotaxis. 2. Measurements on crural fractures.' *Acta Orthop Scand* 1972; **43:** 207–18.

Koskinen EVS. 'The repair of experimental fractures under the action of growth hormone, thyretropin and cortisone.' *Ann Chir Gynaecol* 1959; **(Suppl)**: 90.

Krettek C, Haas N, Tscherne H. 'The role of supplemental lag-screw fixation for open fractures of the tibial shaft treated with external fixation.' *J Bone Joint Surg* [Am] 1991; **73-A**: 893–7.

Lawyer RB, and Lubbers LM. 'Use of the Hoffmann apparatus in the treatment of unstable tibial fractures.' *J Bone Joint Surg* [Am] 1980; **62-A**: 1264–73.

Lindholm RV, Lindholm TS, Toikkanen S, and R Leino. 'The effect of forced inter-fragmental movements on the healing of tibial fractures in rats.' *Acta Orthop Scand* 1970; **40**: 721–8.

Lindholm TS and Törnkvist H. 'Inhibitory effect on bone formation and calcification exerted by the anti-inflammatory drug ibuprofen.' *Scand J Rheumatology* 1981; **10**: 38–42.

Lindsay MK and Howes EL. 'Breaking strength of healing fractures.' *J Bone Joint Surg* 1931; **13**: 491–501.

Lindsay MK. 'Observations on fracture healing in rats.' *J Bone Joint Surg* 1934; **16**: 162–7.

Markel MD, Wikenheiser MA, Chao EYS. 'Formation of bone in tibial defects in a canine model.' *J Bone Joint Surg* [Am] 1991; **73-A**: 914–23.

Mather BS. 'Correlations between strength and other properties of long bones.' *J Trauma* 1967; **7**: 633–6.

Matthews LS, Kaufer H, Sonsdergard DA. 'Manual sensing of fracture stability.' *Acta Orthop Scand* 1974; **45**: 373–81.

McKeown RM, Lindsay MK, Harvey SC, Howes EL. 'The breaking strength of healing fractured fibulae of rats.' *Arch Surg* 1932; **24**: 458–81.

McMaster M. 'Disability of the hindfoot after fracture of the tibial shaft.' *J Bone Joint Surg* [Br] 1976; **58-B**: 90–3.

Mintowt-Czyz WJ and Richards J. 'Evidence of a biphasic healing pattern in tibial fractures.' *J Bone Joint Surg* [Br] 1986; **68-B**: 839–40.

Mølster AO, Gjerdet NR, Alho A, Bang G. 'Fracture healing after rigid intramedullary nailing in rats.' *Acta Orthop Scand* 1983; **54**: 366–73.

Nicholls PJ, Berg E, Bliven FE, Kling JM. 'X-ray diagnosis of healing fractures in rabbits.' *Clin Orthop* 1979; **142**: 234–6.

Nishimura N. 'Serial strain gauge measurement of bone healing in Hoffmann external fixation.' *Orthopaedics* 1984; **7(4)**: 677–84.

Noordeen MHH, Lavy CBD, Shergill NS, Tuite JD, Jackson AM. 'Cyclical micromovement and fracture healing.' *J Bone Joint Surg* [Br] 1995; 77B: 645–8.

Oni OOA, Hui A, Gregg PJ. 'The healing of closed tibial shaft fractures – The natural history of union with closed treatment.' *J Bone Joint Surg* [Br] 1988; **70-B**: 787–90.

Oni OOA, Graebe A, Pearse M, Gregg PJ. 'Prediction of the healing potential of closed adult tibial shaft fractures by bone scintigraphy.' *Clin Orth* 1989; **245**: 239–45.

Oni OOA, Dunning J, Mobbs RJ, Gregg PJ. 'Clinical factors and the size of the external callus in tibial shaft fractures.' *Clin Orthop* 1991; **273**: 278–83.

Panjabi MM, Walter SD, Karuda M, White AA, Lawson JP. 'Correlations of radiographic analysis of healing fractures with strength: A statistical analysis of experimental osteotomies.' *J Orthop Research* 1985; **3**: 212–8.

Pinder IM. 'Refracture of the shaft of the adult tibia.' *J Bone Joint Surg* [Br] 1973; **55-B**: 878.

Potts WJ. 'The role of the haematoma in fracture healing.' *Surg Gynaecol Obstet* 1932; 318–24.

Pugh J and Dee R. 'Properties of musculoskeletal tissues and biomaterials.' in Dee R, Mango E, Hurst LC (eds): *Principles of Orthopaedic Practice*1989 McGraw-Hill: New York

Richards J and Mintowt-Czyz WJ. 'Direct measurement of tibia stiffness using photoelastic links and strain gauges.' in *Monitoring of Fracture Healing by Vibration analysis and Other Mechanical Methods* 1985 Van der Perre, G, and Borgwardt-Christiansen A, (eds), Acco: Leuven

Richards J. 'Stiffness in healing fractures.' CRC Critical Reviews in *Biomedical Eng* 1987; **15(2)**: 145–85.

Richardson JB, Kenwright J, Cunningham JL. 'Fracture stiffness measurement in the assessment and management of tibial fracture.' *J Biomechanics* 1992; **7**: 75–9.

Richardson JB and O'Connor BT. 'Direct fracture stiffness measurement in tibial fractures.' *Int J Orthop Trauma* Supp. 1993; **3(3)**: 72–4.

Richardson JB, Cunningham JL, Goodship AE, O'Connor BT, Kenwright J. 'Measuring stiffness can define healing of tibial fractures. *J Bone Joint Surg* [Br] 1994; **76-B**: 389–94.

Rommens P, Broos P, Gruwez J. 'External Fixation of tibial shaft fractures with severe soft tissue injuries by Hoffmann–Vidal–Audrey Osteotaxis.' *Arch Orthop Trauma Surg* 1986; **105(3)**: 170–4.

Sarmiento A, Schaeffer JF, Beckerman L, Latta LL, Enis J. 'Fracture healing in rat femora as affected by functional weight bearing.' *J Bone Joint Surg* [Am] 1977; **59-A**: 369–75.

Schröder HA, Christoffersen H, Scherff-Sorensen T, Lindequist S. 'Fractures of the shaft of the tibia treated with Hoffmann external fixation.' *Arch Orthop Trauma Surg* 1986; **105**: 28–30.

Sekiguchi T and Hirayama T. 'Assessment of fracture healing by vibration.' *Acta Orthop Scand* 1979; **50**: 391–8.

Slätis P and Rokkanen P. 'The normal repair of experimental fractures. A histo-quantative study of rats.' *Acta Orthop Scand* 1965; 36: 221–9.

Spencer RF. 'The effect of head injury on fracture healing.' *J Bone Joint Surg* [Br]1987 ; **69-B**: 525–8.

Urist MR and Johnson RW. 'Calcification and ossification. IV. The healing of fractures in man under clinical conditions.' *J Bone Joint Surg* 1943; **25**: 375–426.

White AA, Panjabi MM, Southwick WO. 'The four biomechanical stages of fracture repair.' *J Bone Joint Surg* [Am] 1977; **59-A**: 188–92.

Supplementary Bibliography

Anderson LD, and Hutchins WC. 'Fractures of the tibia and fibula treated with casts and transfixing pins.' *Southern Med J* 1966; **59**: 1026–32.

Anglen J, Unger D, DiPasquale T, Herscovici JD, Snoke J, Sanders R. 'The treatment of open tibial shaft fractures using an unreamed interlocked nail – is external fixation obsolete? *J Orthop Trauma* 1993; **7** :163.

Bach AW and Hansen ST.' Plates versus external fixation in severe open tibial shaft fractures.' *Clin Orthop* 1989; **241**: 89–94.

Behrens F and Searls K. 'External fixation of the tibia. Basic concepts and prospective evaluation.' *J Bone Joint Surg* 1986; **68-B**: 246–54.

Bone LB and Johnson KD. 'The treatment of tibial fractures by reaming and intramedullary nailing.' *J Bone Joint Surg* 1986; **68-A**: 877–87.

Briggs BT and Chao YS. 'The mechanical performance of the Hoffmann–Vidal external fixator apparatus.' *J Bone Joint Surg*

1982; **64-A**: 566–73.

Chehade MJ, Pohl AP, Pearc MJ, Nawana N. 'Clinical implications of stiffness and strength changes in fracture healing.' *J Bone Joint Surg* 1997; **79-B:** 9–12.

Clifford RP, Beauchamp CG, Kellam JF, Webb JK, Tile M. 'Plate fixation of open fractures of the tibia.' *J Bone Joint Surg* 1988; **70-B**: 644–8.

Court-Brown CM, McQueen MM, Quaba AA, Christie J. Hughes external fixator in treatment of tibial fractures. J. Royal Soc. Med. 1985;**78**:830–7.

Court-Brown CM, Wheelwright EF, Christie J, McQueen MM. 'External fixation for type III open tibial fractures.' *J Bone Joint Surg* 1990a; **72-B**: 801–4.

Court-Brown CM, Christie J, McQueen MM. 'Closed intramedullary tibial nailing.' *J Bone Joint Surg* 1990b; **72-B**: 605–11.

Court-Brown CM, McQueen MM, Quaba AA, Christie J. 'Locked intramedullary nailing of open tibial fractures.' *J Bone Joint Surg* 1991; **73-B**: 959–64.

Edwards P and Nilsson BER. 'Graphic representation of healing time in fractures of the shaft of the tibia.' *Acta Orthop Scand* 1965; **36**: 104–11.

Ellis H. 'Disabilities after tibial shaft fractures.' *J Bone Joint Surg* 1958b; **40-B**: 190–7.

Ham AW, Tisdall FF, Drake TGH. 'Experimental non-calcification of callus simulating non-union.' *J Bone Joint Surg* 1938; **20-B**: 345–52.

Johner R and Wruhs O. 'Classification of tibial shaft fractures and correlation with results after rigid internal fixation.' *Clin Orthop* 1983; **178**: 7–25.

Klemm KW and Börner M. 'Interlocking nailing of complex fractures of the femur and tibia.' *Clin Orthop* 1986; **212**: 89–100.

Nicoll EA. 'Fractures of the tibial shaft – A survey of 705 cases.' *J Bone Joint Surg* 1964; **46-B**: 373–87.

Oni OOA and Gregg PJ. 'An investigation of the contribution of the extraosseous tissues to the diaphyseal fracture callus using a rabbit tibial fracture model.' *Journal of Orthop Trauma* 1991b; **5(4)**: 480–4.

Reece AT, Oni OOA, Roberts M, Gregg PJ. 'The effects of external fixation on individual osseous tissues during fracture healing.' *J Bone Joint Surg* 1993; **75-B[Supp II]**: 287.

Urist MR and McLean FC. 'Calcification and ossification. II. Control of calcification in the fracture callus in rachitic rats.' *J Bone Joint Surg* 1941b; **23**: 283–310.

Wu J-J, Shyr HS, Chao YS, Kelly PJ. 'Comparison of osteotomy healing under external fixation devices with different stiffness characteristics.' *J Bone Joint Surg* 1984; **66-A**: 1258–64.

Biomechanical Performance of the Standard Orthofix External Fixator and Cortical Screws

6

H.T. Aro and E.Y.S. Chao

Introduction

At the time of its clinical introduction in the early 1980s, the standard Orthofix device was the first modern unilateral external fixator. It was developed for fixation of long-bone fractures and for distraction treatment of limb deformities. Biomechanically, the device was shown to provide fixation stability similar to the Hoffmann–Vidal quadrilateral frame which had been the standard fixation method for two or three decades. Since the original reports of De Bastiani and co-workers (1984, 1986), the Orthofix device has maintained its basic design, indicating the feasibility of its original engineering concepts. The widespread success of its clinical use has inspired and resulted in an increasing armentarium of different modifications of its design and new clinical applications. The original standard Orthofix device, however, remains as a landmark of the treatment modality.

The clinical popularity of the Orthofix device was dictated by its unique mechanical properties and new pin design. It is a unilateral device with a single-frame body and a ball and socket joint at either end to provide easy adjustment of bone fragment alignment. The body contains a telescoping shaft to allow both statically and dynamically controlled axial compression (dynamization) regulated by a body locking screw. The outer end of each ball joint has a pin clamp with five screw seats. The Orthofix half pins (named Orthofix cortical and cancellous screws) are also unique, as their threaded portion is conical (or tapered) in shape, and the shank portion is large (6mm in diameter).

The purpose of this chapter is to characterize the biomechanical performance of the standard Orthofix® External Fixator and its cortical screws. Extensive laboratory studies have been carried out to investigate the static stiffness and fatigue properties of the device and its components. The healing patterns of experimental long-bone fractures stabilized with the Orthofix external fixator have been described. Both in vitro and in vivo studies have also been performed to delineate the biomechanical performance of the Orthofix cortical screws under different loading conditions.

Mechanical Performance of the Standard Orthofix External Fixator

Basic Definitions

An understanding of the basic definitions of structural rigidity or stiffness of bone fragment fixation is essential in evaluating the factors determining the biomechanical properties of a fracture fixation method

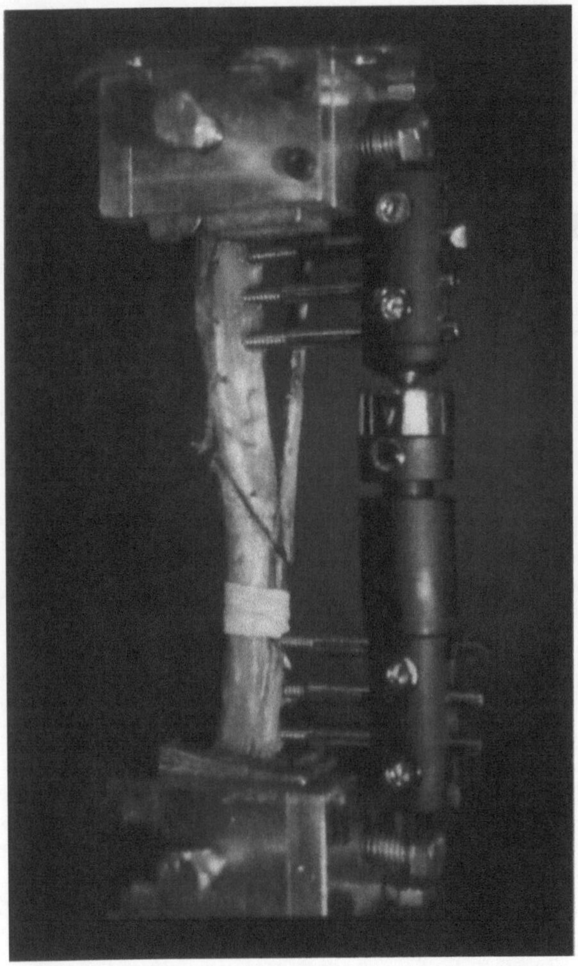

Fig. 6.1 Experimental setup for the in vitro determination of structural rigidity of an Orthofix external fixation system (custom-modified). The fixator has been applied to an osteotomised canine tibia and loaded using a universal mechanical testing device.

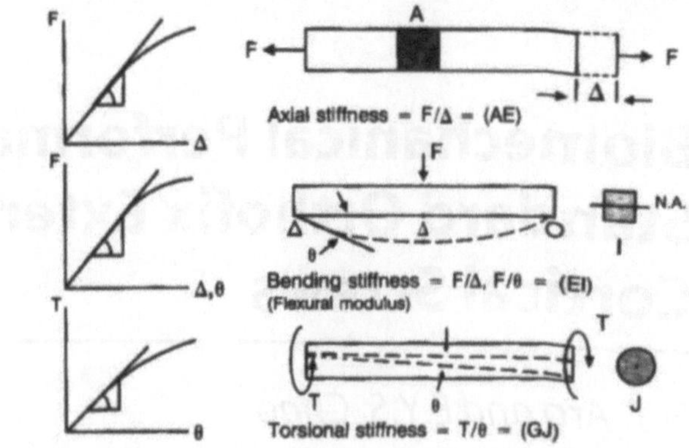

Fig. 6.2 Determination of structural rigidity or stiffness of a fracture fixation device. Using the load deformation curve for each loading mode, the slope of the linear portion of the curve will be used to define the fixation rigidity of an intact bone or the bone fragments fixed with the external fixation device.

(Chao and Aro 1993). Such knowledge is clinically important, not only during the application of the fixation but also when assessing the biological consequences of the selected fixation technique. This knowledge is especially crucial in external fixation, for which many types of frames and fixation configurations are available.

External fixators, designed to treat fractures, must satisfy two fundamental requirements. First, the device should possess adequate fatigue resistance, as the apparatus will be required to stay on the patient under varying conditions of weightbearing for a long period of time. Second, the fixator must possess the ability to realign bone fragments and vary bone fixation rigidity and compression status during the course of treatment. Fatigue resistance and adjustability of fixation stiffness during bone remodelling are equally important for fixators designed for distraction treatment of limb deformities.

Theoretical models have been used to predict the mechanical performance of unilateral or bilateral fixators under any combination of pin and frame parameters (Chao et al 1982, Huiskes and Chao 1986). The structural rigidity (or stiffness) of a fixation device can be accurately determined in vitro using a universal material testing machine. The fixation device is constructed using the recommended application technique on an osteotomised cadaver (Fig. 6.1) or synthetic bone. The bone ends are then loaded under axial compression, bending in two planes, and torsion. During each mode of loading, the load versus deformation curve is recorded and subsequently analysed to define the three basic stiffness parameters: axial, bending (flexural), and torsional. In each load-deformation curve, the slope of the linear portion of the curve is defined as the fixation rigidity or stiffness (Fig. 6.2). Using this testing procedure, it is possible to compare the fixation stiffness of different types of fixation (Chao and Aro 1991).

The rigidity of external fixation can be increased by a number of factors, including increased pin diameter, increased number of pins, decreased side bar separation, decreased pin separation, increased pin group separation, and applying pins in different planes. These variables have different effects on the axial, bending, and torsional stiffness, and by varying these key parameters, it is possible to achieve a desired fracture stability. Pin diameter is the most important parameter influencing fixator rigidity (Chao et al 1983, Huiskes and Chao 1986). At best, the stiffness of a bone-plate or bone-intramedullary nail system can be duplicated in a bone-external fixator system.

In the clinical situation, the overall rigidity of a fixation system is not dependent only on the frame and pins. In an evaluation of the amount of interfragmentary motion and, thereby, the mode of fracture healing, equally important factors are the type of fracture, the accuracy of reduction, the amount of physiological loading, and the characteristics of the pin-bone interface (Fig. 6.3).

In an experimental study (Aro et al 1991), paired canine tibiae were used to demonstrate how the fracture type and the accuracy of fracture reduction affect the fixation rigidity. One bone of each pair was osteotomised and fixed with a custom-modified Orthofix fixator. Osteotomy was performed transversely in five pairs of bones (a model of stable fracture), while an oblique osteotomy (60°) was produced in the other five pairs of bones (an unstable fracture model) (Fig. 6.4). The osteotomised bones were loaded with and without a fracture gap and the rigidity of fixation provided by the fixator was compared with the stiffness of the contralateral intact tibia. The results showed that simulated stable fractures (transverse osteotomies fixed with osteotomy surfaces in contact) behaved like the contralateral intact bones in all loading modes except anteroposterior bending. The presence of a fracture gap principally affected the axial rigidity of the system. The unstable (60° oblique) and stable (transverse) fracture models also showed the main difference in axial rigidity, without significant differences in other loading modes (Fig. 6.5).

During the past few years, circular external fixators have aroused considerable clinical enthusiasm, especially in the treatment of severe intra-articular fractures of the proximal and distal tibia and in reconstructive and lengthening procedures of the limbs (Aronson and Harp 1992, Podolsky and Chao 1993). These devices generally use four pairs of crossed Kirschner-wires (1.5mm to 1.8mm) held under high tension by screws on circular or semicircular ring frames. The wires can be orientated at different angles across the bone, and tension in the pins provides fixation rigidity. Mechanical comparison of one of the early circular external fixators (Volkov–Oganesian device) and conventional external fixators showed low overall fixation stiffness, especially in the axial direction (McCoy et al 1983). Several recent studies

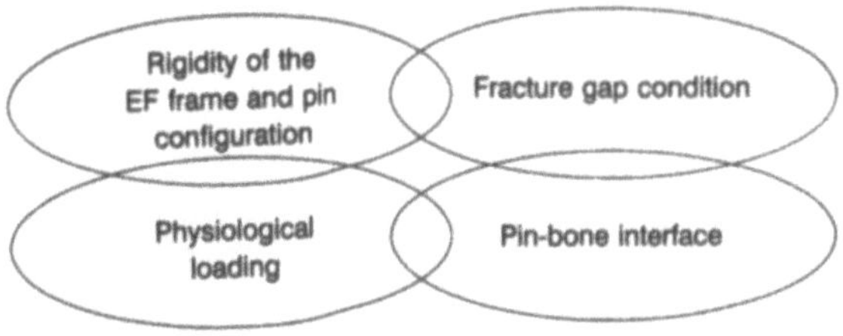

Fig. 6.3 The mechanical milieu (interfragmentary fracture micromotion) and thereby the mode of fracture healing under external fixation is largely determined by four major interacting factors.

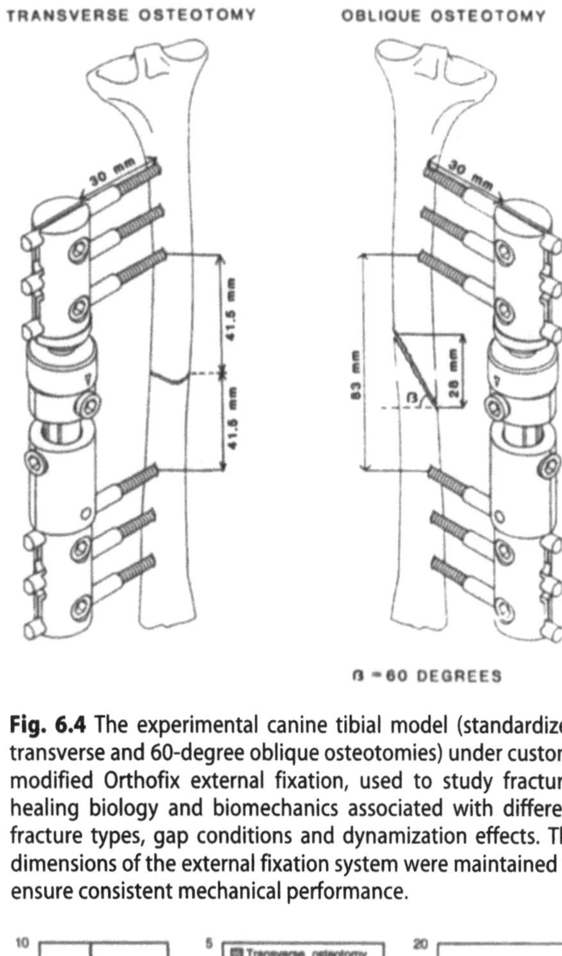

Fig. 6.4 The experimental canine tibial model (standardized transverse and 60-degree oblique osteotomies) under custom-modified Orthofix external fixation, used to study fracture-healing biology and biomechanics associated with different fracture types, gap conditions and dynamization effects. The dimensions of the external fixation system were maintained to ensure consistent mechanical performance.

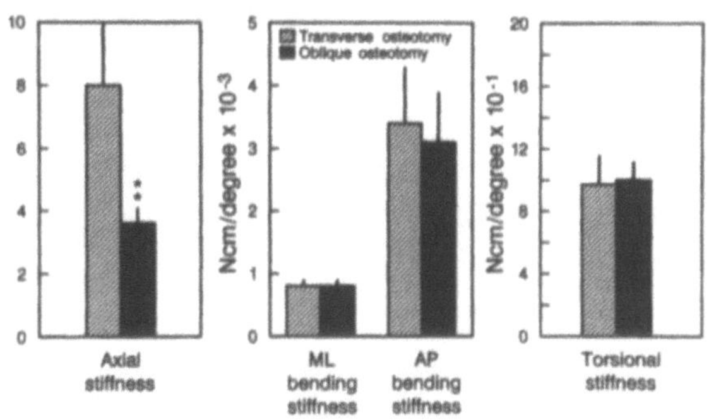

Fig. 6.5 The fixation stiffness of the transverse (hatched bars) and oblique osteotomies (shaded bars) was studied in vitro under different loading conditions of external fixation (custom-modified Orthofix). The axial rigidity of the oblique osteotomy was significantly lower than that of the paired transverse side. The values represent means ± SEM.

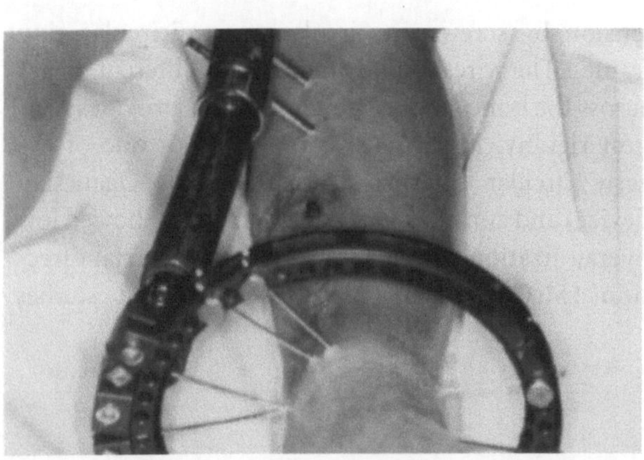

Fig. 6.6 Hybrid Orthofix external device applied to the distal tibia to treat a high-energy pilon fracture with severe closed soft-tissue injury. Applied with proximal cortical screws and a distal ring with tensioned wires.

(Fleming et al 1989, Podolsky and Chao 1993) have shown that the overall stiffness of the Ilizarov device is close to that of unilateral external fixators especially in bending and torsion. Under axial compression, the circular fixators have a nonlinear stiffness behaviour which varies with wire pre-tension (Fleming et al 1989, Podolsky and Chao 1993). The nonlinear stiffness behaviour, reflecting mostly the large deflection of the thin wire, is less pronounced under torsion and bending loads. As expected, the bending stiffness of the circular frame is independent of the loading direction.

Next to wire tensioning, the most important factor affecting the structural stiffness of the Ilizarov device is the diameter of the wire (Podolsky and Chao 1993). Other important factors are the distance between the frame rings and the pin length or the diameter of the frame rings. A disadvantage of this type of fixation, aside from the complexity of the frame and its application, is the possible sliding action of the bone fragments over the wires during functional loading. The use of threaded or olive wires can eliminate such motion, but threads may significantly weaken the wire which must sustain extremely high tension and bending because of pre-tensioning and loading. Contrary to early clinical reports, the circular wire fixators seem to have a relatively high rate of pin-track complications. One solution is to use hybrid external fixators, such as the Orthofix Hybrid Fixator which consists of a ring with tensioned wires which is connected to the standard Orthofix body with one clamp for cortical screws (Fig. 6.6).

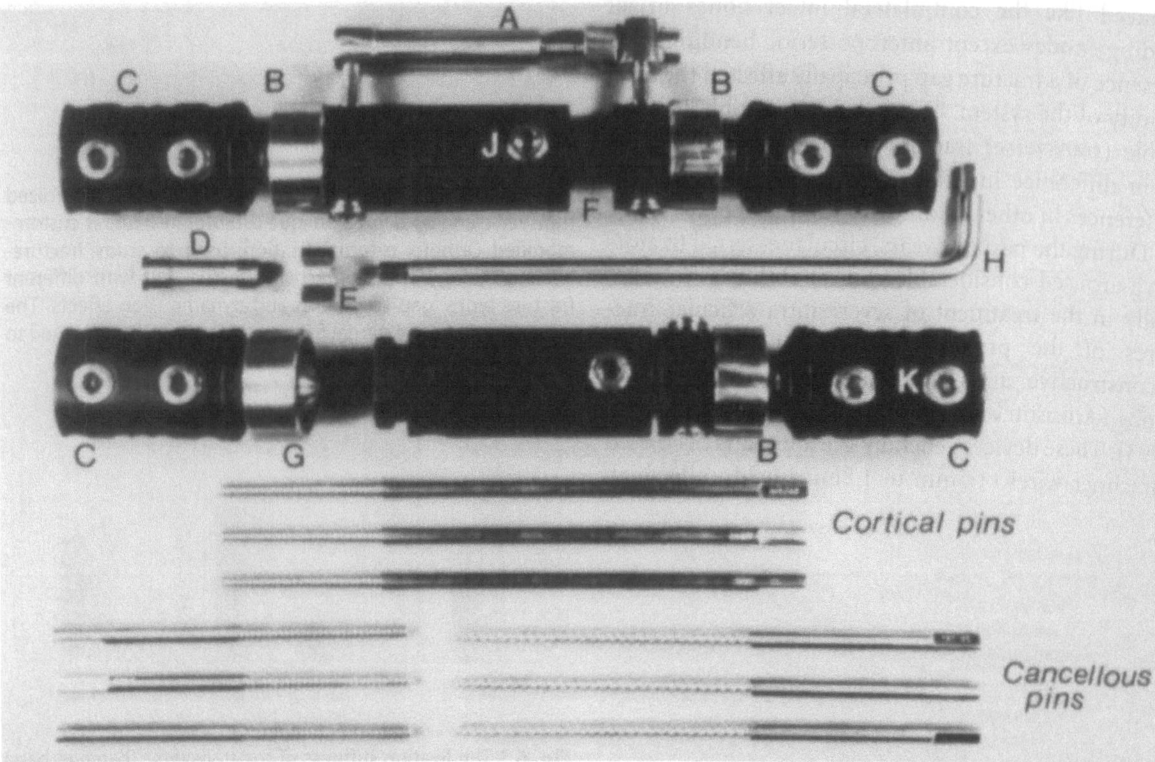

Fig. 6.7 The standard unilateral Orthofix Axial External Fixator and its components and screws (cortical and cancellous pins). **A**: Compression/distraction unit. **B**: ball joint. **C**: straight pin clamp. **D**: ball joint locking cam. **E**: hemispherical bush. **F**: telescoping shaft of the fixator body. **G**: ball joint collar. **H**: Allen wrench. **J**: central body locking nut. **K**: clamp cover screw.

Study Design For Mechanical Testing

Laboratory studies were designed to address several clinically important issues for the mechanical performance of the standard Orthofix device (Chao and Hein 1988), and similar studies were carried out on the small Orthofix fixator (Aro et al 1990). Since the stability of the Orthofix frame is governed by its ball joint structure, the mechanical behaviour of this key component was thoroughly tested. In clinical applications, the central body locking nut of the fixator body, the clamp screws of the pin clamps, and the locking cam of the ball joint may become loose as they are subjected to repetitive loading. The laboratory studies were to establish the scheme for the frequency of retightening needed for these screws. The re-usability of the Orthofix frame and its components was also studied. An appropriate inspection routine for the fixator components was established to ensure safe and effective re-application of a used apparatus.

The studies were designed to analyse the static performance of the Orthofix external fixator in resisting axial compression, bending in two directions, and torsion applied to the ends of bone fragments fixed by the apparatus. The ball joint was tested for its resistance against bending and torsion under varying amounts of tightening torque applied to the locking cam. The performance of the device and its components against fatigue load was also studied. Finally, the mechanical behaviour and potential failure mechanism of each component of the fixator frame subjected to repetitive manual tightening were determined.

A Standard, series 10.000 Orthofix device (24.5cm long from end to end) was used. The fixator consists of: two straight pin clamps and one central body with a telescoping shaft (11.8cm long and extendible by 4.5cm) for axial compression (Fig. 6.7). The main body of the pin clamps is made of medical grade aluminum, anodized to increase its surface hardness. One end of each pin clamp has a spherical ball and an encasing collar, all made of stainless steel. On the central body, each end contains a stainless steel hemispherical bush which is pressed by an eccentric cam to lock with the spherical ball on the pin clamp, thus forming the ball joint. The ball joint allows a total of 37° of angulation and unlimited rotation. The cam position is identified by a pair of markers, one engraved on the cam shaft end (a dot) and the other (a triangle) on the encasing collar (Fig. 6.8). When the two markers are aligned, the ball joint is in its unlocked neutral position. The locking cam starts to lock the

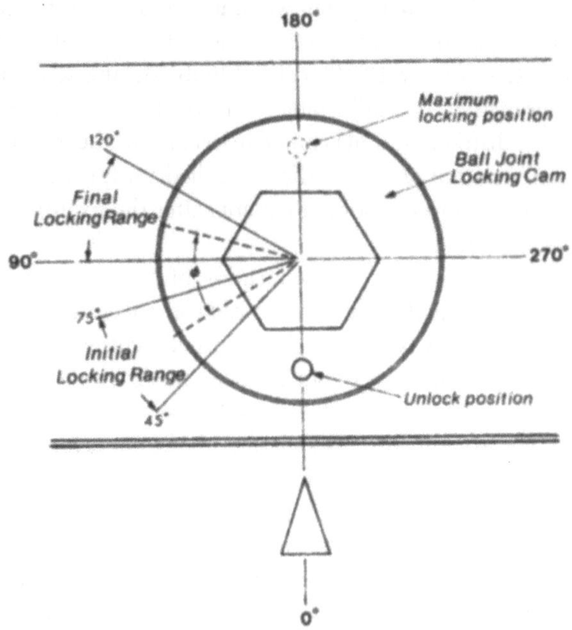

Fig. 6.8 The ball joint locking cam position indicators. Locking position change of the ball joint cam after 400 tightening/loosening torque cycles (24.3 N-m). The mean locking angle shift (∅) was estimated at 45°.

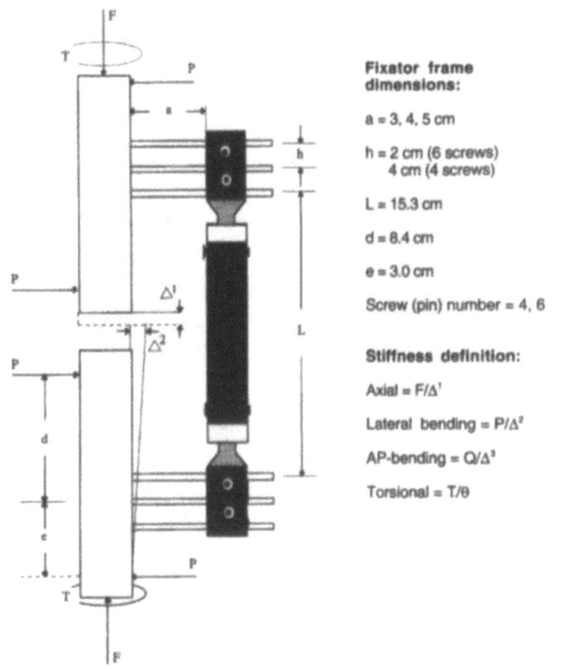

Fig. 6.9 The Orthofix External Fixator frame and bone model dimensions used to test the structural rigidity following the stiffness definition for different loading conditions. Q and Δ^3 are the AP bending force and bone displacement (not shown in the diagram) at the fracture site, respectively. The θ angle is the amount of axial rotation (not shown in the diagram) of the bone model caused by the applied torque, T.

bush and the mating ball when it is rotated 45° to 75° clockwise from its neutral position. The central body can telescope when the central body locking screw is loosened. An adjustable turnbuckle (compression–distraction unit) can be inserted into the locking cam shafts to provide static controlled compression or distraction to the bone fragments after the fixator has been applied.

Consistent and precise location of the pin holes in bone is difficult to achieve in cadaver specimens. For these reasons, a previously described synthetic bone model in the form of square bars, made by casting a plastic padding material, was used in both the static and fatigue experiments. A standard Orthofix frame for tibial application was constructed for testing. The loading configuration, fixator dimensions, and frame stiffness definitions are illustrated in Fig. 6.9. The device was applied to the synthetic bone model and mounted on the MTS testing machine for compression, AP and lateral bending, and torsional loading (Fig. 6.10). In compression and torsion tests, the bone ends were rigidly constrained. Low loading rates of 7.4 N/sec and 1.9 N-cm/sec were used. A gap of 2cm was maintained at the bone ends simulating the fracture site, so that all the applied loads were transmitted to the pins and the fixator frame. The amount of torque exerted on the fixator screws and the cam using the torque wrench provided by the manufacturer was standardised.

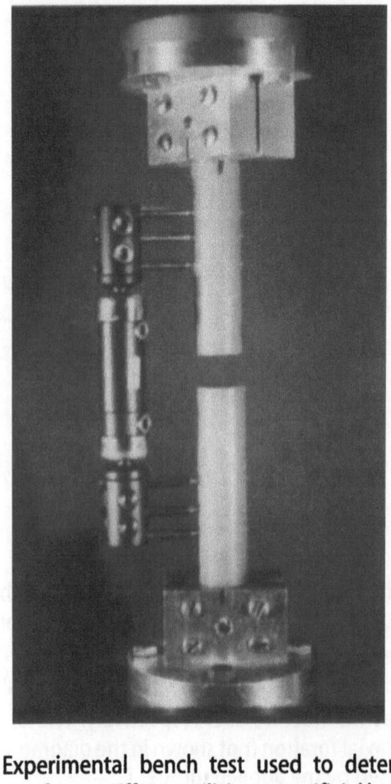

Fig. 6.10 Experimental bench test used to determine the Orthofix fixator frame stiffness utilising an artificial bone model.

Static Frame Stiffness

Based on four identical tests in each loading mode, the overall stiffness of the Orthofix frame is summarized in Fig. 6.11. The stiffness value was higher with six pins as compared to the four-pin configuration under all loading modes except lateral bending, which showed a decrease in stiffness when the pin number was increased. The stiffness values under all loads decreased with increased pin length (pin span 'a' in Fig. 6.9), but this effect was less pronounced under lateral and torsional loads. A comparison between the Orthofix fixator and the standard Hoffmann–Vidal quadrilateral frame was performed with equivalent dimensional measurements (Fig. 6.12). The Orthofix

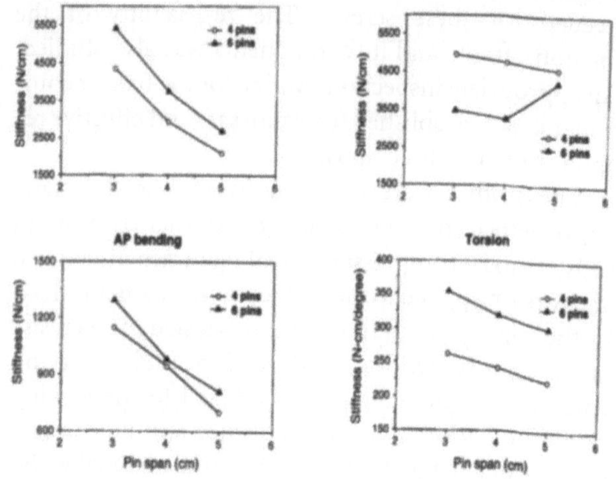

Fig. 6.11 The stiffness of the Orthofix external fixator under different loading modes. The stiffness properties of the fixation were determined both for 4-pin and 6-pin configurations (number of cortical screws) and by changing the distance of the fixator from the bone model (pin span 'a' in Fig. 6.9).

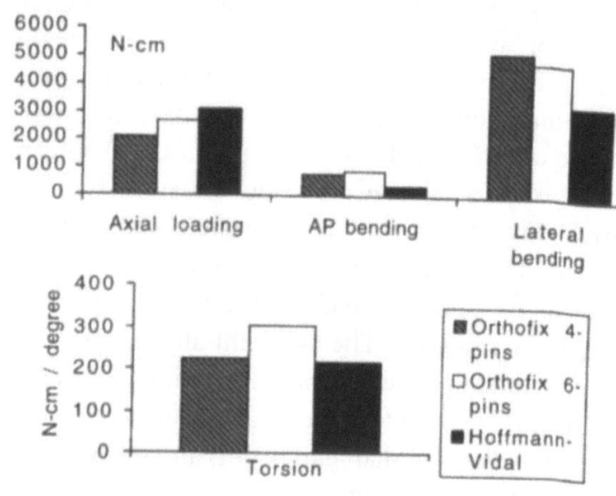

Fig. 6.12 Comparison of the mean frame stiffness of the Orthofix external fixator versus Hoffmann–Vidal quadrilateral frame.

apparatus compared favourably with the Hoffmann–Vidal frame (Hoffmann pins of 4mm in diameter) in stiffness performance, especially in AP and lateral bending. Other studies (Fleming et al 1989) have similarly compared the fixation stiffness of different unilateral and circular fixators (Fig. 6.13). Based on these studies, the Orthofix device and AO fixator with two stacked bars behave similarly whereas Ilizarov fixator has lower stiffness properties in all loading modes except in AP bending.

Performance of Fixator Ball Joint

To quantitate the stiffness and locking strength of the ball joint, the latter was loaded under both bending and torsion (Fig. 6.14). Since ball joint locking strength and rigidity were expected to vary according to cam tightening torque, bending and torsional tests were performed with increasing cam tightening torque from 5.6 N-m to 28.2 N-m in equal increments. A close to linear relationship was obtained between cam tightening torque and ball joint failure strength under both bending and torsional loads (Table 6.1). The failure torque under bending load was slightly higher than that for the torsional load. However, bending stiffness for the ball joint was significantly higher than torsional stiffness under all cam tightening torques. This demonstrates that ball joint performance is dependent on the loading mode applied.

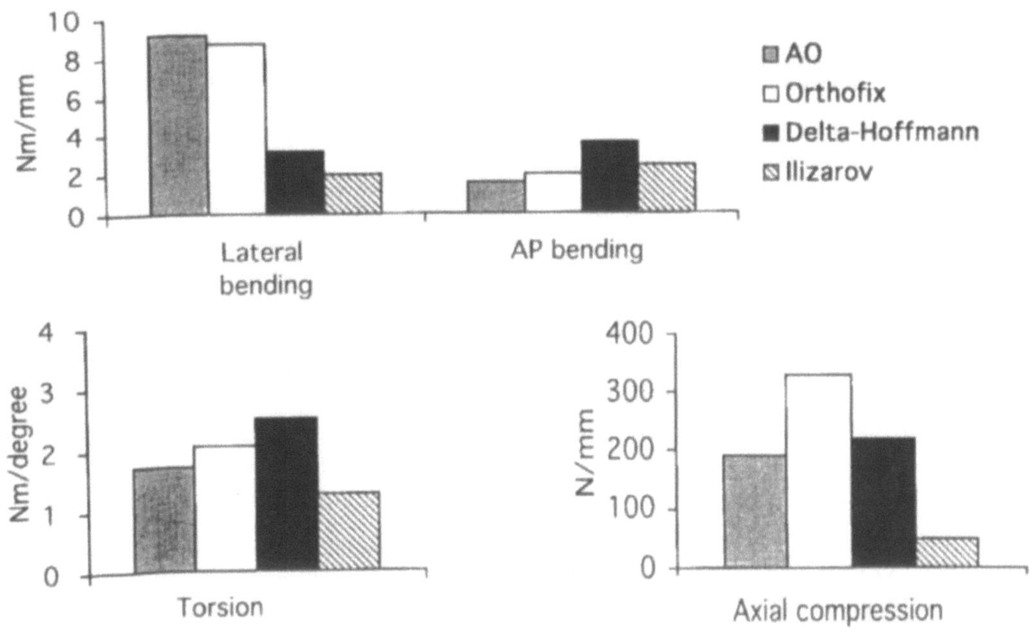

Fig. 6.13 A comparison of three different unilateral external fixators (AO with two stacked bars, standard Orthofix, Hoffmann in delta frame configuration) and Ilizarov fixator (Fleming et al 1989).

Sequentially Applied Cam Torque (N-m)	Bending Test (n = 5)		Torsion Test (n = 4)	
	Failure Strength (N-m)	Joint Stiffness (N-m/degree)	Failure Strength (N-m)	Joint Stiffness (N-m/degree)
5.6	8.5 ± 2.3	16.0 ± 3.7	9.2 ± 1.6	5.2 ± 1.5
11.3	15.6 ± 2.4	21.4 ± 1.5	15.4 ± 2.8	8.5 ± 2.5
16.9	21.4 ± 3.6	24.9 ± 2.1	20.2 ± 3.2	11.1 ± 4.1
22.6	26.8 ± 4.4	27.6 ± 2.7	26.0 ± 2.4	10.7 ± 4.0
28.2	31.9 ± 4.5	28.8 ± 2.7	30.1 ± 4.0	11.8 ± 2.6

Table 6.1 The effect of cam tightening torque on ball joint locking strength and stiffness (Mean ± SD)

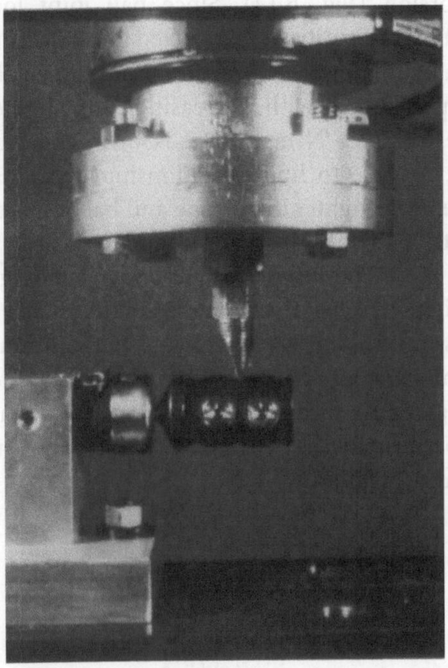

Fig. 6.14 Stiffness and failure strength test of the Orthofix ball joint. The ball joint was loaded both under bending and torsion.

Fatigue Test of Fixator Components

Individual fixator components were studied to determine their fatigue performance. The components examined included the fixator central body locking nut, the ball joint locking cam, and the pin clamp cover screws. Each component was mounted on the MTS testing machine using custom-designed mounting jigs. A low rotation rate (15°/min) was used in tightening the screws and cam until they failed. The rotation versus torque curve was monitored, and a sudden drop in torque value was regarded as component failure. After the static failure test, each component was disassembled and examined to determine the mechanism of failure.

The failure mechanism of the pin clamp cover screws and the fixator central body locking nut was found to be complete yielding of the inner screw socket. The locking cam had two types of failure mechanism: complete rotation of the cam shaft and yielding of the cam inner socket. The failure torques for individual test components are as follows: 60.6 ± 5.0 N-m for pin clamp cover screws, 60.6 ± 3.1 N-m for ball joint locking cams and 38.0 ± 3.1 N-m for fixator central body locking nuts. The clinically applied torques were 40–64 per cent of the failure torques. The mean applied torque obtained in tightening the

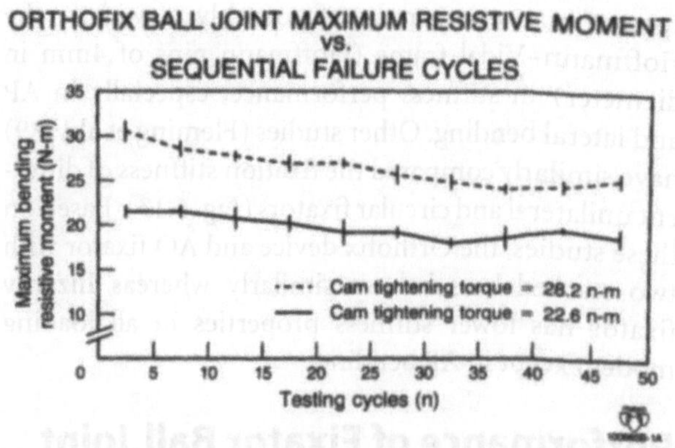

Fig. 6.15 Effect of repeated cam tightening on the maximum resistive bending moment of the Orthofix ball joint. A mean (± SD) of every five testing cycles was presented throughout the entire 50 tightening and bending sequences.

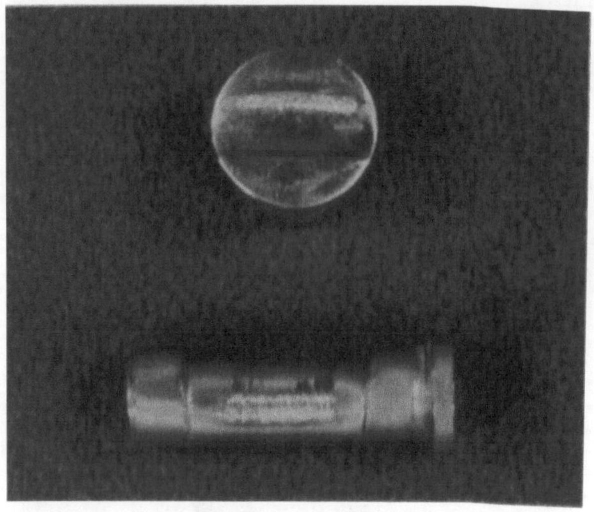

Fig. 6.16 Orthofix ball joint locking cam/bush wear after repeated cam tightening and failure test. The wear marks were located mainly in the edge regions of the articulating surfaces.

locking screw and cam using the Orthofix Allen wrench was 24.3 ± 8.5 N-m among the test subjects (n = 20). This value was slightly higher than the manufacturer's previously recommended torque for cam tightening, which was 22.6 N-m, preset on the torque wrench.

Subsequently, a repetitive tightening test was performed on each specimen as it was rigidly fastened. The corresponding screw, nut or cam was manually tightened to the simulated clinical torque using an instrumented torque wrench. The component was then loosened and retightened, in a cyclic manner, to the same torque level. This testing procedure was repeated for 400 cycles or until the mean clinical tightening torque could no longer be reached. At the end of the test sequence, each component was carefully examined for signs of wear, abrasion, thread or socket deformation, and possible fracture crack formation.

Under the constant applied torque of 24.3 N-m, all pin clamp cover screws survived the entire 400 torque cycles with no apparent failure. However, severe galling and metal particles were found in the aluminum pin clamp screw seat due to frictional wear against the stainless steel screws. The screw socket head also had localized yielding and the threads of the inner pin clamp screw were worn.

All ball joint locking cams survived the entire 400 tightening cycles without major failure. The loosening torque of the locking cam did not change significantly throughout the tightening and loosening sequence. However, after 50 cycles of tightening and bending failure of the ball joint, the failure strength decreased asymptotically to approximately 80 per cent of its original value (Fig. 6.15). The decrease was more significant under higher cam locking torque (28.3 N-m versus 22.6 N-m). Galling and wear were noted on the articulating surface of the cam shaft and bushing (Fig. 6.16).

During the repetitive ball joint tightening test without bending failure, the locking position of the cam migrated gradually from the beginning to the end of the test sequence. The initial locking position for all test specimens ranged from 45° to 75° from the unlocked (0°) neutral position (Fig. 6.8). By the end of the experiment, this locking position had advanced to a range of 90° to 120°, with a mean locking angle shift (Ø) of approximately 45°.

Fatigue Test of Fixator Frame

In fatigue testing of the standard Orthofix device, a cyclic (haversine) axial compressive load of 0 N to 890 N was applied at a frequency of 5 Hz for 2 million cycles. This loading magnitude and duration simulates approximately 2 years of full weightbearing on the fixator. Fixation configuration similar to that used in the static system was adopted. Each component of the fixator was tightened with the instrumented torque wrench to the mean simulated clinical torque. Pin span was adjusted to produce a dynamic bending moment of approximately 26.7 N-m at the ball joint under the maximum applied load of 890 N through the ends of the bone model.

Load and displacement were monitored every 900 cycles by a digital computer interfaced with the MTS testing machine. The time-related change in fixator stiffness was quantifed. In addition, the loosening torque of all locking screws, nuts and cams was examined at 500,000-cycle intervals. These loosening torques were used to evaluate the effect of fatigue loading on the mechanical performance of the fixator components. At the end of each fatigue sequence, all components of each fixator tested were disassembled and inspected for fatigue damage and wear.

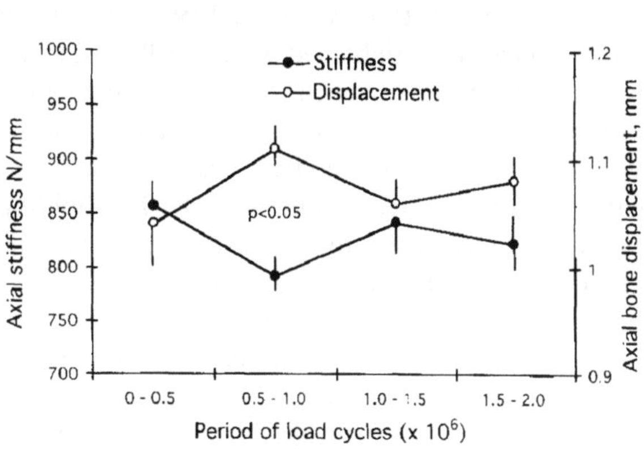

Fig. 6.17 Fatigue test of the Orthofix external fixator frame. The data points (mean ± SD) describe the change of the axial stiffness (closed circles) and the axial bone displacement (open circles) during 2 million loading cycles of the frame.

All four fixators survived the entire 2 million loading cycles without pin fracture or gross failure of the components. There was a small but significant decrease in frame stiffness during the first 500,000 fatigue cycles (Fig. 6.17). This reduction of stiffness could have been attributed to the combination of component loosening, seating of the mating surfaces, and local yielding of the synthetic bone model and/or the pin itself. When the loosening torques were measured for each locking screw and cam at 500,000-cycle intervals, there were no significant changes.

Apparent wear marks were observed in the pin clamp cover screws and the ball joint locking cam and bush. The locking cam/bush surfaces also demonstrated the same wear as that observed in the static test (Fig. 6.16). However, the ball joint surface did not show excessive wear. In spite of these changes, the stiffness property of the entire fixator frame and the loosening torque of the locking cam and tightening screws/nuts did not decrease significantly throughout the fatigue period.

Holding Power of Pin Clamp

The Orthofix device has two pin fixation clamps with five premachined slots for varying the number (from two to four) and location of the bone screws. The holding power of the Orthofix clamp was evaluated by determination of the torque resistance of cortical screws within a clamp (Aro et al 1989). The clamp cover screws were tightened sequentially using an instrumented torque wrench. The applied tightening torque was 24.3 N-m for the Orthofix clamp. Torque resistance of pins within a clamp was also measured with the instrumented torque wrench. The holding power of the Orthofix clamp was tested using eight different pin configurations (4 two-pin configurations, 3 three-pin configurations and 1 four-pin configuration). The pin slots of the Orthofix clamp were numbered from one to five, where number one was the innermost (closest to the ball joint) and number five the outermost (furthest from the ball joint) (Fig. 6.18).

This study showed that the holding power of the clamps is adequate only if certain guidelines are followed at the time of external fixator application. There was a linear correlation between the number of screws placed within an Orthofix clamp and the holding strength of the clamp, as indicated by pin torsional resistance. The holding power of the Orthofix clamp was adequate in symmetric two- and three-pin configurations, which are clinically the most commonly used configurations. However, the pins of

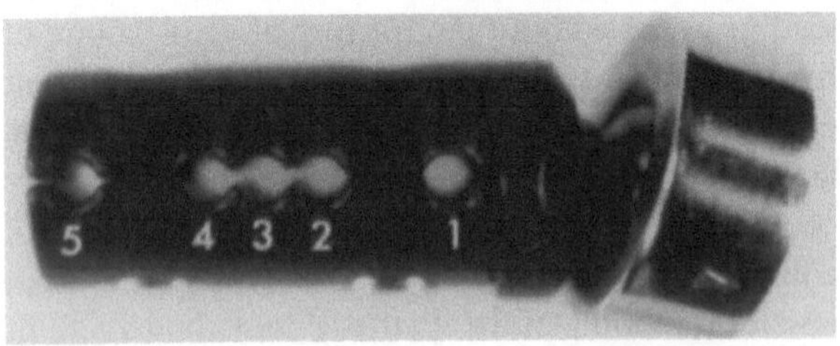

Fig. 6.18 The screw seat arrangement in the Orthofix pin clamp.

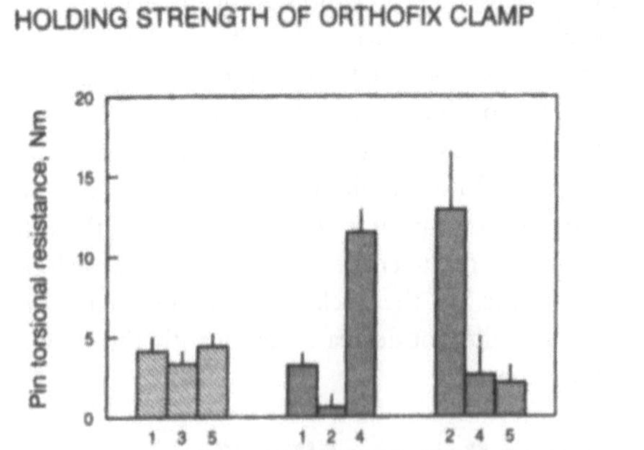

Fig. 6.19 The torsional resistance of pins (cortical screws) in relation to their position in three-pin configurations in the Orthofix clamp. The striped bars represent the symmetric configurations and the solid bars designate the asymmetric three-pin configurations (mean ± SD).

asymmetric two-pin and three-pin configurations (Fig. 6.19), as well as those of the four-pin configuration, showed significant differences in torque resistance. In these configurations, one pin could show high torque resistance while the clamping effect on another pin could be low or absent.

Comments

Although the Orthofix external fixator is a unilateral frame design, it can provide adequate rigidity under different high loading conditions. The use of larger diameter fixation screws is mainly responsible for this performance. The major mechanical advantage of the Orthofix device is its ease of application coupled with the fact that it permits bone fragment alignment, apposition, and compression after screw placement in bone.

The ball joint of the Orthofix device is capable of resisting bending loads comparable to similar structural elements in other types of external fixators. Although its torsional strength is less favorable, such a loading mode remains relatively minor in common fixator applications. The preset torque wrench for tightening the locking cam should be used to ensure consistent performance of the ball joint and at the same time avoid excessive torque application which may lead to premature failure of this key component of the fixator. Since the ball joint has limited strength against torsion and bending, full weightbearing should be matched with the progress of bone fracture union. In unstable fractures, heavy loading should be discouraged; such a high bending moment or torsional load (larger than 30 N-m) occurring at the ball joint may cause it to rotate.

During the Orthofix frame fatigue test, the bending moment exerted at the ball joints of the fixator was approaching its maximum resistive moment. Under this maximal loading condition, the stiffness properties of the fixator did not seem to change throughout the 2 million cycles of fatigue loading when retightening was applied. Such performance was also supported by the nearly constant loosening torque exhibited in pin clamp cover screws, fixator central body locking nut, and the locking cams of the ball joints. The wear that occurred at the locking cam articulating surface did not significantly influence the stiffness property of the frame. These results appeared to reflect the reliability of the device even under severe loading conditions. However, proper initial tightening of the locking cam and periodic retightening were found to be important.

At the end of 400 tightening cycles, the ball joint locking cams had migrated approximately 45° from their initial mean locking position of 60° to the final locking position of 105°. This indicated that there was still 65° of remaining effective cam rotation to provide a positive locking effect before it would become completely dislodged. Such performance is quite encouraging, as the results tend to indicate that the ball joint is still effective, even after a severe repetitive tightening test. Once the ball joint experiences rotational or bending failure even under lower tightening torque, its subsequent locking strength may be reduced due to ball joint surface wear and abrasion.

The present test data suggest that re-usage of the Orthofix device for several consecutive 6-month periods is safe and permissible, provided that careful inspection and routine replacement of the crucial components is performed on the used apparatus before re-application. Between consecutive clinical applications or when the ball joint is known to have failed through bending or rotation, the old locking cam and bush should be replaced to maintain consistent locking strength. When the nut/screw seats on the fixator body and the pin clamp are severely galled, the entire component must be discarded or refurbished.

Fracture Union Mechanisms Under Orthofix External Fixation

It is essential to understand the characteristics of normal bone healing under external fixation. A series of experiments has been carried out for this purpose. These experiments were designed to demonstrate the pattern of healing to be expected with each type of fixation rigidity under standardized healing conditions. The same experimental setup (canine tibial shaft osteotomy) was used throughout, to eliminate other variables such as the extent of soft tissue injury, the variation in fracture surface, the accuracy of reduction, and the type of fracture configuration, all of which are known to influence bone healing under clinical conditions. The use of intra-animal comparisons on analysis also minimized the many inter-animal variables, such as individual differences in age, biological responses, temperament, functional activity, and loading magnitude.

Fracture healing patterns observed when internal fixation devices are used do not cover all the healing modes seen under external fixation. In general, external fixation, by allowing controlled adjustment of fixation rigidity, is an important experimental tool for studying the mechanical factors influencing fracture healing. Thus, the data can be used not only to speculate on possible factors which may enhance fracture union under external fixation, but also to improve the designs of other fracture fixation devices.

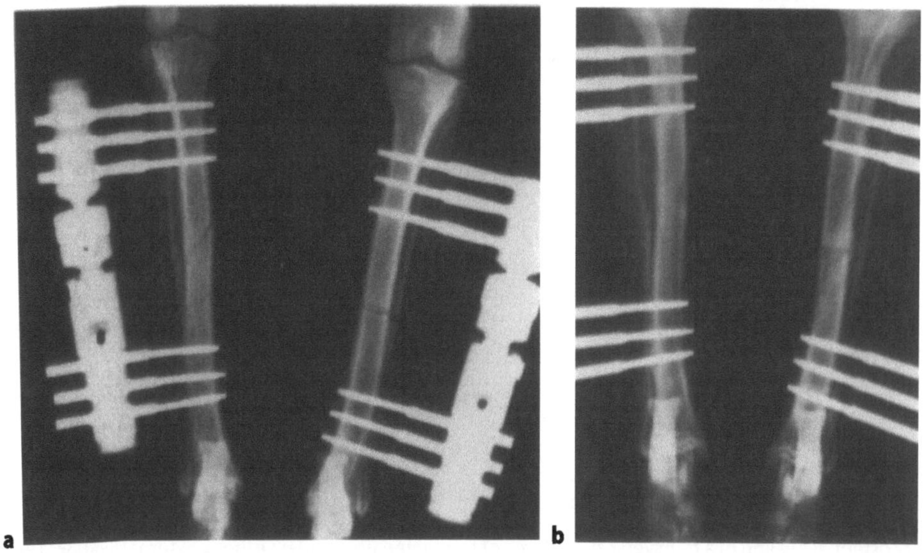

Fig. 6.20 Paired radiographic comparison of the healing of oblique and transverse osteotomies of the canine tibia. Under low loading conditions, the osteotomies healed through primary bone union. Initial AP radiograph on the left and a control AP radiograph at 12 weeks on the right.

Transverse Versus Oblique Fracture Under External Fixation

A highly standardized study (Aro et al 1991) was conducted to compare the healing patterns of transverse and 60° oblique osteotomies of the canine tibia stabilized with custom-modified Orthofix external fixators (Figs. 6. 4 and 6.20). Both osteotomies were reduced in contact but with no static compression. The initial rigidity of the fixation was maintained throughout the bone healing and no axial dynamization of the fixation was performed.

Gait analysis showed that the animals put significantly less weight on the oblique side during the first six weeks of healing. On both osteotomy sides, radiographic callus formation peaked at 6 weeks and decreased thereafter. The amount of periosteal callus was slightly less on the oblique side. Based on paired comparison, the osteotomy bending stiffness at 8 weeks and the osteotomy torsional stiffness at 12 weeks were significantly higher on the transverse side. There was, however, no significant difference in torsional bone union strength at 12 weeks. Both osteotomies showed a significant decrease in local dynamic and static bone scan activity as a function of the healing time. DEXA bone mineral measurements showed no significant differences between the two osteotomies at 12 weeks. Intracortical new bone formation was significantly higher on the transverse side, as a sign of enhanced cortical healing. There was no basic difference in the bone union pattern between transverse and oblique osteotomies. The transverse osteotomies, and occasionally even the oblique osteotomies, showed the growth of secondary osteons across the fracture site (Figs. 6.21 and 6.22). Despite the early cortical healing (fulfilling the classic criteria of primary cortical bone union), the osteotomies had also formed periosteal callus.

This paired comparison of transverse and oblique osteotomies showed that the fracture morphology per se does not dictate the bone union pattern. However, the unstable fracture configuration had a retarding effect on the return of structural stiffness and on the rate of cortical bone repair. It had less effect on the return of bone torsional strength. Naturally, the unstable fracture configurations also increase the chances for failure at the pin-bone interface (pin loosening) with a risk of subsequent loss of stable bone healing conditions.

Constant Rigid Versus Dynamic Compression Under External Fixation

A controlled experiment was designed to study the effects of dynamic axial compression (dynamization) on the healing of stable fractures under external fixation (Aro et al 1990). Bilateral transverse tibial osteotomies were performed and stabilized using unilateral custom-modified Orthofix fixators with an 800 μm gap. The axial constraint of the fixator was released (i.e. axial dynamization was performed) two weeks after osteotomy. The control side in each animal was treated with an identical unilateral external fixator, but the initial axial, bending and torsional rigidity of the fixation was maintained throughout the healing process. In vitro studies had confirmed that

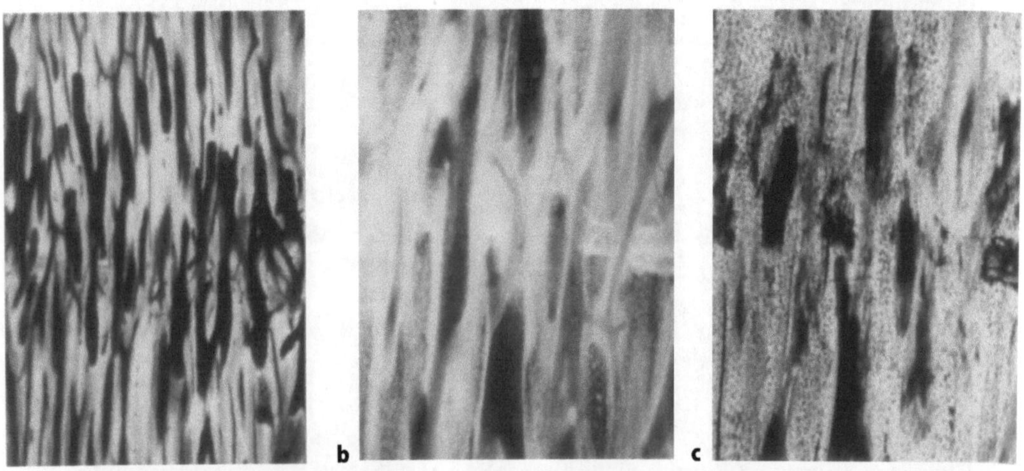

a b c

Fig. 6.21 Primary osteonal healing of a transverse osteotomy of the canine tibia under Orthofix external fixation. The cortical ends were in intimate contact and the osteotomy showed a solid end-to-end (contact healing) with a large number of secondary osteons. The secondary osteons penetrated the original cortical bone across the osteotomy site. **a** Longitudinal microradiograph. **b** The same section studied under ultraviolet light microscopy. **c** Polarized light microscopy of the same section.

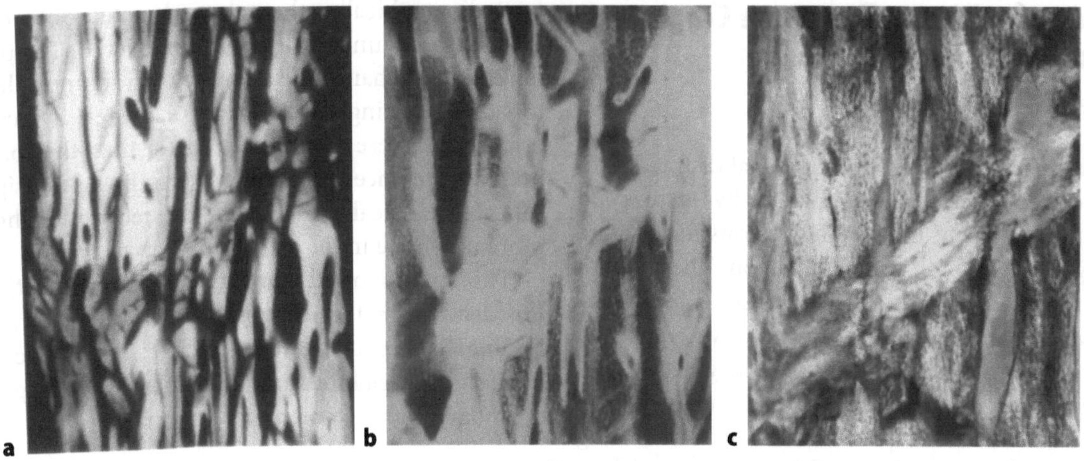

Fig. 6.22 Primary osteonal healing of an oblique osteotomy of a canine tibia under Orthofix external fixation. The osteotomy healed through gap-type osteonal healing. The minimal space between the oblique osteotomy ends was filled by lamellar new bone and the secondary osteons penetrated this new bone to across the osteotomy site. **a** Longitudinal microradiograph. **b** The same section studied under ultraviolet light microscopy. **c** The same section studied under polarized light microscopy, demonstrating the oblique direction of the collagen fibres in gap new bone.

the introduction of axial dynamization (unlocking of the telescoping mechanism in the fixator body) did not alter the fixation rigidity either under torsion or with bending, whereas the axial compressive load was transmitted through the bone (Fig. 6.23). In the rigidly fixed control side, axial loads of less than 200 N were not sufficient to close the osteotomy gap (800 μm) in vitro.

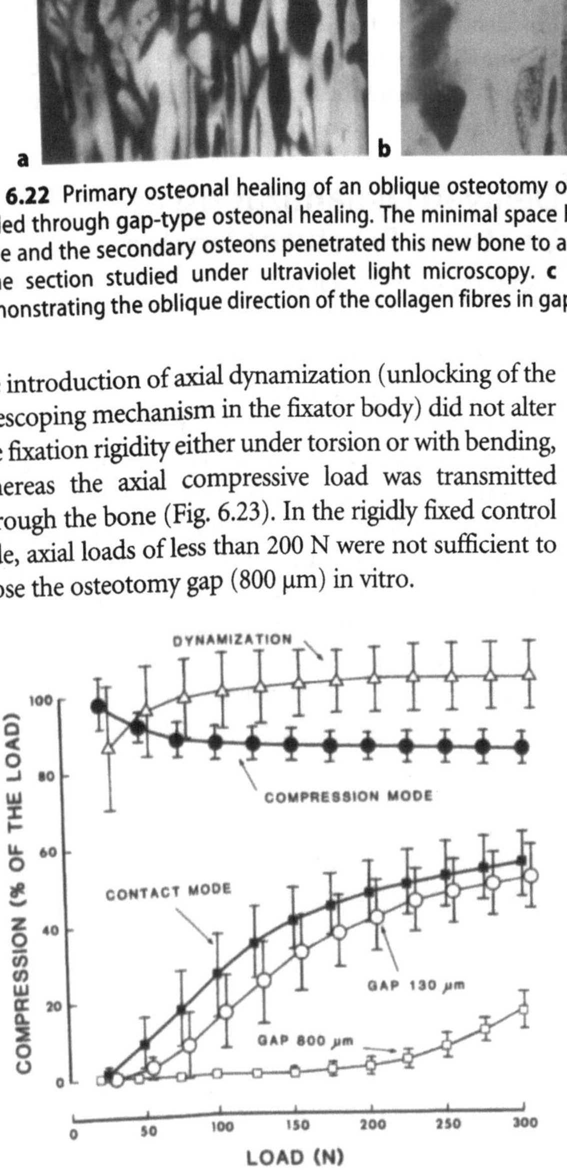

Fig. 6.23 Transmission of axial forces in vitro through the fracture site under the different modes of Orthofix external fixation. Using five pairs of canine transverse tibial osteotomies fixed with a custom-modified Orthofix device, the compression of the osteotomy ends was measured by a thin load washer placed between the osteotomy ends. Release of the telescoping mechanism (axial dynamization) resulted in dynamic compression of the fragments. A gap of 800μm prevented contact at the osteotomy until the load exceed 200 N.

In vivo, dynamization closed the osteotomy gap and induced contact healing of the cortical bone ends with periosteal callus formation. The control bones that were not subjected to dynamization healed through a gap healing mechanism of the cortical bone with or without external callus. In these bones, periosteal callus formation was linearly related to the animal's body weight. The amount of periosteal callus started to decrease earlier on the dynamized side (as a sign of enhanced external remodelling), but the differences in the callus formation and remodelling were not statistically significant. At 12 weeks, both sides showed a high rate of cortical healing through Haversian remodelling, and no statistical differences were observed in the amount of periosteal new bone, formation of intracortical new bone, bone porosity, blood flow to the osteotomy site, or bone scan activity. Intracortical porosity was low on both sides, with minimal formation of endosteal new bone. The torsional strength and stiffness of the dynamized and non-dynamized tibiae were already reaching the level of intact tibiae and no significant differences were found between the two sides.

This study showed that the axial readjustment of external fixation rigidity can facilitate fracture contact and direct cortical bone healing in stable fractures. The results of the rigidly fixed control side showed that rigid external fixation may prevent periosteal callus formation under low loading conditions. The fast mechanical healing of the bones, compared with the previous studies of external fixation, demonstrated the efficiency of osteonal bone healing. Undoubtedly, the stability of the fixation played an important role in achieving this.

Effect of a Large Fracture Gap on Bone Healing Under External Fixation

A fracture gap caused by unintentional distraction of the fracture fragments and augmented by fracture end resorption, is one of the obvious reasons for fracture healing problems with external fixation. The study of Markel et al (1991) examined the use of four non-invasive imaging modalities (quantitative computed tomography, magnetic resonance imaging, single-photon absorptiometry and dual-energy X-ray absorptiometry) in the quantification of bone healing in a delayed fracture union model under external fixation. Bilateral tibial transverse osteotomies were performed and stabilized using unilateral external fixators (Orthofix) with a 2mm gap. The structural, torsional and local fracture callus properties were determined at two-week intervals up to 12 weeks.

Although the indentation stiffness of the fracture callus increased linearly with time, the ultimate torque and torsional stiffness increased more slowly than in comparable fracture models with a smaller fracture gap. The osteotomies gained only about 44 per cent of intact bone strength by 12 weeks. The osteotomies united through secondary bone healing without direct cortical repair. Radiographic callus formation peaked at 6 weeks and declined thereafter. The cortical bone showed a marked remodelling, with high porosity (16.7 per cent) and a relatively low formation of new bone (38.5 per cent) at 12 weeks.

Compared with previous experiments, this study used a fracture union model with an increased osteotomy gap under bilateral stable external fixation. The results demonstrated the detrimental effect of a fracture gap on the healing of fractures under external fixation.

Early Dynamization Under External Fixation

The study of Egger et al (1992) investigated the physiological effects of axial compression under external fixation midway through the fracture healing period in the fracture union model with a significant 2mm fracture gap. Bilateral tibial osteotomies were fixed using custom-modified Orthofix external fixators. The telescoping mechanism of one of the fixators on each animal was released (dynamization) 7 days after osteotomy while the contralateral fixator remained locked as a control.

Radiographically, the released osteotomy closed and increased functional loading occurred. The procedure did not change the amount of fracture callus. In torsional testing at 6 weeks, the dynamized osteotomies were significantly stiffer than the controls but the difference in torsional strength was not significant. Histologically, the released osteotomies showed more new bone in the osteotomy gap region.

This study showed that very early dynamization in this delayed fracture union model improves fracture healing by reducing the fracture gap size and increasing weightbearing, thereby avoiding the secondary fracture union mechanism.

Delayed Dynamization of Unstable Fractures Under External Fixation

Theoretically, axial compression of the fracture site (i.e. axial dynamization under external fixation) can be applied either to encourage early callus formation and thereby secondary osteonal bone union (early dynamization), or it may be used to enhance bone remodelling after early fracture union (delayed dynamization). Stable fractures are suitable for either early or delayed dynamization. In unstable fractures, only delayed dynamization is feasible.

In the study of Aro and Chao (1991), an unstable fracture model of the canine tibia (60° oblique osteotomy with a 2mm gap) stabilized with external fixation (custom-modified Orthofix) was used to determine the effects of delayed dynamization (performed 4 weeks after surgery). In the control osteotomies, external fixation was maintained in the locked mode with the fracture gap throughout the healing period of 12 weeks.

Axial release of the telescoping mechanism (dynamization) resulted in closer contact of the oblique fracture ends, followed by enhanced callus maturation as indicated by the earlier start of external remodelling and by the decreased amount of endosteal callus. The morphological changes were associated with a trend to increased energy absorption at failure during torsional testing. There were no significant changes in paired comparison of torsional strength or stiffness. The unstable fracture model with a large gap resulted in non-osteonal bone healing, regardless of whether the fracture was dynamized or not. The osteotomies gained about 60 per cent of intact bone strength, indicating a slower return than in those with a predominantly osteonal bone healing pattern.

This study showed that even delayed dynamization may close an unintentional fracture gap, with the positive effect of enhanced axial loading on fracture callus remodelling. Delayed dynamization could not, however, reverse the non-osteonal bone union mechanism, demonstrating the importance of immediate fracture apposition in achieving early cortical healing.

Multiple Comparisons of Osteotomy Healing Under External Fixation

Re-analysis of the results of three consecutive studies on fracture healing in the canine tibia under external fixation was performed (Aro and Chao 1993). The re-analysis involved normalization of the radiographic and mechanical data to facilitate intergroup comparisons. As described earlier in this chapter, standardized transverse or 60° oblique osteotomies were performed bilaterally in each dog and stabilized with a custom-modified Orthofix external fixator, applied using six Orthofix cortical screws. The osteotomies were fixed either in contact, with a small 800µm gap, or with a large 2mm gap. A group of transverse osteotomies was axially dynamized at two weeks and a group of oblique osteotomies at four weeks. The healing of the osteotomies was analyzed at 12 weeks. Comparison was also made between operated tibiae and the intact tibiae harvested from control animals.

Normalization of the data was based on the following correlations: the amount of periosteal callus in transverse osteotomies showed a linear relationship (r = 0.778) to the animal body weight. The amount of periosteal callus measured from the radiographs was therefore normalized against the animal body weight in each osteotomy group by dividing the callus area (mm^2) by the body weight (kg). The torsional stiffness and strength of the intact canine tibiae also showed a linear relationship (r = 0.936 and r = 0.915, respectively) to the animal body weight. The mechanical parameters of the healing osteotomies and intact bones were thus correspondingly normalized by dividing the measured values (torsional strength, torsional stiffness, energy absorption and deformation at torsional failure) by body weight.

Sequential radiographic analysis showed that periosteal callus reached its maximum size within six weeks and decreased thereafter. Comparison of the osteotomy groups (Fig. 6.24) showed significant differences both at 6 and at 12 weeks. At 6 weeks, the periosteal callus was largest in oblique osteotomies with a large gap (with or without dynamization). The transverse osteotomies (reduced in contact) also formed a relatively large callus. Animals were loading on the transverse osteotomy side more (a mean difference of 35 per cent) compared with the oblique side during the first six weeks of osteotomy healing.

External remodelling, as indicated by the significant reduction in periosteal callus size between 6 and 12 weeks, occurred rapidly in the transverse osteotomies (Fig. 6.24). The oblique osteotomies showed less

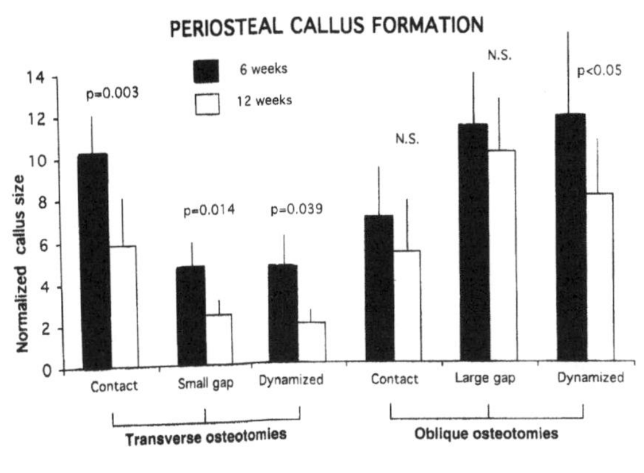

Fig. 6.24 The amount of periosteal callus in healing osteotomies during the maximal callus formation (6 weeks) and at the time of remodelling (12 weeks). The differences between the different osteotomy groups was significant both at 6 and 12 weeks. The p-values shown above the bars describe the statistical significance of the reduction of the callus size between 6 and 12 weeks. The data (mean ± SD) represent the values of the periosteal callus normalized against animal body weight (mm^2/kg).

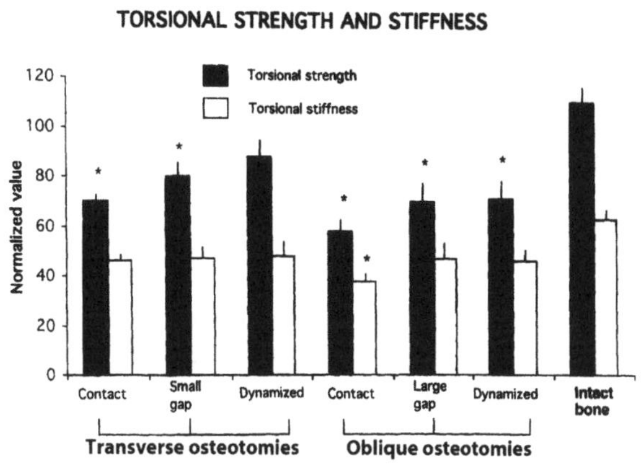

Fig. 6.25 Torsional strength and stiffness of the osteotomies of the canine tibiae healed under external fixation for 12 weeks. The reference values of the intact tibiae are also shown. The asterisks indicate significant differences compared with the intact bone value. The values are normalized against the animal body weight. The bars represent the mean ± SEM, n = 7-8.

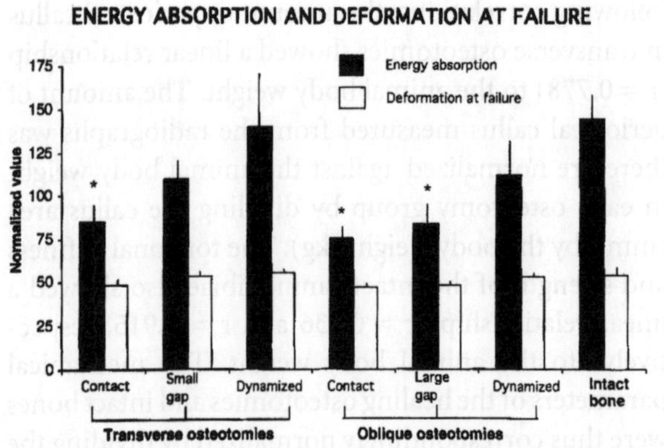

Fig. 6.26 Energy absorption and angular deformation at failure in the torsional test of the canine tibial osteotomies healed under Orthofix external fixation for 12 weeks. The reference values of the intact tibiae are also shown. The asterisks indicate significant differences compared with the intact bone value. The values are normalized against the animal body weight. The bars represent the mean ± SEM, n = 7–8.

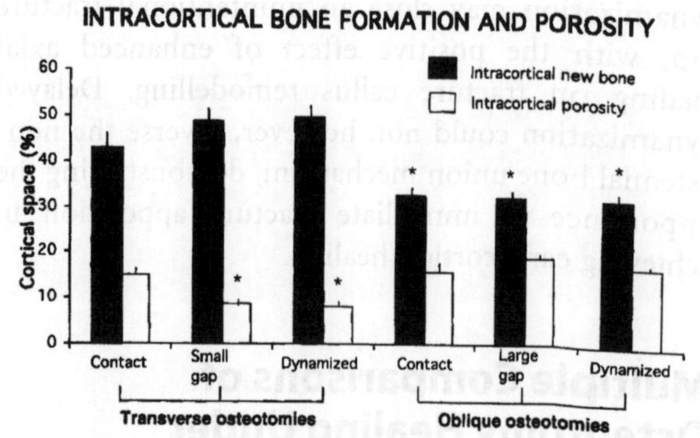

Fig. 6.27 Intracortical new bone formation and porosity in the canine tibial osteotomies healed under Orthofix external fixation for 12 weeks. The asterisks indicate a significant decrease in intracortical new bone formation in oblique osteotomies and a significant decrease in intracortical porosity in transverse osteotomies (small gap, dynamized) compared with other groups of osteotomies. The bars represent the mean ± SEM, n = 7–8.

uniform callus remodelling. Of the oblique osteotomies, only those subjected to dynamization showed a statistically significant reduction in callus size between 6 and 12 weeks (Fig. 6.24), as a sign of enhanced external remodelling.

The torsional stiffness of the healed osteotomies (Fig. 6.25) was reaching intact bone levels by 12 weeks. Only the oblique osteotomies with reduced contact were significantly less stiff than the intact bones (–43 per cent). The torsional strength of the osteotomies was significantly lower (up to –40 per cent) than the intact bone value (Fig. 6.25). Of the different osteotomy groups, only the dynamized transverse osteotomies showed torsional strengths close to intact bones values (difference not significant).

The energy absorption at failure (Fig. 6.26) was also associated with significant differences between the osteotomy groups. The values of fracture energy absorption for dynamized transverse osteotomies, non-dynamized transverse osteotomies with a small gap and dynamized oblique osteotomies approached the intact bone level. The other groups showed significant differences (the variation being between –45 and –49 per cent) in energy absorption compared with intact bones. There were no statistical differences between the osteotomy groups and the intact bone value for deformation at torsional failure (Fig. 6.26).

The amount of intracortical new bone was used as a measure of the formation of secondary osteons and the degree of direct cortical bone healing. Intracortical new bone formation and porosity showed highly significant differences between the osteotomy groups (Fig. 6.27). The transverse osteotomies, independent of fixation mode, showed a high rate of intracortical new bone formation. In transverse osteotomies, new bone accounted for 43.3–49.7 per cent of the cortical space. The oblique osteotomies showed a relatively lower rate of intracortical new bone formation (32.5–33.4 per cent). Intracortical porosity (Fig. 6.27) was lowest (8.2–8.6 per cent) in animals with bilateral transverse osteotomies with a small gap and highest (16.7–19.0 per cent) in the animals with bilateral oblique osteotomies with a large gap. The animals with a transverse osteotomy on one leg (reduced in contact) and an oblique osteotomy on the other leg (reduced in contact) showed no significant differences in intracortical porosity between the two sides (13.9 against 15.8 per cent, respectively), indicating that the osteotomy type per se was not responsible for the difference in intracortical porosity. Intracortical porosity was shown to be related to the periosteal callus formation and its revascularization process.

There were also distinct differences in endosteal new bone formation between the osteotomy groups. The determining factor in endosteal new bone formation was the presence of a significant fracture gap. Transverse osteotomies with a small gap had significantly less endosteal new bone than oblique osteotomies with a large gap (2.5 ± 0.7 mm^2 vs. 16.8 ± 4.2mm^2, p = 0.015).

Classification of Bone Union Mechanisms Under External Fixation

As described, a wide variety of bone healing mechanisms could be achieved with external fixation under controlled conditions. The experiments also delineated the factors governing the mechanism through which bone union will take place under external fixation. The biological and biomechanical pathways to osseous union could be attenuated by changing the axial rigidity of external fixation during the course of treatment. One of the most interesting findings was related to the biomechanical efficiency of different union patterns in restoring the structural properties of the healing bone.

At a given rigidity of external fixation, periosteal callus formation was related to the loading magnitude (dictated by body weight). Under low loading conditions, stable external fixation prevented periosteal callus formation and thus the healing relied on osteonal cortical healing with minimal periosteal and endosteal callus. Axial dynamization of stable fractures resulted in contact of the fracture (osteotomy) ends and facilitated direct cortical healing in the presence of periosteal new bone formation. In unstable fractures,

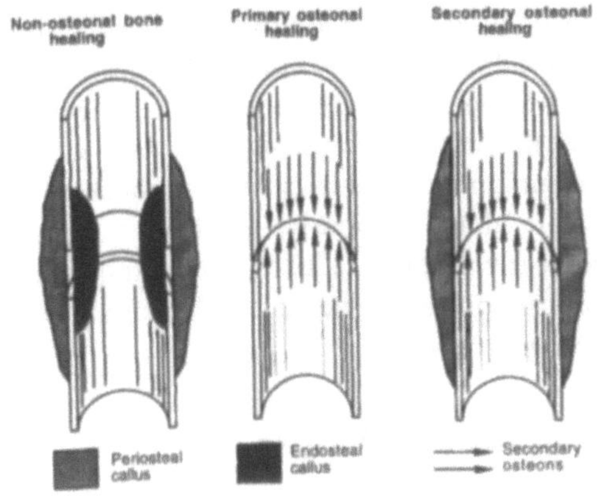

Fig. 6.28 Schematic diagrams illustrating the main fracture healing patterns under external fixation. The non-osteonal bone healing mechanism is characterized by substantial periosteal and endosteal callus formation without early healing of the cortical bone. Primary osteonal healing does not show significant callus formation but the fracture site heals through end-to-end union by means of secondary osteons. Secondary osteonal healing is characterized by periosteal callus formation and direct early healing of the cortical bone by secondary osteons. Both primary and secondary osteonal union may be based on contact healing (illustrated), gap healing, or both. Generally, there are small gaps asymmetrically located around the circumference of the bone cortex and the fracture site heals through the combined contact and gap healing mechanisms.

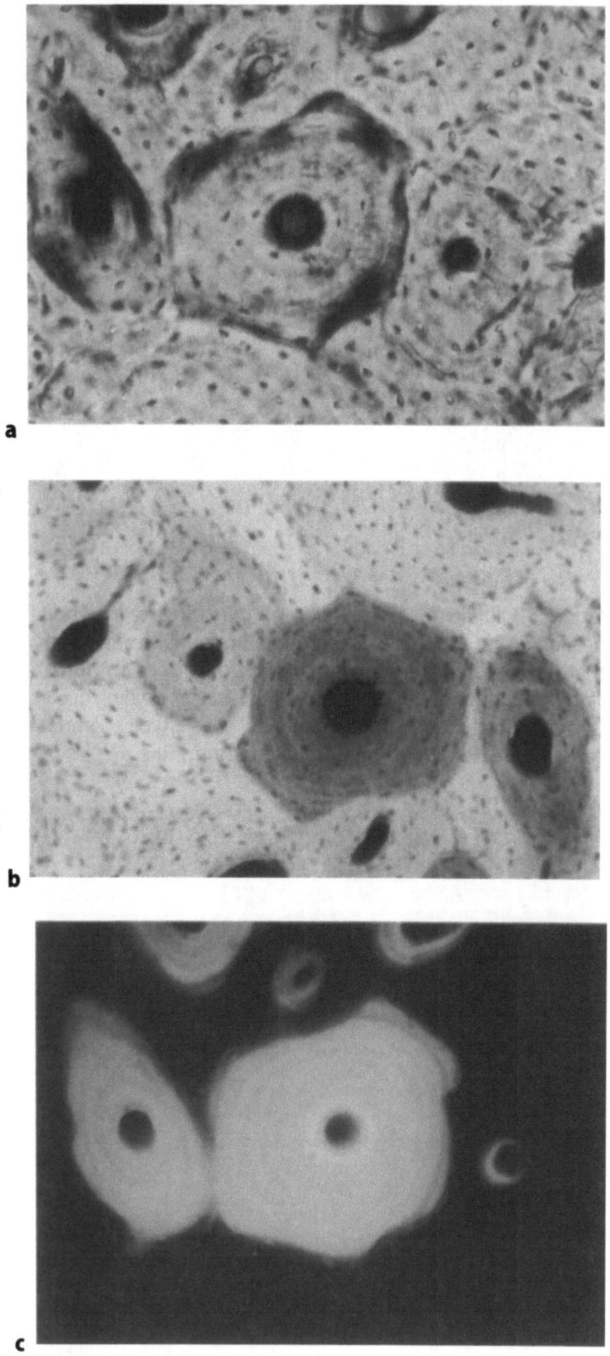

Fig. 6.29 Healing of canine cortical bone by secondary osteons during external fixation. A cross-section of an osteotomized tibia was studied 12 weeks after osteotomy. **a** Under light microscopy, the primary and secondary osteons look the same. **b** Under mircoradiograph, the newly formed secondary osteons show a less dense (dark) structure as a sign of incomplete mineralization. **c** Ultraviolet microscopy demonstrates the presence of labelled (tetracycline, white) new bone around the central canal of the secondary osteons. The new bone of secondary osteons may account for up to 50 percent (Fig. 6.27) of the cross-sectional area of the bone cortex after osteotomy healing.

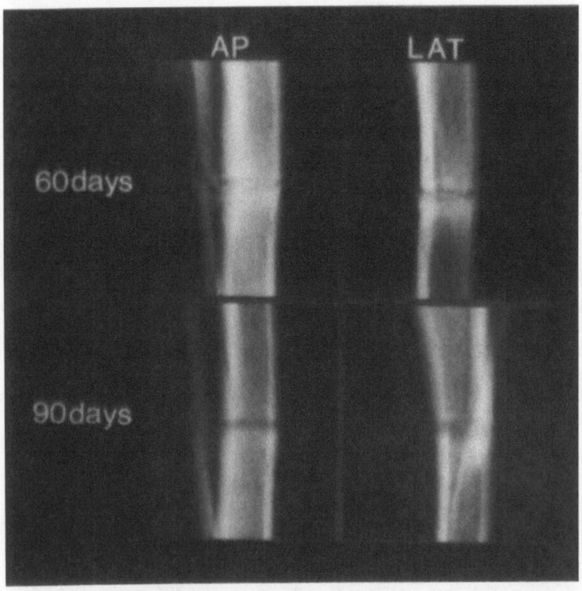

Fig. 6.30 Radiographic features of primary osteonal bone healing under external fixation. Under low loading conditions, the transverse osteotomy of the canine tibia does not form a significant amount of periosteal callus (60 days). Healing occurs through direct cortical bone repair, visible as a typical gradual softening and disappearance of the osteotomy line.

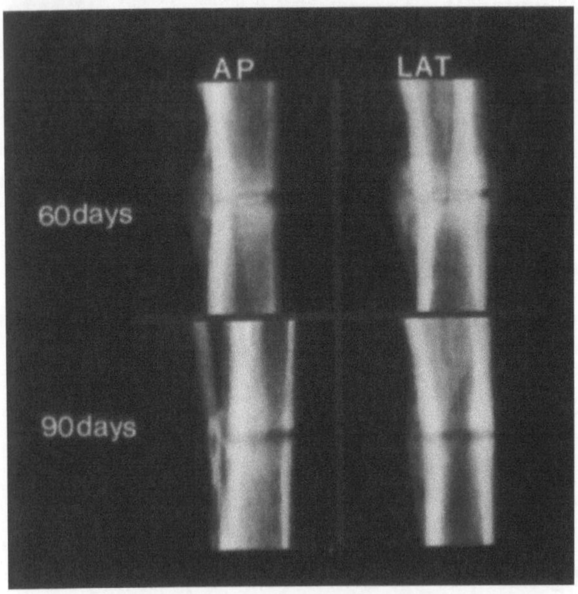

Fig. 6.31 Radiographic features of secondary osteonal bone healing under external fixation. Induced by high axial loading, the transverse osteotomy develops a moderate amount of periosteal callus in the early phase of healing (60 days), followed by a gradual disappearance of the osteotomy line (cortical healing) and simultaneous fairly rapid remodelling of the periosteal callus (diminution of the callus size).

dynamization did not change the non-osteonal pathway of union (periosteal and endosteal callus formation without direct cortical healing).

The results obtained provide a compelling reason for modifying the commonly used classification of bone healing patterns (primary versus secondary bone union). In the modified classification (Aro and Chao 1993), three major types are proposed: non-osteonal bone healing, primary osteonal healing, and secondary osteonal healing (Fig. 6.28). The histological criterion for osteonal healing is the growth of secondary osteons through the cortical bone across the fracture site from one fragment to another (Fig. 6.29). Radiographically, primary osteonal bone healing is characterized by a lack of periosteal callus formation and the gradual disappearance of the fracture line (Fig. 6.30). Secondary osteonal healing is characterized by periosteal callus formation and early cortical bone healing, followed by rapid callus remodelling (Fig. 6.31).

Neither cortical healing alone (the characteristic of the primary bone union mechanism) nor the predominance of periosteal callus formation (the characteristic of the non-osteonal bone union mechanism) seems to be more desirable over the other in the restoration of bone mechanical properties. In contrast, the combination of these bone healing mechanisms, characterized by early cortical healing and concomitant periosteal callus formation (secondary osteonal healing mechanism) would appear to be optimal to meet the time-related mechanical requirements of a healing fracture. One of the advantageous signs of the secondary osteonal union mechanism is rapid remodelling of the periosteal callus. Obviously, the load transmission through early fracture callus is rapidly transferred to the cortical bone as the healing of the cortico-cortical junction progresses.

Clinical Implications

The following conclusions can be applied to clinical practice. Based on the presented data, external fixation per se is not the cause of clinical fracture union problems. The severity of local soft-tissue and periosteal injury, and not the method of fracture fixation, are the main predictors of fracture non-union. In the presence of a healthy vascularized soft-tissue envelope, long-bone fractures heal without delay under stable external fixation. In the presence of severe soft-tissue injury, an externally fixed fracture frequently needs an additional stimulus, such as inductive early bone grafting, for union. If the slow fracture union is caused by unintentional distraction at the fracture site, axial dynamization may be the only additional stimulus needed for union.

The major factors determining the mechanical milieu of a healing fracture, and thereby the mechanisms of fracture union, are the rigidity of the selected fixation device, the fracture configuration, the accuracy of fracture reduction, and the amount of physiological stress induced by functional activity and loading. The critical time for callus formation and osteonal healing of the cortical bone is finite. The preferred type of union mechanism should therefore be determined during the initial stages of fracture treatment.

Anatomical reduction (i.e. axial alignment and close apposition of the fracture ends) should be obtained as early as possible after injury. The goal is to maximize the contact area of the fracture surface and to avoid distraction of the fragments. An external fixation system should be selected according to the anatomical site and fracture morphology to achieve initial fracture stability against bending and torsional forces. Cortical contact of the fracture ends (augmented by static compression, if possible) is essential to improve fracture stability. High fracture stability is important not only for bone union but also for healing of the soft-tissue injury.

The mode of fracture union dictates the further course of patient care. In stable fractures, compensation of any fracture end resorption and improvement of stability can be achieved by means of static compression applied through the fixator body. Under such conditions, the fixation relies on direct cortical bone healing (*primary osteonal bone union*). If such a mechanism of fracture union has been chosen, the external fixator should not be removed prematurely.

With the external fixation of unstable fractures, gradual functional loading results in cyclic fracture micromotion and periosteal callus formation (*non-osteonal healing*). This is the main healing pattern in comminuted fractures incapable of direct cortical bone healing. After the initial healing with periosteal callus, these fractures may benefit from delayed axial dynamization of the external fixator. The procedure may enhance callus remodelling and ultimately prevent refractures after fixator removal.

The combination of cortical healing and periosteal callus formation (*secondary osteonal healing*) seems to optimize the mechanical recovery of a healing bone under external fixation. There are two requirements for such a union mechanism. First, the fracture pattern must be fairly simple to allow accurate reduction and cortical bone contact of the fracture surfaces. The fracture contact is needed for direct cortical healing. Second, periosteal callus formation must be induced by functional loading of the healing bone, i.e. by the early introduction of gradual weightbearing. The question of early dynamization in the induction and promotion of periosteal callus formation still needs further confirmation by carefully executed, prospective, randomized clinical trials.

High-energy fractures usually involve severe periosteal and soft-tissue injury which adversely affects the biological capacity of the bone for union. Associated soft-tissue injuries also limit functional use and loading of the injured extremity. In these circumstances, cancellous bone grafting, performed between 4 and 6 weeks, has been found to be effective in the induction of periosteal callus formation. For these fractures, secondary osteonal healing is the best available goal of treatment. It calls for accurate reduction and stable external fixation of the fracture, repeated debridements and early reconstruction of the soft tissue envelope, followed by induction of the periosteal callus mass by subperiosteal bone grafting.

Selection of an appropriate pin type (cortical vs cancellous bone)
Fracture reduction before pin insertion
Pin insertion through the maximum diameter of the bone (bicortical fixation)
Low-speed predrilling through a drill guide (avoidance of skin, muscle, and bone necrosis)
Creation of stable fracture fixation
Sufficient soft tissue release around pins
Proper care (elevation and early joint motion) of the extremity to decrease oedema
Reduction of soft-tissue motion at skin/muscle-pin interface
Avoidance of excessive loading on the extremity
Regular cleaning of pin sites

Table 6.2 Clinical factors in the prevention of pin-track problems.

Mechanical Performance of Orthofix Cortical Screws

Introduction

The pin–bone interface is most critical for the performance of external fixators. The immediate holding power of external fixation pins is usually good; early pull-out of an external fixation pin is extremely rare. In contrast, loosening of an external fixation pin is not uncommon. A major effort must be therefore be focused on creating and maintaining the best conditions for the performance of external fixation pins.

One common mistake is to assume that the use of unilateral external fixators is easy and that it does not require learning or mastering the surgical techniques. The majority of pin-track complications are related to technical errors of surgery, such as unicortical pin placement. Pin track problems can be controlled, but the established regimens must be followed during insertion and post-operative care (Table 6.2).

The time sequence of events in pin-track sepsis is controversial (Aro et al 1993). First, mechanical loosening of a pin, as a result of thermal bone necrosis or mechanical cortical bone failure, carries a risk of subsequent pin track infection. Second, bacterial colonization from the pin–skin interface to the pin–bone interface may lead to bone resorption and subsequent pin loosening.

Biomechanical aspects of pin–bone interface performance have been studied in detail using both three-dimensional and two-dimensional finite elements (Chao et al 1982, Huiskes and Chao 1986, Huiskes et al 1985). Local pin–bone stresses may reach high levels during weightbearing. Effective precautions should be taken to reduce these stresses considerably, thereby reducing the chances for local bone yielding failure and pin loosening.

Pin geometry and thread design as well as bone thread preparation are critical biomechanical factors in pin performance (Ansell and Scales 1968). Improved cutting technology, with effective chip elimination, is important to minimize the maximum temperatures generated during pin insertion. A pin's inability to remove cut chips efficiently results in increased frictional forces leading to both higher temperatures and increased insertion torques (Wiggins and Malkin 1976). Many factors are involved in efficient bone chip removal during drilling. One of these is the presence or absence of flutes at the pin tips and the various orientations of the flutes. Predrilling is claimed to be the most effective measure to prevent thermal necrosis during pin insertion (Matthews et al 1984). The technique of bone thread preparation is of particular importance when the bone quality is less than optimal for pin insertion.

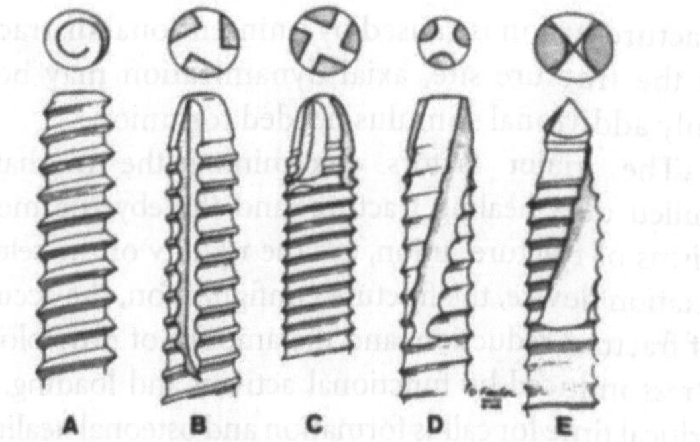

Fig. 6.32 Five cortical screws for external fixation were compared: **A** Orthofix 6/5mm – stainless steel; **B** Hoffmann 5mm – stainless steel; **C** Ace 5mm – titanium; **D** Apex Blunt 5mm – stainless steel, and **E** Apex Sharp 5mm – stainless steel. The geometry of the threaded portions of the screws varied.

The Orthofix cortical screws have many unique properties. The characteristics and performance of these have been examined in both in vitro and in vivo studies.

In Vitro Performance

An in vitro study (Wikenheiser et al 1995) was carried out to compare the mechanical performance of Orthofix screws and four other external fixation pins (Hoffmann, Ace, Apex Sharp, and Apex Blunt) (Fig. 6.32) with respect to insertion torque, pull-out strength, heat generation and microdamage at the pin-bone interface. Pin performance was tested in two models: fresh frozen sheep tibiae and RF-100 foam solid rods. All the studied pins were self-tapping and, except for the Apex Sharp, used predrilling. Thermocouples were used to measure the temperature in the entry and exit cortices as well as inside the pin tip during insertion.

The results showed that pin tip design plays a significant role in relation to insertion torque (Fig. 6.33), heat generation (Fig. 6.34) and pullout strength (Fig. 6.35). High temperatures were measured both within pins and in bone tissue during insertion (Fig. 6.34). The thermocouples placed within the pin tip often recorded temperatures well above the known thermonecrotic value, i.e. 50° C. The insertion torque and temperature curves correlated closely. Pins with a straight flute design generated more heat and had higher insertion torques than helical fluted designs.

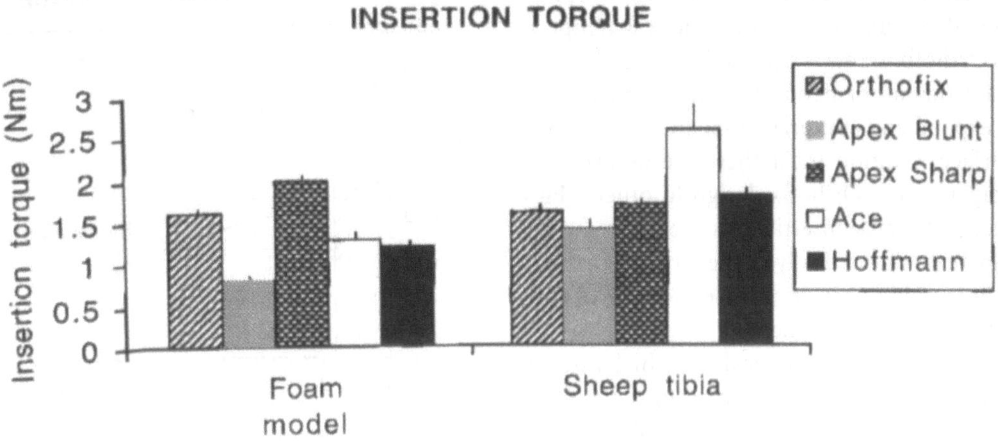

Fig. 6.33 Insertion torques of external fixation screws measured by an instrumented torque wrench. The values represent the mean ± SEM both for an artificial bone model and sheep tibia.

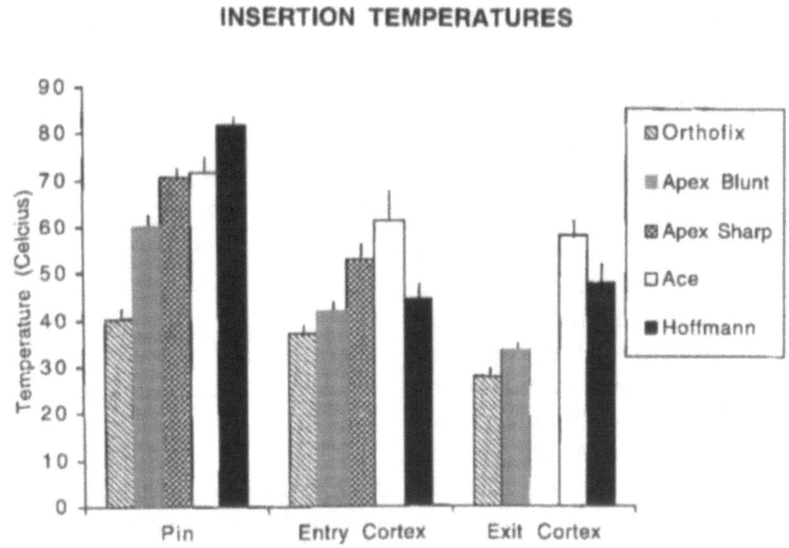

Fig. 6.34 Heat generation during insertion of external fixation screws. The temperature was measured both within the screw tip and in the entry and exit cortices. The values represent the mean ± SEM for sheep tibiae.

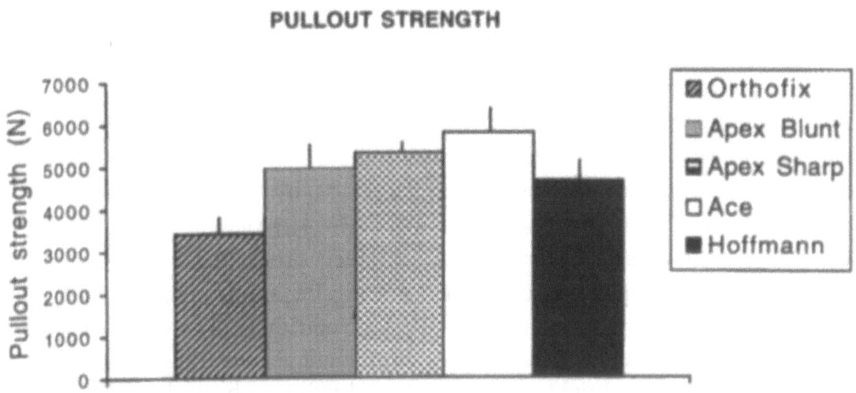

Fig. 6.35 The pullout strength values of Orthofix and four other cortical external fixation screws. The values represent the mean ± SEM for sheep tibiae.

In contrast to the fluted designs, the Orthofix screw demonstrated low insertion torque and low temperature. The Orthofix screw is unique in that it does not cut bone for thread formation but relies on a tapered design to expand and compress bone to form the pin-bone interface. Caution must therefore be exercised when comparing the Orthofix design to others (Figs. 6.33 and 6.34), because insertion torque and temperature will increase dramatically as the tapered Orthofix screw is advanced further once the end-point of clinical tightening has been reached.

Pullout strength is a mechanical test which assesses the immediate holding power of a screw or pin. Pullout strength is greatly influenced by the pilot hole diameter (predrilling) and the difference between the major and minor diameters of the pin. In the test setup, the Orthofix pin had lower pullout strength values than the other pin types (Fig. 6.35). This is interesting because the screw has the largest difference between the major and minor diameters and one would anticipate superior pullout strength. However, in the case of the Orthofix screw, it appears that the other major factor in pullout strength (i.e. pilot hole size) is more critical. The recommended pilot hole size for the Orthofix screw is 4.8mm, and the major diameter of the screw at its threaded tip is also approximately 4.8mm. When the screw is inserted after predrilling, as it penetrates the exit cortex, the pilot hole is a similar diameter to the major diameter of the screw. The tapered design has therefore created threads in the entry cortex, but only partially in the exit cortex, which results in lower pullout strength. As the tapered Orthofix screw is advanced further, the exit cortex will play a greater role in pullout strength once the screw thread/bone interface is created.

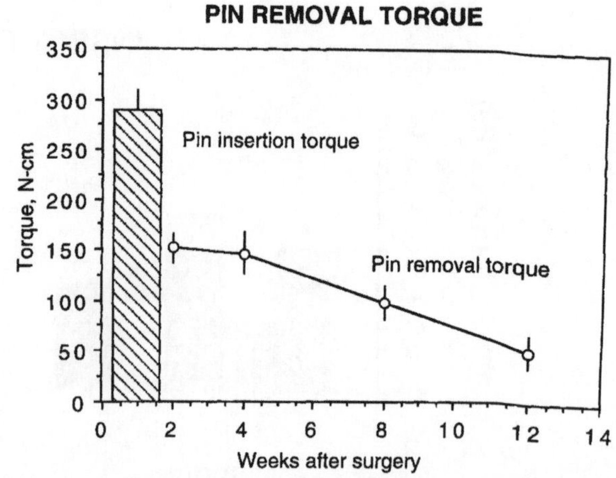

Fig. 6.36 Insertion of Orthofix cortical screws into the canine tibia and the corresponding removal torques. The values represent the mean ± SEM as a function of osteotomy healing time (weeks). The changes between 4, 8 and 12 weeks were statistically significant.

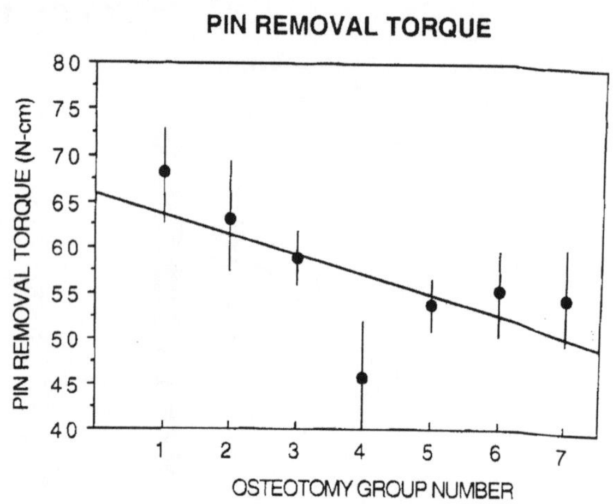

Fig. 6.37 Average removal torques of Orthofix cortical screws in seven different osteotomy groups of the canine tibia 12 weeks after surgery. The values represent the mean ± SEM, n = 7–8. Removal torque values were averaged for all screws (n = 6) in each osteotomy. The groups were: 1. transverse osteotomies in contact; 2. dynamized transverse osteotomies; 3. transverse osteotomies with a small gap; 4. transverse osteotomies with a large gap; 5. oblique osteotomies in contact; 6. dynamized oblique osteotomies, and 7. oblique osteotomies with large gap.

In Vivo Model

The canine model developed for osteotomy healing studies was also used to characterize the nature of cortical bone reactions at the pin-bone interface in association with Orthofix cortical screws. Custom-modified Orthofix external fixators were applied to the tibiae using six tapered Orthofix cortical screws. The screws were inserted after predrilling both cortices with a slow-speed power drill and screw insertion torque was measured. The screws were then tightened until the threaded portion of the screw had penetrated both cortices and the screw was clinically tight. The torque resistance of the screw during the final tightening was measured with an instrumented torque wrench. A transverse or oblique (60°) osteotomy was performed in each tibia and stabilized under different gap conditions (fragments in contact, with a small gap of 800μm, or with a large gap of 2mm).

Free, unrestricted weightbearing was allowed immediately after surgery. Sequential functional evaluations (static and dynamic weightbearing) and radiographic examinations were performed. Anteroposterior and lateral radiographs of the tibiae were examined for the presence of any pin track rarefaction. Rarefaction was defined as a radiolucent line of more than 0.5 mm around a screw at the entry or exit cortex or both. At designated time points, the screw-skin interfaces were examined, the external fixators were removed, and the screw removal torques measured. Pin tracks were then processed and analyzed using quantitative tetracycline histomorphometry and microradiography.

Screw Insertion and Removal Torques

Screw insertion torque was about 20 per cent higher in the tibial shaft than in its proximal and distal metaphyseal regions. Taking into account only the screws with no radiographic changes, the screw removal torques decreased over the time (Fig. 6.36). The percentage reduction of insertion torque value by 12 weeks was uniform among screws in different locations.

The comparison of the osteotomy groups performed at 12 weeks showed highly significant differences in average screw removal torque (Fig. 6.37). The screw removal torques were highest in transverse osteotomies fixed under cortical bone contact and lowest in unstable osteotomy models (in transverse osteotomies with a large gap and in oblique osteotomies).

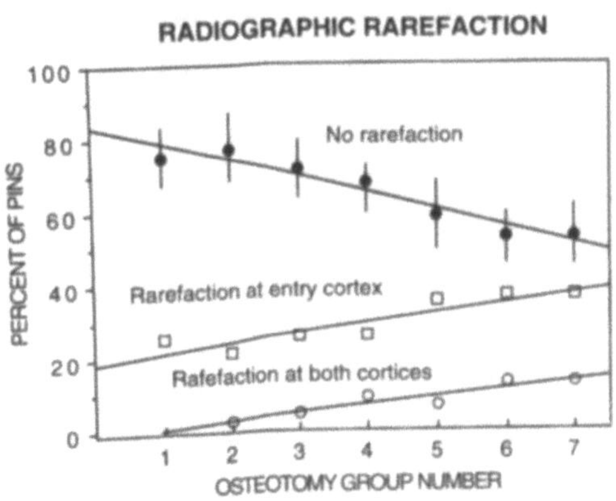

Fig. 6.38 The relative distribution of cortical screws according to their radiographic status at 12 weeks in seven different osteotomy groups of the canine tibia. The data show the number of screws (expressed as percentages) with no rarefaction (filled circles), rarefaction only at the entry cortex (empty square), or rarefaction at both cortices (open circles). The values represent the mean ± SEM, n = 7–8. The groups were: 1. transverse osteotomies in contact; 2. dynamized transverse osteotomies; 3. transverse osteotomies with a small gap; 4. transverse osteotomies with a large gap; 5. oblique osteotomies in contact; 6. dynamized oblique osteotomies, and 7. oblique osteotomies with large gap.

Radiographic Changes Along Screw Tracks

Altogether, 243 screws (65 per cent of the screws analyzed at 12 weeks) showed no radiographic changes, 105 screws (28 per cent) had rarefaction only at the entry cortex, and 24 screws (7 per cent) showed rarefaction at both cortices. The extent of rarefaction varied from a slight radiolucency of the cortical bone to a real radiolucent halo around the screw.

At 12 weeks, the number of screws with radiographic changes was lowest in stable fracture models (Fig. 6.38). In each osteotomy model, rarefaction was most commonly observed only at the entry cortex (Fig. 6.38). Transverse osteotomies reduced under contact had no screws showing rarefaction on both cortices, compared with 8 per cent and 12 per cent in unstable osteotomy models (Fig. 6.38).

Radiographic changes became evident during the first four weeks of osteotomy healing, and the number of screws with changes did not increase significantly thereafter. However, slight rarefaction of less than 1 mm observed at the entry cortex of some screws disappeared over time, and some new rarefaction appeared on other screws between 6 and 12 weeks.

The torque required to remove the screws with entry cortex rarefaction (unstable screws) was approximately 30 per cent lower than that required for screws with no rarefaction (stable screws). Screws with rarefaction at both cortices had low or no resistance to torsion.

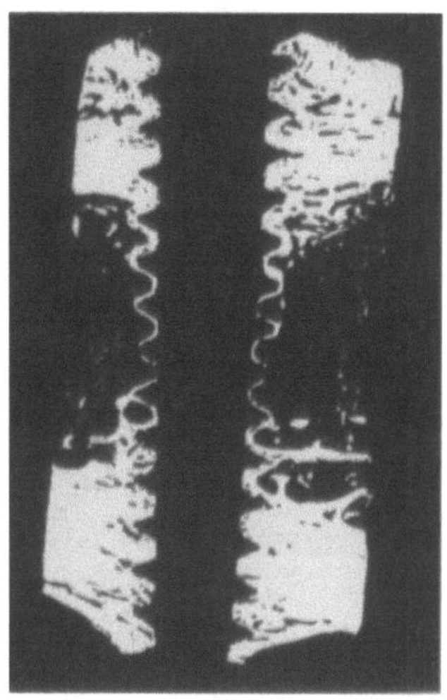

Fig. 6.39 A microradiograph showing the screw track of an Orthofix cortical screw in the canine tibia (12 weeks after osteotomy). The screw track had well preserved bone threads both at the entry cortex and at the exit cortex. The periosteal surface of both cortices as well as the medullary cavity showed newly formed bone threads.

Microradiographic and Histological Findings

Microradiographically, the screws with no radiographic changes showed well preserved bone threads on both cortices (Fig. 6.39). The endosteal and periosteal surfaces as well as the medullary cavity showed newly formed bone threads. The stable screws showed marked intracortical remodelling (formation of secondary osteons) in the vicinity of screw tracks. Secondary osteons were also seen invading into the well preserved bone threads, indicating the process of creeping substitution (Fig. 6.40). The amount of new bone was about 43 per cent of the total cortical bone space both at the entry and exit cortices of stable screws (Fig. 6.41). The corresponding cortical bone porosity (12 per cent) was about four times higher than that of intact canine cortical bone (3 per cent), as a sign of enhanced vascularization.

Screws with radiographic rarefaction at the entry cortices (unstable screws) showed marked porosity and complete or incomplete resorption of bone threads at the entry cortex (Fig. 6.42). The porosity of the entry cortex was increased about two-fold compared with stable screws (Fig. 6.41). The remodelling of the exit cortex showed no significant differences from that associated with the stable screws (Fig. 6.41).

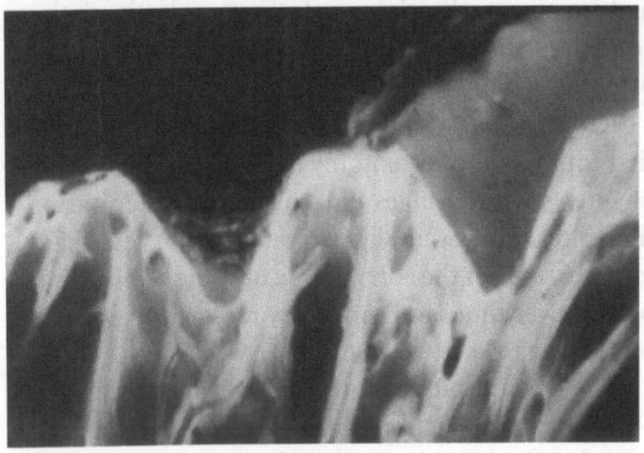

Fig. 6.40 Creeping substitution of cortical bone threads at the screw-bone interface of an Orthofix cortical screw at 12 weeks. The ultraviolet microscopy of a histological section showed new bone formation (tetracycline labeled white new bone) along the screw track and within secondary osteons growing into the bone threads.

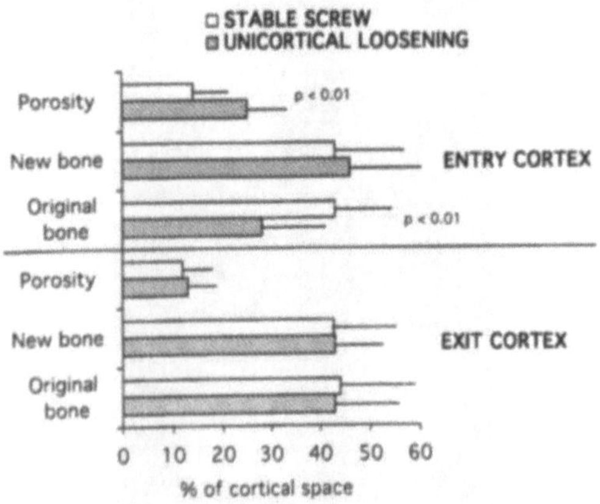

Fig. 6.41 Histomorphometric features of cortical bone remodelling at the entry and exit cortices of Orthofix cortical screws at 12 weeks (the canine tibia). The pins with radiographic rarefaction at the entry cortex (unicortical loosening) showed a significantly increased intracortical porosity at the entry cortex. The bars represent the means ± SEM (n = 14).

Comments

Implantation of any bone screw results in cortical bone remodelling. A similar phenomenon of creeping substitution (Haversian remodelling) was evident in canine cortical bone around external fixation screws. This beneficial biological process replaces any damaged lamellar bone next to the screw and also results in a time-related decrease in screw removal torque. The phenomenon does not seem to be related to the physiological loading of the screw or to the design of the threaded portion of the screw. Coating of external fixation screws with osteoconductive materials such as hydroxyapatite

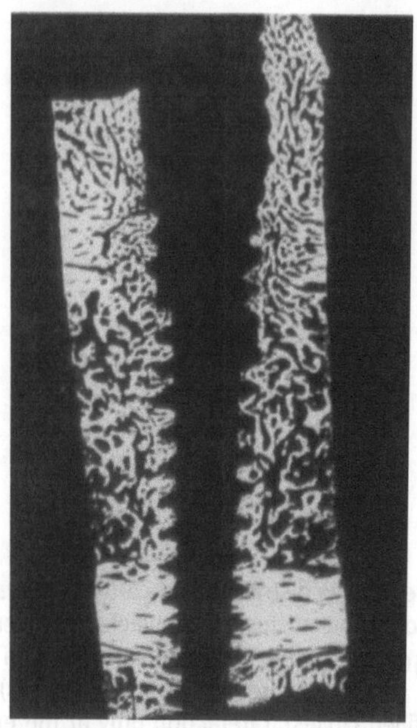

Fig. 6.42 A microradiograph showing the characteristics of an unstable Orthofix cortical screw in the canine tibia (12 weeks after osteotomy). The entry cortex showed a partial loss of bone threads with marked osteoporosis of the cortical bone itself. There is also a marked periosteal reaction at the entry site. The medullary cavity showed new bone formation which had formed well-shaped bone threads.

(Moroni et al 1998a, 1998b) may ideally compensate for the effects of bone remodelling and reverse the time-related decrease of screw anchorage.

The tapered Orthofix cortical screws, originally designed to enable screw tightening during the course of fixation, create radial preloading. As a potential drawback, radial preloading may exceed the limit of bone, resulting in irreversible bone deformation with microfractures. Under highly controlled laboratory conditions, a high insertion torque of a tapered screw, however, was shown not to increase the risk of screw loosening. An obvious explanation is that any cortical bone microfracture caused by radial preloading will be compensated by the high remodelling rate of the cortical bone.

The models simulating heavy loading conditions (unstable, oblique osteotomies and transverse osteotomies with a large gap) demonstrated that immediate weightbearing may cause bone thread resorption and adverse cortical bone remodelling at the entry cortex of fixation screws. Such unicortical screw loosening represents a consequence of micromotion and local bone yielding failure caused by excessive dynamic stresses at the entry cortex of the pin-bone interface.

Interestingly, some of the screws with slight early rarefaction at the entry cortices showed disappearance of the radiographic changes during the period of osteotomy consolidation. This observation suggests possible reversibility of the partial bone thread resorption and cortical bone porosis around external fixation screws after the achievement of bone union. Such a repair phenomenon was not observed in screw tracks with rarefaction in both cortices.

Summary

This chapter has reviewed the results of extensive laboratory studies on the performance of the standard Orthofix external fixator. These studies have delineated (1) the static and fatigue performance of the Orthofix device and its key components in vitro; (2) the healing patterns of experimental long-bone fractures stabilized with Orthofix external fixation, and (3) in vitro and in vivo performance of the Orthofix cortical screws.

The standard Orthofix external fixator is versatile but the orthopaedic surgeon must familiarize himself or herself in detail with its design concepts before applying it. Great attention should be also be paid to mastering the insertion techniques for the Orthofix cortical screws. The larger diameter of these cortical screws is mainly responsible for the adequate rigidity under different high loading conditions.

The Orthofix device and its individual components showed high endurance under fatigue loading. The ball joints of the fixator need proper initial tightening of the locking cam and periodic retightening in order to resist bending and torsional forces. The preset torque wrench for tightening the locking cam should be used to ensure consistent performance of the ball joint and at the same time avoid excessive torque application which may lead to premature failure of this key component of the fixator. Between consecutive clinical applications or when the ball joint is known to have failed through bending or rotation, the old locking cam and bush should be replaced to maintain consistent locking strength.

The biological studies in canine osteotomy models showed consistent bone union under the external fixation, partly reflecting the superior performance of the cortical screws. The pattern of bone union (*Nonosteonal healing, Primary osteonal healing*, or *Secondary osteonal healing*) was dictated by the amount of physiological loading, the fracture type, the fracture gap conditions, and the mode of fixation rigidity. Neither the cortical healing alone (characteristic of the *Primary osteonal healing* mechanism) nor the predominance of periosteal callus formation (characteristic of the *Nonosteonal healing* mechanism) seemed to be more desirable than the other. In contrast, the combination of these two mechanisms of union, (*Secondary osteonal healing*) appeared to be optimal to meet the time-related mechanical requirements of a healing fracture.

Continuous rigid external fixation prevented periosteal callus formation under low loading conditions. The experiments also demonstrated the detrimental effect of a fracture gap on bone union under rigid external fixation. Axial readjustment of the fixation rigidity (axial dynamization) was applied both in stable and unstable fracture models as well as in a delayed fracture union model. Early dynamization facilitated fracture contact and direct cortical bone healing. In unstable fracture models, dynamization was performed late, after the appearance of fracture callus, but it still could close the fracture gap with the positive effect of enhanced axial loading on fracture callus remodelling. The effect of dynamization procedures on the structural properties (torsional strength) of the healing bones was less than expected.

The in vitro behaviour (insertion torque and heat generation) of the Orthofix cortical screw, with its conical shaped threaded portion, differed from that of screws with fluted designs. In the canine model, cortical bone at the interface of the cortical screw tracks showed Haversian remodelling, obviously contributing to the time-related decrease of screw removal torque. High loading conditions caused bone thread resorption and adverse cortical bone remodelling at the entry cortex of the cortical screws. Such unicortical loosening was considered to be the consequence of excessive dynamic stresses and micromotion at the screw–bone interface.

References

Ansell RH, Scales JT: 'A study of some factors which affect the strength of screws and their insertion and holding power in bone.' *J Biomech* 1968; 1: 279–302

Aro HT, Hein TJ, Chao EYS: 'Mechanical performance of pin clamps in external fixators.' *Clin Orthop* 1989; 248: 246–53

Aro HT, Hein TJ, Chao EYS: 'Mechanical characteristics of an upper extremity external fixator.' *Clin Orthop* 1990; 253: 240–50

Aro HT, Kelly PJ, Lewallen DG, et al: 'The effects of physiologic dynamic compression on bone healing under external fixation.' *Clin Orthop* 1990; 256: 260–73

Aro HT, Wahner HT, Chao EYS: 'Healing patterns of transverse and oblique osteotomies in the canine tibia.' *J Orthop Trauma* 1991; 5: 351–64

Aro HT, Chao EYS: 'Effect of delayed dynamization on healing of unstable experimental fracture in the canine tibia.' Transactions of the 36th Annual Meeting of the Orthopaedic Research Society, February 5–8, 1990, New Orleans, Louisiana.

Aro HT, Markel MD, Chao EYS: 'Cortical bone reactions at the interface of external fixation half-pins under different loading conditions.' *J Trauma* 1993; 35: 776–85

Aro HT, Chao EYS: 'Bone healing patterns affected by loading, fracture fragment stability, fracture type, and fracture site compression.' *Clin Orthop* 1993; 293: 8–17

Aronson J, Harp JH Jr: 'Mechanical considerations in using tensioned wires in a transosseous external fixation system.' *Clin Orthop* 1992; 280:23–9

De Bastiani G. Aldegheri R. Brivio LR: 'The treatment of fractures with a dynamic axial fixator.' *J Bone Joint Surg* [Br] 1984; 66B(4): 538–45

De Bastiani G, Aldegheri R, Renzi-Brivio L, Trivella G: 'Limb lengthening by distraction of the epiphyseal plate.' *J Bone Joint Surg* [Br] 1984; 66B: 545–9

Chao EYS, Kasman RA, An KN: 'Rigidity and stress analyses of external fracture fixation devices: A theoretical approach.' *J Biomech* 1982; 15: 971–83

Chao EYS, Hein TJ: 'Mechanical performance of standard Orthofix external fixator.' *Orthopedics* 1988; 11: 1057–69

Chao EYS, Aro HT: 'Biomechanics of Fracture Fixation.' in Mow VC, Hayes WC (eds): *Basic Orthopaedic Biomechanics.* Raven Press, Ltd.: New York, 1991

Egger EL, Gottsauner-Wolf F, Palmer J, Aro HT, Chao EYS: 'Effects of axial dynamization on bone healing.' *J Trauma* 1992; 34: 185–92

Fleming B, Paley D, Kristiansen T, Pope M: 'A biomechanical analysis of the Ilizarov external fixator.' *Clin Orthop* 1989; 241: 95–105

Huiskes R, Chao EYS: 'Guidelines for external fixation frame rigidity and stresses.' *J Orthop Res* 1986; 4: 68–75

Huiskes R, Chao EYS, Crippen TE: 'Parametric analyses of pin-bone stresses in external fracture fixation devices.' *J Orthop Res* 1985; 3: 341–9

Markel MD, Wikenheiser MA, Chao EYS: 'Formation of bone in tibial defects in a canine model.' *J Bone Joint Surg* [Am] 1991; 73-A: 914–23

Matthews LS, Green CA, Goldstein SA: 'The thermal effects of skeletal fixation—pin insertion in bone.' *J Bone Joint Surg* [Am] 1984; 66A: 1077–83

McCoy TM, Chao EYS, Kasman RA: 'Comparison of mechanical performance in four types of external fixators.' *Clin Orthop* 1983; 180: 23–33

Moroni A, Heikkila J, Toksvig-Larsen S, Sten S, Giannini S. 'Hydroxyapatite pins are better fixed. A multicentre, prospective, randomised clinical study.' Presented at the AAOS 1998

Moroni A, Toksvig-Larsen S, Maltarello MC, Orienti L, Stea S, Giannini S. 'A comparison of Hydroxyapatite-coated, Titanium-coated and Uncoated Tapered External Fixation Pins.' *J Bone Joint Surg* [Am] 1998; 80A: 547–54

Podolsky A, Chao EYS: 'Mechanical performance of Ilizarov circular external fixators in comparison with other external fixators.' *Clin Orthop* 1993; 293: 61–70

Wiggins KL, Malkin S: 'Drilling of bone.' *J Biomech* 1976; 9: 553–9

Wikenheiser MA, Markel MD, Lewallen DG, Chao EYS: 'Thermal response and torque resistance of five cortical half-pins under simulated insertion technique.' *J Orthop Res* 1995; 13: 615–9

The Stability of Orthofix External Fixation: a Comparative Evaluation

7

A.H. Broekhuizen

Introduction

External fixation is a well-accepted method for the treatment of open fractures of the lower limb; in contrast, it would not usually be considered as first line therapy for closed fractures of the femoral shaft. This is due in large part to the fact that the forces to which a femoral fixator is likely to be subjected are substantial, particularly during mobilization and weightbearing and this can, in some instances, result in instability of the frame and consequent malalignment or non-union of the fracture (Broekhuizen 1988). Today, many surgeons would prefer, therefore, to use an interlocking intramedullary nail to treat femoral fractures whenever possible.

There remain, however, a number of situations where it would not be appropriate to use an intramedullary nail in association with a femoral fracture. These include severe open fractures; fractures with major comminution; where speed is of the essence, as for example, in polytrauma patients; in children in whom the epiphyses are open, and in a range of other indications such as limb lengthening, non-union and arthrodesis (Fellander, 1963; Ronen et al, 1974; Fraser et al, 1978; Hierholzer et al, 1978; Brooker, 1979; Bordas Sales et al, 1980; Ricciardi 1980; Müller and Witzel, 1981; Hofmann et al, 1982; Hofmann and Probst, 1982; Hurther, 1970; Klemm, 1982a,b; Marti and van der Werken, 1982; Müller et al, 1982; Coppola and Anzel, 1983; Dabezies et al, 1984; Gottschalk et al, 1985; Rööser and Hansson, 1985; De Bastiani et al, 1986; Brug et al, 1988; Murphy et al, 1988; Wentzensen and Evers, 1988; Seligson and Kristiansen, 1989; Shih et al, 1989). In all of these circumstances, external fixation is not only a rational alternative, but it may well be considered the treatment of choice.

The performance of an external fixator in femoral applications must be regarded as the ultimate test of its stability; if it passes this test it may confidently be predicted that it will function satisfactorily in virtually any situation. The question of which fixator to choose, however, is a difficult one, since there are so many available to the surgeon today (Broekhuizen et al 1988 and 1990). While ease of application, overall weight and patient acceptability must be taken into consideration, the surgeon would be expected to be influenced primarily by the stability of the assembly. We have therefore compared the stability of 16 commercially available external fixation systems in an experimental model designed to mimic a fracture of the femoral shaft. While many clinicians may consider biomechanics difficult to understand, its basic concepts must be appreciated by anyone involved in the treatment of muscular and skeletal injuries. We have attempted, therefore, to present the results in a way which reduces the mathematical load, and highlights the clinical relevance of the findings.

Materials and Methods

A total of 16 external fixation device systems was studied (Fig. 7.1A–F, Fig. 7.2G–L, Fig 7.3M–P). These were: the horseshoe shaped Ace–Fischer frame (ACE Medical, Los Angeles CA, USA) in both aluminium and (partial) titanium constructions; the Ace–Hoffmann frame (ACE Medical, Los Angeles CA, USA); the original Hoffmann femoral frame (Jacquet Orthopedie, Geneva, Switzerland); the old AO threaded system designed by Müller and the new tubular AO frame (Mathys, Bettlach, Switzerland); the

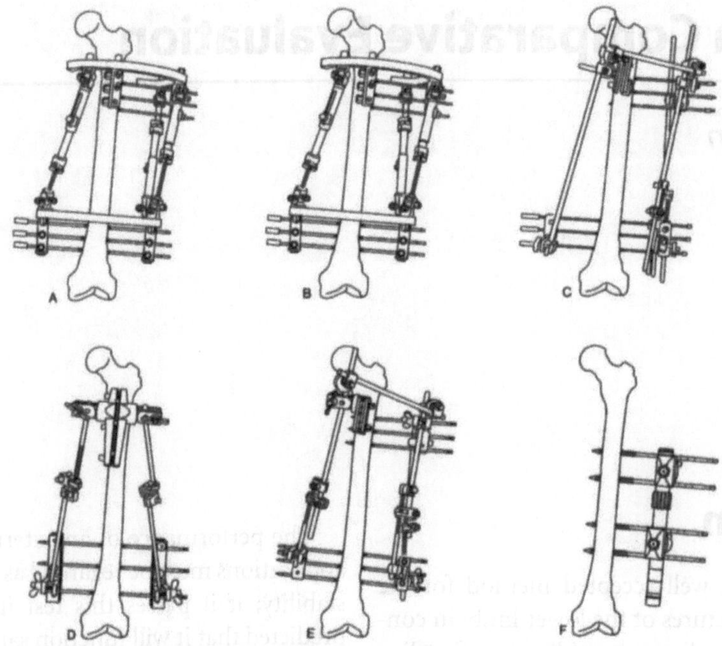

Fig. 7.1 Representative external fixation units (tested in an in vitro study). **A** Ace Fischer femoral frame (anodized aluminium); **B** Ace Fischer femoral frame, made up of anodized aluminium and titanium (horse shoe shaped) rings; **C** The American version of the fixation system originally designed by Raoul Hoffmann, made up of anodized aluminium for use on the femur; **D** Triangular Hoffmann femoral frame (simple triangular) with specially developed large aluminium clamp units. The pins are inserted proximally on the ventral side. **E** Hoffmann femoral frame; **F** MONO-tube (large).

simple triangular variant of the Hoffmann device, the unilateral Hoffmann for the lower leg, suitable for fractures of the femoral shaft in children; the Orthofix dynamic axial fixator (Orthofix, Verona, Italy); a derivation of the system (Murray, 1982; Habboushe, 1984), in which a length of tubing is filled with bone cement; the compact Monofixateur (Orthopaedia, Kiel, Germany); the Wagner device (Mathys, Bettlach, Switzerland); the Shearer System (Thackray, Leeds, England); the AO-Unifix system (Mathys, Bettlach, Switzerland); the MONO-tube-large (Jacquet Orthopedie, Geneva, Switzerland) and the Heidelberg fixator (Zimmer, Swindon, England).

In any comparative evaluation of external fixation devices in an in vivo setting, differences in bone thickness and in the degree of osteoporosis are variables which may distort the true picture. For this reason the various devices studied were applied to identical Perspex rods rather than to bone.

The rods were designed to simulate a fracture of the femoral shaft without bony contact. As far as possible each of the external fixation systems examined was assembled and used in accordance with the manufacturer's instructions. In all but one case three pins were inserted on either side of the fracture; the exception was the Unifix, where two pins only were used on each side. In every instance the thickest available pins were used.

The clinical situations of bed rest, mobilization without weightbearing and physiotherapy to associated joints were mimicked by the successive application of axial, transverse and parallel forces to each system.

Increasing forces up to 160N were employed, as if a leg with a mass of 16kg was suspended from the fixation system (the value for an average adult lower limb is about 10kg). Measurement was made of the displacement of the fragments at the centre of the fracture in response to the forces applied, in order to determine the stability of the fixator–Perspex combinations. Inter-operator variation was assessed by repeated measurements following application of the devices by different surgeons.

For two of the fixators in the series (Orthofix and Hoffmann femoral), the measurements obtained with the frame assembled on Perspex were compared with those recorded when the device was applied to the cadaveric femur of a 73-year-old man. An additional experiment compared in vitro results to in vivo results by repeating the standard measurements in a clinical setting in an anaesthetised patient. The programme of study was completed by determining the weight of each of the 16 fixators assessed.

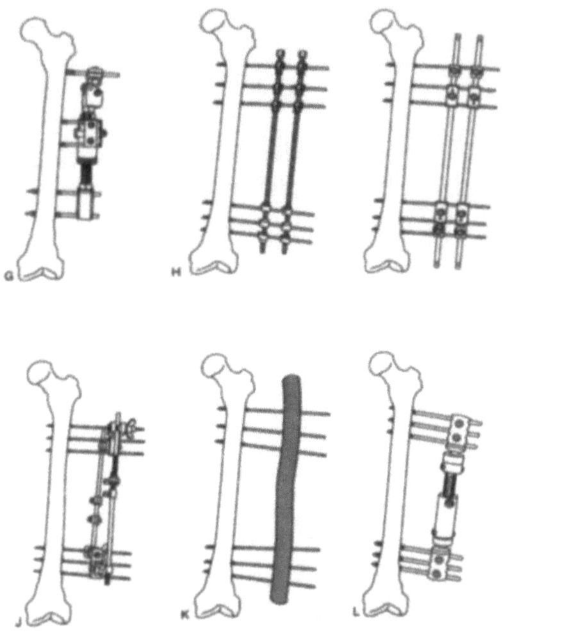

Fig 7.2 Representative external fixation units (tested in an in vitro study). **G** Heidelberg-fixator; **H** AO (ASIF) threaded rod system; **I** AO (ASIF) tubular system; **J** Unilateral Hoffmann fiixator, as used for tibial fixation, mounted on the femur; **K** Simple external fixation constructed using Schanz screws and anaesthetic tubing filled with polymethylmethacrylate bone cement; **L** Orthofix Dynamic Axial Fixator.

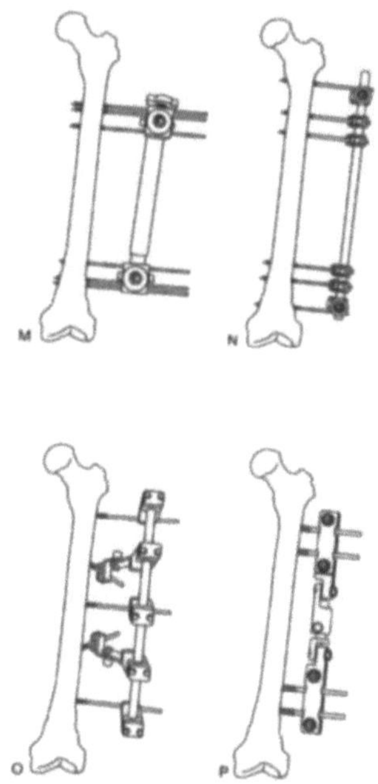

Fig. 7.3 Representative external fixation units (tested in an in vitro study). **M** The Wagner apparatus originally designed for leg lengthening procedures; **N** The Monofixateur; **O** The Shearer fixator; **P** AO-Unifix (the only one tested with two pins on each side).

Results

The amount of displacement of the fragments provoked by an axially applied force was tested with each of the fixators. This is representative of the kind of load to which the fixator would be subjected if the patient was mobilized on two crutches, i.e. in a non-weightbearing situation.

With a stable frame such as the Orthofix, the maximal applied force of 160N resulted in displacement of the fragments by a little over 1mm. At the opposite extreme, the fixator constructed from anaesthetic tubing filled with polymethylmethacrylate bone cement was very unstable, with a load of only 50N producing a displacement of more than 5mm at the fracture site. When parallel and transverse loading of each of the fixators was tested problems were observed particularly with the Shearer, Unifix and Wagner fixators, with slipping of the pins and the clamp units. Where such slipping occurred, a linear relationship was noted in each case between the force applied and resultant movement.

Fig. 7.4 shows the amount of displacement per 10N applied load for each of the systems tested. Repeated problems were encountered with the Wagner apparatus, and the instability of the system was clearly attributable to the fact that the pins could not be mounted securely in the clamps. The fixator constructed from anaesthetic tubing and bone cement broke on numerous occasions during the course of the measurements and with the Unifix and Shearer fixators, slipping pins and clamp units were recorded with both transverse and parallel loading. Recently, new sandblasted pins have been designed for the Unifix in an attempt to improve the grip between ball joints and pins.

Fragment rotation in response to axial, parallel and transverse loading is shown for each of the systems tested (Fig. 7.5). Where devices were unstable, up to 1.6° of rotation per 10N load were recorded. In an adult, this would correspond to 16° of rotation at the fracture site.

To exclude the possible influence of surgical technique, measurements were repeated after application of the devices by different surgeons who had been given similar instruction. Similar results were obtained in each case. There was also little difference in the

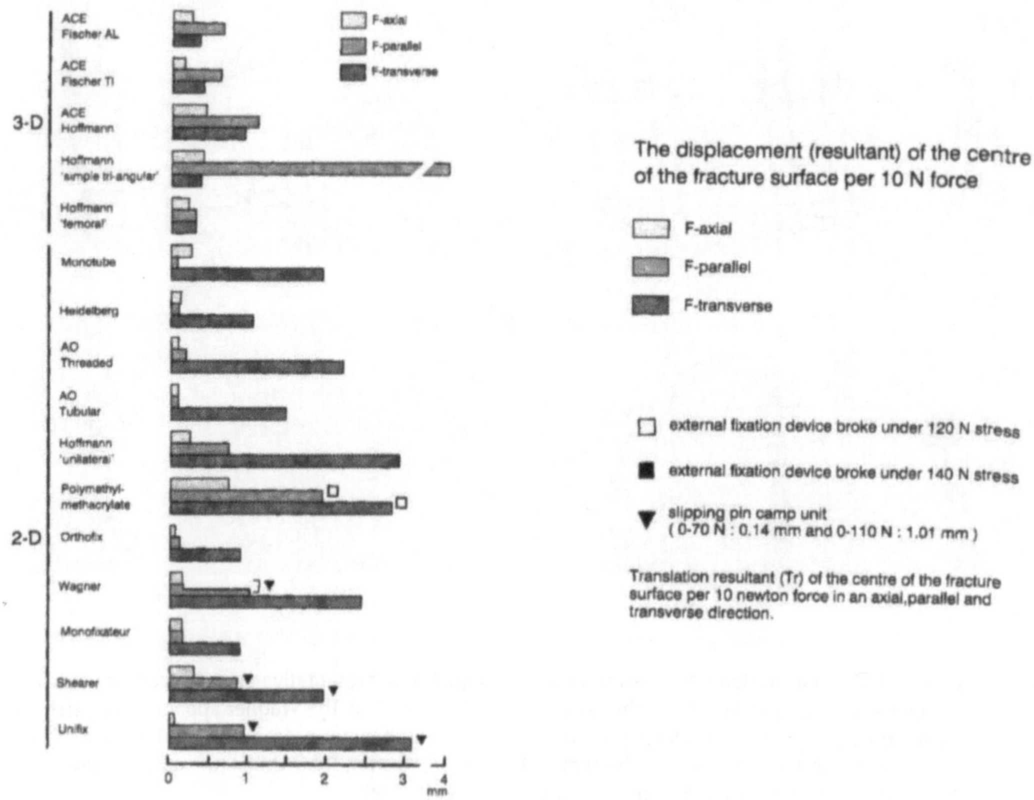

Fig. 7.4 Displacement of fragments in response to a 10N load

measurements recorded when the frames were mounted on the Perspex rods or on the cadaveric femur.

The relevance of the experimental model to the clinical situation was confirmed by repeating the series of in vitro measurements in a 50 year old man with an infected pseudarthrosis of the distal femur following application of the AO tubular frame, which ranked high in the in vitro tests. The frame configuration in this patient was comparable to that applied to the Perspex rods and all measurements were made under general anaesthesia.

Comparable loads were applied to the leg and movements occurring at the fracture site in response to the applied forces were monitored by labelling the fragments with square white markers. No angulation occurred at rest, while under conditions of load, the amount of angulation observed was in consonance with that predicted from the in vitro experiments.

Large differences in weight were recorded for the various fixators studied. These ranged from 400g for the fixator made from anaesthetic tubing and bone cement fixator to 2000g for the Hoffmann femoral frame (Fig. 7.6).

Discussion

It is very evident from the experiments described in this chapter that there are marked differences in the rigidity of the various commercially available external fixators for application to femoral fractures. The "absolute" rigidity conferred by a plate and screws cannot be achieved with external fixation. In our experiments, movements of between 1mm and 4cm and rotations ranging from less than 1° to 16° were observed and can be expected when the devices in question are used to treat fractured femora in adult patients. Primary (or direct) healing of fractures (i.e. without the formation of external bridging callus) thus requires greater stability than can be provided by external fixation.

The results also demonstrate that as far as the ability to withstand axial and parallel forces is concerned, a relatively small, unilateral frame can be at least as stable as a larger, three-dimensional one. Our work suggests, however, that the Wagner apparatus, the Shearer and the Unifix external fixators are not stable enough for

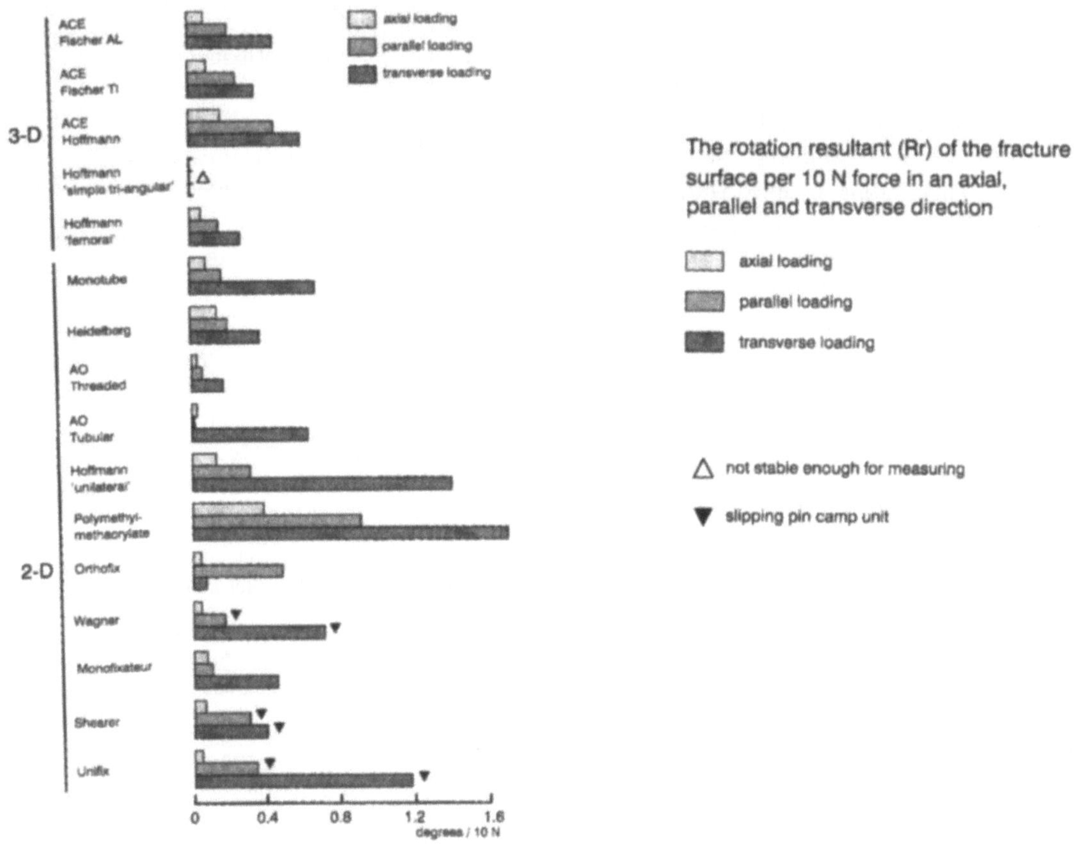

Fig. 7.5 Rotation of fragments in response to axial parallel and transverse loading.

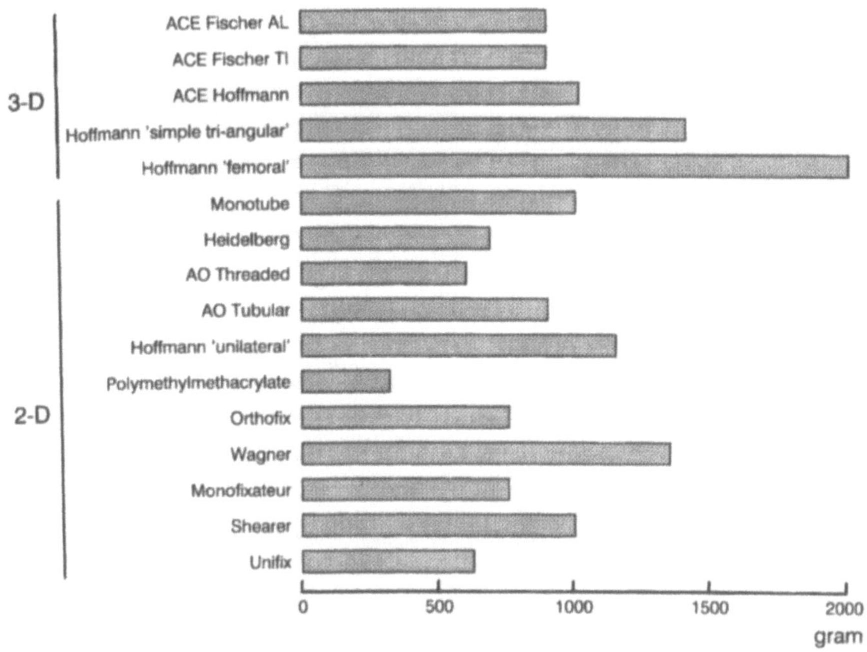

Fig. 7.6 Individual weights of all 16 external fixator units.

the treatment of femoral fractures, as they were unable to withstand the forces to which they would be subjected when applied to the adult femur.

The three-dimensional Hoffmann femoral frame, the two-dimensional Orthofix, the AO tubular frame and the Monofixateur produced the most effective stabilisation. This finding, coupled with the ease and speed with which it can be applied has been sufficient reason for this unit to regard the Orthofix frame as the first choice when faced with the need to externally fix the femur (Broekhuizen, 1990).

Summary

The stability of 16 different femoral external fixators was tested and compared in an experimental model. The weight of the frames varied from 400 to 2000g. Comparative stability also showed wide variation. Movements of between 1mm and 4cm and rotation varying from almost 0° to 16° were measured at the fracture site in the experimental model, which was based upon the geometry of an adult patient. These findings suggest that primary bone-healing would not be expected to occur, since it demands greater stability than can be provided by external fixation. In response to all but transverse loading, a relatively simple two-dimensional (unilateral) frame can confer comparable rigidity to that of a three-dimensional one.

Bibliography

Bordas Sales JL, Collado Fabregas F, Rofes-Capo S et al 'The use of Wagner's external fixator in the treatment of septic fractures of the femoral shaft.' *Rev Chir Orthop* 1980; 66: 501.

Broekhuizen AH. 'Femoral fractures, indications and biomechanics of external fixation.' Thesis, Erasmus University, Rotterdam. 1988 Rotterdam, The Netherlands.

Broekhuizen AH, Boxma H, Snijder CJ. 'Femoral fractures, indications for and biomechanics of external fixation.' *Probl Gen Surg* 1988; 5: 396.

Broekhuizen AH, Boxma H, Meulen van der PA, Snijders CJ. 'Performance of external fixation devices in femoral fractures; the ultimate challenge? A laboratory study with plastic rods.' *Injury* 1990; 21: 145–151.

Brooker AF. 'The use of external fixation in the treatment of burn patients with fractures.' in: Brooker AF and Edwards CC (eds) *External fixation: The current state of the art.* 1979 Williams and Wilkins: Baltimore

Brug E, Pennig D, Gähler R et al 'Polytrauma und femurfraktur.' *Aktuel Traumatol* 1988; 18: 225.

Coppola AJ, Anzel SH. 'Use of the Hoffmann external fixator in the treatment of femoral fractures.' *Clin orthop* 1983; 180: 78.

Dabezies EJ, D'Ambrosia RD, Shoji H et al 'Fractures of the femoral shaft treated by external fixation with the Wagner device.' *J Bone Joint Surg* [Am] 1984: 66A, 360.

De Bastiani G, Aldegheri R, Renzi Brevio L. 'A rational alternative for the external fixation of fractures.' *Int Orthop* 1986; 10: 95.

Fellander M. 'Treatment of fractures and pseudoarthrosis of the long bones by Hoffmann's transfixation method.' *Acta Orthop Scand* 1963; 33: 132.

Fraser RD, Hunter GA, Waddel JP. 'Ipsilateral fracture of the femur and tibia.' *J Bone Joint Surg* [Br] 1978; 60B: 510.

Gottschalk FAB, Graham AJ, Morein G. 'The management of severely comminuted fractures of the femoral shaft, using the external fixator.' *Injury* 1985; 16: 377.

Habboushe MP. 'Al-Rasheed Military Hospital external fixation system for compound missile wounds of bone.' *Injury* 1984; 15: 388.

Hierholzer G, Kleining R, Horstr G et al 'External fixation: classifications and indications.' *Arch Orthop Trauma* Surg 1978; 92: 175.

Hofmann G, Graber M, Probst J. 'Der Oberschenkelschaftbruch im Erwachsenalter: Fixateur externe Methoden und Ergebnisse.' *Hefte Unfallheilkd* 1982; 158: 133.

Hofmann G, Probst J. 'Possibilities of application of the fixateur externe at the femur: indications, results.' *Aktuel Traumatol* 1982; 2: 62.

Hurther E. 'Treatment of lower femoral fractures by external fixator.' *Acta Orthop Belg* 1970; 36; 620.

Klemm K. 'Indication, technic and results using the external fixator in infected fractures and infected pseudarthrosis.' *Langenbecks Arch Chir* 1982; 358: 119.

Klemm K. 'Use of the external fixator in thigh fractures.' in:Uhthoff HK, Stahl E (eds) *Current Concepts of External Fixation of Fractures.* 1982 Springer-Verlag:Berlin

Marti RK, van der Werken C. 'Alternative indications for external fixation according to Wagner.' *Neth J Surg* 1982; 34: 13.

Müller KH, Müller-Faber J. 'External fixation – rare indications, combination of internal and external osteosynthesis technics, secondary operations.' *Langenbecks Arch Chir* 1982; 358: 133.

Müller KH, Witzel U 'The fixateur externe osteosynthesis without osseous support (external distance osteosynthesis) in the lower limbs.' *Arch Orthop Trauma Surg* 1981; 99: 117.

Murphy CP, D'Ambrosia RD, Dabezies EJ et al 'Complex femur fractures: treatment with the Wagner external fixation device or the Grosse-Kempf interlocking nail.' *J Trauma* 1988; 28: 1553.

Murray WP. 'An external fixation system using formable plastic rods.' in: Uhthoff HK and Stahl E (eds) *Current Concepts of External Fixation of Fractures.* 1982 Springer-Verlag: Berlin

Ricciardi L. 'Les fixateurs externes d'Hoffmann–Vidal au niveau du fémur.' *Proceedings of the 7th International Conference on Hoffmann External Fixation* 1980. Montpellier, France, 153.

Ronen GM, Michaelson M, Waisbrod H. 'External fixation in war injuries.' *Injury* 1974; 6: 94.

Rööser B, Hansson P. 'External fixation of ipsilateral fractures of the femur and tibia.' *Injury* 1985; 16: 371.

Seligson D, Kristiansen TK. 'Use of the Wagner apparatus in complicated fractures of the distal femur.' *J Trauma* 1989; 18: 795.

Shih HN, Chen LM, Lee ZL et al 'Treatment of femoral shaft fractures with the Hoffmann External fixator in prepuberty.' *J Trauma* 1989; 29: 498.

Wentzensen A, Evers K. 'Management strategy of multiple fractures of long tubular bones within the scope of polytrauma.' *Aktuel Traumatol* 1988; 18: Suppl 1, 2.

The Influence of Fixator Design on Fracture Repair: the Orthofix Procallus

8

J.C.R. Scott

The Orthofix ProCallus fixator was developed from the original Dynamic Axial Fixator to take account of recent developments in the understanding of the mechanism of fracture repair and the role of micromovement.

History

The original Dynamic Axial Fixator was developed in Verona, Italy. It was the brainchild of Professor Giovanni De Bastiani, Professor of Orthopaedics and Traumatology at the Borgo Roma Hospital in Verona. Having been a professor of Physiology at Padua University, Professor De Bastiani understood the importance of applying basic physiological principles to the management of fractures in his clinic. He was well aware that fractures required to be held in a reduced position by a mechanism which allowed some controlled movement at the fracture site at the appropriate time in the healing cycle. He was also aware that where patients with injuries to the lower limb were prepared to bear weight on their fractures during healing, healing times appeared to be shorter than in those patients reluctant to weightbear.

In the 1970s the use of internal fixation with plates and screws for the treatment of tibial diaphyseal fractures was still popular. Professor De Bastiani did not like this method of treatment, since the complication rate was significantly higher than that associated with conservative management with plaster. It was also clear to him that the use of rigid plates conflicted with many established physiological principles: the rigidity of the system discouraged the formation of callus; extensive stripping of the periosteum deprived the bone ends of their vascularity, and therefore their viability; shielding of the bone from the normal stresses of weightbearing caused disuse osteoporosis, with the risk of later refracture. Finally, and perhaps most important, he was aware of the serious complications which often accompanied the use of plates: deep infection with osteomyelitis and the formation of large sequestra; delayed healing with the need for further surgery as a result of this, and sometimes, the sign of ultimate failure of treatment in a closed fracture –amputation.

In consideration of these facts, he sought a less invasive and less damaging means of treating those fractures which were unsuitable for conservative, non-operative management. This group included fractures which were unstable in plaster, closed fractures with severe soft tissue damage, and open fractures. External fixation seemed to be an excellent alternative, because it involved no further disturbance of the fracture site, and yet provided excellent fixation for unstable or open fractures. Existing fixation systems, however, possessed significant disadvantages. They were generally bilateral or multilateral systems with transfixing bone screws; they were bulky and inconvenient, and they tended to provide a rigid form of fixation throughout the treatment period. In the minds of most surgeons of the time, therefore, the use of external fixation was associated with slow or delayed union[1]. Existing monolateral systems, on the other hand, were not stable enough to prevent malunion.

Professor De Bastiani and his colleagues decided to define the characteristics of a new generation of fixators, which would be monolateral, minimally inva-

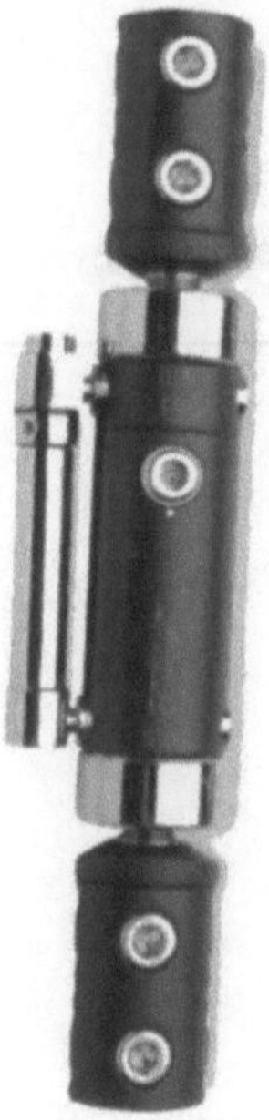

Fig. 8.1 The original Dynamic Axial Fixator devised by De Bastiani.

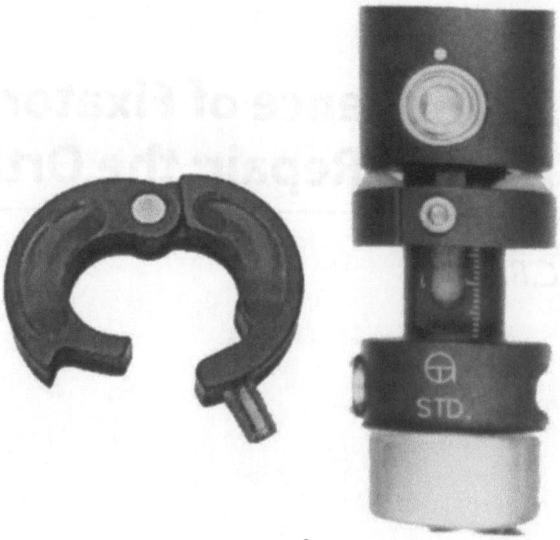

a b

Fig. 8.2 The DynaRing attachment for the original Dynamic Axial Fixator.

sive, easy to use, lightweight and comfortable for the patient but as stable as the multibar Hoffmann when needed, and equipped with the means to modify their biomechanical behaviour during the healing process, in recognition of the changing requirements of the fracture. An engineer, Giovanni Faccioli, incorporated these characteristics into the design of the Orthofix Dynamic Axial Fixator, the DAF (Fig. 8.1). The main features of the fixator are exactly the same today, and are:

1. Strong, rigid monolateral body.
2. Clamps for the bone screws at either end, articulating with the body via ball joints for ease of application and reduction.
3. Non-transfixing, half screws with a tapered thread, and a 6 mm shank; these screws provide excellent bone fixation, but can be removed easily at the end of treatment in the outpatient department due to their conical design.
4. A telescopic facility within the fixator body, to allow for length adjustment during application, and to permit the transfer of axial load from the fixator to the bone at an appropriate stage (dynamization), to stimulate the healing process, and relieve the bone screws of much of the axial load associated with weightbearing.
5. A means of applying compression or distraction at the fracture site where indicated.

The paper in 1984 by De Bastiani et al[2] confirmed that this fixator system could provide excellent fixation for fractures of the femur, tibia and humerus, with good maintenance of position and excellent healing times.

There has been one major modification to the original DAF since 1984. Some surgeons were reluctant to dynamize the fixator because of their concern that shortening might occur. In practice, because the fixator prevents any tendency to translation, torsion or bending, most fractures remain stable even after the body locking nut controlling the telescopic facility is released. For instance, a long oblique fracture may look quite unstable to axial loading. Any shortening of such a fracture, however, must be accompanied by translation, and, if the fracture has a spiral component, torsion. The fixator will prevent this even after the body locking nut is released, and the amount of shortening that does occur will be less than 4–5mm.

Nevertheless, some surgeons were reluctant to accept this, and some fractures are truly unstable. An additional component called the Dyna-Ring was therefore produced. This is a silastic cushion which can be mounted on to the male element of the telescopic body in such a way that some movement and loading can be transferred to the bone without any risk of fracture collapse (Fig. 8.2).

The current advice in the operating manuals for the timing of dynamization is that the body locking nut should be released at 2–4 weeks in stable fractures, and at 6 – 8 weeks in unstable fractures. The Dyna-Ring can be utilized to provide a degree of axial movement on weightbearing at the fracture site in all fractures from some time during the first week following injury until the time for full axial loading is reached.

New Evidence: Animal Studies

Not surprisingly, knowledge of the factors influencing fracture healing has progressed in the years since the publication of De Bastiani's paper in 1984. This has been due in the main to the research efforts of Allen Goodship in Bristol, John Kenwright in Oxford, and James Richardson in Oswestry, all in the United Kingdom. As a result of studies carried out initially in sheep and subsequently in humans, certain basic principles have emerged. The following conclusions can be drawn from the study performed by Goodship on the healing of an osteotomy in sheep, on treatment with external fixation[3]:

1. Some degree of movement at the fracture site, as opposed to rigid fixation, is beneficial for callus formation.
2. The amplitude of this movement is critical for the successful stimulation of callus formation: 2mm of movement was shown to have only limited benefit compared with rigid fixation, while 0.5mm of movement was shown to be highly beneficial, producing both a greater amount of radiological callus, and greater mineralization on chemical analysis of the healing bone.
3. The timing of application of the movement in relation to the injury is important: movement initiated during the first week following fracture has a beneficial effect on fracture healing, whereas movement initiated six weeks after the fracture has no beneficial effect.
4. The type of movement is also critical: it should be rapid rather than slow: movement at a speed of 400mm/sec stimulated fracture healing, whereas movement at 2mm/sec had no beneficial effect, when compared with a "no movement" control.
5. The amount of force applied to produce the movement should not be too great: a force of 200 Newtons was compared with a force of 1000 Newtons, other parameters being kept constant. When compared to a rigid control, the lower force stimulated callus formation, whereas the higher force inhibited it.

New Evidence: Clinical Studies

The above findings were put to the test in a study involving human tibial fractures. Eighty tibial fractures, treated with external fixation, were randomly allocated to a micromotion group or a rigid fixation group. The micromotion group were given applied micromovement of 1 mm at the fracture site for 500 cycles at 0.5 Hz over a 15-minute period. This was applied daily until the patient was weightbearing 20kg. This group healed at an average of 13.4 weeks, compared to 18.1 weeks for the rigidly fixed control group ($p = 0.004$)[4] (Fig. 8.3).

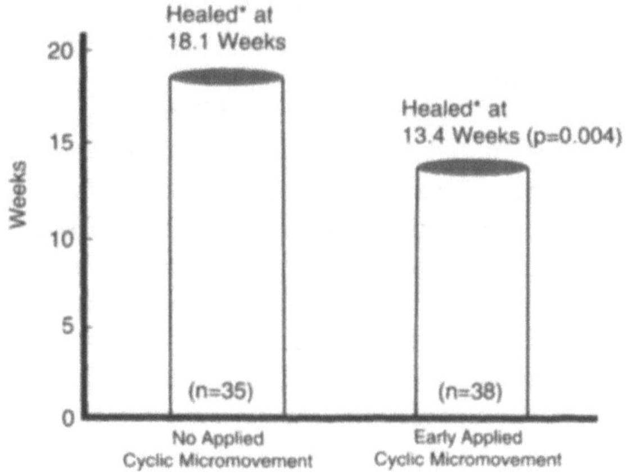

Fig. 8.3 The influence of micromovement on the healing of tibial fractures in adult humans.

Other clinical studies have confirmed the efficacy of dynamization of tibial fractures treated with the DAF. In the study carried out at Nottingham[5], in which 150 tibial fractures were treated with the DAF, the timing of dynamization appeared to be critical for the outcome: all fractures dynamized at less than two weeks united, whereas of the fractures not dynamized until six or more weeks after the fracture, 25 per cent developed a non-union. Looking at it another way, fractures which united were dynamized at an average of 4.1 weeks, but those which developed a non-union were dynamized at an average of 6.1 weeks ($p < 0.05$). Of the 136 fractures which united, the average healing time in this series was 15.4 weeks, and the non-union rate was 9 per cent. This should be compared to a series of 42 tibial fractures treated at the same centre with a rigid fixator without the facility for dynamization. In this group, union was delayed beyond 26 weeks in 55 per cent of cases.[5]

In a study by Foxworthy and Pringle[6], 44 tibial fractures were treated with the DAF. Twenty-two closely matched pairs were studied for timing of dynamization. The group dynamized at 4 weeks or earlier had a significantly shorter healing time than those dynamized later ($p < 0.05$). They conclude:

"...when using the Dynamic Axial Fixator, dynamization should be considered at or before 4 weeks to improve healing rate."

Richardson et al have defined a difference between the phases of dynamization of a fracture.[7,8] They suggest that there are effectively three different mechanical requirements during the healing process. In the initial few days following a fracture, maximum stability is required, to allow the soft tissues to recover as rapidly as possible, and to permit organisation of the fracture haematoma to begin. Towards the end of the first week, "cyclic micromovement" is applied, to stimulate callus formation. This type of motion may be described as one in which the fracture gap opens and closes sequentially (Fig. 8.4). When callus formation is established, and the patient is weightbearing, the body locking nut is released, to allow "progressive loading" of the fracture, to stimulate callus maturation. Progressive loading implies progressive closure of the fracture gap (Fig. 8.5). This is what happens when the central body locking nut of the original DAF is loosened, and is what De Bastiani described as "dynamization".

The work carried out by Richardson and his colleagues demonstrates, however, that cyclic micromovement also occurs with the DAF if the patient is weightbearing in the early stages before the body locking nut is loosened, due to minimal flexion of the bone screws. The amplitude of movement is appropriate to stimulate callus formation, but it does not tend to occur at the optimal time in the healing cycle, because very few patients are prepared to weightbear sufficiently to produce micromovement of more than 0.5mm at the fracture site within the first 7 days following a fracture.

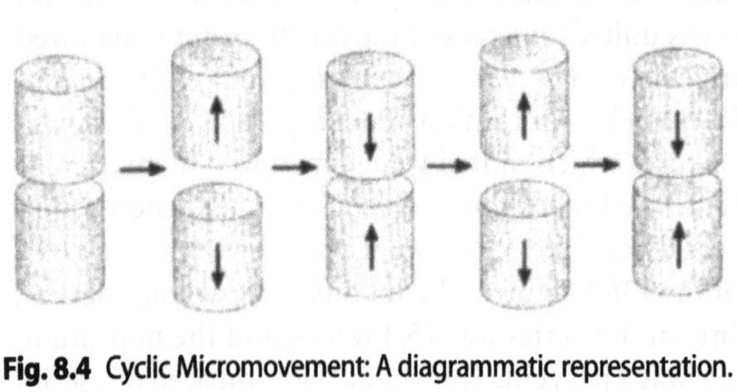

Fig. 8.4 Cyclic Micromovement: A diagrammatic representation.

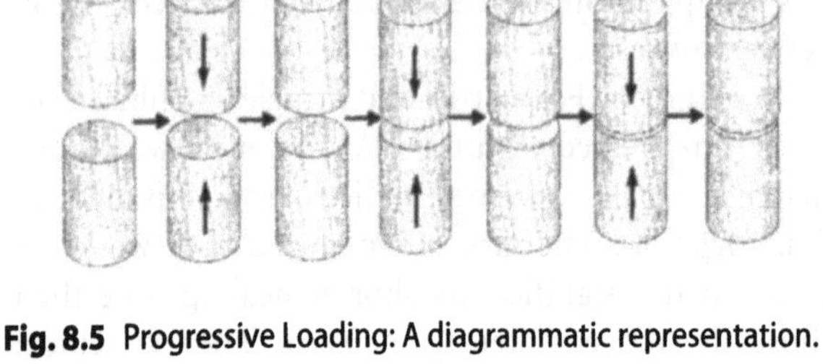

Fig. 8.5 Progressive Loading: A diagrammatic representation.

From reviewing the above work it seems sensible that the term "dynamization" should today be understood to embrace both the micromovement and progressive loading phases of motion at the fracture site.

The ProCallus

With the above studies in mind, the ProCallus fixator was designed to incorporate as much of this new philosophy as possible. The fixator has the following features (Fig. 8.6):

1. A spring mechanism (**a** in figure) to allow movement of up to 3 mm in compression or distraction. This movement is frictionless, and not affected by torsional stress. It is controlled by a micromovement locking nut.

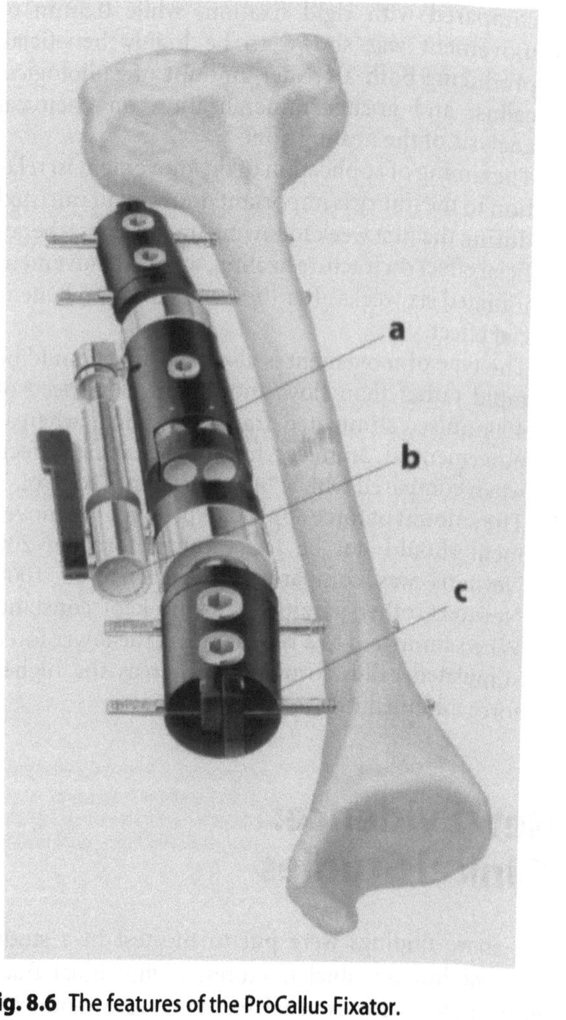

Fig. 8.6 The features of the ProCallus Fixator.

2. A modified compression–distraction unit (**b** in figure), with a lever, called an actuator. This lever operates an asymmetric cam, which distracts the ends of the unit by 3mm when it is moved to its full extent. The movement occurs at a rapid speed even with relatively slow movement of the lever, because of the shape of the cam. This unit is placed into the holes in the cams of the fixator, and is used to apply cyclic micromovement to the fracture. Because of the dampening effect of the bone screws, this movement results in about 1mm of movement at the fracture site.
3. The micromovement mechanism also allows for compressive micromovement on weightbearing. This is achieved when the patient is loading the fracture at least 20kg, and the actuator is removed.
4. A telescopic mechanism, as in the original DAF, which is controlled by a separate body locking nut. This allows the length of the fixator to be altered during application, as with the DAF, and for full progressive loading to be applied at the appropriate time point in the healing cycle.
5. By the use of aluminium bushes, and a redesigned ball, the ball joint is now 30 per cent stronger than in the original DAF. This is useful when treating heavier patients or in unstable fracture configurations. The same torque wrench should be used to tighten the ball joint. Because the bush deforms very slightly when the ball joint is locked, it should be replaced after each use.
6. The screw clamps have been redesigned, so that the use of a template is no longer necessary. The screw clamps have hinged slots (**c** in figure) and will accept either the screw guides or the screws themselves. The hinge at the end of the clamp also has a hole which will accept a 2mm Kirschner-wire. This is useful for pre-positioning the fixator before drilling the screw holes. It should be noted that,

Time from Injury	Healing Stage	Physiological Requirements	Fixator Mode
During Application			• Central Body Locking Nut LOOSENED • Micromovement Locking Nut TIGHTENED
Day 1-7	Inflammation: *Patient bed-bound or non-weightbearing*	Stability	• Central Body Locking Nut TIGHTENED • Micromovement Locking Nut TIGHTENED
Starting at some time between day 1 and 7 and continuing until week 3-6	Callus Formation:	Cyclic Micromovement	• Central Body Locking Nut TIGHTENED • Micromovement Locking Nut LOOSENED
	(a) *Patient non-weightbearing or partially weightbearing up to 20Kg*	• Actively administered using the **Actuator**	**Actuator** used for 10 minutes daily (one full cycle every 2 seconds) for 2-3 weeks, or until partial weightbearing 20Kg. ACTUATOR MUST BE REMOVED AFTER EACH TREATMENT SESSION
	(b) Partial weightbearing 20Kg or more, to full weightbearing	• On weightbearing	**Actuator** is not used once patient is weightbearing 20Kg, and should be removed permanently at this point
Week 3-6 onwards	Callus Maturation: *Clinical evidence of fracture stability; partial weightbearing 20Kg, up to full weightbearing*	Progressive Loading	• Central Body Locking Nut LOOSENED

Fig. 8.7 The ProCallus Fixator: A protocol for use.

when using the metaphyseal clamp, the template is still necessary. This is because the screws are in two separate planes.

7. The fixator is compatible with all the ball jointed modules of the Orthofix Modulsystem. The protocol for the use for the ProCallus fixator is described below (Fig.8.7). This follows all the clinical evidence for the use of the fixator described in the papers referred to above and will allow surgeons to treat fractures in the most favourable mechanical environment at every stage of the healing process.

References

1. Clifford RP, Lyons TJ and Webb JK: 'Complications of external fixation of open fractures of the tibia.' *Injury*, 1987, 18, 174–6
2. De Bastiani G, Aldegheri R and Renzi Brivio L: 'The treatment of fractures with a dynamic axial ficator.' *J Bone Joint Surg*, [Br] 1984, 66-B, No. 4, 538–45
3. Goodship AE: 'Experimental studies of micromotion.' in Coombs, Green and Sarmiento: *External Fixation and Functional Bracing*, 1989 Orthotext
4. Kenwright J, Richardson JB, Cunningham JL, White SH, Goodship AE, Adams MA, Magnussen PA and Newman JH: 'Axial movement and tibial fractures, a controlled randomised trial of treatment.' *J Bone Joint Surg*, [Br] 1991, 73-B, No.4, 654–9
5. Wallace WA and Howard PW: 'A decade of tibial fractures at Nottingham and Derby'. Supplement to *Int J Orthop Trauma*, 1993, 3 (3), 61–3
6. Foxworthy M and Pringle RM: 'Dynamisation timing and its effect on bone healing when using the Orthofix Dynamic Axial Fixator.' *Injury*, 1995, 26, No.2, 117–9
7. Richardson JB, Gardner TN, Hardy JRW, Evans M, Kuiper J-H and Kenwright J: 'Dynamisation of tibial fractures.' *J Bone Joint Surg*, [Br] 1995, 77-B, No.3, 412–6
8. Richardson JB and Kuiper J-H: Scientific poster exhibit, AAOS, Orlando, February 1995.

Part II Orthofix External Fixation in Traumatology

Screw Selection and the Technique of Insertion

9

F. Lavini

Introduction

When using an external fixation fame, account must be taken both of the mechanical stability of the device in the context in which it is being used, and patient compliance. These two aspects have been balanced in the design of the Orthofix Monolateral External Fixation System. A stable assembly requires not only a frame with appropriate mechanical properties, but also an ideal bone–screw interface. The latter depends both upon the suitability of screw design and the formulation of an accurate and reproducible method of screw insertion.

Factors which contribute to the integrity of the bone–screw interface include the material of the screw, the diameter of the screw in relation to the diameter of the bone and the load applied, thread morphology, the relationship between the shape and diameter of the drill used for pre-drilling and the diameter of the screw, and the thermal effects both of the drilling procedure and the insertion of the screws themselves (Lavini et al, 1994). These parameters were used to define the material and characteristics of the Orthofix screws. They are stainless steel (AISI 316L ESR), self-tapping screws, with a conical thread tapering from 6mm to 5mm for the standard range. Two types of thread pattern exist for insertion into cortical bone and cancellous bone respectively.

The present chapter provides information on the selection of appropriate screws for a particular application, and describes the method of insertion for ensuring a stable and problem-free outcome.

Screw Selection

A study of the pre-operative radiographs will provide the following information:

1. The site of application of the screws in a particular segment
2. The number of screws which should be inserted in each segment
3. The type or types of screw to be used
4. The appropriate diameter of the screws
5. The correct overall length and thread length.

The anatomical site will govern the type of screws to be used, and the length of thread to be selected. It will also determine screw diameter and the ideal number of screws per clamp; the bulk of the soft tissues will determine overall length. In a metaphyseal or epiphyseal region, cancellous screws will be used, while cortical screws will normally be used in most other areas. Drills appropriate to the type and diameter of screw selected should be used (see Table 9.1)

The total length of the screw should be such that when the clamp is applied, there will be approximately 2cm between the clamp and the skin surface and the shaft should completely fill the clamp seat. Thread length should be such that about 5mm will remain

Screw Type	Shaft Diameter	Thread Diameter	Drill Size	Application Site
Cortical	6mm	6/5mm	4.8mm	Femur, tibia, adult humerus where diameter >20mm
Cortical	6mm	4.5/3.5mm	3.2mm	Forearm, small bones diameter 12–20mm
Cortical	6mm	3.5/3.2mm	2.9mm	Forearm, diameter 9–12mm metacarpal and metatarsal bones
Cortical	4mm	3.3/3.0mm	2.7mm	Pennig wrist fixator
Cortical	4mm	3.0/2.5mm	2.0mm	Pennig wrist fixator (for metacarpals <9mm diameter)
Cancellous	6mm	6/5mm	3.2mm	Cancellous bone
Cortical self-drilling	6mm	6/5mm	-	Pelvic and pertrochanteric applications
Cortical self-drilling	6mm	4.5/3.5mm	-	Humeral condyles
Cortical self-drilling	6mm	3.0/2.5mm	-	Forearm, diameter 9–12mm metacarpal bones
Mini Cortical self-drilling	3mm	3.0/2.5mm	-	Metacarpal metatarsal bones, phalanges >7mm diameter
Mini Cortical self-drilling	3mm	2.5/2.0mm	-	Phalanges, diameter <7mm

Table 9.1

outside the entry cortex and about 2mm will project beyond the second cortex. As a general rule, two screws are used in each clamp for shaft fractures in the upper limb, while three screws per clamp are used in the tibia and femur.

In addition to screws with a thread diameter of 6mm/5mm and shank of 6mm diameter, which are indicated for femur, tibia and the adult humerus, where the diameter of the bone is greater than 20mm, a range of other thread and shank diameters exists for use in different sites (see Table 9.1). Hydroxyapatite-coated cortical screws are also available for use in situations where the screws are expected to remain in place for extended periods of time, e.g. in lengthening procedures or in osteoporotic bone where the risk of pin loosening and pin track problems is considerable, and increases with time. Laboratory and clinical studies with these coated screws have provided evidence of enhanced security of fixation over prolonged periods and a reduced incidence of pin track infection (Magyar et al, 1997; Moroni, Heikkila et al, 1998; Moroni, Toksvig-Larsen et al, 1998).

A transparent X-ray overlay is available to aid in the selection of appropriate overall length and thread length. Two types are available, one in which screws are shown with a 15 per cent magnification and one in which they are shown with an 8 per cent magnification.

Technique of Insertion

Screws are inserted into the shortest or most difficult fragment first, and it should be noted that the closest screws to the fracture should be at least 3cm from it. A long incision in the skin is required for each screw so

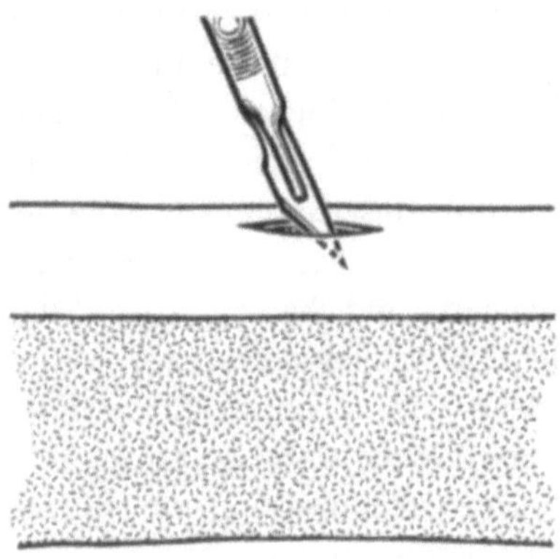

Fig. 9.1 The incision should be long enough to ensure that the skin around the screws will not be too taut.

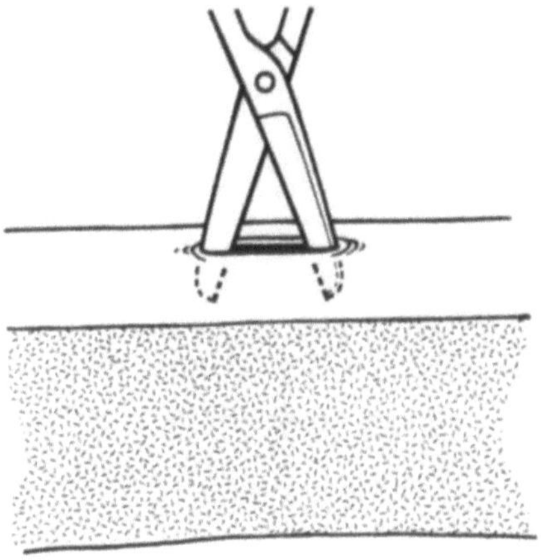

Fig. 9.2 Broad dissection of the underlying fascia will ensure that it will not grip the screws too tightly.

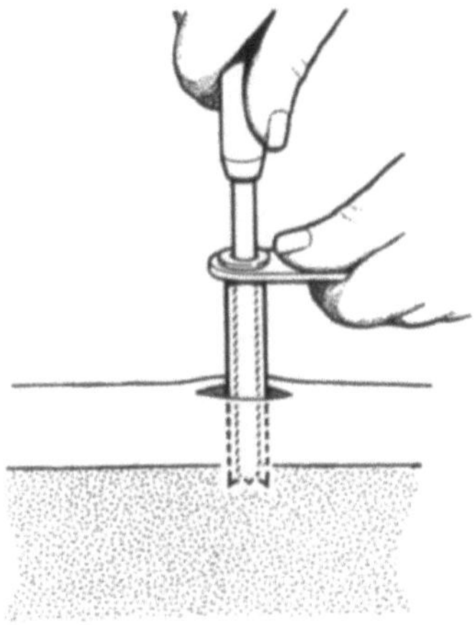

Fig. 9.3 The centre of the bone is located using a trocar and screw guide.

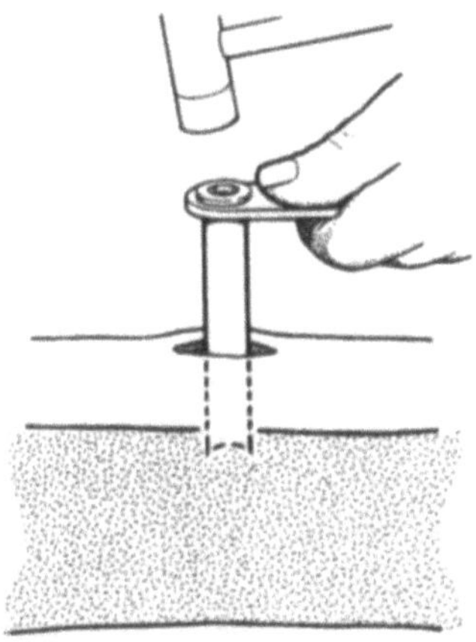

Fig. 9.4 The distal end of the screw guide is engaged in the cortex.

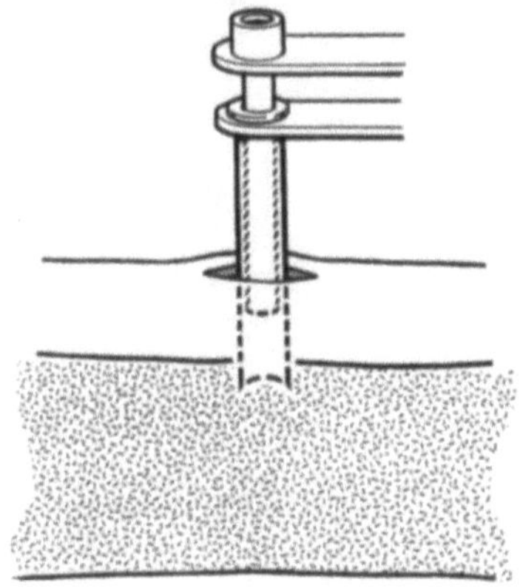

Fig. 9.5 The correct drill guide is introduced into the screw guide.

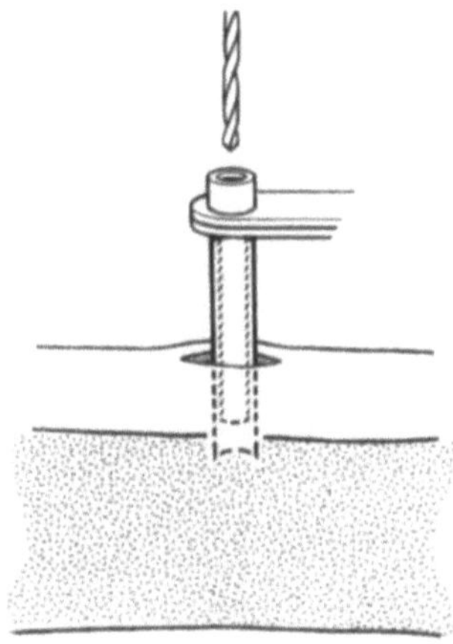

Fig. 9.6 The correct drill bit is inserted into the drill guide.

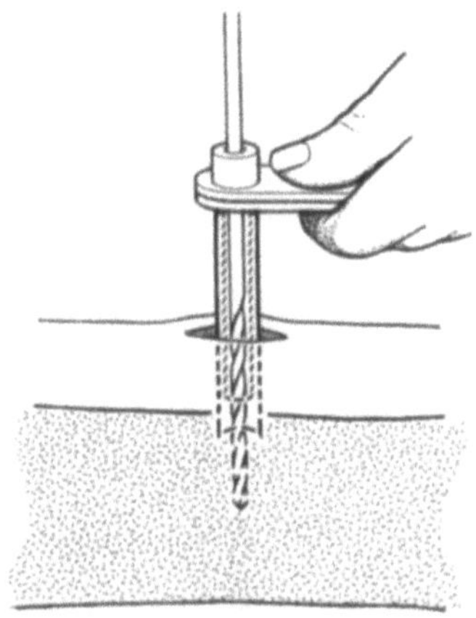

Fig. 9.7 The first cortex is drilled at right angles to the long axis of the bone; drilling is stopped when the second cortex is reached.

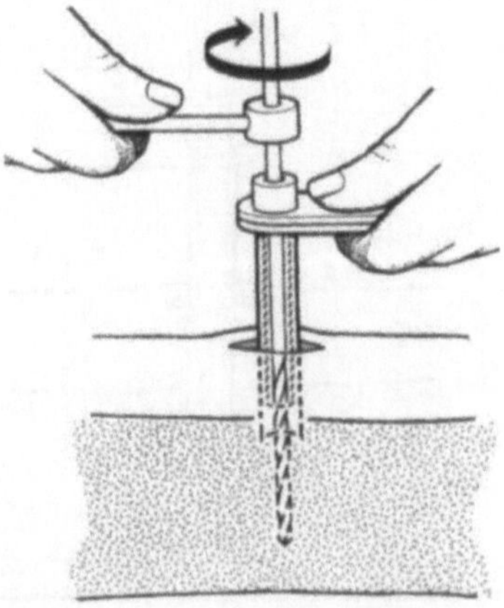

The drill stop is now offset by 5mm to avoid over-n when the second cortex is drilled.

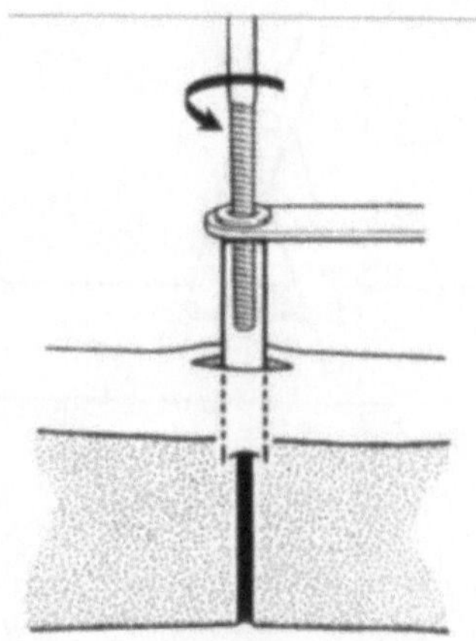

Fig. 9.11 The correct screw is inserted using a T-wrench.

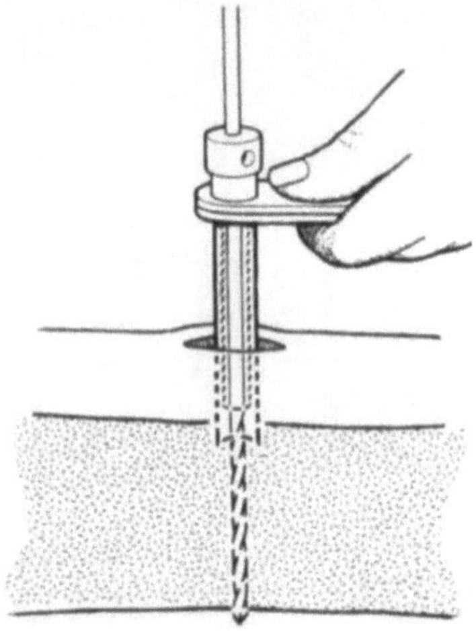

Fig. 9.9 The second cortex is drilled, ensuring that the drill bit penetrates it completely.

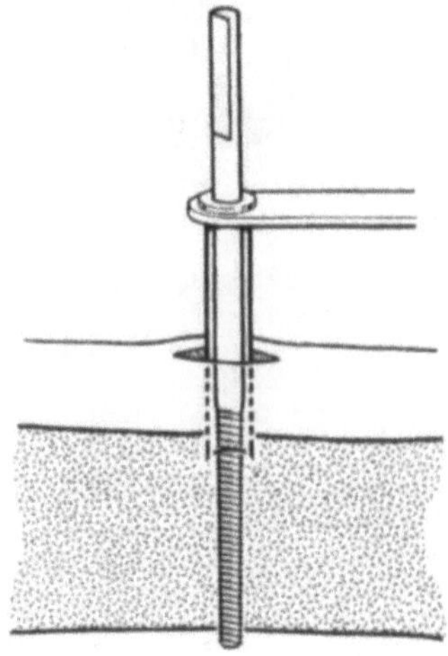

Fig. 9.12 About 2mm of thread should protrude beyond the second cortex.

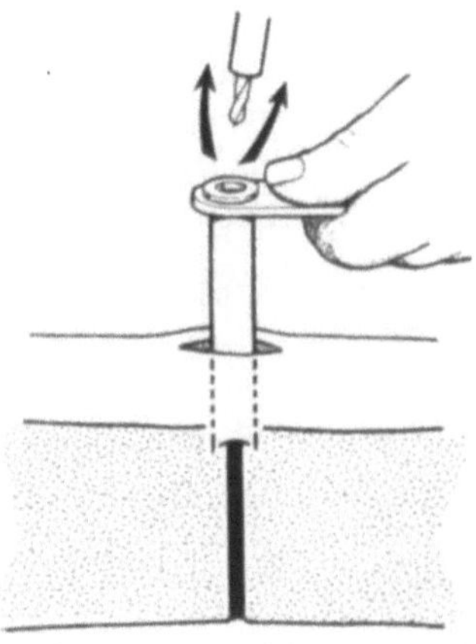

Fig. 9.10 The drill bit and drill guide are removed.

that the skin around the screw is not too taut (Fig. 9.1). The underlying fascia also requires broad dissection (Fig. 9.2) to ensure that it is not taut around the screws, since this could cause discomfort to the patient and limit muscle function.

A screw guide of suitable length is inserted into the incision using a trocar to enable the mid-line of the cortex to be located (Fig. 9.3). It is important to ensure that the screw guide is perpendicular to the longitudinal axis of the bone. Applying gentle pressure to keep the screw guide in contact with the cortex, the trocar is withdrawn, and using a hammer, the screw guide tapped lightly to engage its distal end in the cortex (Fig. 9.4). The correct drill guide is now inserted into the screw guide (Fig. 9.5) and the correct drill bit, fitted with a drill stop, inserted into the drill guide (Fig. 9.6). Care should be taken to ensure that the drill bit is not worn, in order to minimize any thermal effect.

The first cortex is then drilled, and the drill bit advanced to the second cortex, making sure that it is at right angles to the bone (Fig. 9.7). A power drill may be used at speeds not exceeding 500/600rpm. Excessive drill speeds should not be used, to avoid overheating the bone, since this may result in local necrosis and an increased risk of osteolysis. In addition to screw design, drilling time and drilling force are important factors to consider if thermal damage to bone is to be avoided. It has been shown that temperatures generated within the bone are inversely proportional to drilling force and directly proportional to drill-bone contact time (Matthews and Hirsch 1972). The force applied to the drill must be firm, and the time during which the drill is in contact with the bone the shortest possible.

In order to prevent damage to the soft tissues beyond the second cortex, the drill stop (stop collar) should be offset by 5mm before proceeding to drill through the second cortex (Fig. 9.8). Care should be taken to ensure that the drill bit completely penetrates the second cortex (Fig. 9.9). The drill bit and drill guide are then removed, while maintaining pressure on the screw guide handle (Fig. 9.10). The selected screw is then inserted into the screw guide and turned with the T-wrench (Fig. 9.11). Minimal force is required at first, and when the first cortex is engaged, the screw can be tightened with little effort. If excessive resistance is encountered at this stage, it is possible that the screw is not following its pre-drilled path. Under such circumstances, the screw should be withdrawn using the T-wrench and re-inserted along the correct path. An increase in resistance is felt as the screw penetrates the second cortex in normal cortical bone. When inserting screws into cancellous bone or poor quality bone, this change in resistance is not felt and an image intensifier should be used in these circumstances to verify that the second cortex has been penetrated. A further five or six half turns are then normally required to ensure that about 2mm of the screw protrudes beyond the second cortex (Fig. 9.12). As the thread is tapered, re-positioning the screw by turning anti-clockwise *is not possible* since this will loosen it. If there is doubt as to whether the second cortex has been breached, this should be checked by X-ray.

In order to ensure an even distribution of the load between screw and bone in a given clamp, all the screws in a clamp should be of the same type i.e. all cortical or all cancellous. Thus in a clamp overlying a meta-diaphyseal area, all the screws should be cortical. In addition, where two screws only are used in a clamp and, for anatomical reasons, seats 1 and 2; 1 and 3; 3 and 5 or 4 and 5 are used, a dummy screw (a section of shank 50mm long and 6mm in diameter) should be inserted into the free outer seat to equilibrate the pressure of the clamp cover on the screw cluster.

Where it is essential to insert the screws into osteoporotic diaphyseal bone, the number of screws per clamp should be increased i.e. four screws inserted per clamp instead of two or three. In addition, where standard diameter screws are used in osteoporotic bone, the cortical variety should be used but only the entry cortex should be pre-drilled using the 4.8mm drill; the remainder of the screw path should be pre-drilled using a 3.2mm drill to ensure maximal radial load on screw insertion.

In the epiphyseal region, or where the available space for screw insertion is limited (e.g. in the supracondylar area of the humerus, or where screws need to be inserted close to a fracture line), care should be taken to avoid several attempts at drilling the correct path, since this will weaken the bone.

Post-operative management and pin site care are covered in Ch. 11.

Bibliography

Lavini F, Renzi Brivio L, Leso P: 'Biomechanical Factors in Designing Screws for the Orthofix System'. *Clin Orthop* 1994; 308: 63–7

Magyar G, Toksvig-Laesen S, Moroni A: 'Hydroxyapatite-coating of threaded pins enhances fixation.' *J Bone Joint Surg* [Br] 1997; 79B: 487–489

Matthews LS, Hirsch C: 'Temperatures measured in human cortical bone when drilling.' *J Bone Joint Surg* [Am] 1972; 54A: 297–308

Moroni A, Heikkila J, Toksvig-Larsen S, Stea S, Giannini S: 'Hydroxyapatite-coated Tapered Pins are Better Fixed: A Multi-Center Prospective, Randomixed Study'. Presented at the AAOS 1998

Moroni A, Toksvig-Larsen S, Maltarello MC, Orienti L, Stea S, Giannini S: 'A Comparison of Hydroxyapatite-coated, Titanium-coated and Uncoated Tapered External Fixation Pins.' *J Bone Joint Surg* [Am] 1998; 80A: 547–554

The Technique of Wire Insertion

10

M. Saleh

In recent years the concept of hybrid fixation, using combinations of unilateral fixation (cantilever loading) and ring fixation (beam loading) has been recognised as a most effective and biomechanically appropriate means of treating certain types of fractures and deformities. The Orthofix Hybrid Fixation System includes hybrid constructs where, in some instances, rings may be linked directly to a monolateral fixator (Fig. 10.1), while in others, wire-bearing rings are combined with rings bearing specially designed clamps for bone screws in a modular system (The Sheffield Hybrid Fixator, Fig. 10.2). For this reason, a working knowledge of the correct technique of wire insertion is integral to the correct application of these forms of external fixation.

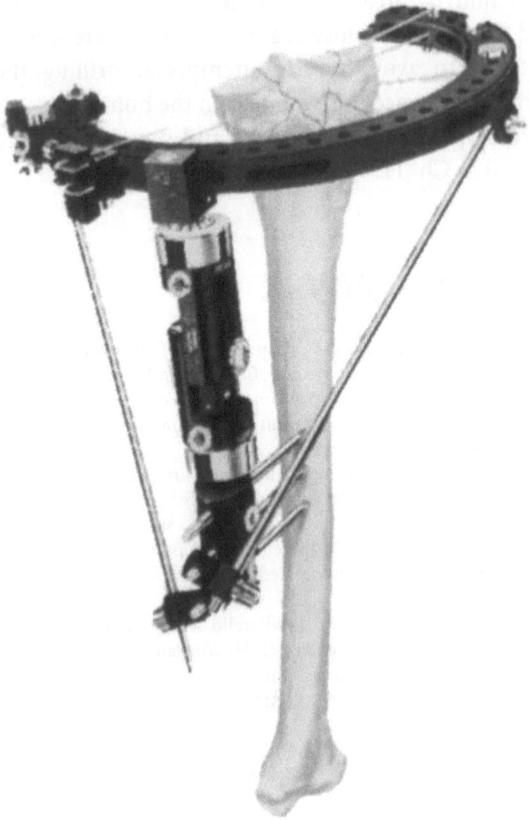

Fig. 10.1 Orthofix Hybrid Fixation: direct linkage of a ring to the ProCallus Fixator.

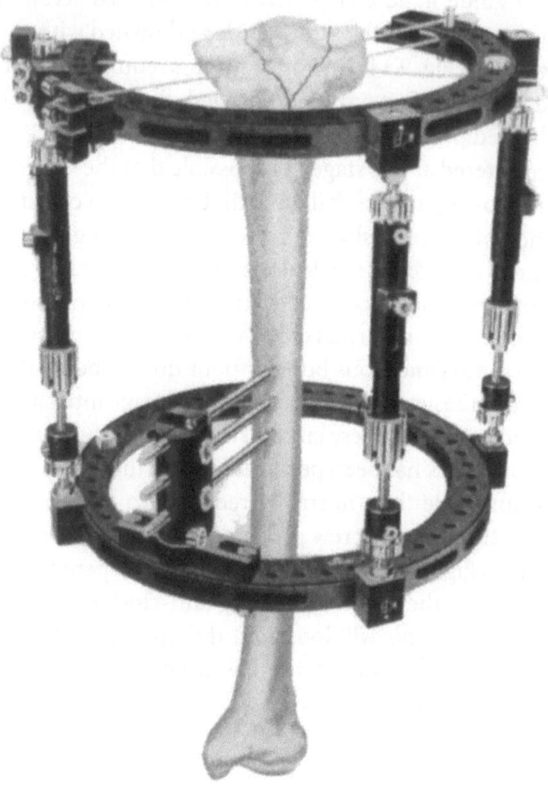

Fig. 10.2 Orthofix Hybrid Fixation: The Sheffield Hybrid Fixator Assembly.

General Principles

When using Kirschner-wires, it is important to ensure that the path they will take will avoid tendons or neurovascular elements. In the region of important neurovascular structures, a 4cm incision should be made, dissecting the tissues down to the bone and inserting the wire under direct vision. Whenever possible, in order to avoid drilling in unprotected soft tissues, wires should be inserted through the side of maximum soft tissue coverage, and pushed on to the bone before commencing drilling. The wire is inserted through the skin and pushed gently to advance it to the bone surface, stretching muscle groups before transfixion. No attempt should be made to insert a wire more than once, since the tip will have become blunt, and as this is the only cutting surface, undesirable heating of the bone may occur. Once the wire has exited from the far cortex the adjacent muscles are stretched, and the wire tapped through the muscles and overlying skin with a small mallet. Some deflection of the wire may be produced during its passage through the limb and care should be taken to avoid this as it may cause abnormal stresses at the wire-bone interface. Since wire-bearing rings in the lower limb will normally be applied to the proximal or distal tibial metaphysis, or to the distal femoral metaphysis, the safe corridors for Kirschner-wire insertion in each of these regions will be discussed, following which, the technique of wire insertion will be described in detail for the upper tibial metaphysis. Wires should be inserted parallel to joints, the first wire being called the "reference wire."

Safe Corridors in the Proximal Tibial Metaphysis

When inserting wires in the proximal tibia, the head of the fibula is an important landmark, since the Common Peroneal Nerve passes posterior to it (Fig. 10.3). Care should be taken to avoid transfixion of this nerve. Where two levels of trans-fibular wires are used,

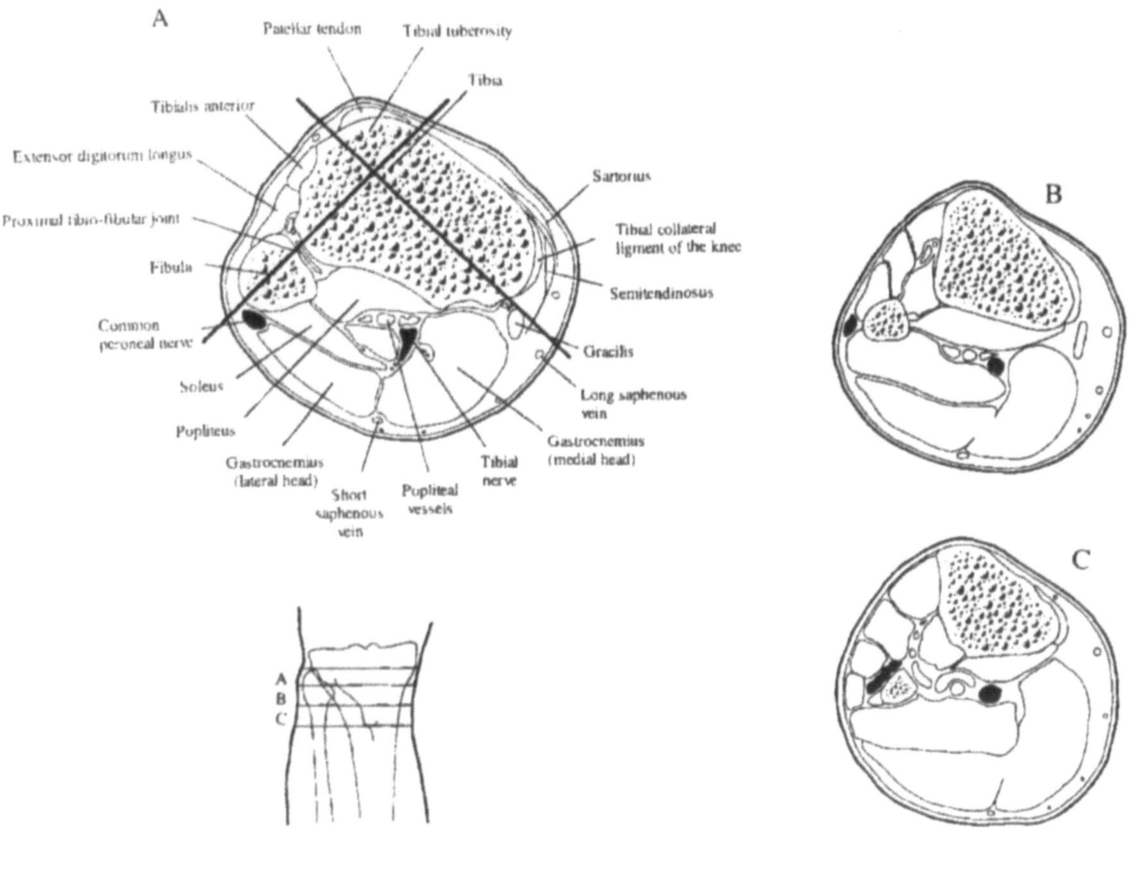

Fig. 10.3 Safe corridors in the proximal tibial metaphysis.

they should either both pass through the head of the fibula, or one should pass through it and one should pass just above its tip. In either case, the upper wire should be sited at least 14mm from the joint line to avoid capsular penetration, and the lower wire must be above the neck of the fibula, where the Common Peroneal Nerve is at risk. The trans-fibular wire must avoid the Patellar Tendon, transfixion of which will cause pain and restricted motion.

The crossing wire, called the medial face wire, is inserted just anterior to the antero-lateral compartment muscles, exiting at the postero-medial border of the tibia, anterior to the Gastrocnemius. It may cause some discomfort if it is too anterior, exiting through the Pes Anserinus, or too posterior, exiting through the medial head of Gastrocnemius. Wires are generally well tolerated and crossing angles of between 60 and 70° may be achieved. Transfixion of muscle leads to discomfort and restricted mobility. Should it be necessary to transfix a muscle, the appropriate joint should be moved to ensure that the muscle is stretched prior to insertion of the wire.

Safe Corridors in the Distal Tibial Metaphysis

See Fig. 10.4. The reference wire is trans-fibular from postero-lateral to antero-medial and is inserted between 5mm and 10mm from the distal articular surface of the tibia. It should pass medial to the Tibialis Anterior Muscle, thus avoiding the anterior tibial vessels. The crossing wire is from postero-medial to antero-lateral, and is inserted directly on to the subcutaneous edge of the tibia, thus avoiding the posterior tibial vessels and nerve. It exits lateral to the tendon of Extensor Digitorum.

If two levels of wires are used, the first trans-fibular wire should be inserted close to the articular surface of the tibia so that the more proximal wire remains close to, or immediately above the level of the inferior tibiofibular joint, in order to avoid the peroneal vessels. All three neurovascular structures are potentially at risk. Transfixion of the extensor tendons must be avoided. Wires are generally well tolerated and crossing angles of between 60 and 70° may be achieved.

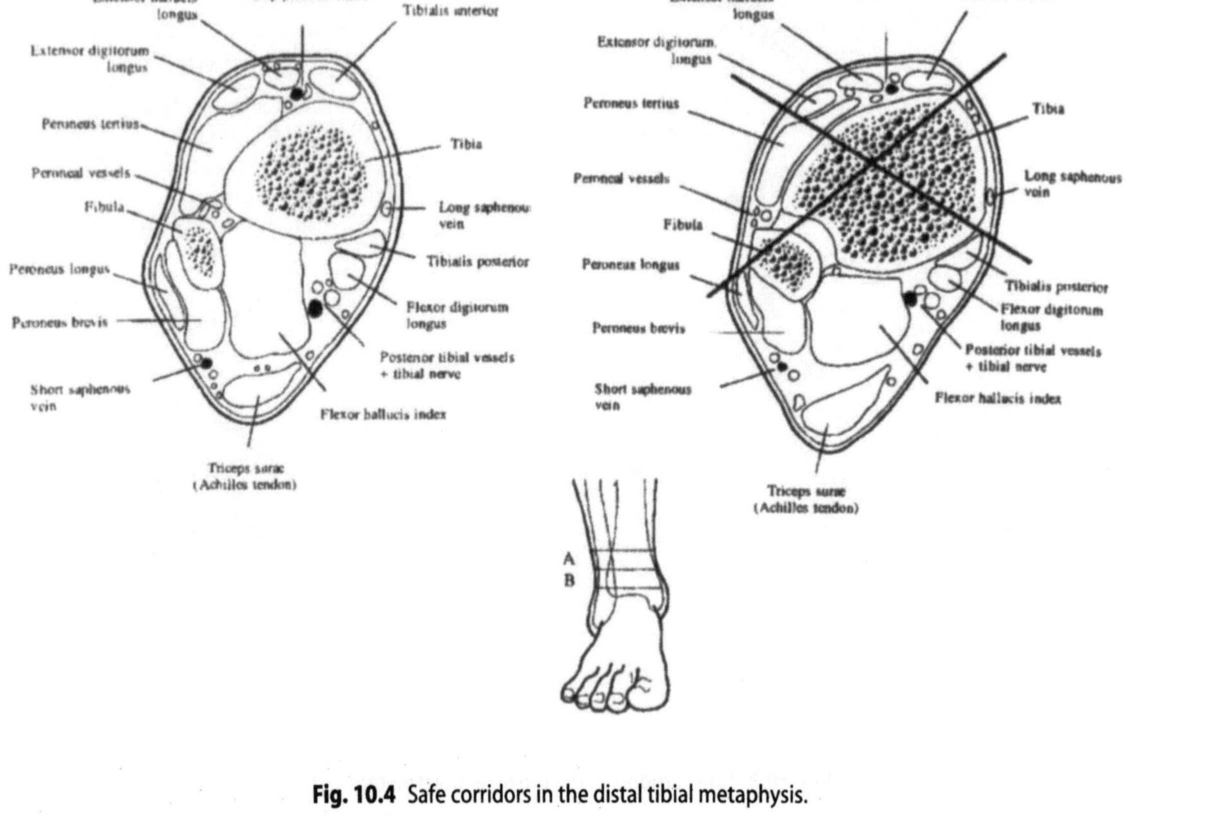

Fig. 10.4 Safe corridors in the distal tibial metaphysis.

Safe Corridors in the Distal Femoral Metaphysis

Wire fixation in the distal femur (Fig. 10.5) is problematic because narrow wire crossing angles produce instability in the sagittal plane and transfixion of the medial and lateral periarticular structures may lead to intractable knee stiffness. Early joint motion may be instituted, but soft tissue movement over the wires may result in discomfort and early loosening.

The first wire should pass from postero-lateral to antero-medial, anterior to the Biceps Femoris Tendon, and the second from postero-medial to antero-lateral, anterior to the Sartorius. The wires should be inserted with the knee extended, and exit through the quadriceps with the knee fixed. Early joint movement should be encouraged. It may be difficult to achieve crossing angles of more than 45°. In general, screw fixation is preferred to wire fixation, except in knee arthrodesis, where improved wire crossing angles may be achieved, as in this situation transfixion of the quadriceps and medial and lateral periarticular tissues is not a problem.

Kirschner-Wire Insertion in the Proximal Tibial Metaphysis

The first wire inserted (trans-fibular reference wire) is a postero-lateral to antero-medial one, through the head of the fibula, running parallel to the tibial plateau and exiting medial to the patellar tendon. It must be inserted below any internal fixation previously applied. It may be introduced either through a Kirschner-wire securing pin, or alternatively, free-hand, using a wire without olive (Fig. 10.6).

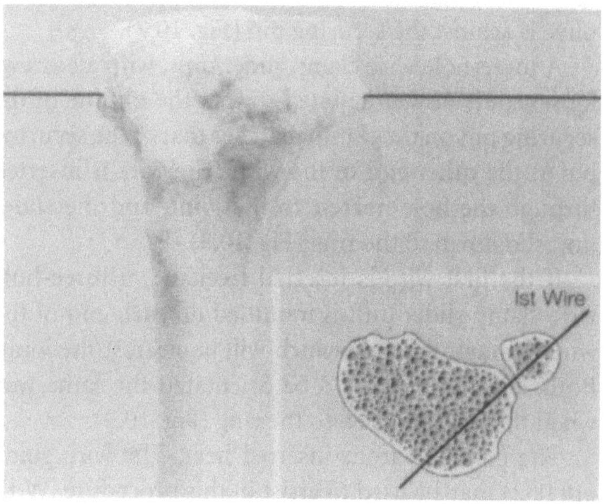

Fig. 10.6 The first (transfibular) wire in the proximal tibial metaphysis.

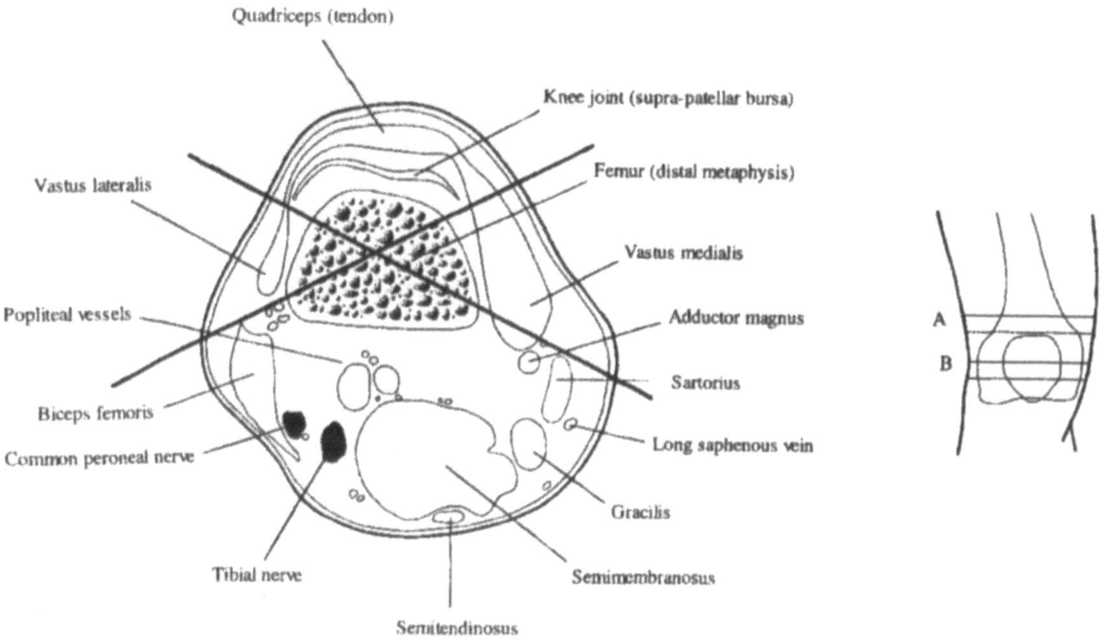

Fig. 10.5 Safe corridors in the distal femoral metaphysis.

Where the wire is inserted through a securing pin, the ring is held in position parallel to the joint surface by an assistant, with the limb centrally placed within the ring. In this case, a wire with peripheral olive should be used. It is easier to insert the first securing pin towards the joint, with the first wire through the hole outside the ring. This allows better visualization of the wire during insertion. The wire is inserted percutaneously or through a small incision (3–4 mm) and pushed down to the bone before commencing drilling, which is carried out at slow speed and with gentle pressure. After it has penetrated the bone, it is tapped through the soft tissues on the far side, until the olive is against the securing pin (Fig. 10.7).

A three-hole wire clamp slider unit, with all screws loosened, is now orientated so that the outline of the securing pin on the clamp matches that of the securing pin at the other end of the wire. The wire is inserted through the hole nearest to the joint, and the slider unit slid down to the ring (Fig. 10.8).

If the first wire is inserted freehand, a three-hole wire clamp slider unit is mounted on each end of the wire through the hole which will be nearest the joint. Both slider units should be orientated the same way when they are attached to the ring (Fig. 10.9).

The parallel wire is inserted next. The wire guide (18.002) may be used to assist in this procedure. With its knob loosened, the sliding support unit of the wire guide is inserted into one of the holes in the ring and its position on the bar adjusted so that one groove in the head of the wire guide is in contact with the wire already in place. The second wire is then kept in contact with the remaining groove in the head of the wire guide during its insertion.The slider unit may be temporarily disconnected from the ring, and then inserted over both wires using the appropriate two holes. The slider unit is then firmly secured to the ring by tightening the appropriate screws evenly with a 3mm Allen wrench (Fig. 10.10).

The ring must now be adjusted so that the limb lies at its centre, since such adjustments can not be made subsequently. Both wires are now tensioned. The wire tensioning device is opened fully and advanced over the wire until it touches the wire clamp slider unit. The handle is now closed and clipped, and the tension read off on the graduated scale. If it is less than 1200N, the wire clamp screw is temporarily tightened using the 5mm Allen wrench and the procedure repeated. Once the correct tension is achieved (i.e. 1200N), the wire clamp screw is fully tightened (Fig. 10.11).

N.B. While tightening the wire clamp screw, it is important not to lever the wire tensioning device to avoid breakage of the Kirschner-wire.

The Kirschner wires are now cut 4cm from the slider unit and bent at both ends. The cut end should be turned in towards the ring to avoid sharp edges

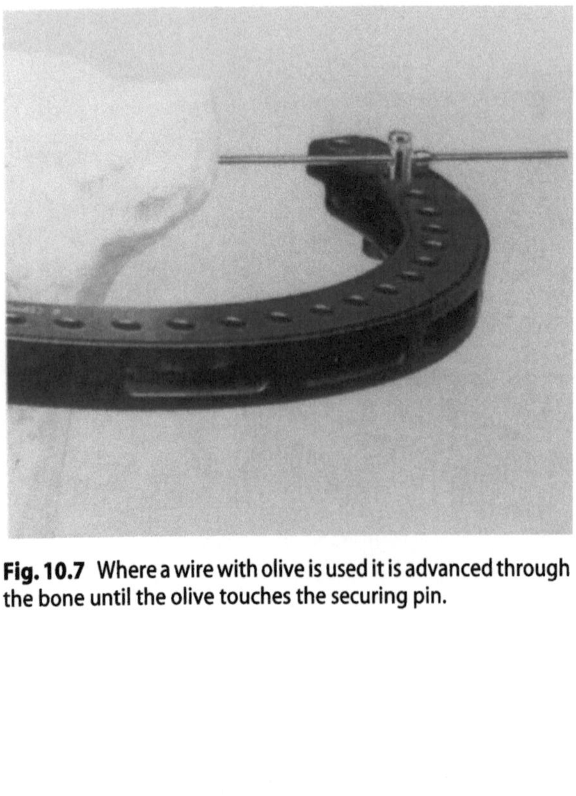

Fig. 10.7 Where a wire with olive is used it is advanced through the bone until the olive touches the securing pin.

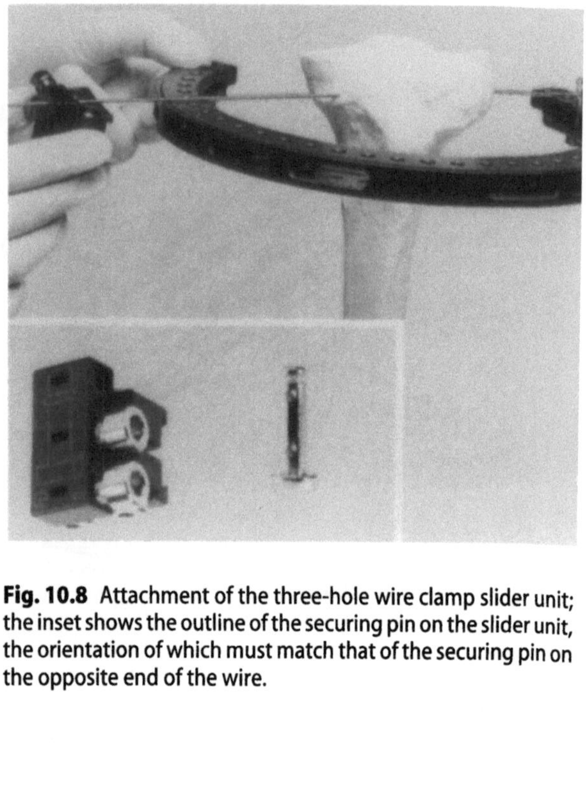

Fig. 10.8 Attachment of the three-hole wire clamp slider unit; the inset shows the outline of the securing pin on the slider unit, the orientation of which must match that of the securing pin on the opposite end of the wire.

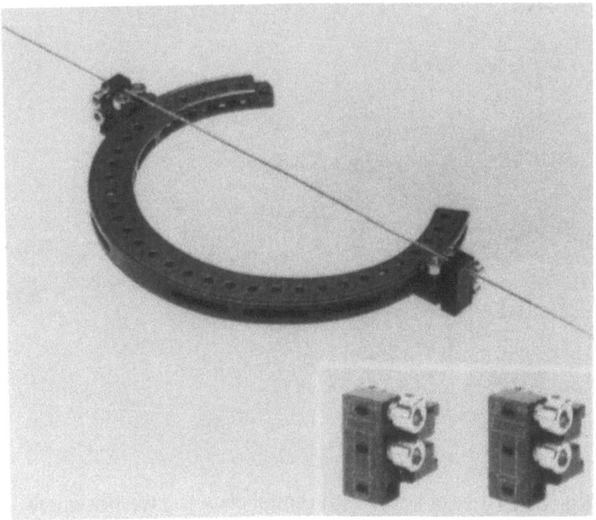

Fig. 10.9 Where a wire without olive is used, two three-hole wire clamp slider units are needed; the inset shows that both slider units must be orientated in the same way in these circumstances.

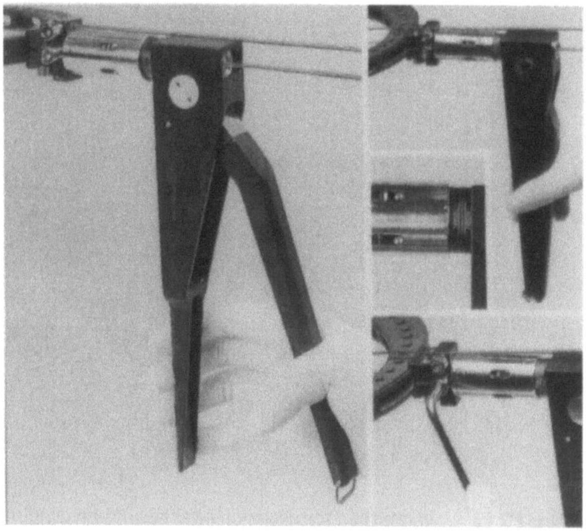

Fig. 10.11 The wire tensioning device in use; insets show the handle closed, the tension scale and final locking of the wire clamp screw once the correct tension has been achieved.

being exposed (Fig. 10.12). Note that if the first wire of a pair is tensioned before the second is inserted, some difficulty may be experienced in guiding the second wire into the appropriate hole in the wire slider unit.

The position and direction of the crossing wires should allow a 60–70° wire separation angle. Ring stability is optimal if the wire crossing angle is as large as possible, and the wires cross in the centre of the tibia. The crossing wires are now inserted, using the technique described above, taking care that the Kirschner-wire securing pin is inserted from the *opposite* surface of the ring from that of the first pair of wires. This will ensure that the crossing wires are not in contact at the bone interface. These wires are now tensioned. Once tensioned, the ring may be considered to be securely attached to the metaphyseal segment. In order to avoid undue stress on a ring, no more than two pairs of wires should be used on one ring (Fig. 10.13).

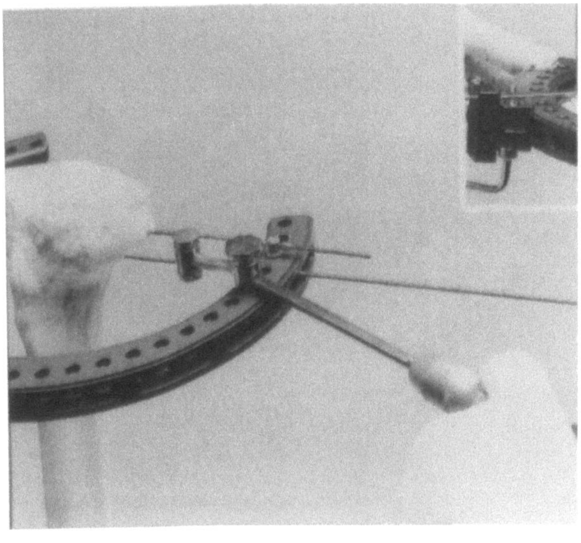

Fig. 10.10 Use of the wire guide to insert the parallel wire; the inset shows the slider unit being secured to the ring.

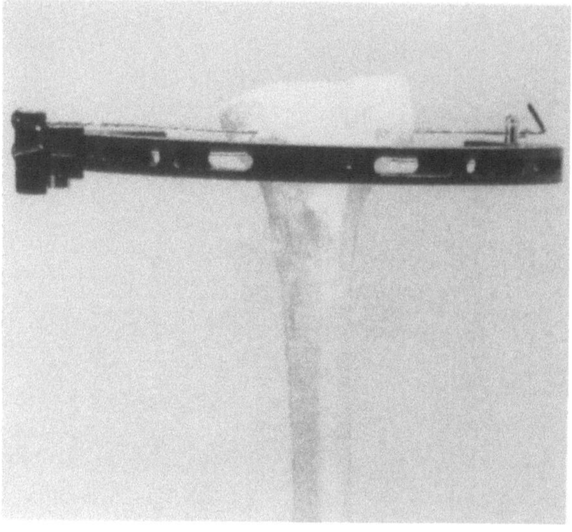

Fig. 10.12 The K-wires are cut 4cm from the slider unit and bent at both ends.

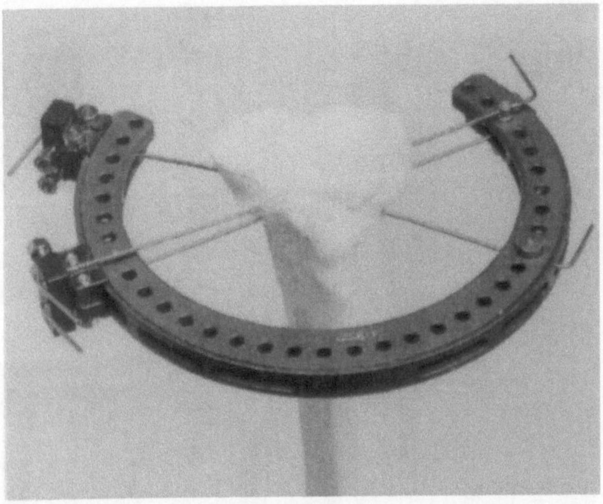

Fig. 10.13 No more than two pairs of wires should be used in one ring.

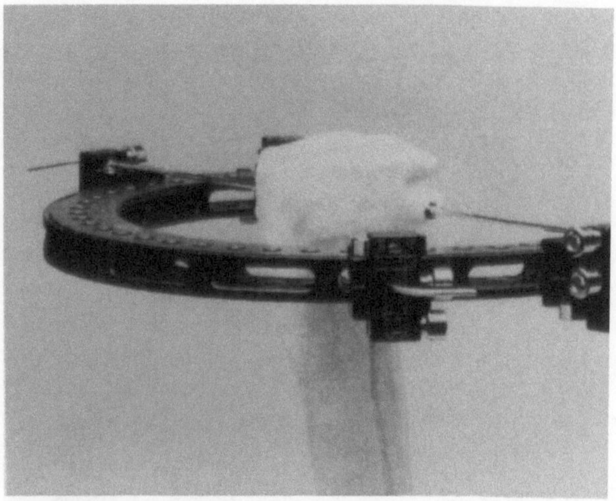

Fig. 10.14 Use of a wire with central olive and washer where large translational forces are anticipated.

Wires with a central olive may be used in conjunction with a washer where large translational forces are anticipated along the line of the wire, e.g. in any situation where there are narrow crossing angles.

The skin must be incised to permit passage of the olive through the soft tissue. Wire tensioning is performed from the side distant to the olive, and tension should be reduced to between 800 and 1000N to avoid excessive pressure on the cortex of the bone (Fig. 10.14).

Pin Track Infection and the Principles of Pin Site Care

11

R.G. Checketts, A.G. MacEachern and M. Otterburn

The Problems

There are many complications of external fixation but by far the most common and most troublesome is pin track infection.[1,4,7,10,11] It is inevitable that where a pin or screw penetrates into a limb and remains in this position for some considerable time, some degree of pin track infection will occur unless extreme care is taken to prevent it. For this reason there has hitherto been a reluctance to use external fixation where alternative methods of internal fixation are available.

The infection rates reported in previous studies are extremely variable, ranging from virtually zero[1] to over 60 per cent[12] (Table 11.1). This great disparity in the reported incidence suggests that the various authors have differing ideas as to what constitutes a pin track infection. It is inconceivable that De Bastiani et al[1] who reported a 0.92 per cent infection rate could be referring to the same type of infection as Edge and Denham,[7] who reported a 42 per cent infection rate.

Most of the reports give the incidence of pin track infection but do not define precisely what is meant by the term. Melendez and Colon[10] describe a classification of pin track infection into four grades but they do not include late complications such as persistently discharging sinuses. MacEachern[11] also suggests classifying pin track infection into four grades. Unless there is a generally accepted method for the definition and classification of pin track infection, accurate comparison of the results from various centres will be difficult if not impossible.

Furthermore, few of the previous reports make any reference to methods of care of the pin sites. If external fixation is to be used successfully in any situation, it is of vital and fundamental importance that the pin sites are maintained in a good state of health. There are no clear guidelines on how pin sites should be cared for, and

	Authors	Year	Incidence
Single Bar Units			
	Burny	1979	30%
	Edge & Denham	1981	42%
	Court Brown & Hughes	1982	27%
Hoffman Double Frame			
	Edwards	1979	37%
	Benum & Svennisen	1982	52%
D.A.F.			
	De Bastiani et al	1984	0.92%
	Melendez & Colon	1982	17%
	Noordeen et al	1995	60%

Table 11.1 Incidence of pin track infection from previous reports

little knowledge of how to deal with infections when they do occur. It seems likely that these are the reasons for the high rates of pin sepsis that have been reported. It is possible that in some cases external fixation has been abandoned prematurely because of pin site sepsis when adequate care could have allowed it to continue.

Classification of Pin Track Infection

Following the suggestions of Melendez and Colon[10] and MacEachern[11] a system of classification of pin track infection has been devised which includes both infections which occur when the fixator is still in place and complications which occur after the fixator has been removed.[5]

Pin track problems and infections are classified broadly as minor or major.[10] Minor infections can be managed on an outpatient basis, they respond to the appropriate treatment and external fixation can be continued. Major infections often require hospital admission, do not resolve with treatment and usually involve more than one pin or group of pins. External fixation has to be abandoned.

Both minor and major infections are divided into three subgroups.

Minor Infections

Grade I: characterized by slight redness around the pin together with a little discharge. These settle with improved pin site care and hygiene. They should probably more correctly be termed problems rather than infections, but should be included in any classification for the sake of completeness, and because if not properly managed they may well progress to a true infection.

Grade II: characterized by redness of the skin, discharge from the pin site and pain and tenderness in the soft tissues (Fig. 11.1). These infections settle with improved pin site care and a short course of the appropriate oral antibiotic which is chosen according to the organism cultured. In almost all cases the organism will be *Staphylococcus aureus*. It is therefore prudent to commence therapy with an anti-staphylococcal antibiotic as soon as soft tissue redness and tenderness appears. The antibiotic may be changed where necessary, a day or two later, if an organism other than *Staphylococcus aureus* is cultured.

Grade III: these infections have the same appearance as Grade II, namely redness of the skin with pain and tenderness in the soft tissues, but fail to settle with improved pin site care and the appropriate oral antibiotic. The affected pin or pins are resited and external fixation can be continued.

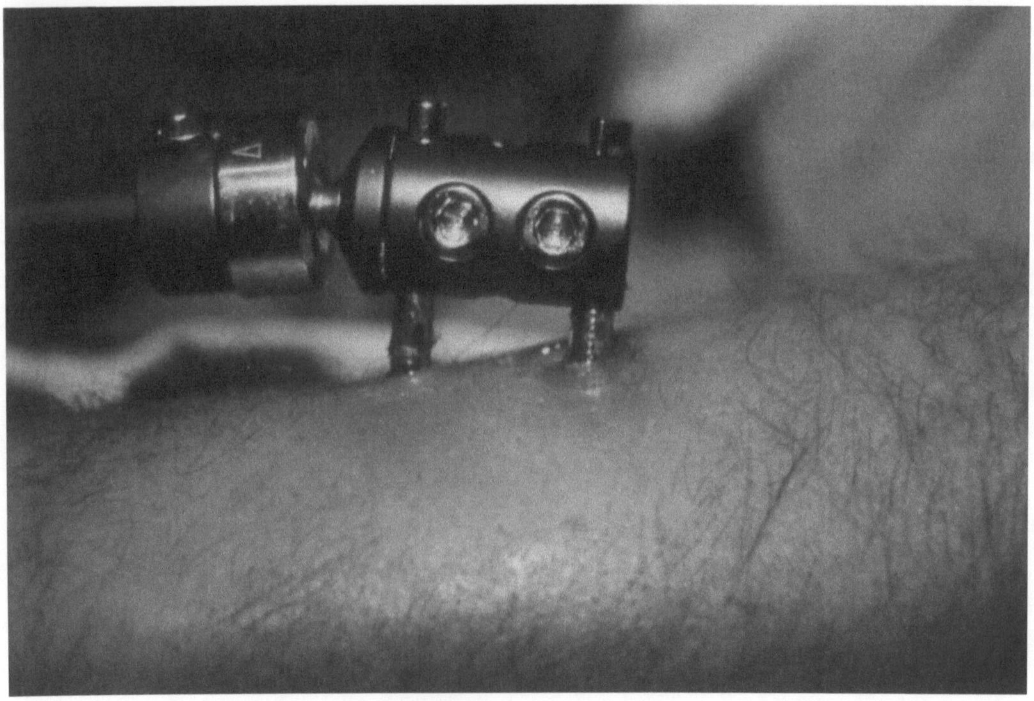

Fig. 11.1 Grade II minor infection. There is a flare and erythema in the skin and discharge around the pin sites.

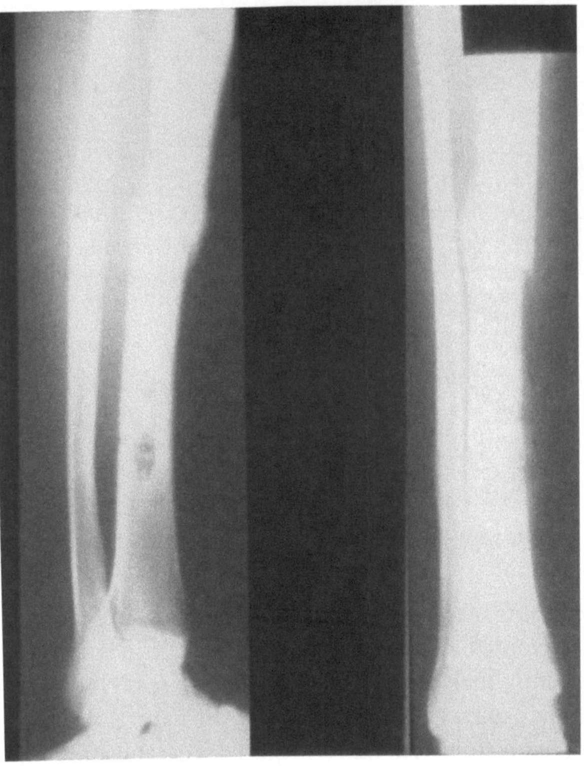

Fig. 11.2 Grade V major infection. Note periosteal reaction on the medial side of the tibia and the osteolysis and sequestrum formation.

Major Infections

Grade IV: severe soft tissue infection involving several pins, sometimes with associated loosening of the pins. Although Grade IV infections are confined to the soft tissues, in view of the extent of the infection, resiting of the pins is impossible and external fixation has to be abandoned.

Grade V: in addition to the soft tissue infection, in Grade V infections there is involvement of the bone. Radiographs will show areas of osteolysis and possibly sequestrum formation. (Fig. 11.2) In such a situation external fixation has to be abandoned, and in most cases the infection then resolves.

Grade VI: these infections occur after fixator removal following completion of treatment. The pin track heals initially, but will subsequently break down and discharge at intervals. Radiographs usually show areas of new bone formation deep to the periosteum with some osteolysis in the cortex and sometimes sequestra, either deep to the periosteum or in the medullary cavity. These infections generally clear with thorough curettage of the pin track under general anaesthetic.

Pin Site Care

If external fixation is to be used consistently and effectively, prevention of infection is imperative. The surgeon, nurses and the patients themselves all have substantial and important parts to play in maintaining the pin sites in a healthy condition. It is only when the problem of infection has been largely overcome that it is possible to use external fixation with confidence in a variety of trauma and orthopaedic conditions.

There are four phases of pin site care: preoperatively; in the theatre; post- operatively whilst the patient is still in hospital, and post-operatively after discharge from hospital.

Pre-operative Care

When it is intended to use external fixation, it is advisable, wherever possible, for the patient and the immediate family to be counselled and the precise nature of the procedure explained. It is useful for the patient to meet other individuals with external fixators so that mutual problems may be discussed informally. Preoperative counselling is usually carried out by a senior nurse or sometimes by a doctor. The problems of pin track infection are discussed and the methods of treatment carefully explained to the patient and the family so that appropriate cleaning and care of the pin sites can begin immediately after surgery.

It is unusual for a patient to reject the use of a fixator, but if it is clear that there will be very little cooperation, it would be wiser not to proceed with external fixation. It is normally found that patients of all ages are keen to learn and carry out the cleaning techniques.

Care in Theatre

In the operating theatre it is the surgeon's responsibility to minimize the risk of pin track infection. First, the skin incisions through which the pins or screws are inserted should be large enough to prevent any soft tissue tethering. Second, drill and screw guides should be used to prevent thermal and other damage to the subcutaneous tissues and muscle planes through which the screws may be passing. The pins or screws should be inserted securely in the bone and should engage both cortices firmly. If the screws are not tight in the bone, they will inevitably start to toggle with joint movement and weightbearing. Loose screws cause damage to the bone and to the soft tissues and this predisposes to pin track infection.

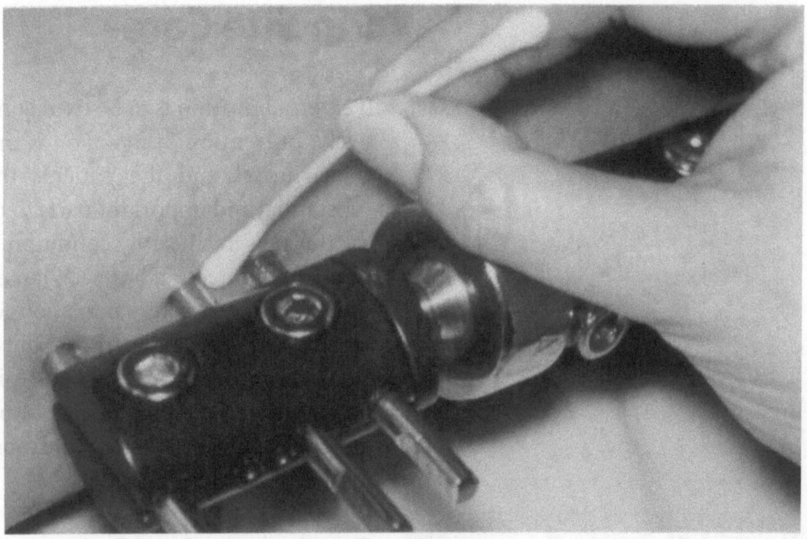

Fig. 11.3 Cleaning of pins and fixator with cotton buds.

At the end of the procedure, just before the patient is taken from the operating table, the surgeon should carefully put the limb through a full range of movements while closely inspecting the pin sites to check that the skin and soft tissues have been adequately released and that there is no undue tension or pressure from the skin or subcutaneous tissues on the shanks of the screws. The surgeon should also check that there is adequate access for pin site cleaning. It is suggested that there should be about 1cm between the skin and the fixator body.

When the patient is returned to bed, it is again important to ensure that the soft tissues are not pushed up against the screws. In particular, where the patient is returned to bed with a femoral fixator in position, it is not uncommon for the soft tissues of the buttock and the posterior thigh to be pushed up against the screws, and if the situation is not carefully monitored, this could, within a few hours, lead to necrosis of the pin tracks and subsequent infection. It is therefore suggested that femoral fixators should be applied a little anterior to the mid-lateral position and that the patient should, if at all possible, be nursed inclined a little towards the non-operated side, by placing a pillow behind the back.

Finally, at the end of the procedure, the pin sites are thoroughly cleaned and an absorbent dressing applied.

Post-operative Care

In the ward it is usual for pin sites to bleed for 24–48 hours. The absorbent dressings are replaced every day until bleeding ceases, and a senior nurse will begin instructing the patient on the technique of pin site cleaning. Antiseptic creams, lotions and sprays are to be avoided. Creams will often cause allergies and frequently make the skin soggy. Iodine spray preparations cause crusting, preventing the natural drainage of tissue fluids. All that is required is careful and thorough cleaning using cotton buds moistened with sterile water. (Fig. 11.3) The first few days after surgery are vital for establishing healthy pin tracks. Patients are encouraged, and indeed required to clean the pin sites themselves, initially under supervision, and discharge from hospital should not be allowed until it is ascertained that the patient is competent in this technique.

It is important to give precise instructions to patients on the techniques to be used so that there is no confusion or misunderstanding on what is required. A new cotton bud should be used for each individual pin site. In addition to the pin site, the shank of the screw and the body of the fixator should be kept scrupulously clean, as this encourages good overall hygiene.

Post-operative, Outpatient Department Care

Following discharge from hospital the patient should return to hospital either daily or on alternate days to ensure that the correct cleaning procedures are being carried out. Once the pin sites have stabilized, the patient returns weekly for the pin sites to be checked by a senior nurse to ensure that the cleaning instructions are fully understood and are being adequately carried out. As time progresses it is often possible to reduce the frequency of the outpatient visits and in many instances it is necessary for the patient to make contact only if there is a problem with the pin sites.

It is useful for there to be one or two named senior nurses to whom the patient can refer at any time should a problem arise. This is important, as it is possible for an infection to develop within 24 hours. In such circumstances prompt treatment will often result in the infection being controlled and thereby prevented from progressing from a minor to a major category.

Patients are taught to clean their pin sites at home with cooled boiled water and cotton buds which can be purchased from any chemist. All patients are taught to recognize potential or definitive infection early, so that appropriate treatment can be instituted promptly. No dressings are applied once the pin sites have stopped bleeding. The patient is permitted to shower, but bathing is not generally recommended. Each patient is given an instruction sheet on pin site care before leaving hospital. (Fig. 11.4)

Incidence

Most reports of pin track infection are retrospective reviews of various external fixation devices and uses. Few prospective studies of pin track infection have been carried out. Checketts et al[5] carried out a prospective study of 353 pin sites over a period of twelve months. The patients were assessed from the time of operation until two months after the fixator had been removed. All the patients were seen weekly by the nursing and medical staff. Of the pin sites, 55 per cent remained trouble free. All the infections which occurred were minor by definition and all of them settled with intensive local care and, where necessary, oral antibiotic therapy. There were no instances of major infection in the twelve-month period and in no case, therefore, was it necessary to discontinue treatment with the fixator (Table 11.2). It was found that the screws closest to the joints (elbow, knee or ankle) were the most frequently affected, presumably because at these sites there was more movement of the soft tissues around the screws. The presence of screw threads outside the skin surface did not increase the risk of infection nor did open fractures have a greater incidence of pin track infection than closed injuries.

Conclusions

Pin track infection cannot be avoided completely but it is essential to minimize it as far as possible by adopting a policy for pin site care which is easily understood by the surgeons, the nurses and the patients themselves. This policy should be rigorously implemented and standardized, in the operating room, in the wards and in the outpatient department.

It is recommended that if at all possible, one individual should be in charge of all aspects of pin site care. This will usually be a senior nurse who has a permanent post in an orthopaedic department. He or she will gain special expertise in all aspects of pin site management and will be in a position to monitor the infection rate in the department and to advise, with authority, all members of the medical and nursing team, and the patients, should a problem or infection arise. It has been shown that simple cleaning with cooled boiled water is effective, provided the care is scrupulous.

According to the classification of pin track infection suggested above, it might be argued that Grade I does not constitute an infection, as often no organism is cultured and antibiotics are not required. This group has been included in the classification however, as in these instances pin site care has been less than perfect. If close attention is not paid to these problems, actual infection will ensue. A more satisfactory term would be Grade I problems, but to avoid confusion they have been classified as Grade I infections.

Excluding Grade I cases, Checketts et al[5] found that the overall infection rate was 18.4 per cent. Like Melendez and Colon,[10] it was found that poor pin site care by the patients, and improper placement of the screws, without adequate soft tissue and skin release, were the most common causes of these problems. Previous reports describing infection rates with external fixation[1,2,3,6,7,8,10,11] are largely meaningless as none of these state what is meant by the term infection or how such problems should be treated. However, Melendez and Colon[10] describe a useful classification which has now been expanded upon and further subdivided so that all the consequences of pin track

	Number of Pin Sites	Percentage
Trouble free	196	55
Grade I	92	25
Grade II	65	18
Grade III	0	0
Grade IV	0	0
Grade V	0	0
Grade VI	0	0

Table 11.2 Twelve Month Prospective Study of 353 Pin Sites with Dynamic Axial Fixators

EQUIPMENT NEEDED.
- Small box or tray to keep equipment together.
- Liquid soap and hand towel – for your use only.
- Cotton buds.
- Small bowl – for cooled boiled water.
- Non-woven swabs.
- Adhesive tape/Elastoplast.
- Polythene/Paper bag – for disposal of used dressings.

Please note If you have dressings on your pin sites:
(a) These should be removed and placed into the polythene/paper bag.
(b) Secure the top and dispose of safely.

NOW COMMENCE PIN SITE CARE –
1. WASH YOUR HANDS THOROUGHLY. Please see overleaf for the correct technique!
2. Clean and check the barrel thoroughly, using cooled boiled water.
3. With cooled boiled water, clean each pin site individually, using the cotton buds or non-woven swabs.
4. All dry crusted material must be removed from the pin site (where the pin enters the skin and the pin. This will take 10 to 15 minutes. **Use new swabs for each pin.**
5. It may be necessary to very gently ease the skin away from the pin in order to achieve this.
6. Dry each pin site using new swabs for each site.
7. Leave pin sites open to the air.
(Dressings are not needed if the pin sites are dry)
8. Clean pin sites twice daily.

IF YOUR PIN SITE BECOMES
(a) Red,
(b) Sore,
(c) Starts to ooze or discharge,
1. Clean as above at least twice daily.
2. Apply a small dry gauze dressing to your pin site.
3. Secure dressing with tape.
4. If after 24 hours the pin site does not return to normal,
Contact – Sister, Fracture Clinic,
Telephone ___________ Extension _______
or the ward you were discharged from.

Fig. 11.4 Patient Instruction Sheet (page 1).

infection, even the long-term ones, can be precisely graded. Melendez and Colon[10] report an overall infection rate of 17 per cent which is comparable to the 18.4 per cent reported by Checketts et al.[5] Thus for the first time it is possible to compare accurately the infection rates from two different centres. The establishment of an effective pin site care policy will enable the medical and nursing staff to have confidence in the use of external fixation and the devices can thus be widely used in the treatment of various fractures and elective orthopaedic procedures.

Poor patient compliance is the most common and most potent aetiological factor in pin track infection.

References

1 De Bastiani G, Aldgheri R, Renzi-Brivio L. 'The treatment of fractures with a dynamic axial joint fixator' *J Bone Joint Surg* [Br] 1984; 66B: 538–45
2 Benum P, Svennigsen S. 'Tibial Fractures Treated with Hoffman's External Fixation' *Acta Orthop Scand* 1982; 53: 471–6
3 Burny FL.' Elastic Fixation of Tibial Fractures: a study of 1421 cases.' in: Brooker AF, Edwards CC. (eds) *External Fixation: the*

THE IMPORTANCE OF THE FOLLOWING TECHNIQUE CAN NOT BE OVER- EMPHASIZED. THE HANDS MUST ALWAYS BE REGARDED AS THE MOST IMPORTANT VEHICLE OF INFECTION. EVERY PART OF THE HAND CAN CARRY INFECTION: THE FINGERTIPS, THUMBS, BETWEEN THE FINGERS AND BACKS OF HANDS AS WELL AS THE PALMS.

USING THE LIQUID SOAP AND RUNNING WATER THE HANDS SHOULD BE WASHED IN THE FOLLOWING MANNER. ON COMPLETION THE HANDS SHOULD BE THOROUGHLY DRIED ON A CLEAN TOWEL.

IF THIS TECHNIQUE IS FOLLOWED CORRECTLY, THE ACTIVITY SHOULD TAKE NO MORE THAN 60 SECONDS.

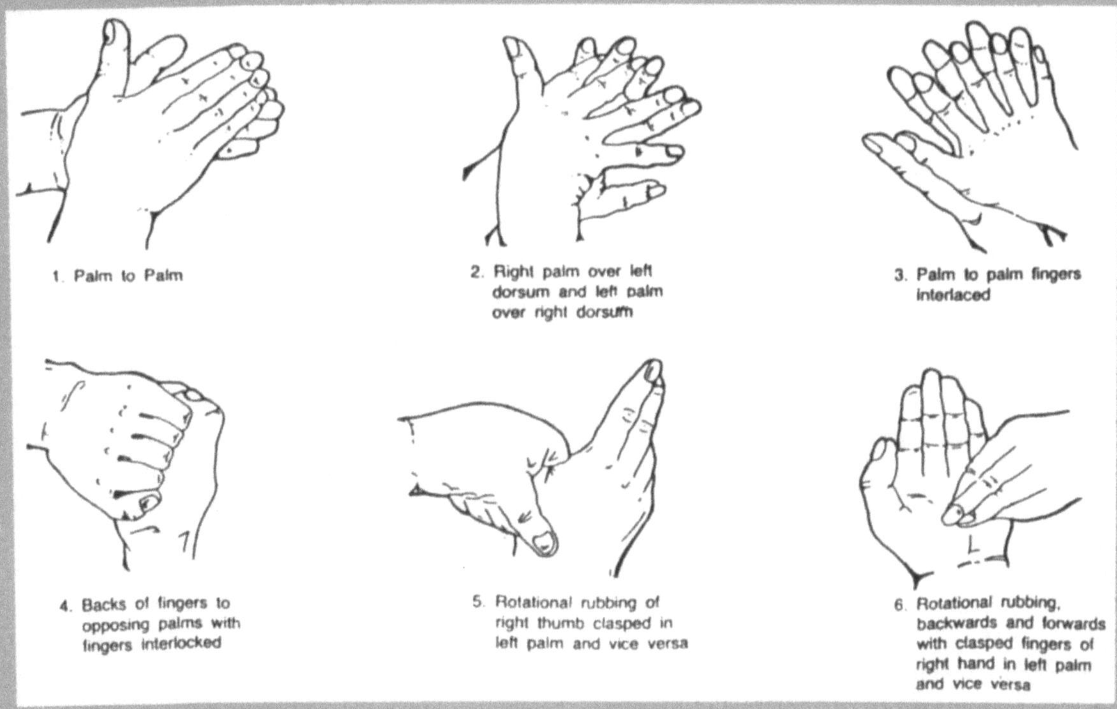

Fig. 11.4 Patient Instruction Sheet (page 2).

Current State of the Art. 1979 Williams & Wilkins: Baltimore

4 Checketts RG, Moran CG, Jennings AG. '134 Tibial Shaft Fractures Managed With the Dynamic Axial Fixator.' *Acta Orthop Scand* 1995; 66(3): 271–4

5 Checketts RG, Otterburn M, MacEachern AG. 'Pin Track Infection: definition, incidence and prevention.' Suppl. *Int J Orth Trauma* 1993; 3 (3): 16–8

6 Court-Brown C, Hughes SPF. 'Experience with the Suktian–Hughes external fixation system.' *J Roy Soc Med* 1982; 75: 949–57

7 Edge AJ, Denham RA. 'External Fixation For Complicated Tibial Fractures.' *J Bone Joint Surg* [Br] 1981; 63B: 92–7

8 Edwards CC. 'Management of the polytrauma patient in a major US centre.' in Brooker AF, Edwards CC, (eds) *External fixation: the current state of the art.* 1979 Williams & Wilkins: Baltimore

9 Green SA. *Complications of External Fixation. Causes, prevention and treatment* 1981 (Thomas, Springfield: Illinois)

10 Melendez EM, Colon C. 'Treatment of Open Tibial Fractures With the Orthofix Fixator.' *Clin Orthop.* 1989; 241: 224–30

11 MacEachern AG. 'External Fixation: past, present and future.' in Bunker TD, Colton CL, Webb JK. (eds) *Frontiers in Fracture Management* 1989 Martin Dunitz: London

12 Noordeen MHH, Lavy CBD, Shergill NS, Tuite JD, Jackson AM. 'Cyclical Micromovement and Fracture Healing.' *J Bone Joint Surg* (Br) 1995; 77: 645–8

SECTION 2 THE UPPER LIMB

Safety Corridors and Structures at Risk in External Fixation of the Upper Limb

12

T. Gausepohl and D. Pennig

Introduction

External fixation in upper limb trauma or orthopaedic surgery demands a specialized knowledge of the anatomical topography. Muscular function and biomechanics of the tendons and bones should be known in detail as well as the neurovascular routes from their origin along the upper arm and forearm to the hand. A minimally invasive technique for the implantation of fixator screws without an extensive surgical approach can only be performed if the surgeon is always aware of the underlying soft tissue structures. It is self evident that any operative technique should start with an anatomical review pointing out the anatomical structures which are at risk.

It is not a simple task to select from the wealth of anatomical data those features which are of basic importance in external fixation. Furthermore, the different fixator systems available on the market, each with their specific pin placement, require different anatomical data. Although it would be ideal to take account of anatomical structures and at the same time satisfy biomechanical demands, in reality this is frequently not possible because the technical construction of the various fixator systems and patients' needs force the surgeon to compromise. This is easy to understand if one considers such different concepts as unilateral fixators, multilateral frames and ring fixators. The latter are primarily designed to provide more stability, especially in the lower extremity, and for three-dimensional corrections after fixator application. From a biomechanical viewpoint, the advantages of ring fixators in terms of stability are tempting. The surrounding soft tissues, however, are largely neglected, with multiple K-wires crossing the extremity in any direction. This often results in soft tissue problems. The same is true for frame constructions which are thought to provide an increased stability compared to unilateral fixators, but in keeping with ring fixators, often do not allow ideal anatomical placement of the fixator screws. In the upper extremity, the argument of an increased stability is less convincing since here, in contrast to the lower extremity, weightbearing is not an essential part of functional recovery. In our opinion a unilateral fixator design provides sufficient stability for early active motion and physiotherapy of the joints and also allows more anatomically acceptable pin placement. The following description of safety corridors in the upper extremity will therefore be limited to unilateral fixation. Starting with the upper arm, pin placement in the humerus, the elbow, the forearm, the wrist joint and the hand will be described.

External Fixation in Fractures of the Humerus

The treatment of humeral fractures with an external fixator even today, is unusual, although some authors (De Bastiani 1984,[1] Ruland 1997)[2] have reported quite good results with this technique. One reason why external fixation in this part of the body is unpopular would appear to be the fear of damaging important nerves and vessels. Another reason is that many fixator systems on the market are not suitable for the use in the upper arm. This is especially true of fixators based on the Ilizarov ring design, not least because they severely compromise comfort by not permitting the patient to rest the arm on the chest for a long period of time.

A major advantage of external fixation over plaster casts is mobility of the adjacent joints. It is self evident that whenever possible fixator screws should not be inserted through muscle bellies which are necessary to allow early active mobilization. In the humerus dorsal or ventral screw placement would severely hinder the elbow joint activity and would inevitably lead to pin track infection. In the humerus, therefore, a lateral approach is advisable.

Subcapital and supracondylar fractures cannot be treated with external fixation. At the proximal and distal ends of the humerus there must be at least enough space to insert two fixator screws. Fig. 12.1 shows fracture zones which can be treated with external fixation and possible screw positions. The black areas in the drawing indicate advantageous screw positions. The grey areas indicate that screw implantation is possible but less favourable. White means that screw insertion should not be attempted in this area. It is thus clear that fractures in the area between the black fields are best suited for external fixation. These are fractures in the distal half of humerus between the insertion zone of the deltoid muscle and the supracondylar region.

Fractures Distal to the Deltoid Tuberosity

Fractures distal to the deltoid tuberosity enable ideal pin positions to be used. The proximal pin group can be inserted into the humerus from its lateral side at the region of the deltoid insertion (Position 1 in Fig. 12.1), the distal pin group can be inserted into the distal humerus in the area of the lateral epicondyle (Position 2 in Fig. 12.1).

The Proximal Pin Group

The region of insertion of the deltoid muscle can be recognized in the X-ray as a slightly prominent rough

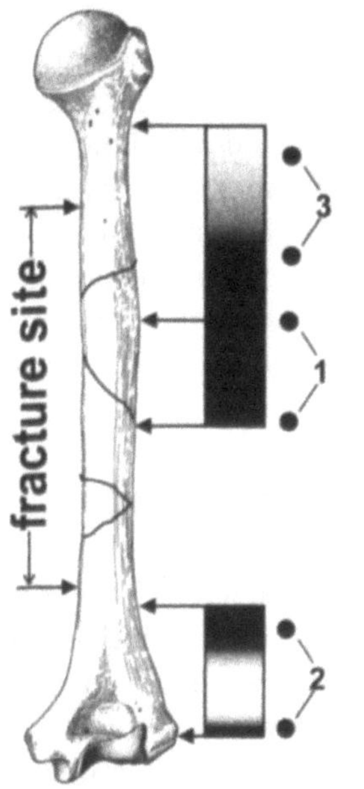

Fig. 12.1 Dorsal aspect of the humerus. On the right side positions for the fixator screws are indicated. Black areas are favourable whereas grey and white areas are less favourable. The arrows on the left side mark the proximal and distal borders for fractures which can be treated with external fixation.

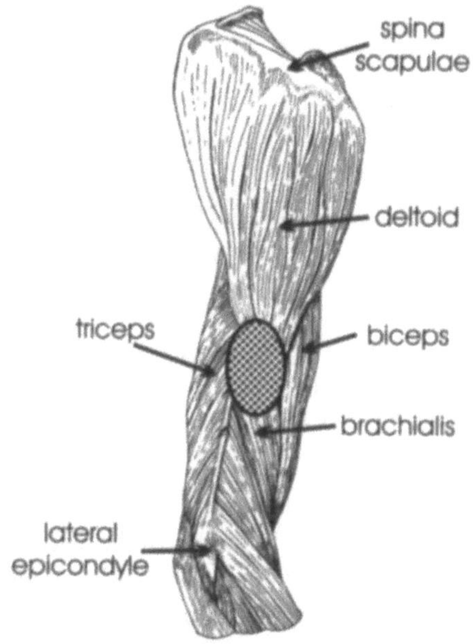

Fig. 12.2 Lateral aspect of the upper arm. The stippled area at the insertion of the deltoid muscle between the lateral triceps and the brachialis muscle indicates a "sweet spot" where the bone can be palpated through the skin. In this area the radial nerve is on the dorsal side of the humerus.

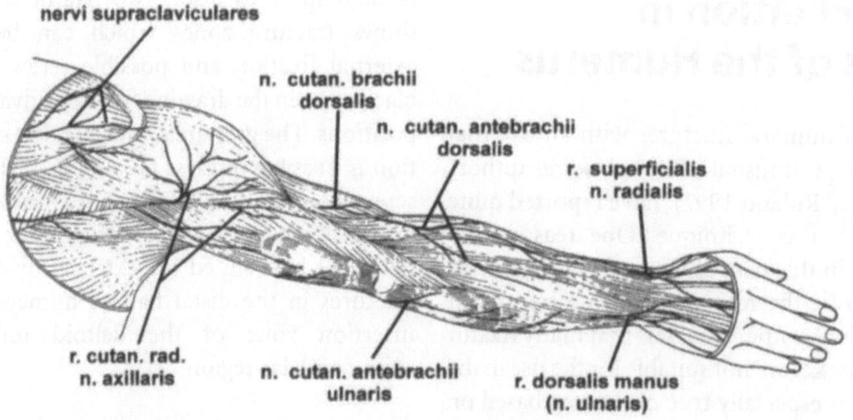

Fig. 12.3 Distribution of the sensory skin branches on the dorso-lateral aspect of the arm.

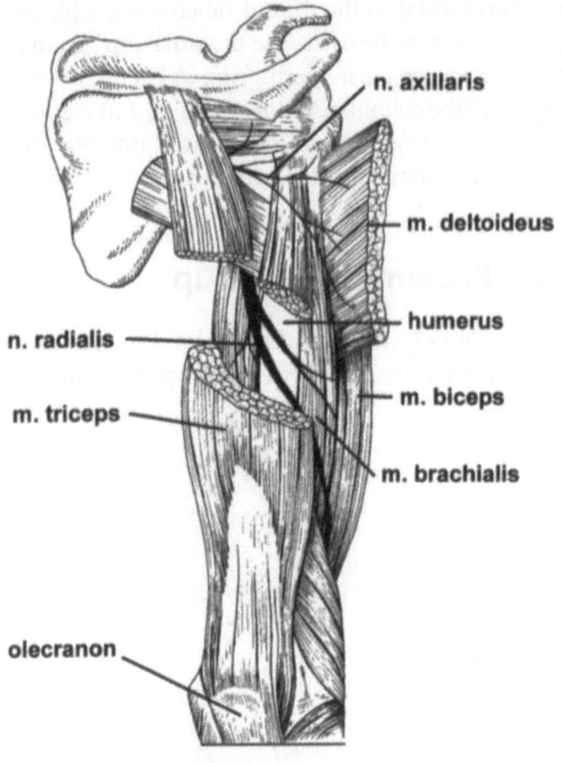

Fig. 12.4 Dorsal aspect of the upper arm with the middle third of the triceps removed. The radial nerve runs in a spiral groove over the dorsal aspect of the humerus.

area, the deltoid tuberosity. It is situated in the midshaft region of the humerus. In the living subject a "sweet spot" can be palpated at the distal end of the deltoid between the ventrally arising brachialis muscle and the lateral belly of the triceps (Fig. 12.2). Because of the thin soft tissue envelope in this area screw insertion is simple and secure. There is enough space between the main flexor belly (biceps) and the extensor (lateral triceps belly) to ensure that active movement of the elbow joint is not compromised. Only muscle fibres at the very origin of the brachialis muscle are affected by the screws in this position.

The skin incision should be at least 3 to 4cm long. With an adequate preparation technique and blunt dissection of the subcutaneous fat layer the sensory cutaneous nerves to the lateral aspect of the upper arm (Fig. 12.3) can be safely preserved. Drill and screw sleeves should be used. If necessary, the bone surface can be exposed using Langenbeck hooks. On the dorsal side of the humerus Hohman hooks are strictly prohibited. In the midshaft region of the humerus the radial nerve – running from its proximal and medial origin in a spiral-like dorsal bone groove to the lateral side – is located on the dorsal side of the shaft (Fig. 12.4). Damage to the radial nerve, therefore, is not likely. If there is any doubt, however, or if the screws need to be inserted more distally, exposure of the bone surface in this area is an easy and safe procedure. Predrilling of the screw holes must be performed carefully since on the medial side the main nerve and vessel route runs close to the bone. Use of a drill stop is recommended.

The Distal Pin Group

Insertion of the distal screws is more complicated. The typical shape of the distal humerus must be taken into account and the screws should not irritate the capsulo-ligamenteous apparatus of the elbow joint. With a careful operative technique, however, secure placement can be achieved. Fig. 12.5 shows cross-sections through the distal humerus. It is clear that insertion of a screw in the area of the olecranon fossa is not advisable as it may lead to damage of the joint capsule (Fig. 12.6a) and may hinder full extension, with the

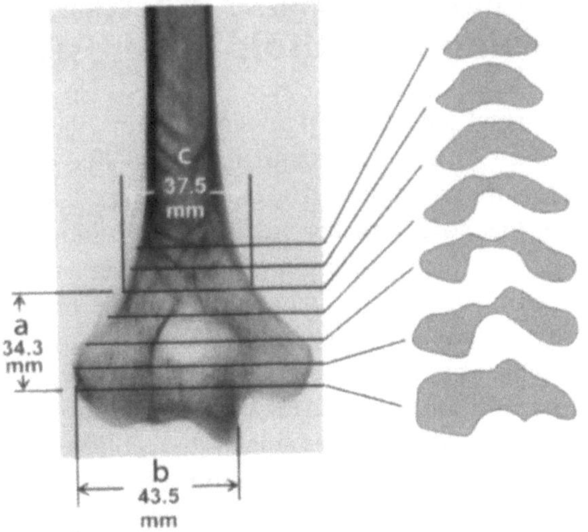

Fig. 12.5 AP X-ray of the distal humerus. Slices cut out of the distal humerus are shown on the right side. The most distal slice is cut out of the humeral condyles – the most distal site for a fixator screw. The more proximal screw of the distal group must be inserted proximal to the olecranon fossa at a mean distance of 34.3mm from the distal screw (see Table 12.1).

olecranon abutting against the screw. Screw insertion should start with most distal screw close to the joint line (Fig. 12.1). Its position is determined by the origin of the lateral collateral ligament (Fig. 12.6b). This screw position is indicated in the drawing (Figs. 12.1, 12.5, 12.6a, 12.6b, 12.7). A more distal insertion would severely hinder flexion and extension of the elbow joint. It is first recommended to insert a K-wire of 1.6mm diameter free hand, and to control the position of this wire under image intensification before the screw hole is predrilled. The second, proximal screw is then inserted at the cranial border of the olecranon fossa. The cross-sections of the humerus in this area (Fig. 12.5) show a more triangular shape. The screw should enter the bone at its radial edge. The average thread lengths required for the distal and proximal screws and the requisite distance between them are noted in Fig. 12.5 and Table 12.1.

Damage to the radial nerve would not be expected since in this area the nerve is already on the ventral side of the bone between the brachialis muscle and the extensor muscle group to the forearm. The "free space" in the distal humerus is indicated in Fig. 12.8. The risk of damage to the radial nerve increases substantially 6cm proximal to the radial epicondyle. Care must be taken not to injure the sensory branch of the radial nerve (n. cutaneous antebrachii lateralis) which reaches the subcutaneous fat layer in the area of the lateral elbow joint. Since the insertion of fixator screws in the area of the elbow joint does not offer much scope for variation it is recommended that the distal pin group is inserted first followed by the proximal screws according to the direction of the distal screws. Fig. 12.1 (Positions 1 and 2) are the ideal positions for the distal and proximal pin groups in fractures distal to the deltoid tuberosity.

	a (mm)	b (mm)	c (mm)
N	16	16	16
mean value	34.3	43.5	37.5
stdev	2.4	2.6	3.4
min	30.0	37.8	30.2
max	38.4	46.8	41.4

Table 12.1 Thread lengths for distal screw cluster in the humerus: b = distal screw thread length; c = proximal screw thread length; a = distance between screws. Minimum, maximum and mean values from 16 cadaveric specimens in each case.

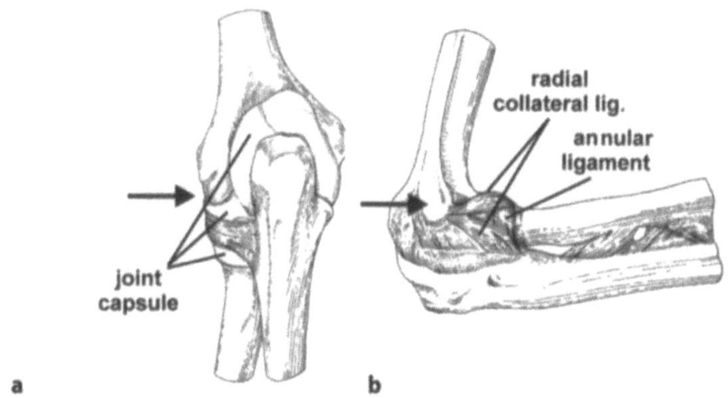

Fig.12.6 **a** Dorsal aspect of the elbow joint. The joint capsule is filled with fluid to elucidate the border of the capsule. The black arrow indicates the position of a fixator screw through the humeral condyles. **b** Lateral aspect of the elbow joint. The soft tissues have been removed except for the collateral ligaments. The black arrow indicates the position of a fixator screw through the humeral condyles.

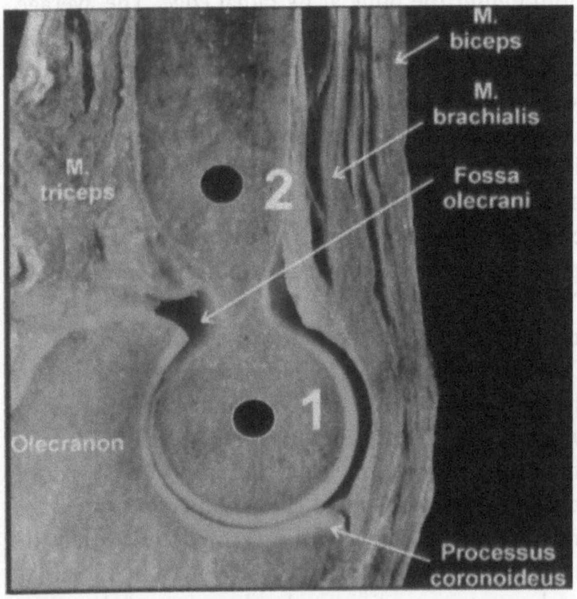

Fig. 12.7 Sagittal section through the elbow joint. The black points indicate the position of the fixator screws. Position 1 is in the centre of the condyles, position 2 just proximal to the fossa olecrani (with kind permission of Prof. Dr J. Koebke, Anatomical Institute, University of Cologne, Germany)

Proximal Fractures or Fractures Involving the Deltoid Tuberosity

As discussed above it is not possible to move the distal pin group to a more proximal position due to the course of the radial nerve. The position of the distal pin group, therefore, remains unchanged (Position 1 in Fig. 12.1). The proximal pin group however must be inserted more proximally according to the fracture site (Position 3 in Fig. 12.1). Unavoidably, the biomechanical conditions are less favorable with an increased distance between the fixator pin groups. This distance should be kept as small as possible with the proximal screws inserted as close to the fracture site as possible. It was demonstrated earlier that the ideal area for screw placement is the region of insertion of the deltoid muscle. Inserting screws more proximally would mean transfixing the deltoid muscle belly. Fig. 12.9 is a coronal section of the proximal humerus demonstrating the increased thickness of the muscle belly and the position of the circumflex artery. Although it is possible to place the fixator screws close to the head of the humerus (at least in the subcapital region), this will increase the risk of pin track infections. Note the posi-

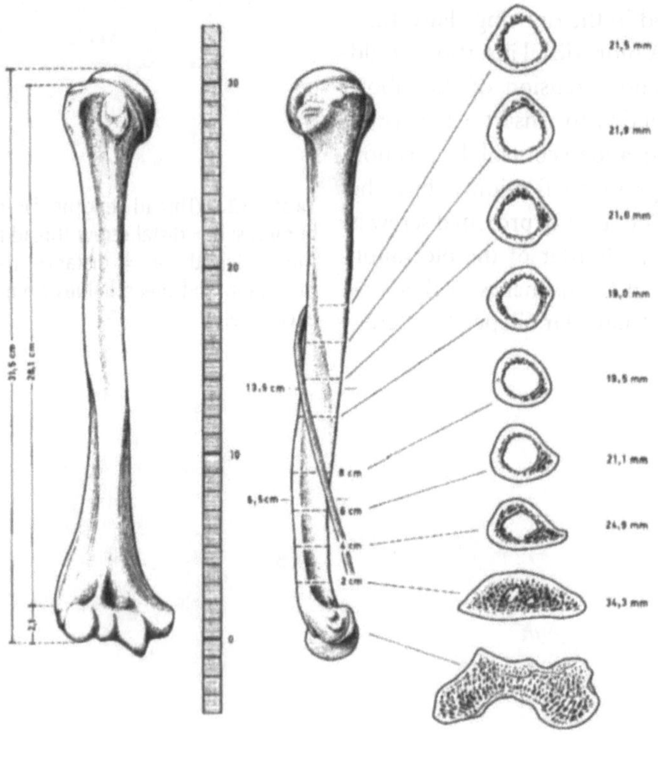

Fig. 12.8 Anterior and lateral aspects of the humerus. The course of the radial nerve is shown on the lateral aspect. It crosses the dorsal border of the humerus at about 13.5cm and the ventral border of the bone at about 6.5cm as measured from the lateral epicondyle. On the right side, slices are shown through different levels of the humerus with the mean latero-medial bone diameter at each level.

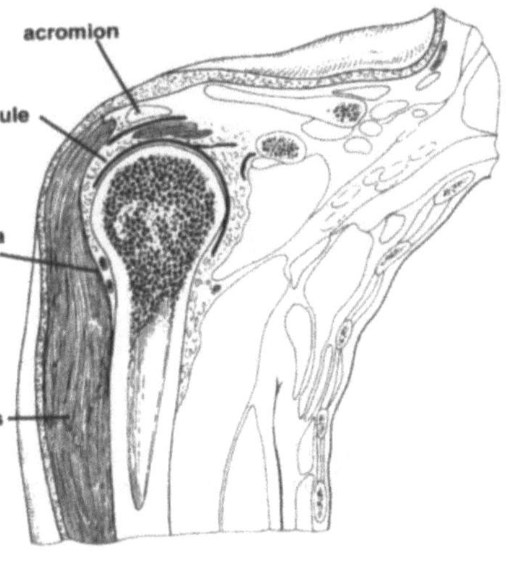

Fig. 12.9 Frontal section through the proximal humerus. Note the position of the nutrient arteries in the subcapital region and the increased size of the deltoid muscle belly in this area.

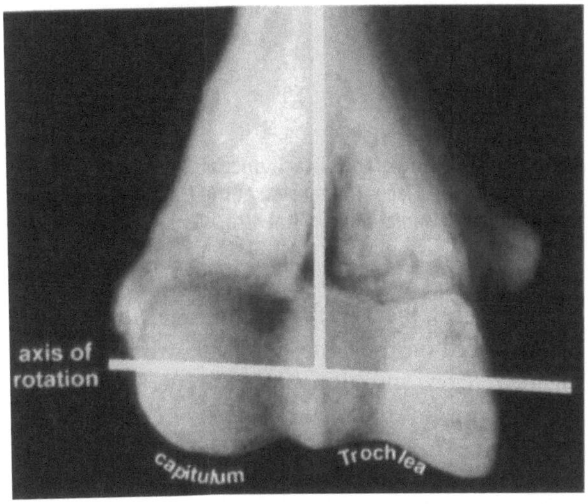

Fig. 12.10 Anterior aspect of the distal humerus. The vertical line indicates the long bone axis. The horizontal line indicates the axis of rotation of the elbow joint.

tion of the nutrient arteries of the humeral head and the narrow layer of fat between the proximal deltoid belly and the humerus in Fig. 12.9, indicating a relative movement between muscle and bone. According to Ruland (1997)[2] the proximal pin group in this case should be inserted more ventro-dorsally at the ventral edge of the deltoid. In this position the risk of damage to the axillary nerve which enters the deltoid belly from the dorsal side is minimal. The course of the axillary nerve is shown in Fig. 12.4.

External Fixation in Dislocations and Fracture Dislocations of the Elbow

Recently joint-bridging fixator systems with motion capacity have been developed for the treatment of dislocations and fracture dislocations of the elbow joint. The anatomical construction of the elbow joint seems ideal in this respect, since from a surgical point of view, the movement between humerus and ulna can be considered as a simple hinge movement. The axis of rotation runs through the centre of the capitulum and the trochlea taking a slightly oblique course according to the carrying angle between humerus and ulna (Fig. 12.10). Clearly, the mechanical hinge incorporated in the fixator must be aligned with the axis of rotation and, therefore, the fixator application is lateral. This is in accordance with the previously discussed lateral approach to the humerus which is most appropriate for screw placement. The humeral pin group can be inserted in the region of the deltoid tuberosity as shown in Fig. 12.1 (Position 1) and Fig. 12.2. In this position the fixator screws are far enough from the injured elbow joint but close enough to provide mechanical stability.

The Ulnar Pin Group

The joint-bridging design of these fixators is based on a proximal pin group in the humerus and a distal pin group in the ulna. Approaching the humerus from the lateral side with the hinge of the fixator system aligned with the rotational axis of the elbow joint also implies insertion of the ulnar screws from the lateral side. From a purely anatomical and topographical standpoint it would be advantageous to use the dorsal side of the ulna for pin placement. This part of the bone can be palpated through the skin over its total length from the olecranon to the ulnar head with no muscles, nerves or vessels between skin and bone surfaces. A unilateral fixator system does not, however, allow insertion of the distal pin group in a totally different direction from that of the proximal screws. But the main disadvantage with screws inserted from the dorsal side into the ulna is discomfort, since the patient is not able to place the arm on a table or a chair rest during the entire period of treatment, and it is patient acceptability which determines the success of a treatment. Lateral insertion of fixator screws into the ulna requires some accuracy. Previous anatomical studies (Gausepohl et al 1997)[3] have demonstrated that the midshaft region of the ulna

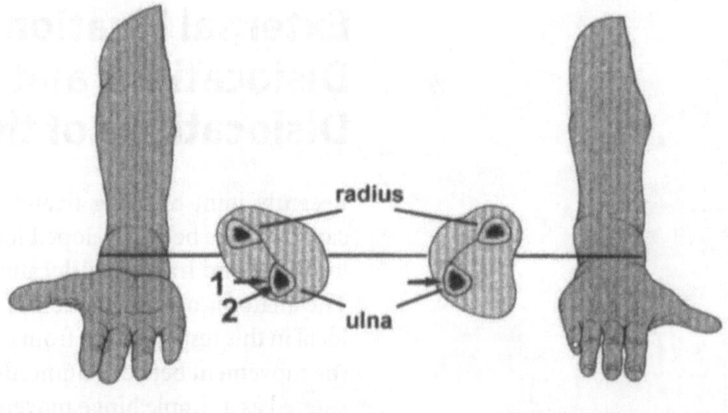

Fig. 12.11 Forearm in pro- and supination. The sections in the frontal plane in pro- and supination demonstrate the movement of the soft tissues during forearm rotation. The black arrows 1 and 2 indicate the direction for fixator screw insertion.

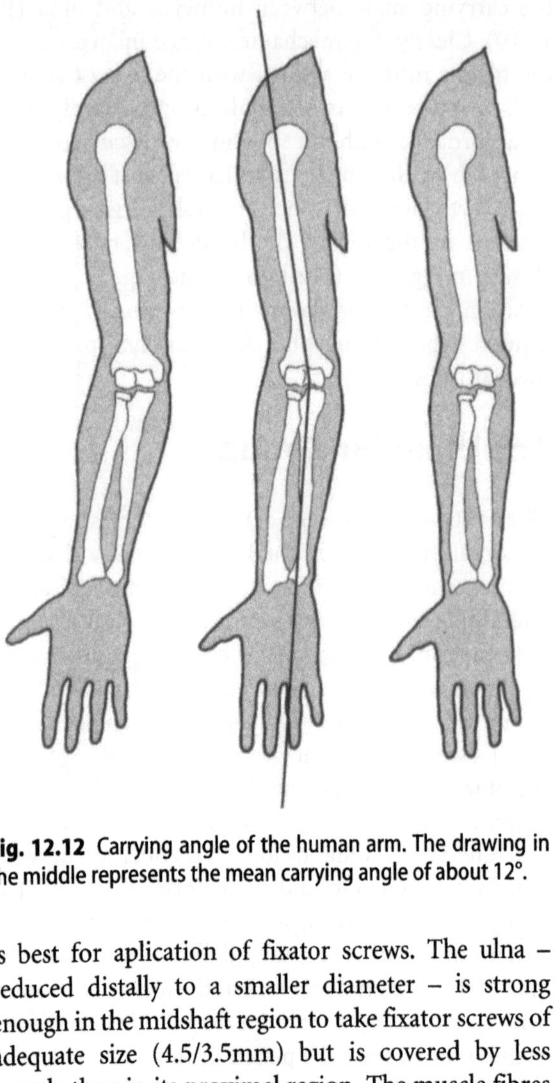

Fig. 12.12 Carrying angle of the human arm. The drawing in the middle represents the mean carrying angle of about 12°.

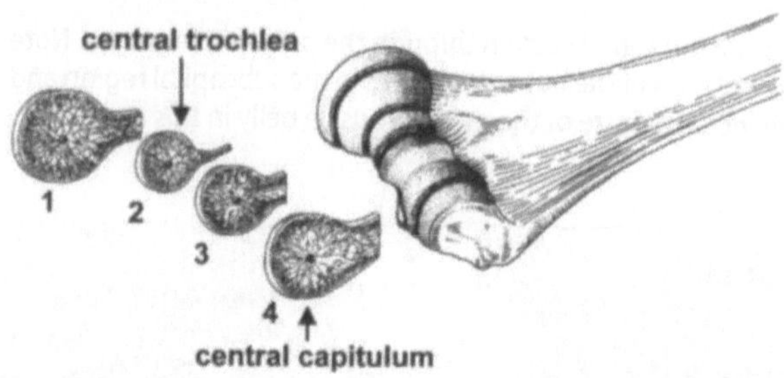

Fig. 12.13 Drawing of the distal humerus. 2mm slices were cut out of the joint surface. 1 ulnar side of the trochlea, 2 centre of the trochlea; 3 radial side of the trochlea; 4 centre of the capitulum.

is best for aplication of fixator screws. The ulna – reduced distally to a smaller diameter – is strong enough in the midshaft region to take fixator screws of adequate size (4.5/3.5mm) but is covered by less muscle than in its proximal region. The muscle fibres (mainly fibres of the extensor carpi ulnaris and the flexor digitorum profundus) originating from the dorsolateral aspect of the ulnar midshaft can easily be pushed aside and the bone surface exposed. There is no nerve or vessel route on this side of the bone but, as in the upper arm, the use of protective screw/drill guides firmly placed on the bone surface is strongly recommended. Screw insertion should be performed with the forearm in the neutral position or in slight pronation. The cross-section in Fig. 12.11 demonstrates the shifting of the forearm muscle bellies with supination and pronation. In pronation there is much less muscle overlying the bone surface. During pro- and supination the radius always stays anterior to the ulna (Fig. 12.11). A humero-ulnar fixator with screws introduced from the lateral side does not, therefore, hinder forearm rotation. In very strong individuals, it is sometimes of advantage to insert the screws at an angle of 10° to 15° dorsally (Fig. 12.11) to prevent the soft tissues rubbing against the screws in full supination. The main step in the operative technique for a joint-bridging fixator with motion capacity is to determine the axis of rotation. Because the injury pattern in dislocations and fracture dislocations displays a high level of instability, the ulna itself and its movement around the humeral trochlea is of no use in determining the centre of rotation. This determination must rely only on the shape of the humeral condyles.

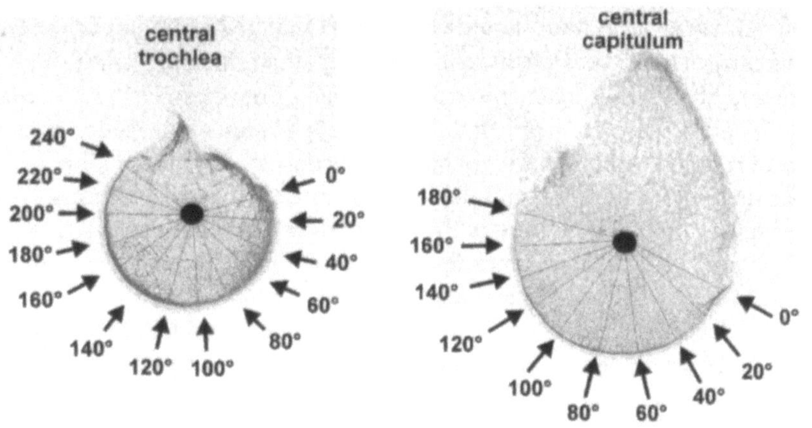

Fig. 12.14 Example of two slices according to Fig. 12.13. The slice on the left side is the central part of the trochlea. The slice on the right side shows the central part of the capitulum. The black point indicates the centre of the circle formed by the joint surface. The joint surface is divided into sectors of 20°. For each of the sectors the true centre was calculated and the radius determined.

In spite of the fact that the main bony movement occurs between the humerus and the ulna, the axis of rotation runs through both the humero-ulna and the humero-radial joints (Fig. 12.10). The latter should not be neglected since a considerable part of the force transmission passes through this joint and thus the radial head plays a major role as a primary stabilizer of the joint. This is mirrored by the frequent involvement of the radial head in the typical injury pattern with subcapital or chisel fractures accompanying dislocations of the elbow joint. If we look at the normal configuration of the elbow joint with a carrying angle of 12°–15° (Fig. 12.12) it is easy to understand that sudden axial pressure, as occurs in a fall on the outstretched arm, will exert distraction forces on the ulnar side and compression forces on the radial side. Placement of the hinge axis of the fixator should take this injury pattern into account, and when applying the fixator it is advisable to allow for a little distance between the humeral capitulum and the radial head to protect the damaged cartilage during the recovery period. In spite of anatomical studies which have demonstrated that the actual movement between humerus and ulna cannot exactly be described as a simple hinge movement but that there are some additional components which allow minimal changes in the position of the flexion and extension axis, from a surgical point of view this is of minor interest. Recent studies from Morrey (1990),[4] London (1991)[5] and our own results have proved that the centre of rotation changes only minimally. Furthermore, the injury pattern must be taken into account. In dislocations or fracture dislocations most of the ligamentous structures are torn with no true guidance provided by the relative positions of the bones. Although the artificially

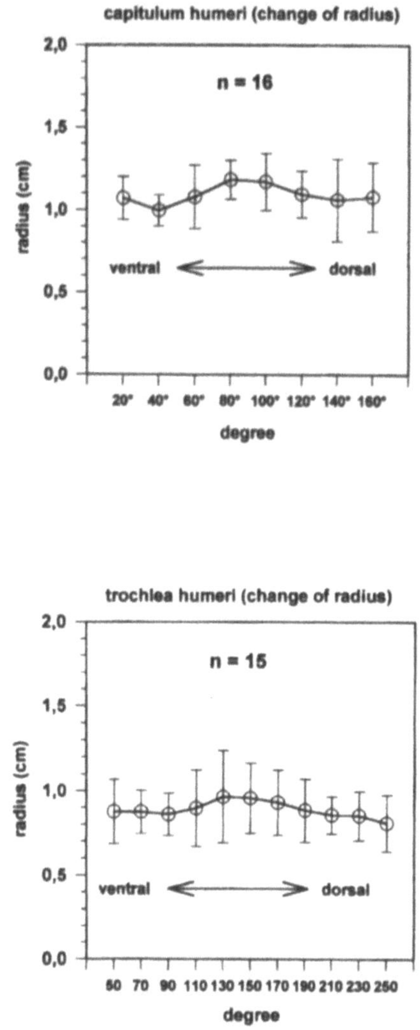

a

b

Fig. 12.15 **a** Diagram demonstrating the change in radius of the capitulum humeri according to Fig. 12.14. **b** Diagram demonstrating the change in radius of the trochlea humeri according to Fig. 12.14.

(by the surgeon) defined centre of rotation should be as close to the natural centre of rotation as possible it is indeed a new centre and the healing ligaments will arrange accordingly. Our own studies have shown that the theoretical centre of rotation running through the middle of the circular shaped trochlea and capitulum only moves in an area of 4 sq. mm in the centre of the condyles. Fig. 12.13 shows slices of 2mm thickness taken out of the centre of the capitulum (slice 4) and the trochlea (slice 2). To determine the instant centre of rotation, segments of 20° were defined along the entire cartilage covered surface (Fig. 12.14). The true instant centre of rotation and the length of the radius was calculated for each of these segments. The graphs in Fig. 12.15 demonstrate the change in the radius for the 2mm slices taken out of the capitulum and the middle part of the trochlea. (unpublished data). There is only a very small change in the length of the calculated radius within the rotational axis. In general it can be seen that in the middle part of the joint the radius is greater than in the ventral or dorsal parts. The schematic drawing in Fig. 12.16 explains this finding. If after application of the fixator the joint is kept in slight distraction to prevent the joint surfaces from rubbing against each other and as a prophylaxis against secondary shrinking of the scar tissue, this change in the rotational centre will be more than compensated for (Fig. 12.16).

To define the centre of rotation intraoperatively, an exact lateral view must be obtained with the image intensifier (Fig. 12.17). The radial and ulnar joint surfaces overlap with a circular shape. The largest circle is formed by the ulnar side of the trochlea (1 in Fig. 12.17). The middle part of the trochlea and the capitulum humeri are of nearly equal size and should symmetrically overlap each other (2 and 3 in Fig. 12.17). The K-wire used to mark the axis of rotation should project as a point in the centre of both circles. This wire normally forms an acute angle with the long axis of the humerus according to the individual carrying angle (Figs. 12.10 and 12.12).

On a lateral X-ray the two humeral fixator screws are in line with the rotational axis of the elbow joint.

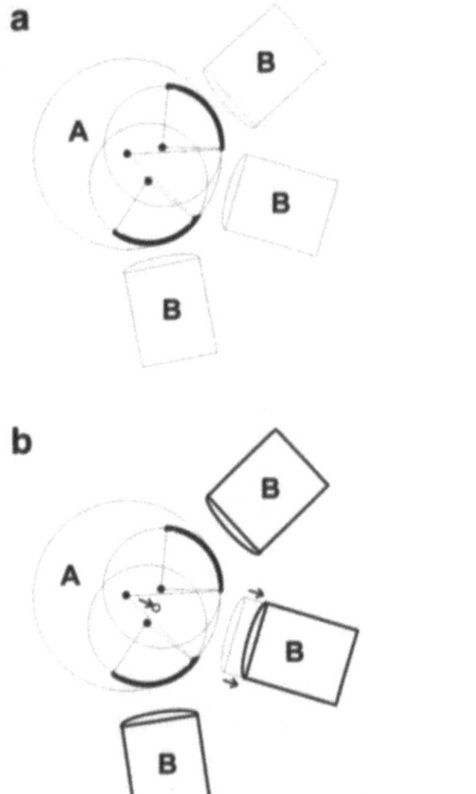

Fig. 12.16 a Schematic drawing. The joint surface in A has 3 different rotational centres. The radius of the middle sector is larger than the others. B is the joint partner. **b** After determination of the rotational centre and application of the fixator a minimal distraction of 1 or 2mm is performed to separate the joint surfaces from one another. The distraction should be performed in a mid-position between flexion and extension.

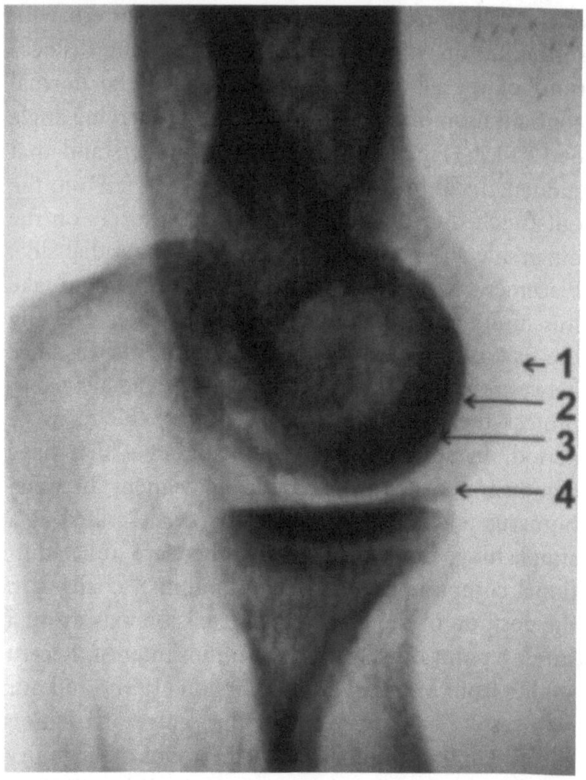

Fig. 12.17 Lateral X-ray of the elbow joint. The circular shaped condyles are symmetrically overlapping each other. **1** ulnar side of the trochlea humeri, **2** outline of the capitulum humeri; **3** outline of the central trochlea; **4** tip of the coronoid process.

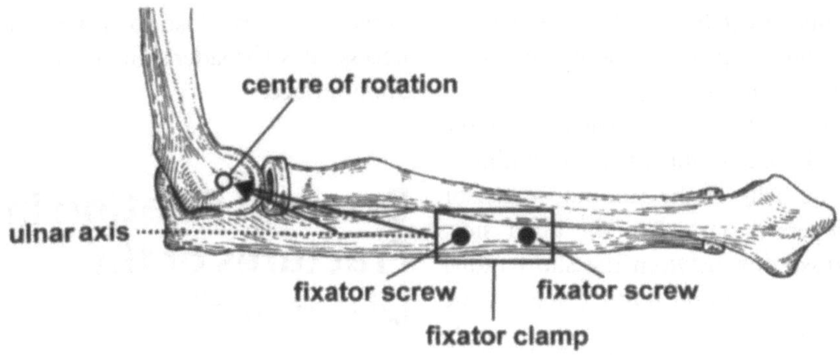

Fig. 12.18 Lateral aspect of the forearm. The position of the fixator clamp and screws in the ulna is indicated. The axis of the ulna lies dorsal to the centre of rotation. The black arrows show the increasing angulation of the fixator module as the fixator clamp is positioned closer to the elbow joint.

The axis of the ulnar shaft lies dorsal to the centre of rotation (Fig. 12.18). It is important to appreciate this because the fixator screws in the ulna must both be inserted through the middle of the bone to achieve maximum purchase. The fixator module coupled to the fixator clamp has then to be angled according to the distance of the fixator screws from the centre of rotation. The closer to the elbow joint the screws are inserted the greater will be the angulation between clamp and ulnar module (Fig. 12.18)

External Fixation in Fractures of the Forearm

Shaft fractures of the forearm are rarely treated with external fixation. A somewhat prolonged healing time requires a longer period of external fixation. The mobility of the elbow joint, which allows not only a wide range of flexion and extension but also a forearm rotation of 160°, results in extensive movement of the soft tissues with most of the muscles crossing two joints. This extensive movement of the soft tissues especially in the proximal forearm is the reason for an increased number of pin track infections which affects the pins in the proximal radius more than those in the ulna. As previously discussed, screw insertion into the ulna can be performed either from the dorsal or the lateral side since there are few muscles covering the bone surface. The proximal radius, in contrast, is totally surrounded by muscles. In the middle and distal thirds of the bone, however, it is possible to find a safety corridor for screw insertion.

In the living subject the dorso-radial position of the extensor muscle group originating at the radial epicondyle of the humerus can easily be recognized with the muscles in tension. These muscles change their position considerably relative to the radius in pronation and supination. Although not recom-

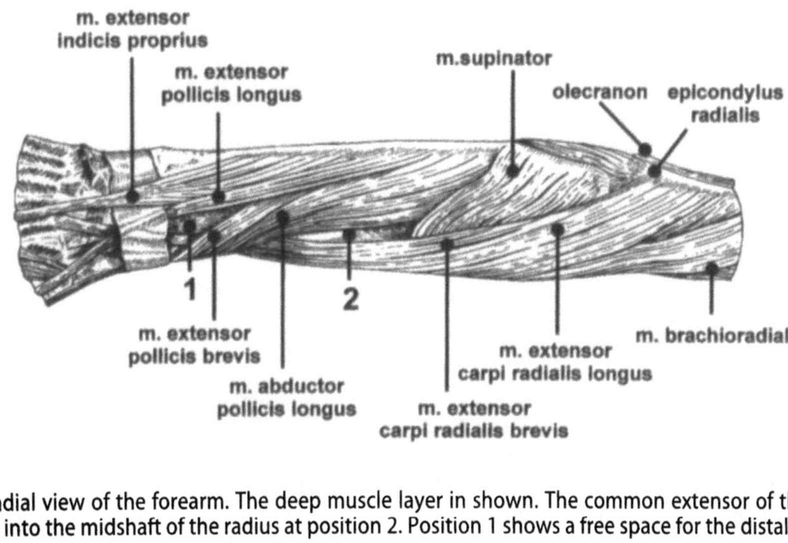

Fig. 12.19 Dorsoradial view of the forearm. The deep muscle layer in shown. The common extensor of the fingers is removed. Screw implantation into the midshaft of the radius at position 2. Position 1 shows a free space for the distal screw.

mended as a routine procedure, if there is a need, insertion of screws into the proximal radius should be performed from the radial side.

In the midshaft region the best approach is from the dorsoradial side in the area of the musculo-tendinous transition zone. The belly of the common extensor muscle for the fingers is pushed to the ulnar side. Following blunt dissection between the short radial wrist extensor and the common finger extensor, the underlying deep layer of the extensor muscles permits insertion of fixator screws between the belly of the abductor pollicis longus and the extensor carpi radialis brevis (Fig. 12.19). The cross-section in Fig. 12.20 demonstrates the safe corridor to the midshaft region of the radius. Note the position of the superficial branch of the radial nerve.

At its distal end the soft tissue envelope of the forearm thins out, with most of the muscles reaching the wrist joint with their tendons. Fig. 12.21 shows the safety corridors to the distal third of the radius. On the dorsal side proximal to Lister's tubercle a trapezoid shaped area free from tendons, nerves and vessels is bordered on the ulnar side by the tendon of the extensor pollicis longus and on the radial side by the tendons of the extensor carpi radialis brevis et longus. The proximal border of this area is formed by the muscle belly of the extensor pollicis brevis (Fig. 12.21). While screw implantation on the dorsal surface of the distal radius is a safe procedure there is another tendon free space more radially. This triangular shaped space – illustrated in Fig. 12.21 – is bordered on the ulnar side by the tendons of the extensor carpi radialis muscles and on the radial side by the tendon of the extensor pollicis brevis. The superficial branch of the radial nerve runs very close to this space (Fig. 12.21) and necessitates a broader skin incision and exposure of the bone surface.

External Fixation in Fractures of the Distal Radius

Extra-articular (Periarticular) Fractures

AO-type A2 or A3 fractures, and in some special cases even type C2.1 fractures, can be treated by external fixation with a radio-radial assembly – i.e. not bridging the wrist joint. The distal pin group is then inserted into the distal fragment if it is long enough to take the screws. The integrity of the dorsal surface at the level of Lister's tubercle should be assessed with the image intensifier. The proximal pin group is inserted from the dorsoradial side using the safety corridor described above, between the bellies of extensor digitorum communis and abductor pollicis longus on the ulnar side and extensor carpi radialis brevis on the radial side (Figs. 12.19 and 12.20). Insertion of fixator screws close to the radio-carpal joint line presupposes a detailed knowledge of the tendon sheaths and the bone dimensions at the very distal end of the radius. In Fig. 12.21 and in the cross-section in Fig. 12.22b the topography of the tendons close to radio-carpal joint line is shown. The cross-sections in Fig. 12.22a,b through Lister's tubercle show the orientation of the fixator screws, both inserted parallel to the joint line. It is not a problem to insert one screw through or a little proxi-

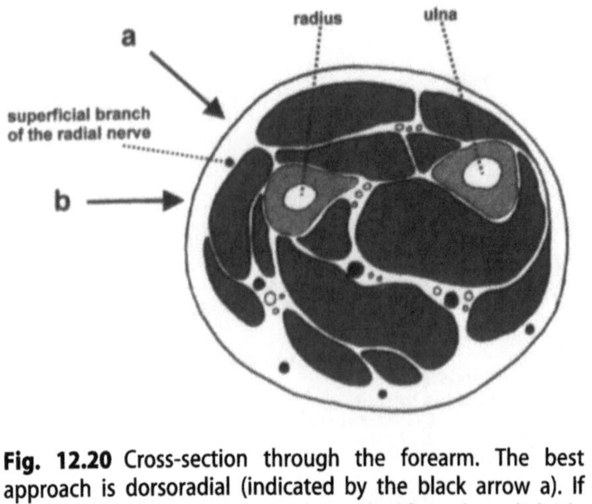

Fig. 12.20 Cross-section through the forearm. The best approach is dorsoradial (indicated by the black arrow a). If necessary the fixator screws can be applied from the radial side (arrow b). Note the position of the superficial branch of the radial nerve.

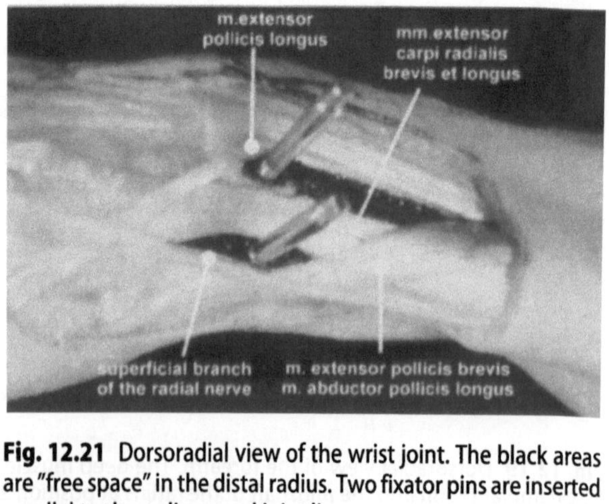

Fig. 12.21 Dorsoradial view of the wrist joint. The black areas are "free space" in the distal radius. Two fixator pins are inserted parallel to the radio-carpal joint line.

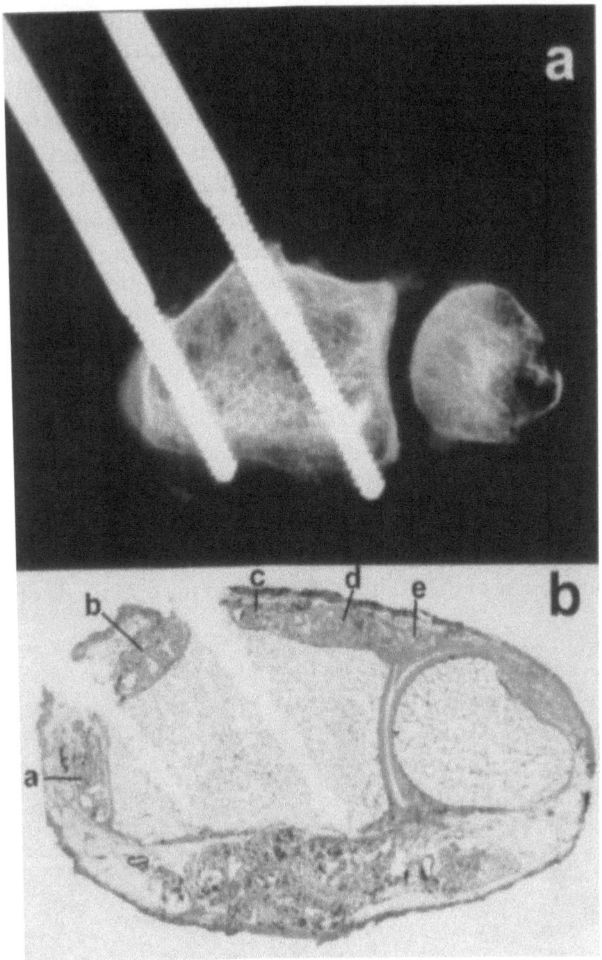

Fig. 12.22 Cross-sections through the distal radius at Lister's tubercle. Note the oblique direction of the screws which is necessary when inserting the fixator pins into the bone. a = m. extensor pollicis brevis; m. abductor pollicis longus; b = mm. extensor carpi radialis longus et brevis; c = m. extensor pollicis longus; d = m. extensor digitorum communis, m. extensor indicis proprius; e = m. extensor digiti minimi.

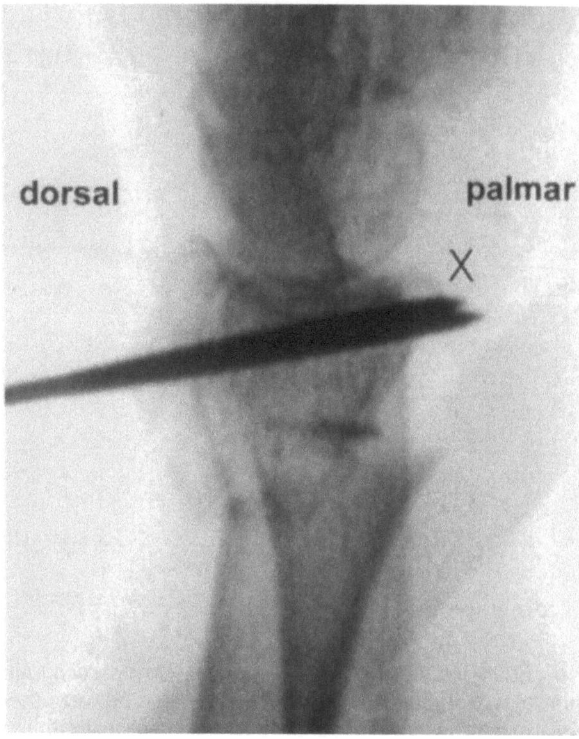

Fig. 12.23 Lateral X-ray of the distal radius and wrist joint. X = palmar lip of the radius. The pilot wires (= 1.6mm K-wires) are inserted from the dorsal surface, aiming for the palmar lip of the radius.

mal to Lister´s tubercle, but it is important to anchor the tip of the screw in the palmar lip of the radius (Fig. 12.23) because here, even in osteoporotic bone, the quality is good enough to permit secure fixation.

Screw insertion should be performed with the aid of an image intensifier and with the distal radius in a lateral position (Fig. 12.23). While the first scew is inserted at Lister´s tubercle, the second screw should be inserted radially. As demonstrated in Figs. 12.21 and 12.22 there is a "free" space between the carpal extensor tendons and the extensor pollicis brevis on the radial side, but both screws must be inserted in an oblique direction as demonstrated in Fig. 12.22. Fig. 12.22b shows a histological cross-section through the distal radius at Lister´s tubercle. The previously inserted fixator screws have already been removed. The "free" space between the tendon sheaths can be identified, making sure that the fibrous canal of the extensor tendons is not damaged. The incision at Lister´s tubercle can be small, provided that the tubercle is clearly identified. With swollen soft tissues in a fracture situation the tubercle can hardly be palpated. Anatomical measurements, however, have shown that the tubercle is almost always situated at the junction between the radial third and middle third of the distal forearm as shown in Fig. 12.24. The radial incision should be larger because the superficial branch of the radial nerve runs close to this area. Blunt dissection and the use of screw and drill guides are advisible to avoid damage to this important sensory nerve.

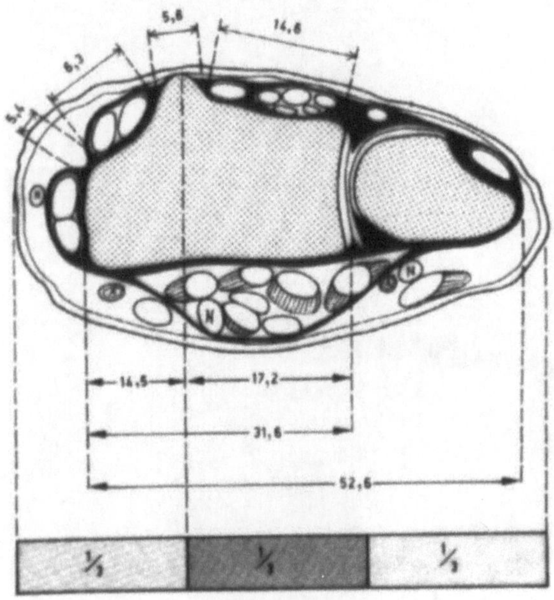

Fig. 12.24 Drawing from a histological cross-section. All intervals are in mm. Lister´s tubercle is situated between the radial and the middle thirds of the total cross-sectional width.

The proximal pin group is inserted into the radial diaphysis in the midshaft region. The dorsoradial screw direction as indicated in Fig. 12.20 should be aligned with that of the distal screws.

Corrective Osteotomies

Corrective osteotomies of the distal radius – especially where hemicallotasis is planned – require a different screw placeent. Pre-operative planing is necessary to determine screw direction. If the dorsal angle is to be corrected the fixator screws must be inserted in a dorso-palmar direction; if radial inclination is to be corrected the screws must be inserted from the radial side. The black arrows in Fig. 12.25 indicate the screw directions in each case. For a dorso-palmar insertion one screw can be inserted through Lister's tubercle as described in the previous section. Since the screw direction is dorso-plamar, however, the second screw must be inserted on the ulnar side of the radius parallel to the ulnar notch. This frequently necessitates opening the fourth extensor compartment which contains the common extensor tendons for the fingers and the extensor tendon for the index finger. Sometimes, however, it is possible to insert the screw between the fourth and fifth compartments (Fig. 12.25). In cases where a tendon in running close to the fixator screw the thread of the screw should be fully inserted into the bone such that the tendon only comes into contact with the polished shaft of the screw. Radial insertion of fixator screws as indicated in Fig. 12.25 is only possible with converging screws. One screw can be inserted dorsal to the extensor pollicis brevis tendon and the other palmar to the abductor pollicis longus tendon (Fig. 12.25). The use of the fixator in corrective osteotomies is more complicated than in acute fracture situations and should be reserved for specialist clinics.

Intra-articular Fractures

In intra-articular fractures of the distal radius the fixator bridges the joint. The distal pin group is inserted into the second metacarpal. The proximal and middle third of the second metacarpal are not overlaid by the extensor tendons to the index finger due to the converging course of the extensor tendons on the dorsal side of

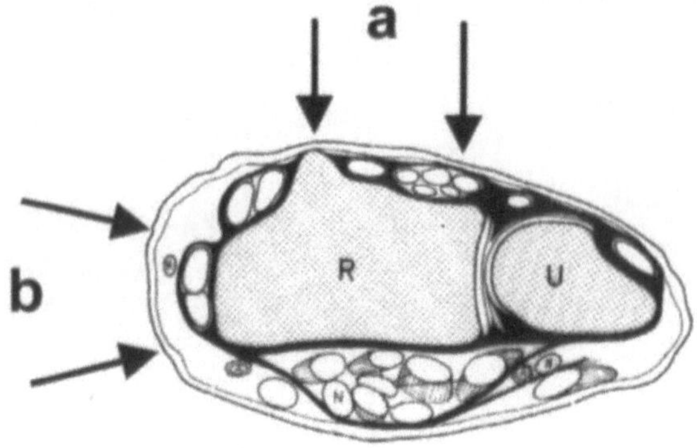

Fig. 12.25 Same drawing as Fig. 12.24. The black arrows indicate the screw insertion points for corrective osteotomies. **a** for correction of the dorsal angle; **b** for correction of radial inclination.

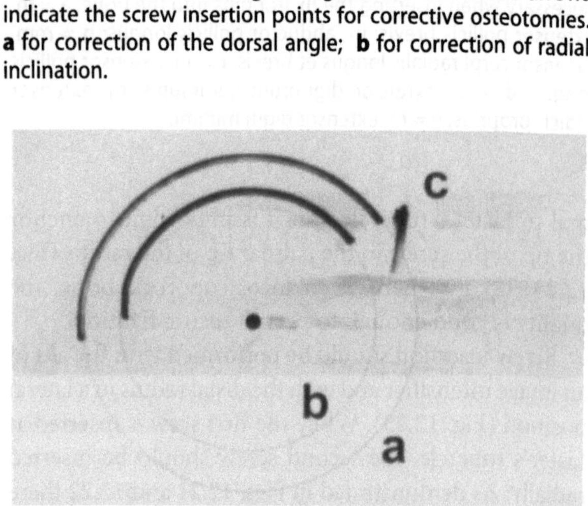

Fig. 12.26 Light trace experiment. A small lamp was attached to the end of a K-wire implanted into the lunate bone and the third metacarpal. Another lamp was fixed to the radius (**c**). **a** metacarpal movement; **b** lunate movement. The centre of both circles is indicated by a black dot and projects to the joint line between capitate and lunate. The wrist is in a neutral position between radial and ulnar deviation.

the hand towards the wrist joint. The fixator screws can therefore be inserted dorsally or dorsoradially. If a fixator which allows mobilization of the wrist joint in extension and flexion during treatment is used, the hinge axis of the fixator must be aligned with the flexion/extension axis of the wrist joint. It is not easy to define a clear flexion/extension axis in the wrist joint but the joint line between the capitate and the lunate bone can be considered as an approximate axis. The fixator hinge axis must therefore be aligned with this joint line perpendicular to the radial shaft. Successful mobilization can only be performed, however, if after reduction of the fracture the hand is in a neutral position between ulnar and radial deviation (Fig. 12.27). Light-trace experiments (unpublished data) provided evidence that flexion and extension of the wrist joint in the neutral position between ulnar and radial deviation defines a fairly constant centre of rotation projecting between capitate and lunate (Fig. 12.26). Aligning the fixator hinge with this axis allows flexion and extension to be performed without tension and therefore without risk of redislocation of the fracture. In ulnar or radial deviation of the wrist this axis changes markedly as indicated in Fig. 12.27. In such cases the wrist joint should not be mobilized until healed.

It is self-evident that the proximal pin group – inserted into the radial diaphysis – should be orientated according to the distal fixator screws. In the middle third of the forearm the superficial branch of the radial nerve (Figs. 12.3, 12.20) leaves the deep muscle layer to reach the wrist joint in the subcutaneous fat layer. Fixator screws in the radial diaphysis should not, therefore, be inserted percutaneously, in order to avoid damage to this important sensory nerve.

External Fixation in the Metacarpals

The use of external fixation in fractures of the metacarpal bones has gained popularity in the last decade. The main advantage of this technique – which in most cases can be performed percutaneously – is the minimal soft tissue damage produced. The gliding layers on the dorsal side of the hand are disturbed only at a few points where the fixator pins penetrate the skin. Extensive adhesions of the gliding layers which are frequently observed as late sequelae after extensive surgery are therefore prevented and the risk of stiffness in the finger joints less likely. But to insert fixator screws percutaneously a detailed knowledge of the anatomical positions of the extensor tendons is mandatory. Previously performed anatomical studies have defined safety corridors to the dorsum of the hand (Gausepohl et al 1998a, b). As demonstrated in Fig. 12.28 there is only minimal risk of transfixing the extensor tendon by percutaneous pin insertion into the second and fifth metacarpal bones. Due to the typical converging course of the tendons towards the wrist joint, especially in the second metacarpal bone, most of the dorsal surface is not overlaid by tendons. The fixator should be applied in a dorsoradial direction. In

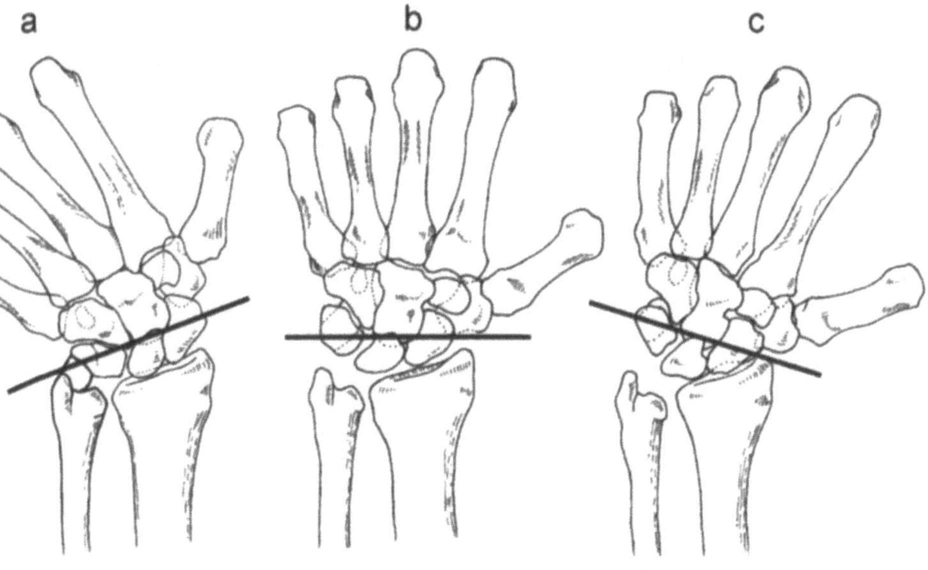

Fig. 12.27 Flexion and extension axis of the wrist joint. **b** = with the wrist joint in a neutral position the rotational axis is perpendicular to the long axis of the radius. **a, c** = The rotational axis changes markedly in ulnar or radial deviation.

the fifth metacarpal the extensor tendon runs on the dorsal side of the bone. The fixator can be applied from the ulnar side. A percutaneous approach to the third and fourth metacarpals is more critical because the pins must be introduced between the neighbouring extensor tendons. In the proximal third of the metacarpals, particularly, a "safety" corridor cannot be defined and a small stitch incision is sometimes unavoidable. Transfixion of the thin connexus intertendinei (Fig. 12.29) between the tendons of the common extensor muscles does not lead to severe loss of movement in the finger joints.

Fractures of the first metacarpal bone can also be treated with an external fixator and the fixator pins inserted percutaneously. As shown in Fig. 12.30 screws can enter the bone between the tendons of the dorsally located extensor pollicis longus and the extensor pollicis brevis and abductor pollicis longus on the palmar side. Even pin insertion on the palmar side of the abductor pollicis longus tendon is possible but this application is less desirable since the ability to rest the hand on a chair or table is compromised.

Fractures close to the base of the first metacarpal (i.e "Winterstein" type) can be stabilized in an extra-articular way, but in fractures involving the saddle joint (i.e. "Rolando" or "Bennett" type) the proximal fixator pins must be inserted into the trapezium (Fig. 12.31).

Although there is enough space in the trapezium to insert two converging fixator pins of adequate size, percutaneous application carries the risk of damage to the superficial branch of the radial nerve and the dorsal branch of the radial artery, both of which overlie the carpal bone in the region of the snuffbox (Figs. 12.30, 12.31).

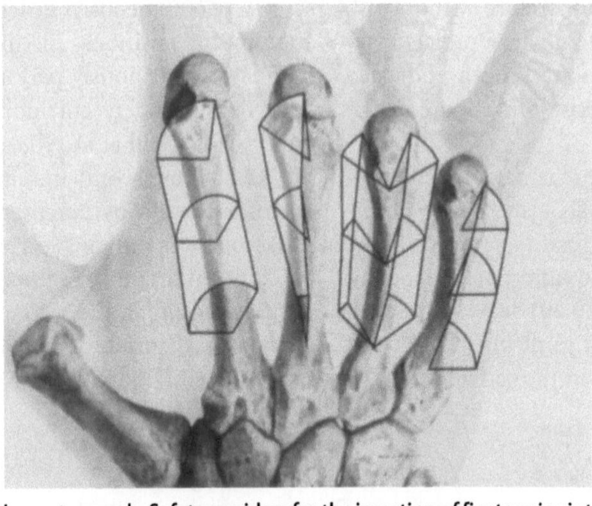

Fig. 12.28 Dorsal aspect of the metacarpals. Safety corridors for the insertion of fixator pins into the metacarpal bones are shown.

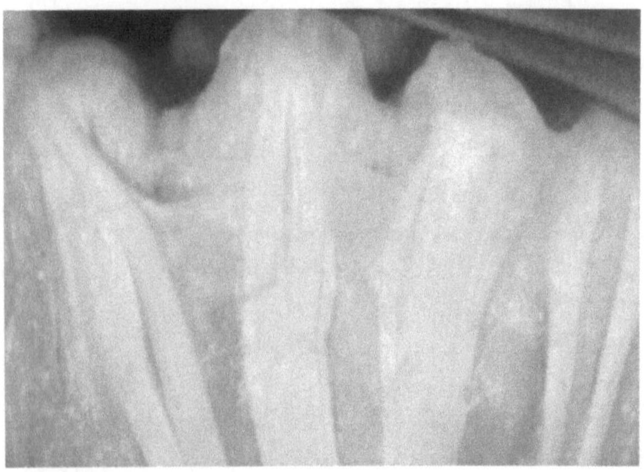

Fig. 12.29 Dorsal aspect of the metacarpus with the finger joints flexed. The skin is removed to demonstrate the position of the extensor tendons. Note the thin connexus intertendinei.

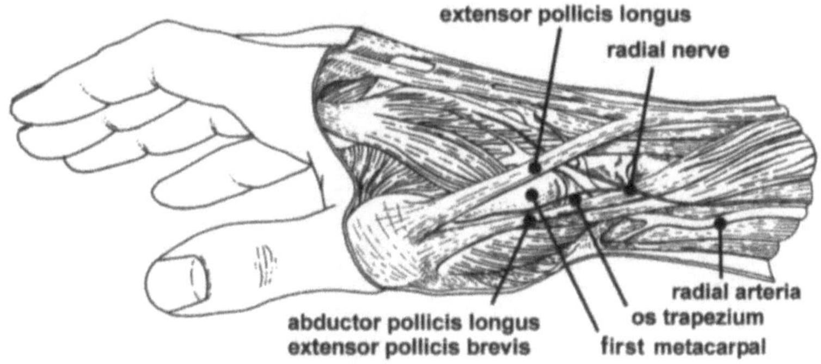

Fig. 12.30 Radial aspect of the wrist and first metacarpal. The skin is removed to demonstrate the "safety corridor" to the first metacarpal. Radial nerve and radial artery cross the trapezium in the snuffbox.

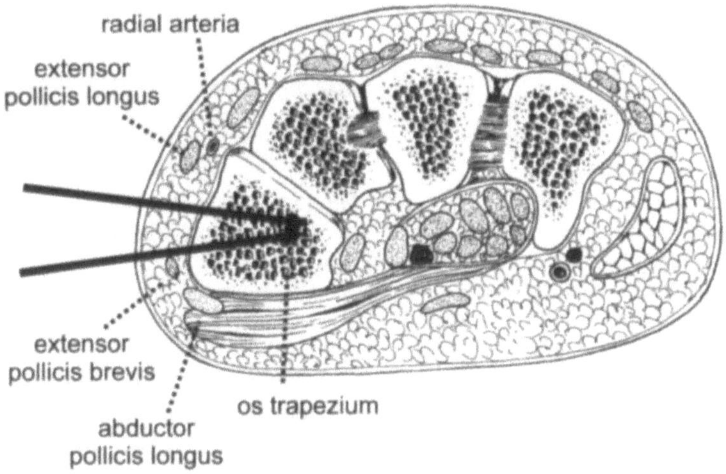

Fig. 12.31 Cross-section through the distal carpus to demonstrate the positions for screw placement in the trapezium.

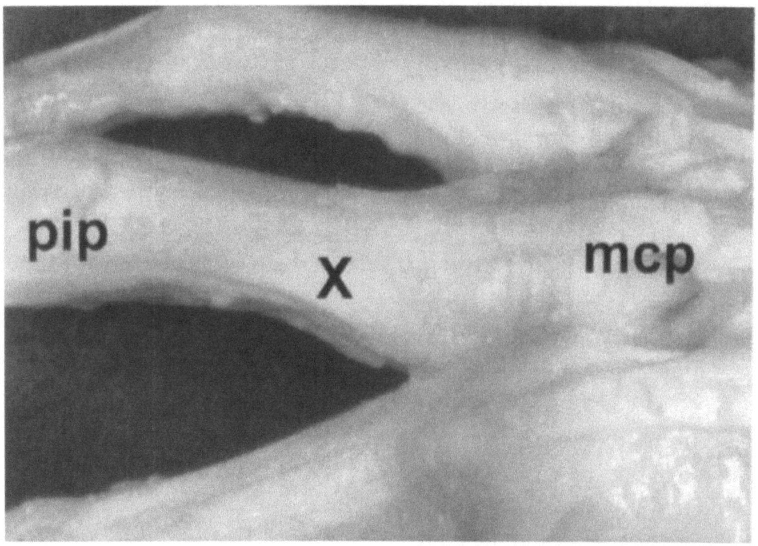

Fig. 12.32 Dorsolateral aspect of the ring finger. The skin has been removed to show the extensor tendon hood (lamina intertendina according to Landsmeer). In the first phalanx fixator pins approaching from the dorsoradial or dorso-ulnar side unavoidably transfix the tendon hood (**x**).

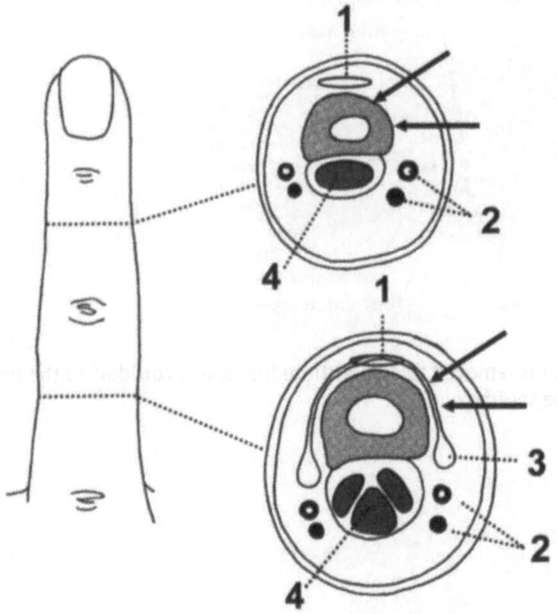

Fig. 12.33 Schematic cross-sections through the first and middle phalanges. The black arrows indicate the orientation of the fixator pins. 1 = extensor tendon; 2 = nerve/vessel bundle; 3 = strong palmar fibre bundle at the palmar border of the extensor tendon hood; 4 = flexor tendon.

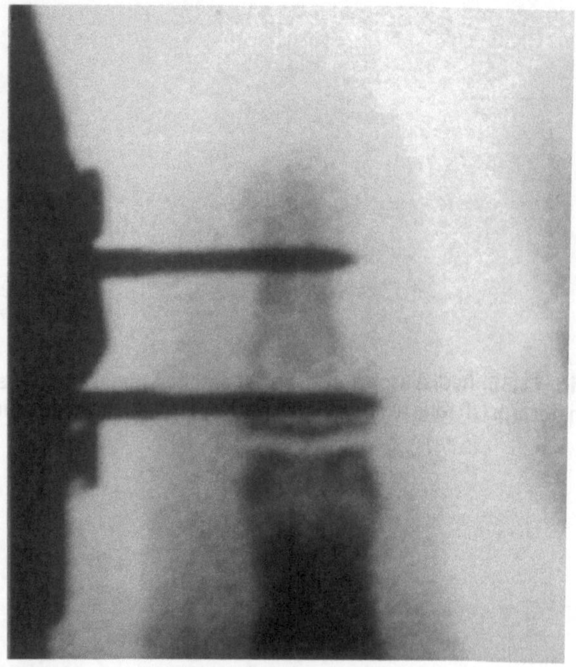

Fig. 12.34 Insertion of two fixator pins (diameter: 1.6mm) into the distal phalanx of the index finger.

External Fixation of the Phalanges

Most of the fixator systems on the market are not suitable for use in the hand. The dimensions of the phalanges especially, dictate the need for a specialized fixator system.

A true safety corridor in the phalanges cannot be found because the anatomical structures are so densely packed. It is self-evident that fixator application should be performed from the ulnar or radial side. In the first phalanx, the extensor tendon hood overlies the proximal two-thirds of the bone, and a fixator pin unavoidably transfixes this structure (Fig. 12.32). Clinical experience and our own anatomical studies, however, have revealed that this disturbs the mechanics of finger movement only minimally (Gausepohl 1998).

In the middle phalanx fixator screws can be inserted from the radial or ulnar side but the dimensions are even smaller than in the first phalanx. Care must be taken not to damage the vascular/nerve bundle on the palmar side. A slightly dorsal orientation of the pins is therefore indicated.

Fixator application to the distal phalanx is rare and a detailed description not required. It is possible, however, to insert two small fixator screws from the radial or ulnar side into the end phalanx as demonstrated in Figs. 12.33, 12.34.

References

De Bastiani G., Aldegheri R., Renzi Brivio L. (1984): 'The treatment of fractures with a dynamic axial fixator.' *J Bone Joint Surg* [Br] 1984; 66B: 538–45

Gausepohl T., Koebke J., Pennig D., Hobrecker S.: 'Anatomische Grundlagen zur Anwendung der unilateralen externen Fixation an Oberarm, Unterarm und Hand.' *Osteosynthese International* 1997; 5: 76–88

Gausepohl T., Lukosch S., Koebke J., Pennig D.: 'Externe Stabilisierung der Mittelhandknochen II-V. Eine anatomisch-klinische Studie.' *Handchir- Mirkrochir- Plast Chir* 1998; 2: 95–108

Gausepohl T., Koebke J., Pennig D., Thiel J.: 'Zur Auswirkung von Implantaten im Mittelhandklnochenkopf und in der Grundgliedbasis auf die Beweglichkeit des Fingergrundgelenkes. Eine anatomische Studie.' *Handchir- Mirkrochir- Plast Chir* 1998; 3: 226–31

Morrey B.F.: 'Post-traumatic contracture of the elbow.' *J Bone Joint Surg* (Am) 1990; 72A: 601–18

London J.T. 'Kinematics of the elbow joint.' *J Bone Surg* [Am] 1981; 64A: 529–35

Ruland O. 'Stellenwert der exernen Fixation in der Behandlung der Humerusschaftfraktur.' Osteosynthese International 1997 5: 94–101

Diaphyseal and Metaphyseal Fractures of the Humerus

13

F. Lavini, A. Donadelli and A. Pizzoli

Introduction

Fractures of the humerus are normally treated conservatively.[1,2] The need for surgical treatment arises in cases where the fracture is difficult to reduce by closed means (e.g. fractures with a butterfly fragment and fractures in obese patients), fractures which have redisplaced following cast treatment, or fractures in polytraumatized patients where bulky forms of stabilization could interfere with nursing care. In addition to the above, there is general agreement that surgery is indicated for unstable fractures, open fractures and fractures associated with major skin and soft tissue injuries which need constant observation and attention.

Available surgical techniques comprise open reduction and internal fixation, intramedullary nailing and external fixation. Rigid fixation by means of a plate and screws requires opening the fracture site, identification of the radial nerve (to avoid damaging it) and is associated with a variety of possible risks including neurological damage, infection, non-union and breakage of hardware. Intramedullary nailing has some advantages, in that it respects the biology of the healing process. However, antegrade insertion has the potential for damaging the rotator cuff, and in retrograde insertion, the diameter of the medullary canal may limit the diameter of the nail that can be inserted, with consequent compromise of the stability. Furthermore, intramedullary nailing is indicated only for fractures of the diaphysis.

Monolateral external fixation can be used to treat both diaphyseal and metaphyseal fractures of the humerus in a minimally invasive way. Percutaneous insertion of the bone screws in well-defined areas avoids the risk of damage to the radial nerve. The excellent bone purchase that can be achieved with correctly inserted screws enables closed manipulation of the fracture to be carried out. Monolateral external fixation is capable of maintaining fracture reduction throughout the entire healing period and allows full mobilization of both the shoulder and the elbow joints during the treatment period. The possible disadvantages are pin track problems which are encountered in a percentage of cases.

De Bastiani et al[3] reported on 40 cases of closed fracture of the humeral diaphysis treated with a classic Orthofix Dynamic Axial fixator. Thirty-nine of these (98 per cent) united with a mean time to healing of 3.4 months. There was a single case of non-union. The overall incidence of pin track infection in 288 fresh fractures of the long bones was 8/1300 pins (0.62 per cent). Cugola et al in 1990[4] reported on 44 fractures of the humeral shaft treated with the Orthofix Dynamic Axial fixator. Results were recorded as excellent in 89 per cent, good in 4.5, fair in 4.5 and poor in 2.3 per cent. Mean time to healing was 3.4 months. There were no cases of deep infection and superficial pin track infection occurred in 13.6 per cent of patients (6/44 patients). This was readily controlled with local application of antibiotics, and in only one case did screws require to be re-sited. Non-union occurred in two cases. In one, healing was achieved in 6.5 months, following application of a functional brace; in the other, despite decorticalization and re-application of the fixator, healing had not occurred at 9 months.

Neumann et al[5] described 27 cases of humeral shaft fracture treated with the Orthofix Dynamic Axial Fixator. Healing occurred in 93 per cent of cases in an average of 13.1 weeks. The incidence of non-union was 3.7 per cent and of superficial pin track infection, 7.5

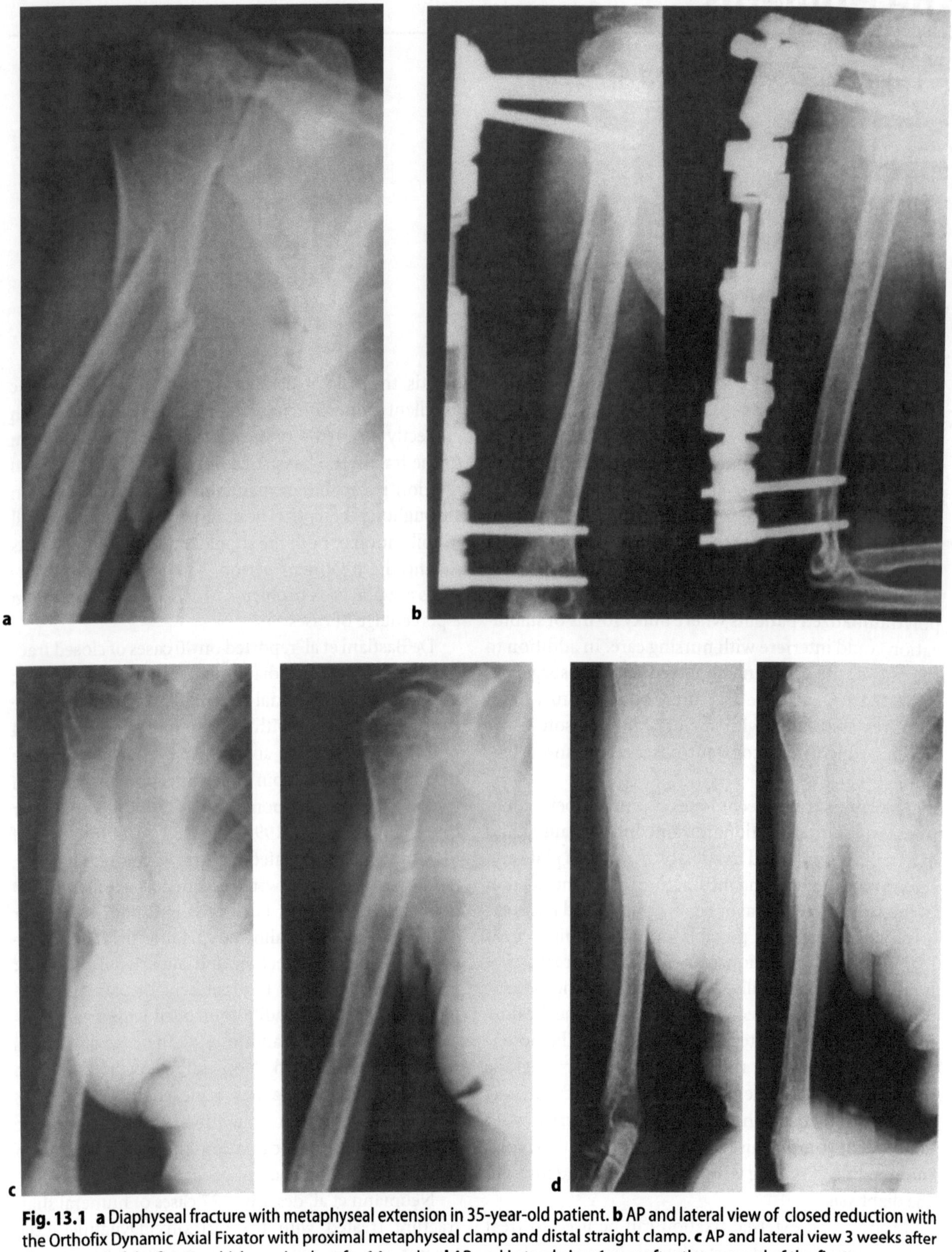

Fig. 13.1 **a** Diaphyseal fracture with metaphyseal extension in 35-year-old patient. **b** AP and lateral view of closed reduction with the Orthofix Dynamic Axial Fixator with proximal metaphyseal clamp and distal straight clamp. **c** AP and lateral view 3 weeks after the removal of the fixator which was in place for 14 weeks. **d** AP and Lateral view 1 year after the removal of the fixator.

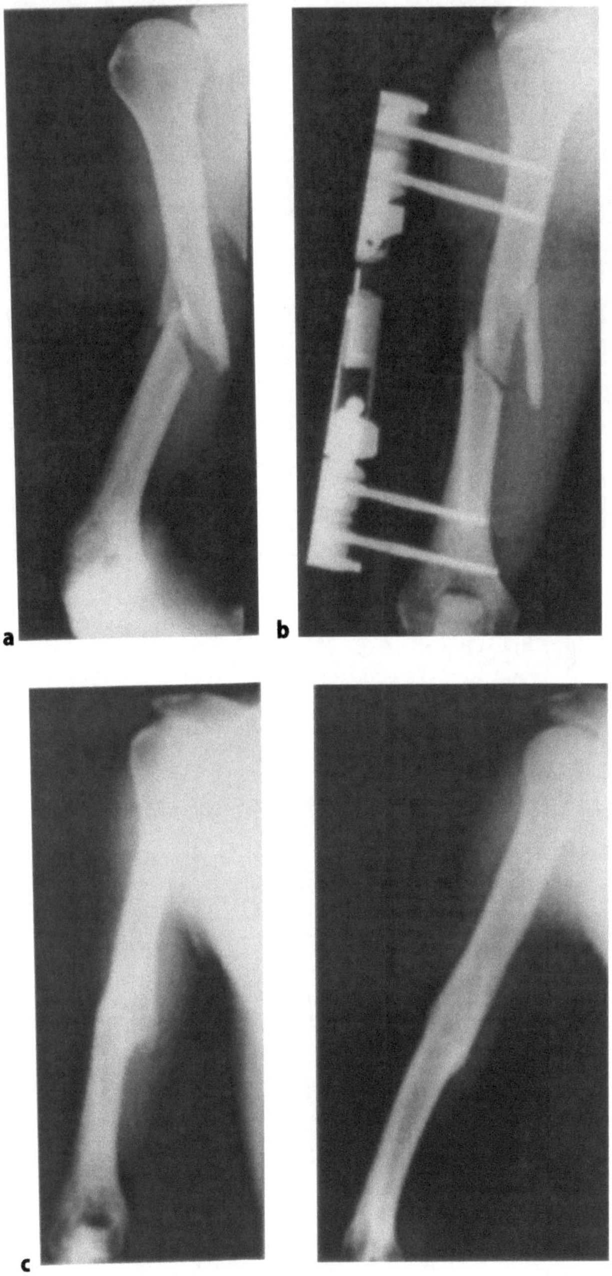

Fig. 13.2 a Closed diaphyseal fracture without radial nerve involvement. **b** Closed reduction using the Orthofix Dynamic Axial Fixator. **c** AP and lateral view 1 year after the removal of the fixator which remained in situ for 11 weeks.

per cent. These authors suggested that the primary indications for the use of external fixation for diaphyseal fractures of the humerus were second and third degree open fractures, and fractures in polytraumatized patients.

The present chapter describes a series of humeral fractures treated by the authors during the period 1990 to 1996.

Patients and Methods

All patients were treated using the standard or short Orthofix fixator (10.000 series) and in a few cases, in patients with a small frame, the small Orthofix fixator (30.000 series). The technique used was identical in all cases. Prior to application of the fixator, the fracture was reduced as completely as possible. This was usually accomplished using traction, with the limb abducted to 90° from the trunk and the elbow flexed at 90°. Reduction was then monitored under image intensification taking particular care to correct any rotational element. The fixator was always applied to the lateral aspect of the limb, and cortical screws were used in every case. All screws were inserted percutaneously through small incisions, using landmarks which, following extensive experience, ensured that no damage would occur to the radial nerve. An open approach may of course be used as an alternative, depending upon surgeon preference.

The first screw to be inserted was the most distal one, approximately 1cm above the lateral epicondyle. Overall screw length and thread length were determined pre-operatively using a transparent X-ray overlay.

In order to reduce the likelihood of the drill slipping on the supracondylar ridge, the authors' practice was to use a small drill diameter initially (3.2mm) and to drill both cortices of the bone under image intensification. This drill was then left in situ with its drill guide and screw guide, and the second of the two distal screws inserted into the third or fourth seat of the clamp template using the 4.8mm drill and following the standard technique (see Ch. 9: Screw Selection and the Technique of Insertion). The 3.2mm drill was then removed and this path re-drilled using the 4.8mm drill. The most distal screw was then inserted. The proximal screw cluster was then inserted into the proximal third of the humerus using the standard technique.

In those cases where the proximal extent of the fracture was very close to the neck of the humerus, screws were inserted into the neck of the humerus itself, in a horizontal plane, using a T-clamp or preferably a Torbay–Garches clamp, which allowed the screws to converge in the humeral neck. In such cases, care was taken to ensure that the second cortex was not penetrated. It was normal practice, in these circumstances, to insert a supplementary screw into the diaphysis, ideally midway between the fracture and the distal screw cluster.

Where the distal limit of the fracture extended into the region of insertion of the distal screws, i.e. within

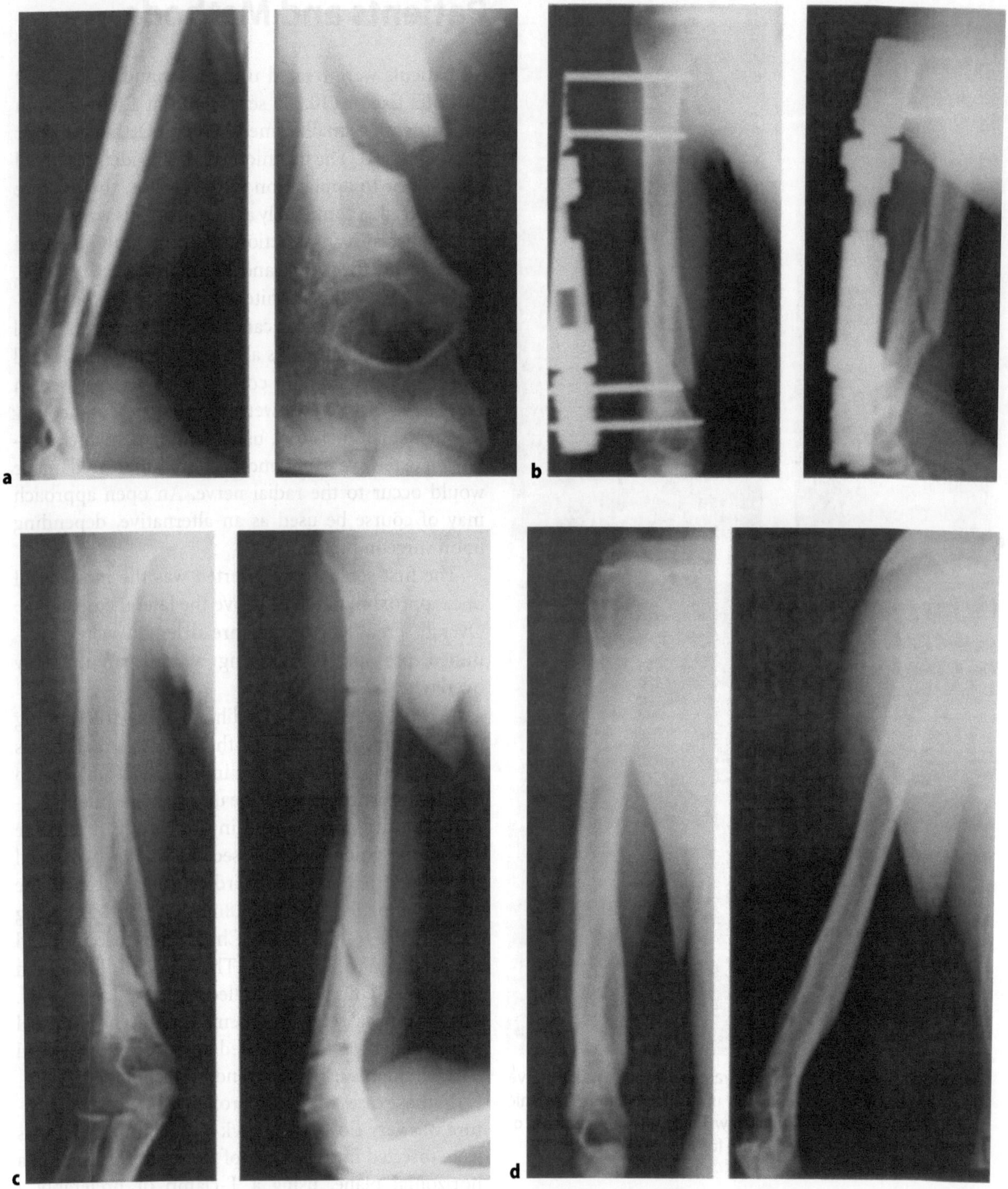

Fig. 13.3 **a** Closed distal diaphyseal fracture in 32-year-old patient. The butterfly fragment is not evident in these pictures. **b** AP and lateral view of the closed reduction with the Orthofix Dynamic Axial Fixator in situ. **c** AP and lateral view 3 weeks after the removal of the fixator which remained in place for 12 weeks. **d** The AP and lateral view 3 years after the removal of the fixator show

4cm of the elbow joint, these distal screws could often still be inserted, accepting the fact that they would be closer together then would normally be desirable. Thus the most distal screw would be inserted at the level of the lateral epicondyle and the more proximal of the two distal screws in the second or third seat of the clamp template. In such cases, some limitation of extension of the elbow joint was accepted while the fixator was in place. In the adult humerus, therefore, all fractures occurring in the region from 4cm below the glenohumeral articular surface to 4cm above the elbow joint were treated with external fixation. Where the fracture involved a large, unstable third fragment, or was bifocal, one or more supplementary screws attached to the body of the fixator were applied. Where non-unions as opposed to fresh fractures were treated, the additional procedure of osteomuscular decortication was carried out.

Following insertion of the screws, the template and screw guides were removed and the definitive fixator applied. Final reduction was then accomplished and ball joints and central body locking nut tightened. It should be noted that where the ProCallus fixator is used, there is no need to use the classic template, since the clamps of the ProCallus itself act as their own template.

Active movements of the elbow and shoulder were encouraged from the first post-operative day. A standard protocol of pin site care was adopted.[6,7] Serial X-rays were taken at three-week intervals to monitor progress. Dynamization using the Dyna-Ring was initiated at two to three weeks, at which time increasing exercise and light lifting were actively encouraged. Full, free dynamization was instituted at approximately six weeks following injury by removal of the Dyna-Ring and unlocking the central body locking nut. In cases where supplementary screws were used, these were removed at four to six weeks from surgery and dynamization commenced following their removal. Once healing was confirmed on X-ray and clinical examination, the fixator and screws were removed as an outpatient procedure.

Functional assessments were carried out between two and three months following removal of the fixator. These included objective assessment of the range of motion at both shoulder joint and elbow joint, on both active and passive movement and whether or not the patient had returned to his or her previous level of activity. The scoring system used for functional assessment is shown in Table 13.1. In addition to these assessments, the healing of the pin sites was evaluated following fixator removal. All patients have been followed up for a minimum of 12 months post-operation.

Results

A total of 25 patients were treated over the period of study. Twenty-two were unilateral, closed, fresh fractures of the humerus, and 3 were non-unions. There were 18 males and 7 females; average age 34 years (range 12–77). Four of the patients with fresh fractures had associated fractures: 2 femoral fractures, both also treated with an Orthofix Dynamic Axial Fixator; one fractured pelvis, treated with an Orthofix and one open fracture of the forearm. One of the patients with a non-union had an associated fracture of the radius.

Healing occurred in all cases. In the patients with fresh fractures the mean healing time was 2.8 months (range 1.5–5 months), while in the case of the non-unions it was 5.3 months (range 4–6 months). Complications were rare. In two instances osteolysis occurred around a screw, one in association with a fresh fracture, and one in a patient undergoing treatment for a non-union. In each case this responded to a short course of antibiotics. In two of the fresh fractures, re-operation with realignment of the fracture was required in the early stages of healing. One patient had a temporary radial nerve palsy as a result of the trauma. This resolved completely in the 6 months following operation. No instance of shortening was observed. Radiological follow up showed no axial deviation and the functional outcome in all cases was very good at the most recent assessment, and is illustrated in Tables 13.2 and 13.3. Illustrative cases are shown in Figs. 13.1–13.3.

Discussion

Closed fractures of the humeral diaphysis/metaphysis usually consolidate readily, regardless of the treatment method employed. Consolidation, however, is not the sole objective in these cases. It is also important to ensure restoration of length, axis and rotation if an ideal functional result is to be obtained. In unstable fractures surgical intervention is the only sure way of achieving this. The present series demonstrates that a minimally invasive technique using a monolateral fixator is able to satisfy this requirement without the risk of deep infection or restriction of range of movement of the shoulder or elbow during treatment. The fact that there were no non-unions following treatment in this series vindicates the use of a closed procedure, even in simple fractures. Superficial, minor pin track infection is the only drawback to the technique, and this occurred in 20 per cent of our patients. These minor problems did not interfere with the treatment programme in any way.

On balance, the advantages of this technique far outweigh the few disadvantages. Based upon our experience, therefore, we would recommend the use of external fixation for unstable fractures, open fractures, fractures in polytraumatized patients, fractures in obese patients, fractures with associated forearm fractures and for the treatment of established, long standing non-unions. Use of external fixation is contra-indicated where there is severe osteoporosis, in fractures that extend beyond the limits of screw placement, or in patients who are likely to find it difficult to cope with routine pin site care.

Range of movement of shoulder and elbow normal; Patient returned to work/former level of activity	Excellent
Shoulder: Less than 20° restriction of abduction, extension, external rotation and internal rotation; Elbow: Less than 15° restriction of flexion, extension, pronation and supination; Patient returned to work/former level of activity.	Good
Shoulder: More than 20° restriction of abduction, extension, external rotation and internal rotation; Elbow: More than 15° restriction of flexion, extension, pronation and supination	Poor

Table 13.1 Scoring System for Evaluation of Shoulder and Elbow Function in Patients with Humeral Fractures (Cugola et al 1990).[4]

Excellent	8
Good	14
Poor	0

Table 13.2 Functional Assessment in Patients with Fresh Fractures (n = 22)

Excellent	0
Good	3
Poor	0

Table 13.3 Functional Assessment in Patients with Non-union (n = 3)

References

1. Balfour GW, Mooney, Vert, Ashby ME. 'Diaphyseal fractures of the humerus treated with a ready-made fracture brace.' *J Bone Joint Surg* [Am] 1982; 64A: 11–3
2. Sarmiento A, Latta LL. *Closed functional treatment of fractures*, 1981 Springer: New York
3. De Bastiani G, Aldegheri R, Renzi Brivio L. 'The treatment of fractures with a dynamic axial fixator.' *J Bone Joint Surg* [Br] 1984; 66B: 538–45
4. Cugola L, Amendola A, Amelio E, Leso P, Lavini F. 'Fratture difisarie dell'omero: trattamento con fissatore esterno assiale (F.E.A.).' *Atti S.E.R.T.O.T.* 1990; Vol XXXII: Fascicolo 1: 13–5
5. Neumann HS, Brug E, Winckler S, Klein W. 'The surgical treatment of diaphyseal fractures of the humerus: stabilisation with plate osteosynthesis, Hackethal nailing, locking nail and external fixation.' *Int J Orthop Trauma* 1993; Suppl to Vol 3 (3); 25–8
6. Checketts RG, Otterburn M, MacEachern G. 'Pin track infection: definition, incidence and prevention.' *Int J Orthop Trauma* 1993; Suppl to Vol 3 (3); 16–8
7. Checketts RG, MacEachern G, Otterburn M. 'Pin track infection and the principles of pin site care.' This book, Chapter 11.

Fractures, Fracture Dislocations and Stiffness of the Elbow: the Elbow Fixator

14

D. Pennig and T. Gausepohl

Introduction

The extraordinary contribution of the hand as the most versatile tool for human development is beyond all doubt. Key to its function is free spatial orientation of the hand in front of the body. The arm can be considered as a lever to bring the hand to an object of interest and to change its position. Its function is integral to the most basic daily living activities, like eating. This clearly points to the importance of the other joints of the arm: the shoulder and the elbow joint. Due to the anatomical structure of the shoulder, stiffness of this joint can be partially compensated for by the scapula sliding on the dorsal aspect of the chest and by movement of the trunk itself. A stiff elbow joint, however, severely compromises hand function since nature provides no compensatory mechanism for flexion and extension – that is, no other mechanism to bring the hand close to or away from the body. A second fundamental function of the elbow joint closely related to hand function is forearm rotation. To fulfill its manifold tasks, the elbow joint consists of three different joints enfolded in one complex capsular apparatus. The combined movement and the high mobility of this joint account for the significant structural complexity of the stabilizing ligaments.

Considering its design and function it can easily be understood that the elbow joint is predisposed to injury. The mechanism of injury may lead to "simple" dislocation of the elbow joint or to a variety of periarticular fracture patterns. The combination of ligament disruption and periarticular fractures creates the most unstable injury pattern. Fracture dislocations, even if treated operatively with open reduction, internal fixation and ligament repair, usually need long arm plaster cast immobilization which is often detrimental to joint function. Treatment of the residual stiffness is difficult and often does not achieve the desired result. This dilemma may be addressed by permitting controlled motion of the joint as soon as possible after injury and operative repair.

Anatomy of the Elbow Joint

The elbow joint has three joint components: humero-ulnar, humero-radial and radio-ulnar (Figs. 14.1a–14.1c). The main movement of the elbow is flexion and extension with both forearm bones moving relative to the humerus. This joint function may be compared to a hinge (Fig. 14.1a). Anatomical studies show additional minor movements of the humero-ulnar joint with a shift of the centre of rotation in full flexion and in full extension. However, in a fracture dislocation with all stabilizing joint components compromised these become irrelevant.

The proximal ulna sits tightly on the trochlea humeri (Fig. 14.1a) and provides the bony stabilization which is assisted by the strong collateral ligaments. The radial head only abuts on the humerus. The only ligamentous structure connecting the humerus with the radial head is a small part of the radial collateral ligament which inserts into the annular ligament. The annular ligament holds the radial head like a sling and with its main attachment on the proximal ulna, maintains the position of the radial head relative to the humerus and the ulna (Fig. 14.1b). These ligaments as well as the distal radio-ulnar joint configuration allow rotation of the radius relative to the ulna. Since the humero-ulnar joint is the main bony stabilizer and the

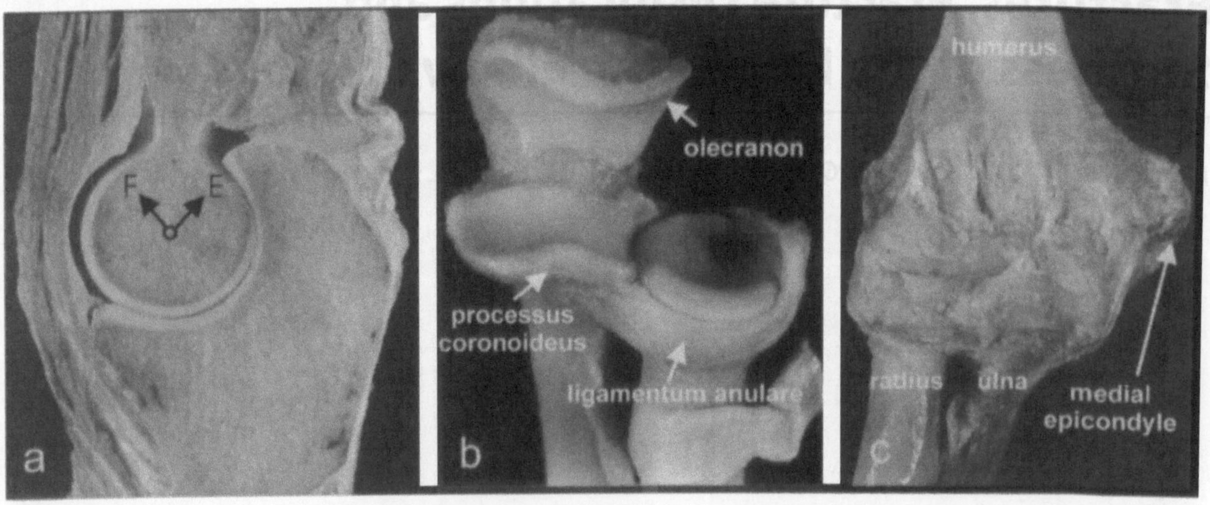

Fig. 14.1 **a** Sagittal cross-section through the humero-ulnar joint. The ring indicates the centre of rotation; in maximum flexion it shifts towards F; in maximum extension it shifts towards E. **b** Ligaments of the proximal radio-ulnar joint. **c** Anterior aspect of the elbow joint ligaments and capsule.

ulnar collateral ligament is the strongest ligamentous structure, humero-ulnar application of a fixator seems advisable. The role of the radial head is to provide a static counterpart for the ulnar collateral ligament. External fixation of the elbow joint has to allow flexion and extension and ideally must not interfere with forearm rotation.

Design of the Humero-Ulnar Elbow Fixator

The Elbow Fixator (Fig. 14.2) consists of two clamps and two links with a central connecting unit (Fig. 14.3a, Fig. 14.3b). The effective length of each link can be adjusted by sliding it back and forth in relation to the central connecting unit. Each link can be individually locked at the desired length by a link locking screw and the two links can be locked at a chosen angle to one another by means of the triangular knob of the central connecting unit (Fig. 14.4). For controlled distraction of the elbow joint a small distractor is available which is placed on the humeral and/or the ulnar link of the fixator (Figs. 14.5a, 14.5b). In acute cases the Elbow Fixator is assembled with the humeral link outside the ulnar link.

To allow mobilization the triangular knob of the central connecting unit is unlocked and a security plate maintains the position of the links. With the link locking screws tightened the elbow joint can be mobilized without any shift of the rotational axis.

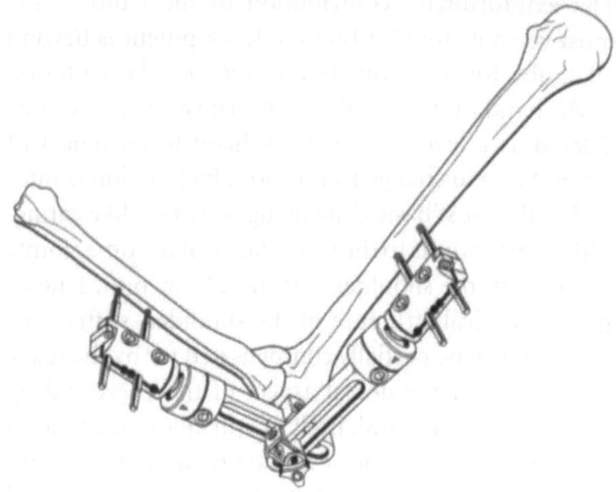

Fig. 14.2 Unilateral humero-ulnar Elbow Fixator in standard configuration.

Application of the Elbow Fixator

Anatomical Aspects of the Lateral Humerus

The humerus is covered anteriorly by the biceps brachii muscle as well as the brachialis muscle. The triceps brachii muscle covers its posterior aspect. The proximal part of the humerus is covered on its anterior, lateral and dorsal sides by the deltoid muscle, which converges on the humerus approximately in the midshaft region. The deltoid muscle being very impor-

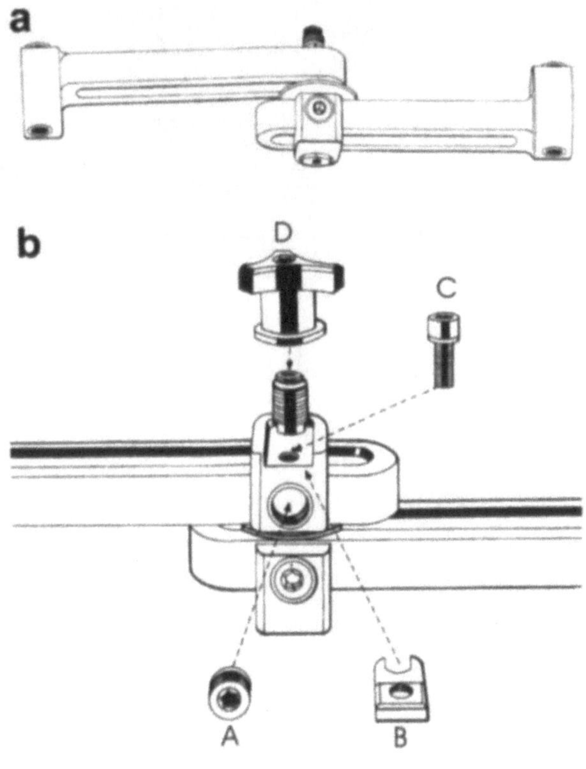

Fig. 14.3 a Two identical links are used; the central connecting unit during assembly. **b** Assembly of the central connecting unit:
A link locking screw
B security plate inserted with its flat surface facing downwards
C plate locking screw
D triangular knob to control flexion/extension

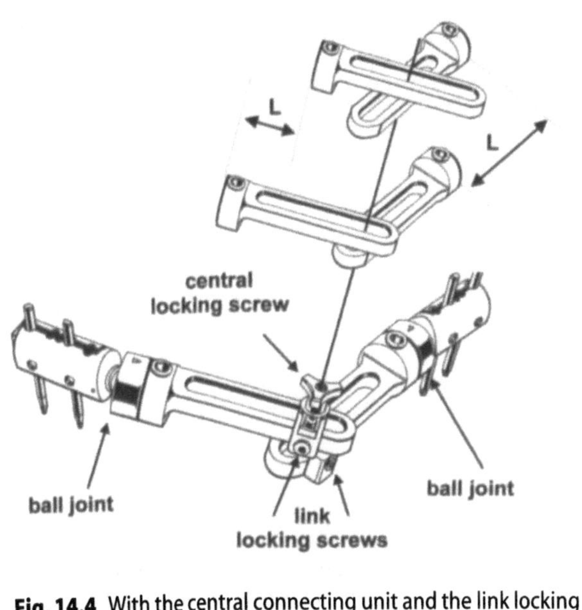

Fig. 14.4 With the central connecting unit and the link locking screws the position of the links relative the each other is determined. This serves to lengthen or shorten the fixator and care has to be taken to allow free rotation of the links on the central connecting unit.

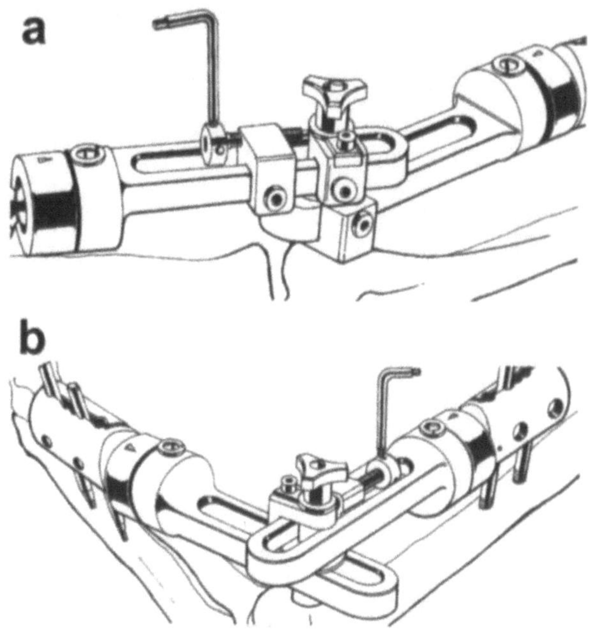

Fig. 14.5 A small distractor placed on **a** the ulnar link, **b** the humeral link.

tant for shoulder function ideally should not be transfixed in order to avoid impairment. At the junction between the proximal and middle thirds of the humerus the neurovasular bundle is on the anteromedial side. The radial nerve crosses from the medial side to the dorsal side and in the distal third of the humerus wraps around the bone towards the anterior aspect of the elbow (Figs. 14.6a, 14.6b).

The humerus itself has a medullary cavity which narrows down in the distal third and in the periarticular portion of the humerus there is no canal at all. In the midshaft of the humerus, the average outer diameter in the frontal (coronal) plane measures from 19–21.5mm (see Fig. 12.8 on p. 108).

The key to application of the Elbow Fixator is proper identification of the rotational axis of the humero-ulnar joint. The patient is positioned supine and a hand table is used. A tourniquet is not applied. Reduction of the displaced elbow is carried out and with the shoulder in internal rotation, the elbow is placed on its medial side. It should be supported by a rolled up towel so that a true lateral view of the elbow joint can be obtained with the image intensifier. The operation must not commence before the image shown in Fig. 14.7a is visible on the image intensifier screen. A 2mm × 150 mm Kirschner-wire is used and the tip is placed in the centre of the circle (Fig. 14.7b). The K-wire is drilled through the lateral condyle in the direction of the X-ray beam. The power drill is discon-

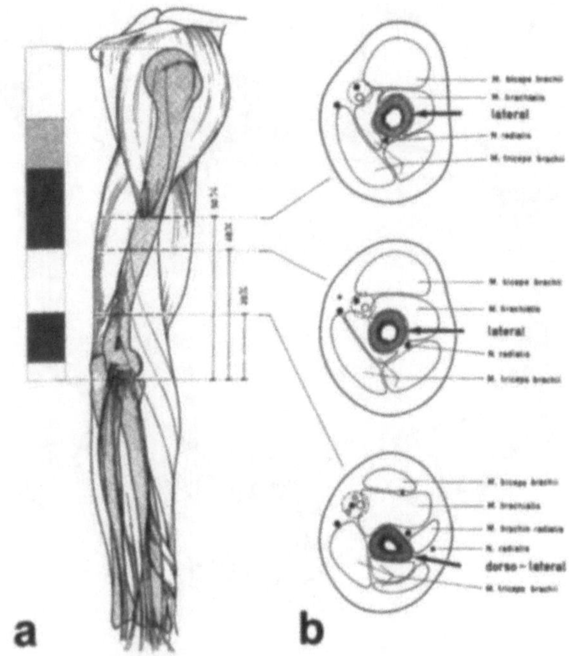

Fig. 14.6 **a** Lateral aspect of the humerus. The figures are based on the full length of the humerus (radial condyle to humeral head). The dark areas on the left side are suitable for pin placement. Please note that in the Elbow Fixator application the lower area around the radial condyle is not used. **b** Cross-section of the humerus at the level of pin insertion (50%/40% of total length). Please note the course of the radial nerve which has to be protected.

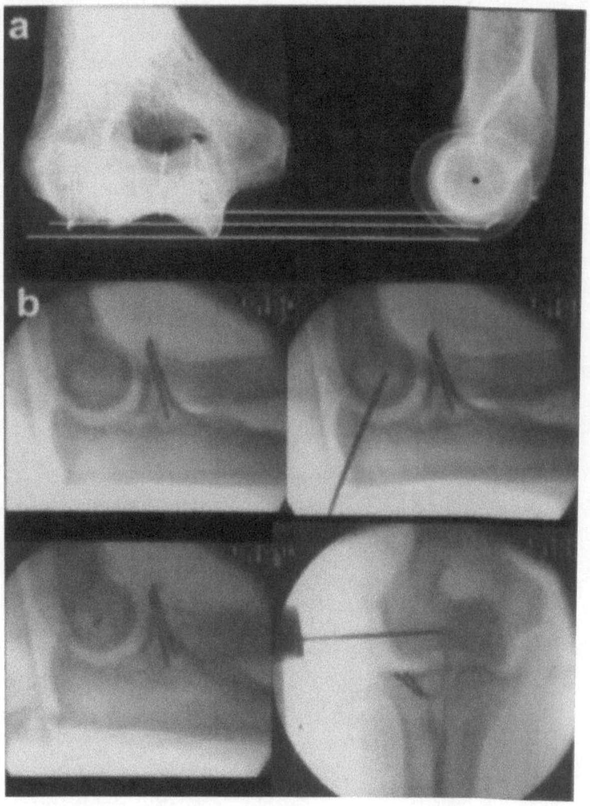

Fig. 14.7 **a** Exact lateral view of the distal humerus with symmetrical superposition of the radial and ulnar articular surfaces. **b** After correct visualization of the lateral aspect of the distal humerus (top left) the 2mm K-wire is placed on the centre of rotation percutaneously (top right). With the K-wire appearing as a dot in the centre it is in line with the rotational axis (bottom left). The AP film shows that only half of the condylar length is penetrated to avoid injury to the ulnar nerve (bottom right).

nected and the position of the K-wire is checked. Provided that the point of entry is the centre of the circle, the K-wire can now be bent until the part protruding from the skin is in the centre of the circle (Fig. 14.7b). This avoids repeated placement of the wire. With the K-wire in the correct position, the fixator is now used as its own template (Fig. 14.8) and the humeral screws are placed first.

Placement of the Humeral Screws

The landmark for the humeral screws is the insertion of the deltoid muscle on the lateral aspect of the bone. This can be felt as a hard spot where the fibres of the deltoid muscle converge. More proximal pin placement within the muscle fibres of the deltoid is not advisable since it negatively affects shoulder function. A more distal placement is dangerous because of the course of the radial nerve. The ideal position for the humeral screws is covered by few fibres of the brachialis muscle. It is advisable to expose the lateral aspect of the humerus through a 4–5cm incision. The anterior cortex of the humerus should be identified and the brachialis fibres displaced posteriorly, which

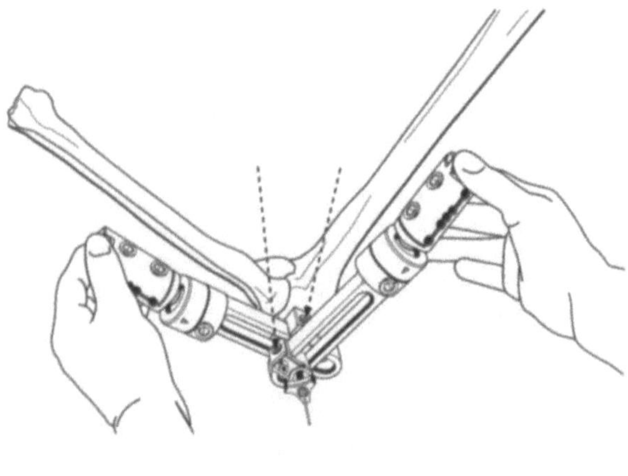

Fig. 14.8 The central connecting unit is slid over the K-wire and the fixator used as its own template for insertion of the screws. Once the fixator has been mounted on the K-wires, the position of the links must be adjusted to ensure that sufficient space will be available for correction and subsequent joint distraction. The link locking screws (see arrows) are provisionally tightened at this point.

will protect the radial nerve and we advise detaching the periosteum to reduce the pain response. With the fixator central unit mounted on the 2mm Kirschner-wire, the screw in clamp seat 1 (most proximal screw) is introduced first. A screw guide with a trocar is inserted and with a 4.8mm drill in a drill guide the bone is drilled (Fig. 14.9). The drill stop may be used to avoid accidental damage to the medial neurovascular bundle. Depending on the soft tissue envelope either a 100/30 or a 110/30 standard Orthofix cortical screw is used (Fig. 14.10). In smaller adults however, the use of a 3.2mm drill is advisable and a 120/20–4.5/3.5mm screw is employed. An outer diameter of the humerus of less than 20mm at the pin insertion site requires use of the smaller screws.

The second humeral screw is now inserted in the fourth seat of the clamp (Fig. 14.11).

The screw guides are removed and the clamp cover locking screws are tightened. The fixator clamp should be positioned at a distance of 15–20 mm from the skin to allow for post-operative swelling (Fig. 14.12).

It is important to leave at least 1cm of sliding capacity in the humeral link especially where the fixator is used in the management of elbow stiffness.

Insertion of the Ulnar Screws

With the forearm in neutral rotation the dorsal aspect of the ulna can be felt through the skin in almost its entire length. Only in the proximal third, distal to the olecranon, the insertion of the flexor digitorum muscle covers it with thin fibres. On the humero-radial epicondyle the extensor carpi ulnaris muscle covers the bone. The ulna has a broad surface on the dorsal side whereas the interosseous membrane inserts into a more pointed part of the bone. The dorsal aspect can be felt easily in the neutral forearm position and the appropriate point of insertion is in the proximal part of the midshaft of the ulna (Fig. 14.13a). The diameter of the bone in this area measures on average 13.4–15.3mm. The radius rotates around the ulna, but due to the thin muscle cover of the dorsal aspect an impingement can be avoided with correct pin placement (Fig. 14.13b).

The distal screws are inserted from the dorsal side into the ulna. The ideal position is the proximal part of the midshaft of the ulna. Stab incisions may be used, but for better identification of the screw sites a 4cm incision is advisable. The screws must penetrate the medullary canal of the ulna for bicortical purchase. The dimensions of the ulna itself make a smaller screw diameter mandatory. Screw insertion is from the

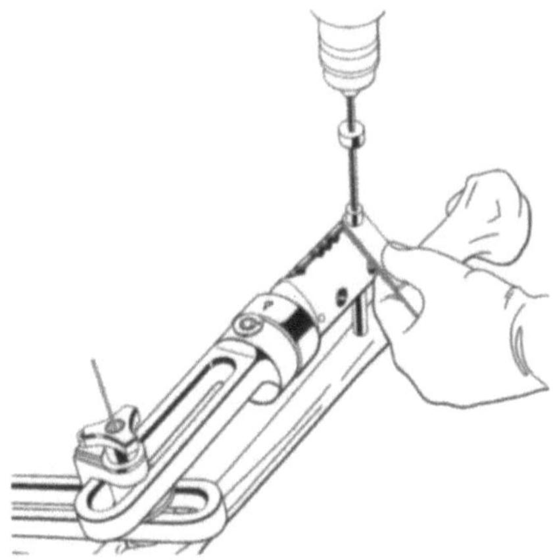

Fig. 14.9 With the triangular knob tightened, the humeral screws are inserted in the frontal plane, at right angles to bone. A screw guide is inserted into the most proximal screw seat of the clamp. A 4.8mm drill guide is used and the bone drilled with a 4.8mm drill bit.

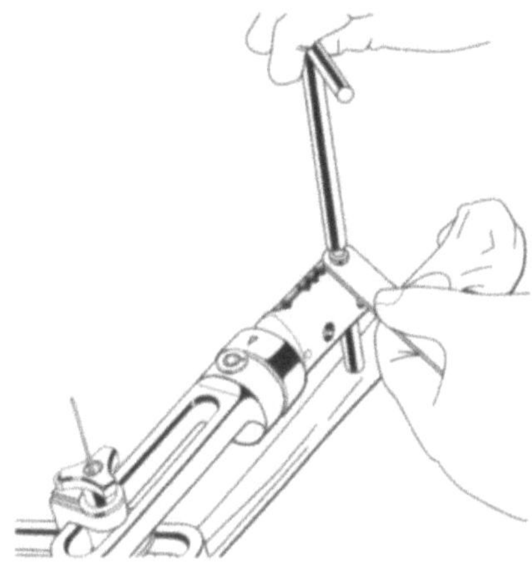

Fig. 14.10 The drill guide is removed and a 6/5 mm, 100/30 or 110/30 cortical screw inserted through the screw guide, using the T-wrench. N.B.: If the humerus is less than 20mm in diameter, the 4.5–3.5mm, 100/20 or 120/20 screws should be used after predrilling with the 3.2mm drill bit through the

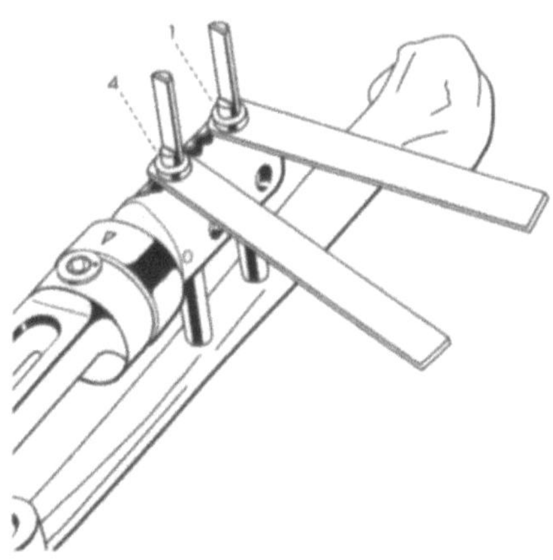

Fig. 14.11 The second humeral screw is then inserted in the same fashion in the 4th screw seat of the clamp.

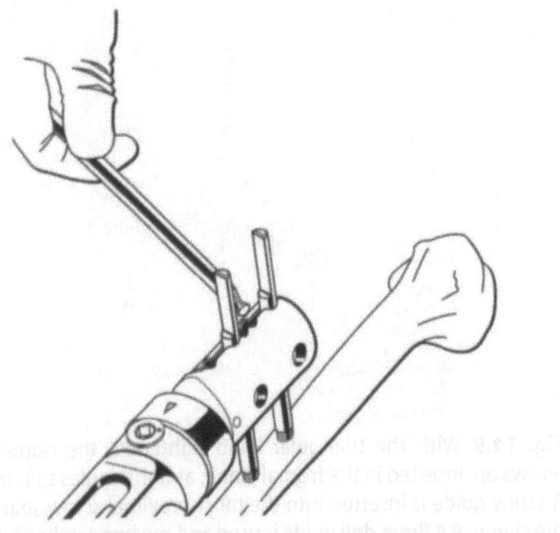

Fig. 14.12 The screw guides are removed and the clamp cover locking screws tightened. The fixator should be positioned at a distance of 15–20mm from the skin to allow for post-operative swelling.

dorsal aspect in the frontal (coronal) plane and the subcutaneous border of the ulna must be identified. The screws are inserted at right angles to the long axis of the bone. It is important that the ulnar screws are placed as centrally as possible in the transverse plane through the medullary canal in order to avoid weakening the bone, and the most distal screw is inserted first. A 3.2mm drill with a drill guide is used through the screw guide in the same fashion as in the humerus (Fig. 14.14). The drill guide is removed and a 4.5/3.5mm 100/20 or 120/20 cortical screw is inserted with a T-wrench (Fig. 14.15). The second ulnar screw is inserted in the same way through the fourth screw seat of the clamp (Fig. 14.16). After removal of the screw guides the clamp cover locking screws are tightened and again the distance from the skin should be 15–20mm (Fig. 14.17). The position of the clamp on the ulnar screws will influence the carrying angle of the forearm in relation to the humerus and this is utilized together with the ball joint for its alignment.

Should it be technically impossible to use a straight clamp, an extended range clamp may be chosen distally to achieve alignment of the fixator with the long axis of the ulna (Fig. 14.18). The extended range clamp gives the surgeon a wider choice of angle for screw insertion in the ulna.

Check of Fixator Alignment

With the humeral clamp and the ulnar clamp cover screws tightened, and the link locking screws, the triangular knob and the cams loosened, reduction of the elbow joint is checked radiographically in the AP plane (Fig. 14.19). At this point the carrying angle of

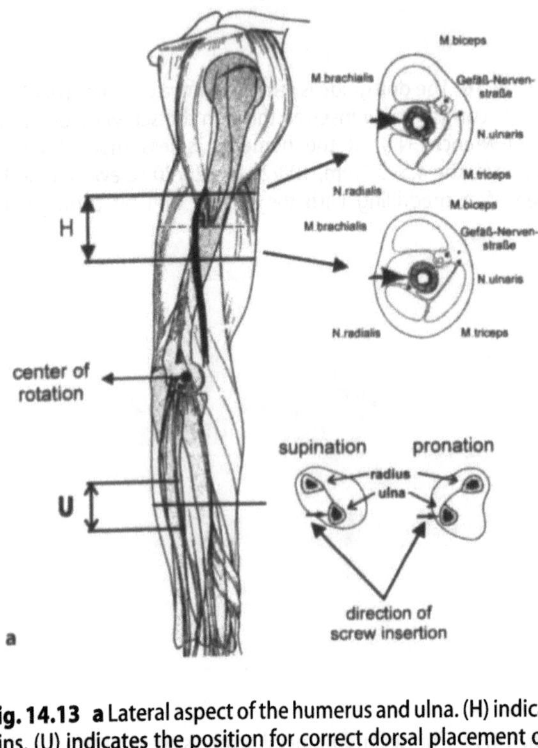

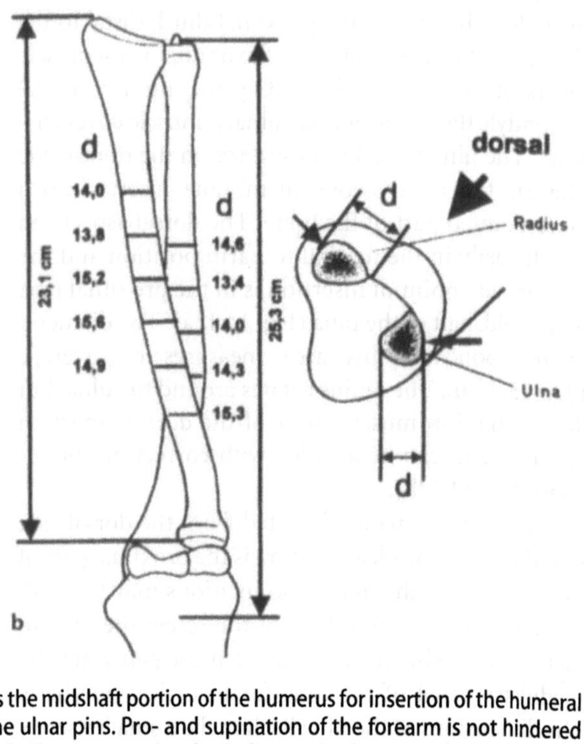

Fig. 14.13 **a** Lateral aspect of the humerus and ulna. (H) indicates the midshaft portion of the humerus for insertion of the humeral pins. (U) indicates the position for correct dorsal placement of the ulnar pins. Pro- and supination of the forearm is not hindered (cross-section on right). **b** Outer diameter of the ulna in the midshaft. The arrow on the ulna indicates the direction of pin insertion.

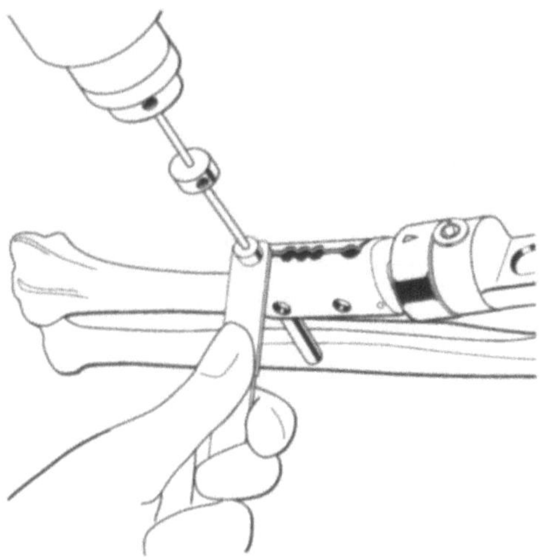

Fig. 14.14 A screw guide is inserted into the most distal screw seat of the clamp. A 3.2mm drill guide is used and the bone drilled with a 3.2mm drill bit. Bicortical purchase is necessary.

the forearm in relation to the humerus may be corrected, and the cam, the clamp position on the screws and the ulnar link locking screw afford a wide range of positions. With the image intensifier the joint line is monitored and the carrying angle is established. The clamp cover locking screws are fully tightened, with the triangular knob tightened first by hand (Fig. 14.20). Use of the Allen wrench on the triangular knob at this point is not possible since the 2mm K-wire protrudes from it. The link locking screws are then tightened followed by the cams (Fig. 14.20). The elbow is now moved from full extension into 100° of flexion and the K-wire monitored throughout this procedure. Bending of the K-wire indicates a poor position of the central connecting unit. Should this be observed, the fixator is taken off the pins and realignment of the 2mm K-wire performed under image intensification.

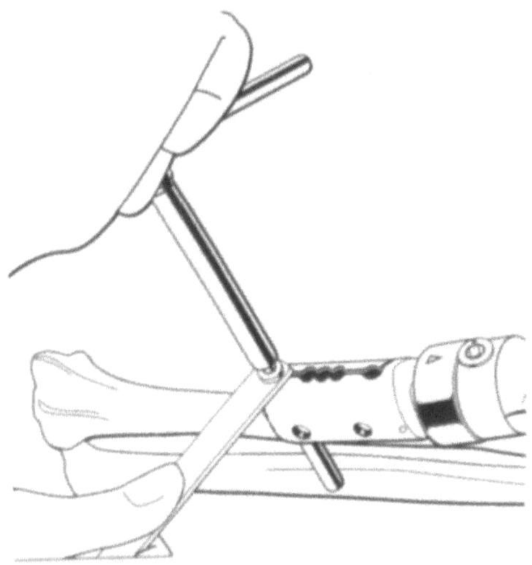

Fig. 14.15 The drill guide is removed and a 4.5/3.5mm, 100/20 or 120/20 cortical screw inserted through the screw guide, using the T-wrench.

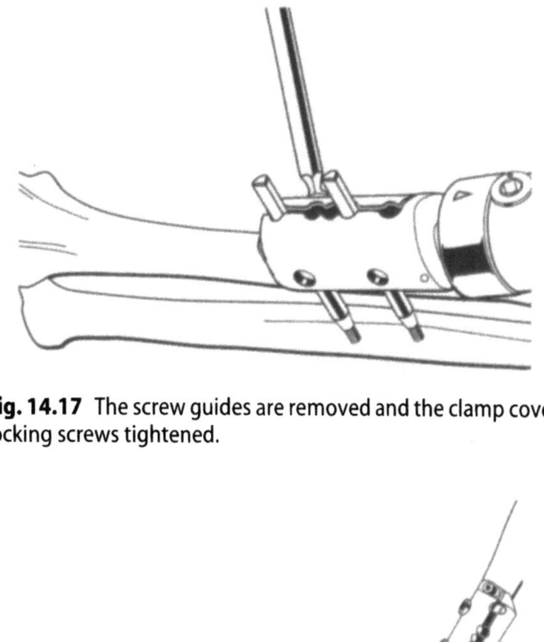

Fig. 14.17 The screw guides are removed and the clamp cover locking screws tightened.

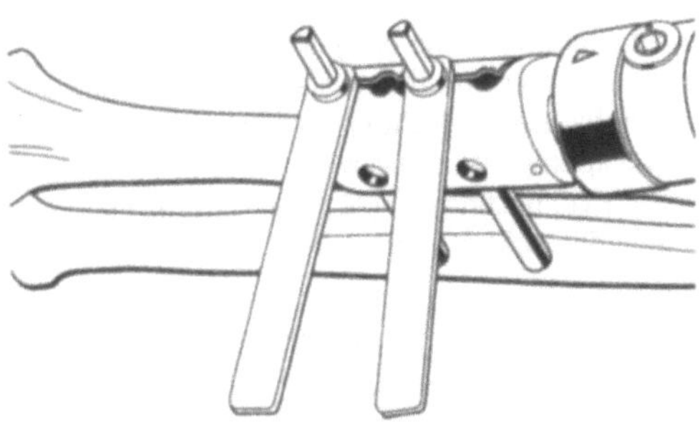

Fig. 14.16 The second ulnar screw is then inserted in the same fashion, in the 4th screw seat of the clamp. Again bicortical purchase is necessary.

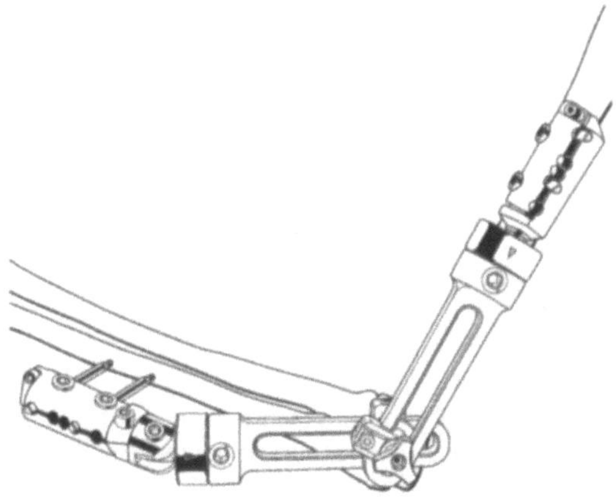

Fig. 14.18 An extended range clamp should be used distally when it is impossible to align a straight clamp with the long axis of the ulna. The extended range clamp gives the surgeon a wider choice of angle for screw insertion in the ulna.

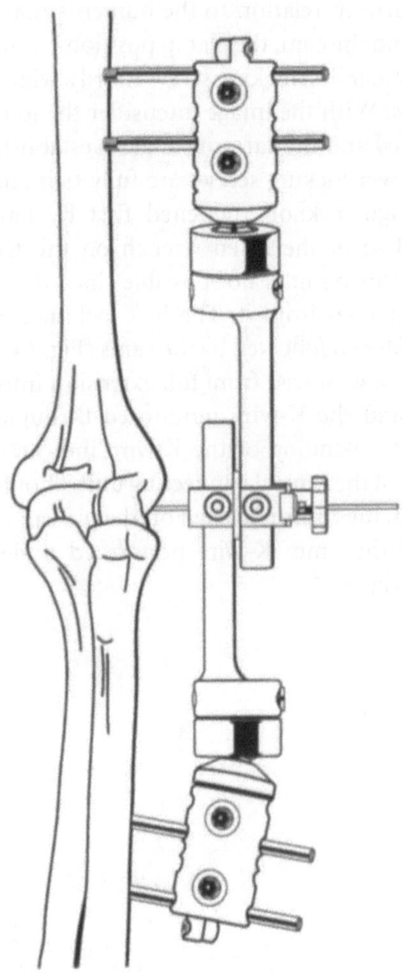

Fig. 14.19 Fixator alignment is now checked in the AP view; the carrying angle is thus determined.

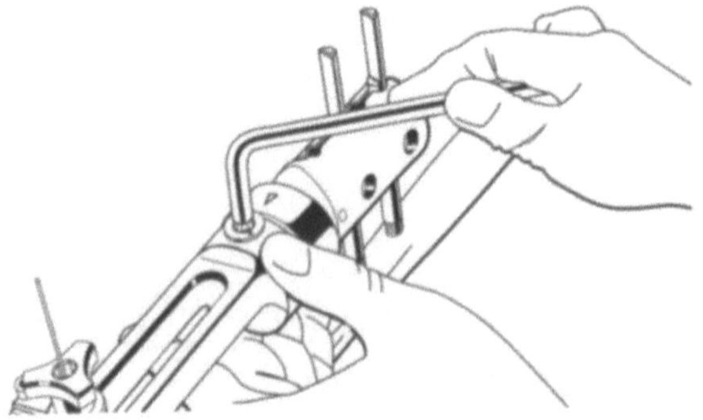

Fig. 14.20 The ball joints are then tightened with the Allen wrench. The triangular knob should be tightened at this point.

The image intensifier is used with the elbow in full extension, 45° and 90° of flexion to check the congruence of the joint line. It must be correctly aligned in all degrees of flexion. If there is asymmetric opening of the joint line the alignment between the fixator and the

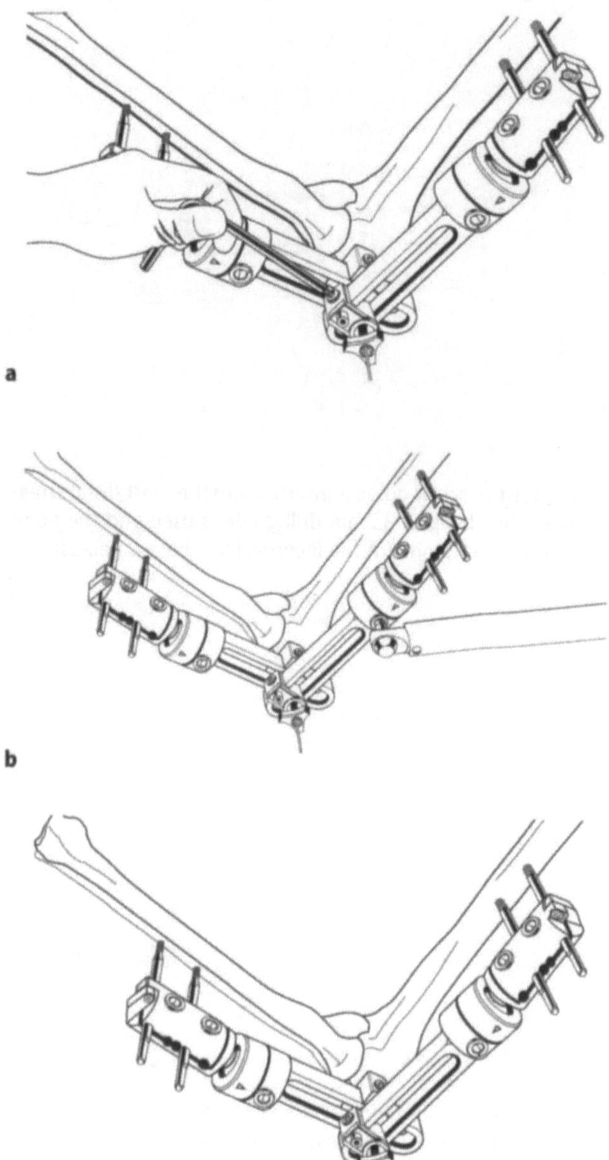

Fig. 14.21 Adjustments may be made by means of the link locking screws and the ball joints, until correct alignment is obtained. **a** Each of the link locking screws is now tightened fully. **b** Final locking of the ball joints is performed using the torque wrench to ensure fixator stability. The torque wrench should only be used to tighten the ball joints. The fixator is locked at an appropriate angle by means of the triangular knob on the central connecting unit (70° of flexion from full extension is recommended). **c** The 2mm K-wire is removed.

bone axis must be confirmed and the position of the central connecting unit checked. Adjustments may be made by means of the link locking screws and the ball joints until correct alignment is achieved. At the end of the procedure all fixator locking screws are fully tightened and a torque wrench is used for the ball joints only. The 2mm K-wire is removed (Fig. 14.21).

The fixator is locked at an appropriate angle by means of the triangular knob of the central connecting unit (70° of flexion from full extension is recommended).

In cases where it is necessary to perform internal fixation procedures on the elbow joint itself, the complete fixator is taken off the bone screws. To facilitate reapplication, the position of the clamp on the pins is marked on both sides of the clamp with an appropriate pen. Only the clamp cover locking screws are now loosened and the fixator removed from the bone screws.

Indications, Supplementary Techniques and Post-operative Management in Acute Cases

Analysis of Instability and Indications

Displacement of the elbow joint in general is caused by a fall on the extended arm. Mechanically, dislocation is explained by an overextension in the humero-ulnar joint with the olecranon abutting on the fossa olecrani. In cadaver specimens it has been shown (Söjbjerg 1989)[1] that the posterior displacement occurs in slight flexion of the elbow, valgus stress and external rotation. Constitutional factors such as a flat semi-lunar fossa may also be important.

When describing elbow displacement the position of the forearm in relation to the humerus is used for definition.

Displacement with or without fracture causes significant damage to the periarticular structures. The direction of displacement indicates to a certain degree which ligaments may have been injured. Anterior displacement is rare and not possible without a fracture of the olecranon. Pure radial and ulnar displacement is also uncommon. Posterior displacement is subclassified as straight posterior, dorso-radial or dorso-ulnar. Most common (80 per cent of cases) is a posterior and posterior-radial displacement. Experimentally, posterior displacment leads to a rupture of the anterior portion of the ulnar collateral ligament (Söjbjerg 1987). Radial ligament injuries are less common and usually affect the annular ligament.

After reduction of a displaced elbow valgus instability is quite common. It has been demonstrated that after resection of the ulnar collateral ligament and joint capsule, a significant valgus instability results whereas removal of the radial head in the presence of an intact ligament causes a lesser degree of instability (Morrey et al 1991).[2] It seems obvious that in posterior radial displacement an injury of the anterior portion of the ulnar collateral ligament and of the annular ligament may be expected. The cadaver study lead to the conclusion that in dislocations not all stabilizing ligaments on the ulnar or the radial side are affected. Clinically, however, in a series of 31 revised elbows there was complete disruption of the medial collateral ligament complex in association with significant valgus instability (Josefsson et al 1987b)[3], but only nine of the 31 elbows redislocated easily under anaesthesia. These results indicate that despite extensive ligament injuries some remaining stabilizing factors exist which may prevent redisplacement.

"Simple" posterior displacement which is stable after reduction should be treated conservatively in a sling for a few days with early mobilization. The main stabilizing factors of the elbow joint seem to be the ulnar collateral ligament complex and the radial head. Injuries involving both structures, therefore, should be considered as highly unstable. The main bony stabilizer on the humero-ulnar side is the olecranon and with a radially or posteriorly displaced elbow in association with an olecranon fracture this should be considered as unstable (Figs. 14.22a–14.22e). The coronoid process is the anterior stabilizer which is increasingly important as the elbow moves into flexion. A displaced coronoid process fracture in association with an elbow dislocation creates instability (Figs. 14.23a–14.23e).

As a general rule the elbow joint should not be immobilized for more than six days. If after reduction and internal fixation of the bony injuries, the surgeon feels that prolonged immobilization is required, an elbow fixator with motion capacity may be included in the management protocol to prevent late disability and stiffness.

Articular Repair, Early Mobilization and Supplementary Techniques

In pure dislocations, the elbow joint is reduced and tested in extension, flexion and valgus stress. If the remaining periarticular structures are competent to control elbow movement without risk of redisplacement, conservative treatment with a short immobilization period of 3–6 days is sufficient. In all cases of elbow injuries with significant soft tissue injury indomethacin 2 × 50 mg per day is used for four

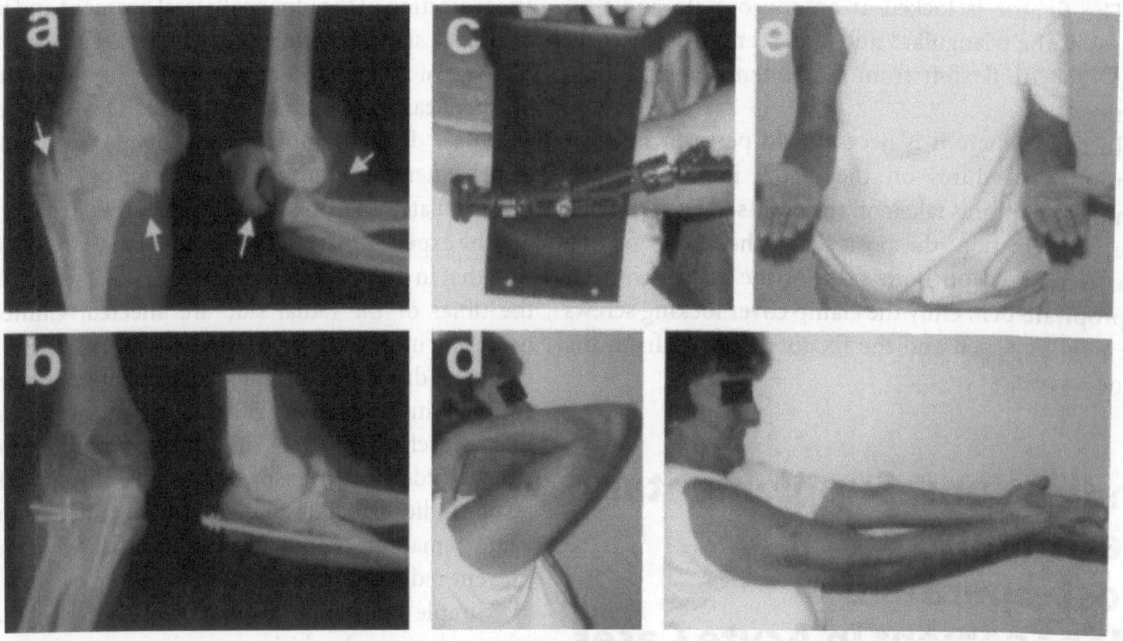

Fig. 14.22 a Dorso-radial dislocation of the elbow with radial head fracture (arrow on the left), AP film; olecranon fracture and coronoid process fracture (arrow on the anterior side right). **b** Internal fixation of the olecranon and the radial head fracture using the Fragment Fixation System. **c** Full lateral X-ray unobstructed by the fixator using a dental film. **d** Flexion and extension 3 weeks after fixator removal. **e** Supination 3 weeks after fixator removal; pronation was unhindered.

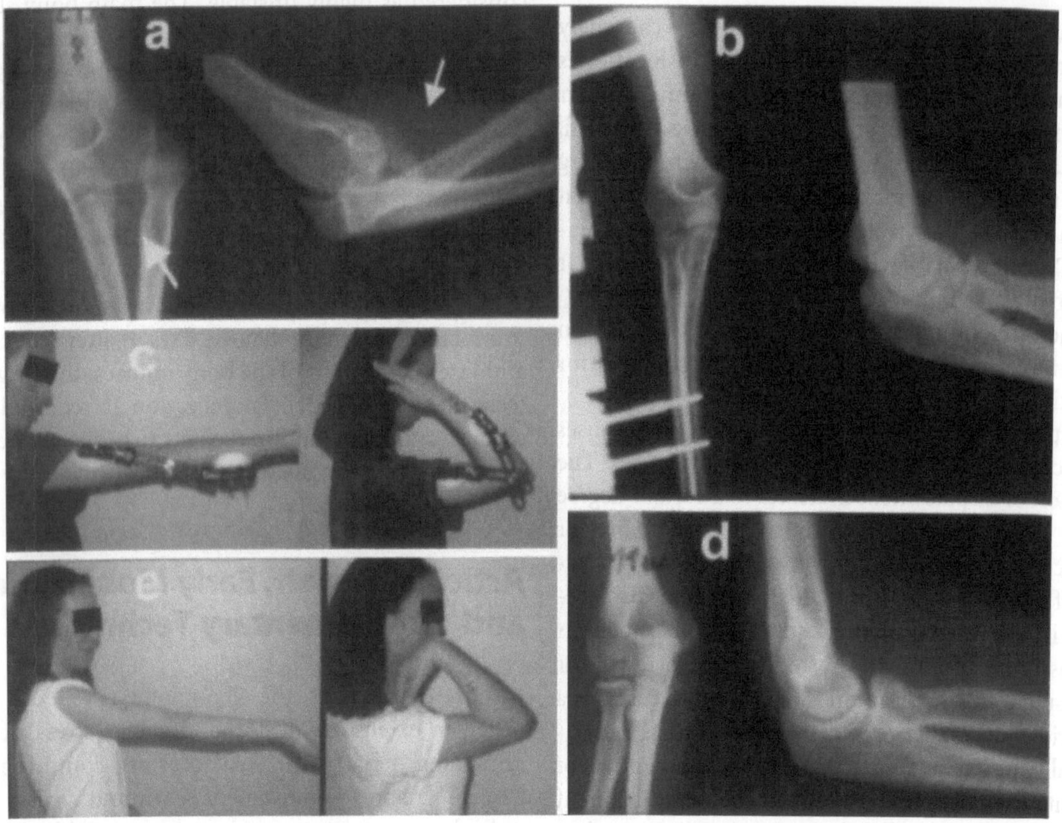

Fig. 14.23 a Posterior displacement in the humero-ulnar joint and proximal radio-ulnar joint disruption. Fracture of the coronoid process and avulsion of the annular ligament in a 21-year-old woman. **b** Closed reduction was performed; the fixator in situ. **c** Extension and flexion 16 days after injury. **d** Joint congruence 11 weeks after injury. Note: no heterotopic bone formation. **e** Flexion and extension 1 year after injury.

weeks to prevent heterotopic bone formation, provided there are no contraindications to its use.

If early mobilization is not possible because of a tendency to redislocate, the Elbow Fixator is applied as described above. There remains the question of whether or not to perform open repair of the ligaments. Even in so-called simple dislocations there is significant injury of the ligamentous structures involved. These, in general, do heal under conservative therapy and early motion. An indication for ligament repair may be present in cases where the repaired ligament(s) will provide the stability to allow early mobilization post-operatively. The instability itself, therefore, is not the indication for open repair, but the necessity to create a stable joint which allows early mobilization. Josefsson et al (1987a)[4] advocated repair of the injured ligaments but could show that their cases with closed treatment in comparison with open repair had a similar functional outcome. Schnettler demonstrated that it is not open repair or conservative treatment which determines the final result but the length of the immobilization period (Schnettler 1993).[5]

We do not routinely perform open repair of the ligaments unless a significant bony avulsion of the ulnar collateral ligament or the radial collateral ligament is present which lends itself to refixation. The effect of early controlled mobilization on periarticular structures is a complex process. The biological response to joint instability is increased fibroblastic activity with formation of fibrosis in an attempt to generate stability. This, however, leads to non-directed and non-functional stabilization, resulting in stiffness.

The concept of transarticular fixation with motion capacity allows controlled restitution of joint mobility. During the first weeks after injury the reparative process requires movement within the normal range to define the working length of ligaments, muscles and capsule. The ligament repair process with increased activity of fibroblasts causes the collagen fibres to line up parallel to the line of tension. A lack of tension would result in disorientation, formation of scar tissue and arthrofibrosis. Haematoma formation and cellular debris causes obliteration of the joint and the formation of fibrofatty tissue within it and is an important factor in the development of joint impairment.

In dislocations the fixator is not only used to provide early controlled mobilization but also helps to maintain an adequate joint space without undue compression of the articular surfaces. To achieve this, the small distractor may be used but in general it is sufficient to perform manual distraction until the joint space appears normal.

When bony structures are involved (olecranon, radial head, coronoid process, capitulum humeri) in the presence of a displaced elbow the articular surface will also have suffered. In these cases we routinely repair the olecranon, the radial head and the capitulum humeri. Due to the impact an articular defect with flake fractures and cartilage abrasions is not uncommon. The repair process in articular fractures starts with a fibrin clot filling the remaining gaps. The cell system available for repair will contain chondrocytes which after several days may create a surface of fibrous cartilage. The fibrin clot repair and the early cellular response must be protected. Early excessive loading of the joint may disrupt the repair process (Buckwalter 1992,[6] 1995[7]) and the fixator, with a certain degree of distraction of the joint, will support the repair. When moving the joint again the articular surfaces must be protected against excessive shear forces. Not only may inadequate loading of articular components lead to redisplacement of the fractures, it may also be detrimental to the repair process.

The role of early mobilization in joint injuries has been studied experimentally in dogs (Behrens et al 1989).[8] Comparing rigid fixation after articular injuries with limited motion it was evident that the latter recovered the proteoglycan content whereas rigid mobilization was associated with further degeneration after functional loading occurred.

To facilitate joint revision and the exposure required for internal fixation, the fixator is temporarily removed. After insertion of the fixator pins in humerus and ulna and alignment of the device in the centre of rotation, the position of the clamps on the pins is marked on both sides. With all other components tightened, the clamp screws are loosened and the device removed. This provides full access to the joint. If an olecranon fracture is present this is dealt with first and the removal of debris from the joint is mandatory. Internal fixation techniques follow the standard protocols and we recommend use of the Fragment Fixation System.

The single most important bony stabilizing structure in ulnar ligament disruption is the radial head, and whenever possible an attempt should be made to restore it. Radial head resection may compromise the repair process of the ulnar collateral ligament. The role of the annular ligament must also not be underestimated. A late consequence of radial head resection, especially in heavy labourers, is incongruence in the distal radio-ulnar joint (Essex–Lopresti deformity). Fractures of the humeral articular surface (capitulum humeri) generally require internal fixation. Unless the coronoid process causes impingement we do not routinely stabilize it. Large exposures and operative trauma may lead to further periarticular damage and result in heterotopic bone formation.

After internal fixation has been completed the fixator is re-applied and care should be taken to unload the joint by distraction as described above.

Post-operative Management

The most important aspect of post-operative management is mobilization. Whereas pro- and supination should be allowed as early as day one after operative treatment, flexion and extension of the elbow should commence after soft tissue healing on day four and is supervised by a physiotherapist. Flexion and extension of the elbow made possible by unlocking the central triangular knob.

As with any external fixation equipment, pin site care is of paramount importance and during the first week pins are cleaned 2–3 times with decreasing frequency during the following weeks. Non-staining mild disinfectants are used. Radiographic control is carried out post-operatively at weekly intervals. A true lateral X-ray may be obtained by insertion of a dental film between the skin and the fixator (Fig. 14.22c). For daily activities full flexion is more important than full extension. The patient is encouraged to use the hand for eating and similar tasks but heavy loading is not permitted. The device remains in situ for six weeks and the progress of elbow joint motion should be recorded. Complications include pin track sepsis which may require removal of the device. With adequate pin site care and the relatively short application time, this complication should not occur. Patients with an allergic response to surgical grade steel should not be treated with external fixation screws. Patients with poorly controlled diabetes or infectious diseases (e.g. HIV) are in general not suitable for external fixation procedures, and the same holds true for the poorly compliant patient.

With incorrect alignment of the central connecting unit, joint subluxation may occur and radiographic control is necessary to confirm alignment. Careful intra-operative control of joint motion under image intensification with the fixator in situ helps to avoid this. If there is subluxation, realignment of the fixator with correct placement of the 2mm Kirschner-wire in the centre of rotation should be carried out.

The correct size of fixator screws must be chosen, particularly in the ulna, to avoid weakening which may cause a fracture at the screw site.

As with any technical equipment, maintainance of the fixator is important and lubrication of the central connecting unit may be necessary to facilitate movement.

The Elbow Fixator in the Mangement of Joint Stiffness: Indications, Supplementary Techniques and Post-operative Treatment

Introduction

To make use of the unique upper limb elbow function requires a stable and painfree joint with an adequate range of motion. Elbow motion has been investigated in healthy volunteers and Morrey and Chao (1976)[9] showed that 90 per cent of daily living activities may be carried out in an arc of motion between 30° and 130° of extension and flexion. Pro- and supination of 50° each was also required. The functions studied included sports and work activities. Most patients will tolerate a loss of extension whereas a loss of the same degree of flexion may be disabling. A total range of motion of less than 100° will therefore lead to impaired upper limb function.

The incidence of post-traumatic elbow stiffness is unknown. It does however seem fairly common, affecting approximately 5 per cent of elbows after injury (Söjbjerg 1996).[10]

In 200 cases of post-traumatic elbow stiffness 38 per cent were related to fracture dislocations of the joint and 20 per cent to elbow dislocation (Mohan 1972).[11] Radial head fractures accounted for 10 per cent of the cases. The injury pattern itself is only one aspect in the development of post-traumatic stiffness, and prolonged immobilization also seems to be an important factor. In our opinion an elbow joint should not be immobilized for longer than one week and in the presence of a significant soft tissue injury, we routinely administer indomethacin provided there are no contraindications.

Post-traumatic elbow stiffness is best classified according to the position of the contracture, as extension or flexion stiffness and an assessment of the function of adjacent joints (shoulder and wrist) is required as well. The causes of post-traumatic stiffness can be divided into intra- and extra-articular, but a mixed pathology is often the reason for limitation of elbow function. Extra-articular causes include muscular and skin retraction, fibrosis of ligaments and capsule, and heterotopic bone formation with bony bridging of the joint. Intra-articular causes include joint obliteration with the formation of fibro-fatty tissue and articular incongruence with secondary degenerative arthritis.

Pathophysiologically, in a stiff elbow the water content of the cartilage increases whereas the proteoglycan content decreases. Radiological narrowing of the joint line is the consequence.

Pre-operative evaluation includes a detailed history of the aetiology of the disability as well as a full clinical examination. When moving the elbow into maximal flexion and extension, gliding of the joint should be palpated. Plain radiographs are necessary and an arthrogram helps to evaluate the remaining joint space. A CT scan and an arthro-CT are also required. The CT helps to decide whether heterotopic bone formation is present and whether it limits the function mechanically. MRI does not seem to be helpful. Diagnostic arthroscopy as a routine measure is not recommended since the joint is tight and iatrogenic injuries to the cartilage may result.

Ulnar, radial and median nerve function should be studied pre-operatively using nerve conduction tests. The ulnar nerve is particularly vulnerable on increased flexion in cases where a lack of flexion has been present for a prolonged period.

Indications

Before operative procedures are carried out on an elbow with limited motion, conservative measures such as physiotherapy and dynamic splinting should be exhausted. We do not advocate manipulation under anaesthesia or a continuous brachial plexus block. This may cause intra-articular damage by avulsion of a cartilage fragment when the fibro-fatty tissue which lines the joint ruptures.

With a range of motion of less than 100° and flexion affected, arthrodiatasis with the Elbow Fixator may be offered to the patient.

Whereas release operations have been described in the literature (Urbaniak et al 1985;[12] Morrey 1990;[13] Söjbjerg 1996)[10] distraction arthroplasty has not been used routinely. It was first described some years ago (Volkov and Oganesian 1975)[14] and has been reported in limited series (Deland et al 1987;[15] Judet and Judet 1978;[16] Regan and Reilly 1993;[17] Regan et al 1991).[18]

Operative Technique

The Elbow Fixator is applied as described above. Each link has to be fitted with a small distractor and when applying the fixator one has to ensure that the capacity of the links is sufficient to permit distraction. The small distractors will move the central connecting unit distally in the humeral link and posteriorly in the ulnar link (Fig. 14.24). Movement of the ulnar link relative to the central connecting unit does not influence the centre of rotation, but the movement in the humeral link requires positioning of the 2mm Kirschner-wire at the proximal border of the condylar ring visible in the lateral X-ray (Fig. 14.25). When distracting along the axis of the humerus, the central connecting unit will move distally into the centre of rotation. Prior to distraction along the humeral link the 2mm K-wire must be removed.

The main benefit of distraction arthroplasty is lengthening of the inevitably shortened ligaments and fibrotic capsule (Fig. 14.26). At the same time the humero-ulnar and the humero-radial joint surfaces will be separated and this helps to protect the cartilage. If the joint is stiff and tight, closed manipulation may lead to excessive loading of the remaining cartilage and further damage to the articular structures may be expected. Since shortening of the ligaments and capsule occurs over a certain period of time the reversal of this process (arthrodiatasis) should be slow as well. Simultaneous distraction along the humeral and the ulnar links will lead to symmetrical distraction of the joint and avoid impingement of either the olecranon or the coronoid process on the capitulum humeri (Figs. 14.27a–14.27c).

The total degree of distraction depends on the resistance of the soft tissues and the humeral distractor is turned a total of 10–12 times (= 10–12mm) while the ulnar distractor is turned 3–5 times (= 3–5mm) clockwise.

To facilitate joint distraction with the elbow fixator, predistraction with a standard Orthofix fixator is routinely performed (for details see Ch. 54). We insert the fixator pins as described above into the humerus and the ulna. A standard Orthofix fixator or a short Orthofix fixator placed on the humeral pins is used with two additional pins in a T-clamp inserted in the olecranon. It is important to align the Elbow Fixator prior to applying the distraction fixator and mark the

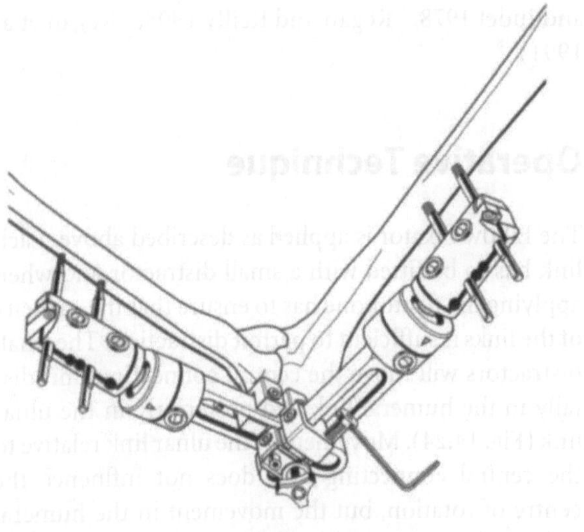

Fig. 14.24 A small distractor is placed on the humeral link to obtain joint distraction. This will shift the axis and requires the K-wire (and therefore the central connecting unit) to be placed 5–7mm proximal to the ideal centre of rotation prior to distraction. In this case, the fixator should be assembled with the humeral link outside the ulnar link, to enable the small distractor to be applied correctly. The humeral link locking screw and the triangular knob are loosened.
A small distractor is also placed on the ulnar link and its locking screw is firmly tightened. When positioning the distractor units, care should be taken to ensure that an adequate length of the distractor screw will be available. The link locking screw of the ulnar link and the triangular knob of the central connecting unit are now loosened, and distraction commenced to unload the cartilage. Initial distraction must be performed during surgery and a normal joint width should be aimed for at this stage. Widening of the joint should be monitored radiographically. Additional surgery may be required to clean the olecranon fossa or the anterior joint compartment, or to remove heterotopic bridges. The ulnar nerve will usually require decompression. Routine anterior transposition is not advocated.

fixator clamp position on the humeral and the ulnar screws. All components of the Elbow Fixator with the exception of the clamp screws must be left locked when temporarily removing the device to apply the distraction fixator. We prefer posterolateral pin insertion into the olecranon for better purchase and better visualization of joint distraction in the lateral view. The standard distractors are used in these cases and we distract 15mm over a minimum of 30 minutes. The standard fixator is then removed and the Elbow Fixator applied. When the Elbow Fixator is mounted, distraction along the humeral and ulnar links is performed as described above. Radiographic control of joint distraction is mandatory prior to moving the elbow into flexion and extension (Figs. 14.28a–14.28c). This movement is performed with gentle force and a total range of

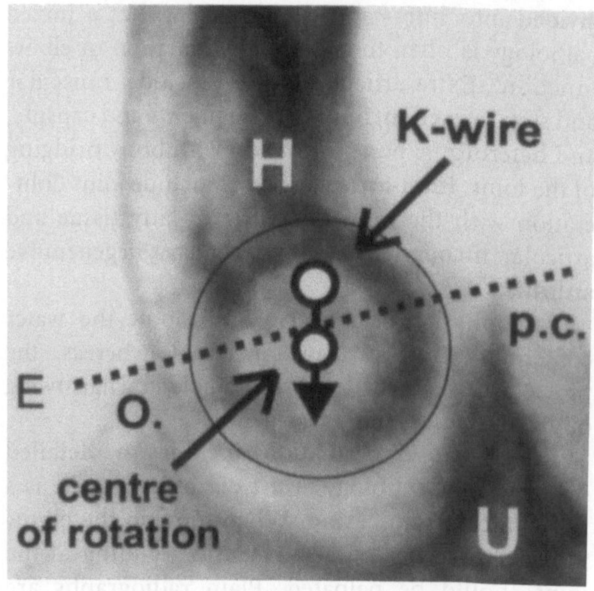

Fig. 14.25 Lateral view under the image intensifier. The true lateral visualization of the condyles is a pre-requisite for K-wire placement. Since the centre of rotation will shift distally during humeral distraction, the K-wire is placed at the proximal end of the condylar ring. E = line from coronoid process (p.c.) to olecranon (o).

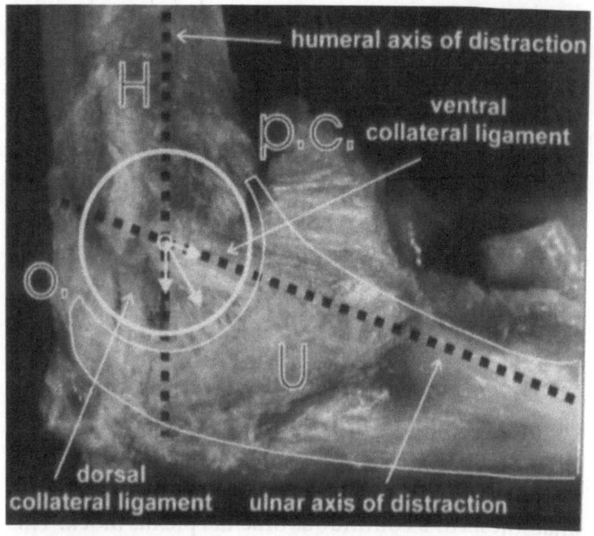

Fig. 14.26 Lateral view of the humero-ulnar joint. The dotted lines indicate the axis of the humerus (H) and the ulna (U). Distraction along the ulnar link lengthens the ventral ulnar collateral ligament; along the humeral link the dorsal ulnar collateral ligament is lengthened. (P.C.) coronoid process; (0) olecranon.

motion of 100° should be aimed for. After intra-operative movement under anaesthesia the fixator is locked. If a lack of flexion was the main problem, the locked position should be between 100 and 120° of flexion from full extension.

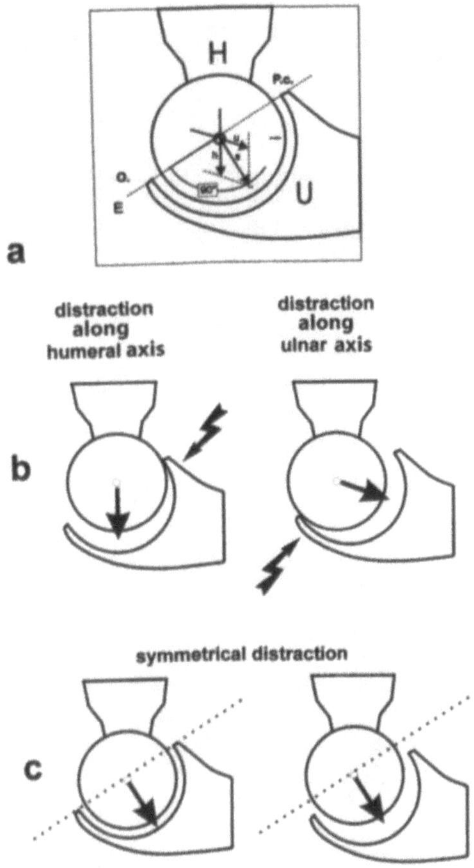

Fig. 14.27 **a** The humeral and ulnar distraction combined lead to symmetrical distraction of the humero-ulnar joint (H Humerus; U Ulna; O Olecranon; E Plane of distraction; P.c. Coronoid process). **b** Distraction along the humeral axis alone leads to impingement of the coronoid process (left), distraction along the ulnar axis alone to impingement of the olecranon process (right). **c** Symmetrical distraction leads to widening of the joint without impingement.

The decompressed ulnar nerve may be affected by increased flexion and immediately post-operatively the patient should be assessed. If dysaesthesia is present the position of the elbow is altered to make it more comfortable for the patient.

The fixator remains in this position for 6–10 days. Whereas intra-operative distraction is described as phase 1, phase 2 is the relaxation phase.

Supplementary Techniques

We do not routinely perform any soft tissue release since the distraction capacity of the fixator will lead to elongation of the shortened structures. CT studies including an arthro-CT will indicate if the joint space is obliterated by bony fragments which then need to be removed through a limited arthrotomy. This is particularly important in cases where the olecranon fossa shows bony apposition. If the fragments are not removed the olecranon will not move into the olecranon fossa during extension. On the anterior side heterotopic bone formation should be removed when bony bridging is identified on the CT scan. Intra-articular fracture malunion has to be evaluated. Since the elbow joint is a non-weightbearing joint only a malunion which affects the movement of the olecranon process, the coronoid process and/or the radial head requires revision. If the joint is subluxed this must be reduced intra-operatively using the small distractors as well as the capacity of the ball joints. It is important to understand that not only posterior subluxation or anterior subluxation may be present but also rotational malalignment between the forearm and the humerus. The CT scan will help to detect rota-

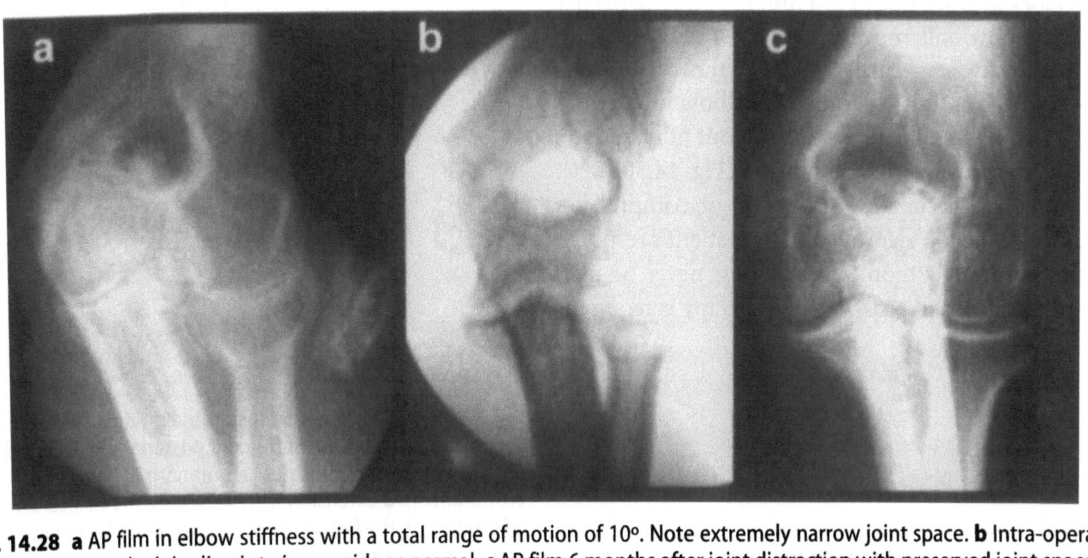

Fig. 14.28 **a** AP film in elbow stiffness with a total range of motion of 10°. Note extremely narrow joint space. **b** Intra-operative distraction. Note: the joint line is twice as wide as normal. **c** AP film 6 months after joint distraction with preserved joint space.

tional malalignment. Posterior subluxation is often associated with malunion and/or shortening of the radial head and the proximal radius. This may require correction to create a stable joint.

Post-operative Management

The relaxation phase to allow the distracted ligaments to respond to forces applied to them lasts 6–10 days. From post-operative day one indomethacin 2 × 50 mg is adminstered provided there are no contraindications. This helps to avoid formation of heterotopic bone and we do not routinely use radiotherapy. After phase 2 (relaxation), phase 3, the mobilization phase, commences with the central connecting unit unlocked (Table 14.1). The patient will require physiotherapy 2–3 times per day and cryotherapy is used prior to physiotherapy. Analgesics may be required prior to the physiotherapy sessions, but we do not advocate the use of continuous brachial plexus anaesthesia. The Elbow Fixator central connecting unit is locked overnight and we alternate the position between the maximum flexion achieved during physiotherapy and the maximum extension. A protocol is helpful to make sure that the elbow will remain one night in maximum flexion and one night in maximum extension (Figs. 14.29a–14.29g). The ulnar nerve must be monitored carefully and any loss of motor function may need intervention. We routinely decompress the ulnar nerve where there is lack of flexion but do not suggest anterior transposition. Nerve conduction tests may be helpful to monitor the ulnar nerve during mobilization.

To increase flexion and/or extension the standard compression–distraction unit is inserted into the cams of the fixator. By turning the compression–distraction screw clockwise at a rate of 2–4 mm (2–4 full turns) per day the elbow will move into flexion (Fig. 14.30a). Counterclockwise turns with the compression–distraction unit will move the elbow into extension. To straighten the Elbow Fixator out fully, spacers are used to reach maximal extension (Fig. 14.30b).

The use of mechanical distraction or compression should never be too vigorous and the patient's response should be carefully monitored. It must never be used alone and active and passive physiotherapy is required.

Distraction phase	intra-operative
Relaxtion phase	6–10 days post-operative
Mobilization phase	5–7 weeks

Table 14.1

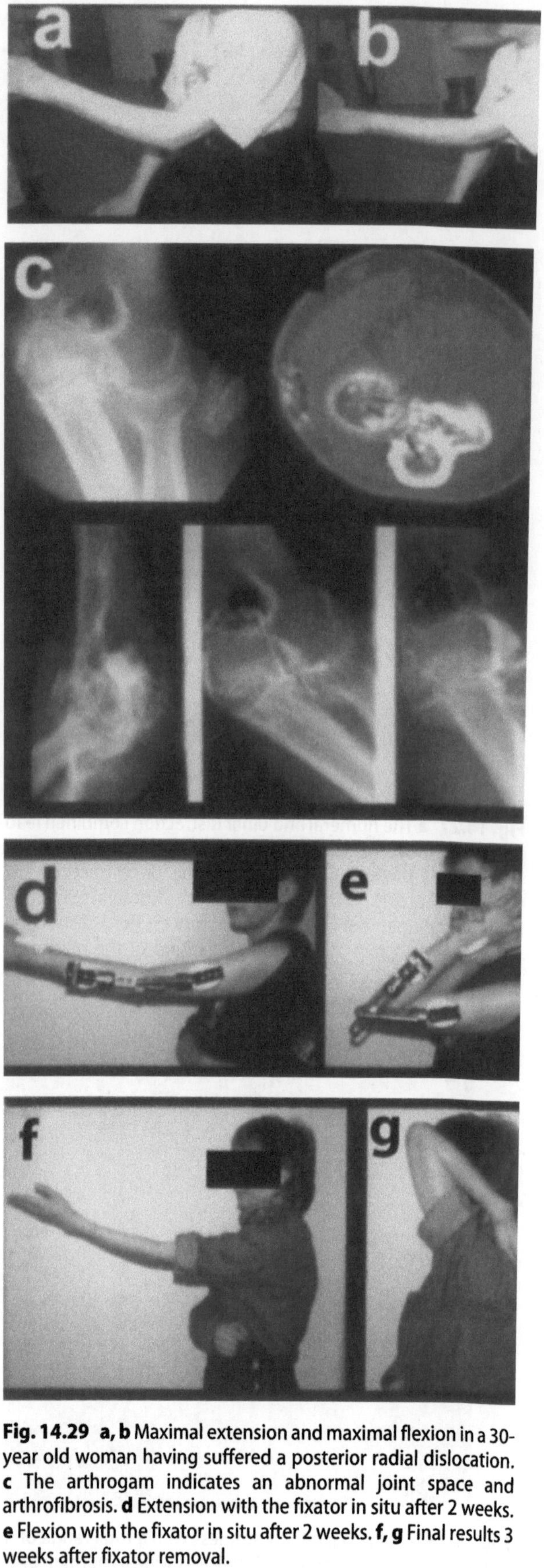

Fig. 14.29 a, b Maximal extension and maximal flexion in a 30-year old woman having suffered a posterior radial dislocation. **c** The arthrogam indicates an abnormal joint space and arthrofibrosis. **d** Extension with the fixator in situ after 2 weeks. **e** Flexion with the fixator in situ after 2 weeks. **f, g** Final results 3 weeks after fixator removal.

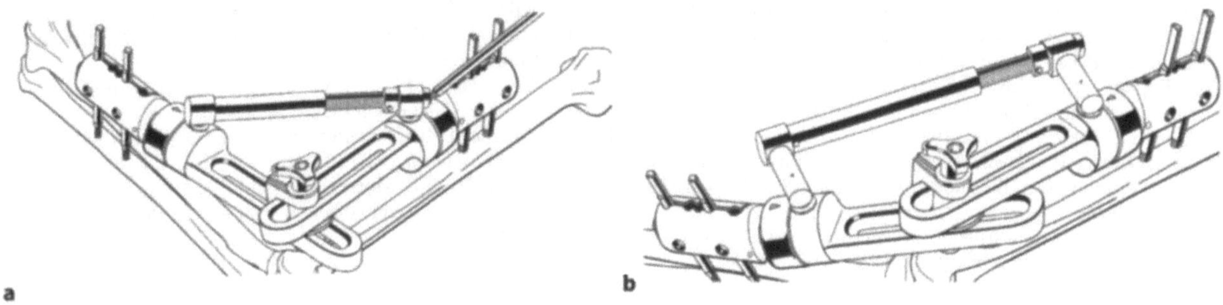

a b

Fig. 14.30 **a** Compression–distraction device inserted in the cams used to increase flexion at a speed of 1–4mm per day. **b** The same device inserted with the spacer to allow full extension.

X-ray control is performed post-operatively and every other week thereafter. The fixator remains in situ for six to eight weeks and a longer period may be required if the response is slow. The target is to reach 100° of motion and flexion is more important than extension. Pin site care is identical to that described for acute cases.

The successful use of arthrodiatasis in elbow stiffness requires considerable clinical experience and is best performed in centres with an appropriate case load. The patient needs to be informed what to expect from the procedure. To achieve a satisfactory result, patient selection is important. Of equal importance is the post-operative management which, ideally, should be carried out in the department performing the operation. The same holds true for pin site care and the department must be familiar with external fixation procedures in reconstructive cases.

References

1. Söjbjerg JO, Helmig R, Kjärsgaard-Anderson P 'Dislocation of the elbow: An experimental study of the ligamentous injuries.' *Orthopedics* 1989; 3(12): 461-3.
2. Morrey BF, Tanaka S, An KN 'Valgus stability of the elbow.' *Clin Orthop* 1991; 265: 187–95.
3. Josefsson PO, Johnell O, Wendeberg B 'Ligamentous injuries in dislocations of the elbow.' *Clin Orthop* 1987b; 221: 221–5.
4. Josefsson PO, Gentz CF, Johnell O et al 'Surgical versus nonsurgical treatment of ligamentous injuries following dislocations of the elbow joint.' *Clin Orthop* 1987a; 214: 165–9.
5. Schnettler R 'Ergebnisse nach Ellbogenluxationen bei konservativer und operativer Therapie.' *Chir Praxis* 1993; 46: 55–6.
6. Buckwalter JA 'Mechanical Injuries of Articular Cartilage.' *Iowa Orthopaedic Journal* 1992; Vol 12:50–7.
7. Buckwalter JA 'Should Bone, Soft Tissue and Joint Injuries be Treated with Rest or Activity?' *Orth Res* 1995; 13: 155–6.
8. Behrens F, Kraft EL, Oegema T 'Biomechanical Changes in Articular Cartilage after Joint Immobilization by Casting or External Fixation.' *Orthop Res* 1989; 7 (3): 335–43.
9. Morrey BF, Chao EY 'Passive motion of the elbow joint.' *J Bone Joint Surg* [Am] 1976; 58A: 501–8.
10. Söjbjerg JO 'The stiff elbow.' *Acta Orthop Scand* 1996; 67(6): 626–31.
11. Mohan K 'Myositis ossificans of the elbow.' *Int Surg* 1972; 57(6): 475–80.
12. Urbaniak JR, Hansen PE, Beissinger SF et al 'Correction of post-traumatic flexion contracture of the elbow by anterior capsulotomy.' *J Bone Joint Surg* [Am] 1985; 67A: 1160.
13. Morrey BF 'Post-traumatic contracture of the elbow.' *J Bone Joint Surg* [Am] 1990; 72A: 601–18.
14. Volkov MF, Oganesian OV 'Restoration of function in the knee and elbow with a hinge distractor apparatus.' *J Bone Joint Surg* [Am] 1975; 57A: 591–600.
15. Deland JT, Walter PS, Sledge CB et al 'Biomechanical basis for elbow hinge-distractor design.' *Clin Orthop* 1987 215: 303–12.
16. Judet R, Judet T 'Arthrolyse et arthroplastie sous distracteur articulaire.' *Revue de Chirurgie orthop*1978; 64:353–65.
17. Regan WD, Reilly CD 'Distraction arthroplasty of the elbow.' *Hand Clin* 1993; 9: 719–28.
18. Regan WD, Korinek SL, Morray BF et al 'Biomechanical study of ligaments around the elbow joint.' *Clin Orthop* 1991; 271: 170–9.

Supplementary Bibliography

Aebi H 'Der Ellbogenwinkel, seine Beziehungen zu Geschlecht, Körperbau und Hüftbreite.' *Acta Anat* (Basel) 1947; 3: 29–284.

Amis AA, Dowson D, Unsworth JH et al 'An examination of the elbow articulation with particular reference to variation of the carrying angle.' *IEEE Eng Med Biol Mag* 1977; 3(6): 76–80.

An KN, Morrey BF, Chao EYS 'Carrying angle of the human elbow joint.' *Orthop Res* 1984; 1: 369–78.

Beals RK 'The normal carrying angle of the elbow. A radiographic study of 422 patients.' *Clin Orthop* 1976; 119: 194–6.

Bennighoff A, Goerttler K. (1980) 'Lehrbuch der Anatomie des Menschen.' in: Ferner H. Staubesand J (eds.) *Allgemein Anatomie, Cytologie und Bewegungsapparat,* Bd.1 Urban 38; Schwarzenberg, München Wien Baltimore.

Bhattacharyya S. 'Arthrolysis: a new approach to surgery of post-taumatic stiff elbow.' *J Bone Joint Surg* [Br] 1974; 56: 567.

Bopp F, Tielemann FW, Holz U 'Ellenbogenluxationen mit Frakturen am Processus coronoideus und Radiusköpfchen-trümmerfraktur.' *Unfallchirurg* 199194: 322–4.

Breen TF, Gelbermann RH, Ackermann GN 'Elbow flexion contractures: Treatment by anterior release and continuous passive motion.' *J Hand Surg* [Br] 1988; 13:286.

Bryan RS, Bickel WHT 'Condylar fractures of the distal humerus.' *J Trauma* 1971; 11: 830.

Cobb TK, Linscheid RL 'Late correction of malunited intercondylar humeral fractures. Intra-articular osteotomy and tricortical bone grafting.' *J Bone Joint Surg* [Br] 1994; 76(4): 622–6.

Costa P, Giancecchi F, Cavazzuti A, et al 'Internal and external fixation in complex diaphyseal and metaphyseal fractures of the humerus.' *J Orthop Trauma* 1991; 17 (1): 87–94.

Dürig M, Müller W, Ruedi TP et al 'The operative treatment of elbow dislocation in the adult.' *J Bone Joint Surg* [Am] 1979; 61(2): 239–44.

Ewald FC (1986) 'Reconstruction of complex elbow problem' in: Tullos HS (ed.) *Instructional course lectures*, vol. XXXV.

Fick R (1911) *Spezielle Gelenk- und Muskelmechanik*, Fischer: Jena.

Fischer O (1887) 'Das Ellenbogengelenk.' in: Braune W, Fischer O (eds) *Untersuchungen über die Gelenke des menschlichen Armes*, Theil 1. Leipzig (XIV. Band der Abhandlungen der mathematisch-physischen Classe der königlich Sächsischen Gesellschaft der Wissenschaften, 81–106).

Fuss FK 'The ulnar collateral ligament of the human elbow joint. Anatomy, function and biomechanics.' *J Anat* 1991; 175: 203–12.

Gausepohl T, Koebke J, Pennig D et al 'Anatomische Grundlagen zur Anwendung der unilateralen externen Fixation an Oberarm, Unterarm und Hand.' *Osteosyn Int* 1997a; 5: 76–88.

Gausepohl T, Pennig D, Mader K 'Der transartikuläre Bewegungsfixateur bei Luxationen und Luxationsfrakturen des Ellenbogengelenkes.' *Osteosyn Int* 1997b; 5: 102–10.

Gausepohl D, Pennig D (1998) 'Luxationen und Luxationsfrakturen des Ellenbogens – Einsatz des Bewegungsfixateurs.' in: *Ellenbogenchirurgie in der Praxis* Meyer RP, Kappeler U (eds) Springer:Berlin.

Glynn JJ, Niebauer J 'Flexion and extension contracture of the elbow: surgical management.' *Clin Orthop* 1976; 117: 289–91.

Green DP, McCoy H 'Turnbuckle orthotic correction of elbow-flexion contractures after acute injuries.' *J Bone Joint Surg* [Am] 1979; 61: 1092.

Gutierrez LS 'A contribution to the study of the limiting factors of elbow extension.' *Acta Anat* (Basel) 1964; 56: 146–56.

Habermeyer P 'Konservative Behandlung von Ellenbogenluxationen.' *Orthopade* 1988; 17: 313–9.

Husband JB, Hastings H 'The lateral approach for operative release of post-traumatic contracture of the elbow.' *J Bone Joint Surg* [Am] 1990; 72: 1353.

Johannsson H, Olerud S (1971) 'Operative Treatment of intercondylar fractures of the humerus.' *Trauma* 11 10: 836–43.

Kapandji IA (1970) *The physiology of joints. Annotaded diagrams of the mechanics of the human joints*, Vol.1, 2. Livingstone: Edinburgh.

Kinast C, Waldström J, Pfeiffer KM 'Konservative und operative Therapie bei Ellenbogenluxation.' *Helv Chir Acta* 1985; 52: 851–4.

Koebke J (1992) 'Funktionelle Anatomie und Biomechanik des Ellenbogengelenkes.' in: Stahl, Zeidler, Koebke et al (eds) *Klinische Arthrologie*, 3. Erg. Lfg. 11.

Lansinger O, Karlsson J, Körner L et al 'Dislocation of the elbow joint.' *Arch Orthop Trauma Surg* 1984; 102: 183–6.

Linscheid RL, Wheeler DK 'Elbow dislocations.' *Am Med Inform Assoc* 1965; 194(11): 113–8.

London JT 'Kinematics of the elbow.' *J Bone Joint Surg* [Am] 1981; 64(4): 529–35.

McKee M, Jupiter J, Toh CL et al 'Reconstruction after malunion and non-union of intra-articular fractures of the distal humerus.' *J Bone Joint Surg* [Br] 1994; 76(4): 614–21.

Mingione A, Barca F (1991) 'Anatomophysiopathology.' in: Celli J (ed) *The elbow traumatic lesions*. Springer:Berlin.

Morrey BF 'Functional anatomy of the ligaments of the elbow.' *Clin Orthop* 1985; 201: 84–90.

Morrey BF (1994a) 'Distraction arthroplasty'. in: Morrey BF (ed) *The Elbow*. Raven:New York.

Morrey BF (1994b) 'Limited extensile triceps reflecting exposures of the elbow', in: Morrey BF (ed) *The Elbow*. Raven: New York.

Morrey BF (1994c) 'Post-traumatic stiffness: distraction arthroplastry' in: Morrey BF (ed) *The elbow and its disorders*. 2nd edn. Saunders: Philadelphia.

Morrey BF, Askew LJ, An KN 'Strength function after elbow arthroplasty.' *Clin Orthop* 1988; 234: 43–50.

Muhr G, Werner E 'Bänderverletzung und Luxation des Ellbogengelenkes.' *Orthopade* 1989; 18: 268–272.

O'Driscoll SW, Horii E, Morrey BF et al (1992a) 'Anatomy of the ulnar part of the lateral collateral ligament of the elbow.' *Clin Anat* 5: 296–303.

O'Driscoll SW, Morrey BF, Korinek S et al (1992b) 'Elbow subluxation and dislocation. A spectrum of instability.' *Clin Orthop* 280: 186–97.

Pauwels F (1965) 'Die Bedeutung der am Ellenbogengelenk wirkenden mechanischen Faktoren für die Tragfähigkeit des gebeugten Armes.' in: Pauwels F (ed) *Gesammelte Abhandlungen zur funktionellen Anatomie des Bewegungsapparates*. Springer: Berlin.

Pauwels F (1973) *Atlas zur Biomechanik der gesunden und kranken Hüfte*. Springer: Berlin.

Pennig D, Gausepohl T (1997) *The Elbow Fixator. Operative Technique*. Operation manual. Orthofix srl: Bussolengo, Italy

Pennig D, Gausepohl D (1998) 'Die posttraumatische Ellenbogensteife – Gelenkdistraktion mit Fixateur externe als Behandlungskonzept.' in: *Ellenbogenchirurgie in der Praxis* Meyer RP, Kappeler U (eds) Springer: Berlin.

Pennig D, Gausepohl D, Mader K (1999) 'Transarticular fixation with motion capacity in fracture dislocations of the elbow.' *Injury* Suppl (in press).

Poigenfürst J, Iselin M 'Die anatomisch konstitutionellen Voraussetzungen der Ellenbogenverrenkung.' *Schriften Unfallheilk* 1965; 68: 57–72.

Ray RD, Johnson RJ, Jameson RM 'Rotation of the forearm: An experimental study of pronation and supination.' *J Bone Joint Surg* [Am] 1951; 33(4): 993–6.

Rydholm U, Tjörnstrand B, Petterson H et al 'Surface replacement of the elbow in rheumatoid arthritis.' *J Bone Joint Surg* [Br] 1984; 66(5): 737–41.

Schwab GH, Bennett JB, Woods GW et al 'Biomechanics of elbow instability: The role of the medial collateral ligament.' *Clin Orthop* 1980; 146: 42–52.

Shahriaree H, Sjadi K, Silver CM et al 'Excisional arthroplasty of the elbow.' *J Bone Joint Surg* [Am] 1979; 81(6): 922–7.

Söjbjerg JO, Ovesen J, Gundorf CE 'The stability of the elbow following excision of the radial head and transection of the annular ligament. An experimental study.' *Arch Orthop Trauma Surg* 1987; 106: 248–50.

Steel FLD, Tomlinson JDW 'The carrying angle in man.' *J Anat* 1958; 92: 315–7.

Steindler A (1964) *Kinesiology of the human body under normal and pathological conditions*, 2nd edn. Thomas Springfield: Illinois.

Tullos HS, Schwab G, Bennett JB et al 'Factors influencing elbow instability.' *Instr Course Lect* 1981; 30: 185–99.

Walker N, Jacob HAC 'Biomechanische Untersuchungen am Ellenbogengelenk.' *Orthopade* 1981; 10: 253–5.

Walter E, Holz U, Köhle H 'Die Indikation zur Operation bei der Ellenbogenluxation.' *Orthopade* 1988; 17: 306–12.

Weizenbluth M, Eichenblat M, Lipskeir E et al 'Arthrolysis of the elbow: 13 cases of post-traumatic stiffness.' *Acta Orthop Scand* 1989; 60: 642.

Weller S, Pfister U 'Die Ellenbogenluxation.' *Akt Traumatol* 1978; 8: 95–100.

Willner P 'Anterior capsulectomy for relief of flexion contractures of the elbow following fracture.' *J Bone Joint Surg* 1948; 26: 71–86.

Wolff J 'Über die Operation der Ellenbogengelenkankylose.' *Berliner klinische Wochenschrift* 1895; 43: 44.

Wolff J 'Zur Arthrolysis cubiti.' *Berliner klinische Wochenschrift* 1897; 46: 1017–8.

Diaphyseal Fractures of the Forearm 15

L. Cugola and A. Atzei

Introduction

Widespread use and acceptance of the AO system of internal fixation has fostered in surgeons a preference for the surgical treatment of diaphyseal fractures of the forearm. This is due not only to the problems involved in achieving and maintaining reduction by conservative means, but also because the latter involves prolonged immobilization and is associated with a fairly high incidence of pseudarthrosis or malalignment. At the present time, therefore, there is little scope for the treatment of these fractures in a plaster cast (with the exception of fractures in paediatric patients), although some authors still recommend attempting a non-invasive treatment in all cases before embarking on a surgical solution.

Even when initial reduction using conservative measures is acceptable, however, it may be difficult to maintain the reduction, and this may lead to a high incidence of unsatisfactory results – 71 per cent according to one author.[1]

The major causes of poor results in these circumstances are: failure to restore the length of the forearm; overlapping of the fracture ends and abnormal axial or rotatory alignment. As a consequence, surgical solutions predominate, and the decision to opt for internal fixation (with compression plates or intramedullary nails) or external fixation, will depend on the type of fracture (open, closed, comminuted, with bone loss) and on the preference and experience of the individual surgeon.

The traditional and established surgical method for the treatment of diaphyseal fractures of the forearm is open reduction and internal plate fixation. This affords stable, though rigid fixation, and bone consolidation occurs by first intention through direct cortical union. Once consolidation has been achieved, however, removal of the hardware is mandatory. This involves a risk of refracture, the incidence of which, according to the literature, is somewhere between 17 per cent and 26 per cent.[2,3,4]

For correct application of the plates, sizeable incisions are needed with extensive associated muscle stripping. In proximal fractures of the radius particularly, this may increase the risk of radial nerve lesions, radio-ulnar synostosis and unsightly scars. In addition, muscle stripping will prejudice the already precarious vascular supply of the mid-distal thirds of both bones of the forearm, and this may lead to delayed or non-union.

Internal fixation with intramedullary nails permits healing of the fracture by second intention with periosteal callus formation, and has a number of advantages over plate fixation. These include: less exposure of the fracture site; the fact that removal of the hardware is often unnecessary following consolidation, and a reduced likelihood of delayed union or non-union, despite the fact that anatomical reduction of the fracture may not be wholly maintained, particularly in respect of rotation. If the nail does not fit snugly within the medullary canal, rotational movements will occur during pronation and supination which may limit the formation of callus and lead to pseudarthrosis, the incidence of which approaches 14 per cent.[5]

In the light of these considerations, external fixation may provide solutions to many of the drawbacks of internal fixation. At the present time, however, the literature contains few reports of studies where external fixation has been used in the treatment of traumatic injuries of the diaphyses of the forearm bones. The authors believe that this may be because:

1. It is not always easy to achieve stable anatomical reduction by closed procedures;

2. The precarious vascular supply to the forearm bones in their mid-distal portion may lead to lengthy healing periods, and the tendency, therefore, is to favour internal synthesis which does not prevent use of the hand;
3. Pronation and supination produce torsion of the radius and this has an adverse effect on the development of callus.

Notwithstanding the above, external fixation has, on balance, more to commend it than internal synthesis. The main advantages are the limited surgical exposure, the reduced risk of serious infection and the absence of unsightly scars, while the disadvantages (in the main more theoretical than real) are:

1. The risk of breakage or infection of the screws;
2. The risk of neurovascular damage.

In addition, external fixation carries an appreciably lower risk of synostosis when compared with internal fixation.

In the literature, apart from a few studies presented in the form of communications at congresses and reporting "encouraging results" with the use of external fixation in diaphyseal fractures of the forearm, the only publications which have defined the efficacy and limitations of external fixation are the reports by Schuind and co-workers (1988)[6] and by De Lee (1981).[7]

Schuind's study,[6] which reviewed 93 patients treated with the Hoffmann external fixator, reported a mean period of stabilization with the external fixator of 13 weeks, with the formation of solid periosteal callus, as a consequence of the elasticity of this type of fixation. Failure of consolidation occurred in 8.5 per cent of patients. There was one case of refracture, but no cases of infected pseudarthrosis or of osteitis, despite the fact that 27.9 per cent of the fractures in this series were open, and open reduction was performed in 57.3 per cent of cases. There were no instances of radio-ulnar synostosis, sympathetic reflex dystrophy or Volkmann's contracture.

In 9.4 per cent of patients an initial loss of reduction was observed due to micromovement at the level of the clamps, and the more pronounced secondary dislocations were easily realigned by closed manipulation under image intensification. In an attempt to reduce the incidence of early loss of reduction, pronation and supination were prevented in the immediate postoperative period, and as a result, early mobilization of the forearm was not permitted. Schuind's experience suggests that this may have been the cause of the pronation-supination deficits encountered in a number of our cases.

De Lee, in his study,[7] suggests that external fixation of the forearm is indicated in open fractures with loss of substance, in infected pseudarthrosis and in association with replantation (as suggested also by Weiland et al).[8]

Materials and Methods

The data presented below describe the authors' personal experience with the small Orthofix Dynamic Axial Fixator (DAF) (model 30.000), which is characterised by the simplicity of its assembly, ease of application, and compact profile.

This method of external fixation was used for the stabilization of diaphyseal fractures of the forearm in 42 patients, 32 of whom were followed up over a mean period of 28.3 months. Tables 15.1 and 15.2 provide details of the type, distribution and treatment methods used. In 30 cases, both forearm bones were fractured, while 10 were isolated fractures of the ulna and 2 were isolated fractures of the radius. There was a total of 30 open fractures: 26 ulna plus radius and 4 isolated ulnar fractures.

In 18 of the cases where both ulna and radius were fractured, both bones were stabilized with the Orthofix fixator; in the remaining 12 cases the fixator was applied only to the radius, ulnar fixation being achieved by means of a K-wire in 7 cases, a plate in 2 cases, and immobilization in a plaster cast without fixation in 3 cases of incomplete compound fracture of the ulna. In two Monteggia fractures, external fixation was used for fixation of the ulna, while stabilization of the radius was achieved by means of a K-wire. Illustrative cases are shown in Figs. 15.1–15.6.

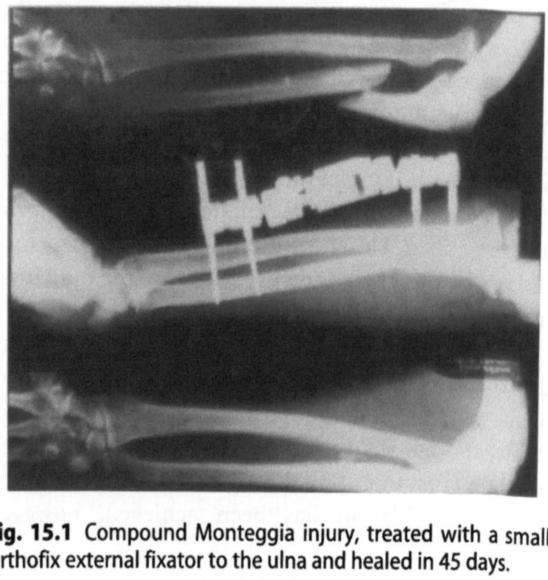

Fig. 15.1 Compound Monteggia injury, treated with a small Orthofix external fixator to the ulna and healed in 45 days.

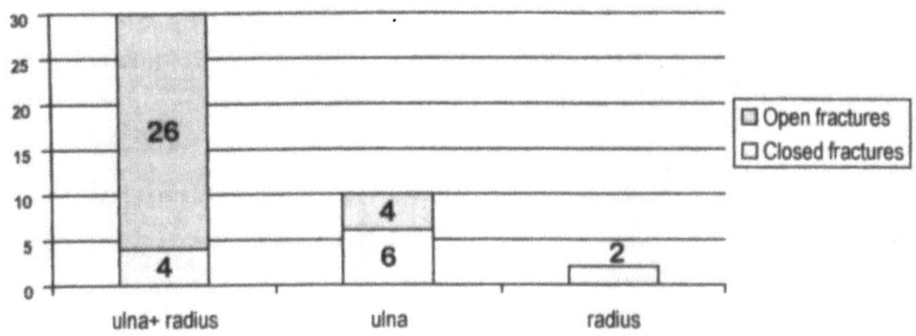

Table 15.1 Fracture Type and Distribution

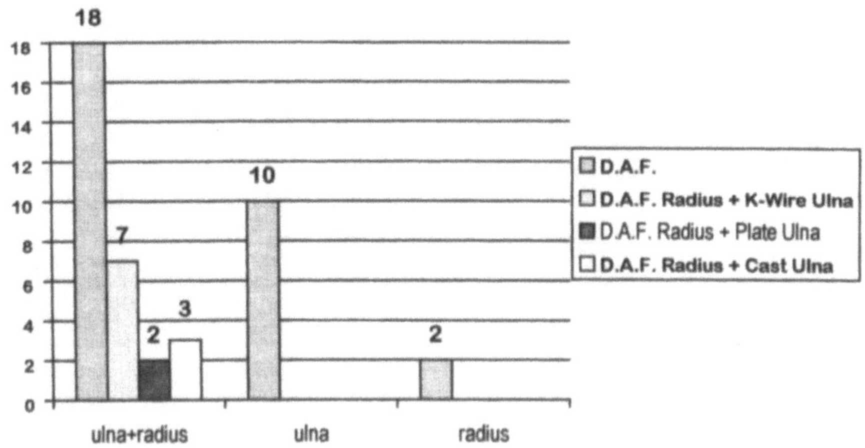

Table 15.2 Treatment

Table 15.2 Treatment

	Excellent	Satisfactory	Unsatisfactory
Healing period	< 6 mths	< 6 mths	> 6 mths
Angular deviation	< 10°	< 10°	> 10°
Shortening	< 1cm	< 1cm	> 1cm
Elbow extension–flexion deficit	< 10°	10°–20°	> 20°
Elbow pronation–supination deficit	< 25%	25%–50%	> 50%

Table 15.3 Classification of results according to Anderson

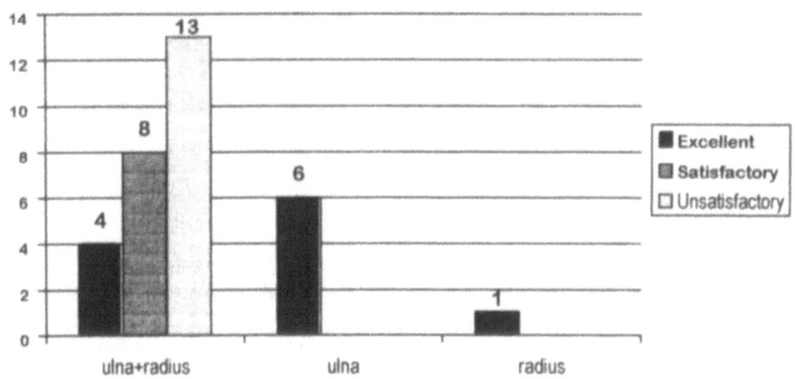

Table 15.4 Results in 32 patients followed up for a mean period of 28.3 months

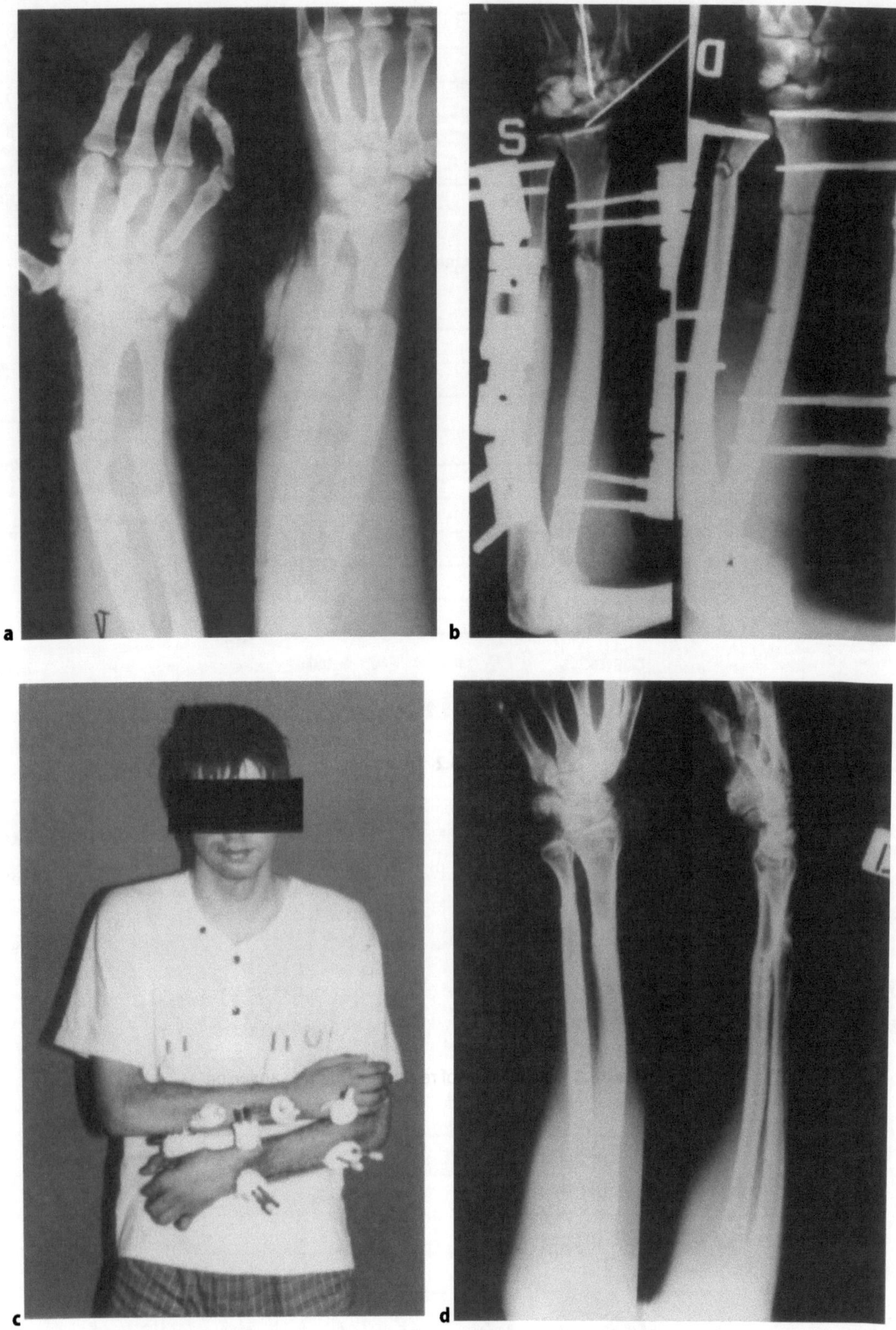

Fig. 15.2 Severe fireworks injury with compound fractures of the bones of both forearms, treated with 4 small Orthofix external fixators. **a** Pre-operative radiographs; **b** Post-operative X-rays showing malalignement of the right ulnar head (corrected during treatment) and temporary fixation of carpo-metacarpal dislocation on the left side; **c** Clinical picture of the patient at the end of treatment; the screws are left in situ for a further week following removal of the fixator to confirm the quality of the callus; **d** X-rays following removal of fixator and screws.

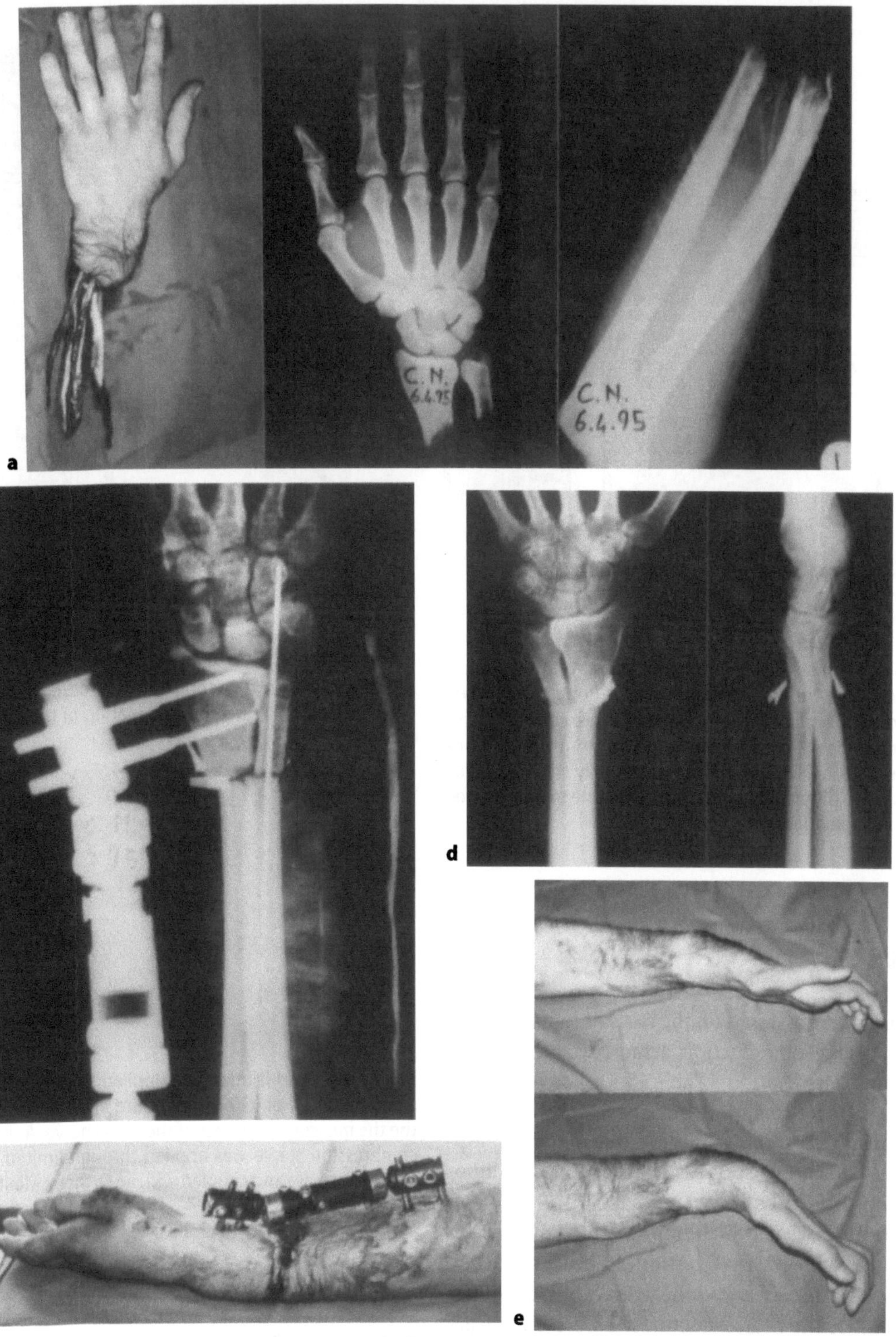

Fig. 15.3 Traumatic amputation of the distal forearm. **a** Clinical and radiological views of the amputation; **b** Bony fixation was achieved using a small Orthofix external fixator on the radius and a longitudinal K-wire in the ulna. Although application of a fixator to the ulna is preferable, external fixation of the radius is frequently used during forearm replantation as it is faster and provides good wrist stability. In this case the forearm was protected with a plaster slab and pronation/supination was not permitted for one month. **c** Clinical picture during treatment: the external fixator does not interfere with wound management; **d** X-rays taken 3 months after replantation showing good healing of the fracture and two vascular clamps which were subsequently removed. **e** Three months after replantation the range of movement of the hand and wrist was still limited: tenolysis and tendon transfer were planned.

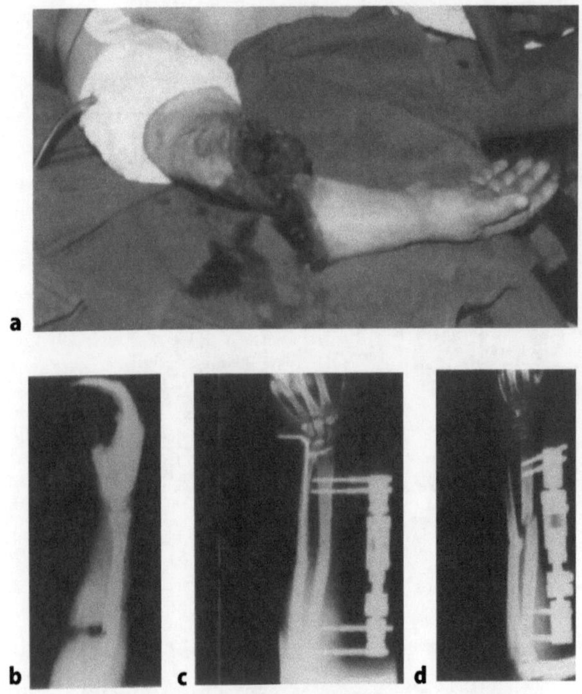

Fig. 15.4 a Crush injury of the forearm. **b** X-rays show compound fracture of radius and ulna. **c** Bony fixation was achieved with a small Orthofix external fixator on the radius and a longitudinal K-wire in the ulna; **d** Two months later, while the ulna has consolidated, the radius not only shows delayed union but also dislocation of the bony ends due to unrestricted pronation/supination.

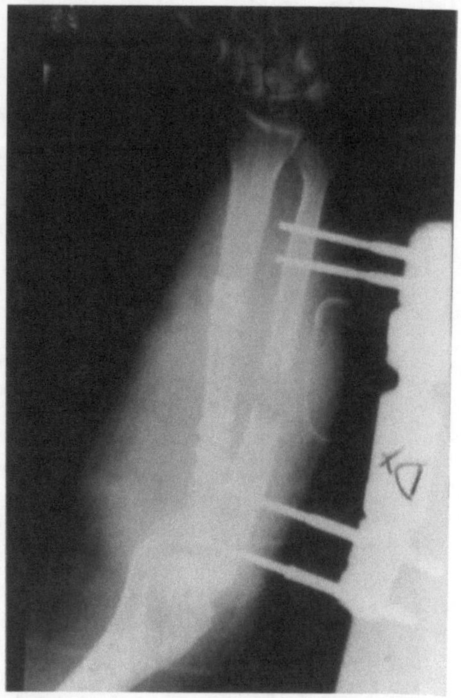

Fig. 15.5 The correct choice in this case of pseudarthrosis; external fixation of the ulna and plating of the radius.

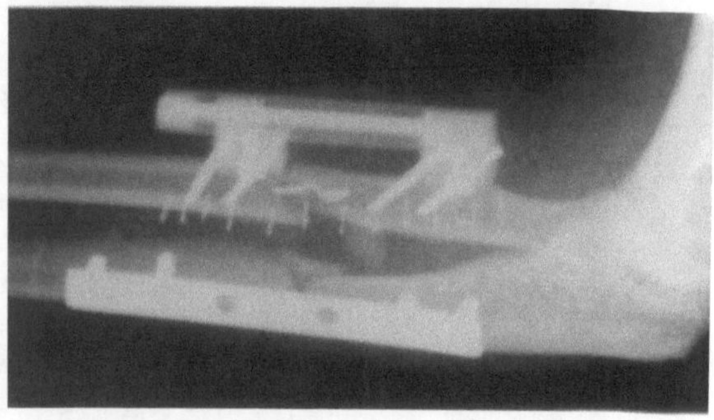

Fig. 15.6 Mixed fixation was applied to the radius in order to avoid exposure of its proximal third and the risk of damaging the the muscular branches of the radial nerve. A shape memory compression staple was applied through limited exposure of the fracture site and coupled with an Orthofix Minifixator of the M 100 series.

Results

The results were assessed on the basis of joint function and the degree of reduction achieved, according to Anderson's classification[9] (Table 15.3). The outcomes, reported in Table 15.4, were unsatisfactory in 13 cases: in 4 as a result of osteomyelitis, in 8 due to the development of pseudarthrosis, and as a consequence of radio-ulnar synostosis in 1.

Of the 18 cases in which both the ulna and radius were treated with external fixation, 13 healed, 4 developed pseudarthrosis and 1 healed with radio-ulnar synostosis. Of the healed fractures, 4 were open fractures which developed osteomyelitis; this resolved over a mean period of 13.1 months, during which time the dynamic axial fixator was kept in place.

Of the 12 fractures in which the dynamic axial fixator was applied to one bony segment only, all but 2 healed uneventfully. Of the 2 which healed with complications, delayed consolidation occurred in 1 case and a 3cm shortening in the other. No cases of refracture occurred following removal of the fixator.

Discussion

The present case series included a substantial percentage of complex fractures, 28 being bifocal or comminuted, and 30 open. Partly as a result of this, the results overall were inferior to those reported by other authors using either internal or external fixation. In this series, 59.3 per cent of outcomes were excellent or satisfactory, whereas Chapman et al[10] and Anderson et al[9] report 80 per cent excellent results; a similar trend was observed in respect of the incidence of osteomyelitis, which was 12.5 per cent in the present series compared to only 2.8 per cent in Chapman's series. The only major advantage seen related to the incidence of refracture, with no cases occurring in the present series as against 22 per cent in Anderson et al's series[9] and in Hidake's series[3] using internal fixation.

In the authors' experience, the factors predisposing to a negative outcome can be identified as:

1. the type of fracture;
2. fractures of both ulna and radius in the same limb treated by different fixation methods;
3. comminuted fractures and those associated with other fractures elsewhere in the same limb.

In keeping with other authors,[7,8] we believe that there is a definite place for external fixation in the treatment of forearm fractures, and especially in:

1. monostotic fractures;
2. open fractures, as first-line fixation treatment, pending possible replacement by another technique, when the soft tissues have healed;
3. open fractures with loss of bony substance, to maintain the length of the segment;
4. replantations.

Unlike Schiund,[6] who advocates blocking pronation-supination in the immediate post-operative period, we did not do this in the present series. In retrospect this was probably unwise. The success of external fixation in closed fractures of the forearm may be related to the limitation of pronation-supination for a period of time to be established on the basis of experience. If this is ultimately proven to be the case, it should be possible to extend the indications for external fixation in the treatment of diaphyseal fractures of the forearm, where it can offer a number of advantages over internal fixation.

References

1. Knight RA, Purvis GD. 'Fracture of both bones of the forearm in adults.' *J Bone Joint Surg* [Am] 1949; 31A: 755–64
2. De Luca PA, Lindsey RW, Ruwe PA. 'Refracture of bones of the forearm after the removal of compression plates.' *J Bone Joint Surg* [Am] 1988; 70A: 1372–6
3. Hidaka S, Gustilo RB. 'Refracture of bones of the forearm after plate removal.' *J Bone Joint Surg* [Am] 1984; 66A: 1241–3
4. Schemitsch EH, Richards RR. 'The effect of malunion on functional outcome after plate fixation of both bones of the forearm in adults.' *J Bone Joint Surg* [Am] 1992; 74A: 1068–78
5. Smith H, Sage FP. 'Medullary fixation of forearm fractures.' *J Bone Joint Surg* [Am] 1957; 39A: 91–8
6. Schuind F, Andrianne Y, Burny F. 'Treatment of forearm fractures by Hoffman External Fixator.' *Clin Orthop* 1991; 266: 197–204
7. De Lee JC. 'External fixation of the forearm and wrist.' *Orthop Rev* 1981; 6: 43–8
8. Weiland A, Robinson H, Futrel JW. 'External stabilization of a replanted upper extremity: a case report.' *J Trauma* 1976; 16: 239
9. Anderson LD, Sisk TD, Tooms RE, Park WI, III. 'Compression plate fixation in acute diaphyseal fractures of the radius and ulna.' *J Bone Joint Surg* [Am] 1975; 57A: 287–97
10. Chapman MW, Gordon JE, Zissimoss AG. 'Compression-plate fixation of acute fractures of the diaphyses of the radius and ulna.' *J Bone Joint Surg* [Am] 1989; 71A: 159–69

The Radius: Distal Metaphyseal and Articular Fractures and Corrective Osteotomies

16

D. Pennig and T. Gausepohl

Introduction

Fractures of the distal radius are common injuries and occur mainly as a consequence of high velocity trauma in younger and low velocity trauma in elderly patients. This may well be the reason for the ongoing controversy regarding treatment. The term distal radius fracture is somewhat incorrect to begin with since the radio-carpal and the radio-ulnar joints are often involved. It is therefore an intra-articular fracture affecting man's most important implement, the hand. External fixation for the treatment of this common injury was introduced by Ombredanne in 1929 who treated adolescents with it. A variety of devices was designed and ligamentotaxis was used to reduce the fracture and maintain the position of fragments.

Considering the heterogeneity of distal radius fractures external fixation should have the options of trans- and periarticular application, controlled adjustment and wrist mobilization with the fixator in place. It is preferable to have a lightweight low profile design which makes a unilateral configuration more desirable. Manipulation to reduce the distal radius fracture should be possible with the device in situ. The fixator should allow not only reduction of the distal radius fracture but also facilitate alignment of the carpus. It therefore seems advantageous to have a double ball joint configuration with dimensions matching the carpal height. Devices bridging the joint with longer or shorter rods only permit indirect reduction and therefore limit the control over the carpal alignment which according to Cooney[1] is of particular relevance for the outcome.

Design of the Pennig II Wrist Fixator

The dynamic wrist fixator allows for periarticular and trans-articular application. The standard configuration is built from a short and a long module with sliding clamps. The centre piece is the double ball joint with dimensions matching the carpal height (Fig. 16.1). The double ball joint allows approximately 180° of flexion and extension (Fig. 16.2), 90° of translation (Fig. 16.3) and 360° of rotation. The fixator clamps allow rotation which adds to the fixator's versatility (Fig. 16.4). In addition to the sliding clamp a compression–distraction module exists (Fig. 16.5). One full turn moves the clamp 1mm.

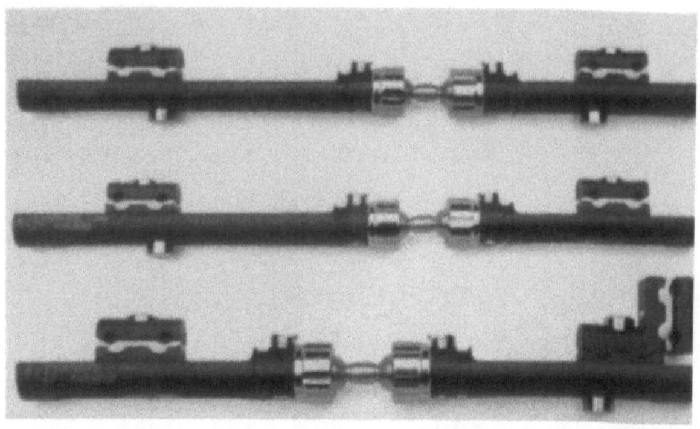

Fig. 16.1 Pennig II wrist fixator. Top: Standard configuration with short and long module and sliding clamps. Middle: Configuration with short compression–distraction module (right) and long module (left). Bottom: Periarticular assembly with T-clamp (right) and compression–distraction module (left).

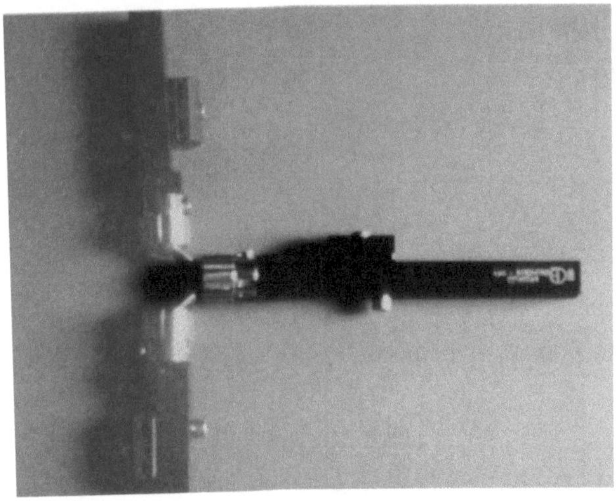

Fig. 16.2 Double ball joint allowing approximately 180° of flexion/extension.

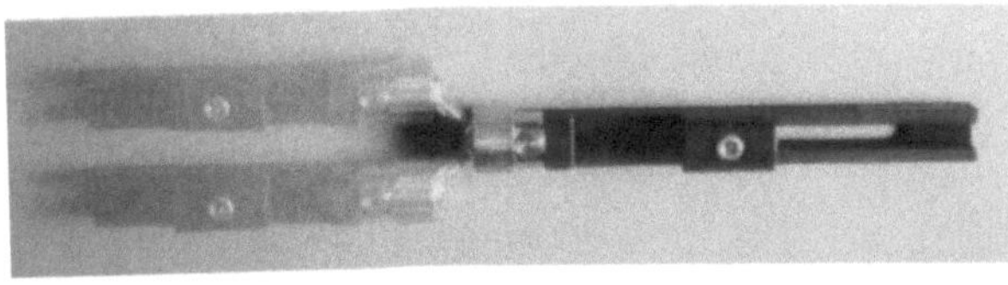

Fig. 16.3 Double ball joint allowing approximately 90° of translation.

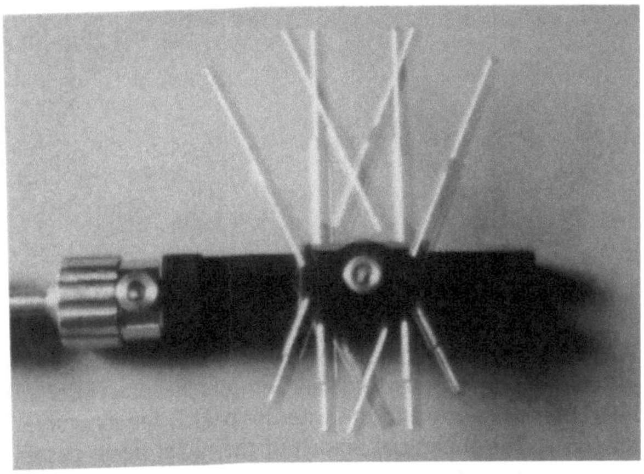

Fig. 16.4 Fixator clamps can rotate which adds to the versatility of the device.

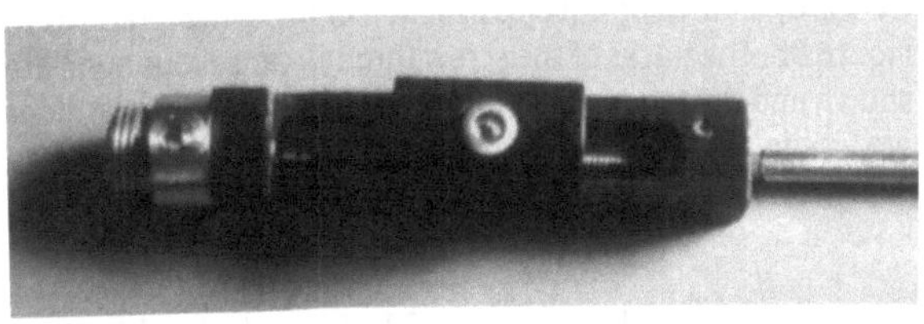

Fig. 16.5 Compression–distraction module. One full turn moves the clamp 1mm.

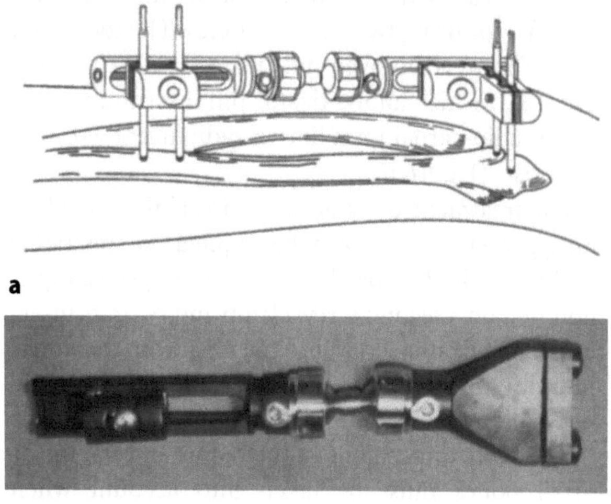

Fig. 16.6 a Periarticular configuration in radio-radial application. **b** Radiolucent T-clamp (X-ray see Fig. 16.17c).

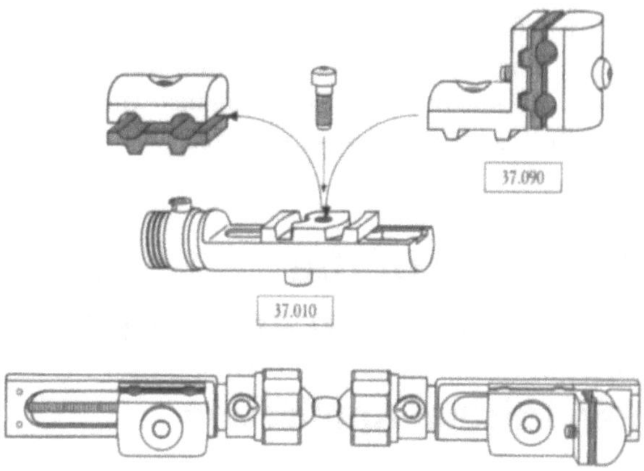

Fig. 16.7 Construction of periarticular fixator. The standard clamp top is exchanged for a T-clamp.

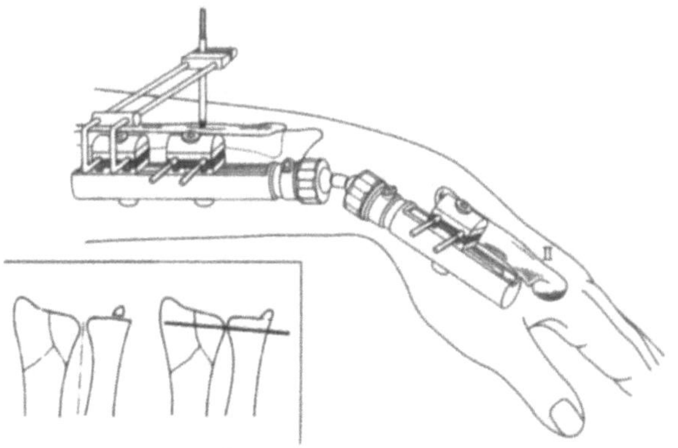

Fig. 16.8 In radio-ulnar instability an ulnar outrigger is introduced on the radial module of the fixator. Inset on left side shows preliminary stabilization of the radio-ulnar joint with a K-wire prior to insertion of a single screw into the ulna from the dorsal side.

The periarticular configuration is built from the same fixator using two short modules. The top of one of the clamps is removed and replaced with a T-clamp (Fig. 16.7) which allows fixator pin insertion parallel to the radio-carpal joint line. A radiolucent T-clamp also exists (Fig. 16.6).

For treatment of radio-ulnar instability an ulnar outrigger (Fig. 16.8) can be applied to the radial module of the fixator. The ulnar outrigger clamp is mounted on a second screw clamp and permits insertion of one fixator screw into the ulna from the dorsal side with the forearm in neutral rotation. This procedure makes pro- and supination impossible.

The bony dimensions in the radius and the metacarpal bones must be taken into account when choosing the fixator screws. In an adult skeleton a 3.3/3.0mm thread diameter is suitable. Two types of screw exist: 70/20mm and 80/35mm. These screws are predrilled with a 2.7mm drill bit. For the smaller skeleton a 3.0/2.5mm thread is available in 70/20mm length. These smaller fixator screws are predrilled with a 2.0mm drill bit. To distinguish the smaller sizes, drills and screws are sandblasted.

Anatomy of the Distal Forearm and Hand

Periarticular Application

In periarticular applications the fixator is mounted from the dorso-radial side. The distal pins are inserted parallel to the joint line again from the dorso-radial side. The landmark here is Lister's tubercle which can be felt under the skin. A 1cm incision is made to identify this tubercle and to avoid any injury to the tendons. Particularly close is the extensor pollicis longus tendon which curves around Lister's tubercle on the ulnar side. We therefore recommend dorso-radial pin insertion to maximise the distance from pin to tendon. Proximal to Lister's tubercle is a small triangle not covered by tendons or muscles. The second screw is inserted in the gap between the first and the second tendon sheath containing the extensor pollicis brevis and the abductor pollicis longus and the extensor carpi radialis longus and brevis. The superficial branch of the radial nerve sits right on top of the first tendon sheath (abductor pollicis longus and extensor pollicis brevis tendon) and must be protected. A 1cm incision is carried out to identify the correct point of insertion (Figs. 16.9a–16.9c).

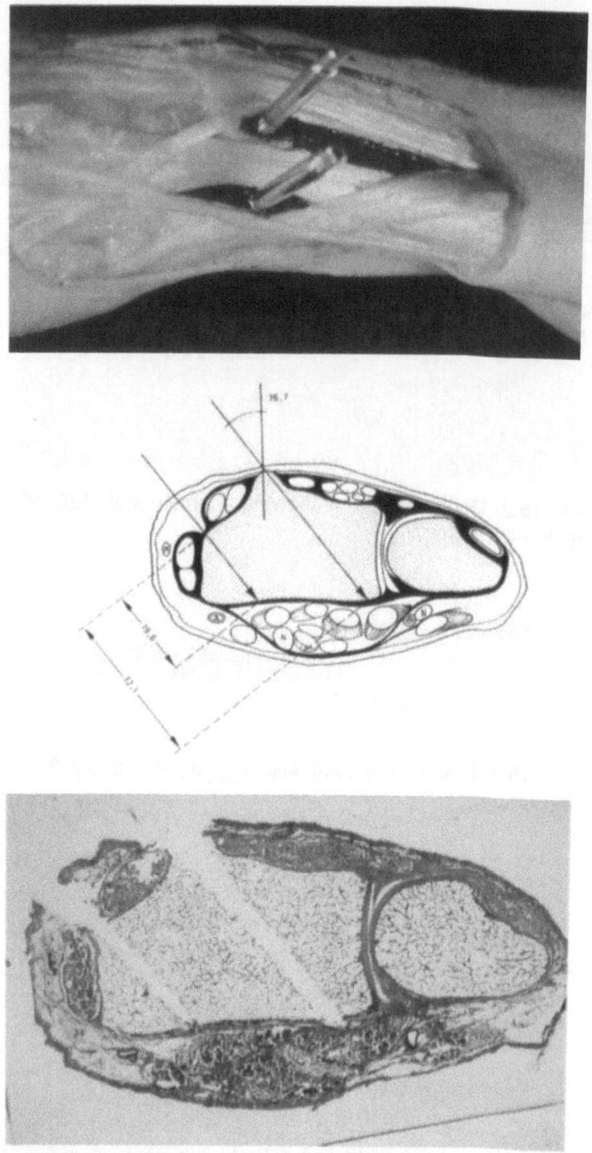

a

b

c

Fig. 16.9 **a** Cadaver specimen. The area of the distal radius suitable for pin placement is dark. The most ulnar pin is inserted into Lister's tubercle and the extensor pollicis tendon curves around it. The superficial branch of the radial nerve passes radial to the most radial pin. **b** Schematic cross-section of the distal forearm at the level of Lister's tubercle. The average distance from cortex to cortex is plotted for pin placement through Lister's tubercle and through the radial styloid (n = 6, CT scans). **c** Histological cross-section of the same region as in Fig. 16.9b. The tracks of the screw through cancellous bone are shown and the tendon sheaths on dorsal, radial and volar sides are visible.

In general the bone can be felt through the skin. The ideal point of entry for the proximal screws is the midshaft radius in a 4–6cm longitudinal gap between the abductor pollicis longus and extensor pollicis brevis muscle on one side and the extensor carpi radialis longus et brevis muscle on the other side. The superficial branch of the radial nerve which must be protected is generally not in danger since its course is radial to the extensor carpi radialis longus et brevis muscle. A 2–3cm incision is made and the periosteum detached to reduce the pain response. When drilling through cortical bone it is mandatory to wash out the drill debris since the little bone chips cause mechanical irritation in the surrounding tissues and may trigger inflammation.

Transarticular Application

External fixators are applied from the radial or from the dorso-radial side. If mobilization of the radio-carpal joint is desired the fixator has to be mounted in the frontal (coronal) plane from the radial side. Dorso-radial application is also a possibility and makes it easier to have an unobstructed AP and lateral view of the distal radius. When applying an external fixator the forearm should be in the neutral position. Placing the hand in pronation may lead to malrotation of the distal radius fragment and the same holds true for placement of the hand in supination.

The average outer diameter of the distal diaphyseal radius is between 13.8 and 15.2mm. The soft tissue envelope on the radial side of the radius generally permits one to feel the bone underneath the skin. For screw placement it is desirable to choose parts of the bone not covered by tendons or muscles. In the more proximal radius the extensor carpi radialis brevis et longus and the extensor digitorum communis muscles are close together. It is however possible to divide the muscles and it is easier to insert the screws from the dorso-radial side. In the middle third there is a gap between the abductor pollicis longus and the extensor pollicis brevis muscles on one side and the extensor carpi radialis longus et brevis muscle on the other side. The space between the two muscle groups is 4–6cm long and seems ideal for radial pin placement. The superficial branch of the radial nerve lies radial to the extensor carpi radialis longus et brevis muscle and is well protected when choosing the dorso-radial approach. In a strict radial approach, however, the position of the nerve has to be respected. It is mandatory to perform an open approach and the nerve should be identified. Complete dissection of the nerve is not recommended; it should rather be covered by surrounding tissue and not be in contact with the fixator pins. The more volar the approach the more risk there is to the nerve. With a strict radial approach in the frontal (coronal) plane the fixator pins will penetrate the extensor radialis brevis muscle either on the dorsal or the volar side. Functionally this is irrelevant in transarticular application of the fixator since these muscles would move the carpus which is immobilized anyway (Fig. 16.10).

The distal pins are placed in the second metacarpal bone and again a dorso-radial or a radial approach in the frontal (coronal) place is possible. The extensor tendon only covers the distal third of the bone and this area should be avoided. Penetration of the extensor hood (MP joint) is not desirable, since this will impair finger function. Due to the oblique course of the index finger extensor tendon the proximal two-thirds of the second metacarpal bone are available for pin placement. The bony landmark for the most proximal screw is a small tubercle which can be felt through the skin on the radial side of the metacarpal II base. The insertion of the extensor carpi radialis longus tendon 5–10mm distal to this tubercle seems to be an ideal place for pin insertion (Fig. 16.10). Due to the bony dimensions the

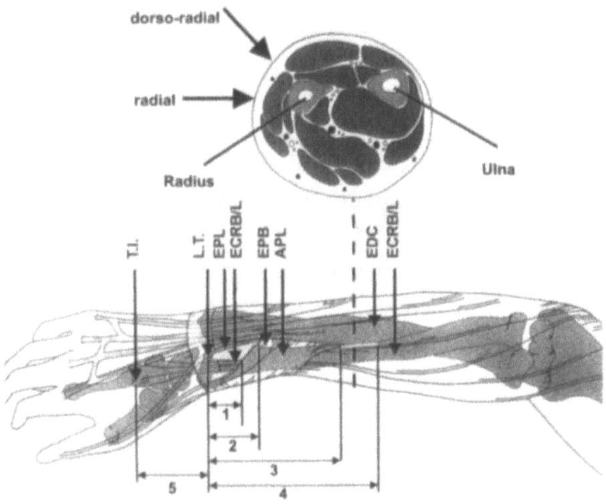

Fig. 16.10 Schematic drawing of the forearm resting on a hand table. The numbers indicate the distances from Lister's tubercle (n = 20). (Arrows indicating dorsal and dorso-radial screw insertion. Nerves in dark grey).

1 = 19.9mm /distance between L.T. and crossing point of ECRB/L and EPB/APL)

2 = 37.4mm (distance between L.T. and crossing point of EDC and EPB/APL and EDC)

3 = 61.8mm /distance between L.T. and crossing point of EPB/APL and EDC)

4 = 102.8mm (distance between L.T. and gap between EDC and ECRB)

5 = 46.8mm (distance between innominate tubercle and L.T.)

T.I. = innominate tubercle; L.T. = Lister's tubercle; EPL = Extensor pollicis longus; ECRB/L = Extensor carpi radialis brevis et longus; EPB = Extensor pollicis brevis; APL = Abductor pollicis longus; EDC = Extensor digitorum communis.

fixator pin should always be smaller than 4mm and the standard pin size is 3.3/3.0mm. For smaller hands a 3.0/2.5mm fixator pin is available. In heavy labourers the interosseous I muscle on the radio-volar side of the second metacarpal bone may be prominent and detaching the fibres for pin insertion is necessary. This muscle inserts on the radio-volar side of the second metacarpal bone.

Operative Technique

Periarticular Application In Distal Radius Fractures

Brachial plexus anaesthesia or general anaesthesia is recommended. Pre-operative preparation of the arm includes shaving of the skin surfaces, and washing of both the forearm and hand with a non-coloured disinfectant. A rolled up towel is placed under the volar side and the forearm held in 30–40° of pronation.

A handtable is used and a tourniquet is mandatory. Lister's tubercle is identified and a 10mm incision is made over it. The bone must be exposed prior to insertion of the first 1.5 or 1.6mm Kirschner-wire. The plane of insertion of this wire is about 40° (35°–45°) to the frontal plane. A template with handle, one screw guide and one pilot wire guide is slid over the K-wire after its position has been checked radiographically (Fig. 16.11).

The second screw guide is now introduced and the second pilot wire guide placed inside. A second 1.5 or 1.6mm K-wire is now inserted parallel to the first, following a 10mm stab incision and exposure of the bone in the area of the radial styloid. During insertion it is helpful to aim for the solid cortex of the volar lip, but care should be take to avoid penetration of the wrist joint (Fig. 16.12).

The template with handle is removed and a radiological check of the positions of both K-wires carried out in two planes. If necessary, one or both K-wires may be re-sited.

When the position of the K-wires is deemed satisfactory, the template with handle, together with screw guides and pilot wire guides, is replaced. The K-wire in Lister's tubercle is then removed together with its pilot wire guide and a 2.7mm drill guide inserted. Predrilling is carried out with the 2.7mm drill bit and an 80/35mm screw inserted (Fig. 16.13). This screw must be advanced very carefully under image intensification in order to avoid over-penetration of the volar cortex. It is important to remember that the screws are tapered in design and cannot be backed out.

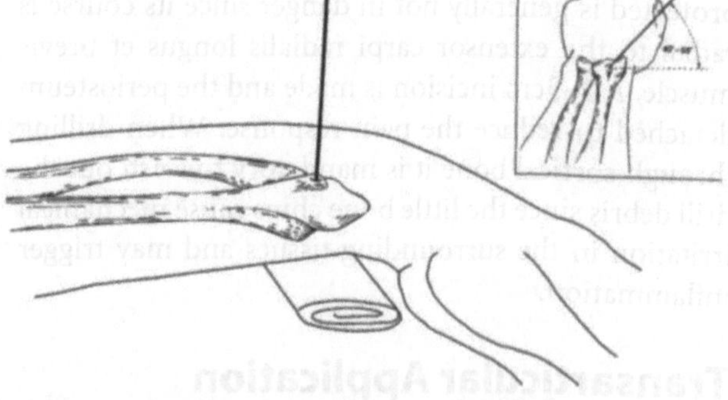

Fig. 16.11 First pilot K-wire (1.5 or 1.6mm) placed in Lister's tubercle at 35 to 45° to the frontal (coronal) plane.

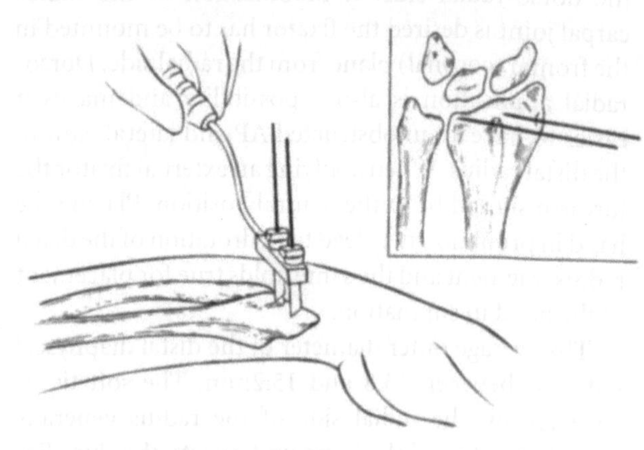

Fig. 16.12 Second pilot wire placed through the radial styloid aiming for the volar lip.

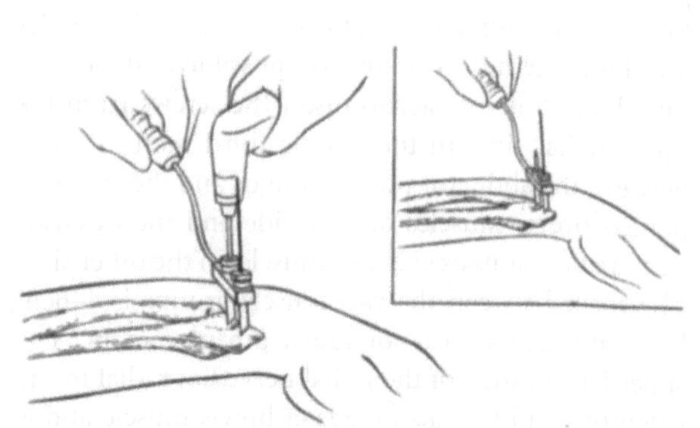

Fig. 16.13 The first pilot wire is exchanged for an 80/35mm screw after predrilling with a 2.7mm drill.

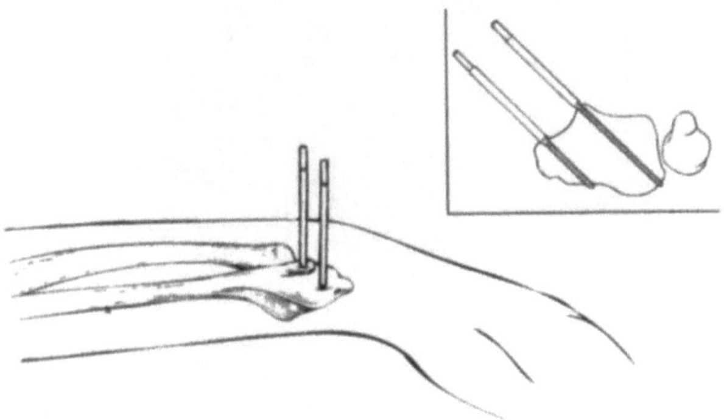

Fig. 16.14 Two periarticular screws in place. Note the longer thread of the screw in Lister's tubercle and the shorter thread of that in the radial styloid (insert on top right).

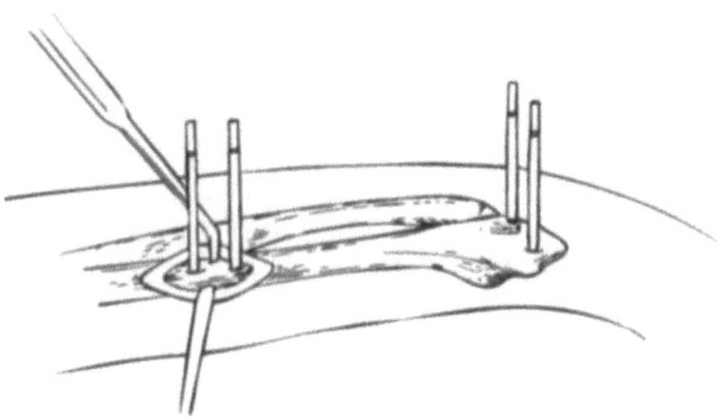

Fig. 16.15 Insertion of screws in the radial diaphysis through an open approach.

The second K-wire is now removed together with its pilot wire guide and drilling for the second screw carried out. Depending upon the size of the radial styloid a 70/20 or an 80/35 screw should be used. A radiographic check at the end of screw insertion is mandatory. The screw should engage the volar cortex securely and penetrate by one thread (Fig. 16.14). Penetration of the radio-ulnar joint however, must be avoided.

Insertion of the proximal screws is carried out at a distance of about 14cm from the distal screws. The fixator may be mounted temporarily on the distal screws with the compression–distraction module placed proximally and the short module with T-clamp, distally. The skin is then marked to indicate the position of the proximal screws and the fixator removed for screw insertion. Alternatively, the cover of the clamp of the compression–distraction module may be replaced with the template/conversion clamp, the fixator mounted to the distal screws and the screw guides inserted into the template/conversion clamp. The proximal screws are inserted through a 25mm incision in order to avoid injury to the superficial branch of the radial nerve. Again, a plane of insertion 45° to the frontal plane is chosen and the appropriate screws inserted after drilling with a 2.7mm drill. In most instances 70/20mm screws will be employed (Fig. 16.15).

The fixator is mounted with the compression–distraction module placed proximally and the short module with T-clamp distally. Where the proximal screws have been applied with the fixator already mounted, the template/conversion clamp should be replaced with the definitive clamp cover. Reduction of the fracture (see page 160 below) is not necessary prior to mounting of the fixator. The templates with handles are now placed over each pair of screws to assist in fracture reduction. Once reduction has been achieved (Figs. 16.16a, 16.6b), all clamp cover and clamp anchoring screws are tightened using the T-wrench or Allen wrench, ensuring that bone screws are seated in the clamp cover slots. Care must be taken to hold the fixator module firmly while tightening to avoid loss of position.

To tighten the double ball joint the cam is turned clockwise until very tight so that the dot rotates a minimum of 90° and a maximum of 170°. If it is rotated in excess of 170°, the ball joint may become loose.

The fixator should be mounted in such a way that it does not obstruct the lateral or AP X-ray (Figs. 16.17a, 16.17b), and the alternative positions possible are illustrated in Fig. 16.18. Fig. 16.17c shows the use of a radiolucent T-clamp to facilitate application of the fixator and improve radiographic control of fracture reduction. Post-operative dressings are applied around the screws but a circular dressing is not recommended. Tightening of the fixator screws should be checked at least once again.

Transarticular Application In Distal Radius Fractures

With very short periarticular fragments or displaced intra-articular fractures, bridging of the joint is necessary. The fractures that can be treated with this technique include AO type B and C fractures, and Frykman type III/IV and VII/VIII fractures.

For the successful application of this technique, the individual characteristics of each case must be taken into account and CT scans may be helpful. Brachial plexus anaesthesia or general anaesthesia is recom-

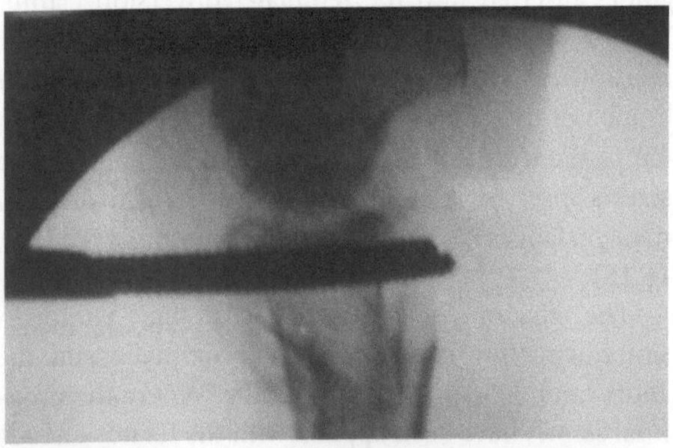
a

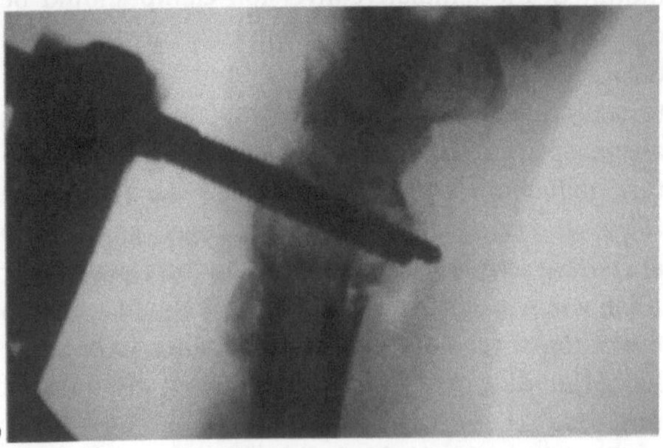
b

Fig. 16.16 a Periarticular insertion of the fixator screws anchoring in the volar lip. Image intensifier view prior to reduction in a 21-day-old fracture. **b** Closed reduction achieved with T-clamp and compression–distraction module.

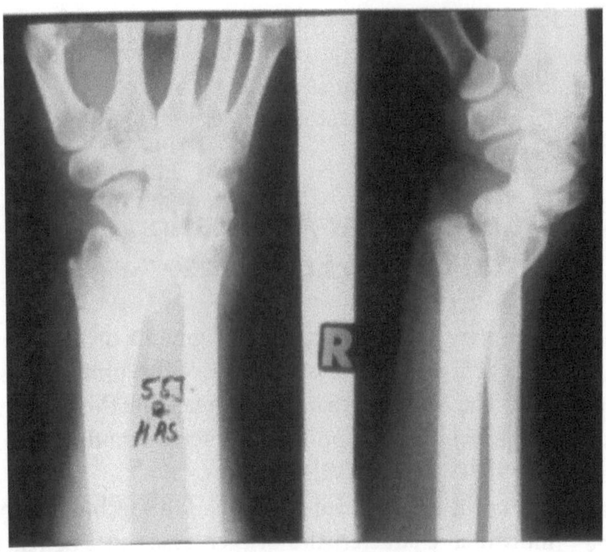
a

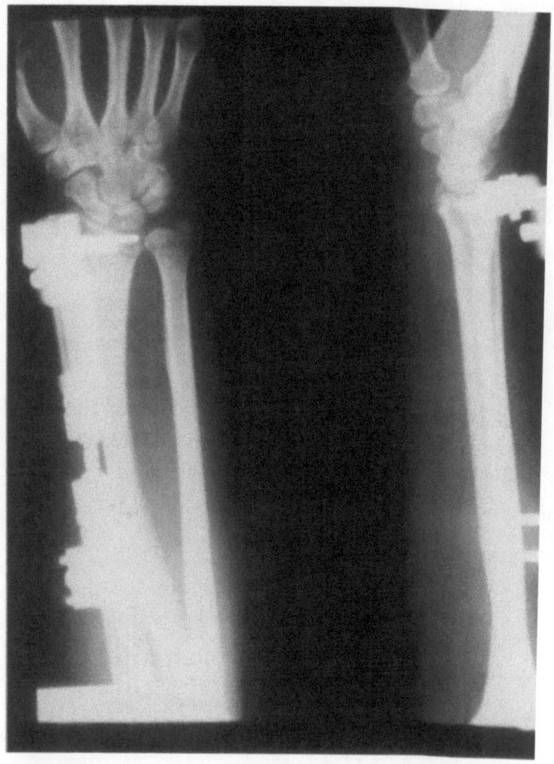
b

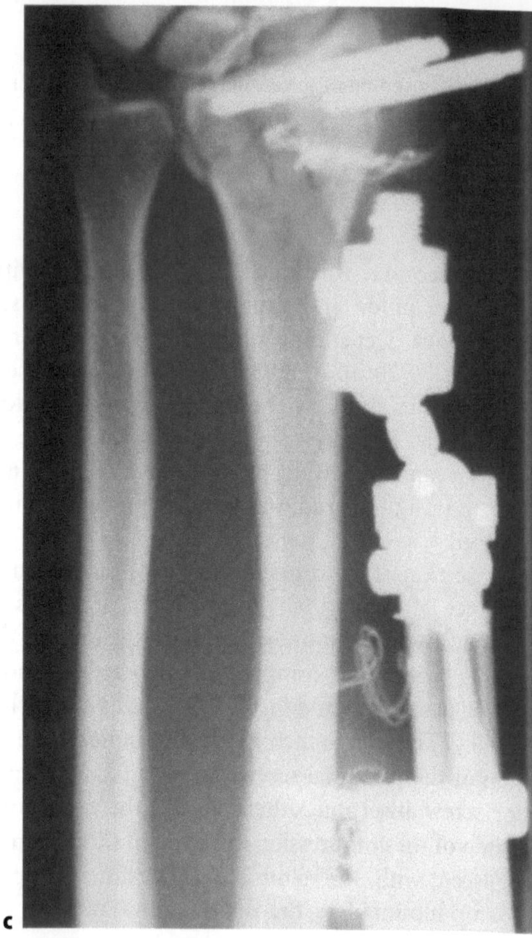
c

Fig. 16.17 a Unstable metaphyseal oblique fracture in a 55-year-old woman. **b** Closed reduction with radio-radial fixator application. **c** X-ray of radiolucent T-clamp in Frykman VI-fracture.

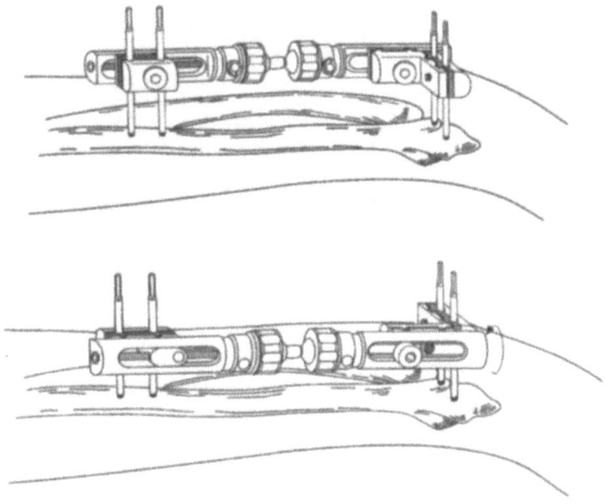

Fig. 16.18 Alternative positions shown to allow an unobstructed lateral or AP X-ray.

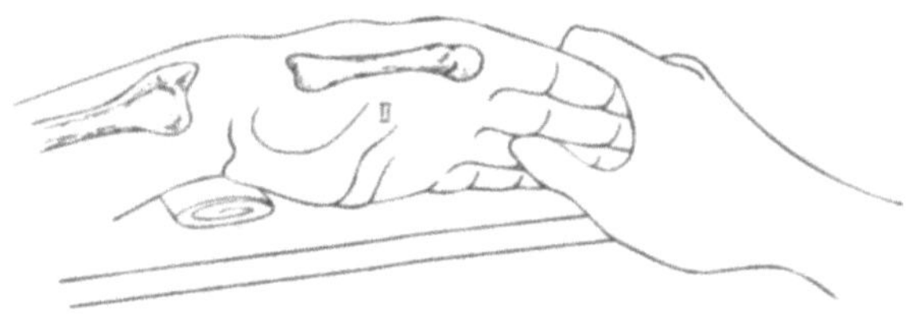

Fig. 16.19 Positioning of the hand. A hand table is used and a folded towel on the ulnar side for support. Note the neutral position of the forearm.

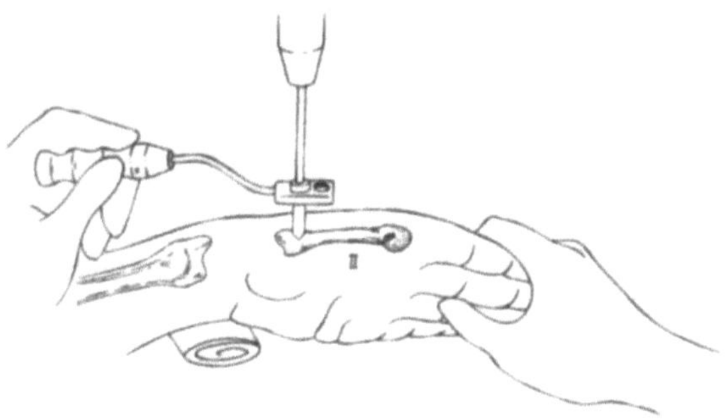

Fig. 16.20 After identification of the innominate tubercle the trocar is used to locate the centre of the bone in the frontal (coronal) plane.

mended. A tourniquet may be used. Pre-operative preparation of the arm includes shaving of the skin surfaces and washing both the forearm and the hand with a non-coloured disinfectant.

A hand table is used. Pre-operative fracture reduction can, but does not have to be carried out. The wrist will usually be placed in moderate (manual) traction, flexion and radial abduction with a folded towel on the ulnar side to support it. The forearm should be in a neutral position (Fig. 16.19). Placing the forearm in pronation may rotate the distal radius fragment and hand and cause malalignment. The fixator is applied to the second metacarpal and the middle/distal third of the radius.

The position of the screws determines the position of the fixator. Screws should be introduced in the frontal plane on the radial side so that wrist mobilization may be implemented at a later stage if desired, without displacement of the fracture fragments, and if applied correctly unobstructed lateral X-rays may be taken. Alternatively, if joint mobilization is not desired, a dorsoradial plane for pin insertion may be chosen.

The proximal metacarpal screw is inserted first, positioned close to the base of the bone in the flare of the tubercle. A stab incision is made and the soft tissue is dissected down to the bone, the centre of which is then located using the trocar within the short screw guide placed through the template with handle (Fig. 16.20).

The trocar is removed and a drill guide inserted into the screw guide. A 2.7mm drill bit is used and both cortices are drilled (Fig. 16.21). When the far cortex is reached, the drill stop is locked on to the drill 5mm above the drill guide. The far cortex is then drilled. This will prevent the drill from damaging the interosseous muscles.

Cortical 3.3/3.0mm thread and 4mm shank diameter, 70/20mm length screws are suitable for most applications both in the metacarpal and the diaphysis of the radius. An 80/35mm screw is also available.

Screws with a smaller thread (3.0/2.5mm) are available. These should only be used in the metacarpal diaphysis when the outer diameter of the bone is less than 9mm. A 2.0mm drill bit is used for the insertion of these screws which have a sandblasted surface.

The proximal screw is inserted into the second metacarpal through the screw guide to a depth of about 10mm (i.e. half the thread length) using the T-wrench (Fig. 16.22).

The longer screw guide is now fully inserted into the template (Fig. 16.23) and the procedure is repeated, starting with a stab incision as before. The second metacarpal screw is then inserted.

Prior to insertion of the screws into the radius, the bone is exposed following a 25mm long incision with the distal radial screw being placed no closer than 40mm to the fracture site. Care should be taken not to sever the superficial branch of the radial nerve or any extensor tendons. Blunt retractors should be used (Fig. 16.24).

The steps described for insertion of the metacarpal screws should now be repeated for the two radial screws (Fig. 16.25).

An image intensifier should be used to verify the position and penetration of the far cortex by all four screws when they have been sited. The screws should not be advanced too far; due to their tapered design, they will become loose if they are backed out.

The fixator should be fully assembled exactly as shown in Fig. 16.26. It is essential that the dot on the cam is facing the threaded neck before each security collar is tightened. Failure to follow this procedure exactly may result in loosening of the collars. The collars are now fully screwed home and, with all other screws loosened, the fixator is applied to the bone screws already in situ, positioning it at a distance of 15–20mm from the skin. Reduction of the fracture is now carried out under image intensification. The two templates with handles with their screw guides in place may be used to manipulate the fragments whilst distancing the surgeon's hands from the radiation beam (Fig. 16.27).

The design of the fixator with its double ball joint is such that the fracture fragments can be manipulated in any plane during reduction. This feature is complemented by the fact that the clamps for the bone screws can both slide and swivel on the fixator module as required. At this point, it is imperative to ensure that the distal ball of the double ball joint is aligned with the centre of rotation of the wrist (the lunate-capitate joint line). Correct positioning can be checked using a K-wire and image intensification. The centre of the anatomical snuffbox is used as a landmark.

Reduction Technique

The classic reduction technique described by Charnley[2] consists of three steps: continuous longitudinal traction together with increased dorsal angulation serves to disimpact the fracture. The Robert–Jones manoeuver brings the distal fragment to the volar side under continuous traction. The last step

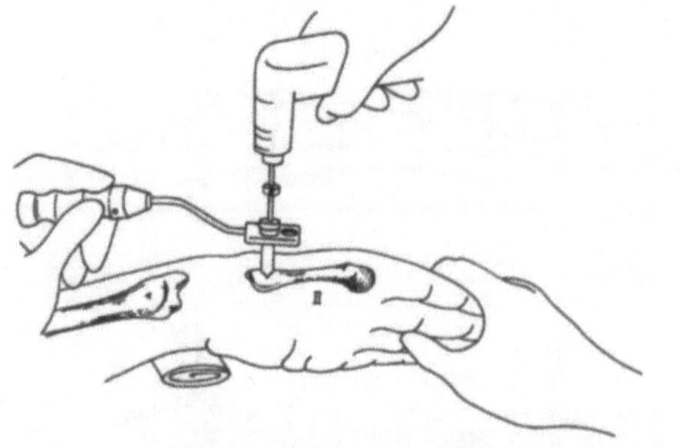

Fig. 16.21 After removal of the trocar drilling with a 2.7mm drill bit.

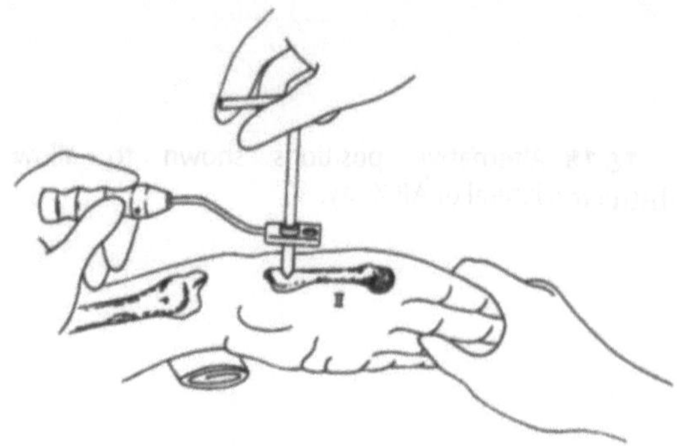

Fig. 16.22 Insertion of the most proximal metacarpal screw (70/20mm).

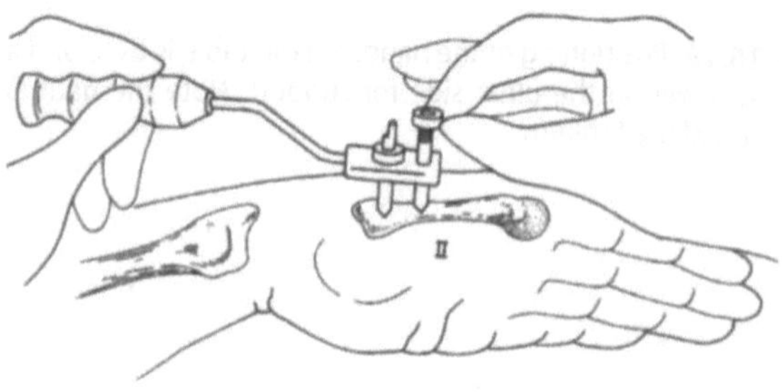

Fig 16.23 Full insertion of the longer screw guide for placement of the second metacarpal screw (70/20mm).

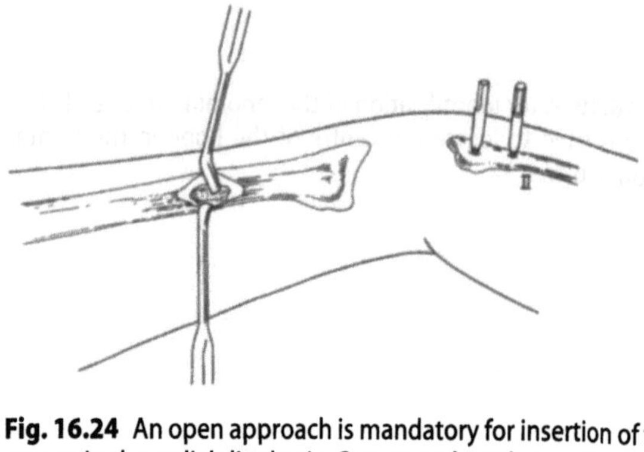

Fig. 16.24 An open approach is mandatory for insertion of the screws in the radial diaphysis. Care must be taken not to sever the superficial branch of the radial nerve.

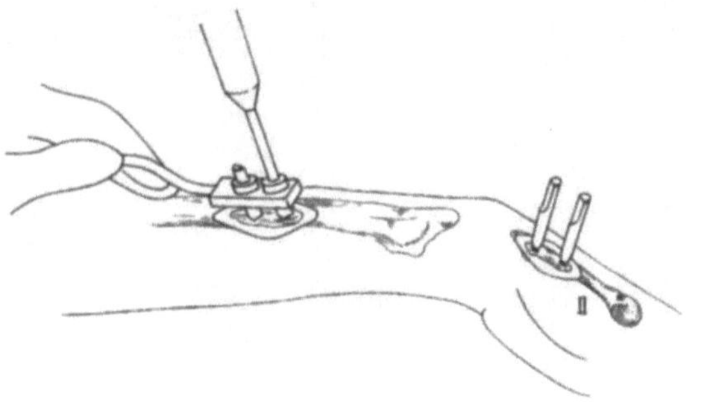

Fig. 16.25 Insertion of the two screws in the radial diaphysis.

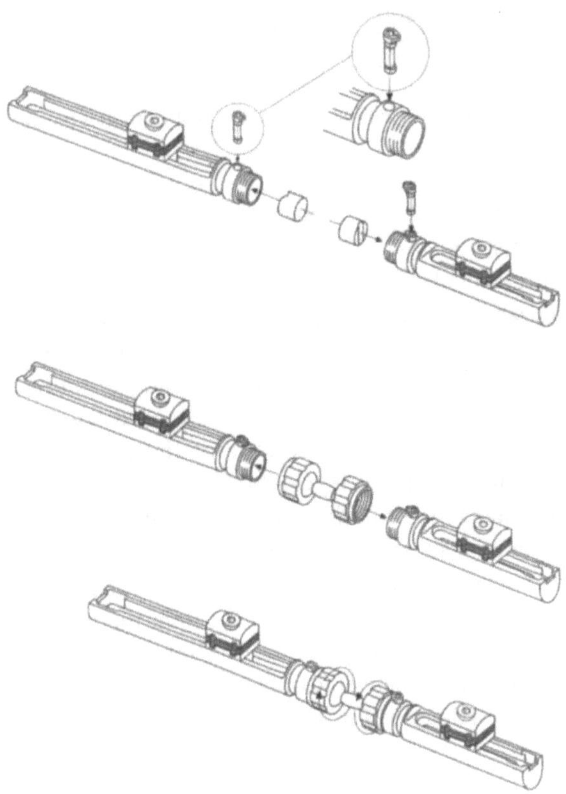

Fig. 16.26 Assembly of a fixator. The collars of the double ball joint must be securely tightened. Prior to tightening the dot on the cam must face the threaded neck.

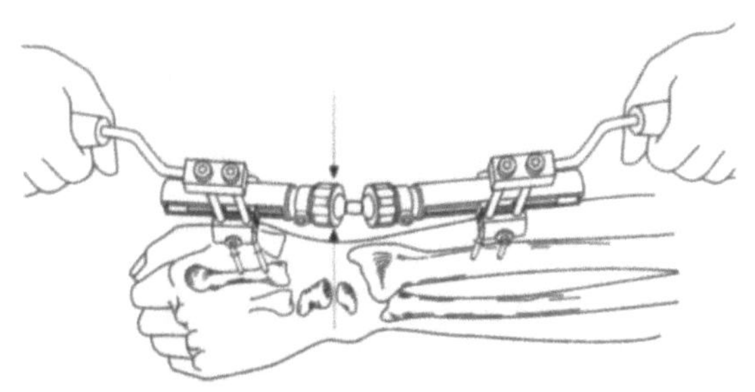

Fig. 16.27 Reduction of the fracture with the use of the templates. This helps to distance the surgeon's hand from the radiation beam. The distal ball joint is on the level of the so-called centre of rotation (the lunate–capitate joint line).

helps to maintain reduction by pronation of the distal fragment. Traction is then stopped. Charnley stated that "some continuous traction must be applied in order to maintain the styloid process of the radius in its reduced position". He obviously recognized the detrimental effect of the pull of the brachio-radialis muscle which inserts on the radial styloid (Charnley 1968).[2]

The reduction technique has not changed significantly since Charnley's first description and the advantages of conservative management should be retained. An external fixator must allow reduction to be carried out with the device in situ.

Reduction in Periarticular Applications

In periarticular applications of the fixator the distal fragment can be controlled well with the two bone screws in place. Here the principles of ligamentotaxis described by Charnley are not valid since direct control over the position with the radio-radial application of the device is possible.

After pin insertion in the distal and the midshaft radius a test reduction is performed. It is of particular importance to avoid rotational malalignment which especially in metaphyseal fractures is indicated by an overriding of the radial styloid as shown in Fig. 16.28. The fixator is applied at a safe distance from the skin (15–20mm) and only the clamp tops are tightened. Reduction is then carried out and it is common to observe sliding of the distal clamp as well as rotation of the screw attaching the T-clamp to the base plate. This indicates the shift of the epiphyseal fragment of the radius and once the correct position is verified under the image intensifier all fixator screws are tightened beginning with the ball joints. Though in theory it is possible to tighten the ball joint by clockwise or counterclockwise movement we recommend clockwise movements, since this is the direction in which all the other screws are tightened. In neglected fractures (2–3 weeks after the injury) the compression–distraction module is helpful. It is mounted on the midshaft radial pins and rotational alignment must be effected prior to tightening of the double ball joints. The only screw remaining loose is the one attaching the T-clamp to the base plate. The compression–distraction module is then used to correct the dorsal angulation and/or to disimpact the fracture. At this point a decision has to be made regarding the indication for cancellous bone grafting (see p. 168). With a substantial mainly dorsal defect this has to be considered. With radio-radial application of the fixator the

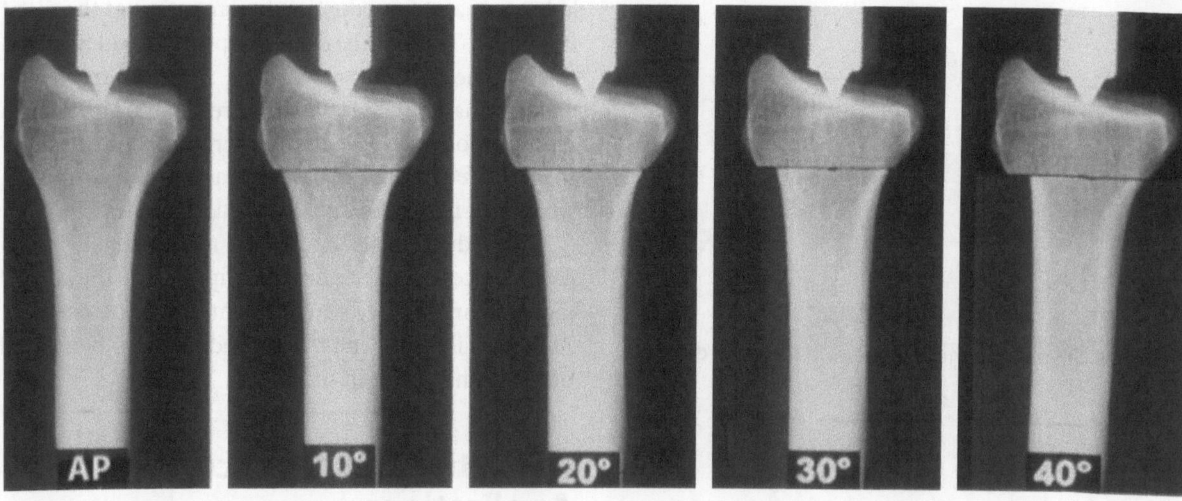

Fig. 16.28 Overriding of the radial styloid may indicate a rotational deformity. The rotation in the cadaver specimen is plotted on the bottom ranging from 10 to 40°.

radio-carpal joint and the radio-ulnar joint remain free to move. If the distal module overrides the wrist joint, dorsal extension will be hindered. This can be avoided by choosing the correct position of the fixator and if necessary, the whole device should be moved more proximally, which can be done without resiting the pins.

Reduction in Transarticular Applications

In transarticular fixator applications the bone screws are inserted in metacarpal II and the midshaft radius. Thereafter a test reduction is performed and a traction X-ray obtained. This will help to identify those cases that will benefit from cancellous bone grafting. Again at this point, it is important to decide whether the intra-articular fracture pattern requires additional stabilization using the Fragment Fixation System. Reduction of the intra-articular fracture may be assisted by arthroscopy but we do not recommend its routine use since the fluid used to flush out the joint will wash out into the soft tissue envelope of the forearm and produce swelling. If closed reduction is possible percutaneous insertion of the Fragment Fixation System is carried out. A limited open approach may be necessary for die punch fragments or volar lip fractures. After reconstruction of the joint the remaining instability is located in the metaphyseal area. The reduction manoeuver to obtain an anatomical position has been described by Gupta (1991)[3] and Agee (1993)[4]

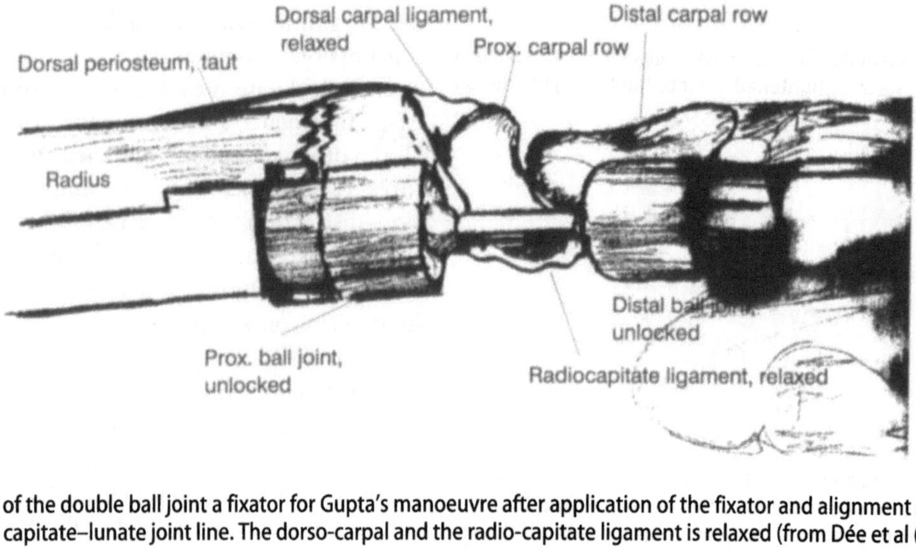

Fig. 16.29 Use of the double ball joint a fixator for Gupta's manoeuvre after application of the fixator and alignment of the distal ball joint on the capitate–lunate joint line. The dorso-carpal and the radio-capitate ligament is relaxed (from Dée et al (1999)[5] with permission).

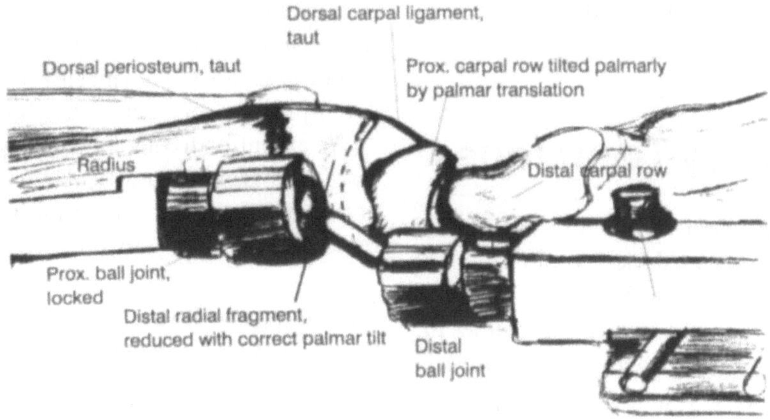

Fig. 16.30 Tightening of the dorso-carpal ligament by transposition of the hand to the volar side. The proximal ball joint is now locked (from Dée et al[5] with permission).

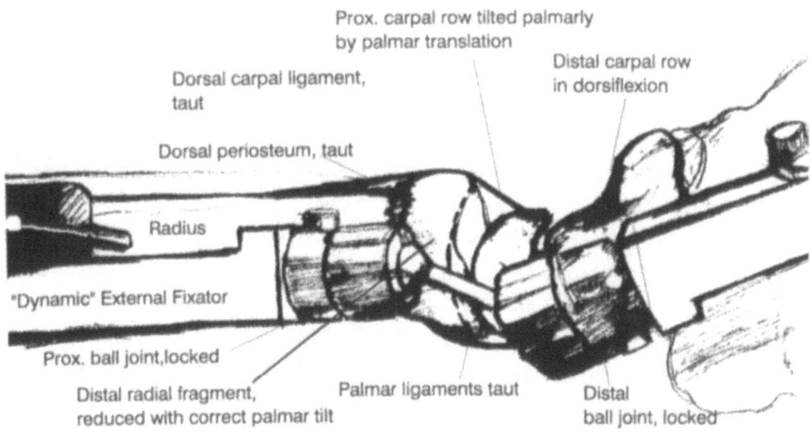

Fig. 16.31 Dorsiflexion in the distal carpal row will tighten the palmar ligaments and maintain reduction (from Dée et al[5] with permission).

as multiplanar ligamentotaxis. The external fixator with the double ball joint within the radio- carpal joint and the carpus lends itself ideally to perform three-dimensional ligamentotaxis. The distal ball joint is set to the so-called centre of rotation of the wrist (capitate-lunate joint line) which brings the proximal ball joint automatically to the level of the radio-carpal joint space. According to Gupta, palmar translation of the carpus serves to restore the anatomical palmar tilt whereas traction through the radio-dorsal ligament and tendon complex adjusts the dorsal fragments. It is not necessary with this technique of volar translation and tightening of the strong volar ligaments to flex the wrist. The short module of the fixator mounted on the second metacarpal may even be extended dorsally for full tightening of the ligaments (Figs. 16.29, 16.30, 16.31). This Gupta manoeuver is based on the observation that flexion in the mid-carpus does not exert any control over the dorsally displaced distal fragment, since the relevant ligaments insert mainly on the dorsal side of the proximal carpal row. A translation and extension of the hand pulls on the much stronger volar ligaments and with longitudinal traction more effectively protects against redisplacement. Overdistraction, however, should never be performed since it triggers a pain response and may contribute to the serious complication of algodystrophy. When flexing the wrist over 20° the pressure in the carpal tunnel is increased, and over 40° the pressure is so high that carpal tunnel syndrome may be the consequence. Measurements during Gupta's manoeuver, however, showed normal pressure in the carpal tunnel. Another side effect of the flexion position (so-called extrinsic–extensor plus position) may be related to the increased carpal tunnel pressure, and finger stiffness is a common observation with this position. With overdistraction the MP joints will not fully flex and MP joint movement is a good indicator, helping to avoid too much tension.

Supplementary Techniques

The first step in using external fixation in distal radius fractures with this particular device consists of bone screw insertion in the second metacarpal and in the radial diaphysis. A trial reduction will then reveal whether the articular surface can be reduced, and pre-operative CT-scanning of the fracture is helpful in assessing radio-carpal and radio-ulnar joint damage. CT scanning also helps in planning the most appropriate approach since a limited exposure is usually performed.

Timing of Surgery

Treatment of distal radius fractures using external fixation within one week of the injury is considered to be acute. Reduction is invariably facilitated by performing the operation within the first few days, since with treatment of distal radius fractures after 14–21 days the incidence of supplemental techniques such as bone grafting is significantly increased. This may be due to the formation of fibrous tissue and early callus. If a distal radius fracture is not reduced for three weeks or more we focus on restoration of the radial length and correction of the radial shift. Percutaneous elevation of the distal radius fragment is attempted with joystick techniques and percutaneous insertion of an osteotome. If this is not possible, in our experience the correction should be delayed until after union. The proliferative callus formation from three weeks onwards usually prevents an adequate reduction and requires large dissections which give rise to post-operative problems as well as prolonged rehabilitation times. In these cases we recommend application of the fixator to secure the normal joint space and proceed to a well-planned corrective osteotomy after 3–6 months.

An exception to this approach is justified in delayed cases with gross intra-articular incongruence. Careful pre-operative planning and a meticulous technique are required for a good post-operative result.

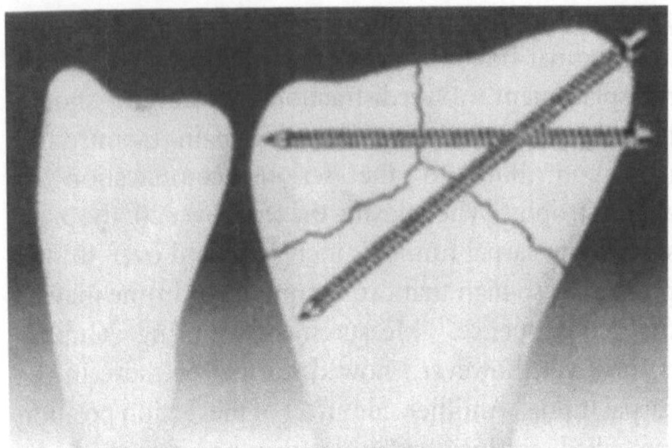

Fig. 16.32 Use of the Orthofix Fragment Fixation System in intra-articular fractures. Medium implants with a thread diameter of 1.6mm are used.

Minimally Invasive Osteosynthesis Techniques (MIOT)

Significant cortical and cancellous comminution in the distal radius on the dorsal and the radial side may lead to late collapse due to resorption of the crushed bone. K-wires acting as bone sutures have enjoyed some popularity but are burdened with problems such as migration, poor purchase and infection. For improved fixation in the distal radius, the Fragment Fixation System is available (Orthofix Srl., Italy, U.K., USA), and serves to eliminate the problem of migration. It combines the ease of insertion of a K-wire with the purchase of a screw (Fig. 16.32).

Supplementary internal fixation is justified whenever there is significant comminution of two or more cortices in the antero-posterior and lateral film. In particular, comminution in the volar aspect of the distal radius creates difficulties for stable reduction. When using implants to improve stability in the distal radius, the use of parallel wires entering from the radial styloid and driven proximally makes little sense biomechanically, and crossed implants seem to be favourable (Figs. 16.33a–16.33c). With an intact volar cortex, a third implant may be added entering from Lister's tubercle and drilled into the volar cortex of the proximal radial fragment.

Supplementary fixation may also be required to stabilize the articular surface. One or two Fragment Fixation System implants can be placed parallel to the reduced joint surface (Fig. 16.34). If there is an articular step-off of more than 2mm or a large enough articular fragment failing to elevate, a limited open reduction may be performed. In this case an implant of the Fragment Fixation System can be used in a joystick fashion to elevate the fragment. The incision depends on the localization of the fragment and whenever possible a dorsal approach is preferred (Figs. 16.35a, 16.35b). Using a bone elevator joint congruence may be restored and stabilization is performed with the Fragment Fixation System. This often leaves a void and to prevent recurrence of the dislocation bone grafting is advisable.

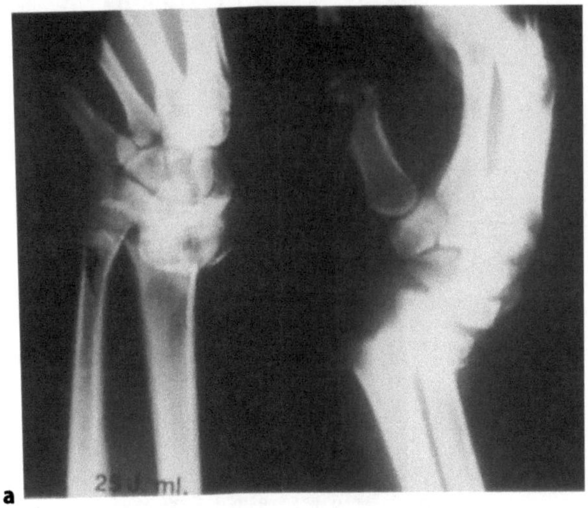

a

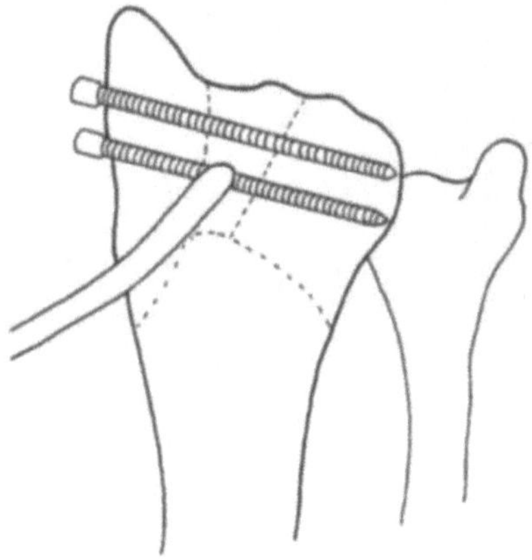

Fig. 16.34 After reconstruction of the articular surface, two medium size Fragment Fixation System implants are used parallel to the joint line.

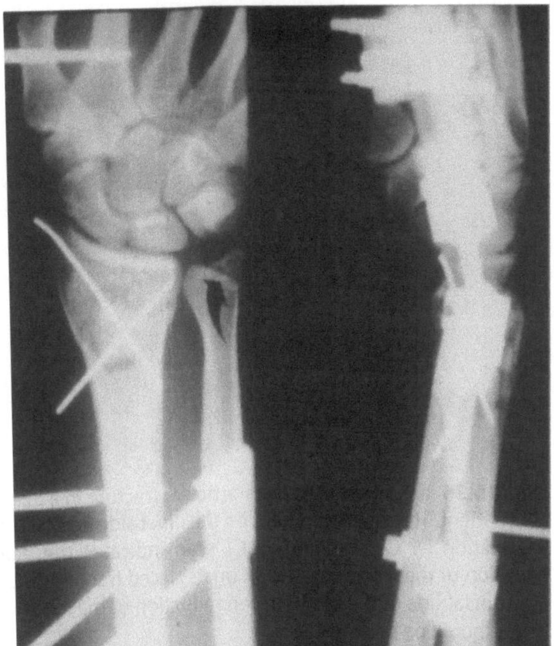

b

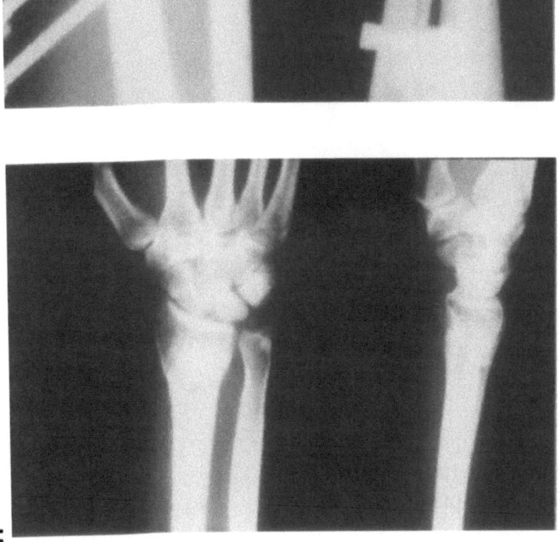

c

With volar lip fractures associated with dorsal comminution it is often impossible to anchor the volar lip fragment in healthy bone. Miniaturized T-, straight and L-plates usually employed in managing phalangeal and metacarpal fractures are best used to address individually the articular fragments. The pattern of articular fragmentation merits careful study and CT scanning is helpful (Figs. 16.36a, 16.36b). Especially in Melone type III, IV and V injuries (Melone (1993),[6] articular reconstruction should be supplemented with miniaturized plates best described as minimally invasive osteosynthesis technique (MIOT).

We usually combine these plates with the medium size Fragment Fixation System implants and washers since the purchase in cancellous bone is better than with a predrilled screw (Fig. 16.37). When applying minimally invasive osteosynthesis techniques a limited volar approach of 3–5cm is performed through the gap between the flexor carpi radialis muscle and the median nerve and it is recommended not to dissect the nerve but to leave adequate soft tissue coverage to protect it from scarring. The pronator quadratus muscle is often damaged and has to be detached from the articular fragments and preserved carefully since it is used to

Fig. 16.33 a Severely comminuted distal radius fracture in a 25-year-old male. Note position of the ulnar styloid, which indicates disruption of the radio-ulnar joint. **b** Closed reduction and crossed insertion of K-wires. The ulnar styloid reduced spontaneously. The radio-ulnar joint disruption is treated with the application of the ulnar outrigger. **c** Final position 8 weeks after surgery. Removal of the fixator and the K-wires 6 weeks after surgery.

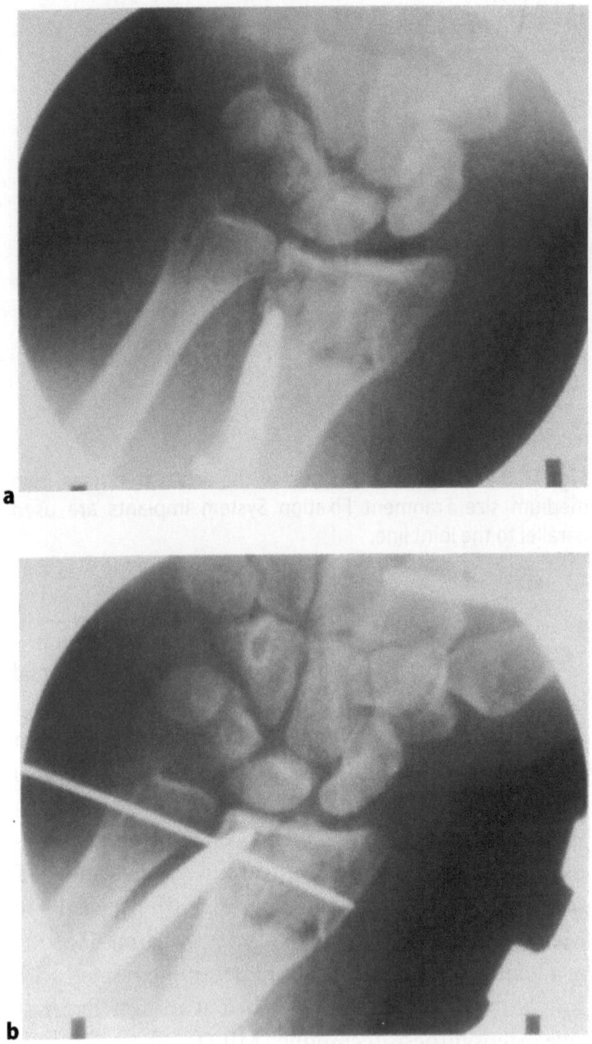

a

b

Fig. 16.35 **a** Limited open approach to elevate a die-punch fragment. Note temporary overdistraction of the joint indicated by the distance between the radius and the scaphoid to facilitate elevation of the fragment. **b** After full correction percutaneous stabilization is performed.

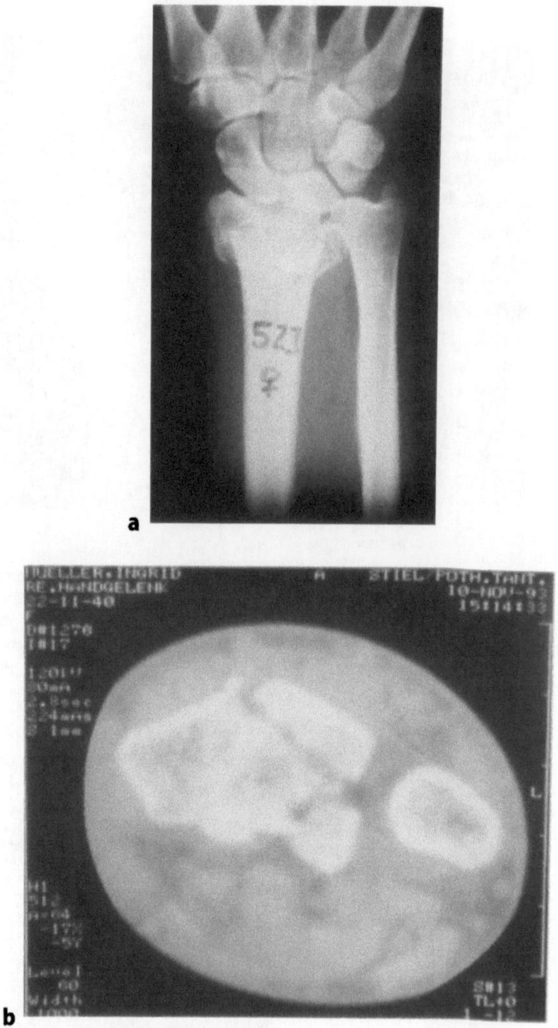

a

b

Fig. 16.36 **a** Comminuted intra-articular fracture in a 52-year-old patient. The radial fragment on the ulnar side merits further evaluation by CT scanning. **b** CT scan indicates the palmar position of the fragment and an undisplaced fracture through the dorsal side of the radius. Open reduction of the radio-ulnar joint should be performed.

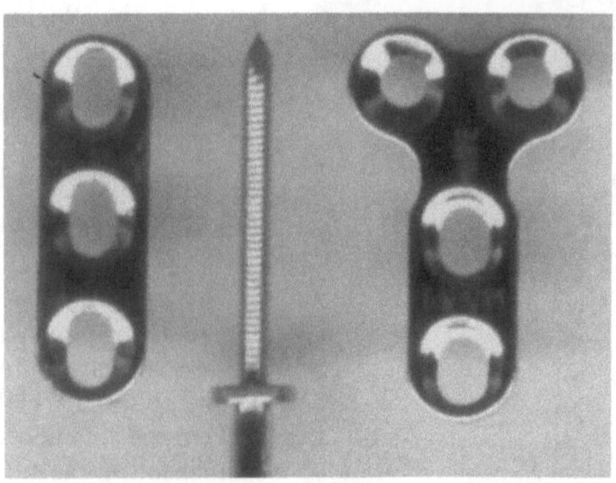

Fig. 16.37 MIOT: miniaturized implants to be used with the medium Fragment Fixation System implants and washers (middle: 1.6mm thread)

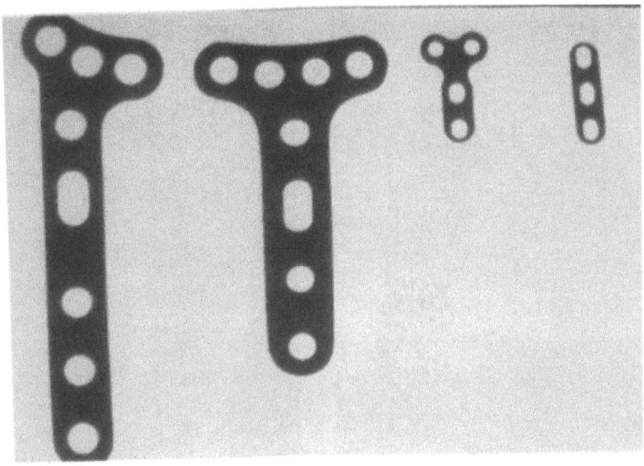

Fig. 16.38 Comparison in size of standard T-plates and MIOT.

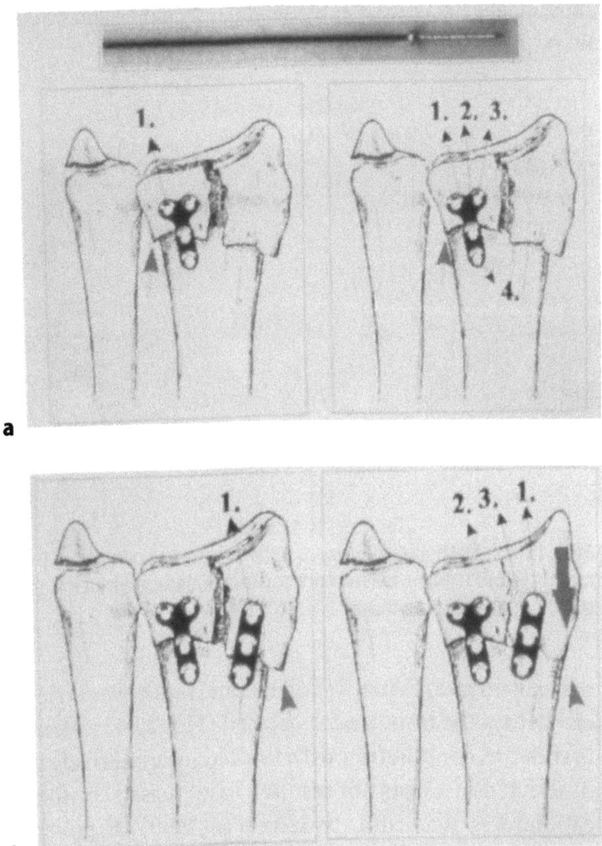

a

b

Fig. 16.39 **a** Operative strategy in volar lip fractures. The MIOT principle consists of application of a T-implant and insertion of one medium Fragment Fixation System implant with washer in position 1. Anatomical reduction of the fragment by pushing it distally. The numbers indicate the sequence of Fragment Fixation System implant insertion. **b** Reduction of the radial styloid with a straight MIOT implant. The numbers indicate the sequence of the Fragment Fixation System implants insertion. The larger arrow indicates the pull of the brachio-radialis tendon which attempts to redislocate and rotate the radial styloid.

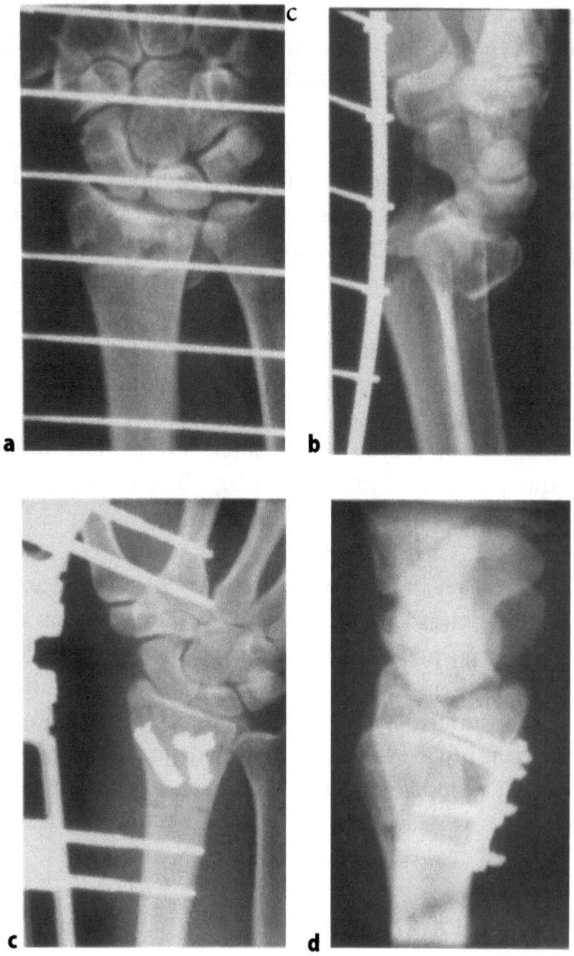

Fig. 16.40 **a** Intra-articular fracture in a 32-year-old woman. AP view. **b** The lateral film indicates fragmentation of the articular surface with the volar lip being displaced. **c** Transarticular application of the wrist fixator. Two MIOT implants in place as illustrated in Fig. 16.39a and 16.39b. **d** Lateral film showing anatomical reduction.

over the implants. The implants used for MIOT are not only smaller in size (Fig. 16.38), they are also significantly thinner since the main stabilizer, the external fixator, is placed outside.

Articular reconstruction usually starts on the ulnar column with the volar medial fragment according to Melone. Commonly, a miniature T-implant is used (Fig. 16.39a). It is particularly important to stabilize the radial styloid fragment since the brachio-radialis muscle with its tendon insertion on the styloid will pull and attempt to redisplace the fragment. A straight miniature implant is best used for the styloid (Fig. 16.39b). Whenever there is a defect in the metaphysis, bone grafting is performed and is best done from the dorsal side. After complete reconstruction of the volar fragments, a reduction is again performed using Gupta's manoeuver which focuses on the volar ligaments. If the dorsal ligaments and tendons help to reduce the dorsal comminution, the fixator is applied and the wound closed over a drain (Fig. 16.40a–16.40d). Should the dorsal articular fragments fail to reduce, a dorsal approach is required and again minimally invasive osteosynthesis techniques are used. It is customary in these cases to add bone graft to reconstruct the metaphyseal defect.

The fixator then serves not only to provide the main stabilizing element but also allows maintenance of the correct joint space. The repair process in articular fractures commences with a fibrin clot filling the persisting gaps. The cell system available for repair will contain chondrocytes which after several days may create a surface of fibrous cartilage. The fibrin repair mechanisms and the earlier cellular response must be protected. Early excessive loading, however, may disrupt the repair process (Buckwalter 1992,[7] 1995[8]) and here the fixator with a certain degree of distraction to keep the normal joint space will help to protect the repair mechanism. When later moving the joint the articular surfaces again have to be protected throughout the repair process. Not only may inadequate loading of articular components lead to redisplacement of the fracture, it also may affect the repair process described above.

Bone Grafting

With initial shortening of more than 10mm on the radial side and more than 5mm on the ulnar side of the radius, one has to expect a substantial structural defect in metaphyseal cancellous bone. In this case the traction X-ray will show a radiolucency after restoration of the radial length and the radial angles (Fig. 16.41). Bone grafting using corticocancellous cylinders is recommended to fill the defect (Fig. 16.42). Harvesting bone from the iliac crest is performed through a 2cm incision using the large bore trephine. This technique has been shown to cause little inconvenience to the patient and a much lower complication rate than open harvesting (Saleh 1991).[9] The usual approach for placement of the bone graft is from the dorsal side in the midline of the radius proximal to Lister's tubercle. After incision and careful retraction of the periosteum, the defect should be tightly packed with cancellous bone chips. The amount of cancellous bone necessary should not be underestimated. A corticocancellous block should finally be fitted in the residual cortical defect. Supplementary internal fixation using the Fragment Fixation System may be required in addition, especially if there is intra-articular involvement. It is best carried out before the bone graft is placed (Fig. 16.43). Bone grafting in conjunction with limited internal fixation in selected cases has not resulted in increased complication rates. According to Seitz et al (1990)[10] the overall results were superior since the technique could demonstrate the maintenance of radial length and articular congruity.

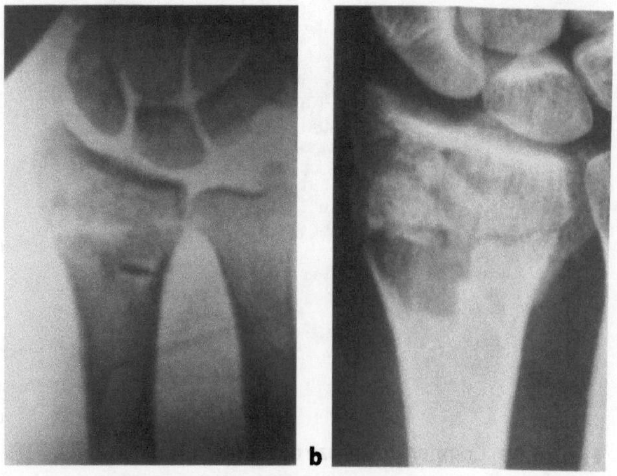

a b

Fig. 16.41 **a** Traction X-ray. Note the wide joint space between the scaphoid, lunate and radius. No significant radiolucency is observed, no indication to graft. **b** The traction X-ray shows a substantial defect proximal to the radial styloid. Filling of this defect is recommended to prevent later collapse.

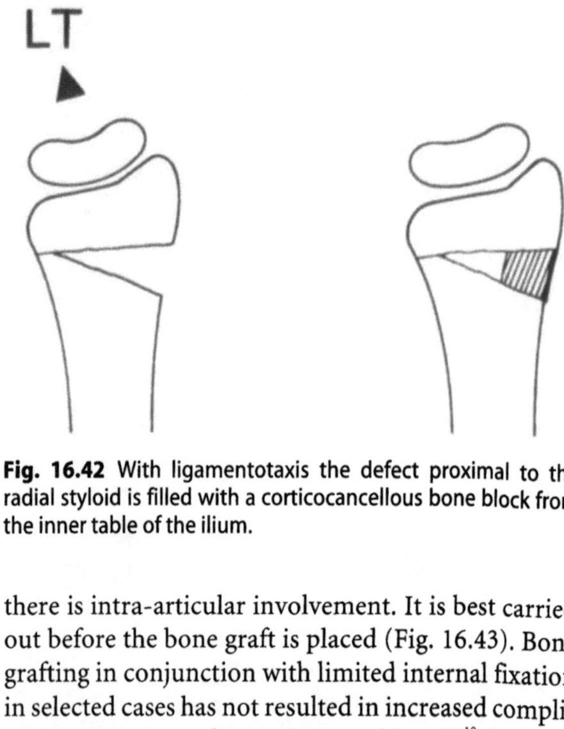

Fig. 16.42 With ligamentotaxis the defect proximal to the radial styloid is filled with a corticocancellous bone block from the inner table of the ilium.

Radio-ulnar Instability

Radio-ulnar instability with a rupture of the interosseous membrane and/or displaced ulnar head should not be overlooked. After reduction, immobilization should be performed in the neutral position

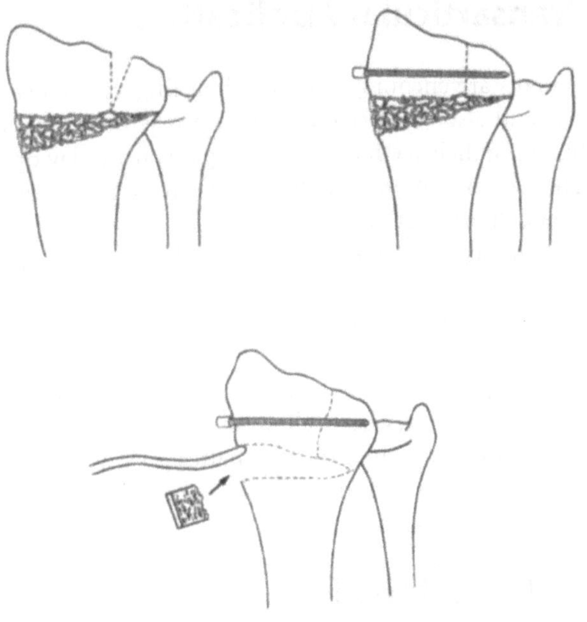

Fig. 16.43 An intra-articular fragmentation and bone defect. The restoration of the articular surface takes precedence. Stabilization with a medium size implant of the Fragment Fixation System. Restoration of the radial angle and filling of the defect with bone chips and corticocancellous bone graft.

with temporary fixation using a K-wire and a long-arm cast. We prefer an ulnar outrigger which is mounted on the fixator with an extra clamp, and approach the ulna from the dorsal side. A single fixator pin is placed in the ulna from the dorsal side after predrilling (Figs. 16.8, 16.33b). This prevents pronation and supination for four weeks after surgery. If there is significant pain during physiotherapy after outrigger removal, it should be replaced and remain in position for another week or two.

Associated Injuries In Distal Radius Fractures

Fracture of the Ulnar Styloid Process

If the styloid does not reduce spontaneously after the congruity of the distal radius has been restored, an interposition should be suspected. A short incision from the dorso-ulnar side should be carried out and the ulnar styloid reduced. Some form of internal fixation such as tension-band wiring, a miniscrew or the Fragment Fixation System may be of use to stabilize the ulnar styloid.

Fracture of the Distal End of the Ulna

A distal metaphyseal fracture or a shaft fracture of the ulna with displacement should be reduced anatomically, which restores the distal radio-ulnar joint. Stabilization using intramedullary wiring or mini external fixation is recommended. A diaphyseal fracture may be treated by intramedullary pinning or plate fixation and, if open, by external fixation. A displaced fracture of the ulna should not be ignored since the distal radio-ulnar joint may be severely affected by a malreduction.

Radio-ulnar Disruption or Injury of the Triangular Fibrocartilage Complex (TFCC)

A disruption of the distal radio-ulnar joint with displacement of the ulnar head must not be neglected. Reduction of the ulnar head and correct positioning in the semilunar notch following reduction of the distal radius fragment is mandatory. The position of the ulnar head in the semilunar notch is temporarily secured with a 1.5mm K-wire. Stabilization is provided either using a long-arm cast or the ulnar outrigger which prevents pro- and supination for a period of four weeks (see also radio-ulnar instability, above). The provisional K-wire is removed at the end of the operation. If reduction of the ulnar head is not possible, the distal radio-ulnar joint should be explored. The triangular fibrocartilage complex may be torn and interposed. If the ulnar disc shows significant damage, a partial or complete resection may be required. If it is undamaged, it is reduced and best held in place with transosseous sutures.

Scaphoid Fractures

Scaphoid fractures occur in less than one per cent of high velocity injuries of the distal radius, but every X-ray must be scrutinized for a scaphoid fracture or other carpal involvement. We routinely stabilize scaphoid fractures in the presence of distal radius fractures preferably using an approach through the anatomical snuffbox. Screw fixation seems advisable.

Scapholunate Dissociation

Scapholunate dissociation indicating an injury of the carpal ligaments may occur in distal radius fractures. The scapholunate interosseous ligament and the radioscapholunate ligament may be involved. It is usually seen in younger patients and a scapholunate diastasis may be visible on the fracture X-ray or after reduction of the distal radius. It is important to be aware of this injury since distraction with external fixation may be detrimental and increase the displacement in the scapholunate joint. In these cases it seems best to use the fixator in a strictly neutral position. In younger patients an acute repair of the ligaments may be attempted but there are very few reports on the outcome. Arthroscopy has been used for diagnosis but since the radiological identification of the problem with stress X-rays is possible, it may not play such an important role. In addition to having the fixator in the neutral position, pro- and supination must be prevented. An ulnar outrigger may be used with neutral rotation of the forearm to allow healing of the ligaments. In these cases the ulnar outrigger should be left in place for six weeks and the fixator should remain in the static mode.

Post-operative Management

Periarticular Application

The wrist joint is mobilized immediately post-operatively. Patients are not permitted, however, to lift or push heavy items.

For pin site care dressings should be changed 2–3 times per week for two weeks and subsequently once a week where there are normal pin sites.

X-ray assessment should be carried out on days 1, 7, 14 and 21 and prior to fixator removal. Retightening of all fixator screws should be carried out on the same days.

As a general rule, the fixator can be removed after 5–6 weeks. However, healing should be confirmed radiologically, since fracture patterns show considerable variation and longer application times may be required in some instances.

Transarticular Application

Patients are encouraged to use their fingers and exercise and also to carry out simple procedures such as brushing their teeth or holding a glass, from day one. They are not allowed, however, to lift or push heavy items. Pin site care is described above.

X-ray assessment should be carried out on days 1, 7, 14 and 21 and prior to fixator removal. Retightening of all fixator screws should be carried out on the same days.

As a general rule, the fixator can be removed after six weeks. However, healing should be confirmed radiographically, since fracture patterns show considerable variation and longer application times may be required in some instances.

Mobilization of Distal Radius Fractures

The value of early active and passive mobilization to avoid post-traumatic stiffness has been accepted in the hip, the knee, the ankle, the shoulder and the elbow. However, there is some reluctance to apply this principle to the distal radius mainly because of fear of redisplacement. With significant intra-articular damage, residual stiffness can be expected if the wrist joint and the adjacent joints remain immobilized for a lengthy period of time. Discussion on the subject of mobilization is not new. In 1893 Lukas Championière[11] initiated the principle of early mobilization of distal radius fractures coining the phrase "le movement c'est la vie". Championière's aim was to avoid the consequences of rigid fixation which in his opinion caused "muscular atrophy, stiffness of joints, proliferation of fibrous tissue, tendon adhesions and oedema formation". Championière applied gentle movement with one hand while stabilizing the fracture with the other. He also found that callus formation was improved by this type of treatment. In his studies he regretted that the residual deformity was significant but had no means to avoid it. Marbaix (1919)[12] could show superior results with Championière's method when compared with delayed mobilization. Early experimental results by Castex in 1891[13] indicated that the pathological–anatomical basis for residual stiffness may be found in the fibrous transformation of muscles, vessels and nerves in the area of a fracture in dogs. These did not occur when the soft tissue envelope around the fracture was massaged. Haematoma formation in the muscular septae of the forearm after distal radius fracture can be interpreted according to

Castex and could explain residual stiffness after prolonged immobilization. Passive mobilization was later discarded by Bardenheuer[14] in favour of an active mobilization. Championière did not agree with active mobilization since he expected a significant displacement of the fracture. He was also afraid of excessive movements since these could be painful. He used a traction bandage to immobilize the fracture itself and mobilized all adjacent muscles and joints. In fractures with significant displacement Bardenheuer discouraged active mobilization, since he aimed at anatomical healing with his newly developed traction bandage.

A recent study failed to demonstrate any benefit from early mobilization (Sommerkamp et al 1994).[15] However, the study is not conclusive, since two different fixators were used, in the static (AO fixator), and so-called dynamic (Clyburn fixator) modes. In addition, the follow-up rate in both groups was less than 70 per cent and there was no well-defined protocol for mobilization of the fixator. Mobilization has been repeatedly accused of resulting in loss of reduction. However, with supplementary techniques the inherent instability of the radial fracture can be controlled and after bone grafting and/or limited internal fixation we have not seen such a collapse.

If controlled wrist mobilization is desired at about three weeks post-operatively, the ball joint aligned with the centre of rotation of the wrist may be loosened by unlocking the cam. This will allow 40–50° of flexion and extension of the wrist. It is essential to ensure that the security collars are fully tightened and this should be checked at regular intervals. The patient should now practise flexion and extension. Provided the fixator has been applied correctly, radial shortening and fracture fragment displacement cannot occur during the wrist movement, because the rotational axis of the fixator is external to the rotational axis of the wrist. If significant pain at the fracture site is reported by the patient on mobilization, the ball joint should be locked for another week after which a further attempt at wrist mobilization may be made.

A study by Rawes et al[16] comparing one fixator system in the "dynamic" versus the static mode (Pennig Wrist Fixator, Orthofix Srl., Verona, Italy) in a randomized, prospective controlled trial showed that the mobilized group had a significantly more mobile wrist with 85 per cent of the range of movement of the opposite wrist. The statically fixed group had 70 per cent wrist mobility. The difference was evident both for intra- and extra-articular fractures. Radiologically, the fracture position was not lost during either form of fixation or after fixator removal. Five out of 32 patients showed disuse osteoporosis and it is interesting that four of these had been statically fixed (Rawes et al 1995).[16]

The role of early mobilization in joint injuries has been studied experimentally by Behrens et al[17] in dogs. Comparing rigid fixation after articular injuries with limited motion it was evident that the latter group recovered the proteoglycan content whereas the rigid mobilization group showed further cartilage degeneration after functional loading occurred (Behrens et al 1989).[17]

Complications of External Fixation

Intra-operative Complications

As with any surgical procedure on the skeleton, preoperative planning of pin placement in relation to the fracture is necessary to avoid complications. Instead of using stab incisions, especially with swelling of the hand and forearm, an adequate incision should be employed. The first interosseous muscle may have to be detached from the metacarpal bone and the bone surface should be clearly visible prior to drilling. Instead of placing both fixator pins in the diaphysis with weakening of the cortical bone, we prefer to place one pin in the proximal metaphysis and one in the metaphyseo-diaphyseal junction. The cross section of the metacarpal bone is significantly reduced in the mid-diaphyseal portion compared to the proximal portion which makes fractures more likely with pins in the diaphysis.

For pin placement in the radius an open approach is mandatory. With identification of the superficial branch of the radial nerve, injury to this structure can be avoided. A blunt dissection is performed to expose the radius and we detach the radial periosteum to reduce pain at the pin sites and ectopic bone formation around the pins. By using an open technique, transfixing tendons is avoided. It is important to position the pins centrally in the bone since eccentric placement may lead to poor purchase and pin loosening. The drill bit should be sharp to reduce heat generated when drilling. Predrilling of fixator pins has been shown to reduce the degree of thermal necrosis which may well contribute to pin loosening. The skin should not be too tight around the pins at the end of the operation and free movement of the skin around the pins should be checked to detect any tethering which may lead to mechanical irritation of the skin and infection.

The fixator pins should be of an adequate size and 3.3/3.0mm seems to combine stable fixation with minimal bone damage and an adequate pin–bone interface. The fixator pins should be placed in such a way that the device can be mounted without obstructing the anteroposterior and lateral X-ray views. If necessary, the fixator may be turned upside down or the position altered in another way to allow assessment of the reduction. If visualization in one plane remains difficult, a dental film may be placed between fixator and skin to obtain an unobstructed view.

Post-operative Complications

Post-operative complications include redisplacement and late collapse, pin-track infections, fractures through the pin sites and reflex sympathetic dystrophy. Late collapse and redisplacement can be avoided by careful assessment of the pre-operative film and a traction X-ray which may reveal a large corticocancellous defect. Supplemental internal fixation using the Fragment Fixation System/MIOT plates and bone grafting are used to avoid a late collapse. The post-operative film should be compared with the one-week control for early detection of slippage of the fracture. Secondary bone grafting may be required in such cases.

Pin-track infection may occur but the risk is minimized by careful pin insertion and meticulous post-operative pin site care. External fixators must not be put on and then ignored, but require active instruction of both the patient and the nursing staff by the attending surgeon. Mild disinfectants should be used for pin site care. Coloured disinfectants have no place since the skin will be stained and inflammation may be obscured. It is important to record the pin site status at each weekly post-operative visit to allow comparison.

Reflex sympathetic dystrophy and post-operative stiffness seem to be related to excessive mechanical distraction and poor positioning of the wrist joint with inadequate flexion and excessive ulnar deviation. By using elevation, cryotherapy and especially a recently developed hand pump which is based on the same principle as the foot pump for reduction of swelling, hand oedema can be treated and avoided (Pennig and Gladbach 1999)[18]. It is important for the patient to make a fist as soon as possible after the operation since this will lead to a more unaffected use of the hand. Circumferential dressing is not recommended and we prefer to use dressing of the pin sites only.

External Fixation In Corrective Osteotomies of the Distal Radius

Introduction

Malunion after a distal radius fracture is not uncommon. The radio-carpal and the distal radio-ulnar joint may be affected. Sequelae are visible deformity, loss of motion, reduced grip strength and pain. The articular incongruence may later result in osteoarthritis.

Unrestricted use of the hand implies full functioning of both radio-carpal and distal radio-ulnar joints and the latter is especially affected in the presence of a rotational deformity of the distal epiphysis. A rotational deformity violates the complex ligament attachments between distal radius, distal ulna and the carpus.

Treatment of malunion should result in complete correction of the deformity. Shortening is a particular problem and when using plate fixation with a volar approach manipulation of the distal fragment and lengthening is technically difficult. The radio-radial application of the fixator dorsally allows angular correction as well as lengthening.

Pre-operative Assessment

Clinical assessment records the visible deformity, the range of motion and grip strength. Standard radiographs of both the affected and the opposite side are carried out. To study rotational deformity which is reflected clinically in loss of supination or pronation, a CT scan of the left and right distal forearm is carried out. On the level of both the volar lip and the distal diaphysis of the radius with its triangular shape a line is plotted and compared with the unaffected side. Pre-operative planning is mandatory (Figs. 16.44a, 16.44b).

Specific Features of the Pennig II Wrist Fixator

Due to the forces encountered in corrective procedures, the Pennig II Wrist Fixator with increased mechanical performance should be used. The wrist fixator assembly for periarticular application consisting of a compression–distraction module and a short module with T-clamp is used. The compression–distraction module is placed proximally and the T-clamp

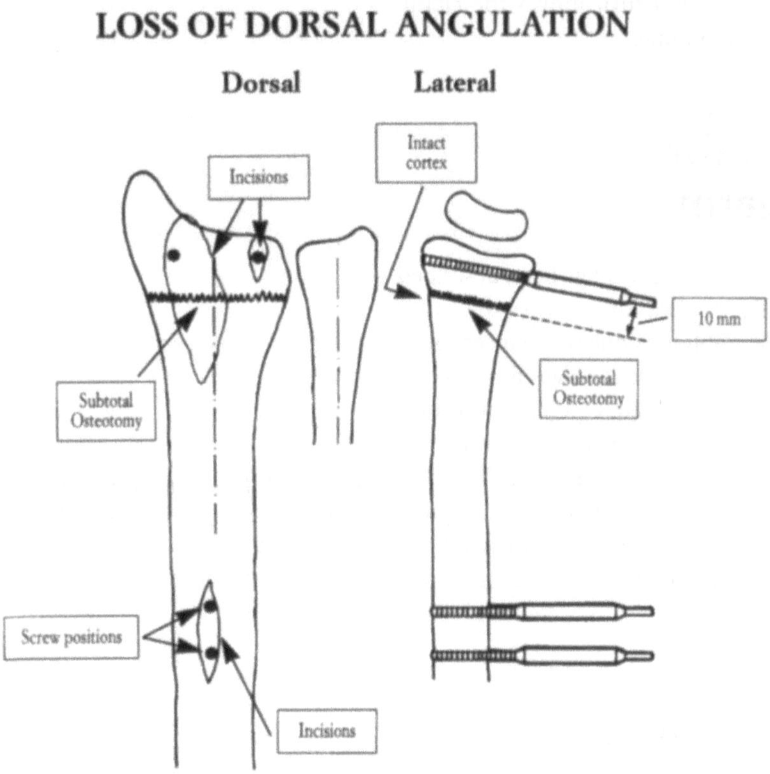

a

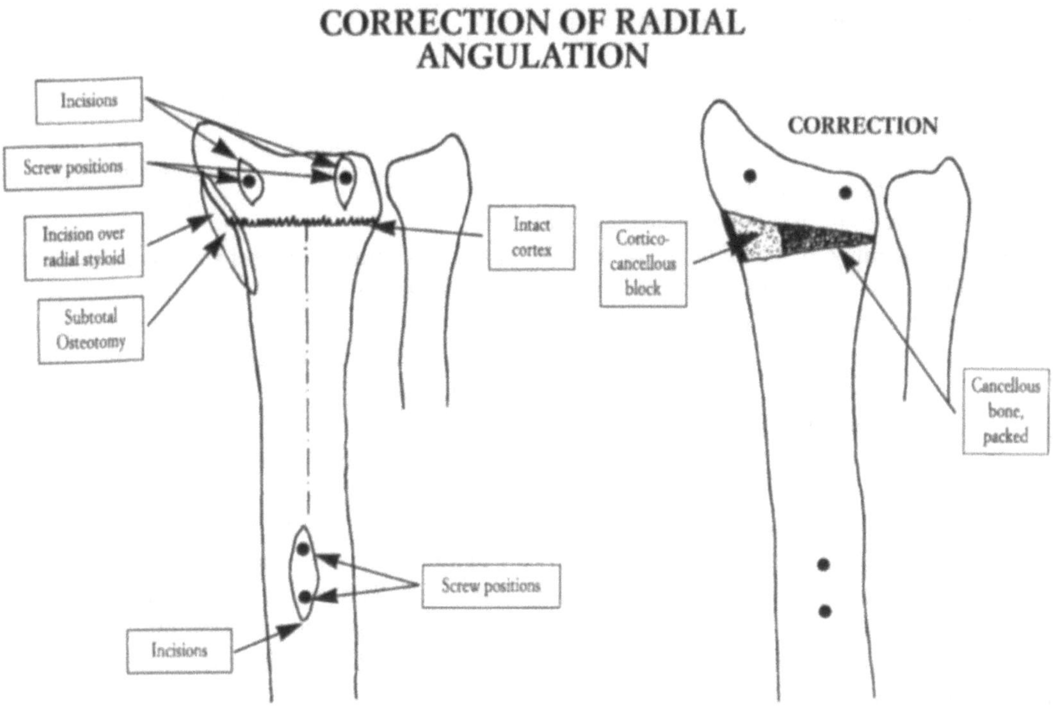

b

Fig. 16.44 **a** Pre-operative planning in loss of dorsal angulation. **b** Pre-operative planning in loss of radial angulation.

distally (Fig. 16.45). One full turn moves the clamp 1mm in the distraction module.

Anatomy of the Distal Forearm

The anatomy of the distal forearm has been described above for periarticular applications. Unlike the situation in fractures where oblique bone screw insertion is performed, in corrective osteotomies dorso-volar bone screw insertion is employed. Open pin insertion is necessary and the landmark is again Lister's tubercle. The second screw is placed on the ulnar side. This part of the radius is covered by the fourth tendon compartment (Fig. 16.46) and care must be taken to avoid any tethering of the extensor digitorum tendons. Open insertion is mandatory.

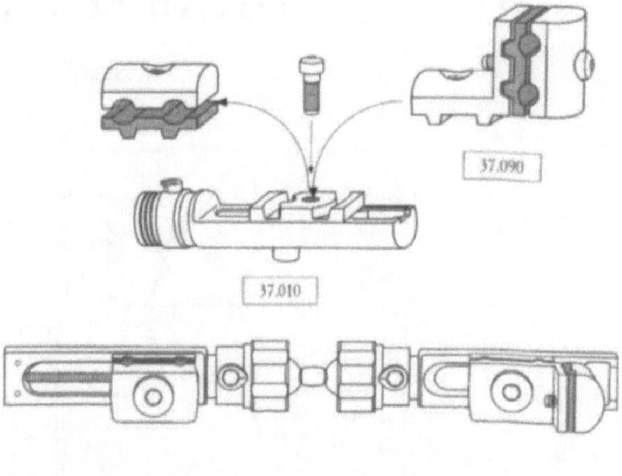

Fig. 16.45 Pennig II wrist fixator with T-clamp distally and distraction–compression module proximally, for corrective osteotomies.

Operative Technique

One Stage Correction and Graft

The operation consists of harvesting of bone graft, selection and insertion of screws, osteotomy, correction and grafting.

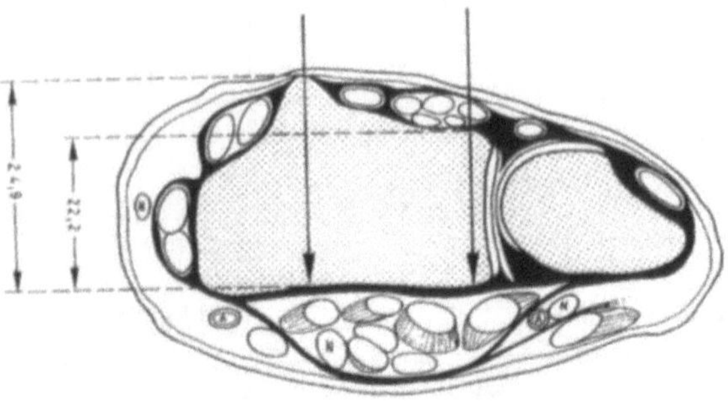

Fig. 16.46 Schematic cross-section of the distal radius through Lister's tubercle. The figures indicate the distance from cortex to cortex at the pin sites (n = 6, measurements by CT scan)

Stage 1: Harvesting of Bone Graft

The bone graft is taken first, before the radius is approached. The size of the graft should be estimated by pre-operative planning. It should be harvested as a corticocancellous block from the inner table of the ilium. A larger piece than necessary is taken together with a supply of cancellous bone chips.

Stage 2: Selection and Insertion of Screws

Depending on the dimensions of the bone and the soft tissues, 80/35 or 70/20 screws are used; thread size 3.3/3.0mm; drill bit 2.7mm. A hand table is used and a tourniquet is mandatory.

The standard procedure consists of insertion of the distal screws first followed by insertion of the proximal screws.

It is important to expose the bone and position the screw guides under direct vision to avoid injuries to tendons and nerves. Drilling must be performed with extreme caution in order to avoid neurovascular injury to structures on the volar side of the radius.

The distal screws should be inserted strictly in the sagittal plane and parallel to the distal radial articular surface. This is ensured by prior placement of pilot wires via pilot wire guides inserted into the screw guides (Figs. 16.47a–16.47c).

A 3–4cm incision is made from the end of the radius proximally. Further dissection should deflect the extensor digitorum tendons to the ulnar side, and the extensor pollicis tendon to the radial side. The first screw is inserted within this incision into Lister's tubercle. A second, 1cm incision is made on the ulnar side of the radius for placement of the second distal screw.

The proximal screws are inserted with the template/conversion clamp temporarily replacing the cover of the straight clamp on the compression–distraction module, as shown in Fig. 16.48.

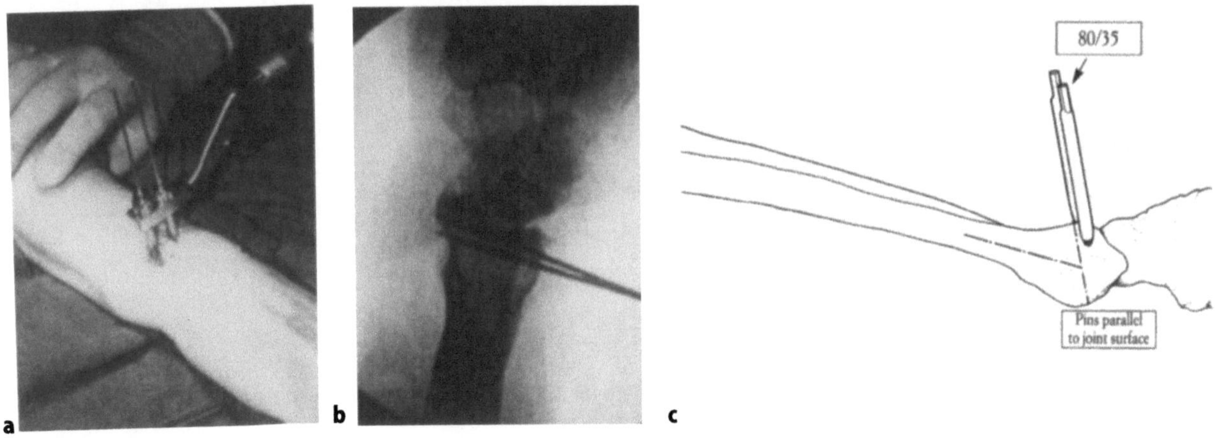

a b c

Fig. 16.47 **a** Use of pilot wires from the dorsal side directed at the volar lip. **b** Radiographic control of correct pilot wire placement. Predrilling for insertion of fixator screws is then performed. **c** Pin placement parallel to joint line.

The fixator is now applied with the distal screws in the T-clamp. The distal clamp should be near the middle of the module, whereas the proximal clamp on the compression–distraction module is moved as close as possible to the ball joint. The fixator is aligned so that both modules are parallel to the long axis of the radius. The position of the skin incision is marked and the fixator is swung aside to allow access.

A 2.5cm incision is made and the diaphyseal radius exposed prior to drilling and screw insertion. The soft tissues are again carefully dissected down to the bone and protected with retractors, special care being taken to avoid damage to the superficial branch of the radial nerve. The longer of the two screw guides is removed from the template with handle and the shorter guide is inserted into the proximal hole of the template/conversion clamp. A drill guide is inserted into the screw guide and the bone is drilled with a 2.7mm drill bit, using the drill stop when the distal cortex is reached, to prevent tissue damage on the volar side. After inserting this screw the longer screw guide is used (Fig. 16.49) for insertion of the second screw. With the image intensifier it is confirmed that all four screws penetrate the opposite cortex. The fixator is now removed to allow free access for the osteotomy.

The type of osteotomy performed will depend upon the correction required. If correction in one plane only is needed, the osteotomy can be subtotal, and the distal fragment turned into position by hinging on the opposite intact cortex. If more than one plane of correction is required, osteotomy must be complete.

The osteotomy is performed through the larger skin incision. The soft tissues are again protected, and a line of 2mm drill holes made about 10 mm proximal to the distal screws, using the drill stop to protect the tissues on the volar side of the radius. The osteotomy is completed with an osteotome. It is opened manually to ensure that it is adequate and the template handles with screw guides in place may be used to provide better leverage.

The fixator is reapplied, ensuring that the modules are parallel to the long axis of the radius. The ball joints and all other screws are loose at this stage.

The osteotomy shown is subtotal, allowing for correction of dorsal angulation only (Figs. 16.50a, 16.50b).

In two- or three-dimensional correction a complete osteotomy is required. It can be performed with the drill initially, using the drill stop to prevent volar soft tissue damage, and completed with an osteotome. The radial anatomy is restored with the help of the templates with handles. The fixator is locked and radial length restored by opening the compression–distraction module.

The centre of the osteotomy is packed with cancellous bone chips and the distal radial fragment is supported by three corticocancellous bone blocks as shown (Fig. 16.51):

Block I: radial side
Block II: dorsal side
Block III: ulnar side

Any remaining gaps in the bone are filled with cancellous bone chips. The osteotomy is closed into the final position, gently compressing the grafts, and the fixator is locked (Figs. 16.52a–16.52c).

The same procedure can be used for the correction of radial shift with shortening. The necessary translation to correct the position can be achieved with the double ball joints loosened, moving the distal fragment as required. Again, it is helpful to slide the screw guides in the templates with handles on to the screws, with the fixator in place, to achieve better control.

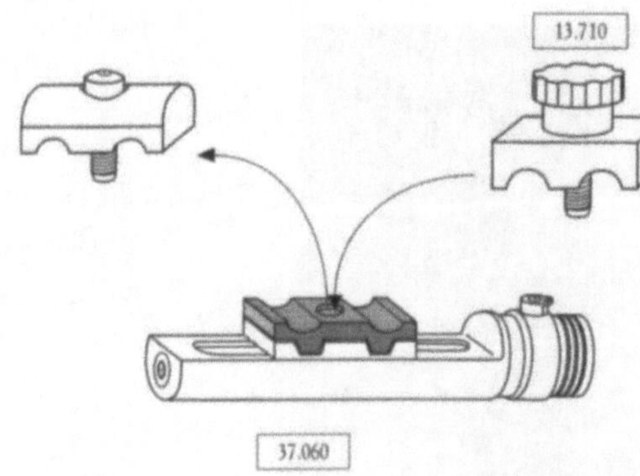

Fig. 16.48 Use of the template/conversion clamp for precise pin placement in the radial diaphysis.

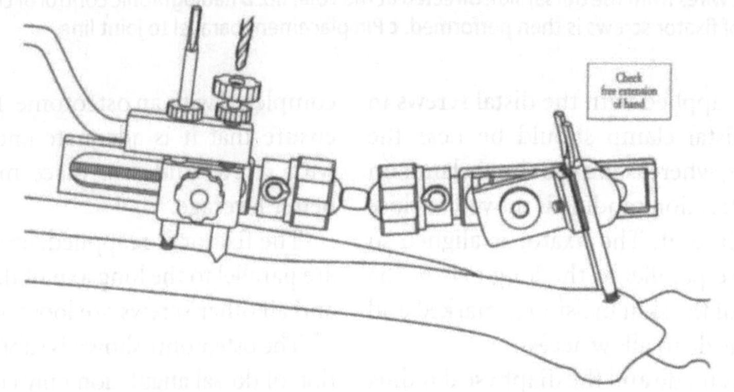

Fig. 16.49 Placement of the proximal screws in the radial diaphysis.

a

b

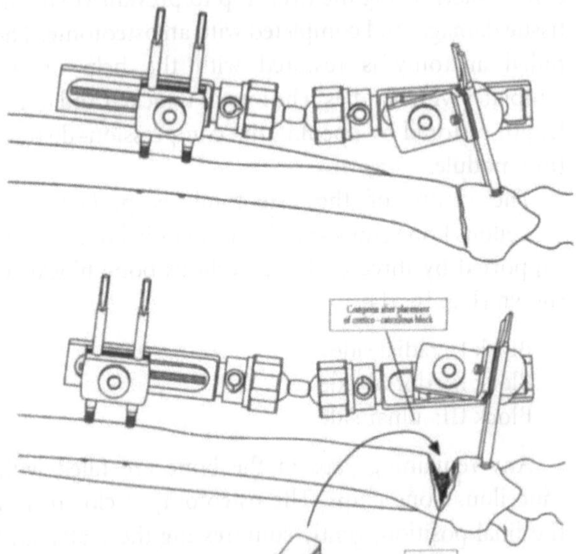

Fig. 16.50 a Incomplete osteotomy for correction of dorsal angulation only. **b** After correction the resulting gap is filled with cancellous bone chips and the corticocancellous bone block. Overcorrection is performed to allow compression of the bone block.

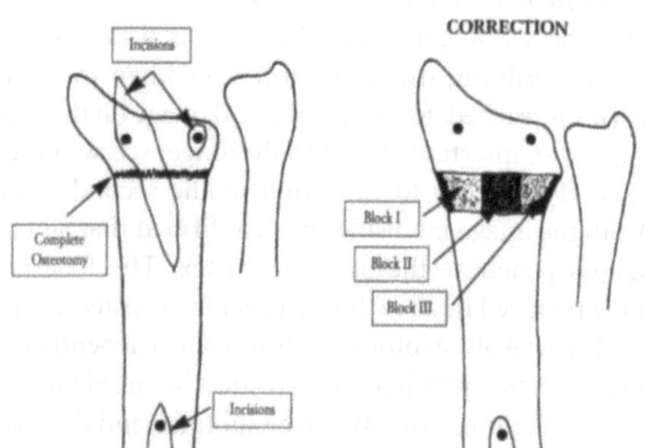

Fig. 16.51 Correction of radial length and angulation. Three bone blocks are used. Overcorrection is performed to allow insertion and compression of the bone blocks.

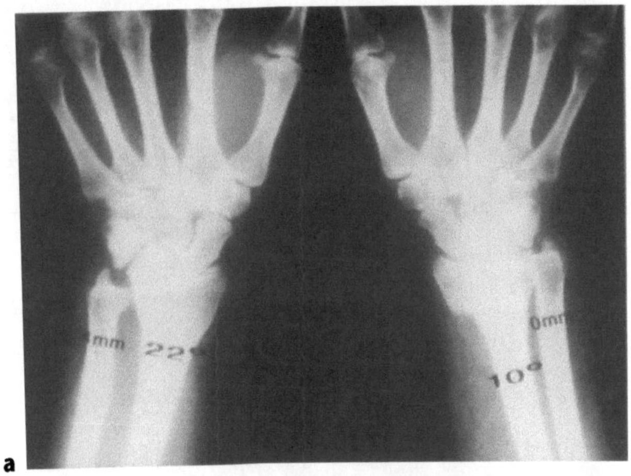

a

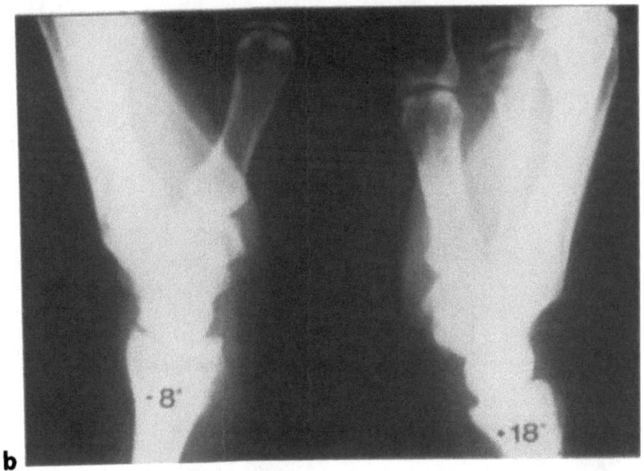

b

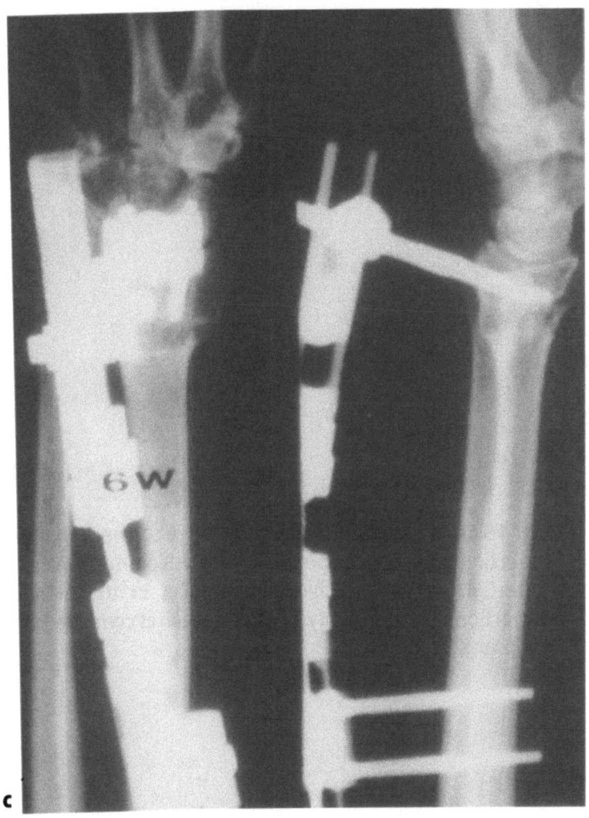

c

To correct malrotation, the degree of rotation is evaluated with the help of a CT scan. The distal pins are inserted at an angle to the proximal pins to reflect the deformity. Following osteotomy correction is performed and the fixator is applied.

The osteotomy wound is closed in layers, and sutures may also be placed in the pin insertion wounds. The fixator is left in place for 6–8 weeks until union is achieved.

Depending on the severity of the deformity and the original injury, the patient may require some physiotherapy to restore function. This should be started immediately, avoiding heavy weights. Because the graft is compressed, the osteotomy is stable and active mobilization of the wrist can normally be resumed within two weeks.

Post-operative management and pin site care are identical with that for fractures and are described above. X-rays are normally taken on days 1, 7 and 28 and again prior to fixator removal.

Gradual Correction: Hemicallotasis

This procedure can be used for the correction of isolated dorsal angulation of the radius only, and the maximum correction possible is approximately 30°.

The screws are placed as described above with careful attention to the alignment of the fixator. In this case the screw on the base of the T-clamp must be positioned over the osteotomy, since the T-clamp will gradually rotate as the osteotomy opens.

The osteotomy is subtotal, through the dorsal, lateral and medial cortices, 10mm proximal to the distal screws, with careful exposure of the bone and protection of the soft tissues. The periosteum, the prime cell source for callus formation, must be preserved.

The osteotomy is carefully opened manually to confirm that it is adequate. The fixator is then applied, with the compression–distraction module proximally and the short module distally. The proximal straight clamp should be positioned at the distal end of the compression–distraction module.

The osteotomy is now closed, and the fixator screws and ball joints are tightened (Fig. 16.53a). The screw by which the T-clamp is attached to the base of the distal clamp is left slightly loose, and the compression–

Fig. 16.52 a, b Radial malunion in a 41-year-old woman with radial shortening, loss of dorsal and radial angulation. **c** Full correction of dorsal angle, radial angle and radial length with bone blocks in place, 6 weeks post-operatively. Fixator was removed 2 weeks later.

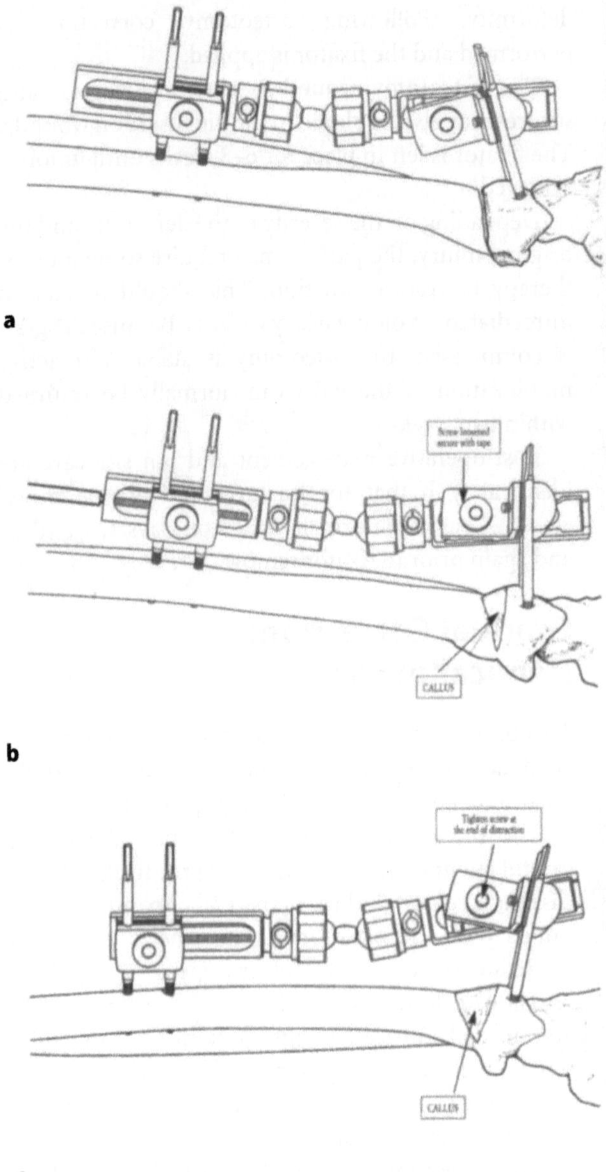

Fig. 16.53 Hemicallotasis for the correction of dorsal angulation. **a** Volar cortex intact. Osteotomy gap closed. **b** After a waiting period of 10 days the osteotomy is opened at a speed of 2mm per day. The distal radial fragment rotates around the bottom screw of the T-clamp. **c** After correction is complete the bottom screw of the T-clamp is tightened.

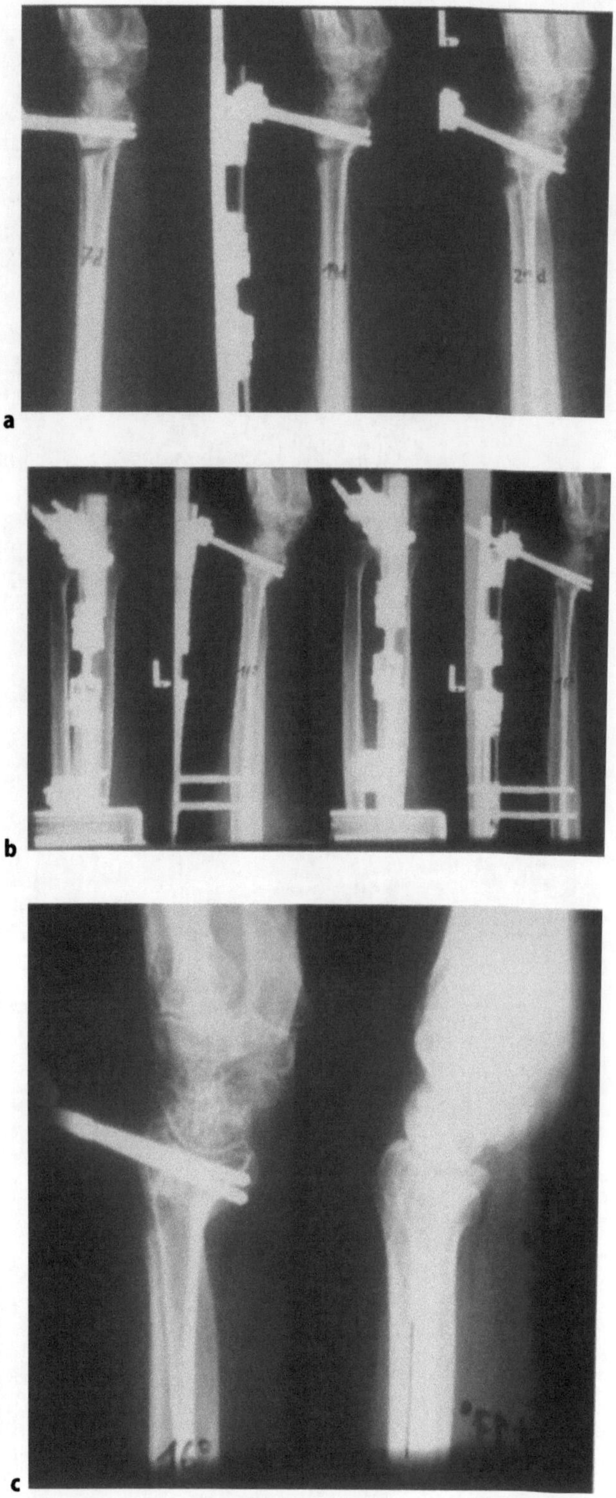

Fig. 16.54 **a** Standard radiographs serve to check the radial correction and correct opening of the osteotomy. **b** After full correction has been achieved the callus in the triangular distraction site has to ossify. **c** Full correction as compared to the opposite side (right).

distraction module used to check that the osteotomy will open correctly. The osteotomy is then closed completely with the compression–distraction module, and put into gentle compression by turning the central screw anti-clockwise. The T-clamp screw is now tightened, and the periosteum and wounds closed with sutures.

The technique of hemicallotasis is now followed as described for other sites. The osteotomy should remain undisturbed for 10 days. At this point the screw holding the T-clamp to the clamp base is loosened slightly. We recommend that this screw is held in place with adhesive tape to prevent further loosening.

Distraction is then started at a rate of 2mm per day in four steps with clockwise turning. The maximum correction possible with this method is approximately 30°. The progress of the opening of the osteotomy should be checked radiographically once a week (Fig. 16.53b). With poor bone stock distraction is performed at a rate of 1mm per day.

When the desired position has been achieved, the T-clamp screw is tightened and the fixator left in position until the new bone has ossified sufficiently and the cortices have formed (Fig. 16.53c). This will occur after two to four weeks (Figs. 16.54a–16.54c). The fixator is then removed. The screws can be left in place for a few days before a final check is made to ensure that the radius has healed.

Post-operative Management

Post-operatively a soft splint is worn for 72 hours and the arm is elevated. Analgesia may be required but we do not recommend the use of continuous brachial plexus anaesthesia.

The post-operative management is identical to that described for fractures but the longer application time has to be taken into account. Successful use of this technique requires meticulous pin site care since resiting of the pins in the distal radius is virtually impossible.

Bony union is confirmed radiographically; in addition to the AP and lateral film oblique views should be obtained. Once healing has been established, a trial removal of the fixator is recommended. The pins may remain in situ for two or three days unless one is absolutely certain of bony consolidation. The patient is instructed not to load the wrist, but physiotherapy is performed throughout the time in fixator and thereafter.

Due to the complex nature of distal radius malunion, restoration of the bony anatomy may only be part of the treatment strategy.

References

1. Cooney WP 'External fixation of distal radial fractures.' *Clin Orthop* 1983 180: 44.
2. Charnley J *Die konservative Therapie der Extremitätenfrakturen.* 1968 Springer: Berlin.
3. Gupta A 'The treatment of Colles' fracture.' *J Bone Joint Surg* [Br] 1991 73B: 312.
4. Agee JM 'Distal radius fractures: multiplanar ligamentotaxis.' *Hand Clin* 1993 9:577–85.
5. Dée W, Klein W, Rieger H 'Reduction techniques in distal radius fractures.' Suppl. to *Injury* 1999 (in press).
6. Melone CP 'Distal Radius Fractures: Patterns of Articular Fragmentation.' *Orthop Clin North Am* 1993 24: 239–253.
7. Buckwalter JA 'Mechanical Injuries of Articular Cartilage.' *Iowa Orthopaedic Journal* 1992 Vol 12:50-7.
8. Buckwalter JA 'Should Bone, Soft Tissue and Joint Injuries be Treated with Rest or Activity?' *Orth Res* 1995 13:155-6.
9. Saleh, M (1991) 'Bone graft harvesting: A percutaneous technique.' *J Bone Joint Surg* [Br] 73-B: 867.
10. Seitz WH, Putnam MD, Dick HM 'Limited open surgical approach for external fixation of distal radius fractures.' *J Hand Surg* [Am] 1990 15A:288-93.
11. Championière JL *Traitement des fractures par le massage et la mobilisation* 1893 Paris
12. Marbaix (1919) see Steinmann F (1919) *Lehrbuch der funktionellen Behandlung der Knochenbrüche und Gelenkverletzungen.* Verlag Ferd. v. Enke: Stuttgart.
13. Castex (1919) see Steinmann F (1919) *Lehrbuch der funktionellen Behandlung der Knochenbrüche und Gelenkverletzungen.* Verlag Ferd. v. Enke: Stuttgart.
14. Bardenheuer (1919) see Steinmann F (1919) *Lehrbuch der funktionellen Behandlung der Knochenbrüche und Gelenkverletzungen.* Verlag Ferd. v. Enke: Stuttgart.
15. Sommerkamp G, Seeman M, Silliman J et al 'Dynamic external fixation of unstable fractures of the distal part of the radius.' *J Bone Joint Surg* [Am] 1994 76A: 1149.
16. Rawes ML, Richardson JB, Hardy JRW et al 'Dynamic versus static external fixation of distal radial fractures: a prospective randomized controlled trial.' *Injury* 1995 26: 140.
17. Behrens F, Kraft EL, Oegema TR 'Biomechanical Changes in Articular Cartilage after Joint Immobilization by Casting or External Fixation.' *J Orthop Research* 1989 7: 335–343.
18. Pennig D, Gladbach B *Use of the AV-Impulse System in the Hand. In: The return of the blood to the heart.* Gardner AMN, Fox RH (eds.) 3rd Edition 1999 (in press)

Supplementary Bibliography

Agee JM, Szabo RM, Chidgey LK et al (1994) 'Treatment of comminuted distal radius fractures: An approach based on pathomechanics.' *Orthopaedics* 17: 115–122.

Asche G 'Stabilisierung von handgelenksnahen Speichenstückfrakturen mit dem Midifixateur externe.' *Handchirurgie* 1983 15: 38.

Clyburn TA 'Dynamic external fixation for comminuted intra-articular fractures of the distal end of the radius.' *J Bone Joint Surg* [Am] 1987 69-A: 248.

Colles A 'On the fracture of the carpal extremity of the radius.' *Journal of Medicine and Surgery, Edinburgh* 1814 10: 182.

Fernandez DL 'Correction of post-traumatic wrist deformity by osteotomy, bone grafting and internal fixation.' *J Bone Joint Surg* [Am] 1982 64: 1164.

Gartland JJ Jr and Werley CW 'Evaluation of healed Colles' fractures.' *J Bone Joint Surg* [Am] 1951 33-A: 895.

Gausepohl T, Pennig D, Mader K 'Principles of external fixation and supplementary techniques in distal radius fractures.' *Injury* 1999 Suppl. (in press).

Jenkins NH, Jones DG, Johnson SR et al (1987) 'External fixation of Colles' fractures'. *J Bone Joint Surg* [Br] 69: 207.

Klein W, Dée W 'Erste Erfahrungen mit einem neuen Handgelenksfixateur zur Behandlung distaler Radiusfrakturen.' *Handchir Mikrochir Plas Chir* 1992 24: 202.

Klein W, Dée W, Rieger HS et al 'Results of transarticular fixator application in distal radius fractures.' *Injury* 1999 Suppl. (in press).

Lambotte A 'Sur l'ostéosynthèse. *La Belgique Medicale* 1908 20: 231.

Lanz U (1987) 'Korrekturosteotomie nach distalen Radiusfrakturen, Technik und Ergebnisse.' in: Buck-Gramcko, Nigst H (eds): *Frakturen am distalen Radiusende.* Hippokrates Verlag: Stuttgart.

Lanz U, Kron W 'Neue Technik zur Korrektur in Fehlstellung verheilter distaler Radiusfrakturen.' *Handchirurgie* 1976 8: 203.

Leung KS, Shen WY, Leung PC et al 'Ligamentotaxis and bone grafting for comminuted fractures of the distal radius.' *J Bone Joint Surg* [Br] 1989 71-B: 838.

Lidström A 'Fractures of the distal end of the radius: A clinical and statistic study of end results.' *Acta Orthop Scand,* 1959 Suppl 41.

McQueen MM, MacLaren A, Chalmers J 'The value of remanipulating Colles' fractures.' *J Bone Joint Surg* [Br] 1986 68-B: 232–3.

McQueen MM, MacLaren A, Chalmers J 'Colles' fractures: Does the anatomical result affect the final functions?' *J Bone Joint Surg* [Br] 1988 70-B: 649–51.

O'Dwyer KJ, MacEachern AG, Pennig D 'Corrective tibial osteotomy for genu recurvatum by callus distraction using an external fixator.' *Chirurgia Degli Organi di Movimento* 1991 76: 355–358.

Ombredanne (1929) 'L'ostéosynthèse temporaire chez les enfants.' *Presse Médicale* Nr. 52

Pennig D *The Pennig Dynamic Wrist Fixator. Operative Technique.* Orthofix Srl., Bussolengo, Italy

Pennig D 'Dynamic External Fixation of Distal Radius Fractures.' *Hand Clinics* 1993 Vol 9: 587–602.

Pennig D, Baranowski D 'Genu recurvatum due to partial growth arrest in the proximal physis; Correction by callus distraction.' *Archives of Orthop Trauma Surgery* 1989 108: 119–21.

Pennig D, Gausepohl T 'External Fixation of the Wrist.' *Injury* 1996 Vol 27, No. 1: 1–15.

Pennig D, Gausepohl T 'Minimally invasive treatment of fractures at the distal end of the radius.' *Jap Journal of Minimally Invasive Orthopaedic Surgery* 1997 No. 5: 39–52.

Pennig D, Gausepohl 'External fixation in the distal forearm: Its use in fractures and malunions.' Instructional Course Lecture. *Jap Orthop Science* 1999 (in press).

Pennig D, Gausepohl T, Lukosch R 'Der Einsatz von Fixationsstiften zur Fragmentstabilisierung in der Handchirurgie.' *Handchir Mikrochir Plas Chir* 1994 26: 270–4.

Pennig D, Gausepohl T, Mader K 'Corrective osteotomies in malunited distal radius fractures. External fixation as one stage and hemicallotasis procedures.' *Injury* 1999 Suppl. (in press).

Salter RB 'The biologic concept of continuous passive motion of synovial joints. The first 18 years of basic research and its clinical application.' *Clin Orthop* 1989 242: 12.

Schuind F, Donckerwolcke M. Rasquin C et al 'External fixation of fractures of the distal radius.' *J Hand Surg* [Am] 1989 14: 404.

Steinmann F (1919) *Lehrbuch der funktionellen Behandlung der Knochenbrüche und Gelenkverletzungen.* Verlag Ferd. v. Enke: Stuttgart.

Vidal J, Buscayret C, Paran M et al (1983) 'Ligamentotaxis.' in: Mears DC (ed): *External Skeletal Fixation,* William & Wilkins: Baltimore.

Youm Y, McMurtry RY, Flatt AE et al 'Kinematics of the wrist I. An experimental study of radial-ulnar deviation and flexion-extension.' *J Bone Joint Surg* [Am] 1978 60-A: 423.

The RadioLucent Wrist Fixator for Distal Radius Fractures

17

D.L. Nelson

Introduction

The RadioLucent wrist fixator (Fig. 17.1) represents a new generation of fixator, based on principles of ergonomics, that is, it was designed primarily with the patient in mind. For this purpose it needed to be low profile, both in height and length, to enable it to pass through the sleeve of a shirt or blouse easily, without the pins or fixator catching on the fabric. It had to be lightweight, since even a small weight at the end of the arm is experienced as heavy by the patient, and it needed to be both rugged and corrosion-resistant, to correspond with current trends in pin site care, which tend to favour patients showering with their fixators in situ.

The RadioLucent wrist fixator is one of the lightest of the unilateral fixators on the market for the distal radius, weighing only 100 grams. By comparison, the Pennig Dynamic Wrist Fixator weighs 135g, the EBI DynaFix 182g, the Agee WristJack 212g, and the Orthofix 30.000 model 264g. The overall length of the fixator is only 13cm but it can expand to 19cm, which is sufficient to accommodate a 195cm (6' 5") patient. Its height is only 15mm, and in conjunction with its pins, it has an overall height above the patient's skin of only 25mm. This short overall length and very low profile allows the patient to dress with ease.

The design of the pins merits particular mention. The RadioLucent fixator's pins are shorter than any earlier pins on the market, yet are sufficient to fit even a 195cm (6' 5") patient, with room to spare between skin and fixator. Pin design was based on a study of the dimensions of the radius and second metacarpal in a series of 50 patients. Pins are available in a range of overall lengths and length of threaded portions. In this way, all types of patient, from very small-framed, short women to very tall, large-framed men can be accommodated, while avoiding extension of the threads beyond the cortices of the bones or above the skin. A radiographic template allows the surgeon to determine pre-operatively the correct sizes of pins to use.

In addition to its extreme light weight and low profile, which are patient benefits, the RadioLucent design team also kept the surgeon in mind. As its name implies, the device is radiolucent, allowing full visualization of the fracture site and carpal bones. The position of the distal radial articular surface, carpal alignment, and scaphoid fractures (see Case 3, below) are easily seen, even if the fixator body is directly over the bones.

The RadioLucent has the same rigidity in its ball joints as the Orthofix 30.000 model, which, overall, is the stiffest external fixator for the distal radius that has ever been produced by any manufacturer. The elegant cam and ball joint design of the Orthofix line was

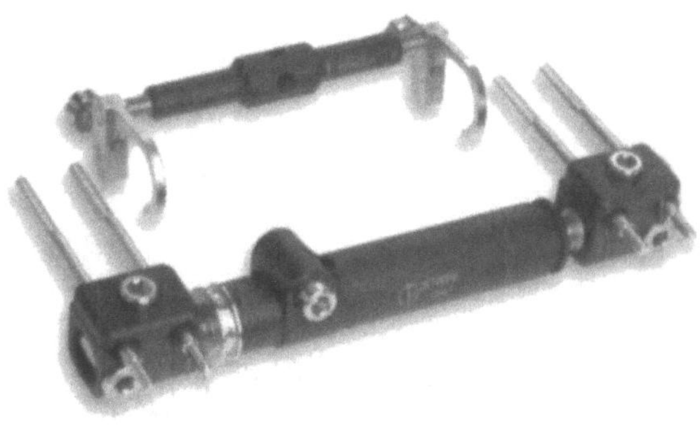

Fig. 17.1 The RadioLucent Wrist Fixator and its detachable compression-distraction unit

retained, while the mobility of the ball joints was increased so that the fixator is capable of a full 60° of angulation in all planes. The cam has been redesigned so that it tightens in only one direction, marked by an arrow on the fixator. There are two benefits to this design: inadvertent loosening is avoided and twice the cam rotation – and hence twice the camming force – is available for the same degree of torque.

The present chapter describes the use of the RadioLucent fixator in three very different fracture problems, as well as current thinking for the associated surgical technique: plane of dissection, plane and technique of pin (screw) insertion, treatment of associated fractures, and other issues.

Materials and Methods

The RadioLucent external fixator has been used in a variety of patients to treat a variety of fracture problems. This chapter will review its use in a comminuted fracture treated by reduction, external fixation and percutaneous pin fixation (Case 1); a complex fracture that required internal and external fixation together with bone grafting (Case 2), and a complex open fracture combined with a scaphoid fracture (Case 3).

Case 1

A 30-year-old, right hand dominant, white, male, self-employed handyman had a motorcycle accident in the mountains injuring his left wrist. X-rays (Fig. 17.2) showed an intra-articular fracture of the distal radius, with widely separated lunate and scaphoid fossae. There was a 75° rotation of the lunate fossa. The distal radius was broken into at least five fragments and comminution extended into the shaft. The distal radio-ulnar joint was disrupted. The scapholunate space was well visualized but not widened, although it was presumed to be injured. Median nerve function was surprisingly entirely intact, despite the energy of the injury.

Closed reduction relieved most of the soft tissue distortion and allowed a further evaluation of the fracture fragments (Fig. 17.3). The distal radius fracture

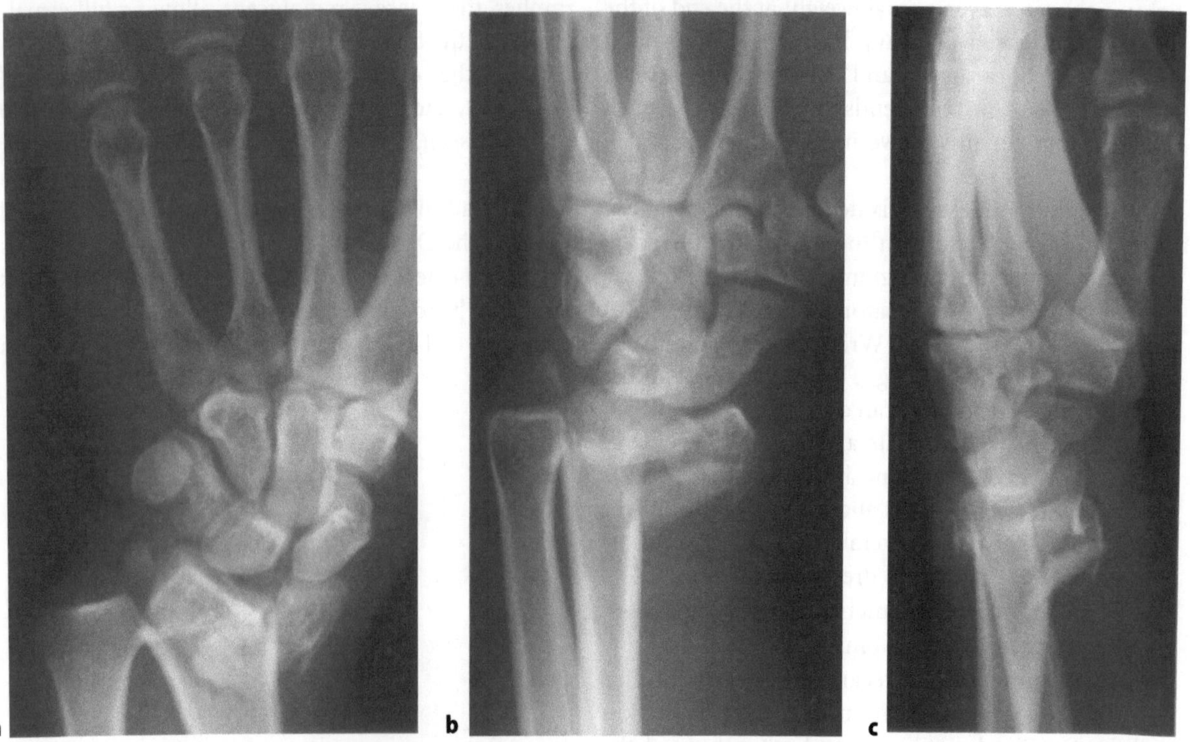

a b c

Fig. 17.2 Case 1: **a** PA view showing severe intra-articular displacement of scaphoid and lunate fossae (lunate die-punch fracture) and disruption of the distal radioulnar joint. **b** Oblique view showing the degree of comminution. Note that the oblique view documents this better than the PA. **c** Lateral view showing a large volar cortical fragment, and many small dorsal fragments. Both the volar and dorsal surfaces are therefore unstable, even if the fracture could be perfectly reduced.

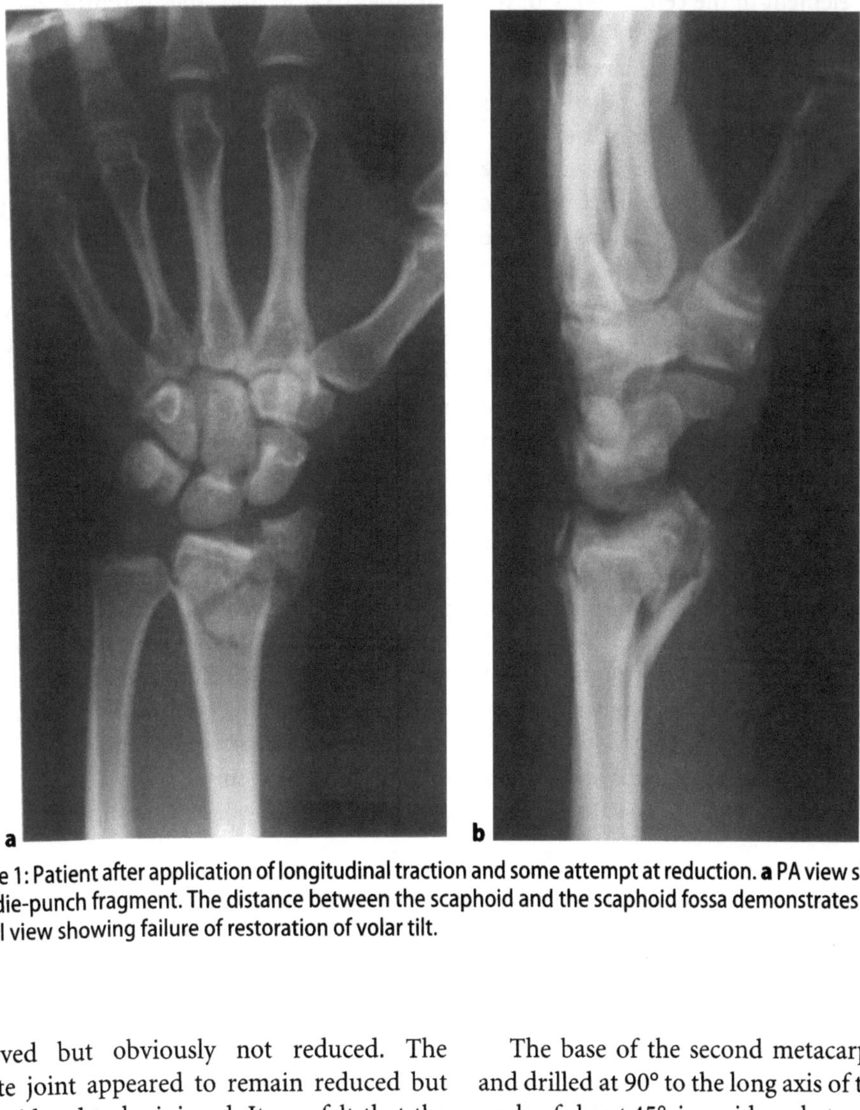

Fig. 17.3 Case 1: Patient after application of longitudinal traction and some attempt at reduction. **a** PA view showing irreducibility of the lunate die-punch fragment. The distance between the scaphoid and the scaphoid fossa demonstrates that this is a traction view. **b** Lateral view showing failure of restoration of volar tilt.

was improved but obviously not reduced. The scapholunate joint appeared to remain reduced but was still considered to be injured. It was felt that the fracture was both irreducible and unstable, and an operative procedure was undertaken two days following injury.

The proximal metacarpal pin was placed first, since it is the only pin which has a uniquely identified site. This pin and the distal metacarpal pin were introduced through an incision some 3cm long along the radial border of the base of the second metacarpal. Percutaneous pin placement carries the risk of nerve or tendon injury, eccentric pin placement or open section defect.[1] Separate stab incisions do not allow optimal visualization of the plane of dissection and do not heal any more quickly than a single incision. Care was taken in making the incision to look for cutaneous branches of the superficial radial sensory nerve. The plane of dissection was between the first dorsal interosseous muscle and the extensor mechanism of the index finger.

The base of the second metacarpal was identified and drilled at 90° to the long axis of the bone and at an angle of about 45°, i.e. midway between the frontal and sagittal planes. An examination of the X-ray indicated that even in this 190cm (6' 3") large-boned male, a thread length of only 15mm was needed. The correct size of pin was selected and inserted. The drill/pin guide was used in drilling and inserting the second metacarpal pin, to ensure that these pins would be parallel and precisely 14mm apart (the spacing in the fixator pin clamps). A mini-C arm was used to verify pin penetration of the opposite cortex, without excess over-penetration.

The distal radial pins were placed next. The RadioLucent fixator was brought into the field. It was used to verify that the pins would not be placed out of the range of extension–compression of the fixator body. The orientation of the fixator was also determined to ensure that the central body locking nut would not overlie the fracture site on the X-ray (it is the only radio-opaque element of the central body of the device).

A 3cm incision was made, with the plane of dissection passing between the extensor carpi radialis longus and extensor carpi radialis brevis, a technique originally propounded by Hill Hastings. The classical plane of dissection, between the brachioradialis and the extensor carpi radialis longus, allows the pins to come into contact with the superficial branch of the radial sensory nerve. In an unpublished study in this laboratory, conducted by the author's associate, Dr Manjit S. Dhillon, it was shown that pins placed in the brachioradialis–extensor carpi radialis longus plane are generally in direct contact with the nerve. In contrast, pins placed in the extensor carpi radialis longus–extensor carpi radialis brevis plane are separated from the nerve by the extensor carpi radialis longus muscle and tendon at an average distance of 8.4mm. This has the additional benefit of placing the fixator at an angle of about 45° between the frontal and sagittal planes, keeping it out of the way on the lateral X-ray. These pins are introduced in a similar manner to the metacarpal pins.

The fixator was then placed on the pins and the pin clamps tightened. The distractor unit was then placed on the fixator and the fracture distracted. Anterior–posterior compression was also performed, to help reduce the fracture fragments. The mini-C arm was used to verify the radial pin placements and fracture reduction. Articular surface reduction was anatomical, so three 0.045 inch K-wires were placed subchondrally in the frontal plane. Two 0.045 inch K-wires were inserted into the radial styloid, one being directed more proximally than the other, attempting to engage the far cortex. Fluoroscopic views did not reveal any metaphyseal voids despite the degree of initial displacement, so bone grafting was not performed.

A 0.062 inch K-wire was introduced, passing from the radius into the ulna, proximal to the distal radioulnar joint and to the cortical comminution, to stabilize the disrupted distal radioulnar joint. Fluoroscopic views were obtained of the scapholunate joint, which appeared reduced on all views. It was therefore decided not to pin this joint, since it would remain reduced for as long as the fixator was in place, which should be long enough for initial healing.

Permanent films were obtained, which revealed that the articular surface was not as reduced as it appeared from the fluoroscopic views. The

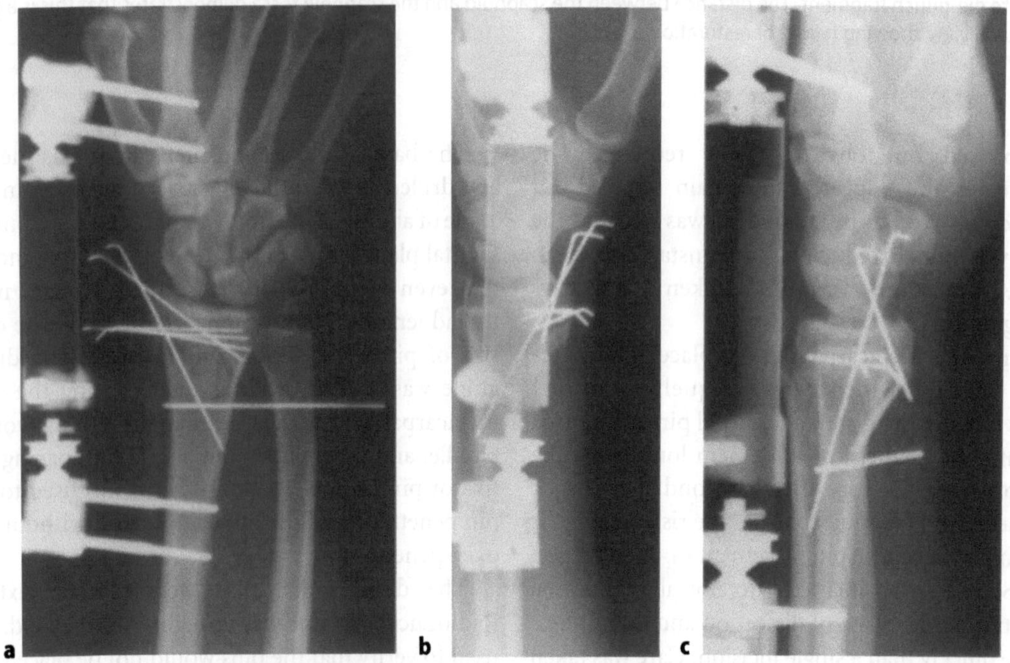

Fig. 17.4 Case 1: Patient after operative reduction, external fixation, and percutaneous pinning. **a** AP view (not a PA view; this is often the easier view to shoot in the OR) shows reduction of articular surface (both the volar and dorsal margins are smooth) stabilized by three horizontal wires and further stabilization of radial styloid fragment by two wires. External fixation alone will not prevent the fragments from subsiding. Note also the stabilization of the distal radio-ulnar joint with a wire that does not pass through the joint cartilage. **b** Oblique view that demonstrates reconstitution of the dorsal and volar cortices. Note the radiolucency of the fixator. **c** Lateral view showing that the lateral angle is about 0°. Note that the dorsal surface is not completely restored, but this is not crucial as long as the fracture is held by an external fixator.

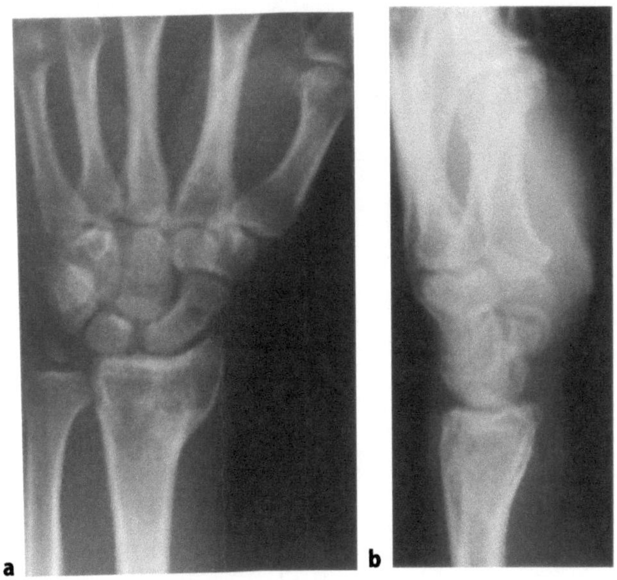

a b

Fig. 17.5 Case 1: Patient at 6½ months after surgery. a PA view showing slight recurrence of the initial deformity (radial tilt of the lunate fossa), despite the subchondral wires. The lower portion of the distal radio-ulnar joint is not perfectly reduced, a fact not shown on earlier X-rays. Since the radiocarpal articular surface is well reduced, an acceptable result overall. b Lateral view showing slight DISI, more than that seen on earlier films.

subchondral wires were removed, a 0.062 inch joystick was introduced into the lunate facet, and the fragment reduced (Fig. 17.4). The K-wires were replaced and permanent films documented the reduction. The incisions were closed with 5–0 nylon.

The patient was started on finger, elbow, and shoulder range of motion exercises. The low profile of the fixator allowed him to slide his arm easily through the sleeves of his clothing.

Fixator and K-wires were removed at six weeks and gentle wrist range of motion exercises commenced. After 3 months, strengthening exercises were begun. The patient returned to light handyman work at 3 months, and his range of motion at 6½ months was flexion: 75°:90° (involved wrist:uninvolved wrist), extension 64°:90°, pronation 80°:80°, and supination 80°:80°. His grip strength was 95:145 lbs. He had no pain on the activities of work or recreation and took no medication for pain relief. His X-ray at 6½ months (Fig. 17.5) showed some minor subsidence of the radial styloid and scaphoid fossa fragment and some minor DISI (Dorsal Intercalated Segmental Instability), but good overall alignment with preservation of

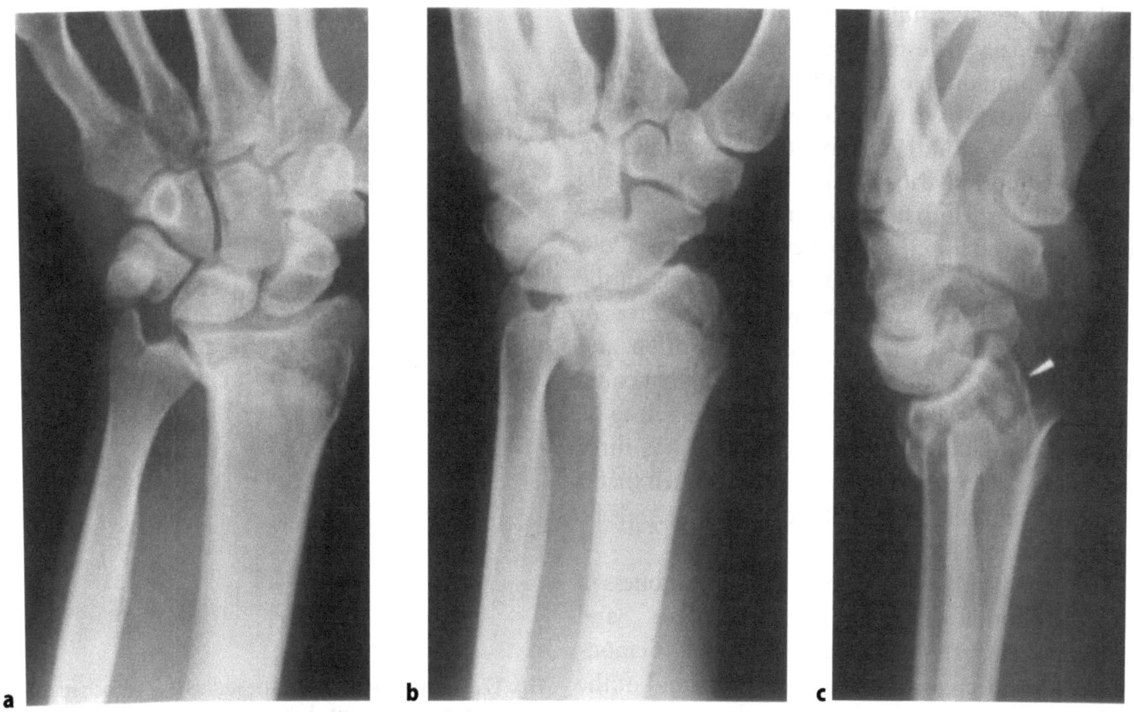

a b c

Fig. 17.6 Case 2: a PA view showing transverse line of the distal radial fracture. The distance between the volar and dorsal margins indicates that the fracture is severely tilted, either in a volar or dorsal direction. Note the variant in the anatomy of the distal radio-ulnar joint. This was symmetrical with the opposite side (not shown). b Oblique view showing intra-articular extensions into the volar and dorsal rims. c Lateral view showing the severe dorsal tilt and dorsal comminution. Note that the intra-articular extensions are not seen. The oblique view is very useful for documenting the intra-articular extension. The volar cortex also has an interposed cortical fragment (fracture line shown by arrow), although it is not displaced.

the joint spaces and good alignment of the distal radio-ulnar joint.

Case 2

A 40-year-old, right hand dominant, white, male, self-employed machinist fell from a ladder at home and injured his left wrist. X-rays in the emergency room showed a complex distal radius fracture, and he was referred for treatment. He did not present until three weeks after the injury. X-rays (Fig. 17.6) were interpreted as showing a distal radius fracture, with a dorsal tilt of 50° and at least two dorsal cortical fragments that were displaced, as well as one volar cortical fragment. There was intra-articular extension of the fracture into the scaphoid fossa of the distal radius. The distal radio-ulnar joint, the ulnar styloid, and the ulnar margin of the proximal lunate demonstrated some longstanding changes suggestive of prior injury and osteoarthritis, although the patient did not recall any symptoms.

The degree of dorsal tilt that implies instability is debated, but there is a general consensus that it is unstable if it is >20°. The dorsal tilt of 50° in this patient implied a significant compaction of the cortical and cancellous bone dorsal to the midplane of the radius. Without a stable dorsal buttress, such a fracture would collapse over time, even if it were successfully reduced initially. The fracture is also unstable when there is comminution of the cortex. In this case, there were fragments broken out of both the volar and dorsal cortices, which would mean that the cortex could not sustain a compressive load even if it were anatomically reduced. It was felt that this fracture should be externally fixed. In addition, due to the degree of dorsal tilt, it was felt that it would require bone grafting. In the author's experience, fractures with this degree of dorsal tilt subside even with external fixation and grafting, so that additional internal fixation that could resist a longitudinally compressive load was felt to be indicated. In addition, since this fracture was three weeks old at the time of presentation, it was felt that it would be unlikely that full correction could be achieved by closed means.

The patient also complained of minor numbness in the distribution of the median nerve, and Semmes–Weinstein monofilament testing demonstrated some decrease in the sensory threshold of the median nerve. It is important to document any median neuropathy prior to surgery, and to document it in a quantitative fashion. Two-point discrimination (sensory density) is not as accurate for this as Semmes–Weinstein monofilament testing (sensory

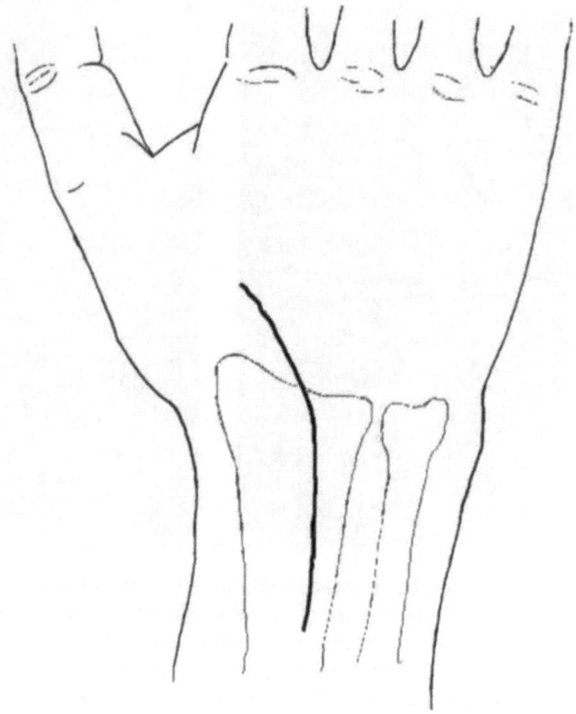

Fig. 17.7 The incision of Ruby, in line with the EPL tendon. This centres the incision directly over the deep dissection.

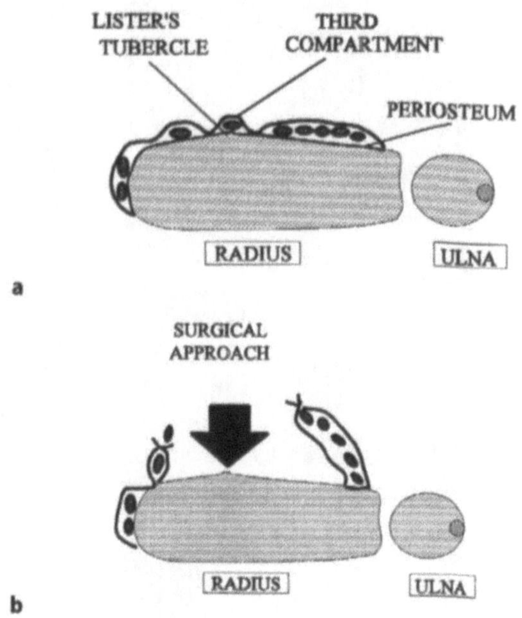

Fig. 17.8 Deep dissection. **a** The radius is approached through the third compartment. **b** If care is taken to stay out of the second and fourth compartments and subperiosteal dissection is maintained, none of the second or fourth compartment tendons will come in contact with either the plate or bony spicules. The EPL is transposed superficial to the extensor retinaculum.

threshold). Non-quantified sensory testing is of very limited usefulness.

The patient was taken to the operating room within a week of presentation. A median nerve decompression at the carpal tunnel was performed initially, due to the pre-operative diagnosis of a median nerve injury (commonly, but not properly, referred to as carpal tunnel syndrome). The wrist would be expected to swell post-operatively, both as a result of the tourniquet and of the operative trauma. Decompressing the median nerve at this time prevents any further compromise of the already injured nerve, which is more than normally sensitive to ischaemia. Exploration of the floor of the carpal canal and proximally, was carried out to verify that there were no fracture fragments within the canal. Median nerve decompression was performed prior to inflating the tourniquet, so as to preserve all of the tourniquet time for fracture fixation.

A RadioLucent wrist fixator was then mounted as described above. Slight distraction was applied, but the wrist was kept in neutral flexion/extension. A dorsal approach per the method of Ruby[3] was made (Fig. 17.7), with the incision in line with the extensor pollicis longus (EPL) tendon. This centres the incision directly over the deep dissection. The distal limb need not follow the EPL, but can be centred if desired. Loupe magnification is useful in watching out for radial sensory nerve branches that may cross the incision.

The radius was approached through the third dorsal compartment (Fig. 17.8) and via subperiosteal dissection of the distal radius. Care was taken to avoid entering either the second or fourth compartments, in order to keep the tendons contained within their compartments. The floor of the compartments (the periosteum) protects the tendons from any hardware that might be inserted, or bone that might protrude from the fracture or bone graft, while the sides of the compartments keep the tendons contained within them. Some authors recommend approaching the distal radius between the second and third, or the third and fourth compartments.[2] It is very difficult, if not impossible, to properly repair the margin of the compartments or maintain proper compartment volume during incision closure. Even with the best of closures the tendons tend to slide out of their compartments and come into direct contact with plate or bone. It is easier never to enter them in the first place than to attempt to repair them later.

After the distal radius had been well visualized by a subperiosteal dissection and the callus removed, the external fixator was used to overdistract the fracture and hold the wrist in about 40° of flexion. The RadioLucent is well suited for this, since its special design allows a full 60° angulation between the two sets of pins. This allowed excellent visualization of the distal radial articular surface, which was approached through a very small (4mm) oblique incision in the dorsal capsule, in line with the orientation of the dorsal ligaments. This does not weaken the joint capsule or interfere with post-operative mobilization.

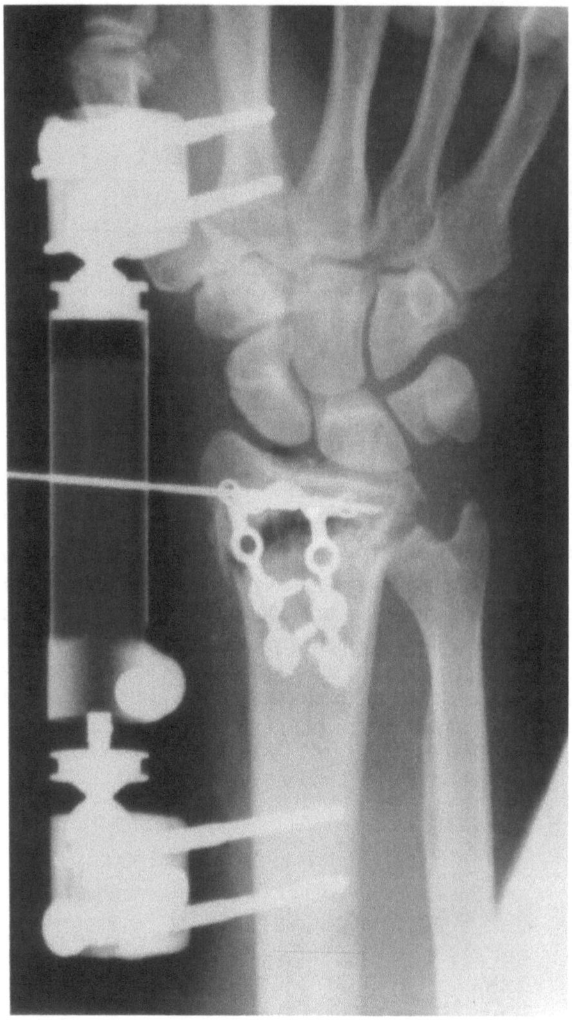

Fig. 17.9 Case 2: Intra-operative X-ray after operative reduction, plate fixation, percutaneous pinning, and external fixation, but before bone grafting. AP view showing reduction of the fracture. Note the volar and dorsal rims are now in proper apposition. The distal radio-ulnar joint was not anatomically reduced, which would have been desirable. Note the void in the metaphyseal bone. The lateral X-ray could not, unfortunately, be located. Restoration of the lateral angle can be inferred from the location of the volar and dorsal rims.

A small arthroscopy probe, appropriate for the wrist, was introduced through the arthrotomy and the intra-articular component reduced. Two 0.035 inch K-wires were then introduced in the coronal plane from the radial side. This both stabilized the fracture for the

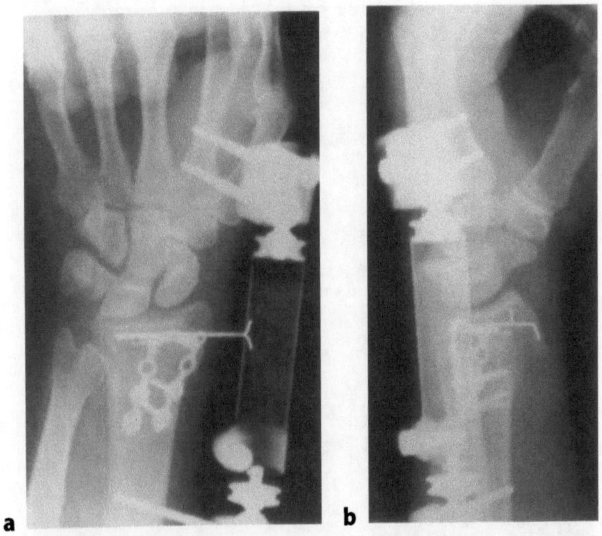

Fig. 17.10 Case 2: Three weeks after surgery. **a** PA view showing a slight change in the relationship between the volar and dorsal rims, implying some subsidence of the lateral angle. Note the filling in of the metaphyseal void noted in Fig. 17.9. **b** Lateral view showing the slight loss of lateral angle. Note how the radiolucency of the fixator aids in the evaluation of the fracture alignment.

future and allowed manipulation of the distal fragments intra-operatively without the danger of displacing this component. Two 0.045 inch K-wires were then inserted in the sagittal plane into the largest of the distal fragments, and used as joysticks to reduce the dorsal angulation following the removal of the callus from between the fracture fragments. Care was exercised when using the joysticks to keep the force on the distal fragments uniform, as the coronal K-wires cannot tolerate very much shear force.

Once reduced, a low-profile plate was placed on the dorsal radius and the joysticks removed. The wrist joint probe was used to palpate the distal articular surface and verify the congruity of the reduction. The wrist was then put into approximately 10° of extension. The range of motion of the fingers was then checked, to verify that full flexion was possible – if it is not, the wrist may be in excessive flexion. Intra-operative radiographs were also taken, to document the reduction of the distal radius, to check the position of the hardware, and to examine carpal alignment and spacing (Fig. 17.9). Note the void in the metaphyseal region. Iliac crest bone graft was tamped into place with a tamp. The final part of the procedure was to verify that the distal radio-ulnar joint was stable.

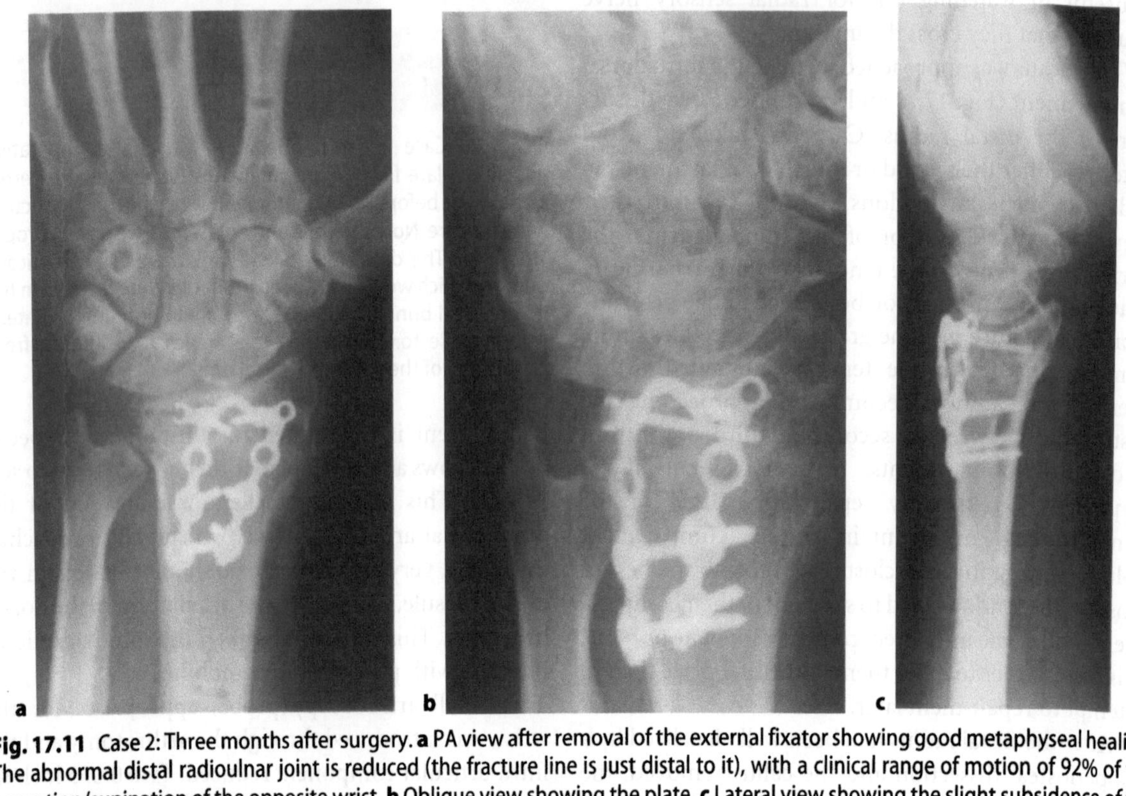

Fig. 17.11 Case 2: Three months after surgery. **a** PA view after removal of the external fixator showing good metaphyseal healing. The abnormal distal radioulnar joint is reduced (the fracture line is just distal to it), with a clinical range of motion of 92% of the pronation/supination of the opposite wrist. **b** Oblique view showing the plate. **c** Lateral view showing the slight subsidence of the dorsal cortex.

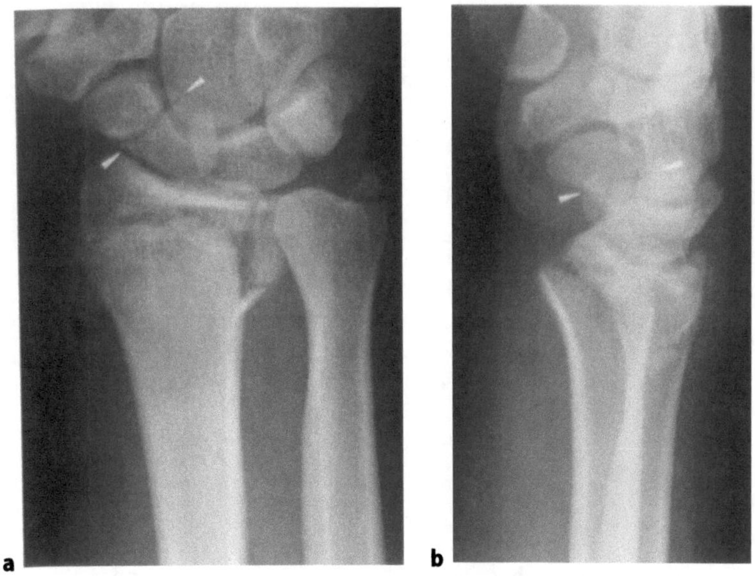

Fig. 17.12 Case 3: Patient at the time of injury.

Closure commenced with repair of the wrist capsule. In this case the arthrotomy was so small and in line with the fibres of the dorsal ligaments, that it did not need repair. The dorsal periosteum was then repaired as well as could be. It is usually found to be so damaged by the injury that the repair is much less than satisfying. The importance of an approach through the third compartment, rather than around it, becomes apparent. The extensor pollicis tendon was left out of its compartment during closure and transposed to a position superficial to the extensor retinaculum, to help avoid rupture. The skin was closed with 5-0 nylon interrupted sutures. A bulky dressing and splint were applied.

The splint was discontinued at one week and finger range of motion exercises begun. There was some slight subsidence evident on the lateral X-ray at three weeks post-surgery (Fig. 17.10) despite the internal fixation and bone grafting. The external fixator was removed at six weeks and gentle wrist range of motion

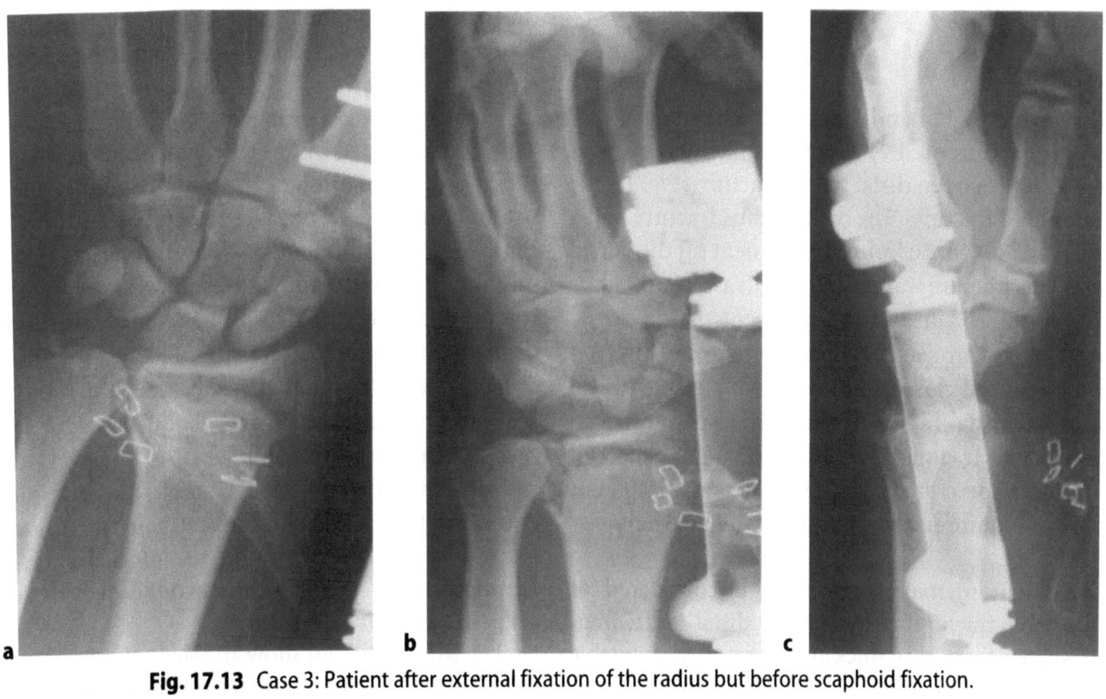

Fig. 17.13 Case 3: Patient after external fixation of the radius but before scaphoid fixation.

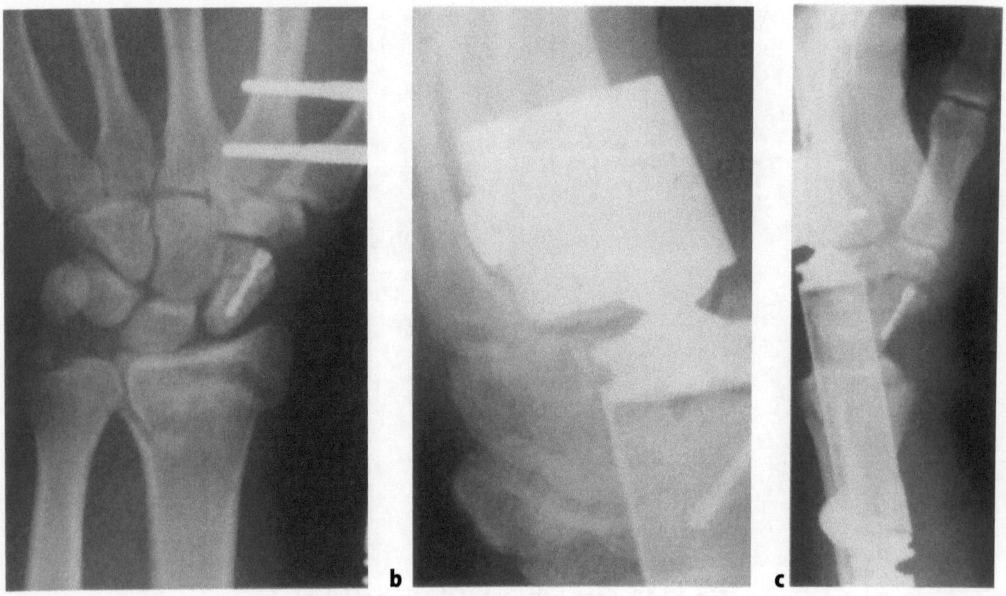

Fig. 17.14 Case 3: Patient after scaphoid fixation with a Herbert screw. **a** PA view showing reduction of the radius and scaphoid. **b** Oblique view with good visualization of the scaphoid alignment despite the overlying fixator. **c** Lateral view showing scapholunate alignment and reduction of the radius.

exercises begun. A follow-up X-ray (Fig. 17.11) at 3 months demonstrated that there was some loss of correction of the dorsal tilt, despite the internal fixation and bone grafting.

The patient returned to work at 3 months, and his range of motion at that time was flexion 50°:85°, extension 50°:90°, pronation 86°:90°, and supination 70°:80°. He had no pain with activities of work or recreation and took no medication for pain.

Case 3

A 30-year-old, right hand dominant, white, male, self-employed labourer fell 20 feet from a ladder. He sustained a Grade I open distal radius fracture (Fig. 17.12) and scaphoid fracture. The distal radius fracture had a dorsal tilt of 20° with a butterfly fragment off the dorsal cortex. This fracture was unstable both as a result of the degree of dorsal tilt and the fragment of the dorsal cortex that had broken out. This fragment can rarely, if ever, be reduced closed to re-establish a stable dorsal cortex. The distal radius in this case also showed an intra-articular fragment involving the ulnar aspect of the radius, as described by Scheck.[4] This last fragment would not require external fixation, if it had been present by itself.

External or internal fixation might be considered for this unstable fracture. However, the distal radial fragment was less than 5mm thick and therefore not suitable for internal fixation. External fixation was chosen as the best option. Additional considerations were the fact that it was an open fracture and that there was a transverse midwaist scaphoid fracture with a radial butterfly fragment. The open fracture itself would suggest that internal fixation should be avoided if external fixation could easily be accomplished. The scaphoid fracture would require internal fixation if an external fixator was applied, or the distraction would prevent the scaphoid from healing. Use of a radiolucent fixator would allow visualization of the scaphoid and carpal alignment during the early healing process.

The patient was taken to the operating room the day of presentation. The stellate open wound was debrided, leaving a skin defect of about 1 × 1cm. This was extended by about 1.5cm on each side, in a radial and ulnar direction, to allow good access to the fracture site. Some dirt and other material was removed from the wound. The fracture was thoroughly irrigated and externally fixed with a RadioLucent fixator. Despite standard positioning of the fixator out of direct lateral plane as described above, it was found to overlie the radius and the scaphoid on the lateral X-ray (Fig. 17.13). Due to the radiolucent properties of the fixator, however, restoration of the distal articular surface of the radius could still be verified and the scaphoid fracture visualized. It was decided not to internally fix the scaphoid until after the third wound debridement, on post-operative day four.

The wound did not show any signs of infection, and the scaphoid was internally fixed with a Herbert screw

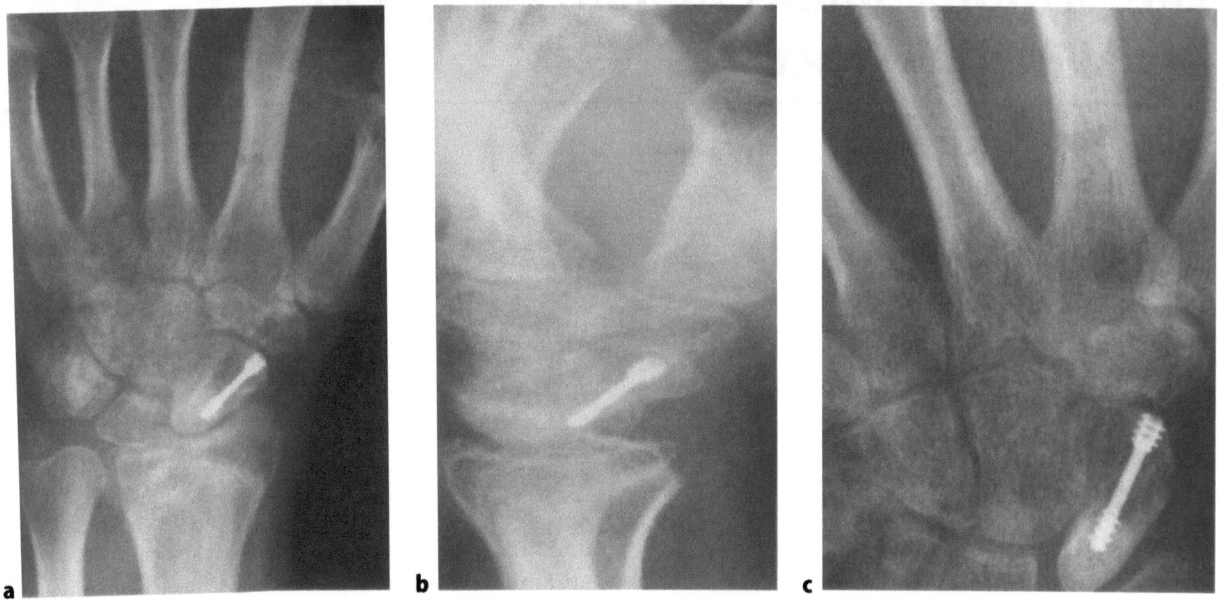

a b c

Fig. 17.15 Case 3: Patient at four months. **a** PA view showing slow healing of the open fracture of the radius and union of the scaphoid, with slight sclerosis of the proximal pole. **b** Lateral view showing good reduction of the radius. **c** Scaphoid view showing union of the scaphoid. The scapholunate interval appears slightly wide. Patient was asymptomatic.

(Fig. 17.14). At the time of the repair, an examination by probe palpation of the distal radial articular surface confirmed that the articular surface was anatomically reduced. If this had not been the case, it could have been reduced at this time and pinned with a subchondral K-wire. The skin was closed primarily.

The wounds healed uneventfully, and the external fixator was removed at six weeks. The patient was placed in a fibreglass thumb-spica to support the scaphoid fracture and started on gentle flexion–extension and pronation–supination exercises. The splint was removed at ten weeks post-injury, but vigorous activities and strengthening exercises were not initiated until three months post injury.

The patient's range of motion at four months was: flexion 45°:75°, extension 50°:80°, pronation 75°:80°, and supination 70°:80° (Fig. 17.15). He had no pain on the activities of daily living and some minor pain on heavy activity. The scapholunate joint, although minimally widened on X-ray, was asymptomatic. He was just returning to work as a self-employed landscape designer.

Discussion

The RadioLucent wrist fixator is the first of a new generation of ergonomically-designed, low-profile, lightweight external fixators. As its name implies, it is radiolucent, allowing full visualization of the fracture site, distal radial articular surface inclination, intercarpal angles, and any carpal fractures.

There have been excellent early results from its use, proving it to be a versatile tool in the treatment of a variety of distal radius fractures, but because it is so new there are as yet no long-term results or large series. Its flexibility intra-operatively is matched by its rigidity post-operatively. The radiolucency of the body is a definite advantage when evaluating fracture reduction and intercarpal alignment. Patients have been very appreciative of the low profile of the fixator, as it has allowed them to dress with ease.

References

1. Seitz WH, Putnam MD, and Dick HM: 'Limited Open Surgical Approach for External Fixation of Distal Radius Fractures.' *J Hand Surg*, 1990; 15A:288–93.
2. Fernandez DL and Jupiter JB: *Fractures of the Distal Radius*. Springer-Verlag:New York, 1966.
3. Weil C and Ruby LK: 'The Dorsal Approach to the Wrist Revisited.' *J Hand Surg*, 1986; 11A: 911–12.
4. Scheck, M: 'Long-Term Follow-up of Treatment of Comminuted Fractures of the Distal End of the Radius by Transfixation with Krischner Wires and Cast.' *J Bone Joint Surg* [Am] 1962; 44-A: 337–51.

The Orthofix Small (30.000) Fixator in Distal Radius Fractures

18

D.L. Nelson

Introduction

The Model 30.000 External Fixator (Fig. 18.1) was the original distal radius fixator designed by Professor De Bastiani. The unilateral design was a significant improvement over the designs of Hoffman (1936) in Europe, and Parkhill (1894) and Anderson (1934) in the United States. This chapter describes its use in a head-injured patient, in whom the use of more modern fixators would have probably resulted in breakage of the fixator.

Materials and Methods

Case History

A 34-year-old, right hand dominant, white male labourer took certain unidentified drugs and drove his motorcycle at high speed into a brick wall. He sustained a closed head injury, pelvic fracture, and comminuted distal radius fracture (Fig. 18.2). He was taken to the operating room after clearance for his head injury, where teams worked simultaneously on his pelvic fracture and his distal radius fracture. A 30.000 external fixator was chosen in view of its strength and robustness. It was anticipated that the patient, due to his lifestyle and his head injury, would tax any fixator to the limit.

The 30.000 fixator was applied first, according to standard techniques, with distal screws in the second metacarpal and proximal screws in the radial shaft. The fracture was then opened. Despite the unloading of the fracture by the fixator, reduction was quite difficult. The number of fracture fragments and their gross instability required the use of multiple wires for provisional fixation. After the distal radius had been reduced, externally fixed, and pinned, the stability of the distal radio-ulnar joint was examined. As expected, it was quite unstable, and a 0.062 inch K-wire was placed across the distal

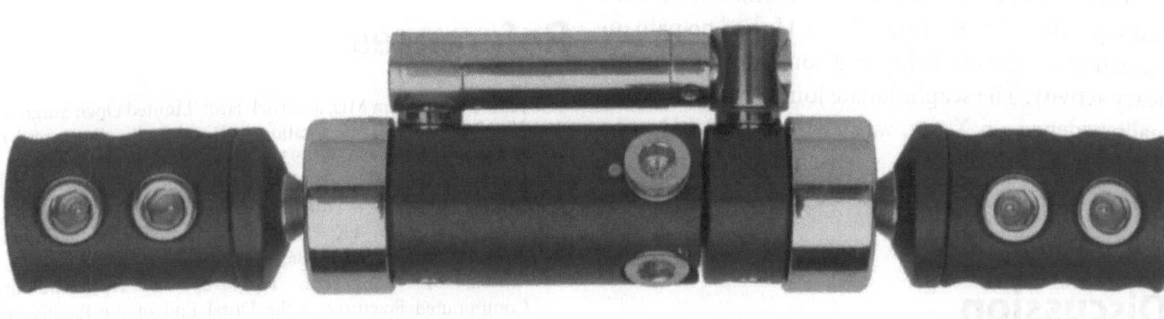

Fig. 18.1 The Model 30.000 external fixator.

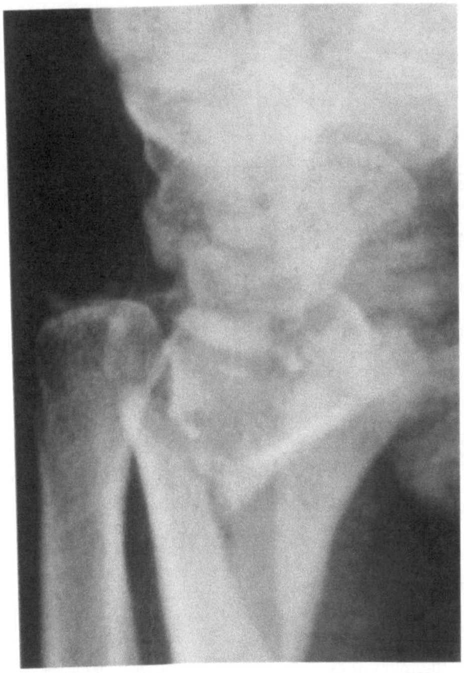

Fig. 18.2 X-ray at time of admission. This lateral view is the only one available, but it documents the comminuted nature of the distal radial articular surface and metaphyseal bone, the proximal extent of the fracture, and the dorsal dislocation of the ulna.

radi-oulnar joint (Fig. 18.3a). A close-up view showed that the radial styloid fragment had a residual rotatory malalignment (Fig. 18.3b).

The patient's mental status post-operatively slowly improved from lethargic and minimally responsive to arousable and uncooperative. He was intermittently combative and would use his injured hand to strike the nurses and the hand therapist. He frequently fell out of bed and had to be restrained. He was transferred to a head injury rehabilitation centre in the early post-operative period.

The patient re-appeared in the orthopaedic clinic five months after surgery, without an appointment or referral. He had recovered to some extent from his head injury and wanted to know if it was time to remove the external fixator! On examination, the external fixator was still in place, together with the sutures from the initial surgery. X-rays showed a healed fracture. The 0.062 inch K-wire was bent (Fig. 18.4), but the fixator was still in excellent condition; the ball joints had not moved, and the cams and screw-clamps were tight. The fixator was removed without incident. The patient's wrist was quite stiff, but range of motion exercises were begun immediately.

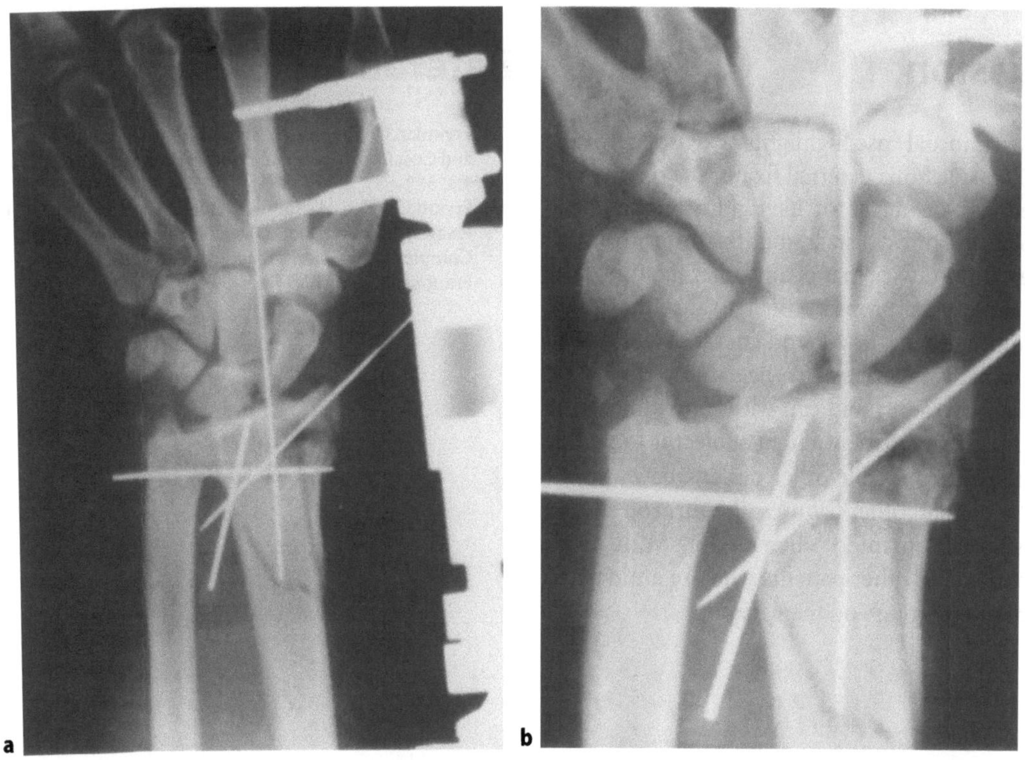

a b

Fig. 18.3 Views following external and internal fixation. **a** PA view showing overall reduction of the fracture. **b** Magnified PA view showing slight rotatory malalignment of the radial styloid fragment but acceptable alignment overall. The K-wire passing axially is securing the proximal radial metaphyseal fragment. It was felt that screw fixation would be difficult to achieve due to the instability of the other fragments, and the rigidity of the fixator allowed provisional fixation with the K-wire alone.

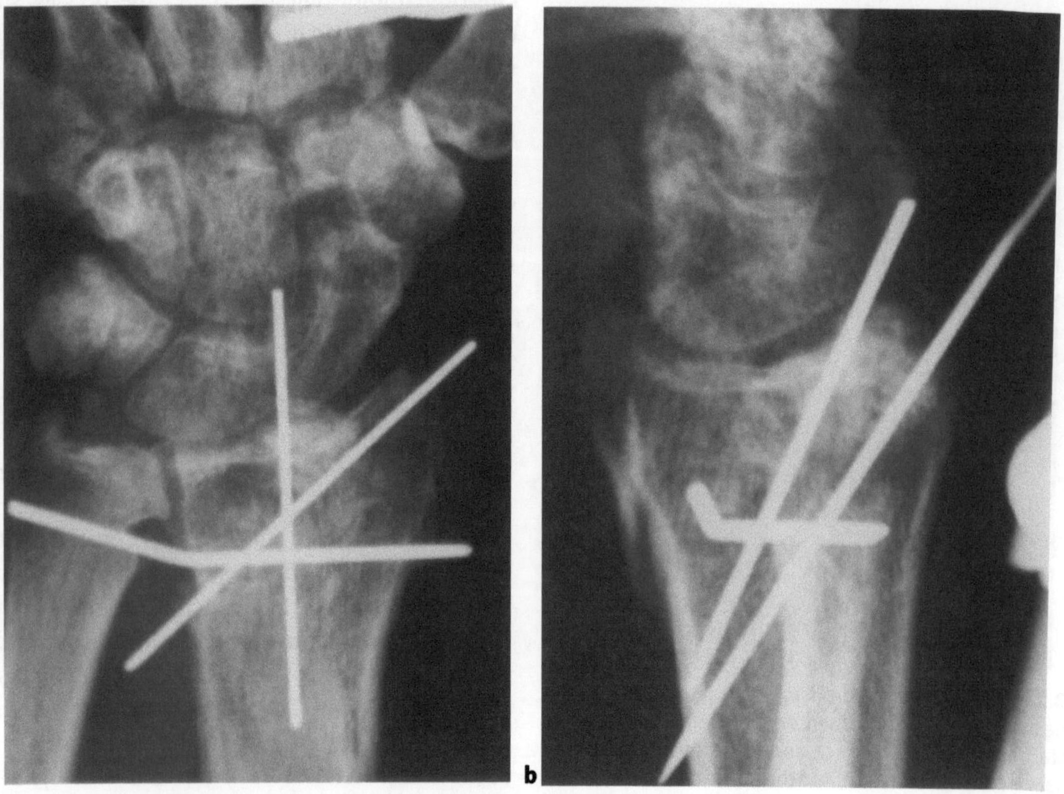

a b

Fig. 18.4 Views at five month post-surgery. a PA view showing the fixator in place (see pin at top) and the bent 0.062 inch K-wire across the distal radio-ulnar joint. b Lateral view showing good alignment.

Discussion

This rather unusual case highlights two aspects of the model 30.000 Orthofix external fixator: its rigidity and its ruggedness. In terms of its rigidity, it has been shown to be the stiffest distal radius fixator, with a stiffness index almost twice that of any other fixator.[1,2] The stiffness index is a property of a fixator that takes account of rigidity in the AP and lateral planes as well as longitudinally. In terms of its ruggedness, the 30.000 is exceptionally robust and can withstand almost any kind of abuse that a patient might subject it to, as this case demonstrated. While other designs have advantages in weight and other features, the surgeon should keep this fixator in mind when dealing with head-injured patients or other patients who are anticipated to be particularly rough on their fixator.

References

1. Frykman GK, and Pettis, JL: 'A Biomechanical, Design Feature, and Cost Comparison of External Fixators.' *Hand Clinics*, 1993; 9:4: 555–65.
2. Frykman GK: 'A Biomechanical Comparison of External Fixators.' in: Nelson, DL, Chairman, Second International Complex Distal Radius Fractures Course, May 12–14, 1994; San Francisco, California.

Metacarpal Fractures, Phalangeal Fractures and Reconstructive Procedures: the Pennig MiniFixator in the Hand

19

D. Pennig and T. Gausepohl

Introduction

Fractures of the hand skeleton are common (Barton 1979;[1] Barton 1984;[2] James 1962).[3] While immobilization for a certain period is necessary, early movement is required to avoid joint stiffness and impairment of tendon gliding. Stable fractures should be mobilized early, whereas unstable fractures may require prolonged stabilization to avoid redislocation or malunion (Swanson 1970[4]; Barton 1979[1]; Buck-Gramcko et al 1986;[5] Bowen et al 1989).[6]

Kirschner wires have enjoyed some popularity in stabilizing fractures of the hand (Edwards et al 1982[7]; Hung et al 1989).[8] With the advent of internal fixation for long bones a miniature version for internal fixation of the hand skeleton was developed (Lister 1978;[9] Heim and Pfeiffer 1982).[10] Both procedures have advantages and disadvantages, with open reduction and internal fixation causing additional soft tissue injury and affecting the gliding tissues (Segmüller 1977;[11] Barton 1979).[1] Periarticular fractures are often difficult to stabilize internally and the implant may have a negative effect on joint capsule ligaments and joint movement.

External fixation has the theoretical advantage of being minimally invasive with the load bearing device being external, but at the same time this is also its disadvantage. Mechanically, external fixation provides adequate stability in the hand (Fitoussi et al 1996).[12] Miniaturized external fixators were described several decades ago, being in the main, small versions of the long bone devices (Asche et al 1979;[13] Asche and Burny 1982).[14] The particular structure of the hand, however, makes the use of a low-profile monolateral device with adapted pin application planes attractive, especially in periarticular fractures (Pennig et al 1995;[15] Pennig et al 1997).[16]

Intra-articular fractures in the hand are particularly difficult to treat because of the joint dimensions and the complex soft tissue envelope. The principle of ligamentotaxis in association with supplementary internal fixation seems to be an alternative to open reduction with internal fixation.

Design of the MiniFixator

The central element of the Pennig MiniFixator is a double ball joint with a single screw locking mechanism embedded in a module 15.5 × 15mm square (Fig. 19.1). The central element connects two threaded bars to constitute (a) short (bars 28.1mm and 18.1mm), (b) standard (both bars 28.1mm) and (c) long (bars 28.1mm and 43.1mm) MiniFixators.

The threaded bars are attached in turn to the clamp modules, of which there are two types: a standard clamp and an L-clamp (Fig. 19.2). The L-clamp is designed to be used when the distance between the bone fixation points is too small to accommodate two standard clamps. Two L-clamps facing one another, as shown in Fig. 19.2b, will permit the insertion of two pairs of wires as little as 6mm apart. In view of this, and because the hexagonal locking screw must always face the surgeon, the L-clamp is available in two models, left (L) and right (R). The standard clamp is normally used for metacarpal or metatarsal bones and the L-clamp for the phalanges.

Compression and distraction are possible using supplementary nuts in association with the threaded bars to move the clamps in the desired direction. The nuts are turned using the 3mm Allen wrench and one full turn of the nut through 360° will compress or distract respectively by one millimetre (Fig. 19.3). The nuts are not generally used in association with fresh fractures.

The clamp modules can each accommodate threaded wires in four different positions. Two wires are sufficient in most circumstances. The wires are specifically designed for use with the MiniFixator to ensure good bone purchase. Standard Kirschner wires are inadequate for the purpose and should not be used. The threaded wires are supplied in two combinations of diameter and length: 2.0mm diameter and 100mm long, or 1.6mm diameter and 70mm long (Fig. 19.4). In both sizes the threaded portion is 15mm long. The wires are trimmed to length following insertion, increasing the versatility of the system and reducing the inventory required.

Before the threaded wires are inserted into the clamp, the dot on the surface of the cam must be aligned with the white dot on the surface of the clamp. This opens up the holes in the clamp, allowing easy passage of the wires. When the wires are inserted into the clamp in a plane along the axis of the bone, they emerge parallel; when they are inserted in a plane at right angles to the diaphyseal axis, they converge (Figs. 19.5a, 19.5b). This is particularly useful when it is necessary to insert wires close to the joint, or into very small fragments. The wires are locked into the clamp by tightening the cam. When wires are inserted into the bone, the clamp will always be stable provided the cam is securely tightened.

Reduction can be carried out with the fixator in situ, using the manipulation forceps; the maintenance of reduction is facilitated by the small number of locking screws, requiring only one size of Allen wrench.

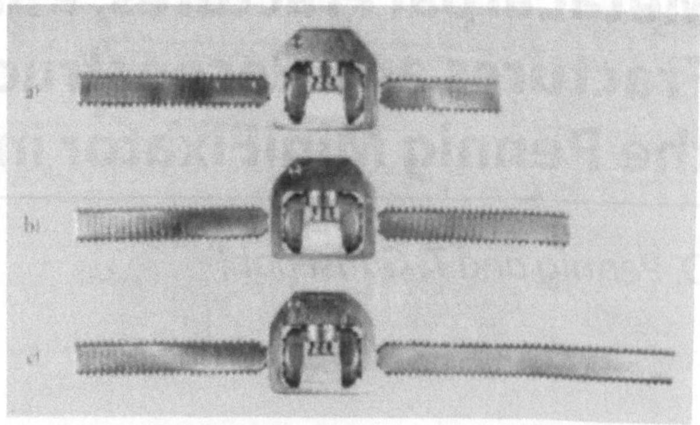

Fig. 19.1 The central element of the Pennig MiniFixator is a double ball joint with a single screw locking mechanism embedded in a module 15.5 × 15mm square. The central element connects two threaded bars to constitute (a) short (bars 28.1mm and 18.1mm), (b) standard (both bars 28.1mm) and (c) long (bars 28.1mm and 43.1mm) MiniFixators.

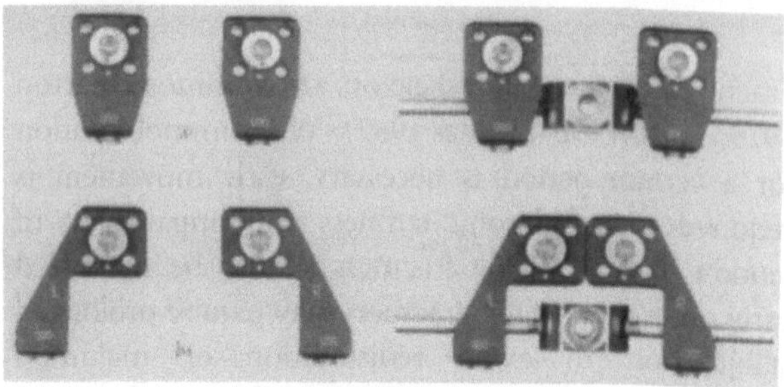

Fig. 19.2 Clamp modules: **a** standard clamp; **b** L-clamp. The L-clamp is designed to be used when the distance between the bone fixation points is too small to accommodate two standard clamps. There is a left and a right L-clamp.

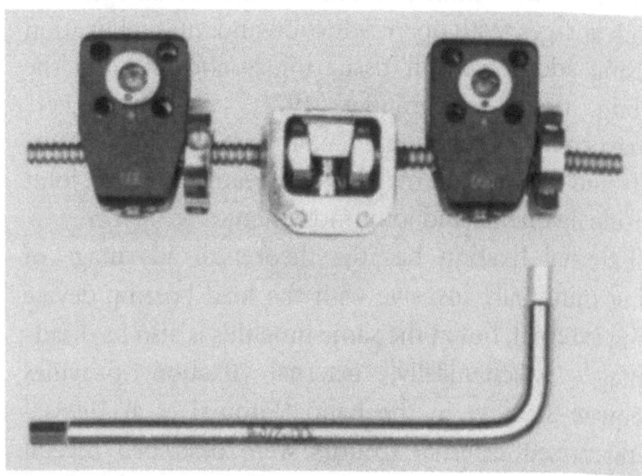

Fig. 19.3 Compression and distraction with the MiniFixator: With the nut outside the clamp compression is performed; with the nut between clamp and ball joint housing distraction is possible.

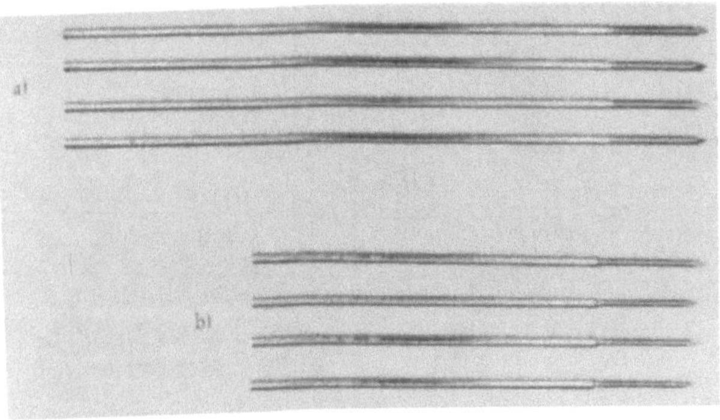

Fig. 19.4 Threaded wires: **a** 2mm thread diameter and 100 mm long ; **b** 1.6mm thread diameter and 70mm long.

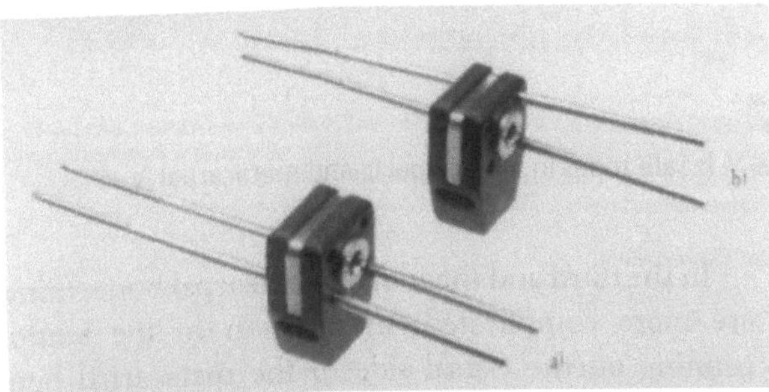

a

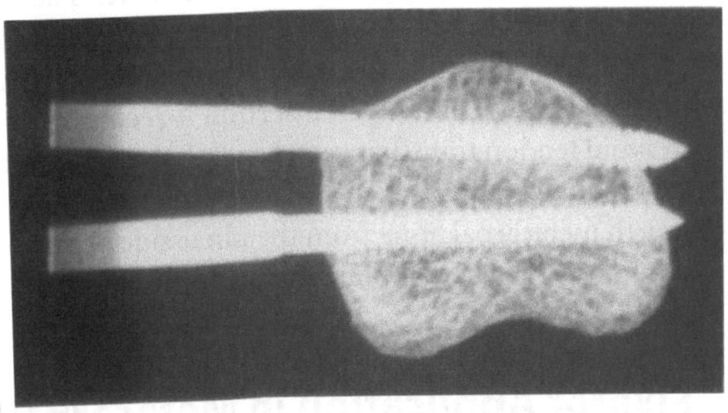

b

Fig. 19.5 **a** The wires emerge parallel when inserted along the axis of the bone (a); wires inserted at right angles to the diaphyseal axis, converge (b). **b** Cross-section of the proximal metaphysis in the proximal phalanx illustrating the convergence of the wires to allow secure fixation of small fragments.

Lengthening and Reconstruction Device

For lengthening or bone transport the ball jointed MiniFixator body is replaced by a lengthening bar. These are supplied in three sizes: (a) short (80mm), (b) standard (100mm) and (c) long (120mm) and are used in association with either standard or L-clamps and 2mm wires, compression–distraction nuts and spacers (See Fig. 19.34). A third wire may be added in each clamp to improve stability especially in osteoporotic bone and in the metatarsals.

Operative Technique

Anatomical Landmarks in Metacarpals

The palm of the hand is not suitable for percutaneous pin placement. On the dorsal side the extensor digitorum tendons from the retinaculum extensorum to the tendon hood partly cover the metacarpal bones. There are considerable variations with increasing frequency from the radial to the ulnar side. The first metacarpal, being part of the thumb, is of extraordinary importance, and is located in its neutral position more to the palmar side. The extensor pollicis longus and the extensor pollicis brevis tendons cover metacarpal I from the dorsal side. Carpo-metacarpal joint I has the radial artery crossing over the area of the trapezoid bone. The superficial branch of the radial nerve crosses in the same area and pin placement in the trapezoid bone requires an open exposure. In the midshaft and distal part of metacarpal I, fixator pins are inserted between the extensor pollicis longus and brevis tendons and this may be done percutaneously.

The second metacarpal bone is covered partly by the extensor tendon. The safe zones are illustrated in Fig. 19.6a and in its distal part the zone is greater than 90° from the dorso-radial side. The angle increases in the middle third and in the proximal third.

When flexing MP joint II because of the connexus intertendinae the tendon is displaced towards the ulnar side and the bone is exposed further. Very distal application in the area of the metacarpal head poses a danger to the extensor tendon hood. Threaded wires inserted proximal to the dorsal tubercle on the metacarpal head have no relevant effects on the MP joint range of motion. With very distal fractures the implant should be inserted dorsally to avoid transfixion of the collateral ligament (Fig. 19.7a). If the fracture is such that more volar placement is required, pin insertion into the metacarpal head should be performed with the MP joint in 90° flexion. The influence on the range of motion of the MP joint is illustrated in Fig. 19.7b. These principles have to be respected in all MP joints.

Most commonly, the fifth metacarpal bone is injured. On its ulnar side there are no tendons to be considered but the dorsal side is nearly completely covered by the extensor tendon of the fifth finger.

Pin insertion is recommended from the ulno-dorsal side and the safe zone is smaller than in metacarpal II ranging from 64° to 69°. There is a considerable variation in the anatomy of this extensor tendon.

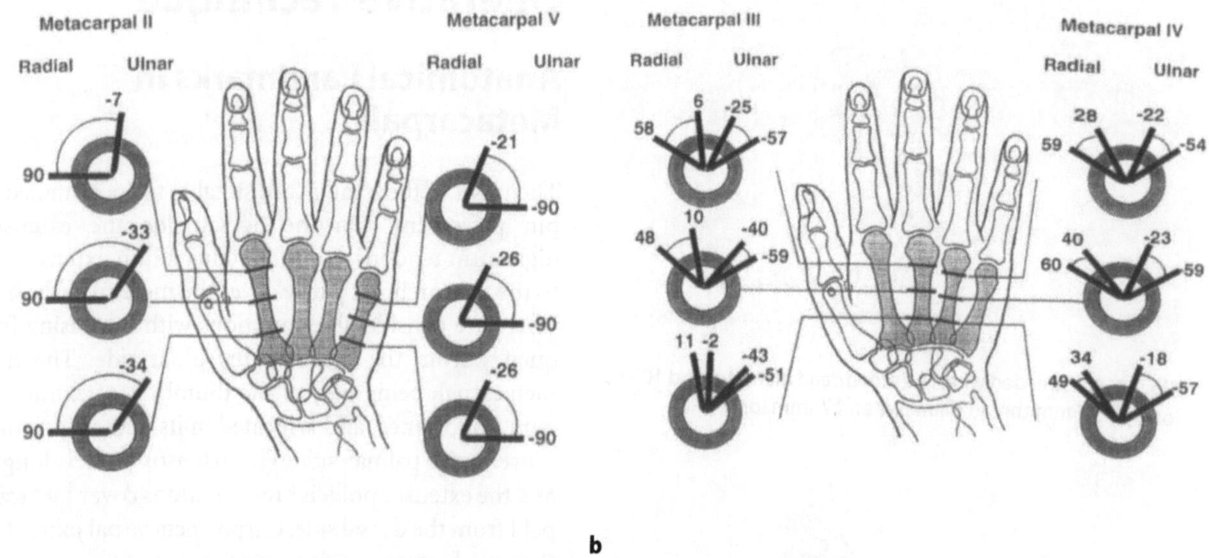

Fig. 19.6 **a** Safe zones in metacarpal II and metacarpal V. **b** Safe zones in metacarpal III and metacarpal IV.

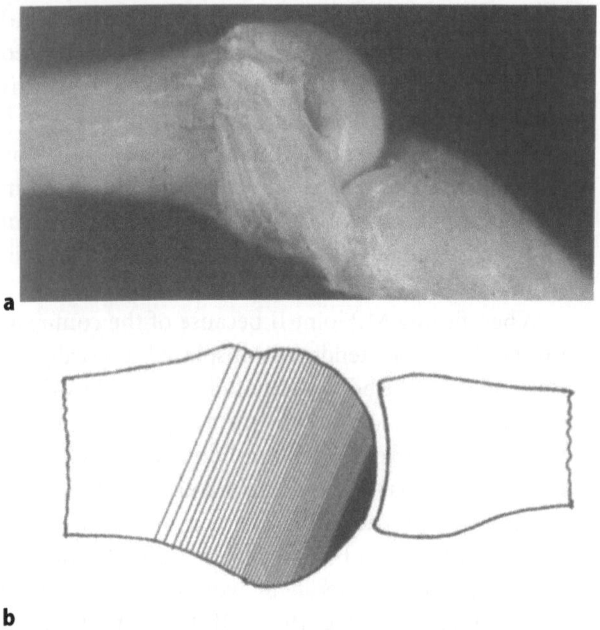

Fig. 19.7 **a** Bone ligament complex of the MP joint in 40° flexion. The collateral ligament on the dorsal side of the metacarpal head crosses over obliquely and inserts at the palmar aspect of the proximal phalanx. **b** Schematic drawing of favourable (lighter) and less favourable (darker) areas of the metacarpal head. A proximal and dorsal insertion is to be recommended from the functional point of view.

In the third and the fourth metacarpal bone, things are more complicated. In addition to the tendon running on the dorsal side of the metacarpal bone there is an adjacent tendon on either side. The safe zone in these bones is much smaller and it becomes exceedingly difficult the more proximal pins are inserted (Fig. 19.6b). Open insertion is recommended to avoid tendon transfixion. In general, the third metacarpal bone is approached from the radial side and the fourth metacarpal bone from the ulnar side. Again, on the fourth metacarpal bone the anatomical variations are significant.

Fixator Application in Metacarpals

Shaft Fractures of the Fifth Metacarpal

For metacarpals the 2mm threaded wires (100/15) are used. A decision must be made, based on the X-rays, as to whether the wires can be inserted in an axial plane or whether they will need to be introduced in a plane transverse to the bone axis. If there is one small fragment, transverse placement of the wires in this fragment is advisable. The minimum distance between a wire and the fracture should not be less than 3mm.

The first wire to be inserted is the one closest to the joint (Fig. 19.8). It is introduced in the frontal plane using power instrumentation and since its thread is not conical it can be backed out if it has been advanced too far. With all applications of the MiniFixator the wires should just penetrate the far cortex protruding no more than one millimetre beyond it to avoid

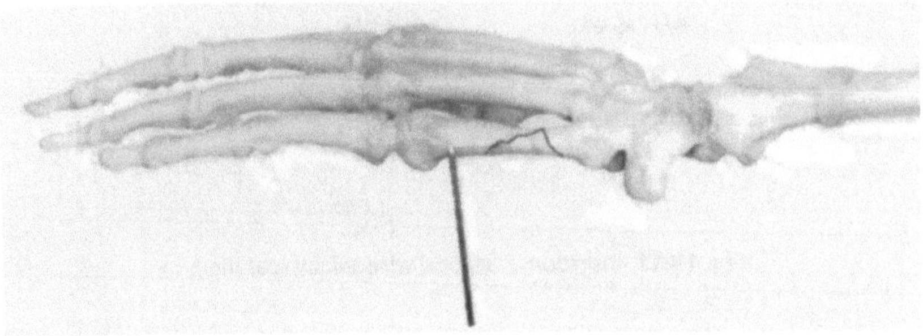

Fig. 19.8 Placement of threaded wires in metacarpal shaft fracture: first wire.

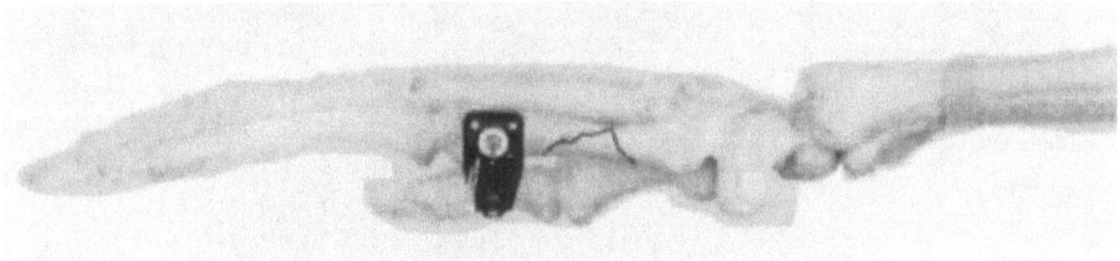

Fig. 19.9 Standard clamp is inserted over the wire.

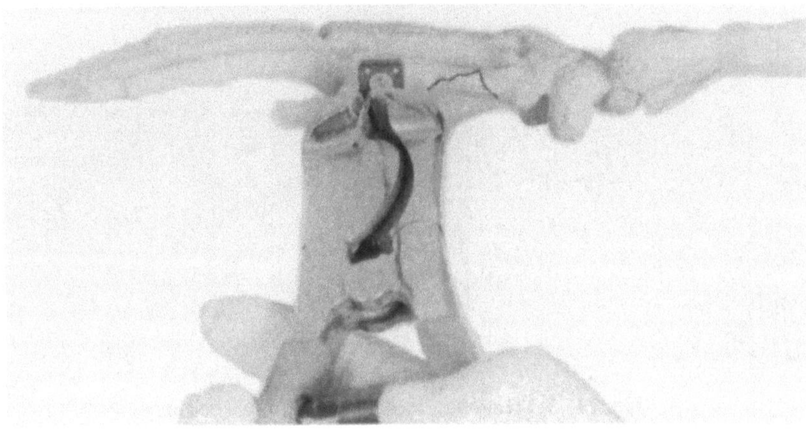

Fig. 19.10 Trimming of first wire.

damage to the adjacent structures. This should be confirmed using image intensification.

A standard clamp is inserted over the wire ensuring that the dot on the surface of the cam is in line with the dot on the clamp surface. The clamp must always be positioned so that the head of the cam faces away from the bone, to allow for subsequent locking of the wires (Fig. 19.9).

As a general rule, the clamp should be positioned about 5–10mm from the skin, to allow for some post-operative swelling. The first wire is then trimmed so that about 5mm project beyond its margin (Fig. 19.10). It should be noted that each wire must be trimmed after insertion, to avoid obstructing the drill during insertion of the next wire.

The second wire is inserted either axially or transversely with respect to the first, according to the length of the fragment (Fig. 19.11). When inserted in a transverse plane the wires converge, so that they can be inserted into very small fragments. The second wire is now inserted under image intensification and trimmed to length.

Depending upon the dimensions of the bone and the site of the fracture, a short, standard or occasionally a long MiniFixator body is selected. One threaded bar is attached to the clamp holding the two wires (Fig. 19.12).

The double ball joint locking cam is then turned clockwise a little so that ball joint movement becomes slightly stiff (Fig. 19.13). The long axis of the fixator can now be aligned with the long axis of the metacarpal which should be reduced clinically. The second clamp is now attached to the other threaded bar.

The second set of wires is now inserted, usually longitudinal to but occasionally at right angles to the diaphyseal axis (Fig. 19.14). When choosing the position for these wires care should be taken to ensure that

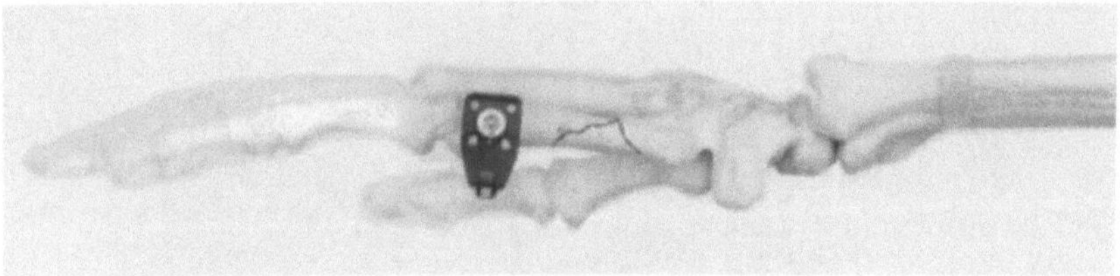

Fig. 19.11 Insertion of second wire axially (parallel).

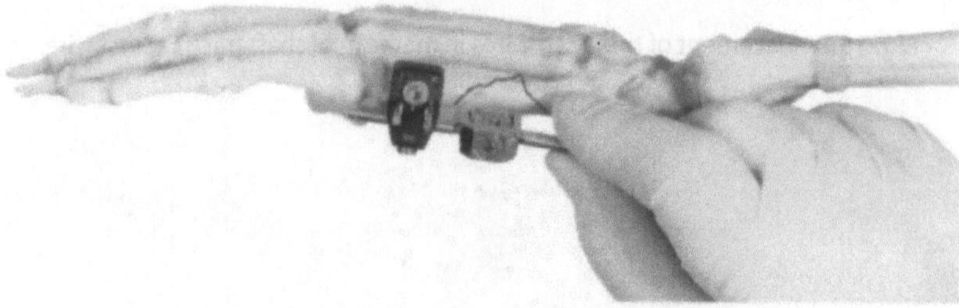

Fig. 19.12 Insertion of a standard MiniFixator body into the clamp.

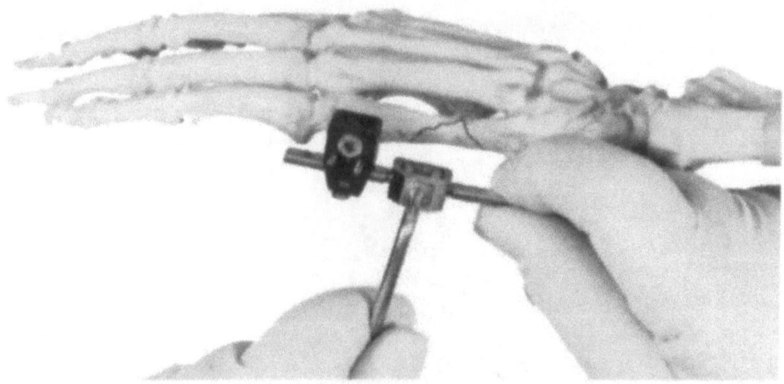

Fig. 19.13 Preliminary locking of the double ball joint.

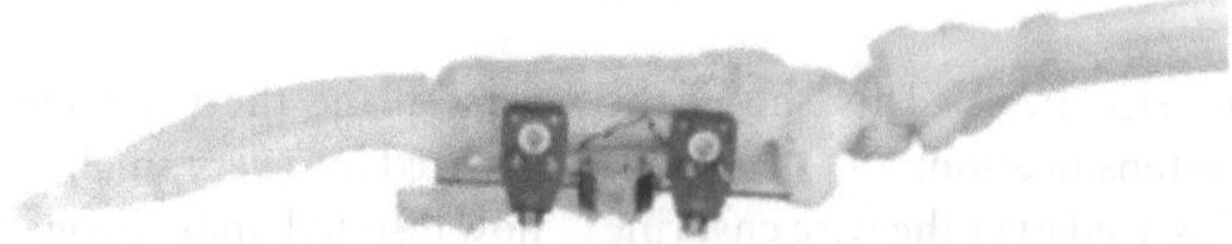

Fig. 19.14 Application of a second clamp and placement of two threaded wires axially.

the clamps have sufficient room on their respective bars to allow for final reduction. This again, is monitored in both planes using the image intensifier.

Once all the wires have been inserted the clamps are locked to them by turning the cam on each firmly (Fig. 19.15). Before final reduction one of the clamps can be locked to its bar with the clamp locking screw, checking that the other clamp has room to move along its bar during the reduction procedure.

With the ball joint fully loosened the fracture is now reduced using traction and counter-traction, taking particular care to avoid any rotational deformities and bearing in mind that in flexion all fingers converge on the topographic location of the scaphoid. The reduction forceps are provided to distance the surgeon's hands from the radiation source. For additional protection, radiation gloves are available and may be worn for this manoeuvre. The forceps grip the clamps to permit manipulation and tightening of the necessary screws after reduction without loss of position.

While the reduction is held (Fig. 19.16) the second clamp is locked to the bar, maintaining the length of the bone. Following this, the double ball joint of the MiniFixator body is locked to control angulation, by turning the cam in the centre of the MiniFixator body clockwise.

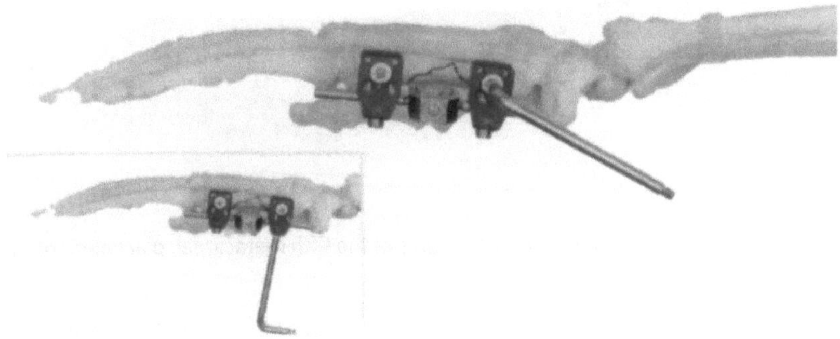

Fig. 19.15 The clamps are locked to the wires by clockwise turns of the cam. Inset: one of the clamps is locked to a threaded bar.

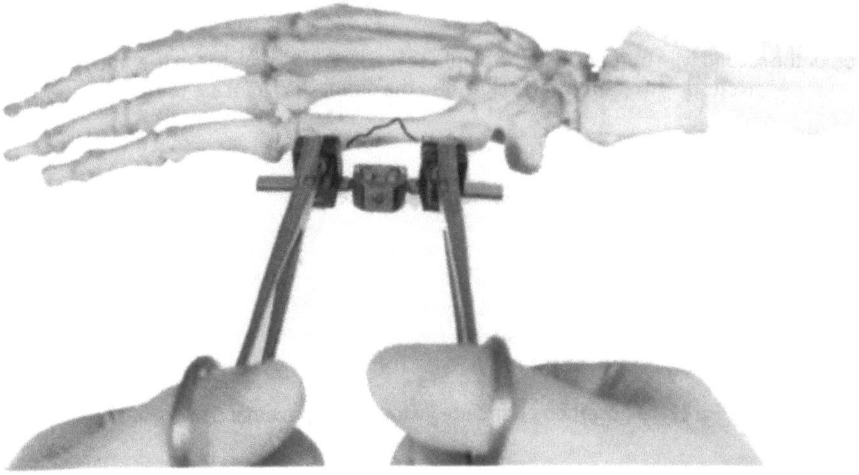

Fig. 19.16 Reduction of the fracture with the assistance of the reduction forceps. The ball joint is completely unlocked and one clamp free to move on the threaded bar.

At the end of the operation a check should be made to ensure that sufficient space has been left between the skin and the fixator (minimum 5mm). The wires are finally trimmed such that 2mm of wire protrudes from each clamp. This helps to prevent the sharp ends of the wires catching in the patient's clothes. A dressing is applied in such a way that the MiniFixator is fully covered. No circumferential dressing is necessary.

The patient is encouraged to move fingers and adjacent joints from the day of operation. It is not possible, however, for the patient to carry out heavy work at this stage.

Subcapital Fractures of the Fifth Metacarpal

The MiniFixator is applied so that in one clamp the wires converge in the small distal fragment. The other clamp is applied in the same manner as described for a shaft fracture of the fifth metacarpal.

The first wire to be inserted is the most volar wire in the distal fragment. This wire is placed in the frontal plane, parallel to the articular surface (Fig. 19.17). If possible, the joint capsule should be avoided. In very distal fractures, however, this may not always be feasible.

The clamp is now slid over the wire and the wire trimmed. The second wire is now inserted in the clamp hole dorsal to the first, so that this pair is in the transverse plane (Fig. 19.18). The second wire will converge with the first as it is being introduced, so that even small fragments can be penetrated by both wires. Convergence of the wires will only occur when the clamp is orientated correctly. If it is mounted back to front, the wires will diverge. Penetration of the wires must be checked in both planes with the image intensifier.

The remainder of the application follows that for shaft fractures of the fifth metacarpal (Fig. 19.19). Rotational deformities very often occur in association with subcapital fractures and particular attention should therefore be paid to ensure correct rotational alignment.

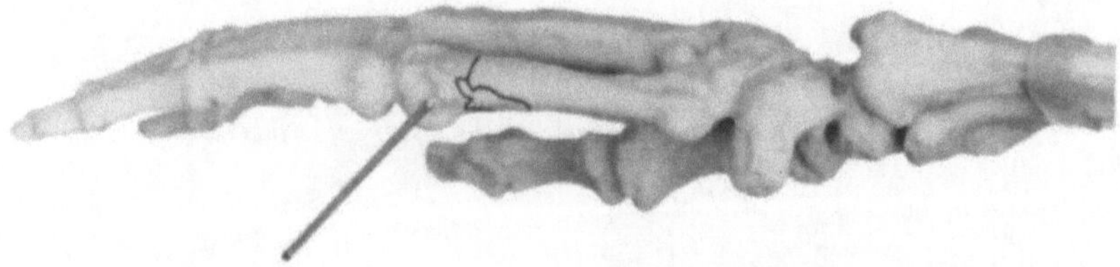

Fig. 19.17 Wire insertion in subcapital fractures of the fifth metacarpal: placement of first wire.

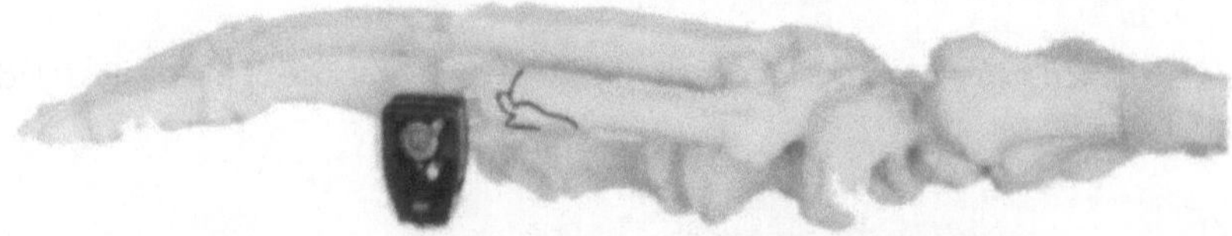

Fig. 19.18 Insertion of the second wire transverse to the diaphyseal axis. Wires converge in the small periarticular fragment. Note: the two clamp holes closest to the double ball joint are used.

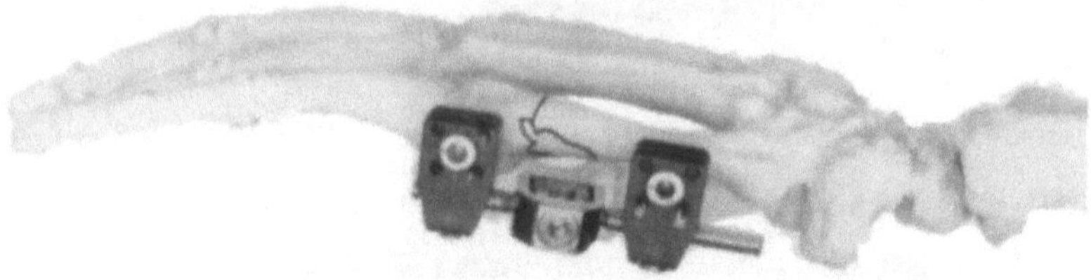

Fig. 19.19 Insertion of threaded wires in the proximal clamp.

Shaft Fractures of the First Metacarpal

Shaft fractures of the first metacarpal are treated in the same way as those of the fifth metacarpal. It is, however, important to avoid transfixion of the extensor pollicis longus and brevis and the abductor pollicis tendons. With open insertion direct visualization of the bone is possible. If a percutaneous insertion is performed the IP joint must move freely at the end of surgery.

With a proximal fracture (Winterstein type) two converging wires are used in the base of metacarpal one. When inserting the threaded wires an open approach is recommended.

Fractures at the Base of the First Metacarpal

A possible indication for use of the MiniFixator is a comminuted fracture of the base of the first metacarpal. In this instance, the fixator is mounted between the trapezium and the shaft of the first metacarpal.

The first wires to be inserted are those in the trapezium. They are introduced in the transverse plane using a semi-open approach in order to avoid injury to the tendons crossing the anatomical snuffbox. Note that in this indication both clamps are applied upside down (Fig. 19.20). The MiniFixator body and the clamp for the shaft of the first metacarpal are attached.

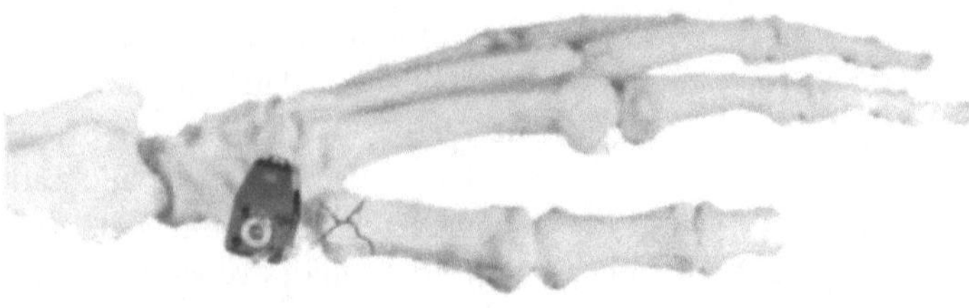

Fig. 19.20 Proximal intra-articular fracture of metacarpal I. Open insertion of two converging wires in the trapezium.

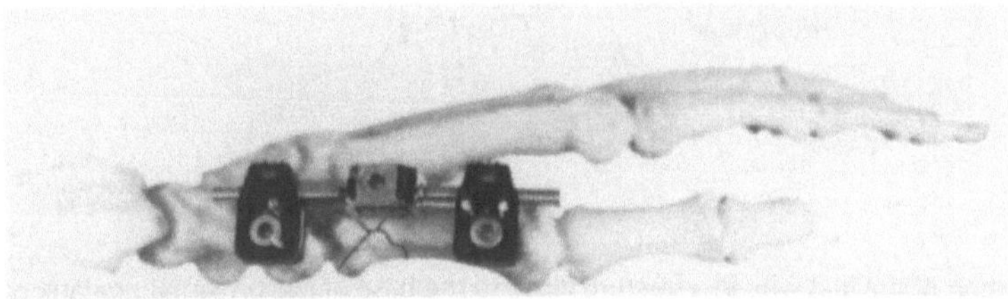

Fig. 19.21 Two parallel wires are inserted into the metacarpal I diaphysis and reduction achieved by ligamentotaxis.

The wires for the diaphysis are inserted in the longitudinal plane (Fig. 19.21) and the deformity corrected by ligamentotaxis. If joint congruence cannot be achieved, open reduction should be carried out and additional internal fixation with screw and/or wires may be necessary.

Fractures of Metacarpals Three and Four

Isolated injuries of metacarpals three and four are uncommon. With fractures involving either metacarpal two or five in association with metacarpal three or four it is best to stabilize metacarpal two or five first. Should this result in adequate reduction of metacarpal three or four, the stability of the reduction should be tested. If stable (which is not uncommon due to the interosseous muscle and the tendon connections), fixation of these metacarpals may not be required. If, however, the fracture is unstable or comminuted, metacarpal three fractures are usually approached from the radial side and metacarpal four fractures from the ulnar side and the fixator is applied as described above. The convergence of the extensor tendons in the proximal part of the metacarpal region usually requires open insertion to avoid tendon transfixion (Fig. 19.6 b).

In all metacarpal applications it is important to insert the wires just into the opposite cortex. Significant penetration of the opposite cortex may result in injury to the neurovascular bundle and the flexor tendons on the volar side. This must be avoided.

Anatomical Landmarks in Phalanges

Only the proximal and middle phalanx have dimensions suitable for external fixation, the distal phalanx is a most unusual indication. The index finger and the fifth finger can be approached from the radial or ulnar sides respectively, without impairing the movement of the adjacent finger. Middle and index fingers are best approached from the dorso-ulnar or dorso-radial sides. Because of the importance of the index finger its movement must not be impaired and in the middle finger a dorso-ulnar application is usually performed. With proximal pin insertion in the proximal phalanx the extensor tendon hood may be transfixed. This does not seem, however, to affect the final range of motion. It is recommended that the threaded wires are inserted with the MP joints in full extension since the extensor hood is displaced volarly in flexion. The volar side of the fingers with the neurovascular bundles is distant from the bone and with the tip of threaded wire sitting in the opposite cortex, injury should not occur.

Fixator Application in Phalanges

Prior to insertion of the first threaded wire reduction of the fracture should be carried out.

The use of the Pennig MiniFixator in the phalanges is somewhat more challenging since the dimensions are so small. At the base of the proximal phalanx 2.0mm threaded wires may be used, but the 1.6mm threaded wires are standard. Wherever possible, bridging of joints should be avoided. If this is inevitable, care should be taken to ensure that overdistraction does not occur, and the joint should be fixed in a functional position.

The L-clamp (Fig. 19.2) was developed to allow fixation of these small bones and it enables the wires to be placed very close to the fracture line in both fragments.

The principles outlined for application to the metacarpal bones are applicable to the phalanges. Wires are placed first in the smaller fragments and a transverse configuration of converging wires is usually necessary. In the proximal phalanx of the index and the little finger, the fixator can be applied in the frontal plane. In the middle and ring fingers, an angle of 45° dorsal to the frontal plane is used. In the distal phalanx, the fracture may be held satisfactorily with only one wire in each fragment. In the other phalanges two wires should be used.

For a fracture close to the base of the proximal phalanx of the index finger, the first threaded wire

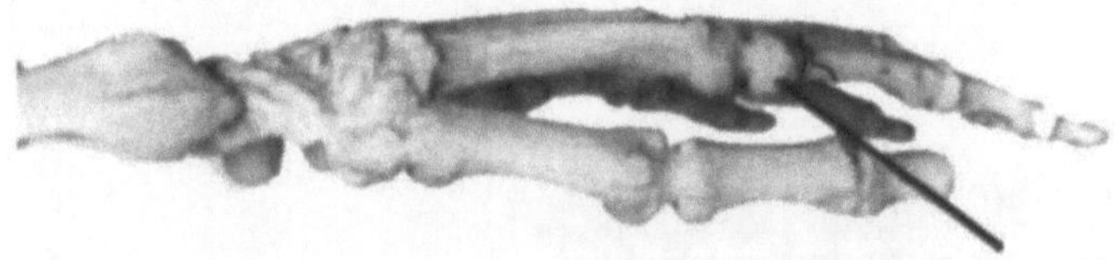

Fig. 19.22 Insertion of the first wire in a fracture close to the base of the proximal phalanx of the index finger.

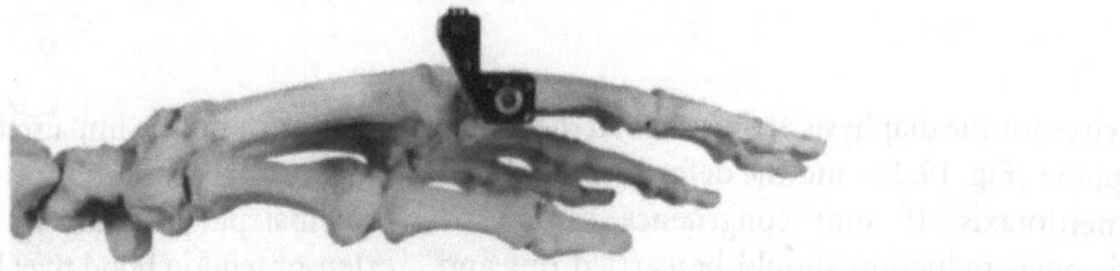

Fig. 19.23 Second wire inserted transversely converging into the small periarticular fragment: Use of an L-clamp.

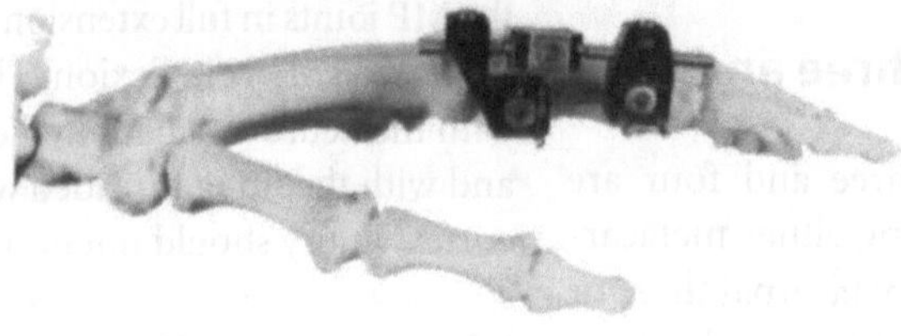

Fig. 19.24 A short MiniFixator is used and a standard clamp serves for parallel threaded wire insertion into the distal fragment of the proximal phalanx.

(2.0mm) is inserted in the frontal plane on the radial aspect of the base of the phalanx.

A standard or L-clamp is applied to the wire, upside down, and the wire is trimmed to length. The second wire is inserted, dorsal to the first. A short MiniFixator body is then mounted and a second L-clamp or, if possible, a standard clamp is attached. The second pair of wires is inserted as described for metacarpal fractures (Fig. 19.22, 19.23, 19.24).

Indications

In addition to conservative treatment for the stabilization of fractures in the hand open reduction with internal fixation has mainly been described. The use of an open approach with plating requires a certain exposure of the fractured bone which might lead to impairment of tendon movement. Where a fracture extends close to a joint plating is challenging. In comminuted fractures there is a risk of disturbing the blood supply of the fragments which may result in delayed union. The MiniFixator system allows effective stabilization of the fracture with closed reduction which is reflected by an average time to union of 5.5 weeks. The "three Rs" of fracture treatment: reduction, retention and rehabilitation, are realized in this concept. Because of the minimally invasive percutaneous application, rehabilitation is facilitated. Stable fractures should be treated conservatively with a short period of rest to avoid immobilization-related problems. If immobilization of an adjacent joint cannot be avoided with conservative treatment of an unstable fracture, use of a MiniFixator should be considered, since transarticular application can be avoided with this technique. Barton's axiom "the best way to make the hand work is to make the hand work" (Barton 1984)[2] is achievable with this method. External fixation in the hand involves fewer soft tissue problems than in the tibia because of the shorter period of application. A more liberal use of the method requires excellent outpatient management, and patient selection is important to reduce the complication rate.

Fracture Management in Metacarpals, Phalanges and Intra-articular Injuries

The classical indications for external fixation are severe open fractures and osteitis. Severely comminuted fractures and fractures with significant soft tissue damage may also be included. Relative indications are closed unstable fractures (Asche et al 1979;[13] Asche and Burny 1982).[14]

When using external fixation the patient must be informed of alternatives, the benefits and risks of conservative management and of open reduction and internal fixation and be warned about fixator specific complications.

External stabilization with a hand adapted minifixator combines the advantage of secure stabilization with a minimally invasive procedure. The reduction itself is performed closed and important elements of conservative fracture management are retained (Pennig et al 1997[16]) (Figs.19.25, 19.26, 19.27, 19.28).

External fixation in the phalanges is technically more demanding. This, however, holds true for internal fixation as well. Use of the 1.6mm threaded wires is recommended (Figs. 19.29, 19.30). Joint bridging should be avoided in extra- and certain intra-articular fractures (Fig. 19.31). It may, however, be necessary in intra-articular fractures where excessive distraction of ligaments and joint capsule must not be applied. The joint should be fixed in a functional position and early physiotherapy is required.

The fixator L-clamp is particularly useful in phalanges and the 1.6mm diameter threaded wires can be inserted very close to the fracture line.

In replantation surgery the fixator is particularly versatile due to the speed of application. The general principles outlined for fractures are followed and the fixator mounted in such a way that the necessary and more important soft tissue management is not hindered. In replantation surgery, the fixator may be expected to remain in place longer than for standard fractures. Whenever the fixator is used for replantation

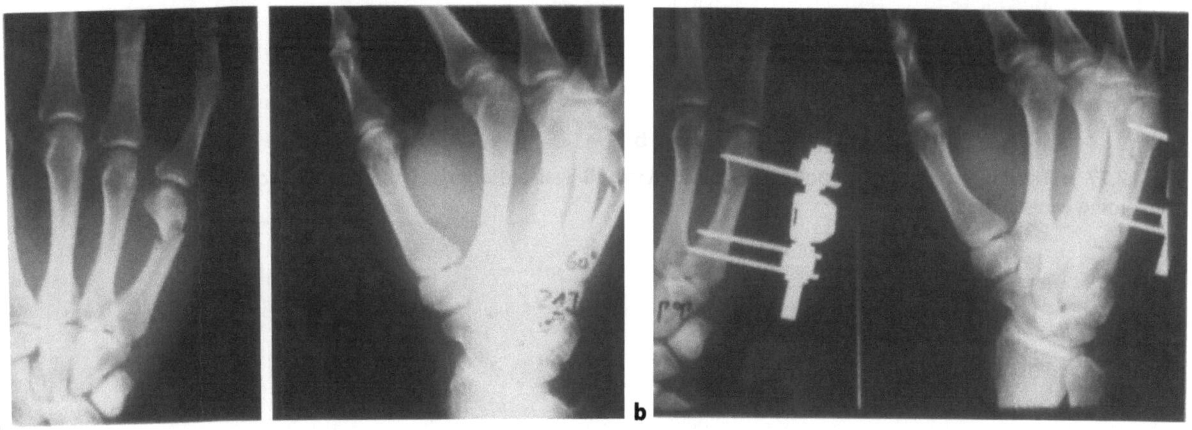

a b

Fig. 19.25 a Subcapital fracture of metacarpal V in a 21-year-old male with severe angulation (60°). **b** Closed reduction with two converging wires in the metacarpal head and two parallel wires in the metacarpal shaft.

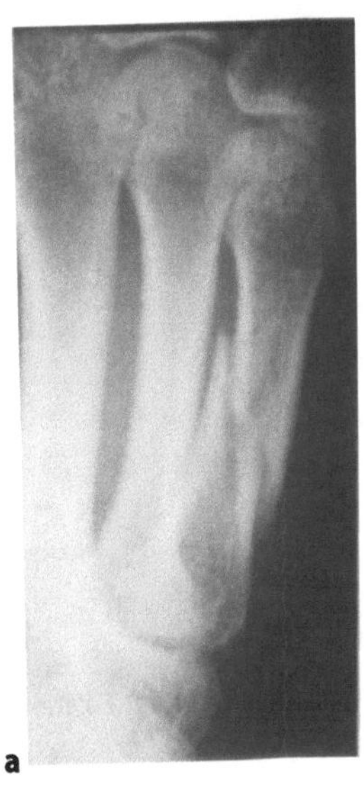

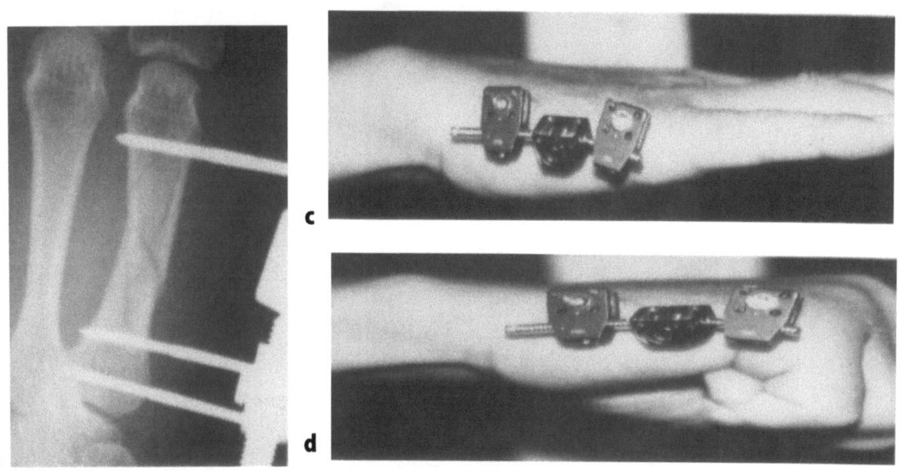

a b c d

Fig. 19.26 a Comminuted unstable metacarpal V shaft fracture in a 30-year-old male. **b** Closed reduction with two converging wires distally and two parallel wires proximally. **c** Extension **d** Flexion at two weeks.

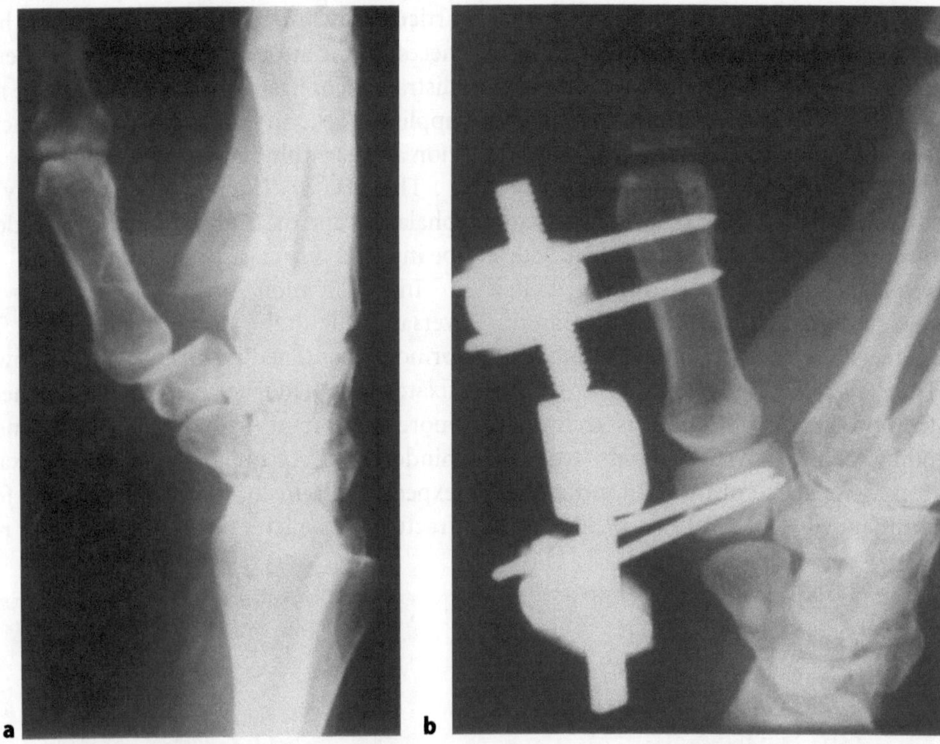

Fig. 19.27 a Dislocation of the first carpo-metacarpal joint in a 30-year-old woman. b Closed reduction after open insertion of two converging wires in the trapezium.

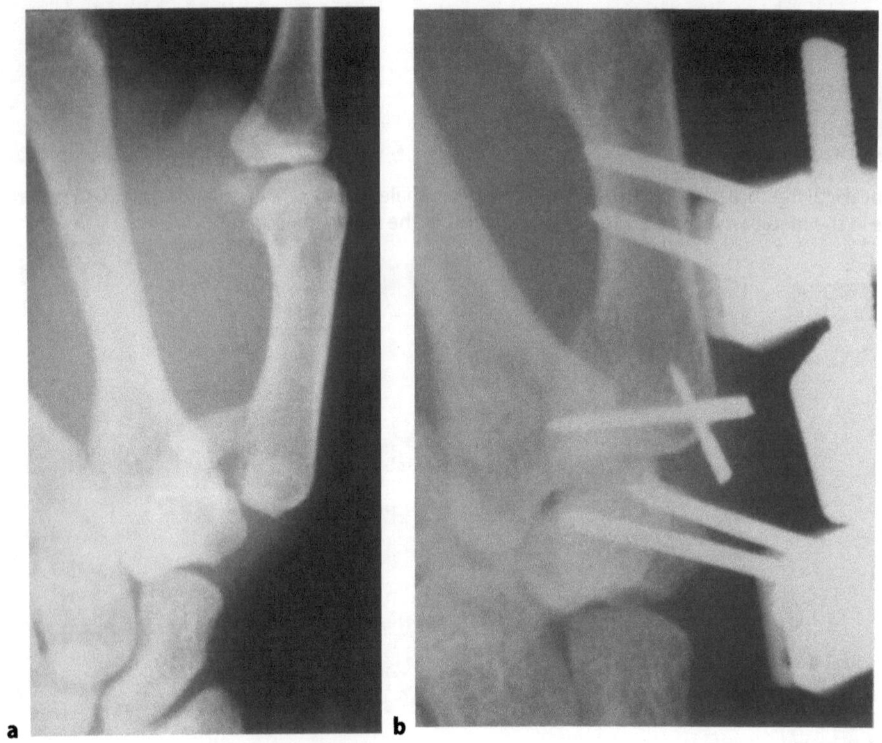

Fig. 19.28 a Bennett type fracture at the base of metacarpal one. b Open reduction and fixation with the Fragment Fixation System. Transarticular application of the MiniFixator.

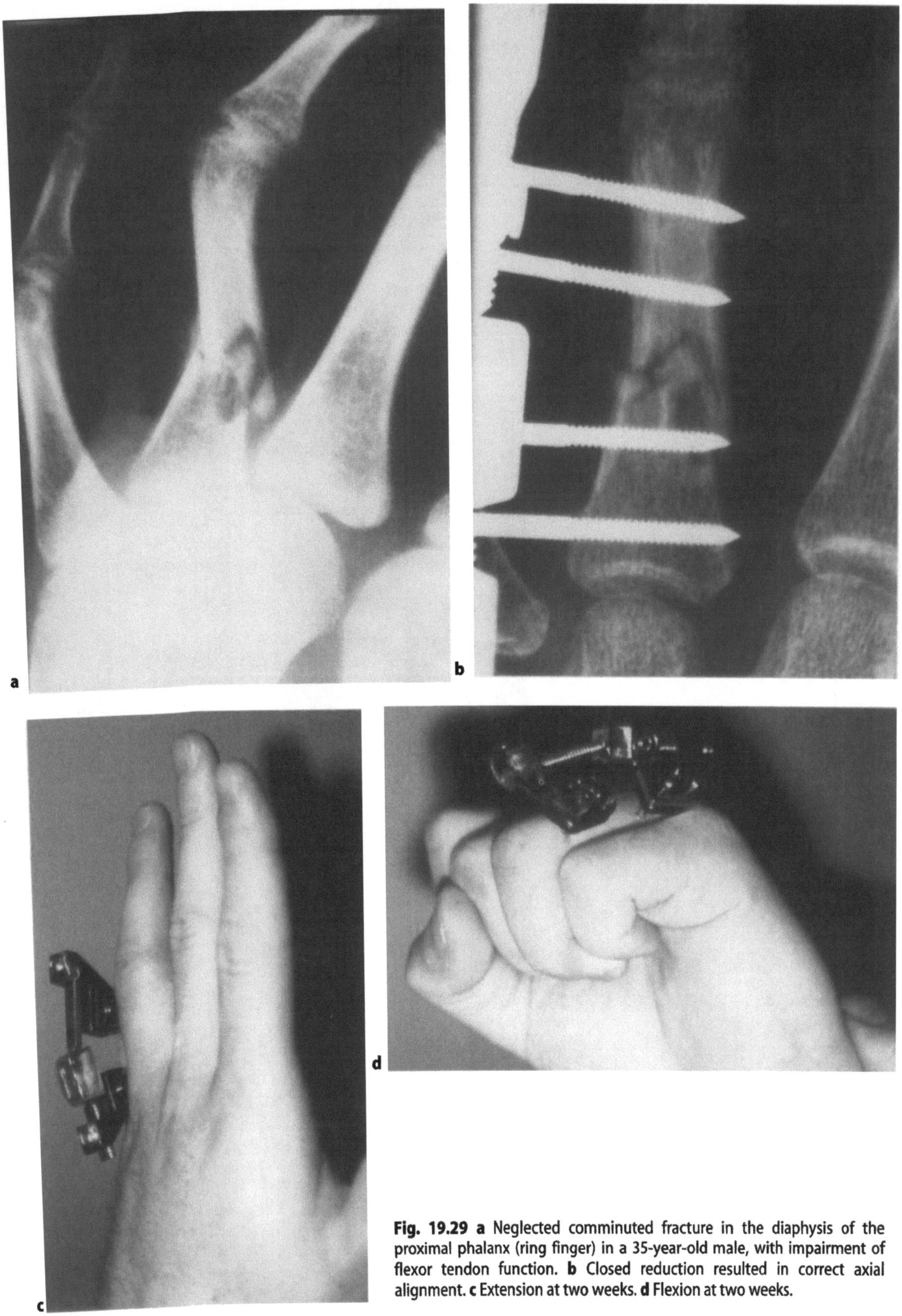

Fig. 19.29 a Neglected comminuted fracture in the diaphysis of the proximal phalanx (ring finger) in a 35-year-old male, with impairment of flexor tendon function. **b** Closed reduction resulted in correct axial alignment. **c** Extension at two weeks. **d** Flexion at two weeks.

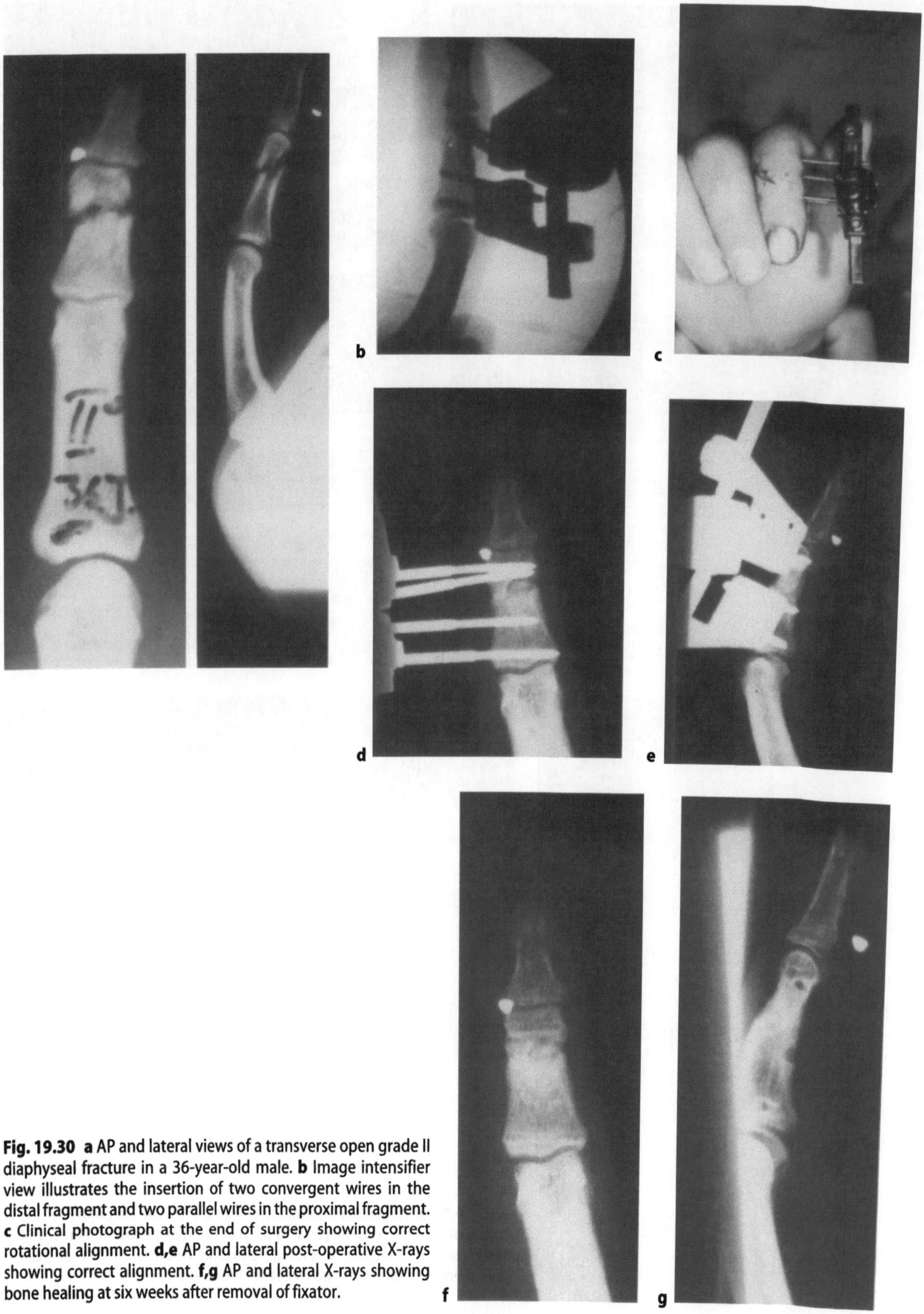

Fig. 19.30 **a** AP and lateral views of a transverse open grade II diaphyseal fracture in a 36-year-old male. **b** Image intensifier view illustrates the insertion of two convergent wires in the distal fragment and two parallel wires in the proximal fragment. **c** Clinical photograph at the end of surgery showing correct rotational alignment. **d,e** AP and lateral post-operative X-rays showing correct alignment. **f,g** AP and lateral X-rays showing bone healing at six weeks after removal of fixator.

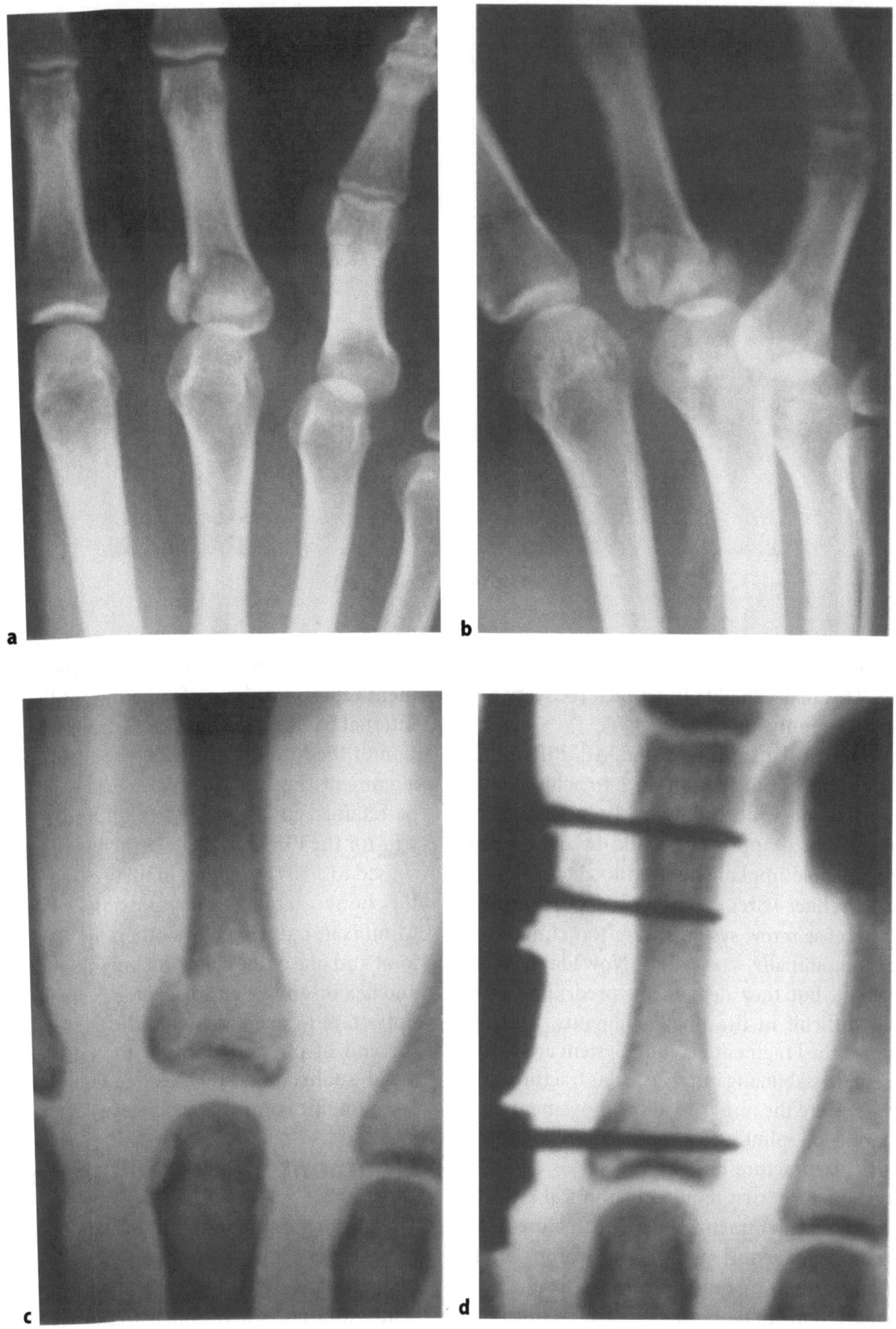

Fig. 19.31 a, b Intra-articular fracture of proximal phalanx in the middle finger of a 36-year-old male. **c** Closed reduction by traction with a clamp placed on the distal phalanx. Note the increased joint space. **d** The reduction of the intra-articular part of the fracture was maintained by a bone clamp and the convergent 1.6mm threaded wires inserted percutaneously in the base of the proximal phalanx. **e** AP view of the reduced fracture. **f** Lateral view. (continued on next page)

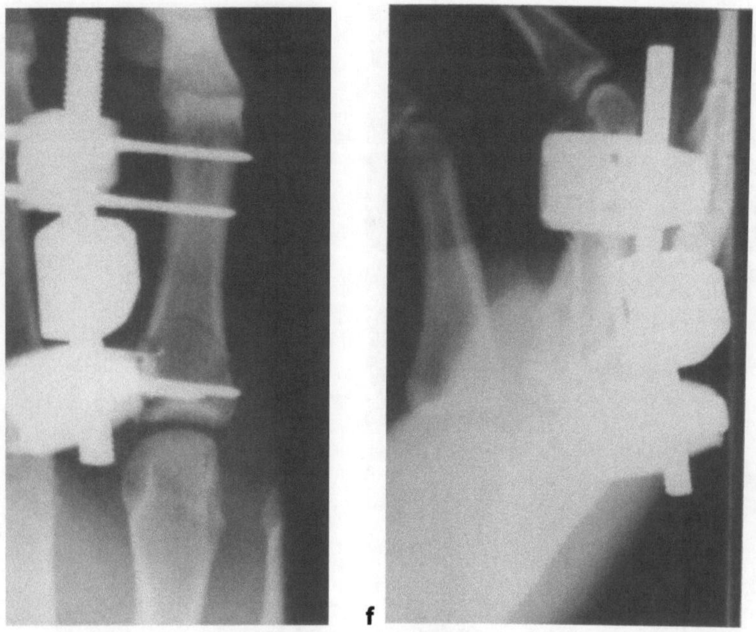

e f

Fig. 19.31 (continued)

surgery, bridging of a joint should be avoided if at all possible. This may expedite functional recovery of the replanted extremity.

In intra-articular injuries of the MP, PIP and DIP joint it is of paramount importance to achieve reduction and fixation which allows early mobilization. If possible a limited approach should be used and the smallest possible implant inserted to retain the fragments. Kirschner-wires have enjoyed popularity but mainly because screw systems were too cumbersome to use and, initially, too large. Nowadays, smaller screws exist, but they depend on predrilling which, again, is difficult in the small fragments. The small implants of the Fragment Fixation System are particularly useful in stabilizing intra-articular fractures of the phalanges. Here the aim is to allow movement after a brief period of splinting (6 days). Combinations of intra-articular fracture lines and meta- or diaphyseal displaced fractures first require anatomical reduction of the intra-articular fracture line. The fracture may be stabilized percutaneously with a bone clamp, and two converging 1.6mm threaded wires in a fixator clamp can be used to maintain reduction. The fixator is then used for the more unstable meta- or diaphyseal fracture. Since the joint is not bridged early motion is possible (Figs. 19.31a–19.31f). Intra-articular fractures with significant comminution making reconstruction virtually impossible, benefit from the principle of ligamentotaxis. Most of these fractures will cause subluxation or complete displacement of the joint. Depending on the extent of the ligament injury, ligament repair may be performed in addition to limited internal fixation. In these cases, transarticular application of the MiniFixator allows restoration of the axial alignment (Fig. 19.32a–19.32e). The MP joint should be retained in 20–40° of flexion and the same holds true for the PIP joints. The principle of ligamentotaxis is used to assist reduction in these cases. Depending on the bony stability it is possible to mobilize the MiniFixator during physiotherapy. The double ball joint and one of the clamp locking screws are unlocked and flexion and extension exercises are performed. It is important to make sure that the fixator is relocked at the end of physiotherapy in the correct position to avoid subluxation. In these cases a more frequent radiographic control is necessary.

Ligament Injuries in the Hand

The most common injury in the hand is the so-called gamekeeper's thumb with a rupture or avulsion of the ulnar collateral lateral ligament of the MP joint. In acute injuries where open repair is chosen, the MiniFixator may be applied from the radial side to metacarpal one and the proximal phalanx. After exposure of the ligament injury the fixator is applied from the radial side and the joint reduced. Radiographic control in conjunction with direct visual control is used to confirm correct joint alignment. Ligament tears can be sutured and the suture will be protected

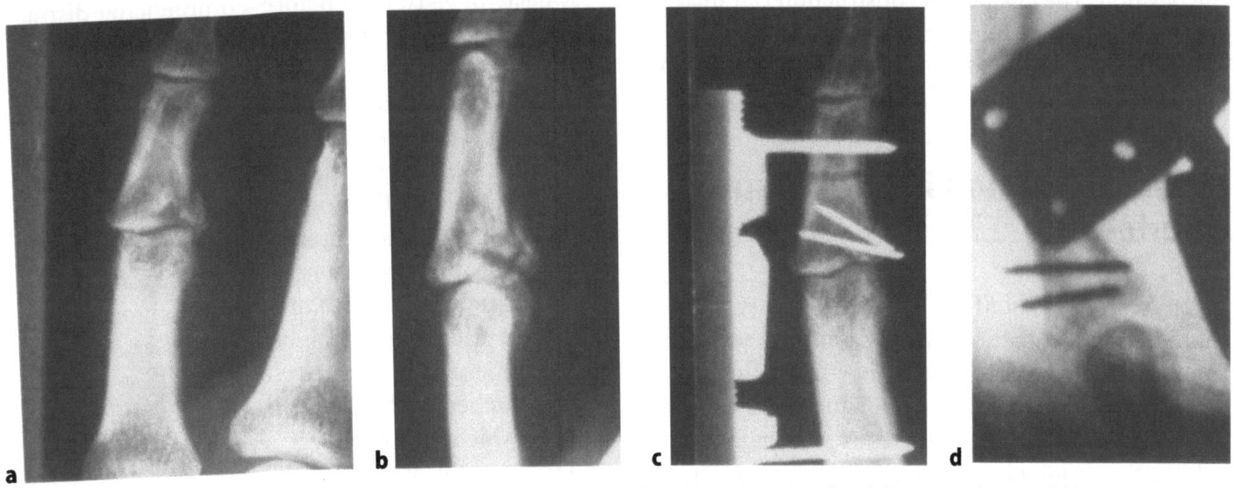

Fig. 19.32 a Intra-articular fracture at the base of the middle phalanx. Note: Rotational malalignment. **b** Lateral film reveals severe palmar comminution. **c** Limited supplementary internal fixation after transarticular fixator application using ligamentotaxis to correct rotational alignment. **d** Lateral film showing satisfactory reduction of the comminuted articular surface.

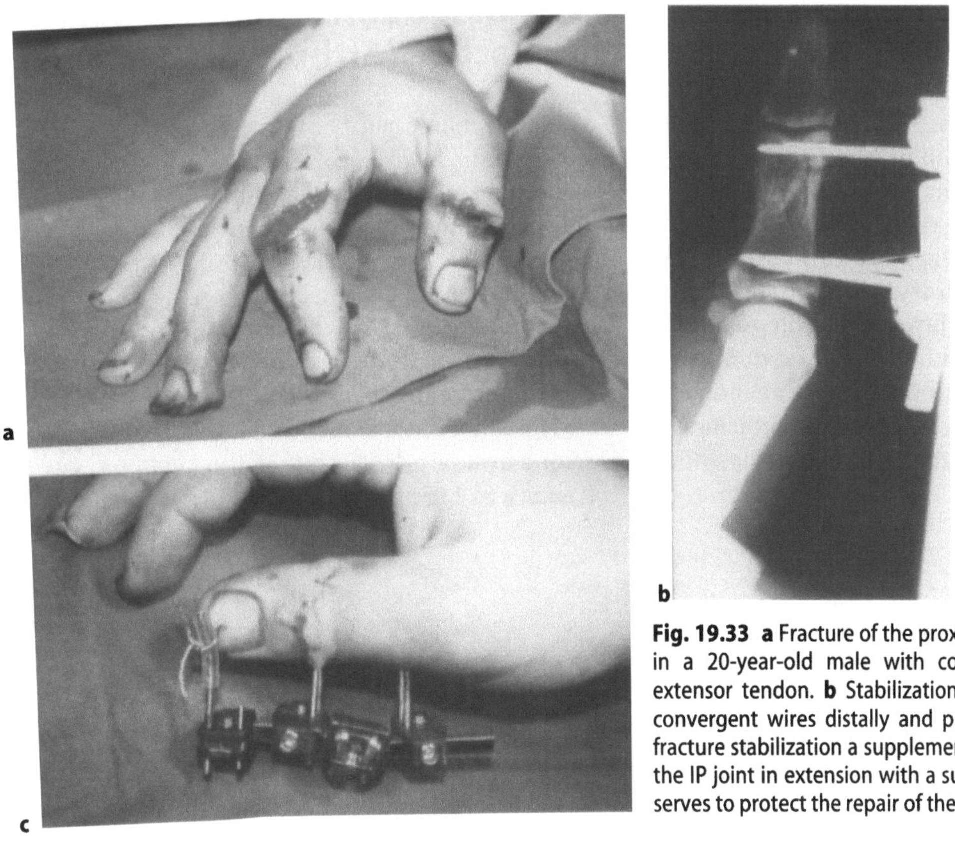

Fig. 19.33 a Fracture of the proximal phalanx of the thumb in a 20-year-old male with complete laceration of the extensor tendon. **b** Stabilization of the fracture with two convergent wires distally and proximally. **c** In addition to fracture stabilization a supplementary clamp is used to hold the IP joint in extension with a suture through the nail. This serves to protect the repair of the extensor tendon.

with the MiniFixator. A flexion position of 15° with the MiniFixator is recommended. Bony avulsions are more stable injuries and after reattachment application of a MiniFixator is not usually required. A thermoplastic splint is used instead.

In neglected cases ligament reconstruction of the ulnar collateral ligament is performed, and a number of techniques are described in the literature. If subluxation is present, the MiniFixator may be applied from the radial side to reduce the joint and maintain the position. The ligament reconstruction can then be performed and the MiniFixator serves to protect the reconstructed ligament complex. Again, 15° of flexion is recommended in the MP joint.

External Fixation in Soft Tissue Injuries

Open dislocations of MP, PIP and DIP joints must be mobilized after reduction. With a significant soft tissue injury present a splint or cast may not be desirable since monitoring of the soft tissue situation is not ideal (Fig. 19.33a–c). Where there is a tendency to subluxation in joint injuries, transarticular application of the MiniFixator should be considered to retain the joint in the correct position.

Lengthening and Segmental Transport

In principle, it is possible to lengthen phalanges, metacarpal and carpal bones. The most common indication, however, is likely to be lengthening of the first metacarpal following amputation of the thumb.

A lengthening bar (Fig. 19.34) with standard clamps or L-clamps is applied in the frontal plane using 2mm wires. A third wire may be added in each clamp to improve stability especially in osteoporotic bone. A metaphyseal or midshaft osteotomy may be performed. A compression–distraction nut and a spacer should be placed on the lengthening bar before the second clamp is applied (Figs. 19.35a–19.35c).

A delay of 7–10 days before commencing distraction is advisable. Distraction is then performed at a rate of 0.5mm per day (one quarter turn of the nut twice a day). Callus formation should be carefully monitored with standard radiographs weekly (Fig. 19.36a–19.36j).

When bone transport is employed for the treatment of bone loss, a lengthening bar with three clamps is used. Two clamps are applied to the larger segment and the osteotomy performed between them, preferably at a metaphyseal site. Note that the segments must be aligned prior to insertion of the wires and application of the lengthening bar.

The numbers of the clamps in Fig. 19.37 indicate the order in which they should be applied. If some shortening is present at the end of transport, the clamp locking nut of clamp 2 is loosened and lengthening continued between clamp 1 and 3.

Soft Tissue Correction and Joint Distraction (Arthrodiatasis)

The distraction capacity of the fixator can be used to widen the web space, for example, between the first and second metacarpal bones, following burns or scarring from other causes (Figs. 19.38a–19.38l). This technique can be used to augment other hand surgery techniques and again, established surgical procedures should be followed. In contrast to bone lengthening procedures, soft tissue correction by distraction can be carried out from day one onwards.

The MiniFixator is mounted between the first and second metacarpals. The rate of distraction is between 0.5mm and 1.0mm per day (a half to one full turn per

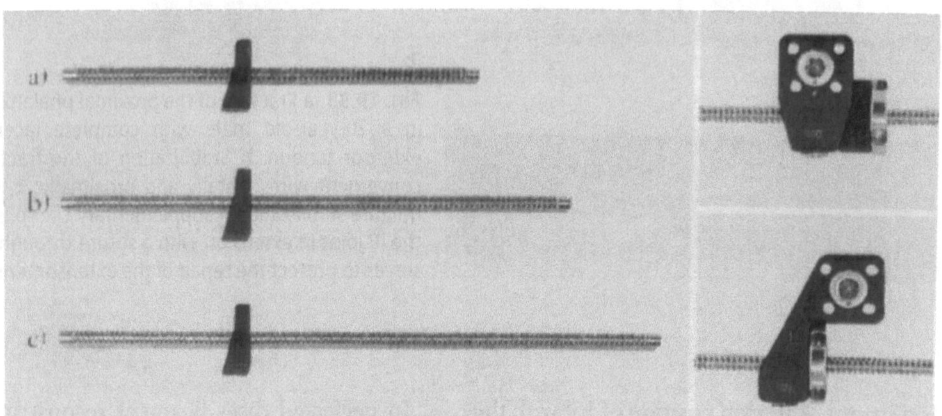

Fig. 19.34 For lengthening or bone transport the ball jointed Pennig MiniFixator body is replaced by a lengthening bar. a) Short: 80mm; b) standard: 100mm; c) long: 120mm. A spacer is used in conjunction with the standard clamp (top right) whereas the L-clamp does not require a spacer (bottom right) for the proper use of the nut.

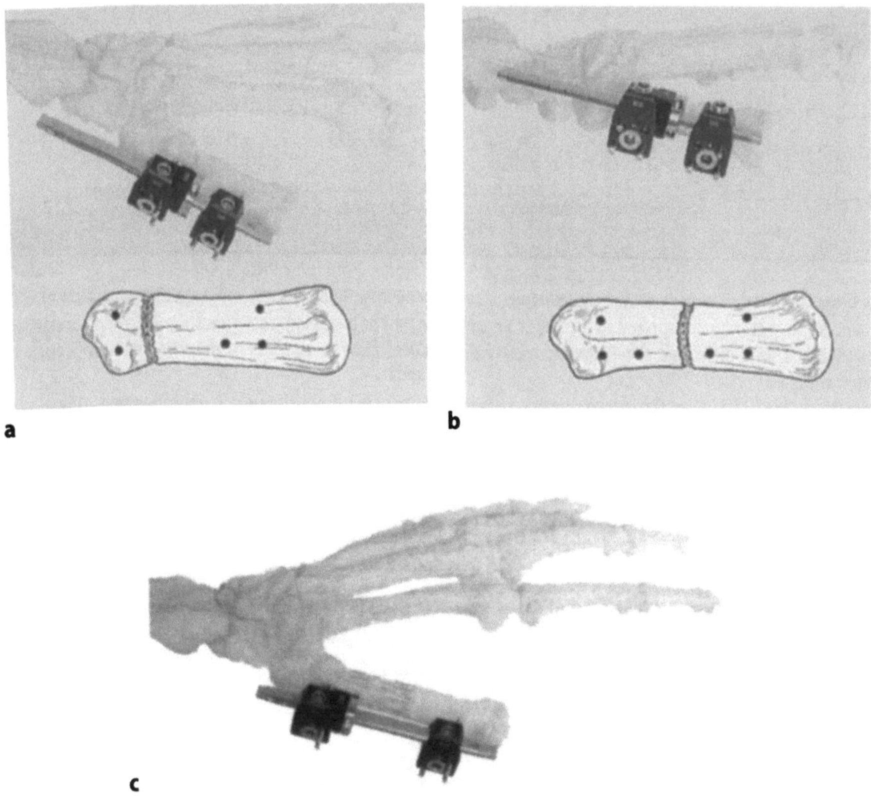

a b c

Fig. 19.35 **a** Use of the lengthening bar in callus distraction of metacarpal one. Proximal metaphyseal osteotomy. **b** Use of the lengthening bar with a midshaft osteotomy. Note that three thread wires per clamp are used. **c** Final aspect at the end of distraction.

day). Substantial scar formation may need to be removed beforehand.

Arthrodiatasis in the MP and PIP joints or the IP joint of the thumb follows the same principles outlined in the chapter on management of elbow stiffness (Ch. 14). Before considering arthrodiatasis in impaired joint function (stiffness) the cause of the stiffness must be determined. If it is a late consequence of a tendon injury, there is no point in distracting the joint without tendon reconstruction. If extensor and flexor tendon function is normal, however, the distraction capacity of the fixator may be used to widen the joint space. In MP, PIP and IP joints a joint space two to three times as wide as normal is aimed for. The fixator is applied in a transarticular manner and the distraction nuts placed between the double ball joint and the clamp. In very stiff joints it may be necessary to apply two fixators, one from either side, to avoid asymmetrical opening of the joint line. After distraction has been performed and a satisfactory joint space achieved, the relaxation phase commences. This lasts 6–10 days and allows the short collateral ligaments and fibrotic capsule to accommodate. The relaxation phase is followed by the mobilization phase, and in cases where two MiniFixators have been applied one device should be removed. Physiotherapy is used to mobilize the joint and the double ball joint and one of the clamp locking screws is loosened during the physiotherapy session. The fixator remains in situ for a total of approximately 6 weeks.

The success rate of this procedure depends largely on the aetiology of the stiffness and the familiarity of the hand-physiotherapist with external fixation equipment.

Contraindications and Postoperative Management

Contraindications to the use of the Pennig MiniFixator in the hand are similar to those for external fixation in general. These include severe osteoporosis, patients who are HIV positive and patients with severe, poorly controlled diabetes mellitus. In addition, in uncooperative or predictably difficult patients, external fixation is not advisable. Careful patient selection will therefore avoid problems at a later stage.

Post-operatively, the arm should be elevated and the patient should be encouraged to keep the arm elevated while walking. A sling, however, should not be used. Routine review of the wire entry sites twice weekly, is advisable. Dressings, in general, are not necessary after two weeks, but the MiniFixator must be protected by a bandage. The patient should not be

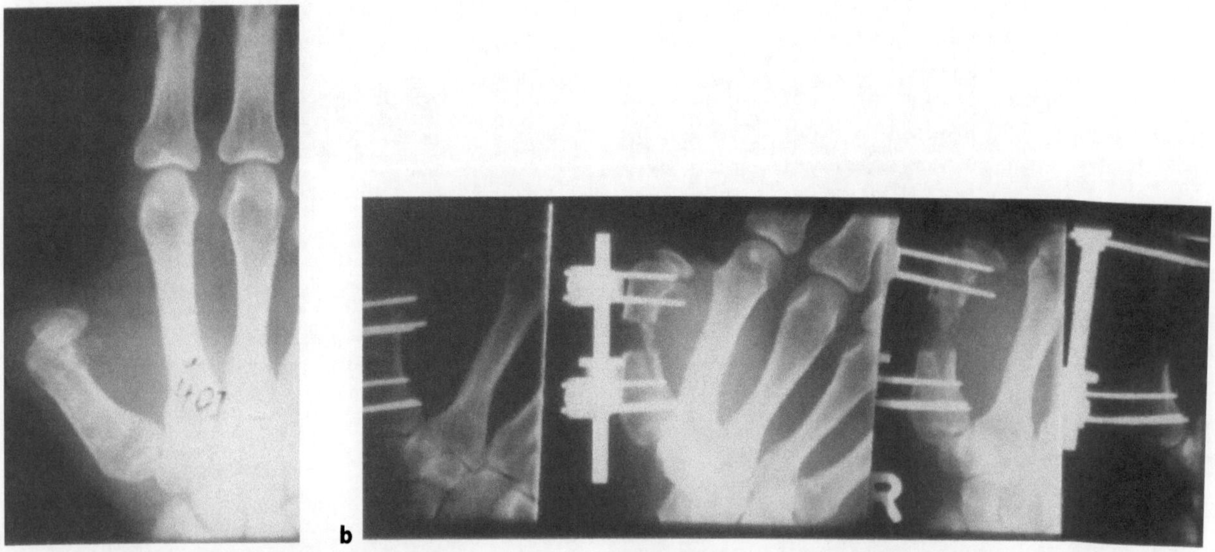

a b

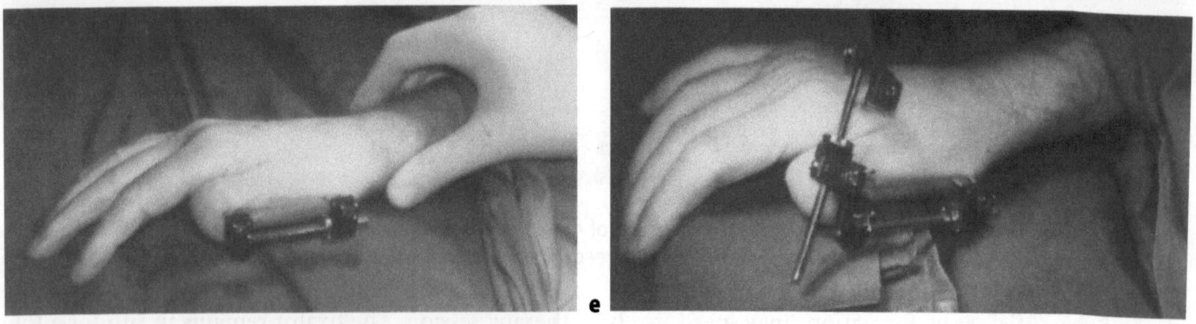

c e

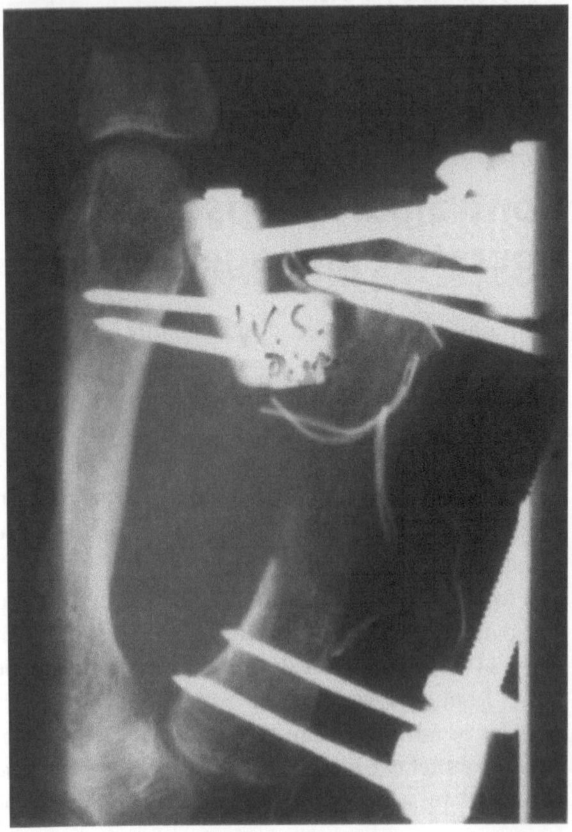

d

Fig. 19.36 **a** Amputation of thumb in a 62-year-old male: 40 years after injury. **b** Callus distraction using a midshaft osteotomy at a speed of 0.5mm per day. **c** Lengthening completed. Note the adduction contracture of the thumb. **d** Metacarpal II to I distraction to widen web space I. The callus is beginning to mature at the end of distraction. **e** Lengthening bar to distract web space I in place.

On next page **f** After soft tissue distraction the web space I is wide; no open soft tissue release performed. **g** Radiographic image of the clinical photograph of Fig. 19.36f. **h** After removal of the lengthening bar between metacarpal II and metacarpal I, the web space is adequate. **i** Final result after callus distraction. **j** Pinch grip with adequate width of web space I and restoration of thumb length.

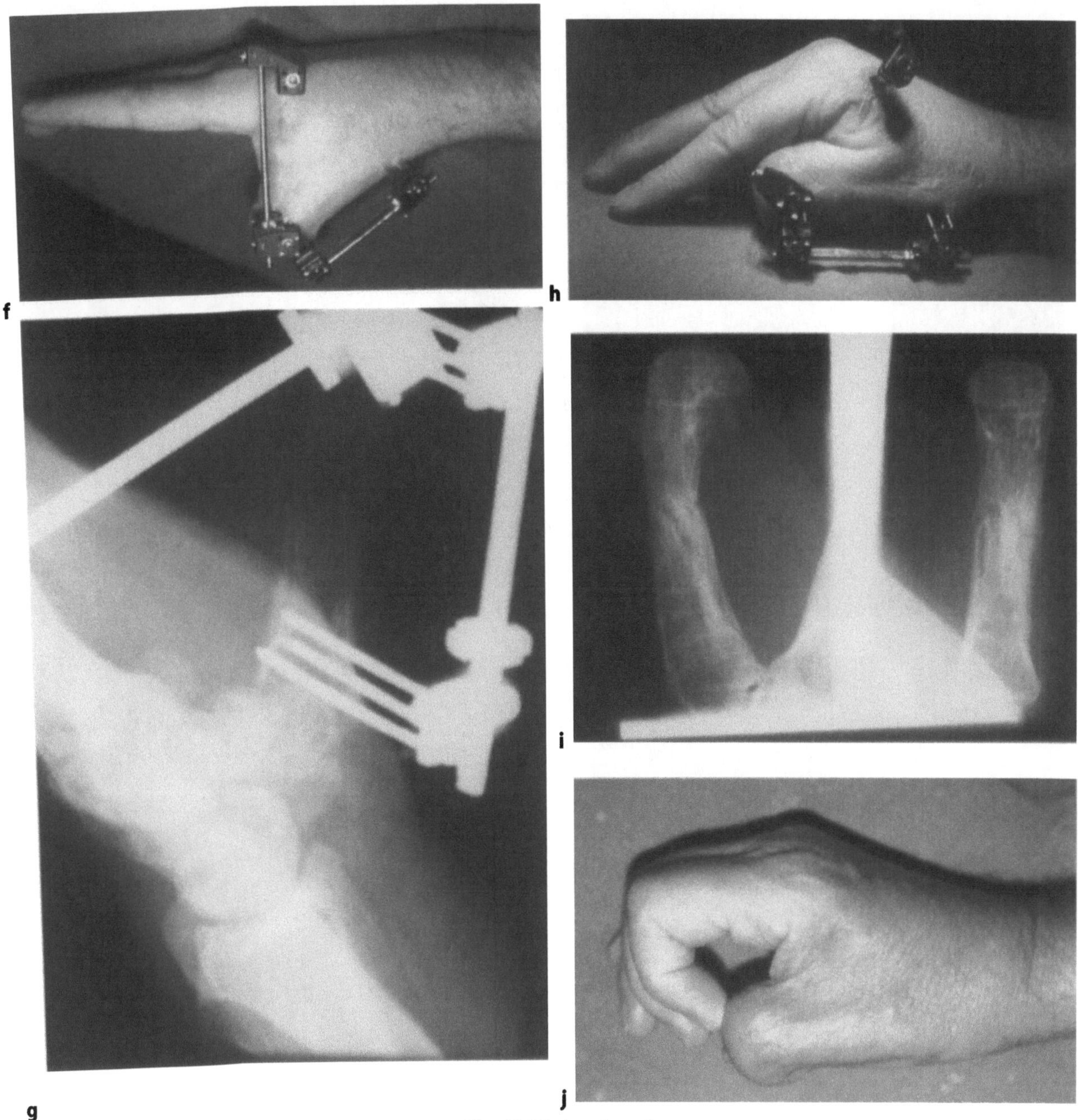

Fig. 19.36 (continued)

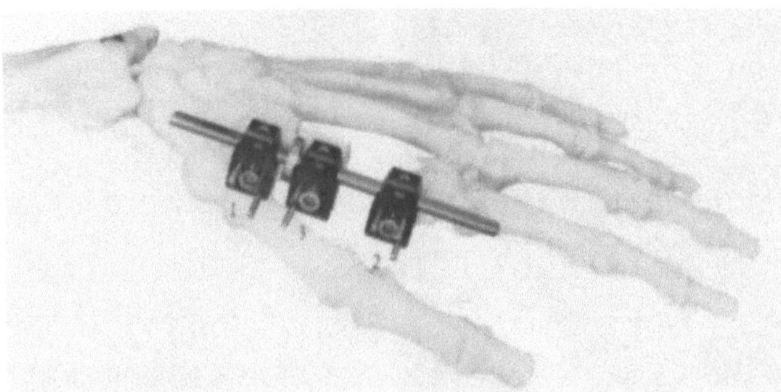

Fig. 19.37 Use of three clamps for segmental transport in segmental defects in metacarpal two. The numbers indicate the sequence of threaded wire insertion in the clamps.

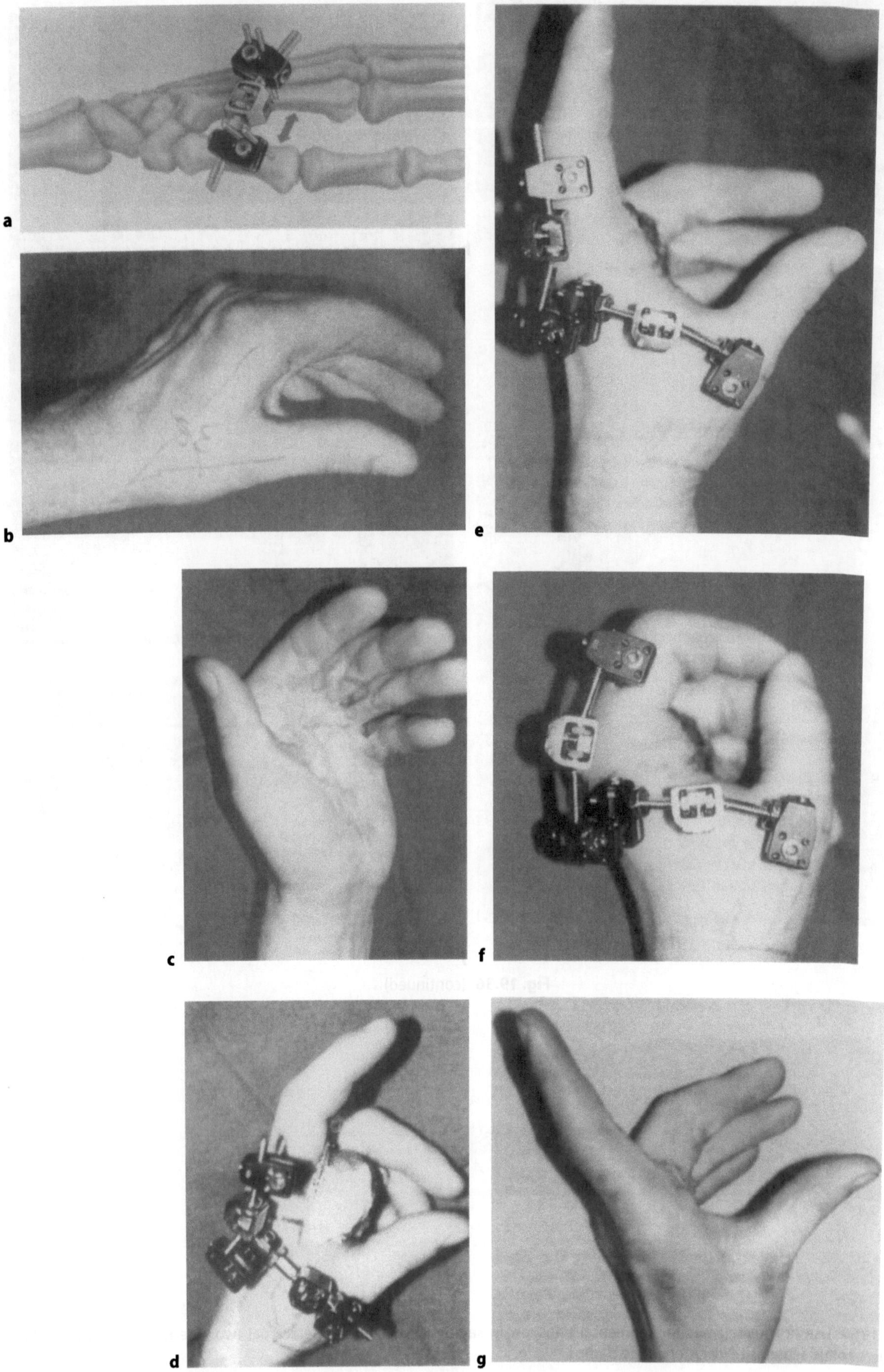

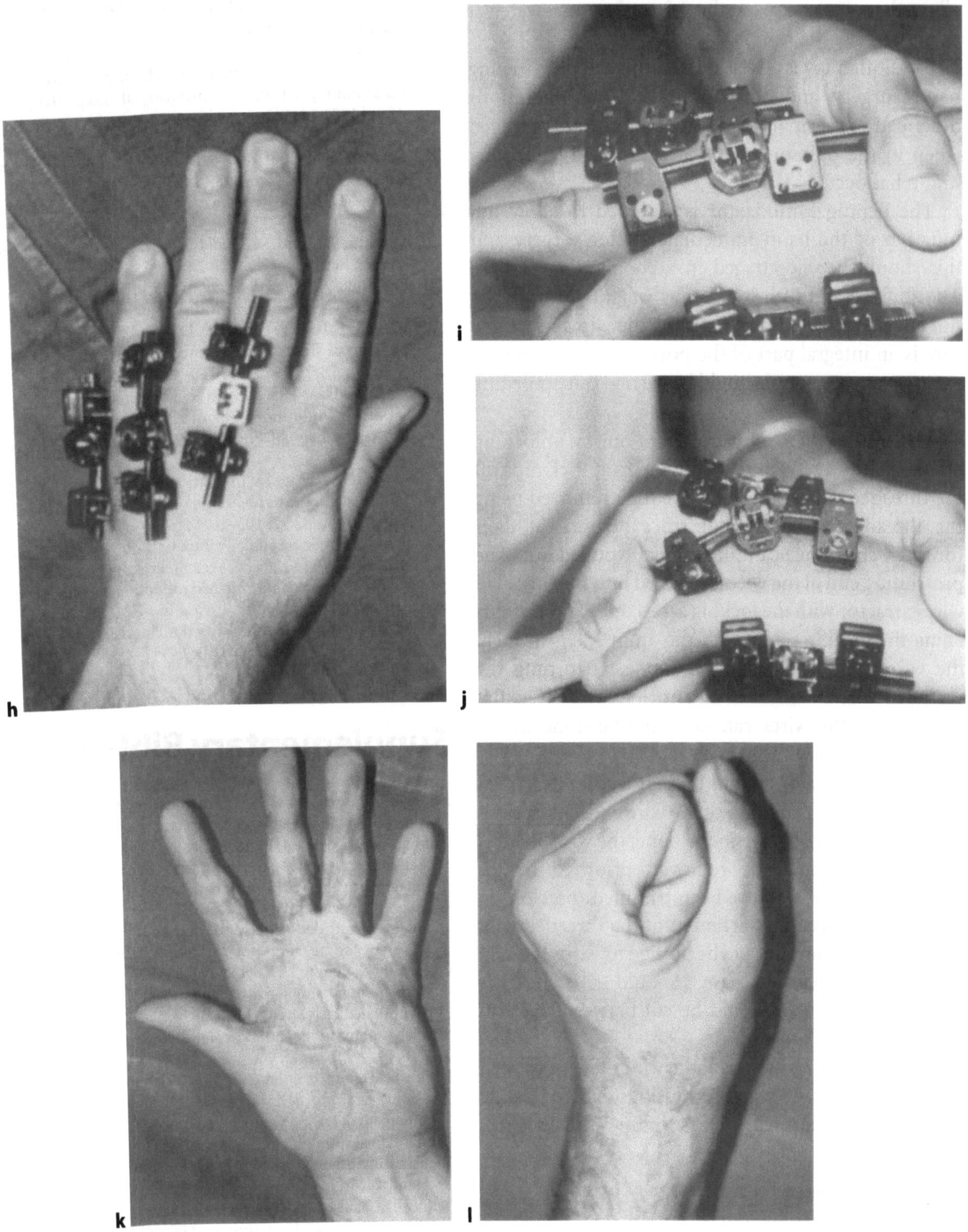

Fig. 19.38 **a** Ball joint MiniFixator used for widening of web space I as an alternative to the lengthening bar. **b** Maximum separation of thumb and index finger 29 years after palmar burn injury in a 30-year-old male. **c** Volar aspect of the hand showing severe contractures and ulnar subluxation of MP joints II, III, IV and V. **d** Application of the MiniFixator to widen web space I after removal of scar tissue and full thickness skin graft on the palmar side. The second MiniFixator between metacarpal two and the proximal phalanx of the index finger is used to reduce the ulnar subluxation of this joint. **e** After distraction with the metacarpal II/metacarpal I MiniFixator, web space I is enlarged. **f** With the double ball joint and the distal clamp unlocked, the MP joint can be exercised. **g** Free extension of the index finger and abduction of the thumb as a final result two weeks after fixator removal. **h** Reduction of the ulnar subluxation of MP joints III, IV and V after removal of scar tissue on the volar side and full thickness skin graft. **i** Unlocking of the double ball joint and the proximal clamp base allows physiotherapy of the MP joint. **j** Flexion with the double ball joint and the proximal clamp base unlocked. **k** Result at six months: Full extension of the fingers and no MP joint subluxation. **l** Full flexion of the fingers six months after the first operation.

allowed to use soap on the wires, but tap water is permitted.

Physiotherapy is advisable for any patient following hand surgery and this applies to the operations described in this manual. The MiniFixator is removed when in the opinion of the attending surgeon bony union has occurred.

The Pennig MiniFixator is designed to allow full function of the hand immediately after surgery and this should be encouraged in a cooperative patient. The shifting and lifting of heavy weights however, is not allowed to avoid overstraining the wires. Wire site care is an integral part of the post-operative management programme and should be carried out according to a protocol.

Removal of the fixator is carried out by unlocking all the fixator screws and sliding the fixator clamps off the threaded wires. The wires are then removed using the threaded wire extractor since because of their threaded ends, they cannot simply be pulled out. The protruding end of the wire is inserted into the threaded wire extractor with the locking screw open. After tightening the locking screw with the 3mm Allen wrench, the wire is removed from the bone by turning the threaded wire extractor in an anticlockwise direction. Removal of the wires can normally be done in the outpatient clinic without analgesics.

When the fixator cannot be removed as described above, due to deformation of the wire ends, or in cases where the wires converge in the bone, the wire or wires in question should be removed prior to fixator removal. If the wires have been trimmed too close to the clamp for secure attachment of the threaded wire extractor, the clamp should be pushed towards the skin to obtain better purchase. Should this not be successful, the wires should be cut between the skin surface and the clamp.

After removal of the wires, the wire sites are washed with disinfectant and a simple dressing applied. Healing of the wire sites normally occurs within 3–4 days.

References

1. Barton NJ 'Fractures of the shafts of the phalanges of the hand' *Hand* 1979 11: 119–33.
2. Barton NJ 'Fractures of the hand' *J Bone Joint Surg* [Br] 1984 66-B: 159–67.
3. James JIP 'Fractures of the proximal and middle phalanges of the fingers' *Acta Orthop Scand* 1962 32: 401–12.
4. Swanson AB 'Fractures involving the digits of the hand' *Orthop Clin North Am* 1970 1: 261–274.
5. Buck-Gramcko D, Hoffmann R, Neumann R *Hand Trauma, a practical guide,* 1986 Thieme Inc. New York (Hippokrates Verlag: Stuttgart).
6. Bowen CVA, Hochan F, Johnston GHF 'Angular deformity in fractures of the fifth metacarpal' *J Bone Joint Surg* [Br] 1989 71-B: 344.
7. Edwards GJ Jr, O'Brian ET, Heckmann MM 'Retrograde crosspinning of transverse metacarpal and phalangeal fractures' *Hand* 1982 14: 141–8.
8. Hung LK, So WS, Leung PC 'Combined intramedullary Kirschner wire and intra-osseous wire loop for fixation of finger fractures' *J Hand Surg*1989 14-B: 171–6.
9. Lister GD 'Intraosseous wiring of the digital skeleton' *J Hand Surg* 1978 3: 427–35.
10. Heim V, Pfeiffer KM *Small fragment set manual.* 1982 Springer-Verlag: Berlin.
11. Segmüller G *Surgical Stabilization of the Skeleton of the Hand.* 1977 Hans Huber: Bern-Stuttgart-Wien.
12. Fitoussi F, Ip WY, Chow SP 'External fixation for comminuted phalangeal fractures, a biomechanical cadaver study' *J Bone Joint Surg*[Br] 1996 21-B: 760–4.
13. Asche G, Haas HG, Klemm K 'The external minifixator: application and indication in hand surgery.' in: Brooker AF, Edward CC (eds) *External Fixation.* 1979 Wilkens & Wilkens: Baltimore.
14. Asche G, Burny F 'Indikationen für die Anwendung des Minifixateur externe, eine statistische Analyse' *Aktuell Traumatol* 1982 12: 103–10.
15. Pennig D, Gausepohl T, Lukosch R 'Externe Fixation zur Unterstützung der Weichteilrekonstruktion in der Handchirurgie' *Handchir-Mikrochir-Plast Chir* 1995 27:264–8.
16. Pennig D, Gausepohl T, Mader K 'Die Anwendung des Minifixateurs bei Frankturen des Handskelettes' *Osteosynthese Intern* 1997 5: 158–65.

Supplementary Bibliography

Foster RJ, Hastings H (1987) 'Treatment of Bennett, Rolando and vertical intraarticular trapezial fractures' *Clin Orthop* 214: 121–9.

Gausepohl T, Koebke J, Pennig D et al (1998a) 'Formänderung der Sehnenhauben bei Streckung und Beugung der Metakarpophalangealgelenke' *Handchir-Mikrochir-Plast Chir* 4: 220–5.

Gausepohl T, Lukosch S, Koebke J et al (1998b) 'Externe Stabilisierung der Mittelhandknochen II vis V. Eine anatomisch-klinische Studie' *Handchir-Mikrochir-Plast Chir* 2: 95–108.

Gausepohl T, Pennig D, Koebke J et al (1998) 'Zur Auswirkung von Implantaten im Mittelhandknochenkopf und in der Grundgliedbasis auf die Beweglichkeit des Fingergrundgelenkes. Eine anatomische Studie' *Handchir-Mikrochir-Plast Chir* 30: 226–31.

Pennig D: *Treatment of Fractures and Deformities in Small Bones. The Pennig Minifixator. Operative Technique.* Orthofix Srl., Bussolengo, Italy

Pennig D, Gausepohl T, Lukosch R (1994) 'Der Einsatz von Fixationsstiften zur Fragmentstabilisierung in der Handchirurgie' *Handchir-Mikrochir-Plast Chir* 26: 270–4.

Pennig D, Gausepohl T, Mader K (1999a) 'External fixation.' in: *Finger Bone and Joint Injuries.* Gilbert A and Brüser P (eds.) Martin Dunitz Ltd: London (in press).

Pennig D, Gausepohl T, Mader K et al (1999b) 'The use of minimally invasive fixation in fractures of the hand – The MiniFixator Concept' *Injury* Suppl. (in press).

Proubasta IR (1992) 'Rolando's fracture of the first metacarpal' *J Bone Joint Surg* [Br] 74-B: 416–7.

Spangenberg O, Thorén L (1963) 'Bennett's fracture, a method of treatment with oblique traction' *J Bone Joint Surg* [Br[] 45-B: 732–6.

Van Niekerk JLM, Ouwens R (1989) 'Fractures of the base of the first metacarpal bone, results of surgical treatment' *Injury* 20: 359–62.

External Fixation in Pelvic Ring Injuries: the Pelvic Fixator

20

D. Pennig and T. Gausepohl

Introduction

Injuries of the pelvic ring are usually seen in multiple trauma victims (Fig. 20.1). The major threat from pelvic ring injuries is blood loss, the source being the fracture surfaces as well as arterial and venous bleeding. Major haemorrhage may be the consequence and be responsible for death due to uncontrollable hypovolaemia. Mortality rates in unstable pelvic fractures range from 8.6 to 22.2 per cent. Open injuries considerably increase the likelihood of a fatal outcome. In the treatment protocol pelvic ring injuries have the highest priority of all skeletal injuries in polytrauma.

Pelvic ring injuries are best stabilized as soon as possible and the golden hour should not pass without adequate management. The benefit of external fixation is its minimally invasive nature and it can be used rapidly (Slätis and Huittinen 1972). In a recent study, major trauma centres in Scotland were assessed regarding their capacity to apply external fixation in the haemodynamically unstable patient with an open book pelvic injury. It was discovered that only 8 out of 31 units were potentially able to perform stabilization of the pelvis within one hour. Resident and non-resident staff with in vivo experience of fixator application were available in 17 out of 31 hospitals. The Orthofix device was the most popular external frame for stabilizing the pelvis (Meighan et al 1998).

External fixation to stabilize the pelvic ring should be available for use not only in operating rooms but also in the resuscitation area and in intensive care

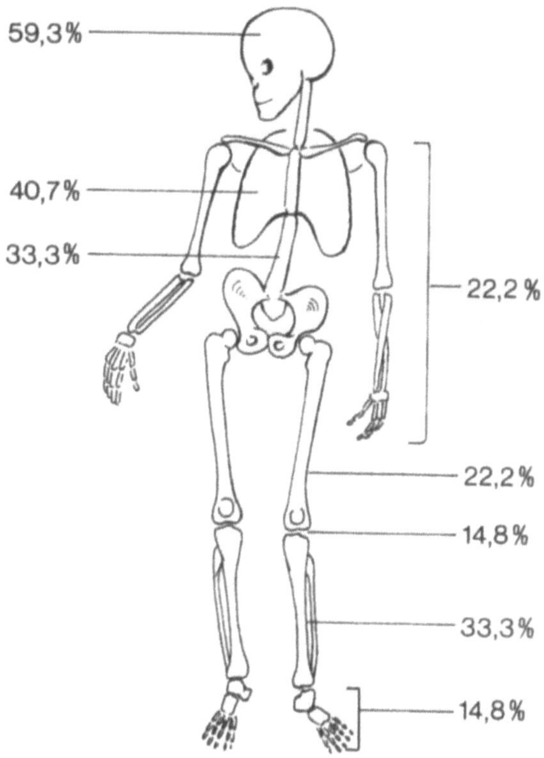

Fig. 20.1 Injury pattern in pelvic ring instability (n = 27; Rieger et al 1991).

units. The Orthofix frame has an application time half that of the Pittsburgh frame and provides greater compression at the fracture dislocation site which may decrease haemorrhage from fracture surfaces (Bell et al 1988).

Biomechanics of the Pelvic Ring

For rational management of pelvic ring injuries it is important to study the basic biomechanics (Pauwels 1965). The pelvic ring posteriorly resembles an arch with the sacrum acting as a keystone (Fig. 20.2). The anterior pelvic ring with the symphysis pubis and the pubic rami are described as a tension band (Fig. 20.3). The strongest and therefore most important structure in the pelvic ring is the posterior complex with sacro-iliac ligaments. Without the ligamentous stabilization a vertical force acting on the pelvis would displace the sacrum posteriorly (Tile 1995).

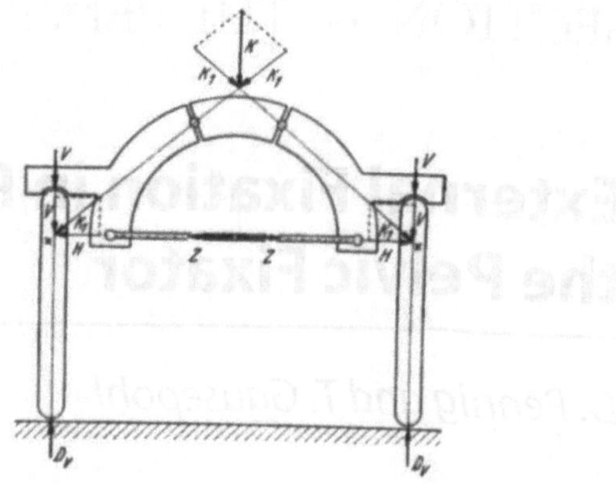

Fig. 20.3 Pelvic ring model according to Pauwels. Z represents the symphysis pubis and pubic rami and acts as a tension band.

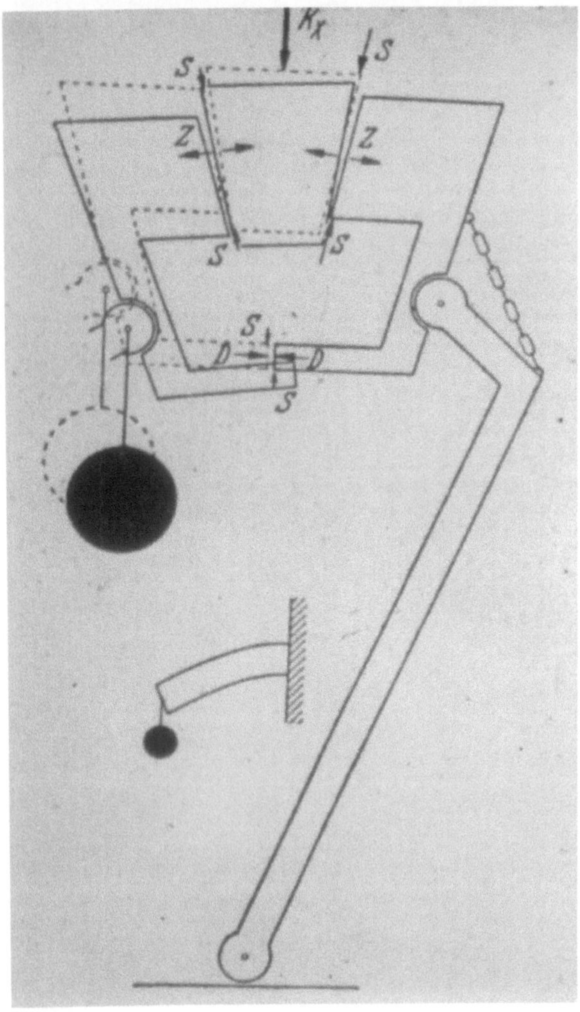

Fig. 20.2 Biomechanical model of pelvic ring according to Pauwels. Displacement of the anterior ring indicates an injury of the posterior ring.

The anterior pelvic ring seems less important but may be an indicator of posterior ligament instability. Widening of the symphysis pubis of more than 2.5cm indicates an injury to the anterior sacro-iliac and sacro-spinous ligaments (Tile 1995). With intact posterior sacro-iliac ligaments this is defined as a stable situation. The major weightbearing areas are the acetabulum, the posterior part of the ilium and the sacrum (Basmizian 1980).

The assessment of pelvic stability is not straightforward. Gross instability may be detected easily but between gross instability and stability there are many gradations. A frequent pattern is external rotation resulting in an open book injury. The lateral compression injuries are less common and the most unstable situations result from shear forces with complete disruption of the posterior ligament complex. Posterior displacement of more than 1cm in any direction indicates complete disruption of the ligamentous structure.

Classification of Pelvic Injuries

Pelvic ring instability was first described in 1859 (Malgaigne) in the double vertical fracture. Pennal in 1961 and Tile in 1995 further analyzed pelvic ring instability and described an A/B/C classification with stable situation A, intermediate situation B and unstable injuries C. This system was recently extended by the

AO/ASIF but their rather complex classification system may prove difficult to use in clinical practice because of a lack of inter- and intra-observer reliability.

A classification system should ideally provide guidelines for management (Pennig 1993). There are two main planes of instability (Fig. 20.4) which are divided into three types.

Type I is defined as an anterior horizontal instability with a lesion of the anterior pelvic ring (symphysis pubis and/or pubic rami) and stretching or rupture of the anterior portion of the sacro-iliac ligaments without displacement of the posterior elements of the pelvic ring (Fig. 20.5a, 20.5b). The pelvic volume is increased and a tamponade effect to stop haemorrhage may not occur. This justifies emergency restoration of pelvic ring geometry by closing the book.

Type II is defined as a posterior instability, IIA being a posterior horizontal instability, IIB a posterior vertical instability. The lesion of the posterior ring consists of a fracture and/or disruption of the SI joint, ilium and/or sacrum. The anterior pelvic ring in these cases has to show no injury or a non-significant one without displacement (Figs. 20.6a–20.6d) and the pelvic volume is not considerably increased. Treatment may be postponed and planned after CT scans show the extent of posterior damage.

Type III, a combination of Type I and II is an antero-posterior instability, IIIA being an antero-posterior horizontal instability, IIIB an antero-posterior vertical instability. The anterior pelvic ring in these cases shows a lesion with displacement of the symphysis pubis and/or the pubic rami. The posterior elements comprise a fracture and/or disruption of the SI joint, ilium and/or sacrum (Figs. 20.7a–20.7d). The pelvic volume may be significantly increased in these cases and emergency reduction is advisable to assist in stopping the haemorrhage. The haemorrhage occurs in the true pelvis and thereafter starts to fill up the retroperitoneum. The volume of the true pelvis is increased when the symphysis pubis and/or the sacro-iliac joint are displaced. For every centimetre of displacement of the symphysis pubis a volume increase of 4.6 per cent; for every centimetre in the sacro-iliac joint an increase of 3.1 per cent has been shown in studies. For combined displacements the volume changes were found to be additive (Moss and Bircher 1996).

The posterior ring is stabilized after 6–8 days with prior CT scanning to show the extent of the injury.

The classification is applied to each hemipelvis with the posterior injury component being used to define the side of the injury.

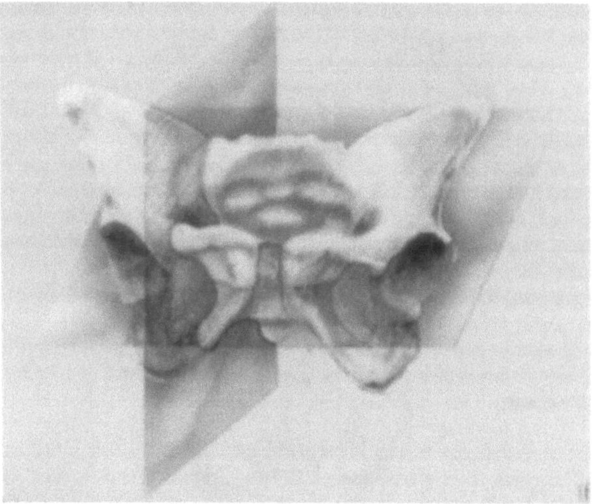

Fig. 20.4 There are two main planes of instability: a horizontal and a vertical plane.

a

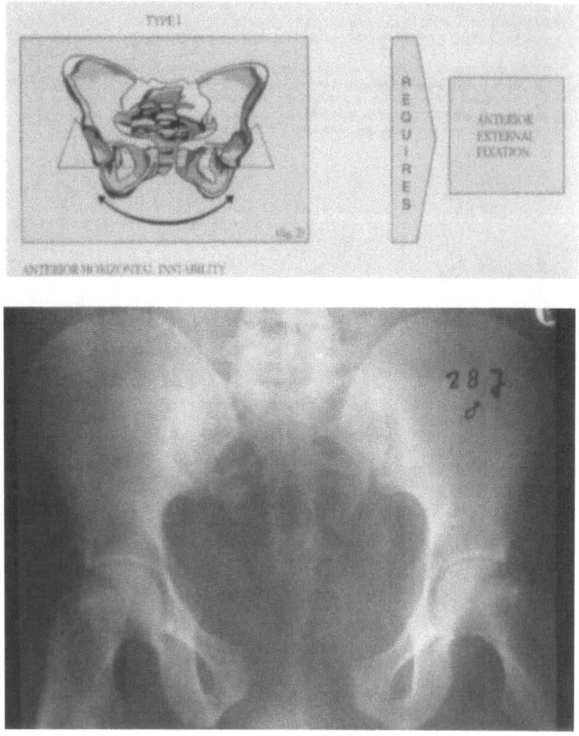

b

Fig. 20.5 a Anterior horizontal instability involving the symphysis pubis and/or pubic rami and also affecting the anterior portion of the sacro-iliac ligaments. **b** Example of a Type I (open book) injury in a 28-year-old male.

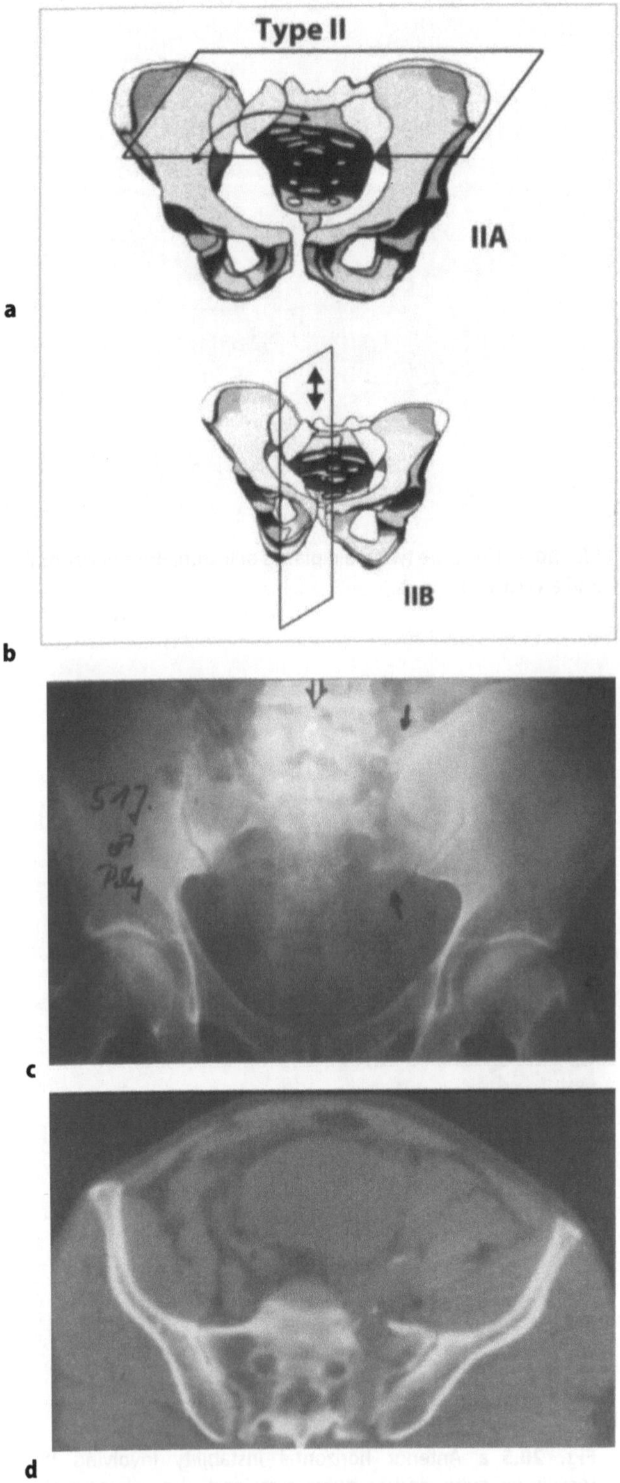

Fig. 20.6 **a** Type II A: Posterior horizontal instability involving the SI joint and/or a fracture of ilium and sacrum. The anterior pelvic ring in these cases shows no or a non-significant injury without displacement. **b** Type II B: Posterior vertical instability. **c** Vertical fracture of the left side of the sacrum in a 51-year-old male patient. The two small arrows indicate the fracture line, the large arrow indicates a burst fracture of L5. Note the intact anterior pelvic ring. **d** CT scan reveals the trans-sacral fracture. Injury to the pre-sacral plexus is common in these cases.

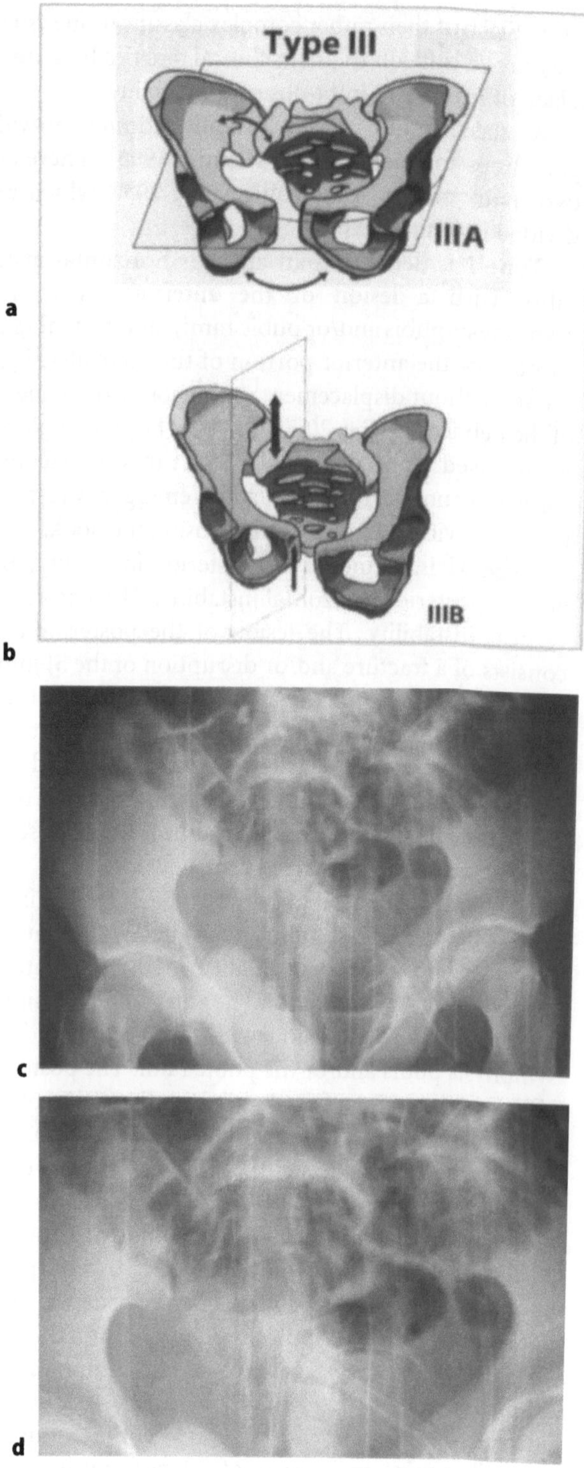

Fig. 20.7 **a** Anterior-posterior horizontal instability, Type III A. **b** Anterior-posterior vertical instability, Type III B. Type III A and B are combinations of Type I and II. **c** Example of a Type III B anterior-posterior vertical instability in a 28-year-old male. **d** The sacrum has been completely destroyed by the impact which results in significant bleeding.

Anatomical Aspects of Pin Insertion

The pelvis is a ring structure composed of sacrum, left and right hemipelvis. Each hemipelvis is formed by ilium, ischium and pubis. The three bones fuse at the tri-radiate cartilage in the acetabulum. The stabilizing factors are the ligaments since the three bones have no inherent stability at all and without the ligaments the pelvic ring would fall apart. For structural stability the posterior pelvic ring is most important. This view is supported by the clinical observation that patients with absence of the anterior strut have a stable link between the spine and the limbs. The posterior and anterior ligaments are the strongest in the pelvis and connecting ligaments (sacro-tuberous and sacro-spinous ligaments) provide further stability in the pelvic outlet. Ilio-lumbar ligaments connect the spine with the sacrum. The inner table of the ilium is covered by the iliac muscle, the outer by the gluteus muscles.

For pin insertion in external fixation the iliac crest and the area between the antero-superior and the antero-inferior iliac spine is available. The iliac crest can be palpated easily but the hemipelvis may be internally or more often, externally rotated. An open approach for pin insertion is advisable (Tile 1995). Close to the antero-superior iliac spine the lateral femoral cutaneous nerve crosses and may be injured by poorly controlled pin placement. For anterior placement a 4–5 cm incision is mandatory. The lateral femoral cutaneous nerve must be protected by Langenbeck retractors and the insertion of the rectus femoris muscle is identified. The capsule of the acetabulum should be respected to avoid penetration of the hip joint. In an anatomical study the most common pin insertion sites (iliac crest and anterior placement) were examined in cross-sections. In 9 hemipelves the distance from the outer to the inner table was measured. A minimum distance of 10mm was considered safe for insertion of 5 and 6mm pins. Fig. 20.8 shows that to only about 2cm below the iliac crest was the minimum width of 10mm available. Between the shaded areas in Fig. 20.8 penetration of the inner or outer cortex may be expected. This results in unicortical purchase of the pin which will not be fully embedded in bone at its distal end. The anterior application with pin insertion on and above the lower anterior iliac spine seems to be safer since a significantly larger area was found with a minimum width of 10mm. For purchase, the depth of insertion is also important and 50mm seems to be in consonance with these measurements (Figs. 20.9–20.11).

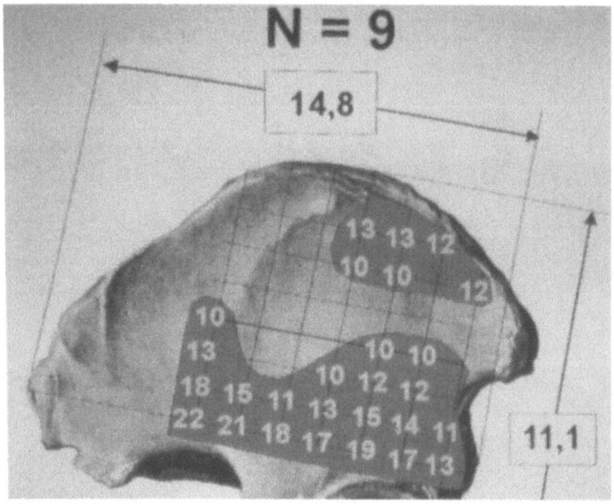

Fig. 20.8 Mean distance between the outer and the inner tables of the ilium. The darker areas indicate a sufficient distance for pin insertion between the two tables (numbers indicate the distance in mm between inner and outer tables). Note that the supra-acetabular region offers a wider cross-section with increased safety for pin placement.

Various insertion sites in cadaver pelves were assessed for the pull-out strength of bone screws. Just below the iliac crest the lowest pull-out force was observed, whereas the supra-acetabular site as used in the lower anterior application had the highest pull-out strength. For external fixation in pelvic injuries this indicates that from a mechanical point of view bone screw placement is more advantageous in the supra-acetabular area (Daum et al 1988).

A study on the effect of screw location on stability in pelvic external fixation compared the superior (iliac crest) and anterior supra-acetabular approach (Kim et al 1998). In Tile Type B injury it was shown that the anterior approach resulted in higher stiffness and reduced sacro-iliac joint separation. This means that an anteriorly applied external fixator better stabilizes the

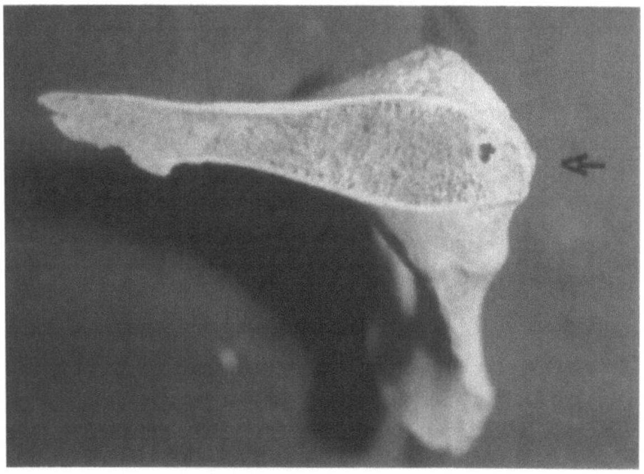

Fig. 20.9 View from the top of the supra-acetabular bone. The arrow indicates the lowest pin insertion site anteriorly.

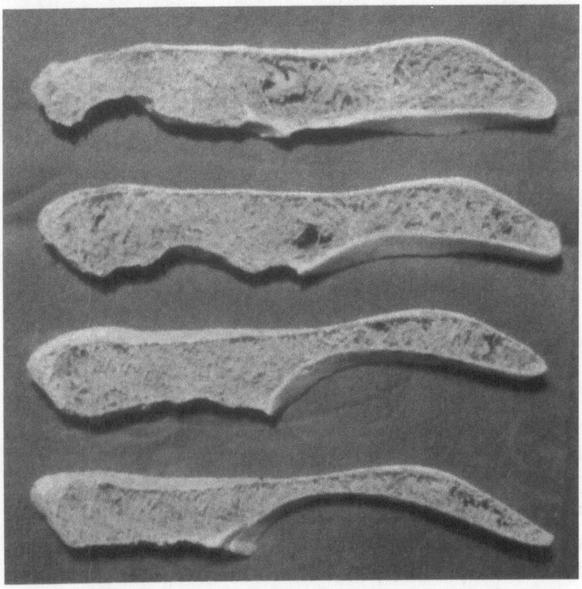

Fig. 20.10 Same view as in Fig. 20.9, 1cm slices starting on the level of the lowest pin (closest to the acetabulum, top piece). The top three slices provide adequate thickness for pin insertion.

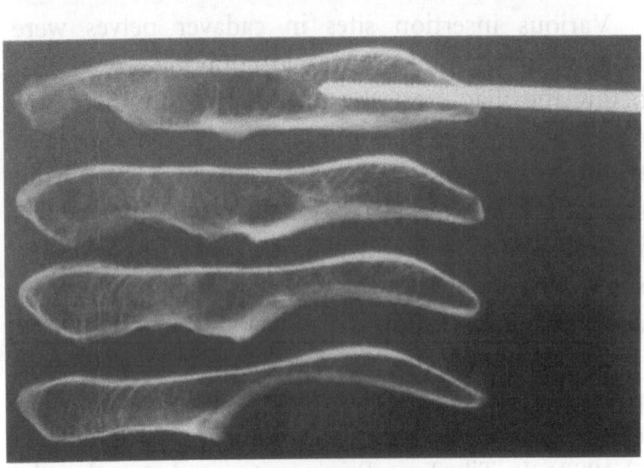

Fig. 20.11 Pin placement in the top slice shown in Fig. 20.10. A 6/5mm self-drilling self-tapping pin is used.

posterior pelvic ring than a device mounted on the iliac crest. The danger to the lateral femoral cutaneous nerve was also evaluated, and the study concluded that anterior location of external fixation screws is a safe and useful technique which provides a 30 per cent increase in stability over the iliac crest approach (Table 20.1).

	iliac crest		anterior	
type	AO-tubular	Orthofix	AO-tubular	Orthofix
Tile B	143.9	163.3	201.2	203.2
Tile C	no significant difference (p = 0.05)			

Table 20.1 The effect of screw location on stability of pelvic fixation (Kim et al 1998). Values shown are in Newton metres.

Pre-operative Management

A patient with a pelvic injury is usually polytraumatized and has to be resuscitated without delay. The anaesthetist's effort in resuscitating the patient requires the presence of the trauma or orthopaedic surgeon during the first hour of the patient's management. A simple and rapid way to stabilize the pelvis provided both femora are stable is to flex the hip and knee at 90° and wrap the two legs together with an elastic bandage. This will support the pelvic structure and also increase the venous return from the lower limbs. It is, however, only a temporary measure.

After obtaining an accurate history from the physician on site or the ambulance attendants, a physical examination is carried out. In Apley's algorithm the first step is to look. The patient has to be undressed and wounds must be carefully scrutinized. The detection of bleeding from the genitalia or rectum is vital. In the absence of leg fractures, rotation and shortening are indicators of pelvic ring displacement.

Apley's "feel and move" is also used in the pelvis. The contour of the pelvis should be palpated and the hemipelvis is carefully rotated at the antero-superior iliac spine and the iliac crest to detect abnormal movement. External rotation of the femora while palpating the iliac crest may be helpful to detect rotation of the hemipelvis. The symphysis pubis should be felt and a large gap indicates disruption. Traction should be applied with an intact limb to detect gross instability. In the conscious patient a neurological examination to determine injury to the lumbo-sacral plexus is performed. The most commonly injured nerve root (L 5) merits particular attention.

A standard X-ray of the same format as used by the anaesthetist for the chest is then obtained. With an image intensifier vertical displacement may be studied. Based on clinical examination and standard X-ray the surgeon is in a position to decide if emergency stabilization of the pelvic ring is necessary. CT studies, although readily available in most departments and an absolute necessity in an accident unit, may delay the resuscitation and therefore do not play such an important role in the first "golden hour". However, for further planning after emergency stabilization a CT study is mandatory.

In positioning the patient, ready access of the image intensifier to allow AP imaging of the pelvis must be ensured pre-operatively and the patient is moved on to the operating table if necessary. The patient should be in the supine position and the lower abdomen and proximal femora are shaved and disinfected. Draping

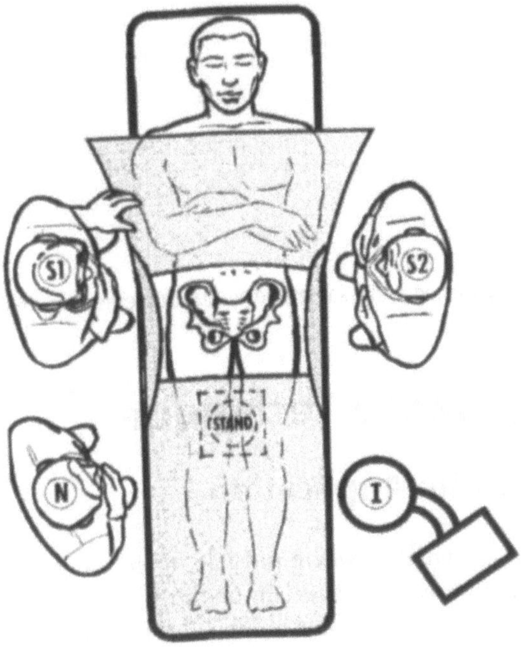

Fig. 20.12 A patient in the supine position. S1 and S2 are the position of the surgeons, N the nurse and I the image intensifier.

is then carried out, leaving free access from the umbilicus to the pubic area. The image intensifier (I) is positioned opposite the surgeon (S1) who should begin with the uninjured side. One assistant (S2) is required and the scrub nurse (N) should work from the same side as the surgeon. The legs of the patient should be accessible to allow an unscrubbed assistant to help with the reduction (Fig. 20.12).

Design of the Pelvic Fixator

Standard Configuration

The fixator consists of two primary links with ball joint attachments. The primary links are joined via a connector unit which comprises: a connector post, a grooved bush and a self-retaining cam.

To ensure that the clamps for the bone screws are correctly aligned when the fixator is assembled, the links must be presented to one another as shown in Fig. 20.13, one with the step beneath the collar facing upwards, and one with the step facing downwards. When assembling the fixator, the connector post is inserted into the two primary links and the grooved bush applied over it. The self-retaining cam is inserted with its pin facing downwards, from the side of the larger groove. If the pin at the extremity of the cam is not facing downwards, insertion of the cam is not possible. Slight rotational movement of the self-retaining cam may be needed to introduce it fully.

When a **supplementary link** is used, the two primary links are attached to the same side of the supplementary link with the step beneath the collar of each primary link facing the same direction (Fig. 20.14). For **independent screw placement** a straight bar with rotating clamps and a connecting ball joint module is available.

The components provided in the pelvic fixator kit allow for the entire spectrum of external fixation management.

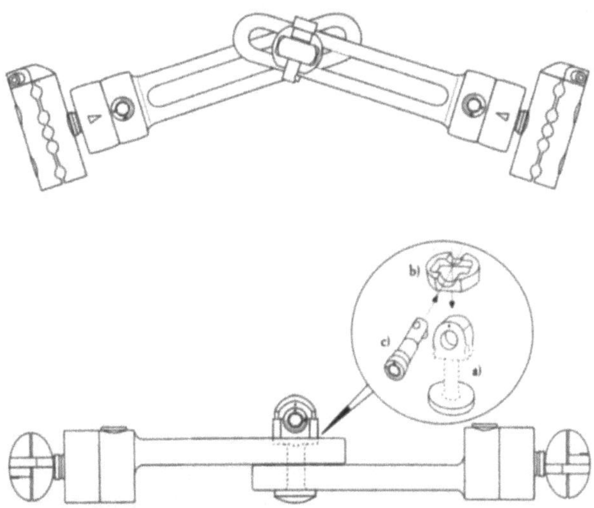

Fig. 20.13 The fixator consists of two primary links with ball joint attachments. The primary links are joined via a connector unit which comprises (a) a connector post, (b) a grooved bush and (c) a self-retaining cam.

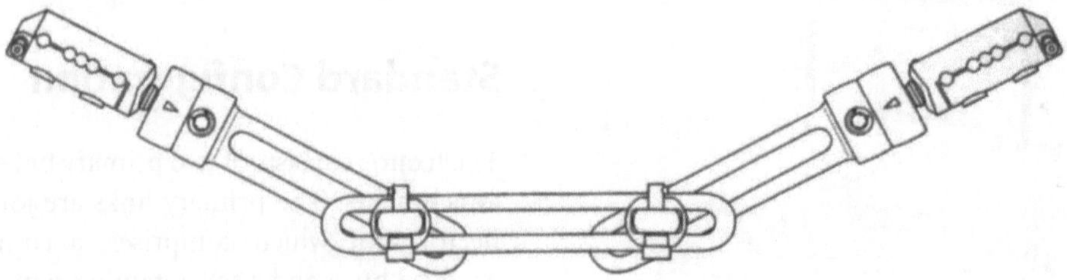

Fig. 20.14 When a supplementary link is used the two primary links are attached to the same side of the supplementary link with the step beneath the collar of each primary link facing the same direction.

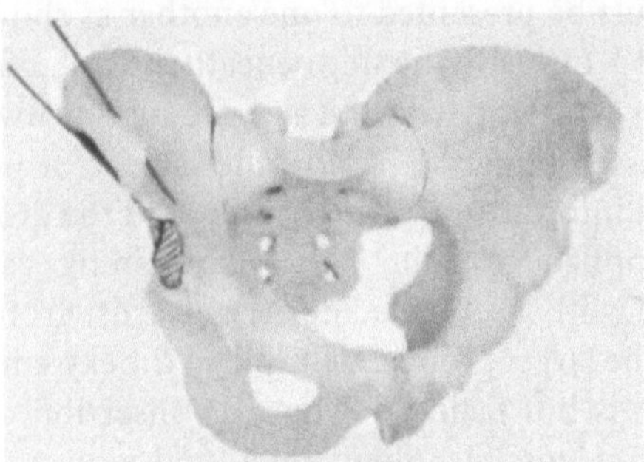

Fig. 20.15 A K-wire is used on the inner and the outer table of the ilium to identify orientation of the hemipelvis. The shaded area is the pin insertion site.

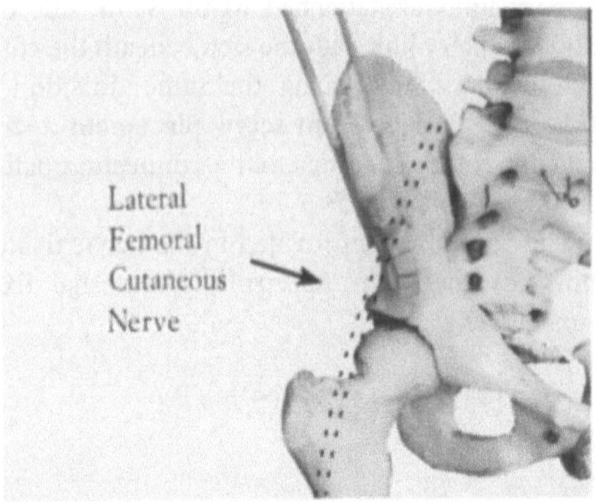

Fig. 20.16 The lateral femoral cutaneous nerve crosses in the proximal part of the incision.

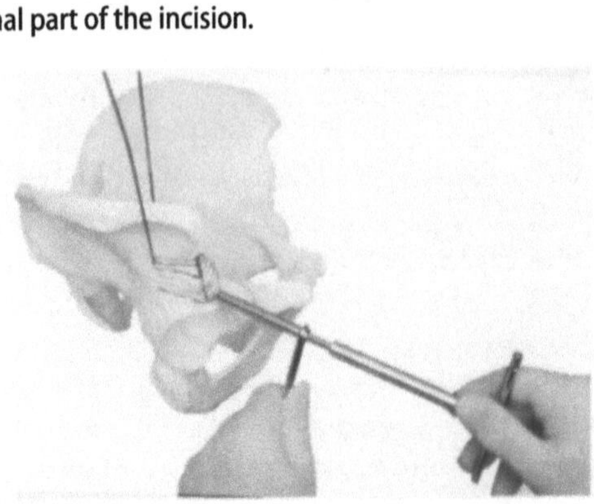

Fig. 20.17 Orientation of the first screw in the supra-acetabular bone.

Operative Technique

Anterior Application

It is advisable, where possible, to commence with the uninjured side, especially on the first few occasions that the external fixator is applied. The landmark for screw insertion is the anterior superior iliac spine which can be easily palpated.

To establish the orientation of the hemipelvis, which may be significantly rotated externally (most likely) or internally, a pair of Kirschner wires (1.6mm) should be used. The first K-wire is inserted from the iliac crest along the inner table of the ilium, while the second K-wire is inserted along the outer table of the ilium (Fig. 20.15).

Once the position of the hemipelvis has been established, a short, 3–4cm incision should be made, starting just below the anterior superior iliac spine. The lateral femoral cutaneous nerve must be protected from injury, by means of Langenbeck retractors (Fig. 20.16). The bone should be exposed and the screw guide for the first bone screw inserted down to the bone, taking account of the orientation provided by the two K-wires (Fig. 20.17). The inclination of the pelvis in a supine patient must be considered as illustrated in Figs. 20.18a–20.18c.

The screws should be inserted between the inferior and the superior iliac spines and more on the inferior side, starting with the screw at the level of the anterior inferior iliac spine. Screws should be angled slightly upwards to avoid penetration of the acetabulum and to allow the fixator body to be positioned in line with the anterior pelvic ring (Fig. 20.19).

A self-drilling, self-tapping screw with its long axis in the sagittal plane should be hammered through the cortex with gentle taps and then screwed home with the T-wrench. It is of the utmost importance not to force the screw in any direction, but rather to let it find

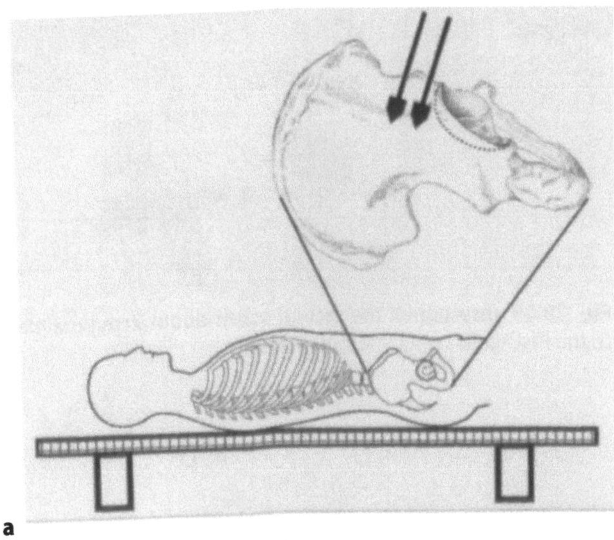

a

Fig. 20.18 a Note the inclination of the hemipelvis in the supine patient. b The two K-wires are shown of the left side. Insertion of the fixator pins must not be at right angles to the operating table because of the inclination of the hemipelvis. c This shows the correct insertion angle taking into account the inclination of the hemipelvis.

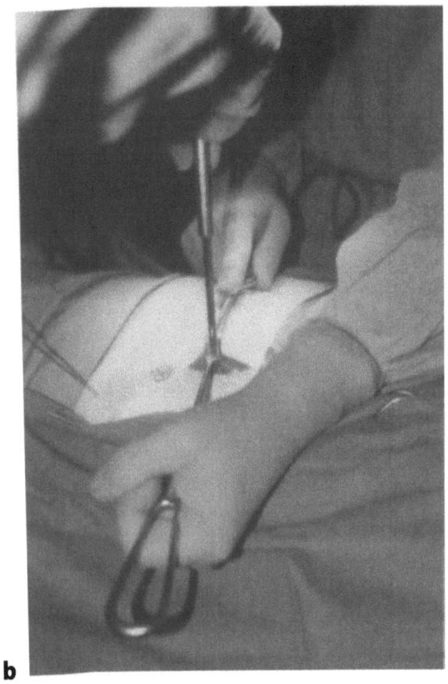

b

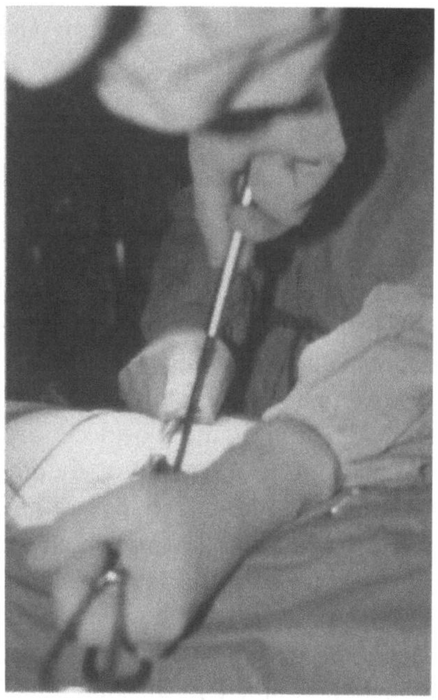

c

its way between the inner and outer tables of the ilium. The depth of insertion is 40–50mm, which is almost the entire thread length (Fig. 20.17).

The first screw in its screw guide is now housed in the first seat of the T-clamp. The second screw should be placed about 2cm proximal to the first screw, which will correspond to the third or fourth clamp seat (Fig. 20.19). It is important to make sure that the screw tip is not forced outside the pelvis. After a certain amount of practice, it may be preferable to insert the screws parallel to one another in both planes, freehand. In young patients (16 years and under), the use of a drill (3.2mm) to penetrate the hard cortex to a depth of 1cm may be necessary. If a drill bit is used, this power instrument should be handled with extreme care and a drill guide must be employed to protect the soft tissues.

When both screws have been inserted into the first hemiplevis, the procedure is repeated for the opposite hemipelvis. When choosing screw direction in the injured hemipelvis, its rotation must be taken into account and a reduction may be obtained by applying lateral force in open book injuries (Type I). Once the second pair of screws has been inserted, both pairs should be grasped firmly to ensure that they will be able to withstand the loads exerted upon them by the fixator during the process of reduction. Should there be any doubt about the appropriateness of screw placement, an X-ray must be taken at this stage (Figs. 20.20a. 20.20b).

T-clamps should be mounted on each pair of screws at a similar distance from the skin. The fixator is now applied and reduction carried out. To ensure that the clamps for the bone screws are correctly aligned when the fixator is applied, the links must be presented to one another as shown, with the steps beneath the collars pointing in opposite directions (Fig. 20.21).

To assist reduction, which in most cases implies internal rotation of the injured side, the legs may be used to gain leverage. Reduction can be accomplished with the manipulation forceps, which distance the surgeon's hands from the X-ray beam (Fig. 20.22).

With the ball joints and connector unit cam unlocked, reduction of virtually all types of pelvic displacement can be achieved under image intensification.

The nature of the fixator with its ball joints and sliding links is such that it was possible to simulate all of the examples of pelvic displacement in Figs. 20.23–20.26 starting from the neutral position. After reduction has been achieved the connector unit cam and the ball joint are tightened with the Allen wrench (Fig. 20.27).

It is important to make sure that the minimal distance between the fixator and the skin in all circumstances is more than 5cm, to allow for bowel distension which commonly occurs during intensive care management of these patients. Should it be necessary, the fixator can be adjusted to take account of abdominal distension by loosening the clamp screws and moving it away from the pelvis, following which the clamps screws are re-tightened. Final locking of the ball joints is performed with the torque wrench (Fig. 20.28). A Type I (open book) injury is shown in Fig. 20.29a. Closed reduction resulted in an anatomical position of the symphysis pubis (Fig. 20.29b). Fig. 20.30 illustrates the fixator application in an butterfly fragment involving both pubic rami. Plating would require a large exposure and closed reduction seems favourable.

Iliac Crest Application

If it is desired to use this approach, there are certain technical aspects to be considered. Whereas the iliac crest itself has a width of 10–15mm, immediately below the iliac crest the width of the bone is often less than 5mm (see Fig. 20.8). The likelihood of penetrating either the inner or the outer table is therefore considerable. In addition to the above, mention has already been made of the fact that the reduction of

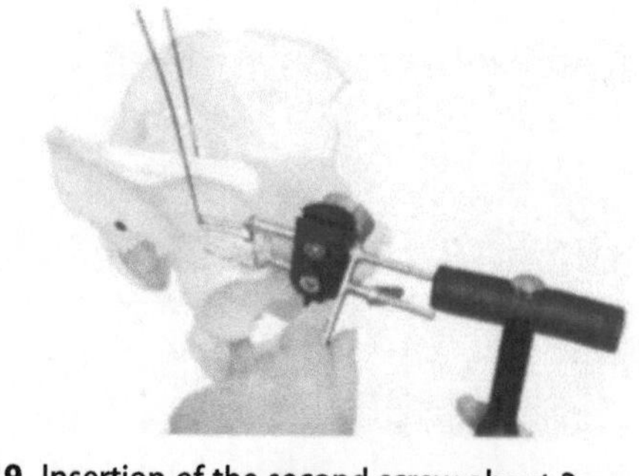

Fig. 20.19 Insertion of the second screw about 2cm proximal to the first screw using a template clamp.

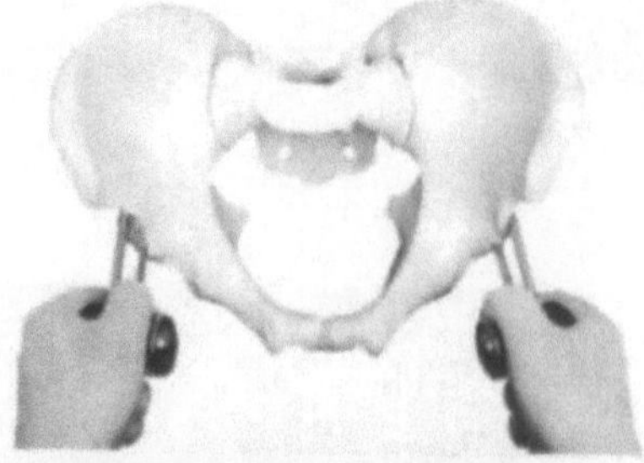

a

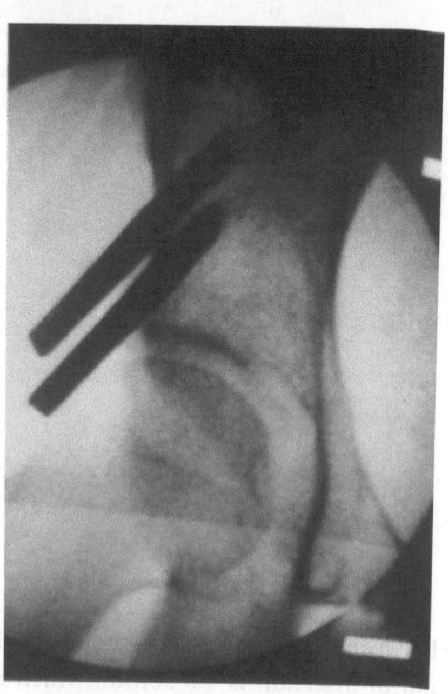

b

Fig. 20.20 a After insertion of two pins on both sides these are tested for stability first without and thereafter with the T-clamps mounted. **b** Radiographic check of correct pin placement in the AP film.

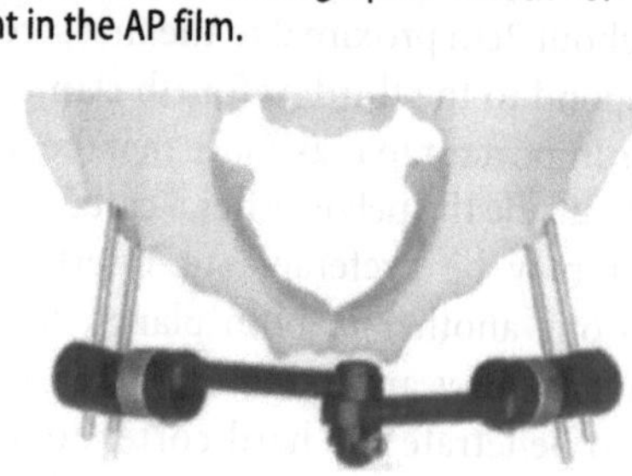

Fig. 20.21 Mounting of the fixator unit.

pelvic displacement from the top rather than the front is more cumbersome and may be compared to closing a book from the top or the front (Figs. 20.31a, 20.31b). Biomechanically there also seems to be a distinct disadvantage when compared to the anterior approach (Kim et al 1998). The pull-out strength of bone screws in the supra-acetabular bone is significantly higher than that in the area of the iliac crest (Daum et al 1998).

Straight Clamps

Screws (220/50) should be inserted at an angle of 45° to the long axis of the body through a 3–4cm incision over the iliac crest. The first screw is inserted 1.5–2.0cm posterior to the anterior superior iliac spine, through a screw guide (Fig. 20.32). The straight clamp is then mounted on the screw guide and the second screw inserted about 2cm posterior to the first (Fig. 20.33). Because of the hardness of the iliac crest, especially in younger patients, the path for the screws may be predrilled using a 3.2mm drill bit. The procedure is then repeated on the opposite site. The fixator is applied and reduction carried out (Fig. 20.34).

Independent Screw Placement

Since the iliac crest is a curved structure, one may wish to have the option of placing screws other than parallel to one another in a straight line. Thus, one may choose to insert screws in the centre of the crest where there is superior bone stock and at angles which will allow them to find the ideal path between the inner and the outer tables of the ilium. This may be achieved using

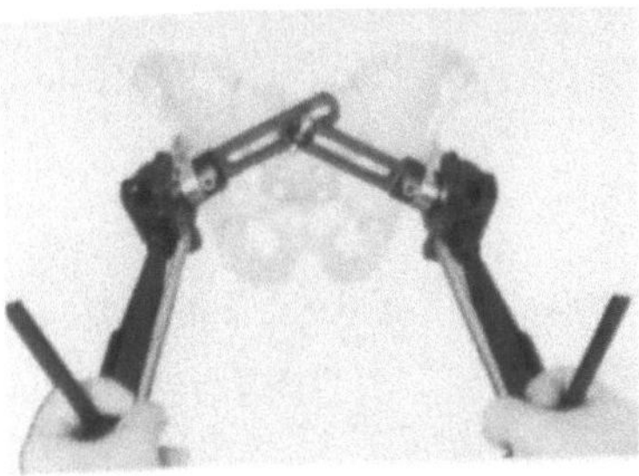

Fig. 20.22 Use of the manipulation forceps.

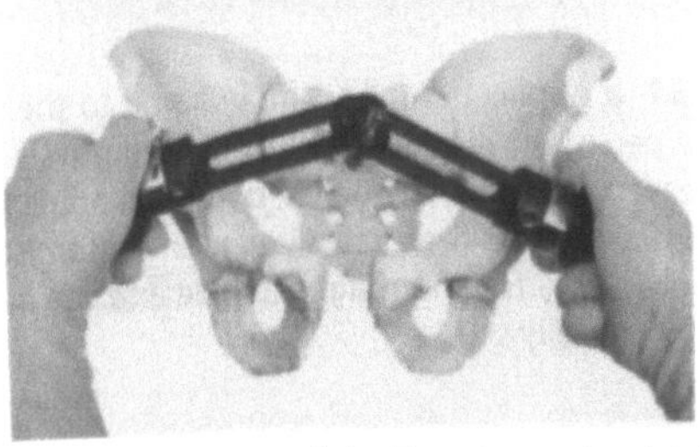

Fig. 20.23 Simulation of the Type I open book injury.

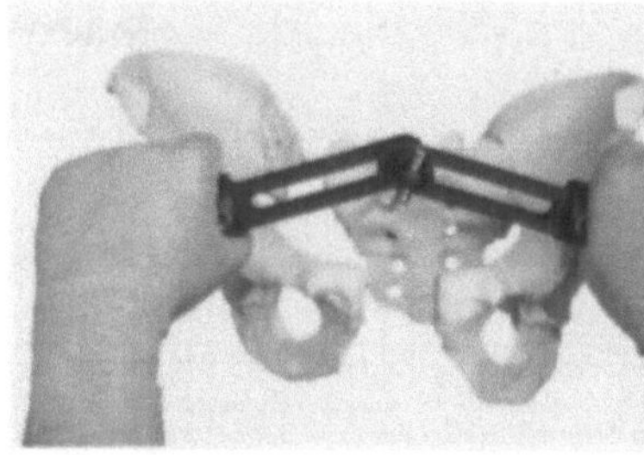

Fig. 20.24 Simulation of the Type III A anterior-posterior horizontal instability.

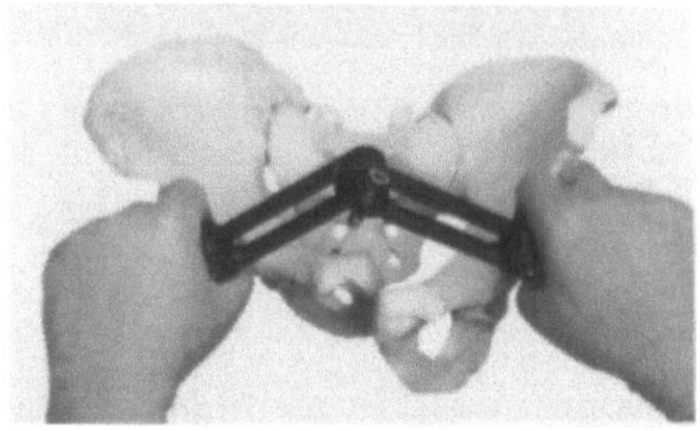

Fig. 20.25 Simulation of the Type III A with internal rotation of the hemipelvis (anterior-posterior horizontal instability).

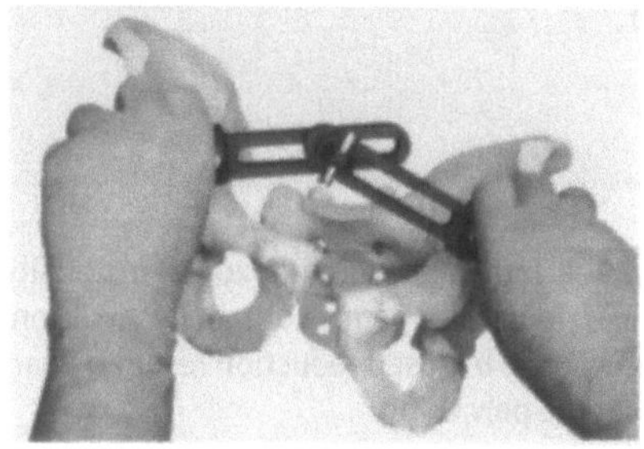

Fig. 20.26 Simulation of the Type III B injury (anterior-posterior vertical instability).

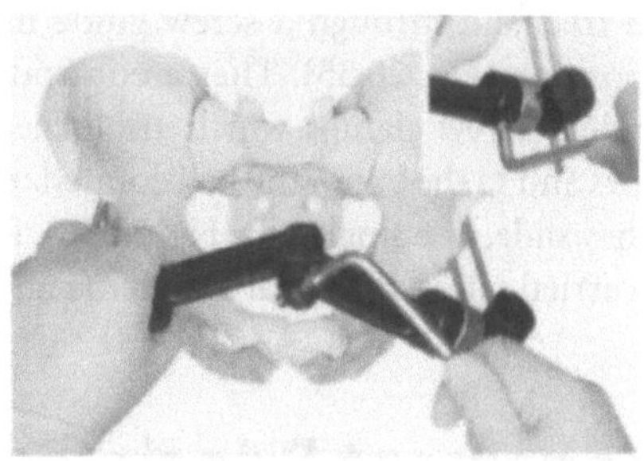

Fig. 20.27 Locking of the connector unit and the ball joint with an Allen wrench.

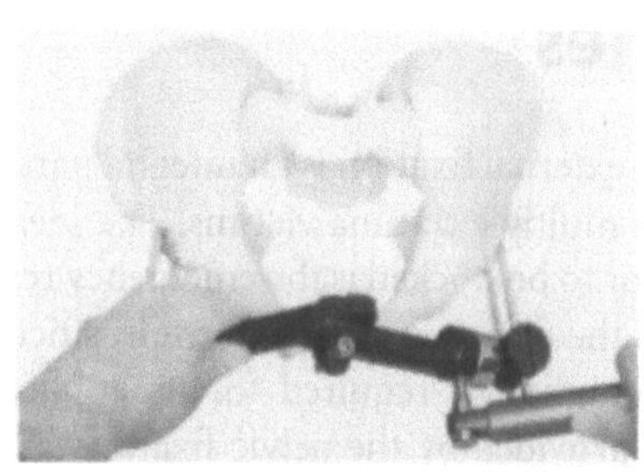

Fig. 20.28 Locking of the ball joints with a torque wrench.

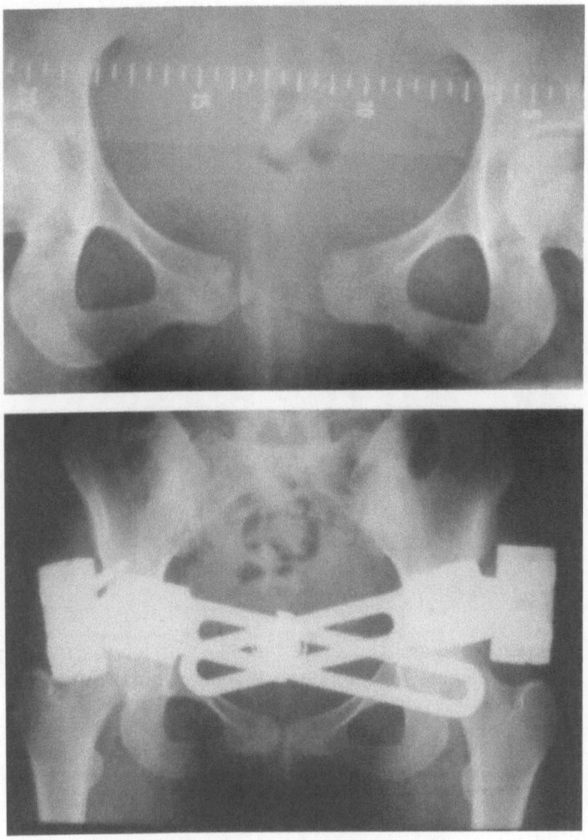

a

b

Fig. 20.29 **a** Type I (anterior horizontal instability) injury in a 28-year-old female patient. Note bony avulsion of the left symphysis pubis. **b** Closed reduction resulted in an anatomical position of the pelvic ring.

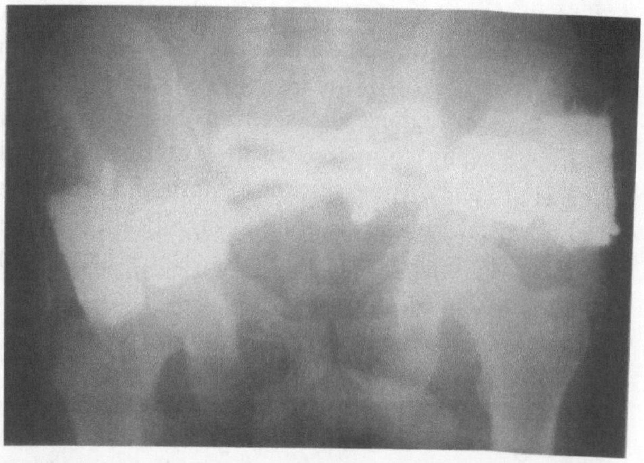

Fig. 20.30 Anterior fixator application in a butterfly fragment involving both pubic rami. Closed reduction was performed with anterior fixator application.

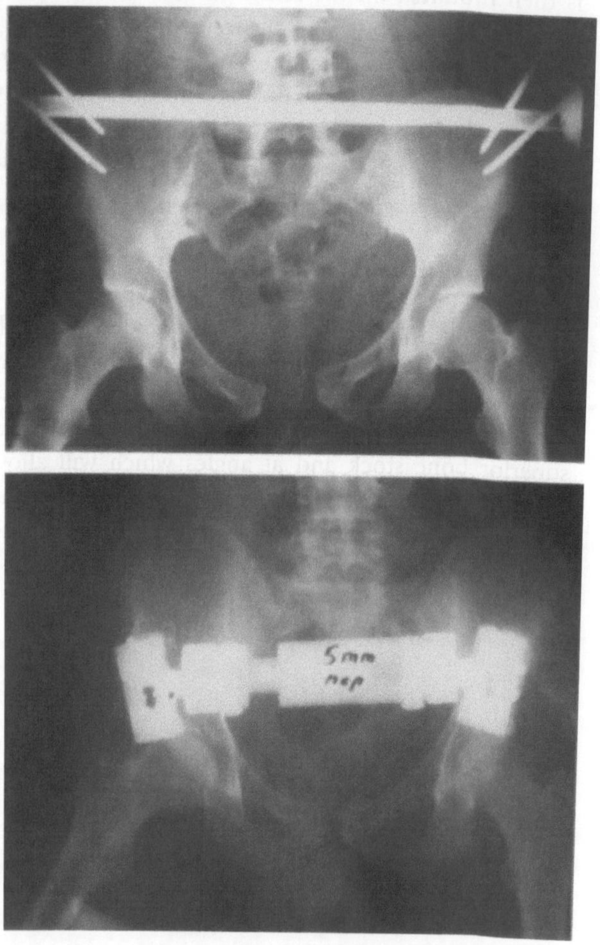

a

b

Fig. 20.31 **a** Application of a simple frame to the iliac crest. Note the persistent displacement of the symphysis pubis and the increased volume of the pelvis. **b** Anterior application of an Orthofix 10.000 series fixator resulted in an anatomical position of the pelvic ring. Haemorrhage stopped and the patient was haemodynamically stable.

ball-jointed modules for independent screw placement. Where these modules are used, screws are inserted freehand through a screw guide in the preferred position (Fig. 20.35). They are introduced into independent screw clamps which are locked both to the screws and to the bar of the ball-jointed module on which they slide, by a single nut (Fig. 20.36). Reduction is then carried out in the usual manner (Fig. 20.37).

Management Principles in Posterior Pelvic Ring Injuries

Anterior external fixation is an integral part of resuscitation in multiple trauma victims. The ideal place for the fixator to be stocked is the emergency resuscitation area and the device is suitable for this, since no power instrumentation is required for its application. The stability provided by the pelvic fixator was proven in mechanical studies (Bell et al 1988) and its three-dimensional reduction capacity has been demonstrated. The fixator in the anterior position, however, only replaces the tension band effect of the pubic rami and the symphysis pubis. It cannot control a significant posterior instability and for this, the steps outlined below must be followed.

To assess posterior pathology, CT scanning (Fig. 20.6d) and examination under fluoroscopy are mandatory. CT scanning does not necessarily have to be carried out on the day of injury but should be performed over the next few days. At this point it is important to decide whether the patient can be dealt with within the receiving institution, or if referral is advisable.

Without familiarity in fixation of the posterior pelvic ring, the results in vertically or horizontally unstable posterior injuries will be less favourable. The CT scan should encompass the full range from the fifth lumbar vertebra downwards. Injuries of the posterior ring may involve the SI joints, vertical fractures of the sacrum and/or an intra-articular fracture of the ilium. All of these injuries require techniques which are illustrated in Figs. 20.38–20.43.

Posterior surgery should not be delayed for more than six to eight days. If delayed any longer, bone formation will commence, especially in those cases where head injury is present. Under such circumstances, reduction of a vertical displacement or a horizontal displacement may become exceedingly difficult. The resultant leg length discrepancy and/or the neurological complications encountered will significantly influence the outcome.

Post-operative Management

During the immediate post-operative period, haemoglobin levels and haemodynamics should be carefully monitored, which is routine in multiple trauma vic-

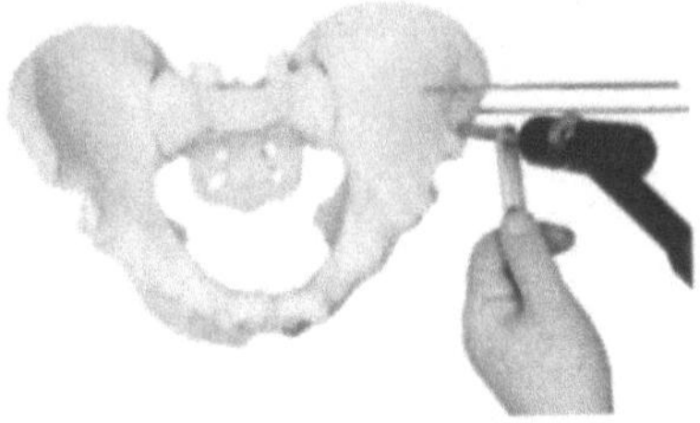

Fig. 20.32 Iliac crest application. The shaded area indicates the most suitable position for pin placement. The two K-wires facilitate orientation.

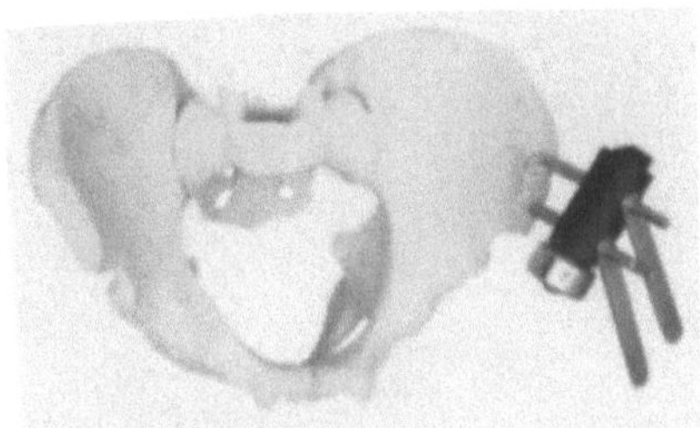

Fig. 20.33 A straight clamp is mounted and the second pin inserted.

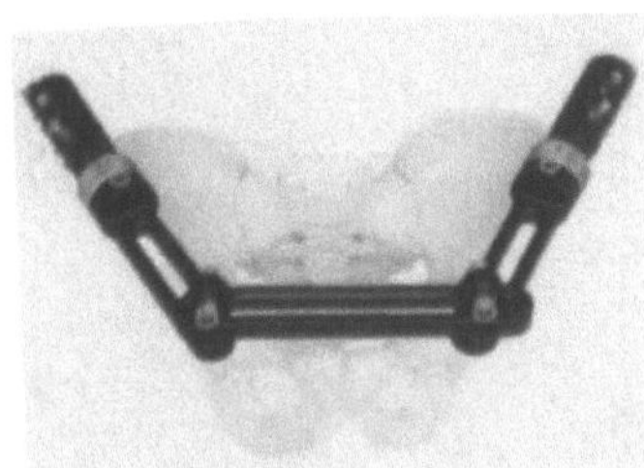

Fig. 20.34 After the repetition of the procedure in the opposite side the fixator with a supplementary link is applied and reduction carried out.

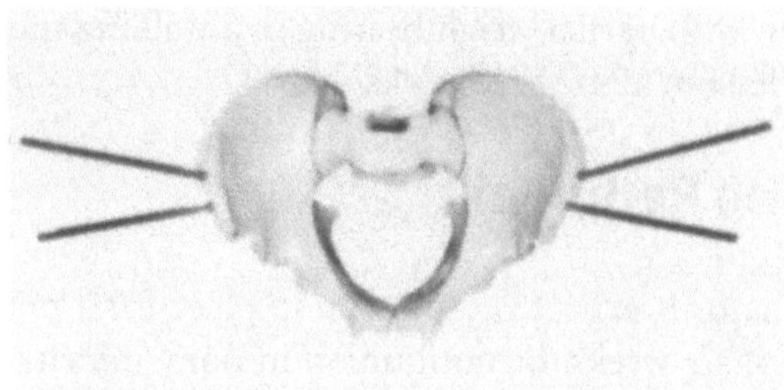

Fig. 20.35 Application with ball jointed modules for independent screw placement. Four screws have been inserted with free choice of pin orientation.

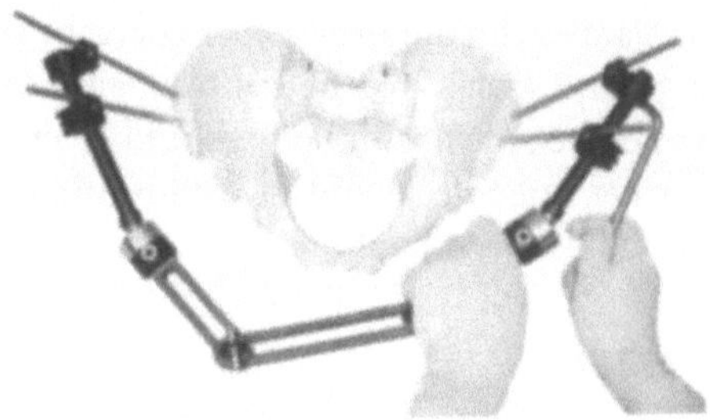

Fig. 20.36 Mounting of the independent screw clamps and a pelvic fixator with a supplementary link.

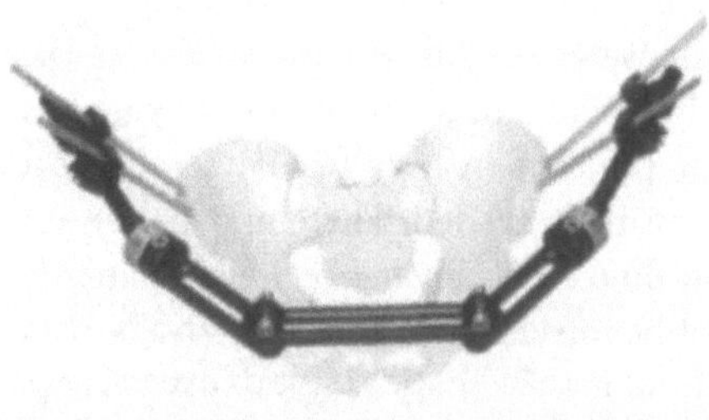

Fig. 20.37 Reduction is carried out in the usual manner.

tims. Should the patient continue to lose blood and other sources of bleeding have been excluded, arteriography should be carried out early (within six hours of fixator application) (Fig. 20.44).

Under ideal circumstances the angiography suite should be equipped with the means of embolizing the ruptured vessels. The value of MAST trousers has not been proven under these circumstances, and adverse effects have been reported. If the patient requires to be turned on either side, preference is given to the uninjured hemipelvis.

Since physiotherapy should be started on day one in these patients to help to prevent the sometimes lethal complication of deep vein thrombosis, there will be considerable movement of the skin around the screws. Daily changes of dressing are initially necessary and the incision should be checked to determine whether it is generous enough, or whether it rubs against the screws. If this is the case, it must be enlarged. Physiotherapy should continue with the patient being allowed to sit up, if possible, after one week and mobilization with partial weightbearing in a walking frame is carried out after three weeks.

Frame Removal

The fixator is expected to remain in place for a minimum of six weeks, or until union in bony injuries of the anterior pelvic ring, and for nine weeks in lesions of the symphysis pubis. At the end of the treatment period the fixator body is removed first, leaving the screws with the clamps in situ. Mobilization is continued and if no pain or discomfort is experienced by the patient, clamps and screws may be removed after one week. If pain persists, the fixator body should be reapplied for a further three weeks and a weightbearing X-ray on either limb is carried out.

Pin Site Care

The visible parts of the screws and surrounding skin should be cleaned on the day following application of the Pelvic Fixator and at least once a day thereafter. Only sterile water should be used for this purpose. A dry absorbent dressing with additional gauze is used around the pin sites. After a few days, when they are dry, no dressing is needed. There may be some drainage of clear fluid especially in overweight patients. This should not be mistaken for infection and is not a true complication. It may be the result of excessive patient mobility and subsequent irritation of the tissues

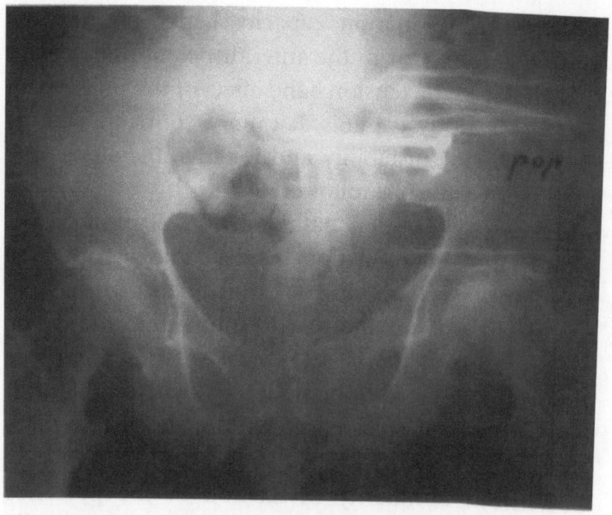

Fig. 20.38 Posterior screw placement in the case shown in Figs. 20.6c, 20.6d. The screws should not be overtightened to avoid nerve root entrapment in the sacral fracture.

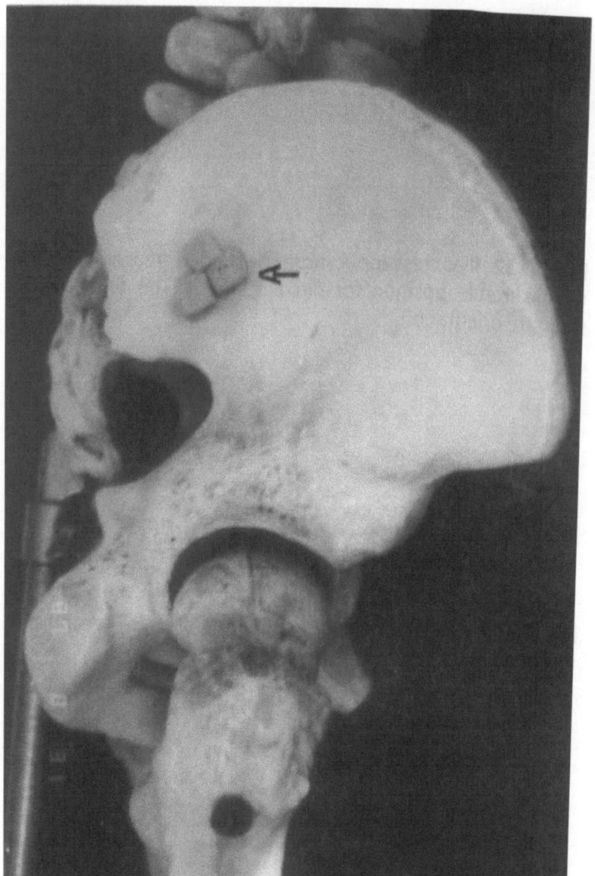

Fig. 20.39 The screws shown in Fig. 20.38 are inserted in the area indicated by the arrow.

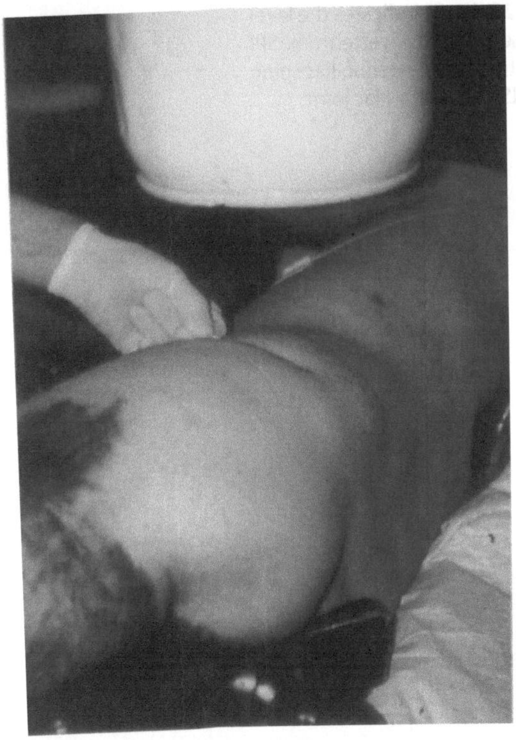

Fig. 20.40 Lateral decubitus position with the patient on the uninjured side. K-wires are used to identify S1 in the lateral film.

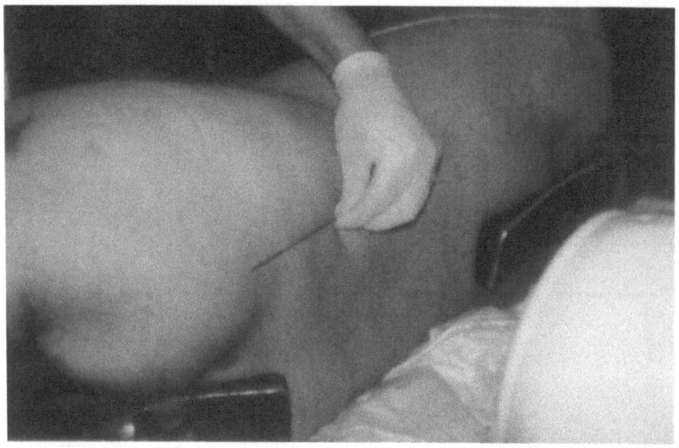

Fig. 20.41 With the image intensifier providing an AP view the SI joint level is identified with help of a K-wire.

A. INTRA-OPERATIVE COMPLICATIONS	
Injury to the lateral femoral cutaneous nerve or a branch of the circumflex artery.	This may be avoided by using blunt dissection down to the bone and protecting structures at risk with Langenbeck retractors.
Poor purchase of the bone screws in the pelvis.	The screw/s should be removed and resited.
Inadequate reduction of the pelvic pelvic ring achieved.	Assess for posterior pelvic ring pathology (CT scan), and if this is absent, check for possible interposition of bladder or other soft tissues in the symphysis pubis.
B. POST-OPERATIVE COMPLICATIONS	
Insufficient distance between fixator body and skin, a situation which, if not corrected, could predispose to pressure sores in regions of contact.	Loosen clamp screws and slide fixator away from skin surface. Retighten clamp screws to establish fixator in its new position
Pin track infection.	Enlarge skin and soft tissue incision around screw/s involved and follow established procedures for Pin Site Care.
Bone osteolysis at pin site.	Remove and resite screw.
Pain during mobilization.	Check for posterior pathology (CT scan). Decrease weightbearing temporarily.
Signs of peripheral oedema and pain.	Check for deep vein thrombosis and if present treat accordingly.
Colostomy required, increasing the risk of contamination of pin sites by faecal organisms.	Protect pin sites at all times with appropriate dressings.
Draining sinus after screw removal.	Surgical exploration and debridement of the sinus.

Table 20.2 Possible complications and recommended actions

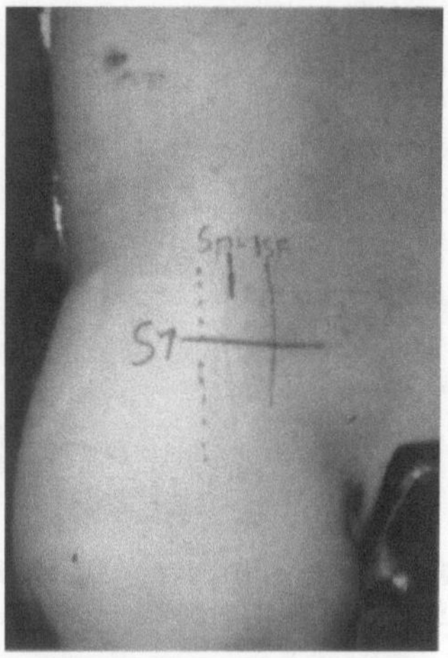

Fig. 20.42 S1 indicates the level of the first sacral vertebrum. SPI identifies the posterior iliac spine and ISF the sacro-iliac joint.

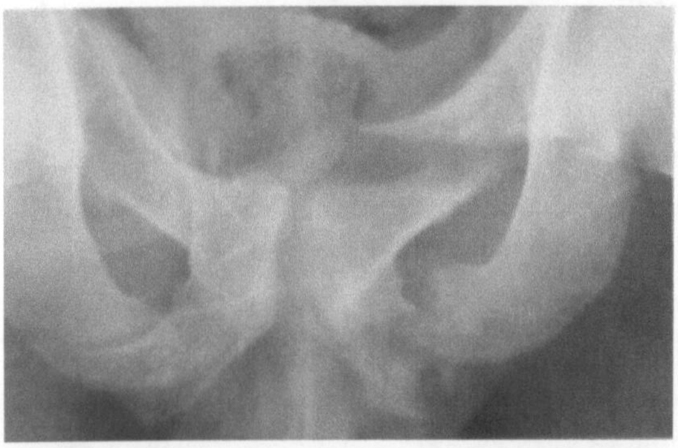

a

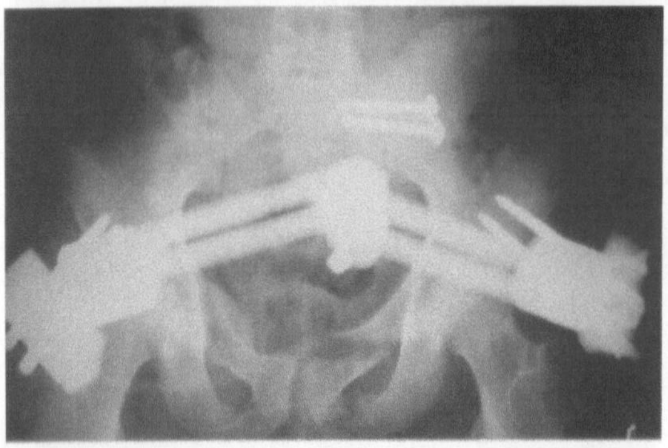

b

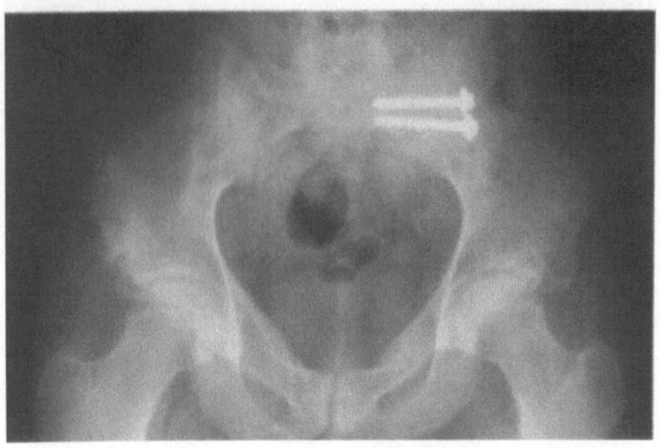

c

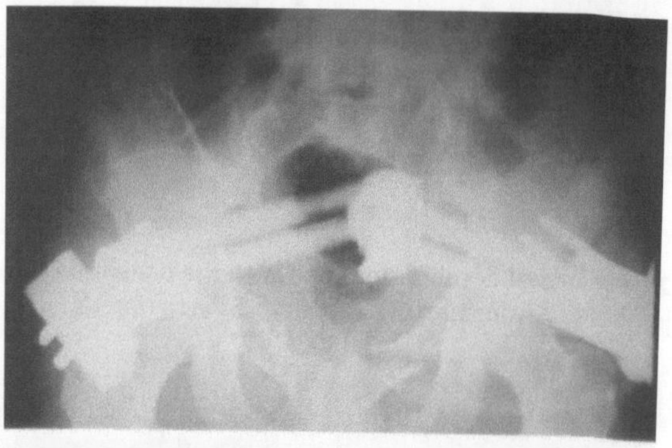

d

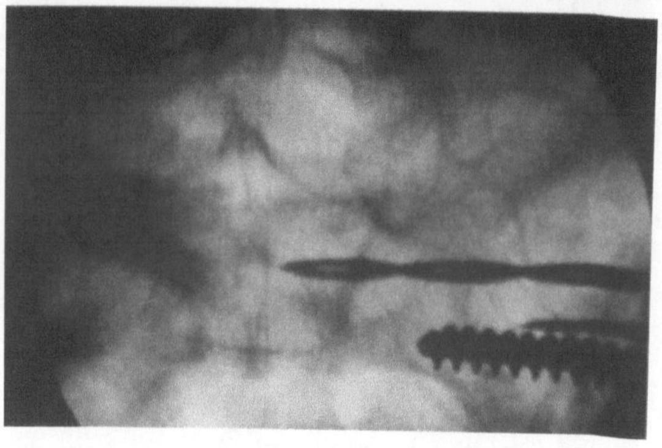

e

Fig. 20.43 **a** Type III A anterior-posterior horizontal instability in a 32-year-old male. Note the butterfly fracture of the pubic rami. The sharp spike of the left pubic ramus has perforated the bladder and the small intestine. Rupture of the urethra was present. **b** Anterior application of the fixator and stabilization of the pelvic ring. **c** Image intensifier view for posterior fixation in the case shown in **a** and **b**. In the centre a 1.6mm K-wire is present. The lower screw has been inserted in the direction of S1 and the upper screw is about to be inserted. The use of cannulated screws does not seem to provide an advantage since the passage of the drill cannot be felt through the outer table of the ilium, the inner table and into the sacrum. During this procedure the fixator components were loosened. **d** Position of the posterior screws above the foramen of S1. Note the position of the butterfly fragment. **e** Bony union of the anterior pelvic ring occurred after six weeks. One year follow-up shows anatomical reduction of the pelvic ring.

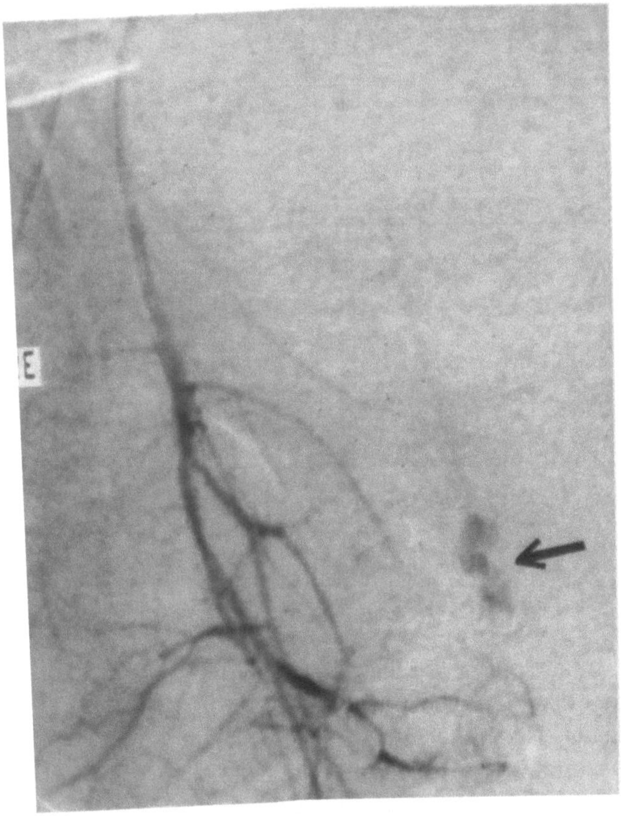

Fig. 20.44 Angiogram in a haemodynamically unstable patient four hours after anterior fixator application. The arrow indicates bleeding from the right obdurator artery.

around the screws. Normal care on pin cleaning is required.

When inflammation is seen and the exudate is purulent with the skin around the screw red and warm, a bacteriological swab should be taken and the appropriate antibiotic given for about a week. In the presence of a colostomy, the pin sites should be supervised very closely to detect any signs of incipient infection which, if it occurs, should be treated aggressively. Weightbearing should be restricted until resolution has occurred.

References

Apley AG, Solomon L (1993) *Apley's system of orthopaedics and fractures* (7th ed). Butterworth-Heinmann Ltd.: Oxford.

Basmizian JV (1989) see Grant.

Bell AL, Smith RA, Broon TD et al 'Comparative Study of the Orthofix and Pittsburgh Frames by External Fixation of Unstable Pelvic Ring Fractures.' *J Orthop Trauma* 1988 2(2): 130–8.

Daum WJ, Tencer AF, Cartwright TJ et al 'Pull-Out Strengths of Bone Screws at Various Sites About the Pelvis – A Preliminary Study.' *J Orthop Trauma* 1998 2(3): 229–33.

Kim WY, Hearn TC, Seleem O et al (1998) 'Effect of Screw Location on Stability of Pelvic External Fixation' – Abstract presented on the OTA Meeting 1998.

Malgaigne JF (1859) *Treatise in Fractures.* Lippincott: Philadelphia.

Meighan A, Gregory A, Kelly M et al 'Pelvic fractures: the golden hour.' *Injury* 1998 29(3): 211–213.

Moss MC and Bircher MD 'Volume changes within the true pelvis during disruption of the pelvis ring. Where does the haermorrhage go?' *Injury* 1996 27, Suppl.1: 21–3.

Pauwels F (1965) *Gesammelte Abhandlung zur funktionellen Anatomie des Bewegungsapparates.* Springer Verlag: Berlin.

Pennal GF, Tile M, Waddell JP et al 'Pelvic disruption: Assessment and classification.' *Clin Orthop Relat Res* 1980 151: 12–21.

Pennig D 'The place of anterior external fixation in the stabilization of pelvic ring disruptions.' Suppl. 1993 *Int J Orthop Trauma* 3(3): 44–8.

Slätis P, Huittinen VM 'Double vertical fractures of the pelvis.' *Acta Chirurg Scand* 1972 138: 799–807.

Tile M (1995) *Fractures of the Pelvis and Acetabulum* (2nd ed.). Williams & Wilkens: Baltimore.

Supplementary Bibliography

Buchholz RW 'The pathological anatomy of Malgaigne fracture dislocations of the pelvis.' *J Bone Joint Surg* [Am] 1981 63-A: 400–404.

De Bastiani G, Aldegheri R, Renzi-Brivio L 'The treatment of fractures with a Dynamic Axial Fixator.' *J Bone Joint Surg* [Br] 1984 66-B: 538–45.

Grant (1980) *Method of Anatomy* (4th ed). Wilkens & Wilkens: Baltimore.

Haeske-Seeberg H (1988) Inaugural Dissertation, Westfälische Wilhelms-Univesität Münster.

Hesp WL, van der Werken C, Keunen RW et al 'Unstable fractures and dislocations of the pelvic ring: results of treatment in relation to the severity of injury.' *Netherlands J Surg* 1985 37: 148–52.

Martin JG, Nepola JV, Marsh JL 'The treatment of unstable pelvic injuries with the Orthofix external fixator.' Suppl. *Intern J Orthop Trauma* 1993 3(3): 49.

Mears DC, Fu FH 'Modern concept of external skeletal fixation of the pelvis.' *Clin Orthop* 1980 151: 65.

Müller-Färber J, Müller KH 'Die verschiedenen Formen der instabilen Beckenringverletzungen und ihre Behandlung.' *Unfallheilkunde* 1984 87: 441–5.

Pennig D, Renzi-Brivio: *Pelvic Applications. Fractures and Disruptions of the Pelvic Ring. Operative Technique* Orthofix Srl., Bussolengo, Italy.

Pennig D, Gladbach B, Majchrowski 'Disruption of the pelvic ring during spontaneous childbirth. A case report.' *J Bone Joint Surg* 1997 79-B: 438–40.

Pennig D, Klein W, Brug E (1989) 'Pelvic ring disruptions.' in: *External Fixation and Functional Bracing.* Coombs R, Green S, Sarmiento A (eds.) Orthotex: England.

Rieger H, Pennig D, Brug E el al 'Beckenringverletzungen und Bauchtrauma.' *Unfallchirurg* 1991 94: 110–5.

Schweiberer I, Dambe LT, Klapp F 'Die Mehrfachverletzung: Schweregrad und therapeutische Richtlinien.' *Chirurg* 1978 49: 608–14.

Tile M 'Pelvic ring fractures: should they be fixed?' *J Bone Joint Surg* [Br] 1988 70-B: 1–2.

SECTION 4 THE LOWER LIMB

Proximal Femoral Fractures: the Pertrochanteric Fixator

21

E. Alcivar A.

Introduction

While it has now been demonstrated convincingly that mortality rates following trochanteric fractures of the femur can be dramatically reduced when surgical, as opposed to conservative treatment is employed, (Kennedy et al 1957; Evans 1949; Riska 1970; Dahl 1980), recent attention has tended to focus mainly on internal methods of fracture stabilization such as the sliding hip screw, or an intramedullary device such as the Gamma nail. While both of these techniques produce acceptable results, a number of problems associated with their use have been reported in the literature (Wolfgang, Bryant and O'Neill 1982; Nunn 1988; Simpson, Varty and Dodd 1989, Davis et al 1990, Bridle et al 1991; Halder 1992; Mahaisavariya and Laupattarakasem 1992; Fornander et al 1994).

Fractures of this type frequently occur in elderly osteoporotic patients with concomitant medical disorders, who are unable to tolerate lengthy periods of anaesthesia or any appreciable blood loss. External fixation, therefore, represents an attractive alternative, since it offers a less invasive and potentially more rapid means of stabilization. Several reports of the use of external fixation have appeared in the literature over the years (Scott 1957; Gotfried et al 1985; Dhal et al 1991). Encouraged initially by the work of Scott, this clinic has used external fixation as the treatment of choice for these fractures since 1960. The initial work was carried out by the father of the author, Eduardo Alcivar Elizade, and continued by the author.

In all, four devices have been used over a period of more than 30 years. We initially used the Roger Anderson Fixator. This fixator had a simple design which enabled two screws to be placed in a convergent fashion along the femoral neck, and two screws in the femoral shaft. The device could be applied rapidly and convergent placement of the proximal scews prevented redisplacement of the reduced fracture. The device was flimsy in its construction, however, and early mobilization of heavier patients was not always possible. The first 950 cases in the unit were treated using this fixator.

We next used the conventional Hoffmann fixator with two parallel screws introduced along the femoral neck and two into the femoral shaft. This device was somewhat more robust, and was used to treat 180 patients, but it was felt that its stability could be further improved. This led the author to produce an improved design incorporating a three-component clamp (Fig. 21.1) which would permit the introduction of up to 6 screws into the femoral neck, and incorporated a stout rod to confer even greater strength. This device represented a major improvement in stability, but while it was used successfully in the next group of 189 patients it was still not ideal. In the case of both the conventional Hoffmann and the author's improved design, parallel placement of the screws along the femoral neck meant that some degree of loss of reduction was possible, and while in the author's design up to four screws could be placed in the femoral shaft, all of these were committed to a single plane of introduction which might not always have been the most appropriate one in a given patient.

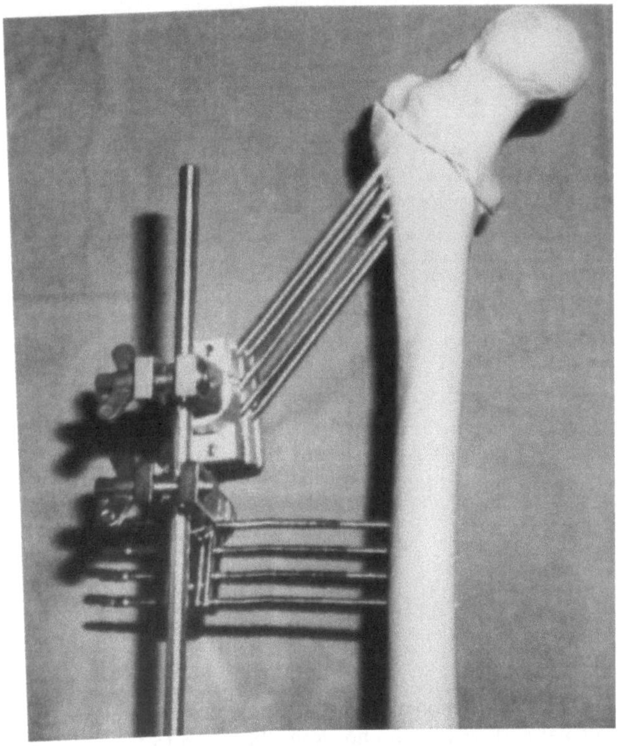

Fig. 21.1 Author's original model.

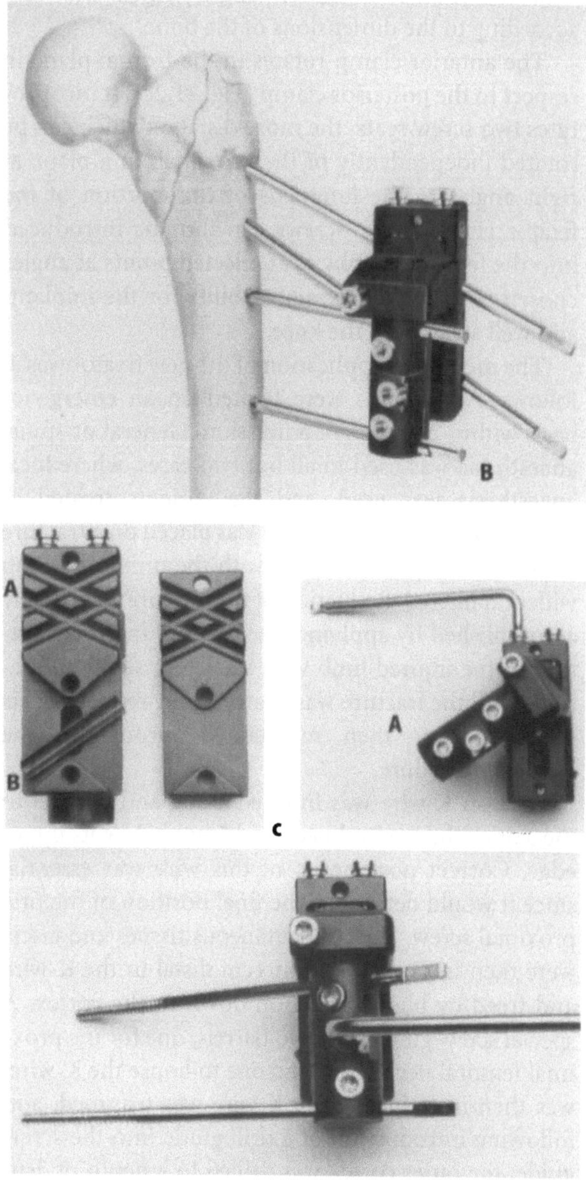

Fig. 21.2 **a** The pertrochanteric fixator with anterior (A) and posterior (B) clamp components. **b** The posterior clamp with two fixed seats at 115° to the longitudinal axis (A) and one swivelling seat (B) to permit convergent placement. **c** Movement of the anterior clamp in the frontal plane is controlled by locking screws. **d** Rotation of the distal screw seat of the anterior clamp in relation to the proximal seat is controlled by a locking screw.

Problems inherent in the stability or versatility of the devices used initially, led the author to collaborate in the design of new fixator (Orthofix srl, Verona, Italy) for the treatment of pertrochanteric fractures, which addressed the shortcomings in the earlier models used. The present chapter is a preliminary report on the results obtained with this new fixator.

Patients and Methods

Patients were deemed suitable for treatment with external fixation if they presented with stable pertrochanteric fractures, if they were polytrauma victims, in poor physical condition or of limited resources. In addition to the above, which were considered to be absolute indications, we also often employed external fixation in patients with unstable trochanteric fractures, subtrochanteric fractures, patients with associated fractures of the distal femur and patients whose religious convictions proscribed the use of blood transfusions. Obesity, residence in rural areas far from medical supervisory services, obviously poor levels of self-care, cutaneous disease in the region where screws would be inserted and extreme osteoporosis were considered as contraindications to use of the technique.

The new fixator (Fig. 21.2a) is compact and unobtrusive. It comprises a posterior clamp and an anterior clamp. The former has two fixed screw seats machined at an angle of 115° to the longitudinal axis, and one swivelling screw seat (Fig. 21.2b). Thus one screw is introduced along and parallel to the femoral neck, while a second screw is placed such that it will converge with the first at a chosen angle, which will vary according to the dimensions of the bone.

The anterior clamp rotates in the frontal plane in respect to the posterior clamp (Fig. 21.2c). It incorporates two screw seats, the more distal of which can be rotated independently of the proximal, in a plane at right angles to the long axis of this portion of the fixator (Fig. 21.2d). Screws can thus be introduced into the femoral diaphysis at selected points at angles chosen to provide maximal stability for the implant, and well away from the knee.

The method of application of the new fixator was as follows. All patients were treated on an emergency basis within 24 hours of admission. General or spinal anaesthesia was used in all but two cases, where local anaesthesia was used, and the patients treated as ambulatory cases. The patient was placed on a fracture table in the supine position, with the uninjured limb widely abducted. Reduction of the fracture was usually accomplished by applying traction and internal rotation to the injured limb with the leg in slight abduction, until the fracture was anatomically reduced. This reduction was then maintained throughout the surgical procedure.

A 2mm K-wire was inserted along and parallel to the axis of the femoral neck and 5mm below its upper edge. Correct positioning of this wire was essential since it would determine the final position of the first proximal screw. Skin, subcutaneous tissues and fascia were then incised at a point 1cm distal to the K-wire and freed by blunt dissection down to the cortex. A special screw guide with two barrels, one for the proximal femoral neck screw and one to house the K-wire, was then introduced, The K-wire was trimmed, and following introduction of a drill guide into the screw guide, the outer cortex was drilled to a depth of 3cm under image intensification. The first screw was then inserted and advanced under image intensification until the threaded portion had passed through the fracture line and the tip was no closer than 1cm to the articular surface (Fig. 21.3a). In osteoporotic bone, care was taken to ensure that this screw was in contact with the superior cortex of the femoral neck. The correct position of the screw was then confirmed in two planes under image intensification.

After removal of the screw guide and K-wire, this screw was housed in one of the fixed screw seats in the posterior clamp of the fixator, the choice of seat depending upon the thickness of the neck. A trocar inserted into the swivelling seat was then used to identify the position for the second femoral neck screw. Following an appropriate incision the second screw was then inserted so that it converged slightly with the first, within the head of the femur, keeping it close to the inferior cortex of the femoral neck (Fig. 21.3b). When both screws had been introduced, the posterior clamp locking screws were tightened, leaving a gap of about 2cm between the fixator and the skin.

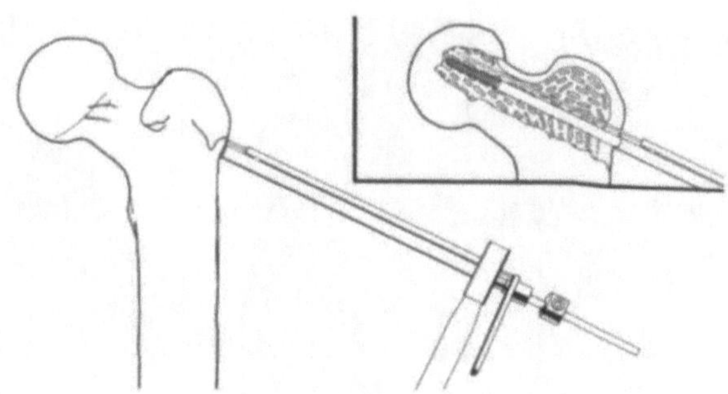

a

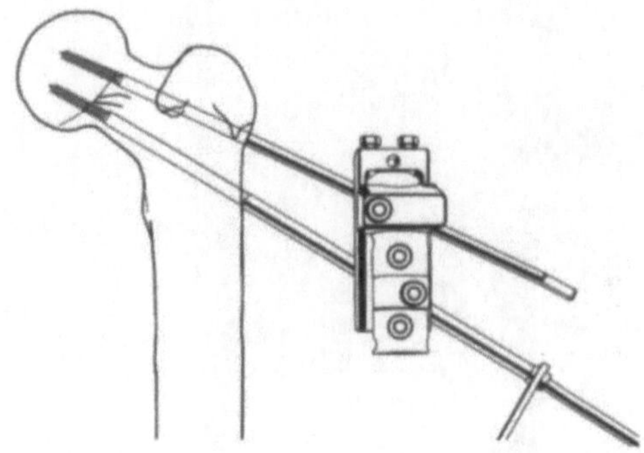

b

Fig. 21.3 a Insertion of the first proximal screw parallel to the femoral neck with its tip no closer than 1cm to the articular surface. **b** Insertion of the second proximal screw to converge slightly with the first in the femoral neck.

The anterior clamp of the fixator was then positioned for introduction of the screws in the femoral shaft. These screws are ideally introduced at right angles to the long axis of the bone, but depending upon bone quality, can be introduced at an angle to it. The fact that the anterior element of the fixator could be rotated in relation to the posterior element meant that regardless of the angle of insertion, they could always be inserted into the central portion of the diaphysis. The proximal diaphyseal screw was introduced first in the normal way (Fig. 21.4a). The distal diaphyseal screw was then inserted, following further axial rotation of this section of the anterior clamp in relation to the proximal diaphyseal screw, if necessary (Fig. 21.4b).

Once all four screws had been positioned, and maintenance of fracture reduction confirmed, all locking nuts were well tightened. Traction was released, and flexion and extension of the knee and hip performed to ensure the absence of skin tethering around the screws. Following skin suture where indicated, dry dressings were applied around the screws.

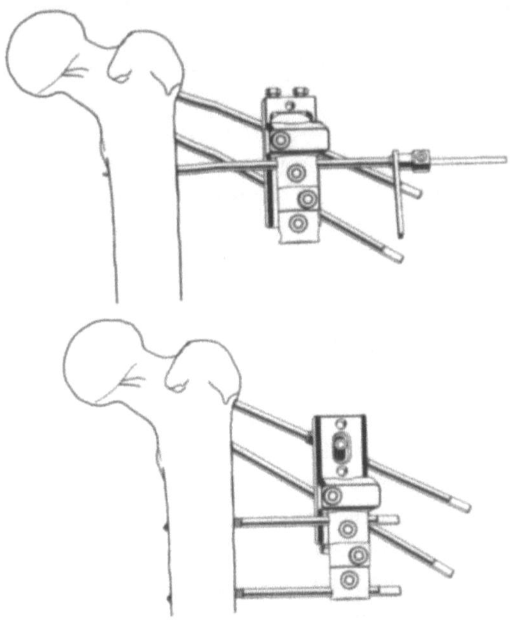

a

b

Fig. 21.4 a, b Insertion of the distal screws in the femoral diaphysis.

Post-operative management

Patients were allowed out of bed on the first post-operative day to use a commode. On the second post-operative day they began a structured programme of physiotherapy leading to the reacquisition of full ambulatory activity. All patients were allowed to weightbear to the extent that they were able to tolerate it, from the outset, unless their fracture was very unstable, in which case our policy was to wait until radiological signs of fracture healing were observed. Patients were instructed in the principles of pin site care prior to discharge from hospital.

Results

A total of 56 patients have been treated with the fixator to date and complete follow-up data are available on 43 of these. Many of these patients were considered to be high risk patients for any kind of surgical intervention due to their poor general state of health, and for this reason external fixation was considered the most appropriate form of surgery for them. There were 34 females and 9 males; their ages ranged from 62 to 102 years (mean 73 years). The Boyd Classification was used to describe the fractures (Boyd and Griffin 1949): there were 27 Boyd I, 14 Boyd II, 2 Boyd III and 0 Boyd IV.

Surgical and post-operative data are shown in Table 21.1 from which it can be seen that operating times were short and blood loss negligible. Patients were invariably discharged home in under a week. Data from the follow-up period post-discharge is shown in Table 21.2. Clinical and radiological union occurred in 3-4 months in all but one case, in whom a non-union developed. Mean shortening of the treated limb was 1.6cm. The nature and incidence of post-operative complications is illustrated in Table 21.3. The commonest post-operative complication was transient disorientation, which resolved rapidly. Antibiotics were not given routinely. Superficial wound infection occurred in 28 per cent of patients and these all

Mean time from admission to surgery	15 hours
Mean duration of surgery (range)	24 minutes (17–34 minutes)
Blood loss during surgery	nil
Mean blood replacement	1 unit
Intra-operative complications	1 (broken drill bit)
Mean period of hospitalisation (range)	3 days (0–6 days)

Table 21.1 Surgical And In-Patient Data

Mean time to partial weightbearing (crutches)	17 days
Mean time to clinical and radiological healing (range)	105 days (67–127 days)
Mean time with fixator in place	103 days

Table 21.2 Data From the Follow-Up Period Post-Discharge

Temporary post-operative disorientation	13 (30.2%)
Phlebitis	2 (4.7%)
Screw protrusion through femoral head	2 (4.7%)
Malunion	1 (2.3%)
Non-union	1 (2.3%)
Superficial infection1	12 (28%)
Shortening > 2cm	5 (11.6%)

Table 21.3 Post-operative complications

resolved with improved pin site care, coupled with oral antibiotics where indicated. More persistent infections disappeared when screws were finally removed at the time of fracture consolidation. There were no instances of deep wound infection in this series and no patients required re-operation for their fracture.

At most recent follow-up 24 patients (56 per cent) were walking without the help of crutches or cane; 14 (33 per cent) required some form of walking aid and 5 (12 per cent) were non-ambulant. Typical cases are illustrated in Figs. 21.5, 21.6 and 21.7.

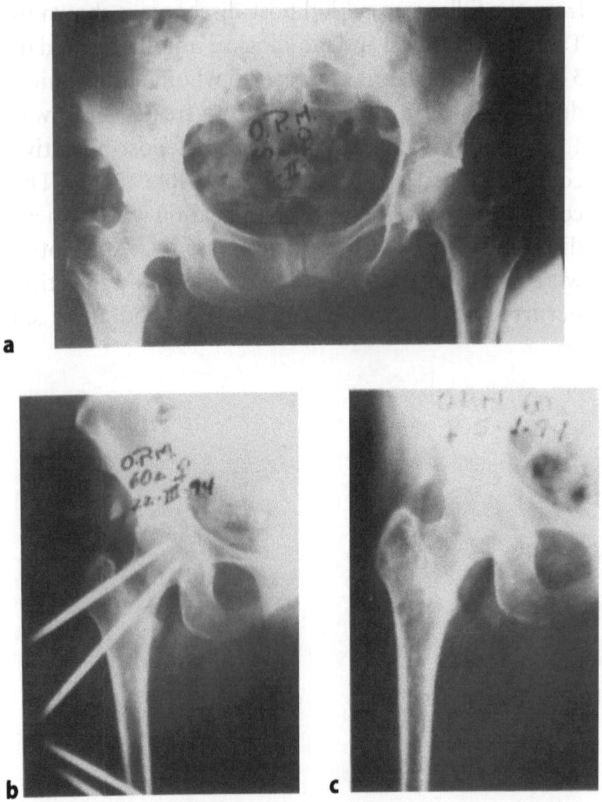

Fig. 21.5 a Female patient aged 60 with a Boyd I intertrochanteric fracture of the right femur. **b** Radiographic appearance 45 days post-operation. The position of the screws within the femoral neck is ideal and signs of consolidation are apparent. **c** Final result 3 months post-operation after removal of the fixator. Patient is fully weightbearing and asymptomatic.

One patient in this series died within the first month following operation (2.3 per cent), 3 patients had died within three months of operation (7.0 per cent) and 6 (14 per cent) within six months of operation.

Discussion

The fact that union almost always occurs in pertrochanteric fractures regardless of whether surgical or conservative treatment is used, coupled with the very low incidence of avascular necrosis of the femoral head, may account for the rather complacent attitude generally adopted towards this common and difficult fracture. Mortality rates provide clear evidence to demonstrate that surgical rather than conservative treatment should almost always be the logical choice, and some form of sliding hip screw, or the more recently introduced Gamma nail are popular choices. While producing acceptable results in the majority of patients, these techniques are not without their problems. In the case of the sliding hip screw, failure of fixation has been reported in 10 to 20 per cent of cases (Wolfgang, Bryant and O'Neill 1982; Nunn 1988; Simpson, Varty and Dodd 1989), most commonly cutting out of the screw from the femoral head (Davis et al 1990), while fracture of the femoral shaft has been reported in association with the Gamma nail (Bridle et al 1991; Halder 1992; Mahaisavariya and Laupattarakasem 1992; Fornander et al 1994), often necessitating additional major surgery.

Both techniques are normally associated with more than 250ml of blood loss during operation and with operating times of the order of 60 minutes. In one series of 105 trochanteric fractures treated with the Gamma nail and 104 treated with a standard compression hip screw device (Fornander et al 1994), mean blood loss associated with stable and unstable pertrochanteric fractures was 275ml and 315ml respectively for patients treated with the Gamma nail and 280ml and 530ml for those treated with a compression hip screw. Mean operating times for the same groups were 68 and 71 minutes for the Gamma nail and 49 and 72 minutes for the compression hip screw. In this same study mean duration of hospitalization was 17 days for patients treated with the Gamma nail and 16 days for patients treated with a compression screw. In the series reported by Bridle et al (1991),

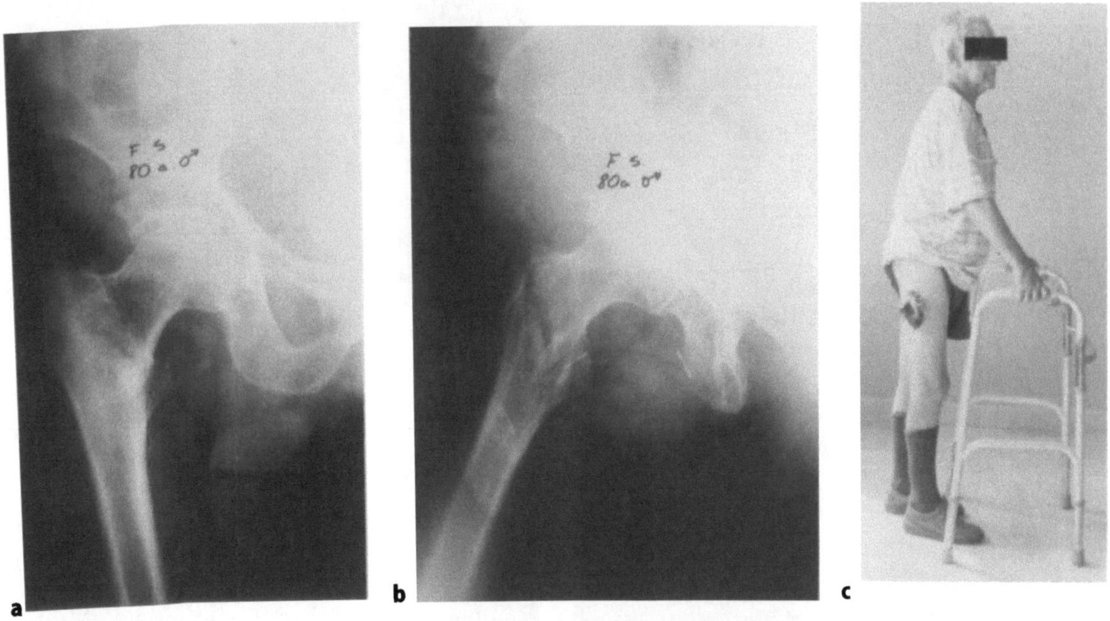

a b c

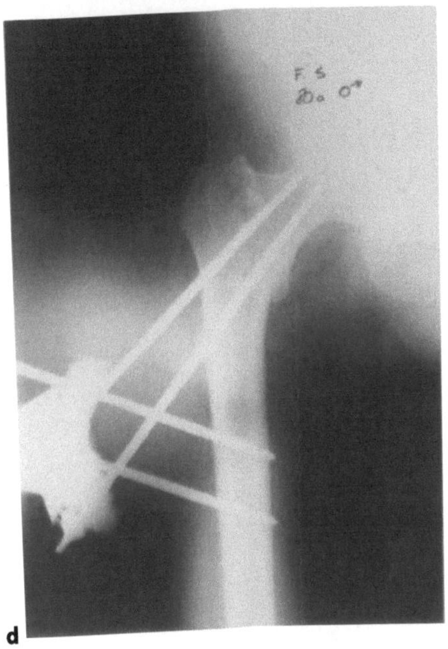

d

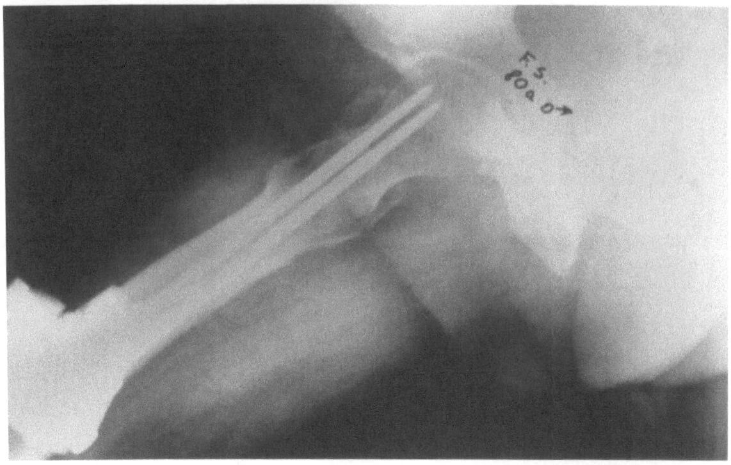

e

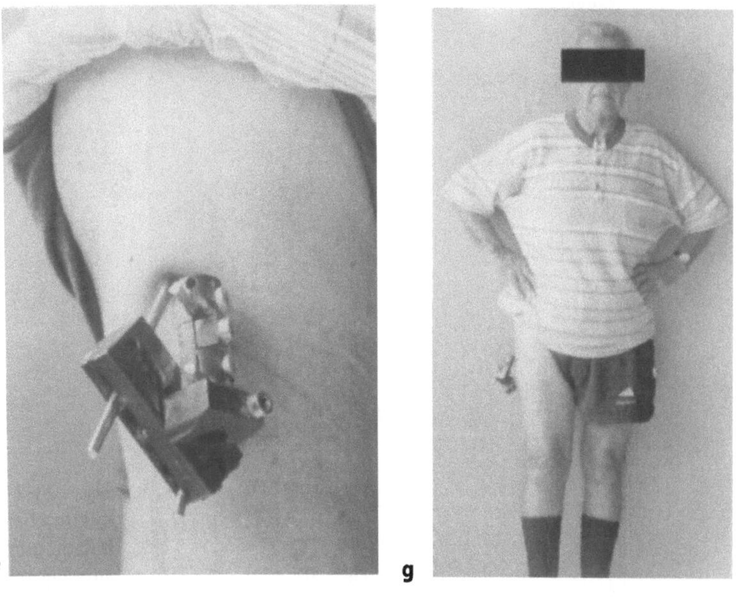

f g

Fig. 21.6 a, b Male patient aged 80 with a Boyd I intertrochanteric fracture of the femur. **c** Patient partially weightbearing 15 days post-operation. **d, e** Radiographic appearance one month post-operation with evidence of consolidation. **f,g** Patient fully weightbearing one month post-operation.

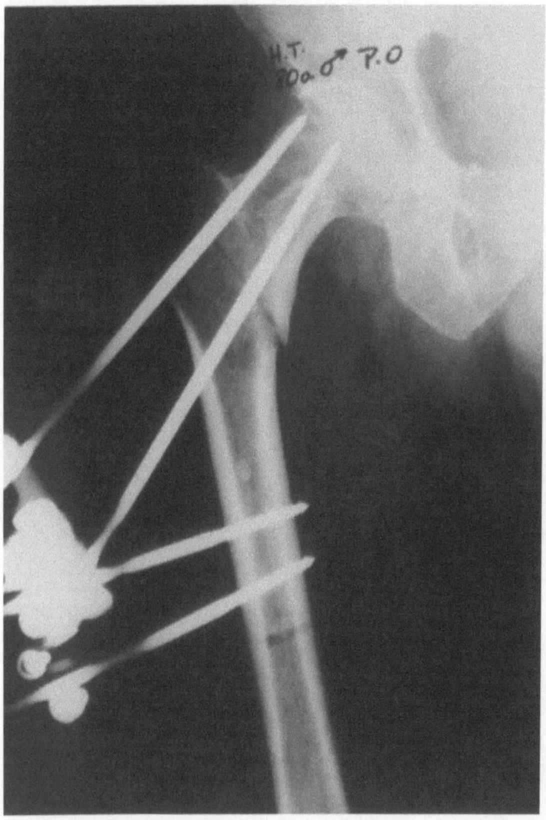

a

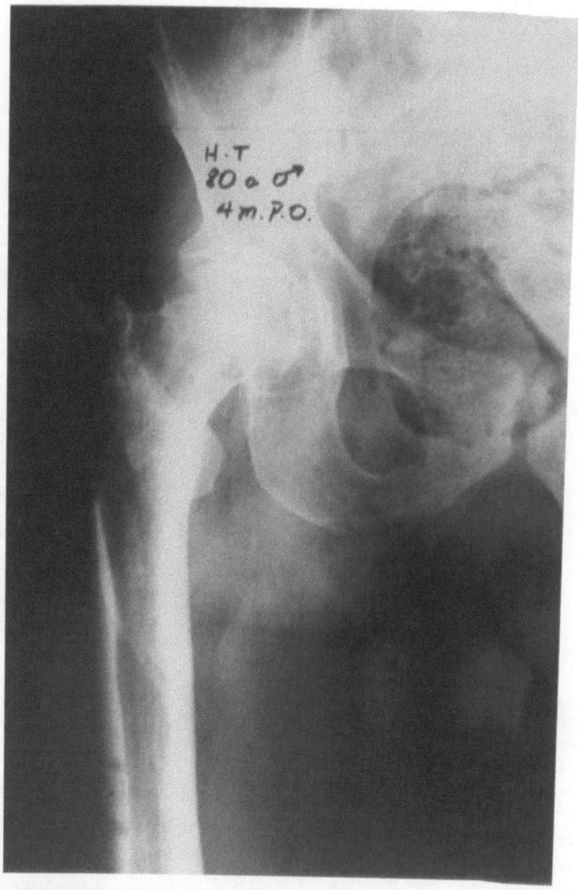

b

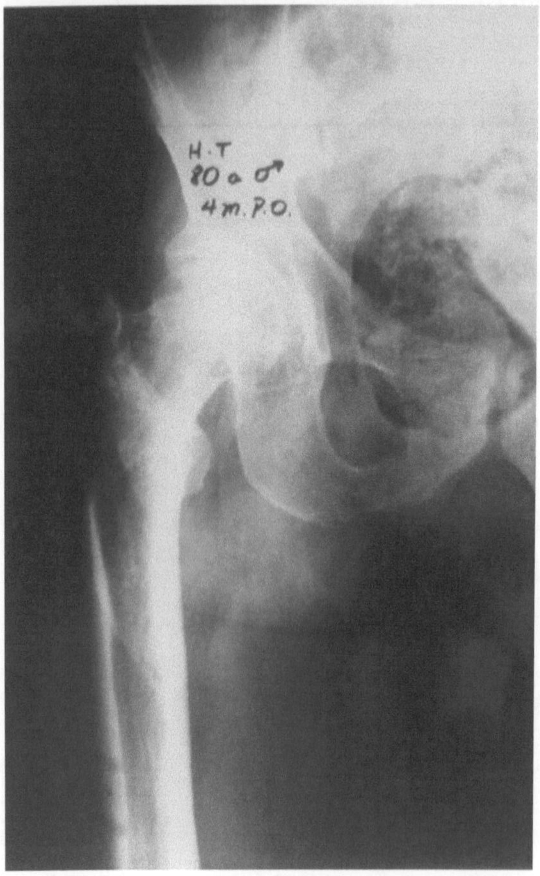

c

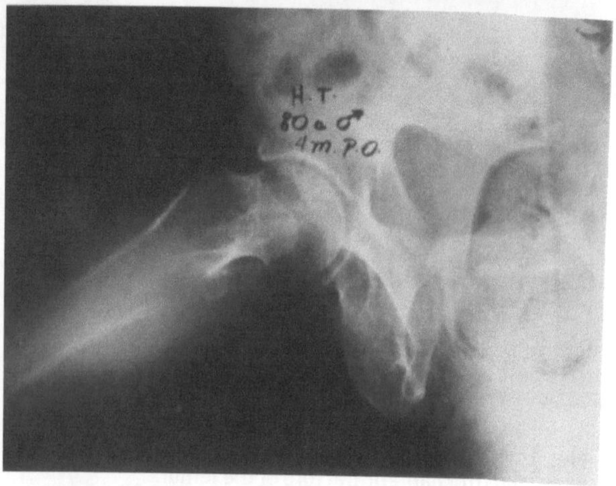

d

Fig. 21.7 a Male patient aged 80 with a Boyd I intertrochanteric fracture of the femur. Postoperative X-ray. **b** Radiographic appearance 2 months post-operation showing virtually complete consolidation. **c, d** Final result at 4 months post-operation, following removal of the fixator.

hospital residency was considerably longer, averaging 37 days for patients treated with the Gamma nail and 39 days for patients treated with the dynamic hip screw.

Compared with these findings, the early results with the new external fixator are very encouraging. Blood loss during the operation was negligible since the procedure is minimally invasive, and mean operating time was 24 minutes. Mean duration of hospital stay was only 3 days, which has important cost-saving implications. While superficial pin track infection occurred in 28 per cent of patients, this was readily controlled, and did not necessitate early removal of the fixator, or prejudice the outcome in any instance. No patients in this series required re-operation for their hip fracture.

Of particular interest are the mortality figures recorded with the new fixator compared with those reported for internal fixation techniques and for other forms of external fixation. The six-month mortality figure was only 14 per cent for the new fixator, which compares very favourably with the figures reported in association with alternative techniques.

This fixator has a number of additional advantages inherent in its design. The ability to introduce screws in a convergent mode close to the cortices of the femoral neck provides good stabilization and prevents collapse at the fracture site. In addition, the angle at which the femoral shaft screws are inserted can be varied to provide the maximum stability. The position of the distal screws high in the femoral shaft ensures complete mobility of both hip and knee throughout the treatment period. The device is very compact and this encourages partial weighbearing at an early stage. We further believe that the minimally invasive nature of the operation compared with internal fixation procedures means that patients experience less pain in the early post-operative period, and this may be an additional factor which contributes to the pattern of early partial weightbearing.

The elderly, high risk patient with a pertrochanteric fracture places a heavy burden on health services already under severe pressure. Any form of treatment which has the potential to conserve resources and enable the patient to be returned to the community in a speedy and safe manner is thus well worthy of consideration. Our initial experience with a new and novel form of external fixation suggests that this form of treatment may confer particular benefits in this patient population, and merits further prospective study comparing it directly with other commonly used treatment modalities. It has also prompted us to use this form of treatment in increasingly younger individuals as its potential has become apparent.

References

Boyd HB, Griffin LL. 'Classification and treatment of trochanteric fractures.' *Arch Surg* 1949; 58: 853-66

Bridle SH, Patel AD, Bircher M, Calvert PT. 'Fixation of intertrochanteric fractures of the femur.' *J Bone Joint Surg* [Br] 1991; 73-B: 330–4

Dahl E. 'Mortality and life expectancy after hip fractures.' *Acta Orthop Scand* 1980; 51: 163-70

Davis TRC, Sher JL, Horsman A et al. 'Intertrochanteric femoral fractures: mechanical failure after internal fixation.' *J Bone Joint Surg* [Br] 1990; 72-B: 26-31

Dhal A, Varghese M, Bhasin VB. 'External fixation of intertrochanteric fractures of the femur.' *J Bone Joint Surg* [Br] 1991; 73-B: 955–8

Evans EM. 'The treatment of trochanteric fractures of the femur.' *J Bone Joint Surg* [Br] 1949; 31-B: 190–203

Fornander P, Thorngren K-G, Tornqvist H et al. 'Swedish experience with the Gamma nail versus sliding hip screw in 209 randomised cases.' *Int J Orthop Trauma* 1994; 4: 118–22

Gotfried Y, Frish E, Mendes DG, Roffman M. 'Intertrochanteric fractures in high risk geriatric patients treated by external fixation.' *Orthopedics* 1985; 8: 769–74

Halder SC. 'The Gamma nail for peritrochanteric fractures.' *J Bone Joint Surg* [Br] 1992; 74-B: 340–4

Kennedy JC, McFarlane RM, McLachlin AD. 'The moe plate in intertrochanteric fractures of the femur.' *J Bone Joint Surg* [Br] 1957; 39-B: 451–7

Mahaisavariya B, Laupattarakasem W. 'Cracking of the femoral shaft by the Gamma nail.' *Injury* 1992; 23: 493–500

Nunn D. 'Sliding hip screws and medial displacement osteotomy.' *J R Soc Med* 1988; 81: 140-2

Riska EB. 'Factors influencing the primary mortality in the treatment of hip fractures.' *Injury* 1970; 2: 107–15

Scott IH. 'Treatment of intertrochanteric fractures by skeletal pinning and external fixation.' *Clin Orthop* 1957; 10: 326–34

Simpson AHRW, Varty K, Dodd CAF. 'Sliding hip screws: modes of failure.' *Injury* 1989; 20: 227–31

Wolfgang GL, Bryant MH, O'Neill JP. 'Treatment of intertrochanteric fracture of the femur using sliding screw plate fixation.' *Clin Orthop* 1982; 163: 148–58

The Impact of External Fixation of Femoral Fractures on Mortality and Morbidity in Polytrauma Patients

22

E. Brug, S. Winckler, M. Püllen and W. Klein

Introduction

In the late 1970s it was generally accepted that the patient with multiple injuries was too ill to undergo surgical stabilization of a long bone fracture in the period prior to admission to the Intensive Care Unit. Priority in the resuscitation phase was given almost exclusively to ensuring that respiratory and cardiovascular function was restored and maintained, by intubation and fluid replacement. An exception to this rule was the emergency treatment of uncontrollable massive bleeding from large vessels in the extremities, which if ignored, would render useless any concomitant treatment for shock.

The first phase of surgical treatment in Wolff et al's scheme for the management of polytrauma victims,[1] was generally reserved for initial life-saving measures, i.e. attention to intracranial, thoracic and abdominal injuries, together with other injuries which, if left untreated, were recognized either to have a prejudicial effect on outcome, or could lead within a few hours to irreversible local damage. These included second and third degree open fractures, vascular lesions with ischaemia and irreducible dislocations, where the risk of local dermal pressure damage and the rapid development of oedema make the 6-hour time point a critical one in terms of ischaemic tolerance and the risk of infection.[2,3] Patients with femoral fractures were not considered to fall into any of these categories, and were frequently put in traction, sometimes for several days, prior to surgical treatment to stabilize them. These fractures were often treated definitively in the second surgical phase after the patient had been in the Intensive Care Unit for some days.

It was gradually recognised, however, that untreated injuries of the extremities in general, and of the femur in particular, had a major influence on morbidity and mortality in the polytrauma patient. Apart from the obvious risk to adjacent vessels and nerves from the constant movement of the bone fragments, various cellular components and humoral agents were shown to be released[4] which had the potential to produce life-threatening systemic complications. These included damage to the renal tubular system due to the accumulation of myoglobin and impairment of the microcirculation due to the release of thrombokinase.

The most sinister, however, were the lung complications which were frequently observed to occur in polytrauma patients with femoral fractures, and included fat embolism[5] and the Adult Respiratory Distress Syndrome. Riska et al[6] observed that long bone fractures were associated with the development of fat emboli in the lungs, and that where such fractures could be treated by early operative fixation, clinical fat embolism could be prevented. Goris[7] showed that where femoral fractures were stabilized as early as possible, post-operative complications, especially lung complications, were reduced, and mortality decreased, while Seibel et al[8] demonstrated clearly that where polytrauma patients were treated in traction for a period of time prior to surgical stabilization of their femoral fracture, both lung problems and the cost of care were increased in comparison with patients who underwent early surgical stabilization.

By the early to mid 1980s, therefore, a plea was being made for the earliest possible stabilization of femoral fractures, and Johnson et al[9] in 1985 suggested that "The early stabilization of spine, pelvis and long bone fractures should now be considered part of the initial resuscitation". It was also appreciated that after the first 24 hours following injury the patient was often not fit for surgery, and might well not be again for a further two weeks or more. It was becoming clear, therefore, that if major complications and a prolonged recovery period were to be avoided, femoral fractures should be operated upon during this first 24-hour period if at all possible. Aware of the changing climate of opinion at this time, our own policies were adapted to meet the challenge. To determine what effect such changes in our treatment programme had produced, we carried out various retrospective analyses on the polytrauma patients with femoral fractures admitted to this unit over the period 1976 to 1992. In particular, we wished to know whether the earlier stabilization of these fractures was contributing to a reduction in mortality and morbidity (which latter we defined as duration of intensive care, artificially assisted respiration and unconsciousness).

Results of the Survey

In the period between 1976 and 1992 some 1313 polytrauma patients were treated in the unit, 529 of whom had sustained 658 femoral fractures. The two-compartment injuries predominated, with intracranial injuries in 61 per cent of patients and thoracic cavity injuries in 28 per cent.

Between 1976 and 1983, 755 patients with polytrauma were treated, of whom 267 had unilateral or bilateral femoral fractures. Of a total of 330 femoral fractures, 218 (66 per cent) were treated surgically, using plates in 60 per cent, nails in 30 per cent and other methods in 10 per cent. In 32 per cent of the patients it was either not possible to operate in view of their general condition, which precluded a lengthy osteosynthetic procedure, or they were fractures in children, for whom surgery was not indicated. In 2 per cent of patients, primary amputation was indicated (Fig. 22.1).

In 1984 we introduced the Orthofix Dynamic Axial Fixator[3,10] (Orthofix, Verona, Italy) into the unit, and this radically influenced our treatment of femoral fractures. We initially used it as an alternative to plating, which is a particularly time-consuming form of osteosynthesis, but in 1985 expanded its use to

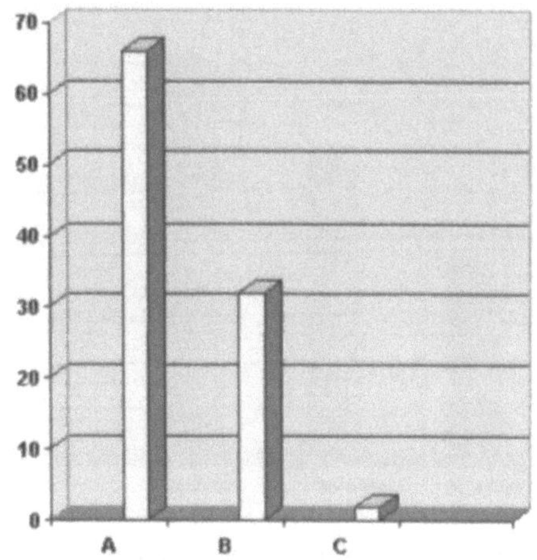

Fig. 22.1 Type of management of femoral fractures in polytrauma, 1976–83 (n = 330). A = Plate, medullary nail, conventional fixator; B = Conservative treatment; C = amputation.

embrace the treatment of closed fractures, if for whatever reason nailing, (which was our preferred form of treatment), was not possible. Between 1984 and 1992, therefore, our treatment pattern for femoral fractures in polytrauma patients showed a marked change. Of 328 patients in this category, 41 per cent were treated by means of some form of nailing; 33 per cent were stabilized using the Orthofix fixator and only 7 per cent with plates (Fig. 22.2). In all those cases treated using the Orthofix fixator complete healing occurred and no change of stabilization method was ever required.

It was further noted that during the period 1976-1983 it was possible to operate in the first 24 hours (i.e. prior to admission of the patient to the intensive care

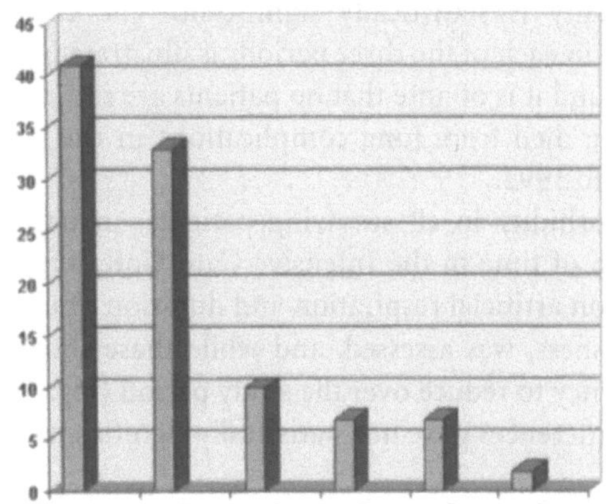

Fig. 22.2 Type of management of femoral fractures in polytrauma, 1984–92 (n = 328). Percentage of patients treated by each method. A = Locking nail, other medullary nail; B = Orthofix Fixator; C = Conservative treatment; D = Other; E = Plate; F = Amputation.

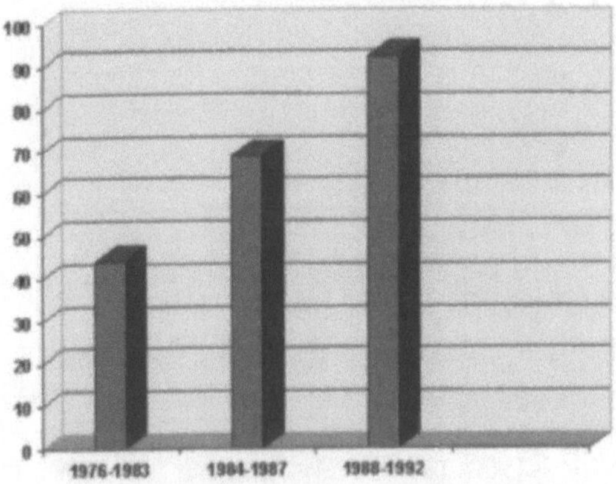

Fig. 22.3 Percentage of polytrauma patients with femoral fractures who could be treated surgically in the first 24 hours following injury during the periods 1976–83, 1984–87 and 1988–92.

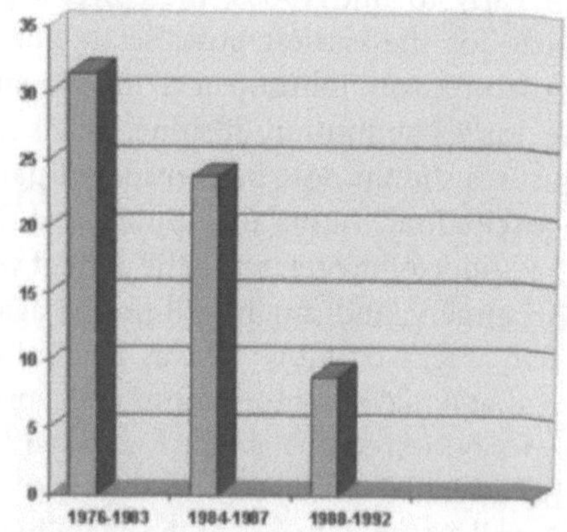

Fig. 22.4 Mortality as a percentage of the polytrauma patients with femoral fractures, treated during the periods 1976–83, 1984–87 and 1988–92.

unit) on only 44 per cent of those femoral fractures requiring surgery.[11] A further 23 per cent were treated between the second and the fifth day and 21 per cent between the sixth and the fourteenth day following injury. In the period between 1984 and 1987, which represented our period of initial experience with the Orthofix fixator, 68.8 per cent of femoral fractures could be treated within the first 24 hours, while during the period between 1988 and 1992, this figure rose to 92.3 per cent[12] (Fig. 22.3).

An analysis of mortality rates and cause of death was also carried out. The mortality rate fell progressively between 1976 and 1992: 84/267 (31.5 per cent) of polytrauma patients with femoral fractures died in the period 1976-83; 32/137 (23.7 per cent) between 1984 and 1987, and only 11/125 (8.8 per cent) between 1988 and 1992 (Fig . 22.4). This reduction in mortality is statistically significant. The cause of death in each of the three periods is illustrated in Fig. 22.5, and it is of note that no patients are recorded as having died from lung complications in the period 1988 to 1992.

Morbidity in all surviving patients, in terms of length of time in the Intensive Care Unit, length of time on artificial respiration and duration of unconsciousness, was assessed, and while these showed a tendency to reduce over the study period (Fig. 22.6), the differences were not statistically significant.

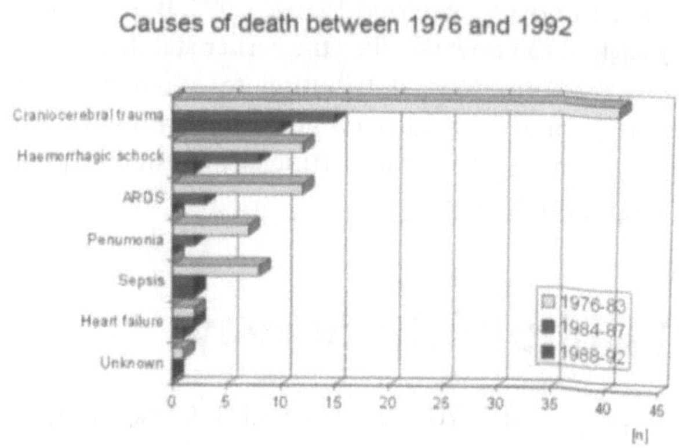

Fig. 22.5 Causes of death between 1976 and 1992. A = Unknown; B = Heart failure; C = Sepsis; D = Pneumonia; E = ARDS; F = Haemorrhagic shock; G = Craniocerebral trauma.

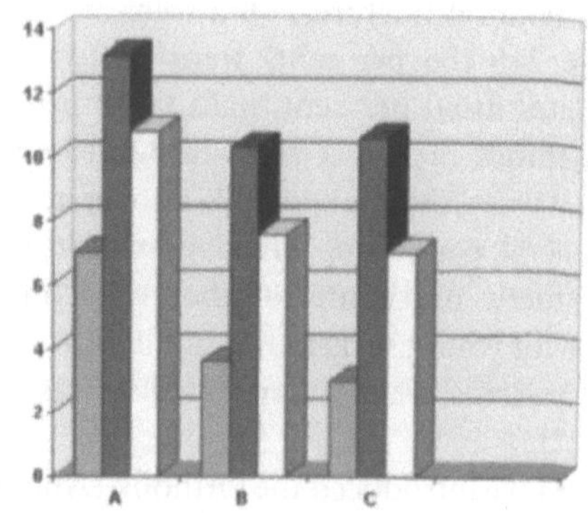

Key: Grey = 1976-83, Black = 1984-87, White = 1988-92

Fig. 22.6 Morbidity in surviving patients. A = Time in ICU (days); B = Time on artificial respiration (days); C = Time unconscious (days).

Discussion

The risk to the polytrauma patient of leaving a femoral fracture untreated while other, seemingly more pressing issues are dealt with first, has in recent years been shown to be considerable, both in terms of the effect upon mortality rates and on the incidence of complications. In addition to the threat posed to adjacent vessels and nerves by an insufficiently immobilized femoral fracture, the likelihood of serious respiratory problems and damage to the renal tubular system and to the microcirculation are all increased and contribute to a possibly fatal outcome. Thus, stabilization of the fracture by osteosynthesis, undertaken as soon as possible, and ideally, within the first 24 hours following injury and prior to transfer of the patient to the Intensive Care Unit, is of crucial importance.

In the period between 1976 and 1983, plating was performed in 60 per cent of all of our polytrauma cases with femoral fractures undergoing surgery, while 30 per cent were treated by intramedullary nailing. Both of these treatment modalities can be time-consuming, and the additional trauma they cause, coupled with the not inconsiderable surgical time involved, frequently did not justify their use in the first 24 hours following injury. Our retrospective analysis of patients treated during this period shows that only 44 per cent had their femoral fractures stabilized on the first day. In the remainder, surgery was performed two or more days after injury, when the patient would already have been in the Intensive Care Unit, and at an additional risk from possible contamination. We were receptive, therefore, to the idea of a method which could provide early, stable fixation of these fractures in a less invasive fashion than the conventional techniques currently available.

In 1984, the Orthofix Dynamic Axial Fixator was introduced into our unit. The advantages of this device in a polytrauma setting were immediately apparent to us. It could be rapidly applied with negligible additional blood loss; it was minimally invasive compared with both plating and nailing; there was no interference with the fracture site; post-operative correction could be performed without the need for further general anaesthesia; the stability it conferred was such that it could be used as definitive treatment until healing of the fracture had occurred,[13,14] and it did not require a second operation for removal of the device at a later date – simple removal of the bone screws could be effected as an office procedure. It had the added benefit that complications, apart from superficial pin site infections, were rare.

Our analyses demonstrate that the introduction of the Orthofix fixator had a major influence both on our treatment protocol for femoral fractures in the presence of polytrauma and on the incidence of associated mortality. In particular, we were now able to operate on many femoral fractures very close to the time of admission, and prior to their transfer to the Intensive Care Unit, whereas previously we would have deferred surgical intervention for one or several days due to the severity of concomitant injuries. In the period 1984-1992, following inception of its use, 81.3 per cent of femoral fractures were treated within the first 24 hours. If the most recent period of evaluation was considered, i.e. 1988-92, this figure rose to 92.3 per cent. Conversely, the incidence of mortality fell by 48 per cent (from 84/267 patients to 43/262 patients) between the period 1976-83 and the period following our change of policy (1984-92). As can be seen in Fig. 22.5, it is noteworthy that in the last period of study, from 1988 to 1992, no patient died as a result of pulmonary complications.

With the introduction of improved intramedullary nailing systems in the mid-1980s, we would generally consider the latter to be the best method for stabilizing femoral fractures. There remain, however, many cases where the patient's overall condition would contraindicate nailing in the first 24 hours, e.g. where the circulation is unstable, where the patient is a poor anaesthetic risk, where there are existing respiratory problems (although this remains controversial),[15,16] where there is severe craniocerebral, pelvic or visceral trauma or where an open fracture is associated with major soft tissue damage. In such instances external fixation in general, and the Orthofix fixator in particular, which can be applied rapidly and with minimal additional trauma, is, in our opinion, the treatment of choice.

References

1. Wolff G, Dittmann M, Frede KE. 'Klinische Versorgung des Polytraumatisierten.' *Chirurg* 1978; 49: 737–44.
2. Brug E. 'Dringlichkeit der Versorgung von Extremitätenverletzungen beim Polytrauma.' in: Peter K, Lawin P, Jesch F (Hrsg): *Der polytraumatisieret Patient.* Thieme: Stuttgart, New York, 1982.
3. Brug E, Klein W, Grünert. 'Die Behandlung der offnen Frakturen mit dem Fixateur externe - unter Berücksichtigung der dynamisch-axialen Fixation 'Orthofix'.' *Der Chirurg* 1987; 58: 699–705.
4. Hutchins PM, Macnicol MF. 'Pulmonary Insufficiency After Long Bone Fractures.' *J Bone Joint Surg* [Br] 1985; 76B: 835.
5. Allardyce DB, Meek RN, Woodruff B, Cassim MM, Ellis D. 'Increasing our knowledge of the pathogenesis of fat embolism; a prospective study of 43 patients with fractured femoral shafts.' *J Trauma* 1974; 14: 955–62.

6. Riska EB, von Bonsdorff H, Hakkinen S, Jaroma H, Kiviluoto O, Paavilainen T. 'Primary Operative Fixation of Long Bone Fractures in Patients with Multiple Injuries.' *J Trauma* 1977; 17: 111–21.
7. Goris RJA, Gimbrere JSF, van Niekerk JLM, Schoots FJ, Booy LHD et al 'Early Osteosynthesis and Prophylactic Mechanical Ventilation in the Multitrauma Patient.' *J Trauma*, 1982; 22: 895–903
8. Seible R, LaDuca J, Hassett JM, Babikian G, Mills B, Border DO, Border JR. 'Blunt Multiple Trauma (ISS 36), Femur Traction and the Pulmonary Failure Septic State (PFSS).' *Ann Surg* 1985; 202: 283–93.
9. Johnson K, Cadambi A, Seibert GB. 'Incidence of Adult Respiratory Distress Syndrome in Patients with Multiple Musculoskeletal Injuries: Effect of Early Operative Stabilization of Fractures.' *J Trauma* 1985; 25: 375–84.
10. De Bastiani G, Aldegheri R, Renzi-Brivio L. 'The Treatment of Fractures with a Dynamic Axial Fixator.' *J Bone Joint Surg* [Br] 1984; 66B: 538–45.
11. Brug E, Pennig D, Gähler R, Haeske-Seeberg H. 'Polytrauma und Femurfraktur.' *Akt Traumatol* 1988; 18: 930–4.
12. Winckler S, Brug E. 'Der Stellenwert der Femurfraktur beim Polytrauma.' in: *Die dynamisch-axiale externe Fixation*; Neumann H-S, Klein W, Brug E (Hrsg). Hans Marseille Verlag GmbH: Munchen 1993.
13. Broekhuizen AH, Boxma H, Meulen van der PA, Snijder CJ. 'Performance of external fixation devices in femoral fractures; the ultimate challenge? A laboratory study with plastic rods.' *Injury* 1990; 21: 145–51
14. Broekhuizen AH. The stability of external fixation systems for the treatment of femoral fractures – a comparative evaluation. This book, Ch. 7.
15. Pape H-C, Kolk MA, Paffrath T, Regel G, Sturm JA, Tscherne H. 'Primary Intramedullary Femur Fixation in Multiple Trauma Patients with Associated Lung Contusion – A Cause of Posttraumatic ARDS?' *J Trauma* 1993; 34: 540–8.
16. Bosse MJ, Mackenzie EJ, Riemer BL, Brumback RJ, McCarthy ML, Burgess AR, Gens DR, Yasui Y. 'Adult Respiratory Distress Syndrome, Pneumonia, and Mortality following Thoracic Injury and a Femoral Fracture Treated with Either Intramedullary Nailing with Reaming or with a Plate.' *J Bone Joint Surg* [Am] 1997; 79A: 799–809.

Supracondylar and Intercondylar Fractures of the Femur

23

F. Ali and M. Saleh

Introduction

Distal femoral fractures pose a difficult problem for the surgeon with significant complication rates and generally unsatisfactory results.[1,2] These fractures usually result from a high energy injury in the young or a fall in the elderly. As a result, they are typically comminuted or involve osteoporotic bone. The spectrum of injuries is so great that no single implant has been found to be suitable for every case.

Prior to the 1970s non-operative management was the treatment of choice.[2,3] As surgical techniques and implants have improved, operative fixation has gained widespread acceptance. Open reduction and internal fixation can be achieved using condylar plates and screws or intramedullary nails. Intercondylar and intra-articular extensions of these fractures can be managed by these implants alone or may be supplemented by additional screw fixation. These techniques include the use of the condylar blade plate,[4,5,6] the dynamic condylar screw and plate[7,8] and the condylar buttress plate.[9,10] Intramedullary fixation may involve antegrade nailing[11,12,13] or retrograde nailing as with the supracondylar femoral nail.[14,15] Flexible and semi-rigid nails e.g. the Zickel nail, have a limited place in the management of these fractures.[16] A total knee replacement including a modular distal femoral component can be used in an elderly patient with gonarthrosis.[17]

The sucess of the treatment depends very largely on the effectiveness of the distal femoral fixation, and this in turn depends on the amount and quality of available bone stock. Using external fixation, support may be taken across the knee, thus neutralizing the effect of the lower limb lever arm and augmenting the distal femoral fixation.

There has been very little published on the management of these fractures using an external fixator. Current opinion is that the use of external fixation is limited mainly to the management of severe open fractures.[18] The results of a retrospective study on the use of external fixation in the treatment of distal femoral fractures are presented below. This is the first report describing the use of limited internal fixation to reconstruct the articular surface combined with external fixation. The advantages and limitations of this method of treatment are then discussed.

Materials and Methods

For the purpose of this study a distal femoral fracture was defined as a fracture involving the distal 9cm of the femur on X-ray.

Between 1988 and 1997, 13 distal femoral fractures were treated by external fixation in the Limb Reconstruction Service at the Northern General Hospital in Sheffield. All fractures with severe comminution or intra-articular extension were included in the study. Simpler or non-articular fractures were treated by other methods and as such were not included. Those with injuries to the same limb (e.g. a floating knee) were excluded from the study. There were 7 male and 6 female patients. Average age was 45 years with a range of 19 to 74 years. Eight fractures resulted from a road traffic accident, four from a fall and one patient was kicked by a horse. Most of the data were extracted from the case notes. Patient satisfaction, however, was determined by interview, either in the clinic or over the telephone. The average follow-up time was 30 months (range 15–52 months).

The AO/ASIF classification described by Müller was used in the study to classify the fractures based on radiographic appearance.[19] There were 4 type A3 fractures, 1 type C1, 5 type C2 and 3 type C3 fractures. Seven fractures were open and 6 were closed. Two of the compound wounds were grade II, three were grade IIIA and two were grade IIIB. Two of these patients had multiple injuries. All cases were admitted under the same consultant (MS) although more than one surgeon was involved. The monolateral fixator (Orthofix srl, Verona) was used in all cases. If the knee joint was crossed, connection to the tibia was via a ring system.

Two or three screws were inserted into the distal fragment (Figs. 23.1a–c). In 7 cases the articular fracture was reduced and fixed either percutaneously or open, with 6mm cannulated lag screws, the external fixator being used to neutralize the fracture. In cases where the distal fragment was short or of poor bone stock the fixator was taken across the knee (Figs. 23.2a–f). In 6 cases the fixator was extended across the knee to protect the distal fixation. The average time for which a fixator spanned the knee was 5.5 weeks (range 3 to 12 weeks). In general, the fixator was left in place until the fracture had united.

Clinical results were assesed using the criteria of Schatzker and Lambert and modified by Mize et al (Table 23.1).[20] The time to independent weightbearing out of fixator was the clinical parameter used to assess union. This was determined from the case notes. The radiological appearance was assessed to confirm this. Knee range of movement was obtained from the case notes and a full range of movement defined as 0° to 135° of flexion.

Operative Technique

A detailed pre-operative plan is made, since there is very little room to insert both cancellous screws and external fixator pins. Via a limited incision the fracture is reduced under direct vision and imaging. The fracture is held with a tenaculum forceps and guide wires are inserted in the optimal positions for the cannulated screw fixation. The skin is temporarily closed. Stab wounds are made and under radiological control 3.2mm drill bits are inserted in the position of the external fixator screws. The drill bits are then removed and the skin flaps reopened. 6mm cannulated cancellous screws are then inserted over the guide wires. The skin is closed and the external fixator pins

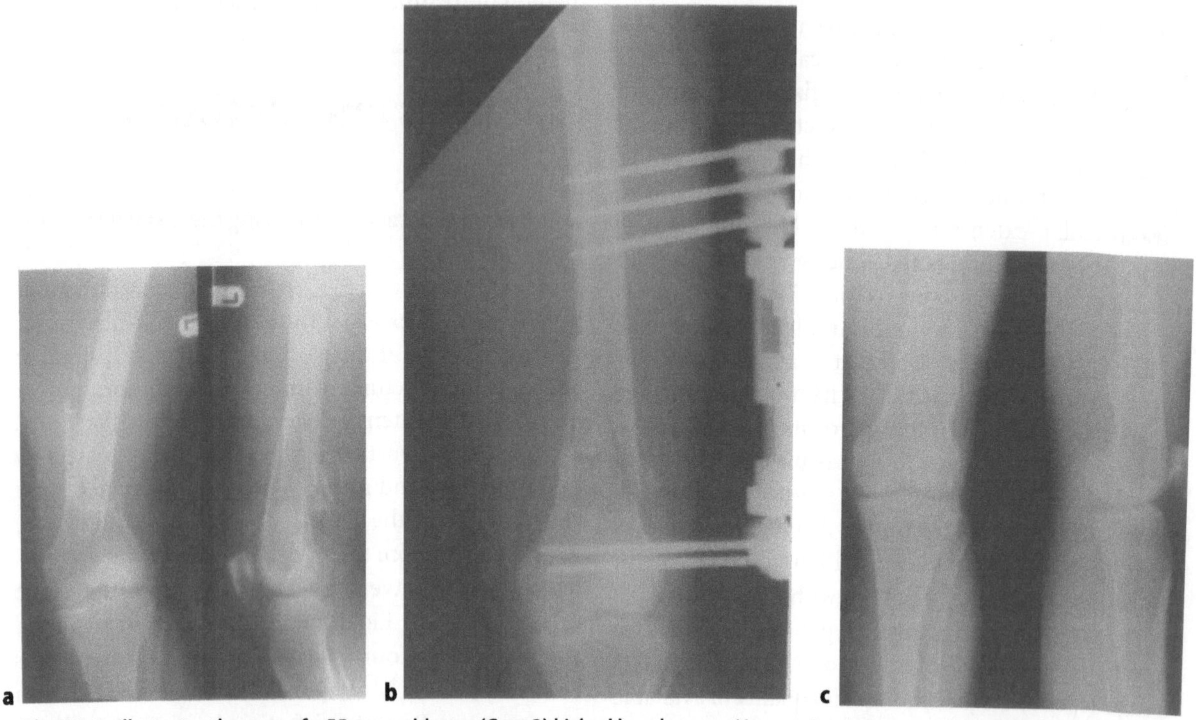

Fig. 23.1 Illustrates the case of a 55-year-old man (Case 3) kicked by a horse. **a** He sustained an open Type A3 fracture. **b** This was reduced and held by an external fixator with two screws in the metaphysis. The fixator did not cross the joint. **c** Union after fixator removal four months post-injury.

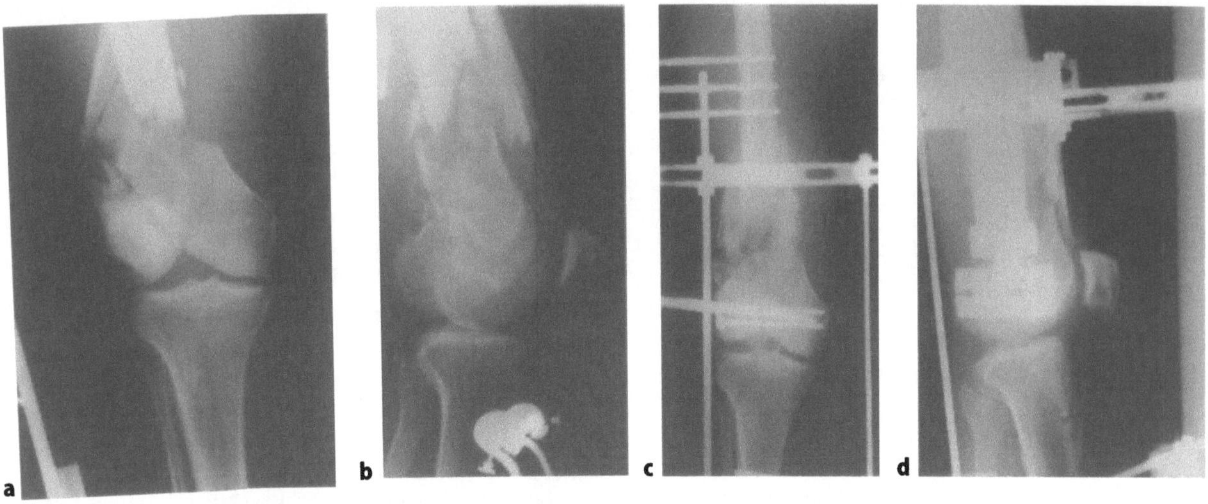

a b c d

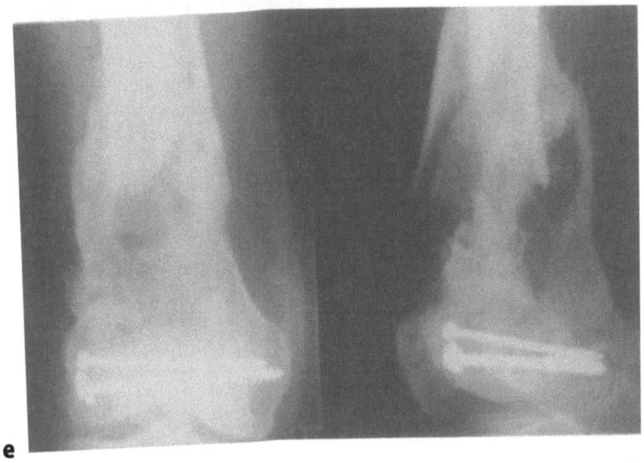

e

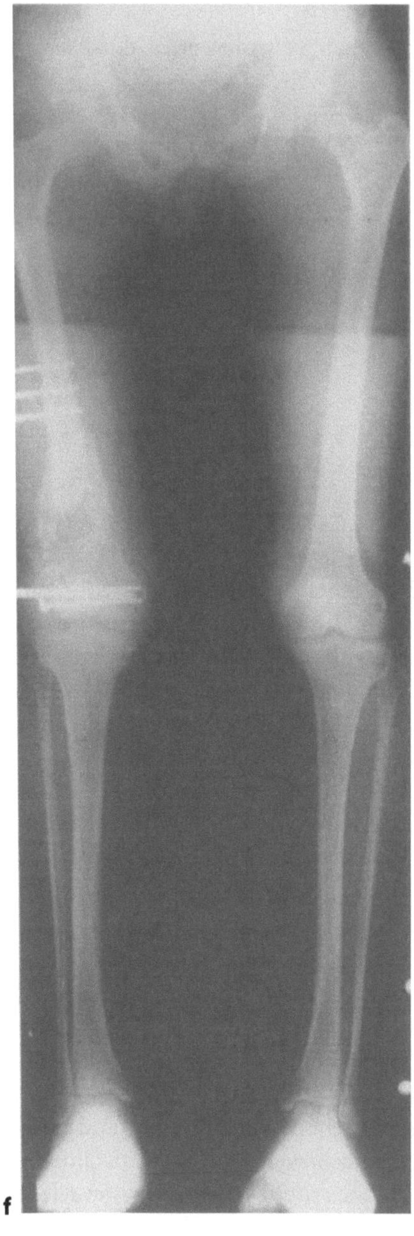

f

Fig. 23.2 Illustrates the case of a 35-year-old man (Case 7) involved in a road traffic accident who sustained a closed Type C3 fracture (**a, b**). He was treated using two cancellous screws to reconstruct the articular surface of the femur, followed by an Orthofix fixator with T-clamp. **c, d** Fixation was taken across the knee using the Sheffield Hybrid Fixator Assembly. **e** The situation four months post-injury after frame removal. **f** The alignment at three months just before frame removal.

are placed through the previously made stab incisions and attached to a metaphyseal clamp. Two or three cortical screws with long screw shafts are inserted into the proximal femoral diaphysis and connected to the distal screws by a short or standard-bodied fixator (Fig. 23.1b). Note that when the knee is not crossed the diaphyseal pins are inserted with the knee flexed, and the fascia lata released. If the knee is crossed, the present technique utilizes a preconstructed hybrid frame consisting of two 2/3 rings connected by three appropriate length threaded bars and, if neccessary, hinges. This is attached to the femoral diaphyseal screws and the proximal tibial screws by use of the Sheffield clamp (Fig. 23.3).

Excellent

All of the following: loss of flexion of less than 10°, full extension, no varus, valgus or rotational deformity, no pain and perfect joint congruence.

Good

Not more than 1 of the following: loss of flexion >20°, loss of extension >10°, varus or valgus deformity of more than 10° and minimal pain.

Fair

Any two of the criteria listed in the previous category.

Failure

Any of the following: Flexion to 90° or less, varus or valgus deformity >15°, disabling pain regardless of X-ray appearance, and joint incongruence.

Table 23.1 Clinical results of treatment of distal femoral fractures (Mize et al)

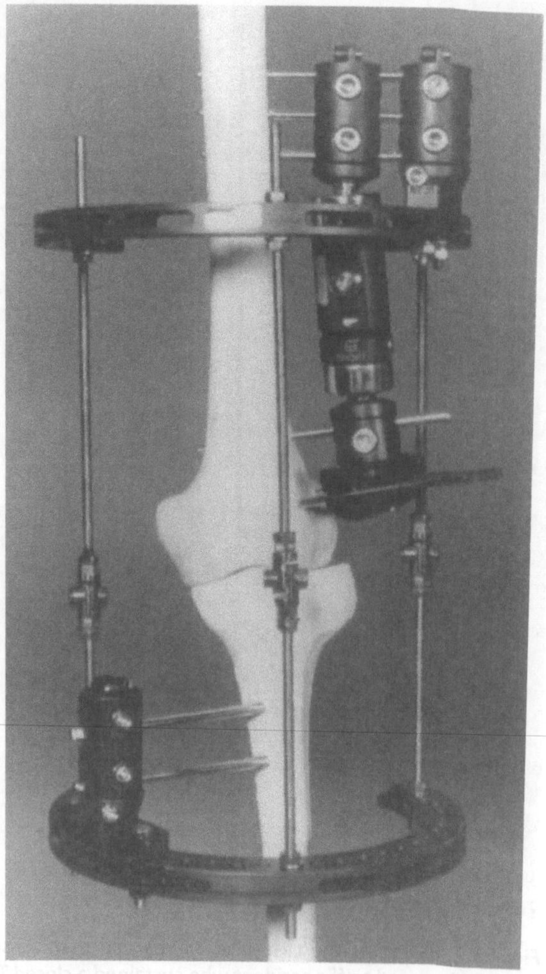

Fig. 23.3 Fixator crossing the knee joint. Diaphyseal screws and proximal tibial screws are connected to the hybrid system by Sheffield Clamps.

Results

In 12 out of 13 patients the fracture united (Table 23.2). The single patient whose fracture did not unite was a 38-year-old male who was involved in a road traffic accident and sustained a grade IIIB open fracture with severe soft tissue damage and bone loss. The fracture eventually united, however, following exploration of the non-union site, bone grafting and further treatment in another external fixator crossing the knee joint. The average time to union in the other patients was 6 months with a range of 3 to 13 months.

The average range of movement (ROM) of the knee was 100° of flexion with a range of 30–135° (full ROM). The average range of movement when the knee was crossed was 85° compared to 110° when the knee was not crossed with the fixation. There was no difference in the range of movement between the open and closed group. Four patients achieved a full ROM. Evaluation of the results using the criteria of Mize et al revealed 9 good to excellent results and 4 failures. Of the failures, 2 were purely due to a ROM of less than 90°. The other two were due to pain, deformity and a decreased ROM. Only one of these failures was in the open group.

The principal complication noted was non-union in one patient. Five patients had minor pin tract infections which settled with regular cleaning and antibiotics. One patient had loosening of the pins and had the fixator removed at 6 weeks (Case 2). Subsequent management in a cast brace led to a good result. Four patients required manipulation under anaesthesia to improve the ROM. Two of these subsequently required a quadricepsplasty. Patients were interviewed by one author (FA) either in the clinic or by telephone. Ten patients said that overall they were satisfied with their final result, but three said they were unhappy, the main reason being persistent pain.

Discussion

The management of supracondylar fractures of the femur remains controversial. Most studies over the past thirty years have attempted to compare the results of surgical versus non-surgical methods. Open reduction and internal fixation using a variety of devices remains the most frequently reported surgical method. However, no internal fixation method has repeatedly achieved satisfactory results in the management of the more complex fractures.

In a review of all the published articles on this subject we found that most centres have used external fixation only as a temporary device for the initial management of fractures and soft tissues in open wounds.[1,21,22] It has also been used in the multiply injured patient when the overall condition does not permit early definitive fixation.[18] Seligson reported on the use of the Wagner Apparatus in managing 5 cases of open fractures. He commented that this method involves the use of less metal and less extensive exposure than internal fixation devices; wound access is easy and ambulation is usually easier.[23] Use of the Ilizarov fixator has been reported in 4 patients in a German series. This technique was found to be technically difficult, however, and was associated with a high complication rate.[24]

The largest series published was that by Noer and Christensen[25] who treated 17 supracondylar fractures with the Orthofix Fixator. Good results were obtained, with all fractures uniting and patients mobilized after 16 days. This study only involved Type A2 and A3 fractures. No fractures treated had intercondylar extensions and the knee was not crossed by the fixator.

On reviewing the clinical results we found that 69 per cent of our patients had a good to excellent result using the Mize criteria. This compares to 71 per cent reported by Sanders et al[8] using a DCS and side plate and 52 per cent by Merchan et al[26] using a condylar blade plate. It contrasts, however, to other studies where better results have been obtained, e.g. 94 per cent by Dazinger et al[27] using the supracondylar nail and 81 per cent by Siliski et al[6] using the blade plate. The reason for this is that our study group comprised, in the main, patients with severe soft tissue injuries and comminution, while in many of the other studies this was not necessarily the case.

The average range of movement in this study was 100° of flexion. This was comparable to the range of movement obtained in other studies using various

Patient	Age	Sex	Follow-up (months)	Mech Injury	Open / Closed	AO class	Fixator Type	Cross knee? How long?	Time to union (months)	Final ROM	Complications	Clinical resultes (Mize)	Patient response
1	29	M	38	RTA	C	C2	monolateral, 2 screws	Y, 4 weeks	6	5–100	required quadricepsplasy	good	satisfied
2	74	F	24	fall	C	C2	monolateral	N	6	10–100	loose, fixator removed	good	satisfied
3	55	M	23	kicked	O	A3	monolateral	N	3.5	full	none	excellent	satisfied
4	19	M	30	RTA	O	A3	monolateral	N	5	full	bone graft 3/12. 3cm short	good	satisfied
5	34	M	52	RTA	C	C2	monolateral, 2 screws	Y, 12 weeks	7	0–100	shortening	failure	satisfied
6	31	M	30	RTA	O	C2	hybrid, 2 screws	Y, 3 weeks	7	0–100	none	good	satisfied
7	35	M	15	RTA	C	C3	hybrid, 2 screws	Y, 4 weeks	3	0–70	none	good	satisfied
8	54	M	22	RTA	C	A3	monolateral	N	6	full	none	good	satisfied
9	38	M	27	RTA	O	A3	monolateral	Y, 4 weeks	nu	5–90	non-union; shortening	failure	unhappy
10	45	F	40	fall	C	C3	monolateral, 1 screw	N	3.5	0–90	none	good	satisfied
11	55	F	30	fall	O	C1	monolateral	N	13	full	none	good	unhappy
12	48	F	26	RTA	O	C2	monolateral, 2 screws	N	6	0–30	required quadricepsplasy	failure	unhappy
13	64	F	31	fall	O	C3	monolateral, 3 screws	Y, 6 weeks	6	0–60	none	failure	satisfied

Table 23.2 Results of all patients

devices.[6,13,27] The average range of movement was less when we crossed the knee with the fixator as opposed to when we did not. The knee was only crossed, however, in the more severe injuries where the distal fixation needed to be reinforced. Four of our patients needed manipulation under anaesthesia and two of these required quadricepsplasty. The fact that we crossed the knee with the fixator in three of these four patients could be a contributory factor here. In addition, the external fixator pins may transfix the lateral periarticular tissues distally and the fascia lata proximally. This can, however, be minimized by inserting the proximal screws with the knee flexed and avoiding the use of transfixion wires.

There was one non-union in our study. The average time to union in the other patients was 6 months. This is slightly longer than in most other published results[4,27,28,29] but, again, it must be remembered that the patients treated in the present series had much more complex injuries than those in the other studies described.

The use of an external fixator has many theoretical advantages in helping to promote union. In the distal femur the cortex is thin, and there is a widened medullary cavity with cancellous bone. In addition, the distal fragment is usually short. All these features make stable fixation difficult to achieve. Also, because the fracture site is so close to the knee joint, movement of the knee allows movement at the fracture site. By using an external fixator, and especially by crossing the knee joint, we were able to achieve a more stable fracture fixation. The concept of cross-joint fixation is not new. Kuntscher described a technique of driving a K nail across the knee joint in supracondylar fractures in order to achieve a good fixation.[30]

Compared to open methods of treatment, negligible soft tissue dissection or periosteal stripping is performed.[23,27,31] The soft tissue envelope and the periosteal blood supply is thereby undisturbed. Intramedullary nails may also offer this advantage but there is a certain amount of periosteal stripping when inserting a supracondylar nail using the open technique. It has also been reported that intramedullary nails, especially reamed, proximally inserted nails, may damage the endosteal blood supply and hinder union.[23]

The threat of infection has been one of the major problems in the management of cases of this kind due to the high energy nature of some of these injuries, with soft tissue damage and open fractures. Added to this, the extensive periosteal stripping, soft tissue dissection and prolonged operative times may all contribute to the incidence of infection seen with internal fixation methods. In recent reports this has ranged from zero to 5.9 per cent.[3,4,6,7,13,27]

There were 7 open fractures in our study. There were no cases of osteomyelitis. Siliski reported 2 cases of osteomyelitis in 20 open fractures when using the blade plate.[6] External fixation offers the advantage that metalwork is not applied directly to the fracture site. In addition, wound access and management is easier in open fractures when a fixator is in place. A possible criticism is that external fixation pins are intra-articular. Notwithstanding this, no deep infection and no septic arthritis was seen in the present series.

External fixators have the ability to maintain length and alignment whilst spanning a zone of comminution or bone loss. In addition they allow for lengthening of the limb with little additional intervention. Frequently there is shortening, due either to bone loss from a compound injury or to intentional shortening at the fracture site in order to promote union. Proximal lengthening can be performed during the course of treatment using the external fixation system.

The limitation of this study is that it is a retrospective analysis of an uncontrolled population. More than one surgeon was involved although all the patients were under the care of the same consultant (MS). The small number of patients in the series precludes a statistical analysis of the differences. However these results can be used as a comparison with other reports.

Conclusion

While comparing results among various studies can be difficult because of a lack of standardized reporting criteria and small numbers, the results of the study suggest that although there may not be significant differences in the clinical results and the union rates obtained, the use of external fixation does have a place in the management of the more complex distal femoral fractures, especially those associated with open wounds, soft tissue injury, bone loss and comminution. The absence of deep infection and other serious complications so far, is encouraging.

References

1. Johnson KD, Hicken G. 'Distal Femoral Fractures.' *Orthop Clinics North Am* 1987; 18(1): 115–132.
2. Neer C, Brantham S, Shelton M. 'Supracondylar Fracture of the Adult Femur: A study of one hundred and ten cases.' *J Bone Joint Surg* [Br] 1967; 49A: 591–613.
3. Connolly JF, Dehne D, La Follette B. 'Closed Reduction and Early Cast Brace Ambulation in the Treatment of Femoral Frac-

tures. Results of one hundred and forty-three fractures.' *J Bone Joint Surg* [Am] 1973; 55A: 1581–99.

4. Healy WL, Brooker AF. 'Distal Femoral Fracture: Comparison of Open and Closed Methods of Treatment.' *Clin Orthop* 1983; 174:166–71.
5. Shelton ML, Grantham SA, Neer CS, Singh R. 'A New Fixation Device for Supracondylar and Low Femoral Shaft Fractures.' *J Trauma* [Am] 1974; 14: 821–35.
6. Siliski JM, Mahring M, Hofer HP. 'Supracondylar Intercondylar Fractures of the Femur.' *J Bone Joint Surg* [Am] 1989; 71A:95–104.
7. Giles JB, DeLee JC, Heckman JP, Keever JE. 'Supracondylar-Intercondylar Fractures of the Femur treated with a Supracondylar Plate and Lag Screw.' *J Bone Joint Surg* [Am] 1982; 64A: 864–70.
8. Sanders R, Regazzoni P, Rüedi T. 'Treatment of Supracondylar-Intercondylar Fractures of the Femur using the Dynamic Condylar Screw.' *J Orthop Trauma* 1989; 3:214–22.
9. Johnson KD. 'Internal Fixation of Distal Femoral Fractures.' *Inst Course Lect* 1989; 38:437–48.
10. Sanders R, Swiontkowski M, Rosen H, Helfet D. 'Double Plating of Comminuted Unstable Fractures of the Distal Part of the Femur.' *J Bone Joint Surg* [Am] 1991; 73A: 341.
11. Leung KS, Shen WY, So WS et al 'Interlocking Intramedullary Nailing for Supracondylar and Intercondylar Fractures of the Distal Part of the Femur.' *J Bone Joint Surg* [Am] 1991; 73A: 332.
12. Wu C, Shih C. 'Interlocking Nailing of Distal Femoral Fractures.' Acta Orthop Scand 1991; 62(4): 342–45.
13. Wu C, Shih C. 'Treatment of Femoral Supracondylar unstable Supracondylar Fractures.' *Arch Orthop Trauma* 1992; 111:232–36.
14. Iannacone WM, Bennett FS, De Long WG, Born CT, Dalsey RM. 'Initial Experience with the Treatment of Supracondylar Fractures using the Supracondylar Intramedullary Nail: A Preliminary Report.' *J Orthop Trauma* 1994; 8:322–7.
15. Lucas SE, Seligson D, Henry SL. 'Intramedullary Supracondylar Nailing of Femoral Fractures. A preliminary report of the GSH Supracondylar Nail.' *Clin Orthop* 1993; 296:200–6.
16. Zickel RE, Hobeika P, Robbins DS. 'Zickel Supracondylar Nails for Fracture of the Distal End of the Femur.' *Clin Orthop* 1986; 212: 79–88.
17. Freedman EL, DJ, Johnson EE. 'Total Knee Replacement including a Modular Distal Femoral Component in Elderly Patients with Acute Fracture or Non-union.' *Journal of Orthopaedic Trauma* 1995; 9(3): 231–7.
18. Wiss DA. Fractures about the knee. Rockwood C.A. and Green D.P. (eds) *Fractures in Adults*, Lippincott-Raven 1996, 1972–99.
19. Müller M, Nazarian S,Koch P, Schatzker J. In: *A Comprehensive Classification of Fractures of Long Bones.* Springer-Verlag: Berlin, 1990, 138–47.
20. Mize RD, Bucholz RW, Grogan DP. 'Surgical Treatment of Displaced, Comminuted Fractures of the Distal End of the Femur.' *J Bone Joint Surg* [Am] 1982; 64A: 871–9.
21. Iannacone WM, Taffet R et al 'Early exchange intramedullary nailing of distal femoral fractures with vascular injury initially stabilized with external fixation.' *J Trauma* 1994; 37(3): 446–51.
22. Ronen GM, Michaelson M, Waisbrod K. 'External Fixation in War Injuries.' *Injury* 1974; 6(2): 94–8.
23. Seligson D, Kristainson TK. 'Use of the Wagner Apparatus in Complicated Fractures of the Distal Femur.' *J Trauma* 1978; 18(12): 795–9.
24. Van der Werken C, Meeuwis JD et al 'Treatment of femoral fractures with the Ilizarov Fixator' (German). *Unfallchirurg* 1992; 95(11): 534–6.
25. Noer HH, Christenson N. 'Distal Femoral Fractures treated by External Fixation with Orthofix' (Danish). *Hgeskrift Laeger* 1993; 155(35): 2699–702.
26. Merchen E, Maestu P, Blanco R. 'Blade Plating of closed displaced Supracondylar Fractures of the Distal Femur with the AO system.' *J Trauma* 1992; 32:174–8.
27. Danziger MR, Caucci D, Zecher SB et al 'Treatment of Intercondylar and Supracondylar Distal Femoral Fractures using the GSH Supracondylar Nail.' *The American Journal of Orthopedics* 1995; 24(9): 684–90.
28. Schatzker J, Horne G, Waddell J. 'The Toronto Experience of the supracondylar Fracture of the Femur 1966–1972.' *Injury* 1974; 6:113.
29. Stewart MJ, Sisk TD, Wallace SL Jr. 'Fracture of the Distal Third of the Femur. A Comparison of Methods of Treatment.' *J Bone Joint Surg* [Am] 1966; 48A: 784–807.
30. Kuntscher GB. In: *Practice of Intramedullary Nailing* (Translated). Springfield, IL: Charles C, Thomas, 1967, 234-58.
31. Foster TE, Healy WL. 'Operative Management of Distal Femoral Fractures.' *Orthopaedic Review* 1991; 20(11): 962–9.

High Energy Tibial Plateau Fractures

24

J.L. Marsh

Introduction

Tibial plateau fractures are common and can be treated with a variety of techniques. They are usually the result of low energy trauma, most commonly a valgus-directed force producing split, split depression, or local compression fractures of the lateral plateau. Tibial plateau fractures from high energy mechanisms such as axial loading, motor vehicle accidents, and pedestrian versus motor vehicle accidents are less common and, unlike low energy tibial plateau fractures, frequently have severe associated soft tissue injuries which include contusions, fracture blisters, communicating open wounds, compartment syndrome, and neurovascular injury.[19] The management of this subset of tibial plateau fractures is complex, and will be the subject of this chapter.

Outcome of Tibial Plateau Fractures

The treatment of tibial plateau fractures by a variety of techniques generally leads to a favourable outcome. Treatment options include non-operative methods such as traction, casting, and cast bracing;[2,6] surgery designed to reduce and stabilize the fracture through limited approaches such as arthroscopically assisted, percutaneous fixation,[10] and external fixation[4,14,17,20] and open surgical approaches with fixation with plates and screws.[9,11,21] Indeed, it is hard to find a technique of treatment that has not been reported to achieve generally excellent results for the majority of patients.

Several authors have identified treatment factors that maximize the chances of a favourable outcome.[8,12,14] Angular alignment of the leg is one of the most important.[8,12,14,19] Limbs that heal in angular malalignment usually have weightbearing forces directed over the most severely injured tibial condyle which leads to arthrosis and progressive deformity. Coronal plane stability of the knee plays a role in alignment. Malreduction of the medial and lateral tibial condyles in relation to one another may result in leg malalignment. Condylar widening or condylar slope in the coronal plane allows the femoral condyle of the affected side to be unsupported, producing malalignment.[8] Malaligned limbs generally have coronal instability from residual bony deformity since late collateral ligament laxity is unusual.[15]

Regardless of the treatment technique the menisci must be preserved since they have a chondral protective effect which improves the outcome in patients with tibial plateau fractures. One study comparing operative and non-operative treatment techniques found that the worst results after tibial plateau fractures occurred in surgically treated patients where the meniscus had been excised.[9]

Complications of treatment must be avoided to obtain good results. Wound breakdown or infection of the knee or proximal tibia have repeatedly been shown to lead to a poor outcome in a high percentage of patients in whom these complications occur.[13,21]

Two factors have generally been held to be of critical importance in producing optimal outcome. These are an exact articular reduction when displacement is more than a certain number of millimeters and early motion of the injured knee. Careful review of the literature discloses that although surgical indications are frequently based on reducing fractured plateaus that are displaced more than a few millimeters, there is actually little evidence that articular step-offs negatively affect outcome.[8] The same is true of early motion. There are good results reported for techniques that stress early motion, and also for techniques that immobilize the knee for many weeks.[5,7] These reports cast doubt on the critical importance of these factors.

Most of the reported results of treatment include only low energy fractures, or only a few high energy fractures. There is very little reported information which focuses on the results of treatment of high energy fractures. The difference in osseous and soft tissue injury patterns between these two tibial plateau fracture categories indicates that the outcomes achieved and the treatments required might well be different.

High Energy Fractures of the Tibial Plateau

What are high energy fractures of the tibial plateau? Several authors have pointed out the types of soft tissue injuries and fracture patterns that indicate that greater energy was absorbed in the area of the proximal tibia during the production of the fracture.[14,18,19] The fracture patterns include bicondylar fractures, fractures with the shaft disassociated from the condyles, tibial shaft fractures with proximal extensions into the plateau, and certain medial tibial plateau fractures. Associated soft tissue injuries such as bruising or contusion, a communicating open wound, or tibial plateau fractures associated with compartment syndrome or vascular disruption, indicate high energy fractures. Using the AO Classification, the high energy fractures are some B patterns (medial side), and many of the C patterns. In the Schatzker classification, the high energy fractures are mostly Schatzker VI, with some Schatzker V and IV. In the Tscherne and Goetzen classification of soft tissue injuries associated with closed fractures, the associated soft tissue injury would be Grade II or III.[18]

There are very few reported case series so the factors that relate to outcome for high energy tibial plateau fractures are less well defined. In the author's experience, if the patient has a good condylar reduction, accurate angular alignment and satisfactory knee stability, the outcome will probably be favourable. In these fractures, the incidence of surgical complications is much higher, and the potential negative impact on outcome of these complications is greater.[13,21] There are no data to indicate that the articular reduction measured in millimeters of displacement or the achievement of early motion have a strong bearing on outcome.

There are fewer treatment methods available for high energy tibial plateau fractures. The severe soft tissue injury, limb instability and major fracture displacement preclude some treatment techniques. Traction followed by cast bracing may fail to achieve condylar reduction, and there may be difficulties in obtaining accurate shaft alignment.[2] Even if a satisfactory reduction is obtained, a long period of hospitalization is required. Treatment by open reduction and plate fixation in skilled hands can restore alignment and stability to the injured proximal tibia. Although good results have been reported, medial and lateral plating is often required, and the nature of the soft tissue injury may lead to a totally unacceptable risk of surgical complications. If these complications occur they may be devastating for the patient.

Recently, external fixation has emerged as a popular method of treatment for high energy fractures of the tibial plateau.[4,13,14,16,17,19,20] and in many authors' opinions has become the treatment of choice. External fixation offers the possibility for indirect reduction and stabilization and accurate alignment without soft tissue stripping. These are very attractive features in this injury subset.

External Fixation of the Tibial Plateau

A variety of external fixation techniques using different frames has been reported. These frames can be applied for stabilization after an aggressive open approach to reduce and fix the fracture. Alternatively, they can be used in conjunction with a philosophy which limits soft tissue dissection in the area of the fracture, and where reduction is obtained by indirect methods using distraction, percutaneous manipulation of fractured fragments and the assistance of the fixator itself. Regardless of the frame chosen, access to the soft tissues must be maintained. Some knee motion is desirable, but in the most severe injuries, a period of cross knee external fixation is necessary. The surgeon must have as a priority excellent fixation of the proximal tibia. In some cases, however, this can be difficult due to the presence of small comminuted fragments close to the joint.

Satisfactory results have been reported with the use of both ring and wire fixators and monolateral frames with pin fixation in the proximal tibia. The vast majority of proximal tibial fractures can be treated with either technique. Wires can stabilize smaller fragments closer to the joint, but the stability of fixation that can be obtained with carefully applied proximal pins and a monolateral frame can be surprising. With either technique, solid proximal purchase is required. The surgeon should be aware that joint sepsis secondary to proximal pins or wires has been reported with both types of frames.[14,16,20]

External fixation techniques have been used almost exclusively for high energy fractures. The use of external fixation is not indicated for routine split, split depression and local compression fractures. Less than 5 per cent of all tibial plateau fractures in the author's practice are treated with external fixation.

Technique of Monolateral External Fixation of Tibial Plateau Fractures

This section will describe the goals of treatment and techniques that the author has used in the treatment of high energy tibial plateau fractures using a monolateral frame and proximal pin fixation; wire fixation has only rarely been necessary, and mostly in reconstruction cases.

Goals

The aims are to reduce the condyles to one another underneath the femoral condyles, avoiding tilt, and avoiding widening. Reduction of the joint surface itself is a secondary goal that is often accomplished percutaneously or through limited approaches based on an anterior fracture line. Extensile incisions or tibial tubercle osteotomies are never performed. After the condyles have been reduced, the shaft is aligned and stabilized beneath the reduced condyles using the fixator without an open approach. These goals should all be accomplished with limited soft tissue dissection. The frame should not be removed until the fracture is healed.

Timing

The timing of application of the frame is variable and will depend on the injury. Emergency frame application is indicated in open tibial plateau fractures and fractures associated with compartment syndrome, arterial injury, and severe displacement where the skin is compromised. These fractures are routinely treated with cross knee fixation initially. Knee spanning frames provide provisional stability and realign the limb; they can be rapidly applied with little preoperative planning.

Frame applications on the same side of the knee are rarely applied as an emergency procedure. Preoperative planning with the aid of a transverse computerised tomographic scan (CT), is very important. Fractures are provisionally splinted, radiographic studies obtained, planning completed, and surgery performed on an elective operating list within a couple of days of injury. Patients treated as an emergency on the night of injury with a cross-knee frame may have this changed to a below-knee frame at a second operation if the fracture pattern permits.

Set up

The frame is applied on a split-leg radiolucent table under biplanar fluoroscopic control (Fig. 24.1); traction is not required. The opposite hip and knee are flexed out of the plane of the operative limb in a leg holder. This makes the biplanar fluoroscopic control easier. Accurate limb alignment is facilitated using a limb alignment grid in conjunction with fluoroscopy.

Condylar Reduction and Fixation

The condyles must be reduced and stabilized prior to applying the fixator. Condylar reduction is assisted by manual traction, a femoral distractor, or distraction through a frame previously placed across the knee. A varus or valgus force opposite to that of the major injuring force may assist in reduction. Large pointed reduction forceps applied percutaneously to the medial and lateral condyles help to obtain accurate condylar alignment followed by compression (Figs. 24.2, 24.3). To assist in fragment manipulation, awls or elevators may be applied percutaneously or through a small, carefully chosen open approach. If an open approach is selected, it is based on a major anterior fracture line to allow visualization of the joint through the fracture line. This direct approach to the fracture limits soft tissue stripping. Arthroscopy is never used in these high energy cases.

After reduction has been obtained and fluoroscopic evaluation indicates that it is satisfactory, the major fracture lines between the two condyles are fixed with 6.5mm cannulated screws. These screws are applied perpendicular to the major fracture line in an orientation determined during preoperative planning. These screws should be placed as close as possible to subchondral bone for optimal purchase, and to leave room for more distal application of external fixation pins (Figs. 24.4, 24.5). In most cases, two screws are sufficient, but occasionally more are needed. Washers may be necessary to optimize purchase in the soft cortex over proximal cancellous bone.

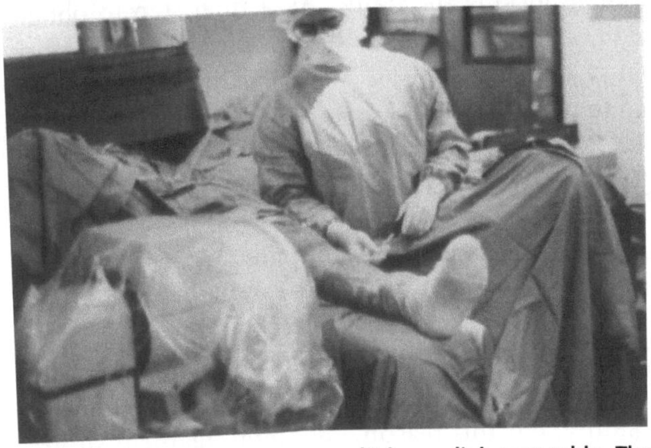

Fig. 24.1 Positioning is on a split-leg radiolucent table. The patient is in the supine position with the injured leg in extension. The opposite side of the table is dropped and the opposite leg placed in a lithotomy holder. This facilitates obtaining biplanar fluoroscopic images, which are critical to this procedure.

Fixator Application

The external fixator is used to reduce, accurately align, and stabilize the shaft beneath the reduced condyles. The type of frame chosen is important. An adjustable monolateral frame with ball joints and a telescopic body (Orthofix) allows fine tuning of axial alignment without soft tissue stripping (Fig. 24.5). Later in the course of treatment, axial dynamization assists in the maturation of callus at the metaphyseal/diaphyseal junction and protects the pin bone interfaces. A disadvantage of this frame construction using a proximal T-clamp is the fact that the direction and orientation of the proximal fixation pins are dictated by the design of the T-clamp. The author feels, however, that the advantages outweigh this disadvantage. Although there are clamp modifications now available that allow converging, and more versatile pin placement, the author has not found these to be necessary in the cases he has treated.

Careful fluoroscopic visualization should allow pin application into the 1:4 or 2:5 positions of the proximal T-clamp. This pin spread is preferred in order to obtain optimal fixation. The first pin should be applied "freehand" after having planned its location to accommodate a second pin in the desired clamp position. The pins should be applied beneath the previously placed cannulated screws, which will keep them as far from the joint as possible. The pins are orientated either from anterior to posterior, from anteromedial to posterolateral or from medial to lateral. The direction chosen is based on the pre-operatively determined location of the major condylar fracture lines, a consid-

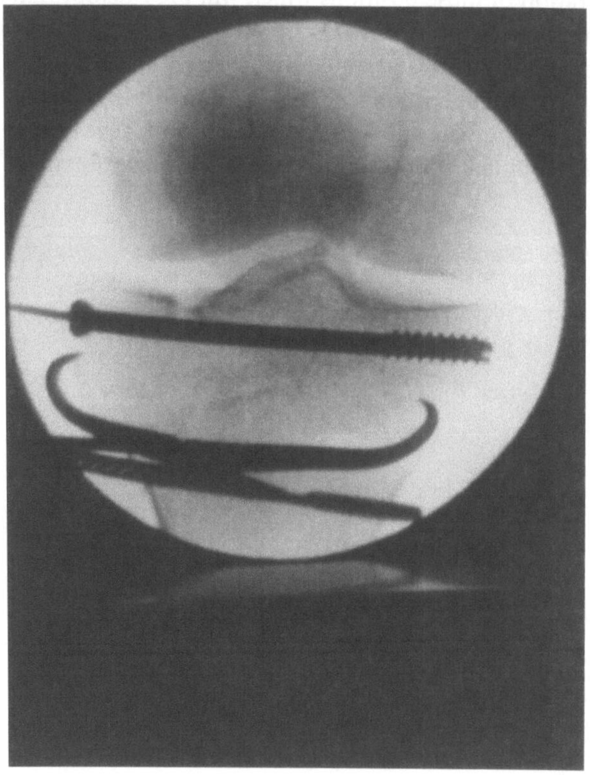

Fig. 24.2 An AP fluoroscopic view of a bicondylar tibial plateau fracture with a large tenaculum reduction forceps in place, during placement of a 6.5mm cannulated partially threaded screw in the subchondral region.

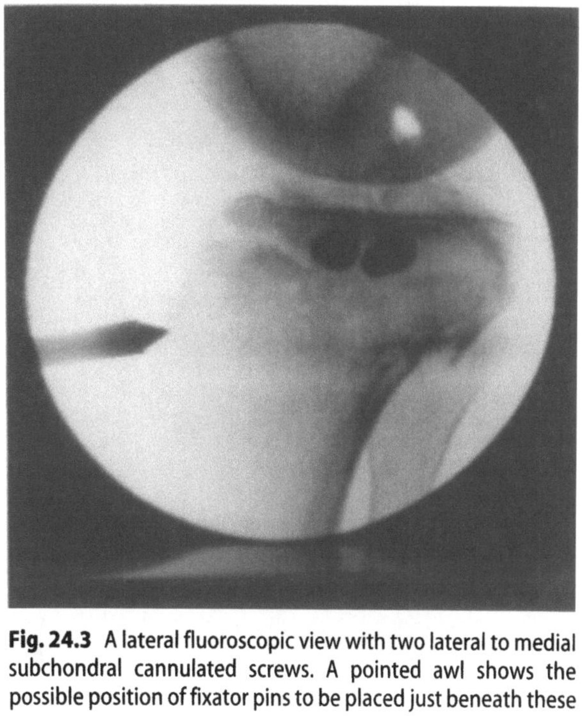

Fig. 24.3 A lateral fluoroscopic view with two lateral to medial subchondral cannulated screws. A pointed awl shows the possible position of fixator pins to be placed just beneath these screws.

eration of those positions which will provide optimal purchase for the external fixation pins, and the intra-operative appearance under fluoroscopy.

After application of the proximal pins, distal cortical pins are applied in a straight clamp. The frame is mounted and accurate axial alignment obtained prior to locking the frame. As a final step to obtain additional stability, the author often applies a further pin at approximately 90° to the main cluster, using a pin to pin clamp.

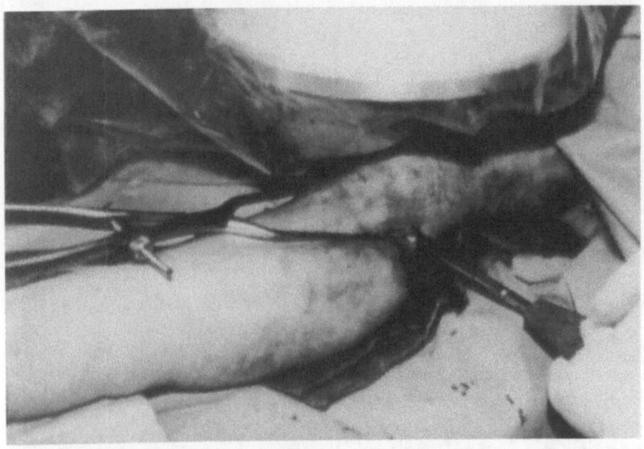

Fig. 24.4 The largest tenaculum reduction forceps which are available on most pelvic sets span the medial lateral width of the knee and hold the reduction. The fluoroscope and placement of a cannulated screw are demonstrated.

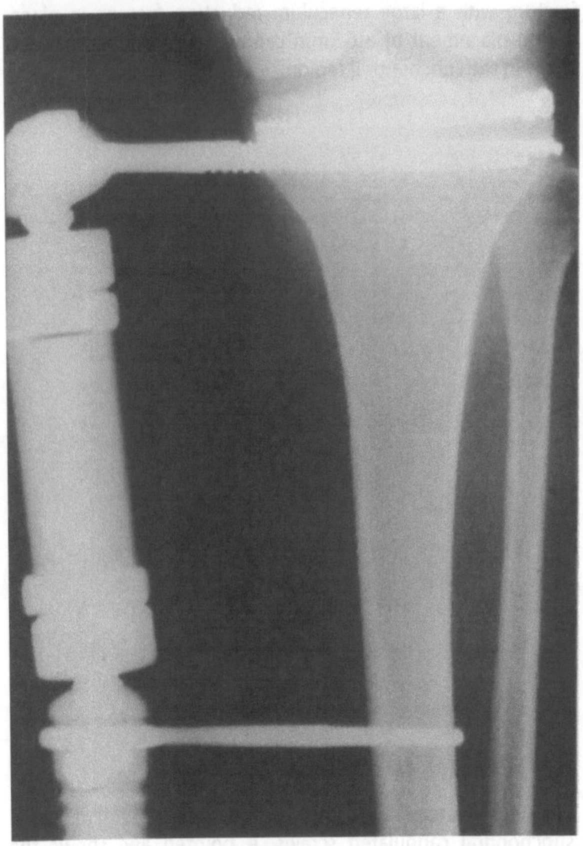

Fig. 24.5 This AP radiograph shows the position of subchondral cannulated screws and the fixator pins beneath these screws.

Ligament and Meniscal Injuries

Ligament and meniscal injuries are common in tibial plateau fractures.[1] In these high energy fractures, collateral ligaments generally stay attached to the bony fragment, and condylar reduction and fixation will therefore usually restore medial and lateral stability. For this reason, collateral ligament suture is not required. Injuries to the anterior or posterior cruciate ligaments on the major fracture fragments are addressed when the major condylar fragments are reduced and do not require further intervention. If one of the cruciate ligaments is avulsed on a bony fragment that is not reduced during the major reduction, a limited arthrotomy is required for screw or suture fixation. Intrasubstance lesions of the cruciate ligaments are not addressed in these high energy tibial plateau fractures. In the author's experience, late reconstruction has rarely been necessary.

Meniscal injuries frequently occur in association with these high energy fractures. The exact incidence is uncertain. The author does not routinely visualize the joint during surgical repair of these fractures. At follow-up none of the patients in this series was found to be symptomatic from meniscal injuries.[14] Meniscal injuries that occurred must either have healed during treatment or not affected the outcome in relation to the other injuries to the knee.

Post-Operative Protocol

Patients are allowed twenty kilograms of weightbearing (Fig. 24.6). The knee is supported in a knee immobilizer, which is fashioned around the frame. Patients are taught to perform a very gentle range of motion knee exercises, but these should not be at the cost of producing proximal pin inflammation. Most patients can increase weightbearing in conjunction with dynamization of the frame at about 4–6 weeks after injury. The exact timing will depend on the fracture pattern. Frame removal is effected at an average of 12 weeks after injury. If the patient is able to ambulate with full weightbearing in the frame, this is a good sign of union. Most patients do not require protection after frame removal.

Cross Joint Fixation

In open fractures or those with associated compartment syndrome, which require emergency surgery, cross joint fixation is often performed temporarily on the night of the injury. The frame can then be revised to a below-knee frame at a subsequent surgery for the management of open wounds or a fasciotomy site. Temporary spanning fixation of this kind may be in place for from one or two days, to one or two weeks.

Occasionally fractures may require longer periods of cross joint fixation. These are fractures which are severely comminuted, have the major metaphyseal disruption very close to the joint, or have a large joint depression component (Fig. 24.7). A very severe soft tissue injury is another indication for longer spanning fixation. Cross knee fixation for 3–6 weeks allows healing of the soft tissues, provisional stabilization of small comminuted fragments, and sealing of large joint depression cavities that communicate with the joint. In these cases, attempts to obtain definitive fixation on the same side of the knee leads to an unstable construct, proximal pin sepsis, and secondary joint sepsis through communicating joint depression cavities.

The cross knee frame should be applied as the first step in the procedure since it will distract the joint, assisting in condylar reduction. The frame is applied directly anteriorly, to provide optimal control of the forces across the knee. It should span the entire injury zone, and care must be taken to avoid the suprapatellar pouch during proximal pin insertion. A double coupling clamp may be necessary to construct a long enough frame. Reduction and cannulated screw fixation of the articular surface is performed as previously described, with the frame in place.

The cross knee frame is converted to a below-knee frame at 3–6 weeks after injury. Range of motion knee exercises are commenced at that time. In the author's experience these severely injured knees are able to recover a satisfactory range of motion after this period of immobility.

Results

The results of treatment of high energy tibial plateau fractures by external fixation using several different external fixators have been documented in the recent literature.[4,13,14,17,20] In all of these series there are 25–35 per cent open fractures, 10–20 per cent compartment syndromes, and predominantly Schatzker VI fractures with a significant percentage of AO Type C3 fractures. The duration of external fixation has most commonly been reported to be between 12 and 16 weeks. Considering the high energy nature of these fractures and the complexity of treatment, relatively few complications have occurred. Non-union occurs in less than 5 per cent of fractures, angular malunion in 10 per cent or less, and deep infection over the proximal tibia in less than 5 per cent of cases.

The results of treatment of 21 high energy tibial plateau fractures using the exact techniques and fixator described in the previous section have been previously reported.[14] There were 14 closed and 7 open fractures. One patient had a vascular injury, and 4 had compartment syndrome. Four patients were treated with cross knee frames, and 17 with frames on the tibial side of the knee only. The average duration of external fixation was 12 weeks. One patient only had a bone graft to the proximal tibia.

In all patients the proximal tibia healed without an additional procedure. Only 3 of the 21 patients had an angular malunion greater than 6°. Nineteen of the 21 knees achieved at least a 115° arc of flexion/extension. There was no difference in the range of movement between the 17 patients treated with external fixation on the same side of the knee and the 4 patients who were treated with cross knee external fixation.

Patients were followed up for an average of 38 months post- injury. On a 100 point knee score they averaged 87 points, (range 55–100 points) Sixteen of them were rated "good" or "excellent". The 7 patients who had knee instability on physical examination reported no functional handicaps secondary to this instability. Sixteen knees had no evidence of radiographic arthrosis, and only one had severe arthrosis. These patients scored close to age-matched controls on the SF-36 general health status instrument. Considering the severity of the injury, we considered the results excellent, and these knees appear to be doing well over time.

There were complications in this series related to the proximal pins which negatively affected patient outcome. Infection of proximal pins or wires are common complications when treating tibial plateau fractures by external fixation.[14,16,20] Seven of these 21 patients required antibiotics for inflammation of proximal pins, 2 of which led to knee joint infection. Due to the close proximity of pins and wires to the knee joint, septic arthritis is a concern with these techniques, and has been reported in other series. Septic arthritis has been seen to occur after both pin fixation and wire fixation of the proximal tibia.

Direct communication with the joint is one possible cause of joint infection. Capsular reflections extend for 15mm below the joint.[3] A wire or pin penetrating these

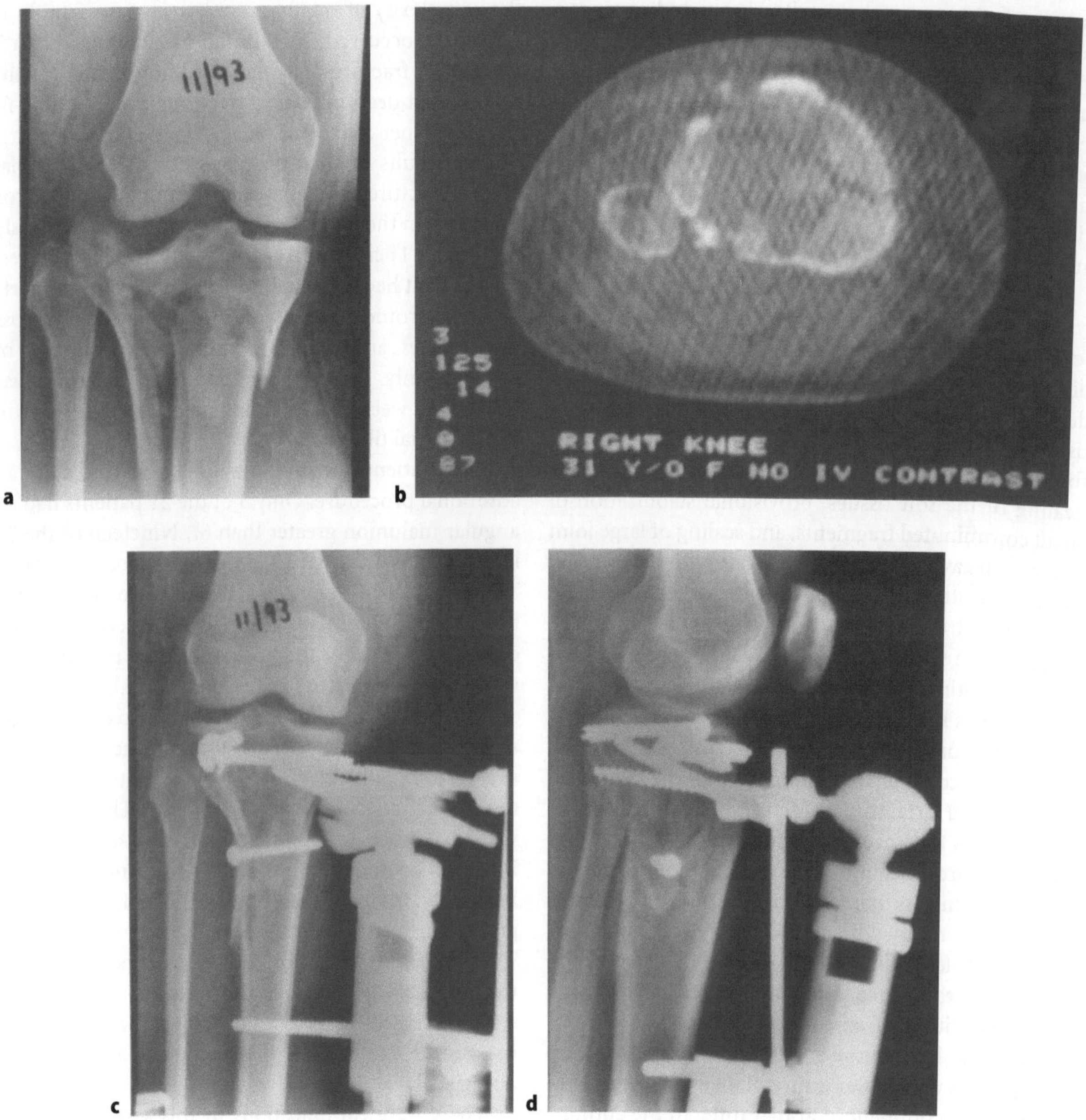

Fig. 24.6 Case 1: A 34 year-old female sustained ipsilateral injuries to the right tibial plateau and right tibial plafond in a motor vehicle accident. She was managed in traction for four days, and then underwent reduction and external fixation of both the tibial plateau and the tibial plafond through limited approaches. **a** An AP radiograph shows a markedly displaced proximal tibial plateau fracture involving both the medial and lateral condyles, which does not easily fit into any of the common fracture classification systems. The shaft is disrupted from the proximal tibia. **b** A transverse CT scan taken just below the level of the joint shows a coronal fracture line of the medial condyle and severe lateral joint depression. **c, d** AP and lateral post-operative radiographs show the position obtained after reduction and fixation with three screws and a monolateral external fixator placed anteromedially. Reduction was obtained by a combination of traction, reduction forceps, and a short extra-articular anterolateral approach. No bone grafts were used. **e** This full length AP view of the tibia shows the alignment of the limb after reduction and fixation and the position of the two external fixators. **f** This is a clinical photograph taken three weeks post-operatively, showing the proximal tibia fixator as well as well as the articulated fixator used for the tibial plafond. An out of plane accessory screw was placed from medial to lateral and attached to the proximal cluster of the articulated fixator for the tibial plafond. If the tibial plafond fracture had not been present, this would have been attached to one of the clusters of the tibial plateau fixator. **g, h** 22 months post-injury an AP standing radiograph of both knees and a lateral radiograph of the affected knee show sound fracture union and good maintenance of the joint space.

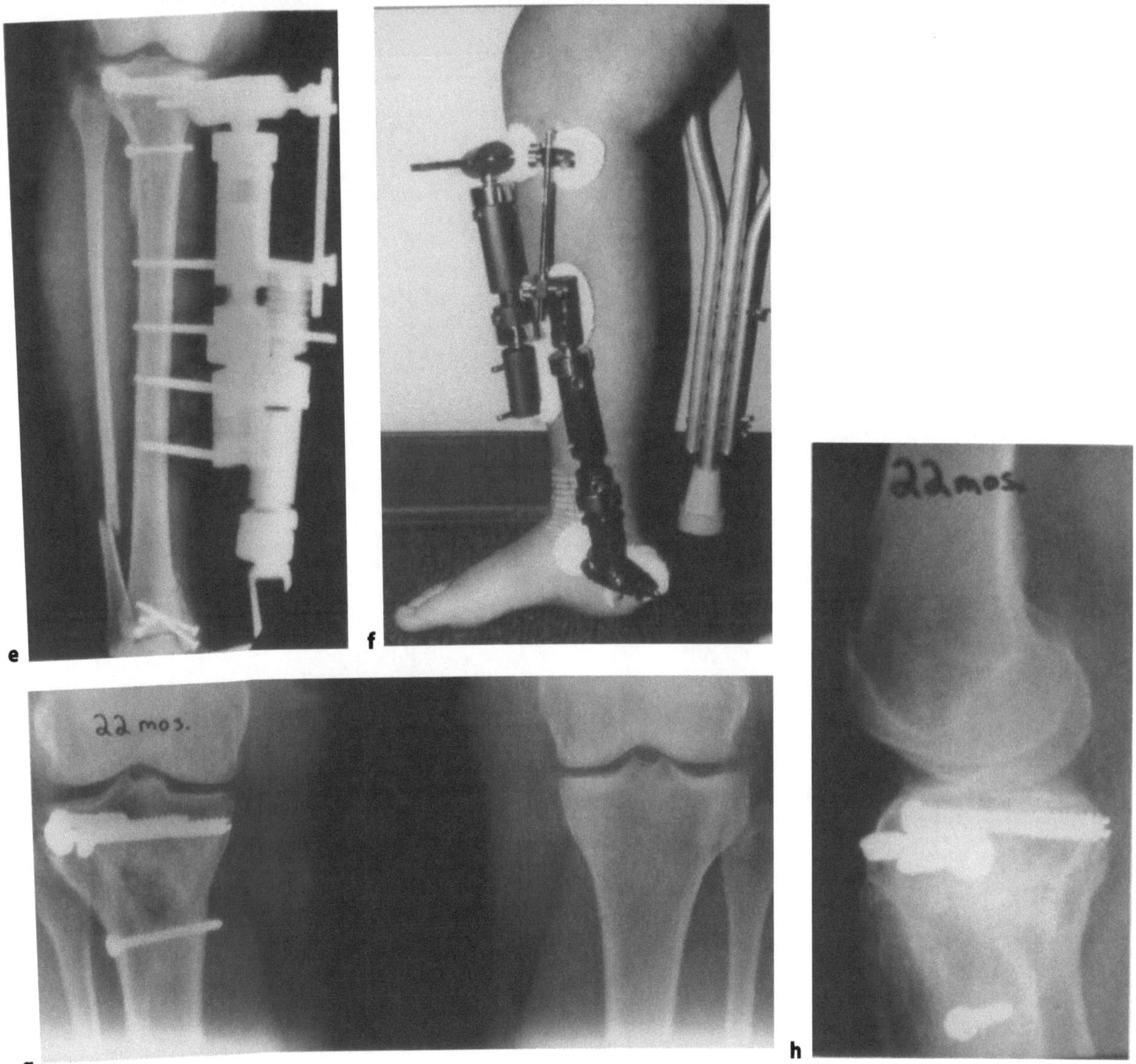

Fig. 24.6 (continued)

capsular reflections can result in direct communication with the joint. Alternatively, infection can occur through fracture lines communicating with the joint. In the author's view, the greatest potential for knee sepsis occurs in the high energy fractures associated with severe injuries to the soft tissues, particularly when there are large joint depression cavities that communicate proximally. Poor proximal fixation contributes to proximal pin or wire loosening and potential sepsis.

To minimize the risk of septic arthritis, the surgeon should aim to obtain excellent stability and should not accept poor fixation of the proximal tibia. Pins or wires should be kept at least 15mm from the joint. Post-operative knee range of motion exercises should be gentle, to avoid proximal pin inflammation. In the post-operative period, knee effusions should always be considered as potentially septic, and where clinical suspicion exists, the diagnosis should be confirmed by aspiration. In proximal tibia fractures with severe soft tissue injury, and especially in fracture patterns where proximal fixation would be difficult to obtain, with large joint depression cavities communicating with the joint, cross knee fixation is indicated. The results did not reveal any obvious disadvantages associated with a 3–6 week period of cross knee fixation, which removes communicating pins or wires from zone of injury.

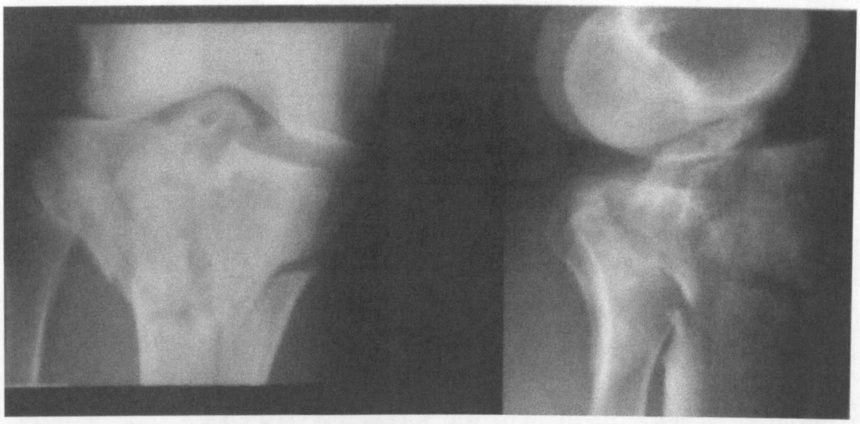

a

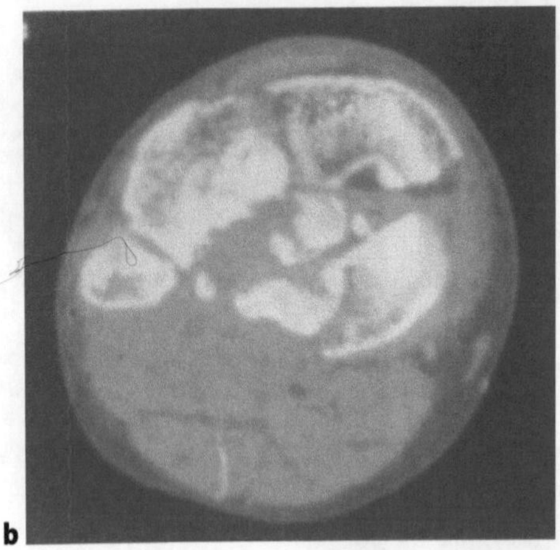

b

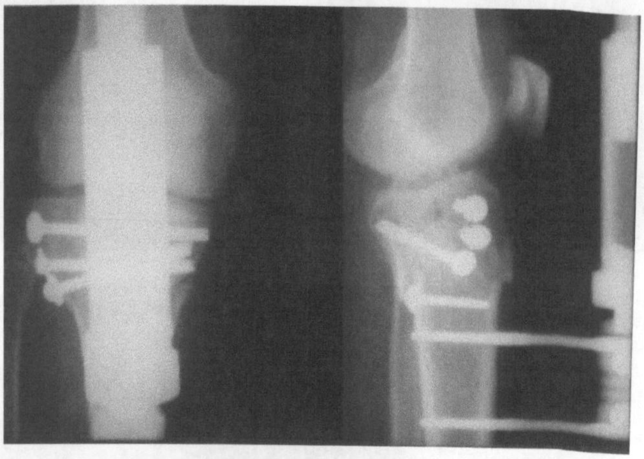

c

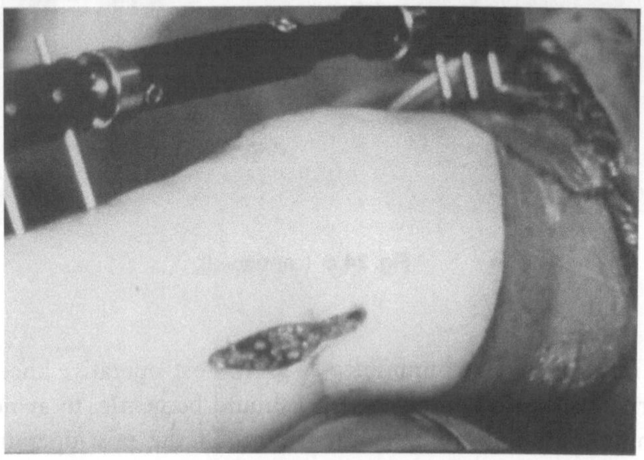

d

Fig. 24.7 Case 2: A 42 year-old construction worker fell 12 feet and sustained a high energy tibial plateau fracture as an isolated injury. He was treated by initial cross knee fixation for 5 weeks, which was then converted to below the knee fixation. Reduction was achieved after the initial application of the cross knee frame by a combination of percutaneous approaches and a posteromedial extra-articular approach. **a** AP and lateral radiographs show a severely comminuted proximal tibia fracture. In the AO Classification this would be a Type C3 fracture. **b** A transverse CT scan shows the comminution of the proximal tibia with one major lateral fragment and two major medial fragments. **c** An AP and lateral radiograph after cross joint external fixation and screw fixation of the proximal tibia, showing satisfactory reduction. **d** This clinical photograph shows the cross knee fixator, as well as the incision made for the posteromedial approach. **e** At 5 weeks the patient was returned to the operating room and the cross knee fixator was revised to a fixator on the proximal tibia only. The fixator screws were placed from anterior to posterior, and beneath the most proximal cannulated screw. **f** This clinical photograph shows 90° of knee flexion eight weeks after injury and three weeks after revision to a below the knee fixator. The original posteromedial incision has healed. **g, h** AP and lateral radiographs taken 5 years after injury show union and only mild degenerative changes. His range of motion was 0–125° and he complained only of weather-related pain.

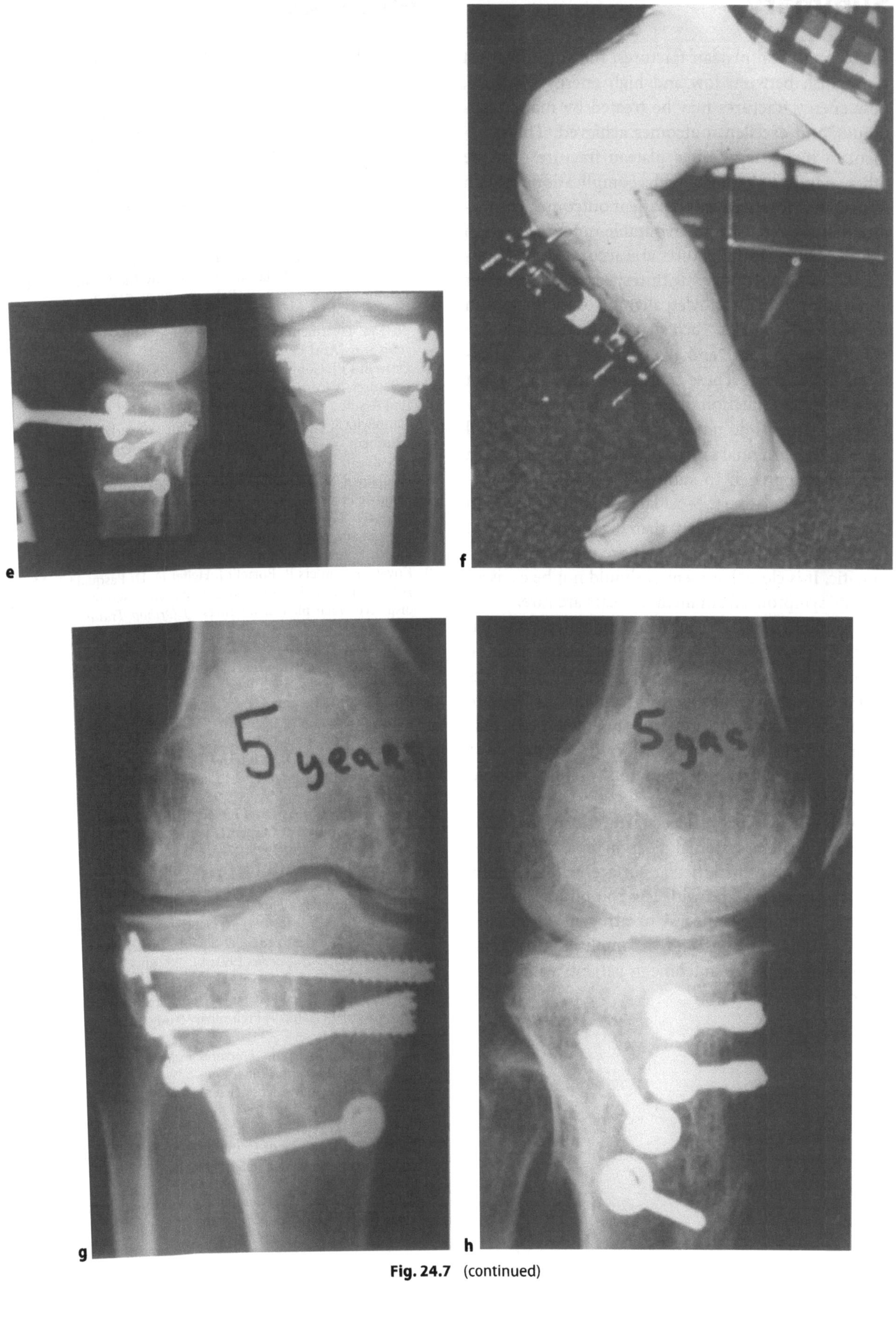

Fig. 24.7 (continued)

Summary

In treating tibial plateau fractures, the surgeon must distinguish between low and high energy fractures. Low energy fractures may be treated by many techniques, and excellent outcomes achieved. The treatment of high energy tibial plateau fractures, on the other hand, is fraught with complications which impact in a negative way on patient outcome. The factors that are related to a favourable outcome in high energy tibial plateau fractures are: accurate repositioning of the tibial condyles with respect to one another and to the femoral condyles; aligning of the shaft with the reduced condyles, such that the final limb alignment is near neutral, and avoidance of the complications of treatment. These factors are more important than an exact reduction of the articular surface. Early knee movements do not appear to be necessary in all cases to obtain a final satisfactory range of motion. An aggressive approach to suture of the collateral ligaments is not necessary. Most late instabilities relate to bony malalignment rather than ligamentous laxity. Ligament instabilities that occur are often not symptomatic. It is clear that menisci should not be excised, but late symptoms from meniscal tears are rare.

To obtain optimal results with monolateral external fixation, good fixation in the proximal tibia must be obtained with the proximal fixator screws. Ball joints and a telescopic body assist in obtaining accurate alignment. If good fixation cannot be obtained, cross knee fixation should be considered. In the most severely injured proximal tibias, this will help to avoid septic arthritis.

High energy tibial plateau fractures can be treated with monolateral external fixation and cannulated screw fixation of the articular surface, with generally satisfactory results and with few complications. This technique minimizes the risk of iatrogenic surgically-induced complications and accomplishes the goals required to optimize outcome in patients with severe proximal tibia fractures.

References

1. Bennett WF, Browner B. 'Tibial Plateau Fractures: A Study of Associated Soft Tissue Injuries.' *J Orthop Trauma* 1994; 8: 183–8.
2. DeCoster TA, Nepola JV, El-Khoury GY. 'Cast Brace Treatment of Proximal Tibial Fractures: A Ten Year Follow Up Study.' *Clin Orthop* 1988;231: 196–204
3. DeCoster TA, Stevens M. 'Safe Extra-Capsular Placement of Proximal and Distal Tibial External Fixation Pins'. Presented at the International Congress on Advances in the Ilizarov Method Commemorating 10 Years in the USA, Houston, Texas November 7–9, 1996.
4. Dendrinos GK, Kontos S, Katsenis D, Dalas A. 'Treatment of High-Energy Tibial Plateau Fractures by the Ilizarov Circular Fixator.' *J Bone Joint Surg* [Br] 1996; 78-B: 710–7.
5. Drennan DB, Locher FG, Maylahn DJ. 'Fractures of the tibial plateau. Treatment by closed reduction and spica cast.' *J Bone Joint Surg* [Am] 1979; 61-A: 989–94.
6. Duwelius PJ, Connolly JF. 'Closed Reduction of Tibial Plateau Fractures: A Comparison of Functional and Roentgenographic End Results.' *Clin Orthop* 1988; 230: 116–26.
7. Gausewitz S, Hohl M. 'The significance of early motion in the treatment of tibial plateau fractures.' *Clin Orthop;* 1986; 202: 135–8.
8. Honkonen S. 'Indications for Surgical Treatment of Tibial Condyle Fractures.' *Clin Orthop* 1994; 302: 199–205.
9. Jensen D. 'Tibial Plateau Fractures: A Comparison of Conservative and Surgical Treatment.' *J Bone Joint Surg* [Br] 1990; 72-B: 49–52.
10. Koval KJ, Sanders R, Borrelli J, Helfet D, Di Pasquale T, Mast JW. 'Indirect reduction and percutaneous screw fixation of displaced tibial plateau fractures.' *J Orthop Trauma* 1992; 6: 340–6.
11. Lachiewicz PF, Funcik T. 'Factors influencing the results of open reduction and internal fixation of tibial plateau fractures.' *Clin Orthop* 1990; 259: 210–5.
12. Lansinger O, Bergman B, Korner L, Anderson G. 'Tibial Condylar Fractures: A 20 Year Follow Up.' *J Bone Joint Surg* [Am] 1986; 68-A: 13–9.
13. Mallik AR, Covall DJ, Whitelaw GP. 'Internal Versus External Fixation of Bicondylar Tibial Plateau Fractures.' *Orthop Rev* 1992; 21(12): 1433–6.
14. Marsh JL, Smith ST, Do TT. 'External Fixation and Limited Internal Fixation for Complex Fractures of the Tibial Plateau.' *J Bone Joint Surg* [Am] 1995; 77-A: 661–73.
15. Moore TM, Meyers MH, Harvey JP. 'Collateral Ligament Laxity of the Knee: Long-Term Comparison Between Plateau Fractures and Normal.' *J Bone Joint Surg* [Am] 1976; 58-A: 594–8.
16. Murphy CP, D'Ambrosia R, Dabezies EJ. 'The small pin circulator fixator for proximal tibial fractures with soft tissue compromise.' *Orthopaedics* 1991; 14: 273–80.
17. Stamer DT, Schenk R, Staggers B, Aurori K, Aurori B, Behrens FF. 'Bicondylar Tibial Plateau Fractures Treated with a Hybrid Ring External Fixator: A Preliminary Study.' *J Orthop Trauma* 1994; 8: 455–61.
18. Tscherne H, Gotzen L. *Fractures with Soft Tissue Injuries.* Springer-Verlag: Berlin, 1984.
19. Watson J T. 'High-Energy Fractures of the Tibial Plateau.' *Orthop Clin North Amer* 1994; 25: 723–52.
20. Weiner LS, Kelley E, Yang E, Steuer J, Watnick N, Evans M, Bergman M.'The Use of Combination Internal Fixation and Hybrid External Fixation in Severe Proximal Tibia Fractures.' *J Orthop Trauma* 1995; 9: 244–50.
21. Young MJ, Barrack RL. 'Complications of Internal Fixation of Tibial Plateau Fractures.' *Orthop Rev* 1994: 149–54.

Proximal Metaphyseal Fractures of the Tibia

25

L. Renzi Brivio

Introduction

Fractures in the proximal region of the tibia may involve the metaphyseal area alone, or both the metaphysis and the joint itself. Where there is very severe comminution of the articular surface, as in AO type C2 and particularly AO type C3 fractures, it is becoming common practice to bridge the joint with an external frame using the principle of ligamentotaxis to achieve gross reduction and to combine this with minimal internal synthesis to re-establish the joint surface.[1,2]

In C1 fractures on the other hand, where the articular surface is not comminuted, and in A2 and A3 fractures which involve only the metaphysis, internal synthesis with a plate and screws is often used.[3,4,5,6] In recent years, however, there has been a tendency to move away from the use of extensive internal synthesis, especially in the tibia, in view of the associated problems. Interest has therefore focused on less invasive methods of stabilizing these fractures, and in particular in the use of closed reduction and external fixation, with or without minimal internal fixation.[7,8,9]

In A2 and A3 fractures, where only the metaphysis is involved, unisegmental external fixation alone is capable of stabilizing the fracture and maintaining this stability throughout the entire healing period. Where the fracture line involves the joint surface, as for example in a C1 fracture, it may be considered as a combination of two separate fractures, (a) that which must be reduced for anatomical reconstruction of the joint surface (the articular fracture), and (b) that involving the metaphysis, where fixation will not of itself influence the reduction of the articular surface (the metaphyseal fracture) (see Fig. 25.1), and a different approach is indicated for each of these.

The simple articular component may be stabilized by means of minimal internal synthesis using one or more lag screws. Where there is no displacement of the elements of the joint surface, reduction can be achieved in a closed manner; where there is displacement, however, anatomical reconstruction of the joint surface should be obtained, and this may necessitate a limited open approach to the joint surface, or the use of arthroscopy. Once the joint surface has been restored, the metaphyseal component of the fracture can readily be stabilized using a monosegmental external frame, in a closed procedure.

The present chapter describes the use of the Orthofix Module system in the treatment of types A2, A3 and C1 fractures of the proximal tibia with reference to the use of the Metaphyseal clamp, the Torbay-Garches clamp and the T-clamp.

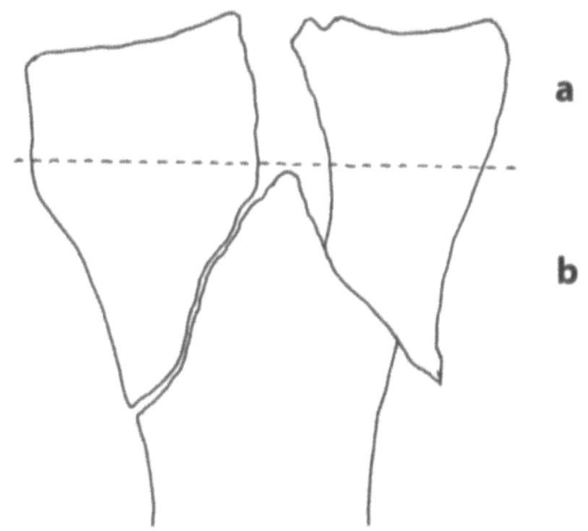

Fig. 25.1 A C1 fracture of the proximal tibia which may be considered as two separate fractures: **a** The articular fracture; **b** The metaphyseal fracture.

Methods and Materials

Use of the Metaphyseal Clamp

The metaphyseal clamp allows screw placement in both epiphyseal and metaphyseal areas in a biplanar configuration. It consists of two parts:

1. A component with four seats for horizontal placement of screws in the epiphyseal region of the bone.

2. A component with two seats for vertical placement of screws in the meta-diaphyseal region of the bone. This portion can be rotated to permit screw placement in the centre of the bone where there is superior bone stock, and it is locked in the desired position by means of a rotation locking screw using a polyhedral Allen wrench. Note that the configuration of screw seats in the clamp takes account of the relative positions of the diaphyseal and metaphyseal axes (Fig. 25.2a).

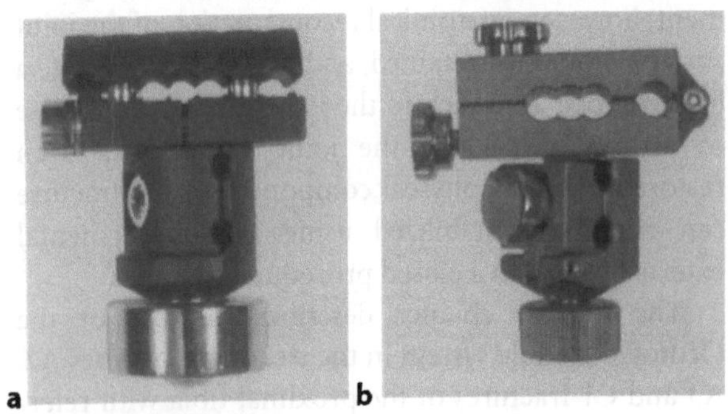

Fig. 25.2 The Metaphyseal clamp. **a** The definitive clamp; **b** The dedicated template.

In A2 and A3 Fractures

This clamp may be used in A2 and A3 fractures where there is sufficient space (i.e. at least 3cm) between the articular surface and the upper limit of the metaphyseal fracture, to permit introduction of the horizontal screws and at least one of the vertical screws (Fig. 25.3). Application may be either medial or antero-medial. The screws used in conjunction with the metaphyseal clamp are usually cancellous screws. Total screw length and length of the threaded portion will be determined preoperatively using a transparent X-ray overlay.

The first screws to be inserted are normally the epiphyseal (horizontal) screws and these should be introduced parallel to the plane of the joint under image intensification. Whether the anterior or the posterior screw is inserted first, care must be taken to ensure that there is adequate room for insertion of the second screw. A dedicated clamp template (Fig. 25.2b) exists, and this is used together with screw and drill guides in the normal fashion. Following application of the horizontal screws, one or two vertical screws are inserted, depending upon the space available. The vertical portion of the clamp template is rotated in the horizontal plane to identify the ideal position for optimal bone purchase (Figs. 25.4).

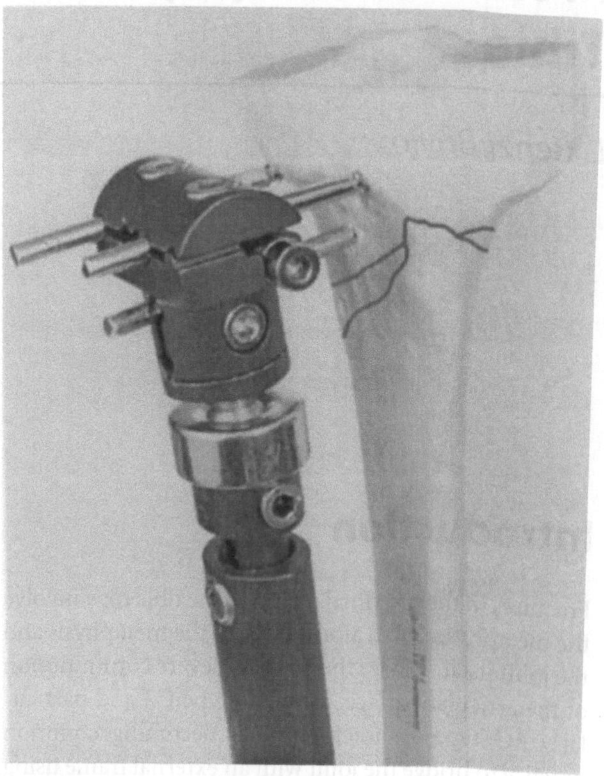

Fig. 25.3 Sawbone model showing the Metaphyseal clamp applied to a fracture of the proximal tibia.

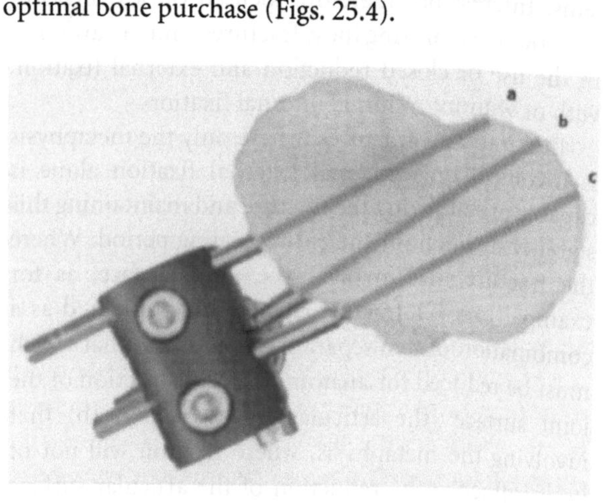

Fig. 25.4 View from above showing the horizontal screws in place (a, c), and one possible position (b) for insertion of a vertical screw.

Once the proximal screw cluster has been inserted, gross reduction of the fracture is achieved under image intensification and maintained during insertion of the distal screws. These (diaphyseal, cortical) screws are now inserted using either a classic template attached to the metaphyseal clamp template (where the 10.000 series is used), or a ProCallus body/straight clamp attached to the definitive metaphyseal clamp. When all the screws have been inserted and the definitive fixator applied, final reduction of the fracture is achieved and final tightening of both ball joints and the central body locking nut performed.

In C1 Fractures

The metaphyseal clamp may be used in some C1 fractures where the metaphyseal fracture is sufficiently distal to allow application of the clamp proximal to it. The articular fracture is reduced first. Where there is no displacement of the articular surface, as demonstrated pre-operatively by CT scan or tomography, stabilization may be achieved in a closed manner using one or two lag screws, inserted under image intensification. Where there is displacement of the articular surface, congruence must be restored by appropriate manipulation of the fragments either through a limited open approach, or under arthroscopic control. Once the articular fracture has been stabilized, the metaphyseal clamp is applied as described above, and the remainder of the assembly attached in the normal way (Fig. 25.5).

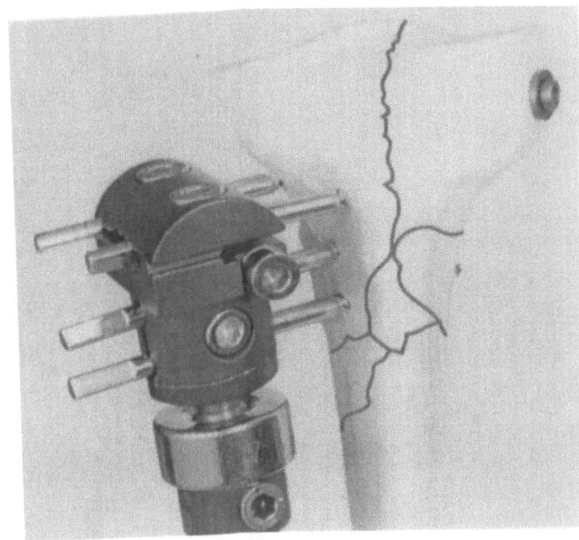

Fig. 25.5 Sawbone model to illustrate use of the Metaphyseal clamp in a C1 fracture of the proximal tibia where congruity of the articular surface has been restored using a lag screw prior to application of the clamp.

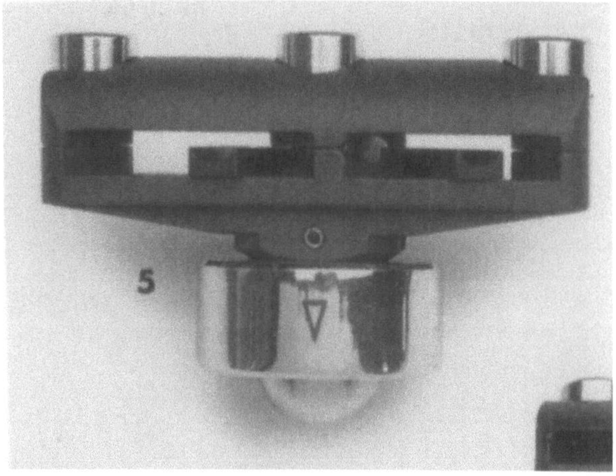

a

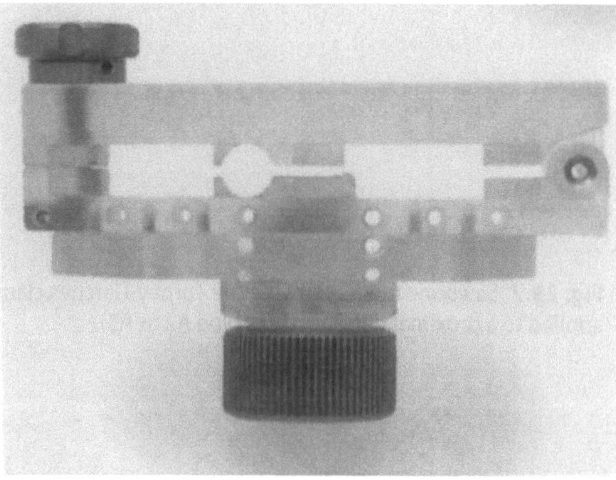

b

Fig. 25.6 The Torbay-Garches clamp which allows screws to be introduced in a convergent mode in A2 and A3 fractures where there is limited space. **a** The definitive clamp; **b** The dedicated radiolucent template.

Use of the Torbay-Garches

This module allows screws to be inserted in a convergent mode in the horizontal plane in the epiphyseal region. It consists of an elongated T-clamp with two outer swivelling screw seats and one intermediate, fixed screw seat. It has a dedicated template which is radiolucent (Fig. 25.6a, 25.6b).

In A2 and A3 Fractures

This clamp is used in A2 and A3 fractures where there is limited space between the articular surface and the upper limit of the metaphyseal fracture. Cancellous screws are used in the epiphyseal region, following the standard insertion technique, and should be introduced parallel to the plane of the joint surface under image intensification (Fig. 25.7). It may be applied medially,

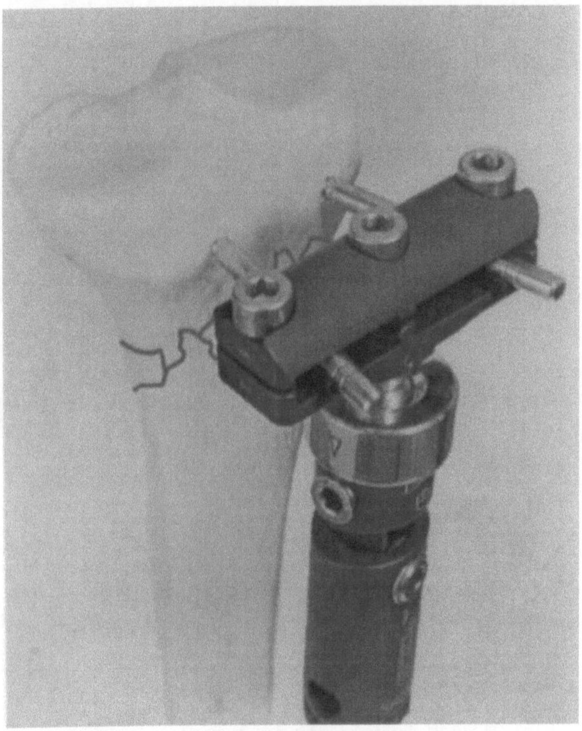

Fig. 25.7 Sawbone model showing the Torbay-Garches clamp applied to a proximal tibial fracture (Type A2 or A3).

antero-medially or anteriorly, depending upon the nature and location of the associated soft tissue injuries.

In the medial and antero-medial applications, the posterior screw is normally inserted first, and two screws are usually sufficient for most applications. In medial applications, the posterior screw is inserted parallel to the posterior cortex (Fig. 25.8a). This screw is then positioned in an appropriate seat of the radiolucent clamp template to allow the anterior screw to be introduced through the widest possible thickness of bone.

In antero-medial applications, the posterior screw is inserted obliquely, through the postero-medial half of the tibial plateau, but parallel to the joint surface. As for medial applications, the template is mounted on this screw and the anterior screw is inserted just medial to the patellar tendon, through the antero-lateral half of the tibial plateau (Fig. 25.8b). In anterior applications, the screws are inserted in a convergent mode, lateral and medial to the patellar tendon, using the outer, swivelling screw seats (Fig. 25.8c). Care should be exercised in this application to avoid over-penetration of the screws into the popliteal fossa, with the risk of damage to vascular structures.

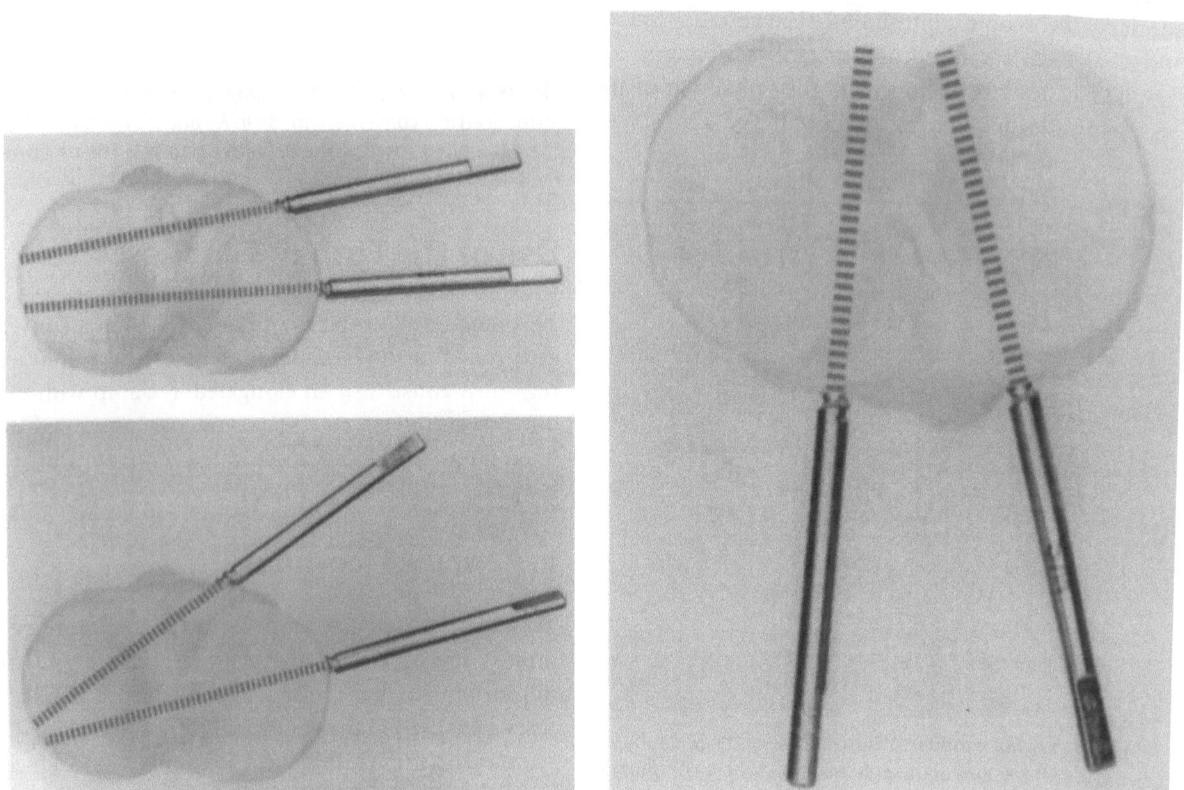

a b c

Fig. 25.8 Shows position of the bone screws when the Torbay-Garches is mounted: **a** medially; **b** antero-medially; **c** anteriorly.

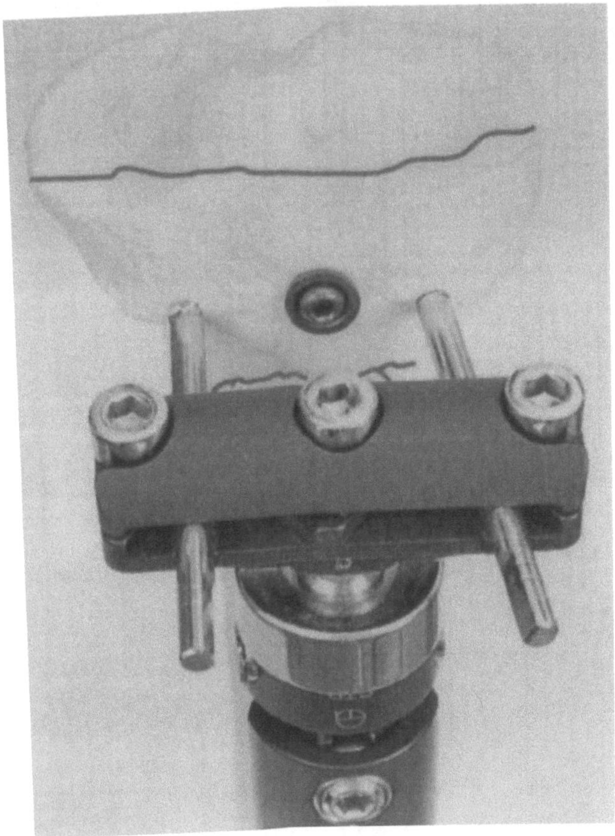

Fig. 25.9 Method of application of the Torbay-Garches in a C1 fracture where space is limited. Initial stabilization of the articular fracture with Kirschner-wires in the planned positions for the bone screws is followed by the insertion of a lag screw in the same plane as the wires. The latter are then replaced with the bone screws.

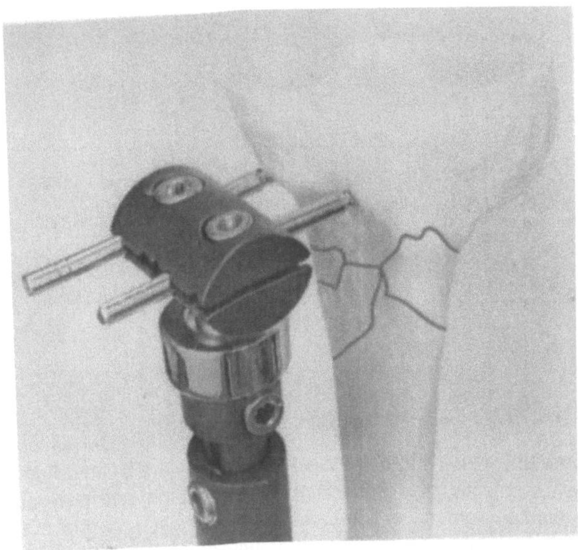

Fig. 25.10 Sawbone model showing the T-clamp applied to an A3 proximal tibial fracture.

Once the proximal screws have been positioned, alignment of the fracture should be verified under image intensification and maintained during insertion of the distal (diaphyseal, cortical) screws. These are now inserted in the standard manner using either the classic template in combination with the Torbay-Garches clamp template (where the 10.000 series is used) or a ProCallus body/straight clamp attached to the definitive Torbay-Garches clamp. When all the screws have been inserted and the definitive fixator applied, final reduction of the fracture is achieved and final tightening of both ball joints and the central body locking nut performed.

In C1 Fractures

Reduction of the articular fracture must be achieved initially, and stabilized using one or more lag screws. These lag screws must, as far as is possible, be perpendicular to the line of the articular fracture when viewed from above. The proximal screws of the fixator assembly should be placed in a plane immediately below the lag screws, and parallel to the joint surface. In situations where space is very limited, use of only one lag screw is recommended, since the proximal screws of the fixator will need to be inserted in the same plane as this lag screw (Fig. 25.9). In these circumstances, once the articular fracture has been reduced, either via a closed, or limited open manner, it is helpful to stabilize it by means of two Kirschner-wires inserted in the planned positions for the fixator screws. The lag screw is then introduced between the two wires to compress the articular fracture, and the wires subsequently replaced by the fixator screws.

Once the proximal screws have been applied, the metaphyseal fracture is stabilized as described for A2 and A3 fractures above.

Use of the T-Clamp

Where the Torbay-Garches clamp is not available, the standard (10.000 range) T-clamp may be used for the same indications (A2, A3, C1 fractures). This clamp, however, does not allow positioning of the proximal screws in a convergent mode, since its screw seats are fixed in a parallel relationship to one another (Fig. 25.10).

Typical case examples are illustrated in Figs. 25.11 and 25.12.

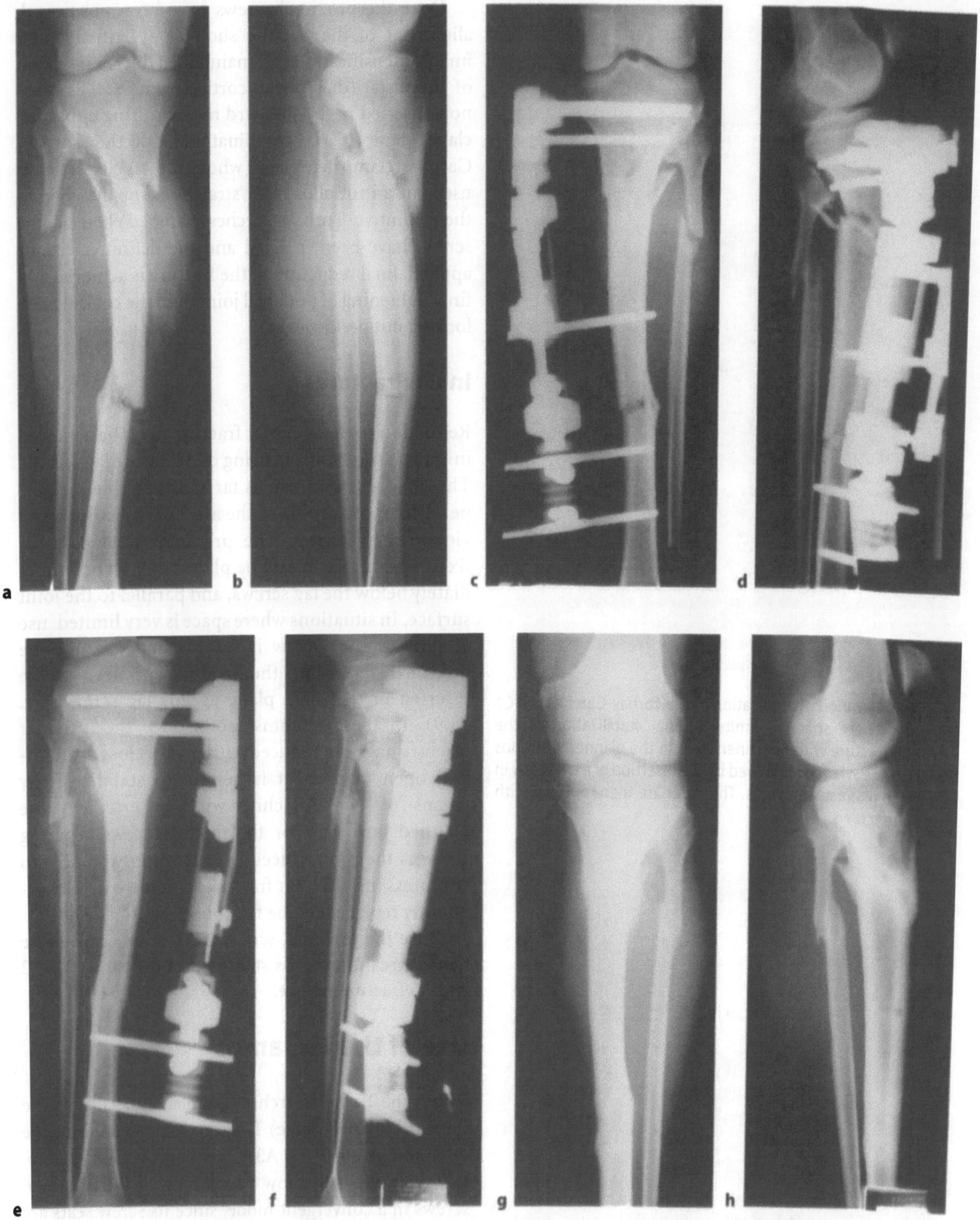

a b c d e f g h

Fig. 25.11 **a** Bifocal fracture of the tibia: A3.1 fracture of the proximal tibia plus a mid-diaphyseal fracture. AP view. **b** Lateral view. **c, d** AP and lateral views two weeks post-operation; the Metaphyseal clamp has been used to stabilize the metaphyseal fracture. A supplementary screw has been inserted into the long, unstable middle fragment. **e, f**. AP and lateral views at 3 months post-operation; the supplementary screw has been removed. **g, h** AP and lateral views at 5½ months post-operation; all hardware removed and both fractures solidly healed.

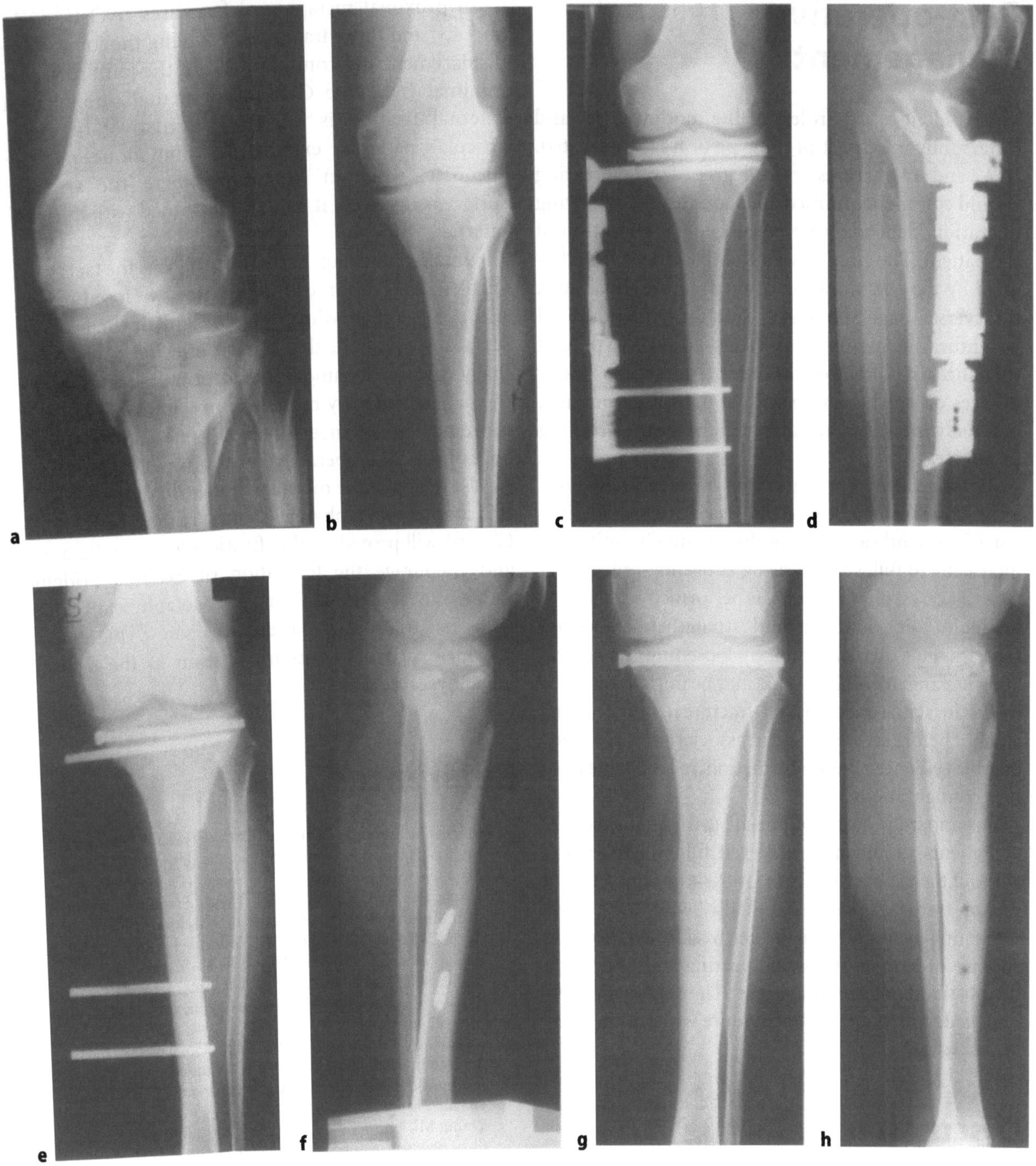

Fig. 25.12 **a** C1.2 fracture of the proximal tibia; AP view. **b** Following foot traction to reduce fracture. **c, d** AP and lateral views immediately post-operation showing lag screws in place to secure articular component and fixator with T-clamp to stabilize metaphyseal component. **e, f** AP and lateral views at 3 months post-operation immediately following removal of the fixator. All screws still in situ. **g, h** AP and lateral views 3 weeks after removal of the fixator. Fracture healed, lag screws still in place.

Post-operative Management

This is identical regardless of the module used, and differs only in respect of the type of fracture treated. In A2 and A3 fractures, some degree of weightbearing should commence immediately, on the day following operation, depending upon the general condition of the patient. The amount of weightbearing will be dictated by the configuration of the fracture. In simple, transverse metaphyseal fractures, unlimited weightbearing may be permitted according to patient tolerance. In oblique or comminuted fractures, lesser degrees of weightbearing will be permitted initially, gradually increasing to full weightbearing as healing progresses.

In articular fractures, patients are completely non-weightbearing for at least eight weeks, after which time partial weightbearing may be gradually initiated, increasing to full weightbearing as healing proceeds.

In all cases, physiotherapy is performed regularly to maintain joint function and strengthen associated muscles. Full dynamization, by loosening the central body locking nut of the fixator may be initiated at three weeks in stable metaphyseal fracture configurations and not before six weeks and in association with radiographic evidence of callus formation, in less stable fracture configurations.

A standard protocol of pin site care is followed.[10,11]

Patients should have achieved full weightbearing without the use of crutches before fixator removal. The fixator frame is removed initially, with the screws remaining in situ for one further week to confirm the absence of pain on full weightbearing and to exclude the possibility of minor collapse. The screws are then removed as an outpatient procedure without the need for anaesthesia.

Discussion

In fractures of the proximal tibia there is a growing tendency to move away from the use of major internal synthesis with plates and screws. These methods involve wide exposure of the fracture site with stripping of the periosteum and consequent damage to the vascular supply, necrosis of bony fragments and the potential risk of deep infection. In many such instances the use of intramedullary nails may not be appropriate, particularly where the fracture is close to the joint or where the articular surface itself is involved.

In proximal metaphyseal fractures (AO types A2 and A3) and those fractures involving the joint where displacement and comminution of the joint surface is minimal (AO type C1), unisegmental, monolateral external fixation is a viable alternative. In extra-articular patterns, external fixation alone may be adequate, while in situations where the articular surface is involved, it may be combined with minimal internal synthesis.

A major advantage of this approach is the fact that it enables stabilization of the fracture by closed means, and even in cases where realignment of the articular surface is required, this can be effected using minimally invasive techniques. Additional advantages for the patient are early mobilization with a full range of movement at the knee joint at all times and the avoidance of a second operation for removal of hardware.

Use of any of the modular attachments described in this chapter (Metaphyseal Clamp, Torbay-Garches, T-Clamp) will provide stable fixation for these fractures and encourage the formation of external bridging callus. Where space permits, the Metaphyseal Clamp, with its triangular pattern of screw placement, provides particularly secure fixation in the difficult metaphyseal region.

References

1. Marsh JL, Smith ST, Do TT. 'External Fixation and Limited Internal Fixation for Complex Fractures of the Tibial Plateau.' *J Bone Joint Surgery* [Am] 1995; 77-A: 661–73.
2. Marsh JL. 'High Energy Tibial Plateau Fractures: Treatment with Monolateral External Fixation.' This book, Ch. 24.
3. Burrl C, Bartzke R, Coldewey J, Muggler E. 'Fractures of the tibial plateau.' *Clin Orthop* 1979; 138: 84–93.
4. Mallik AR, Covall DJ, Whitelaw GP. 'Internal versus external fixation of bicondylar tibial plateau fractures.' *Orthop Rev* 1992; 21: 1433–6.
5. Moore TM, Patzakis MJ, Harvey JP Jr. 'Tibial plateau fractures: definition, demographics, treatment rationale, and long-term results of closed traction management or operative reduction.' *J Orthop Trauma* 1987; 1: 97–119.
6. Young MJ, Barrack RL. 'Complications of internal fixation of tibial plateau fractures.' *Orthop Rev* 1994; 149–154.
7. De Bastiani G, Aldegheri R, Renzi Brivio L. 'The treatment of fractures with a dynamic axial fixator.' *J Bone Joint Surg* [Br] 1984; 66-B: 538–45.
8. Smith ST, Marsh JL, Found EF. 'External fixation for severe tibial plateau fractures.' *Orthop Trans* 1992–3; 16: 631.
9. Weiner LS, Kelly M, Yang E, Steuer J, Watnick N, Evans M, Bergman M. 'Treatment of severe proximal tibial fractures with minimal internal and external fixation' (Abstract) *J Orthop Trauma* 1991; 5: 236–7.
10. Checketts RG, Otterburn M, MacEachern G. 'Pin track infection: definition, incidence and prevention.' *Int J Orthop Trauma* 1993; Suppl Vol 3 (3); 16–18.
11. Checketts RG, Otterburn M, MacEarchern AG. 'Pin track infection and the principles of pin site care.' This book, Ch. 12.

Diaphyseal Fractures of the Tibia: Defining the Place of External Fixation

26

J.R.W. Hardy and J.B. Richardson

Introduction

The management of tibial diaphyseal fractures is frequently rationalised into a simple regimen of one type of treatment for all injuries. Any treatment modality, however, has the potential for post-treatment complications. This means that the clinician should have both an understanding of the risks and benefits of a treatment and the necessary skills to apply it. The availability of a variety of treatments which can be applied in appropriate situations avoids the dependence upon a single treatment policy with its attendant complications.

In the 200 or so publications on tibial fracture management each year, high energy injuries receive the most attention and low energy injuries the least. For this reason treatment patterns for low energy injuries vary throughout the United Kingdom. There is only one published algorithm that describes and explains the optimal use of external fixation in the management of these fractures (Hardy et al 1996).

Fractures of the tibia commonly arise from sporting activities (Cattermole et al 1996), road traffic accidents (Court-Brown CM and McBirnie J 1995) and industrial accidents (Wu Y-S and Zhang F-B 1994). A proper diagnosis involves eliciting the symptoms and signs of both bone and soft tissue damage. Radiographs are essential but diagnosis of the soft tissue injury requires a good history of the mechanism of injury, early examination of the leg and ultimately, examination under anaesthesia in some cases. The soft tissue injury is often largely ignored and yet it is an excellent guide to the selection of those patients who require more than a conservative approach.

The first assessment in a treatment algorithm for a tibial diaphyseal fracture should consider whether the wound is open or closed. It is accepted practice that compound wounds should be treated differently from closed wounds (BOA/BAPS 1993), regardless of the bony injury, and the Gustilo classification should therefore be considered in any algorithm (Gustilo and Anderson 1976, Gustilo et al 1984).

Unlike residual deformity of the femur, residual deformity of the tibia is much more noticeable. The image-conscious patient is looking for as little functional loss and deformity as possible. Shortening in excess of 1cm tends to be unacceptable, particularly where the fractured limb was congenitally the shorter of the two limbs before fracture. A deformity of greater than 10° is noticeable clinically (Nicoll 1964). The effect on the line of weightbearing through the ankle joint depends on the level of the deformity; a high fracture has a greater effect than a low fracture. The axial stability of a fracture should therefore be taken into account in determining the method of immobilization. Only one algorithm classifies fractures in terms of axial stability (Hardy et al 1996) although this can often be inferred from the AO/ASIF classification (Müller et al 1991).

The healing of a fracture depends upon the patient's age, the tissue damage at the time of fracture (Ellis 1958a, Court-Brown et al 1990a, Oni et al 1988a, Weissman et al 1966, Nicoll 1964, Keating et al 1991), and the method of immobilization of the fracture site. This algorithm applies to patients over the age of skeletal maturity only. Treatment of patients under the age of 16 is limited because of the importance of avoiding damage to the growth plates. The use of plaster casts and external fixation techniques only are recommended for the treatment of diaphyseal fractures in children, which often heal without complication (Ellis 1958a, Weissman et al 1966).

Diagnosis of the severity of injury to the soft tissues is most difficult. The soft tissues include skin, fat, muscle, tendon, artery, nerve, and periosteum. The periosteal, or soft tissue hinge, as described by Sir John Charnley (Charnley 1961), is as important in the tibia as it is in the radius. The diagnosis of the presence of an intact periosteum cannot be inferred from the initial history and examination but can be deduced on examination under anaesthesia.

Bony injury depends on the magnitude of the injuring load, the rate and type of loading, the local structure of the tibia, the material properties of the bone, and the soft tissues. The same energy may produce a different pattern of injury in an elderly osteoporotic individual and an athletic young person. The pattern of bone injury tells the surgeon something about the type of load that caused the fracture. A spiral fracture results from indirect injury and is caused by a torsional force. It has been estimated that it requires 50 per cent less force to break the bone in torsion than in bending (Oni et al 1988b). A simple transverse fracture occurs with a bending load, and an oblique fracture occurs with bending while the bone is in compression. With a rapid rate, or higher magnitude of loading comes comminution of the tibia and concomitant fracture of the fibula. Low energy injuries of the tibia heal on average in 16 weeks when time to independent weightbearing is considered. High energy injuries take much longer to heal (Ellis 1958a, Court-Brown et al 1990a, Court-Brown et al 1991). The pattern of the fracture predicts not only its severity but also its axial stability.

The Closed or Gustilo Type 1 Undisplaced Fracture

Patients with a history of a low energy insult, no deformity, little bruising over the shin, an axially stable fracture, an intact fibula, and an undisplaced fracture are usually treated conservatively in plaster with early load-bearing through the injured limb. Those that are compound should be treated as recommended below.

The Closed or Gustilo Type 1 Displaced Fracture

Integral to deciding the management of a patient with a displaced fracture is the diagnosis of the state of the periosteal hinge (Charnley 1961). Following an injury which causes displacement, the periosteum is divided either over a part, or over the whole of its circumference. Diagnosis of periosteal injury in the closed fracture should take place under general anaesthesia as the periosteum is well innervated and movement in the acute stages causes pain. The tibia should be reduced before assessing the state of the periosteum.

An intact fibula usually implies a low energy injury. One should beware the oblique tibial fracture with an intact fibula which often slips into varus, or proceeds to a hypertrophic non-union because the fibula holds the fracture gap apart. These fractures should be reduced perfectly. The fibula can be used as a fulcrum, the fracture gap opened and the ends of the bones guided into perfect reduction using image intensification. If under anaesthesia the varus returns with an applied axial load, then the fracture is unstable and fixation is required. If external fixation is used then the fibula must be divided.

If, following a high energy injury, reduction is found to be easy, and the fracture once reduced is distractible, a circumferential tear of the periosteum should be suspected. Accurate and maintained reduction is important to maximise the healing potential of the fracture (Ellis 1958a). Transverse high energy injuries with no soft tissue hinge are difficult to treat in plaster cast, because early weightbearing causes deformity. Other patterns of closed, bony injury with a circumferential periosteal tear are associated with shortening and deformity on weightbearing. It is not known if these patients are best treated by open reduction and internal fixation with dynamic compression plates, closed intramedullary nailing, or external fixation. External fixation in these circumstances may be an acceptable method of immobilization. However, post-operative management becomes arduous because the pin sites must be maintained clean and uninfected for long periods. In these patients intramedullary nailing should be considered unless the patient's occupation involves working on the knees.

Tibial fractures that are difficult to reduce usually have a partially intact periosteum (Charnley 1961). The longer the time elapsing between injury and attempted reduction, the more difficult the reduction, because the soft tissues contract. Early and definitive management of a diaphyseal fracture is always recommended. When reduction is prevented by an intact periosteum in a shortened transverse fracture, it is easiest to overcome by recreating the deformity that occurred at the time of injury. This is the same principle as that used to reduce children's distal forearm fractures (Rang 1984). When reduction has been achieved, the site of the periosteal hinge can be

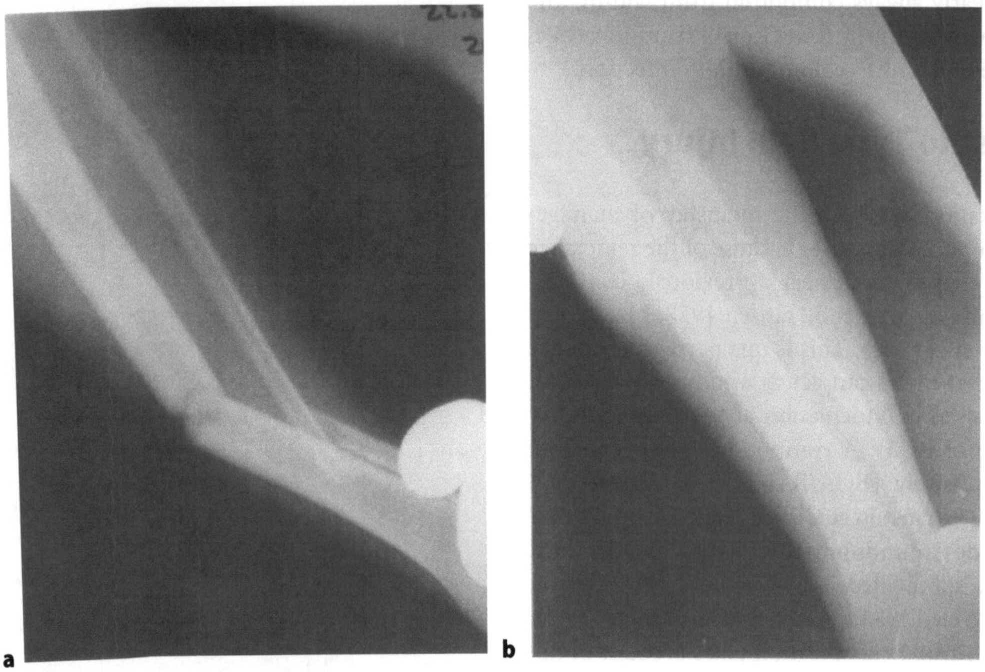

a b

Fig. 26.1 Diagnosing the site of the periosteal hinge under anaesthesia, shown on radiographs. **a** The tear in the periosteum is on the medial surface. **b** A varus force demonstrates an intact lateral surface periosteum. This fracture was unstable to an axial load and for this reason was treated by external fixation.

deduced by attempting to displace the fracture in anterior, posterior, medial and lateral directions (Fig. 26.1). After reduction, axial stability should be assessed by applying an axial load of at least 20kg to the foot.

A reduced, axially stable fracture with an intact periosteal hinge is best treated with a plaster cast. The periosteal hinge is used to maintain the reduction in plaster by using the plaster to provide two points of pressure against a third fulcrum, opposite the intact periosteum. Early weightbearing is usually rewarded by appearance of callus beneath the intact periosteum first (Fig. 26.2). The patient with this pattern of injury may be encouraged to bear weight as early as comfort allows.

If the applied axial load demonstrates that the fracture is unstable with respect to shortening, then walking in plaster is likely to cause similar shortening (Watson 1994). If, however, the same patient has a demonstrably intact periosteal hinge, the likelihood of the fracture healing within 16 weeks is high. These patients benefit from external fixation which maintains length and allows them to weightbear. A modern unilateral frame, such as the Orthofix, which permits the early application of cyclic micromovement, permits sufficient movement at the fracture site to encourage callus formation.

The skin lesion of a compound Gustilo Type I fracture should be treated as for all compound fractures. There is usually no contamination, however, as the

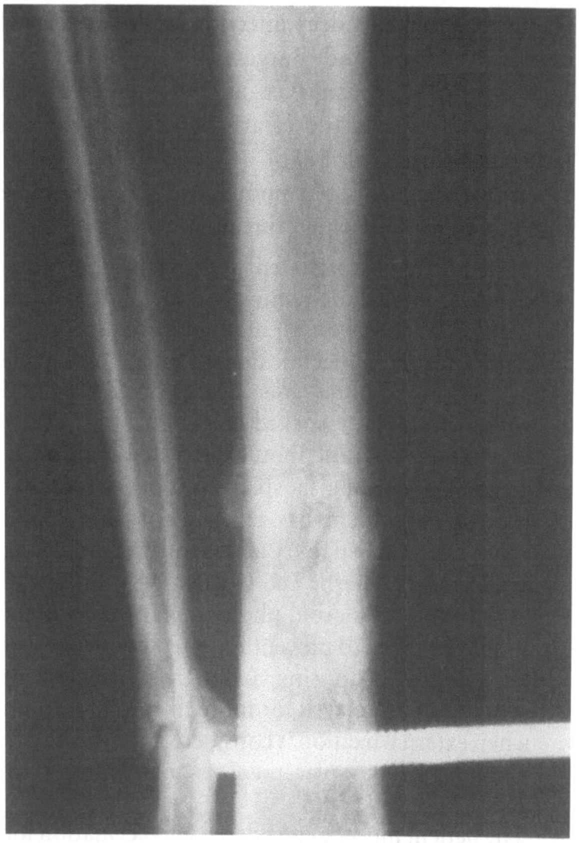

Fig. 26.2 Radiograph of the same patient as in Fig. 26.1 demonstrating that callus has appeared on the side of the intact periosteum first.

wound is nearly always compound from within, and methods involving the introduction of fixation devices into the site of fracture seldom result in infection.

The Gustilo Type II–III Injury

External fixation has been the mainstay of management of compound fractures because of the reluctance to leave foreign material near a previously contaminated wound (Clancey and Hansen 1978, Marsh et al 1991, Baker et al 1992). This is due partly to evidence indicating that metal can act as a nidus for bacterial infection caused by inoculation at the time of injury (Andriole et al 1973). A compound wound must be treated aggressively (BOA/BAPS 1993, Gustilo and Anderson 1976, Gustilo et al 1984). The Gustilo classification divides wounds into three 'types' and the third type is now subdivided a–c (Gustilo and Anderson 1976, Gustilo et al 1984, Gustilo and Gruninger 1987). The revised Gustilo classification takes account of the mechanism of injury, the degree of soft-tissue damage, the fracture configuration and wound contamination (Gustilo et al 1990). Type II and III compound injuries are associated with substantial periosteal stripping and tend to be the result of high energy injuries. They are often complicated by deep infection as well as delayed union (Anderson and Burgess 1943, Gustilo and Anderson 1976, Gustilo et al 1984, Gustilo and Gruninger 1987, Gustilo et al 1990, Dellenger et al 1988a, Dellenger et al 1988b).

The management of compound wounds should be based upon the following principles:

1. Basic fracture management at the scene of the accident should include removal of obvious contaminants from the wound, attempted reduction (to reduce further ischaemic tissue damage), splintage of the injured bone, and coverage of the wound with an iodophore-soaked dressing.
2. A compound wound should be treated as an emergency. On arrival at hospital, and once resuscitation of the patient has taken place, the wound should be swabbed to try and identify the infecting organisms (Tscherne and Gotzen 1984, Robinson et al 1989). A Polaroid photograph of the wound should be taken to prevent repeated uncovering of the iodophore dressing. Operative management should not be delayed for more than 6 hours, and when external fixation is considered, pre-operative planning of pin placement is mandatory (Fig. 26.3).
3. The patient must be considered for vaccination for tetanus, and intravenous antibiotics should be begun immediately, to treat the likely contami-

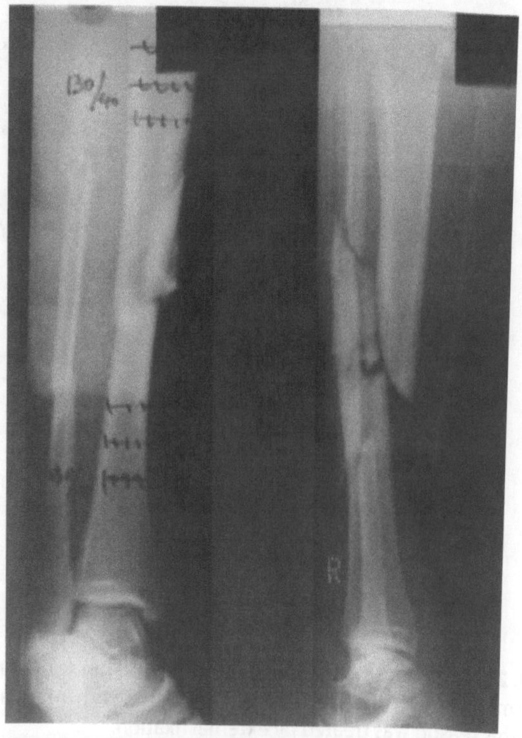

Fig. 26.3 Pre-operative planning of pin placement ensures that pins are placed more than 2.5cm from the fracture site so as not to interfere with the fracture haematoma, and that the correct length of pin is used.

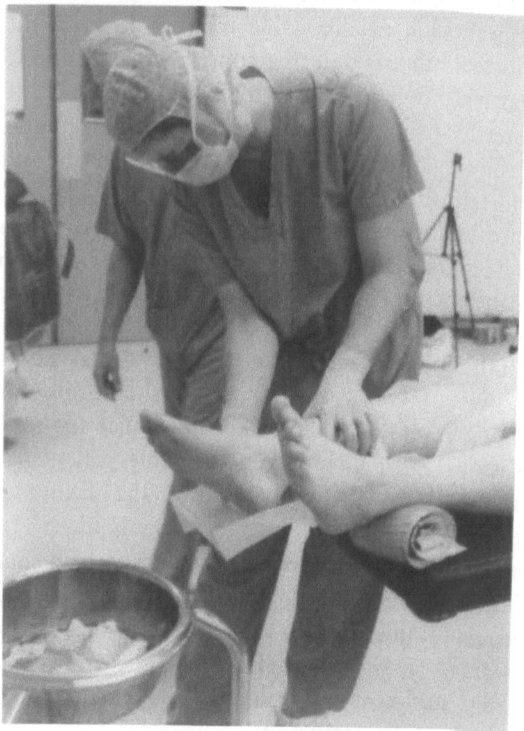

Fig. 26.4 A social clean of the surrounding skin before the operation is as important as aseptic precautions during the operation.

nating organisms. Antibiotics are continued for 3 days and changed depending upon the results of bacterial culture (Wilkins and Patzakis 1991).

4. On arrival in theatre, with the wound covered, the limb should be cleaned of dirt with a large sterile gauze soaked in chlorhexidine solution (Fig. 26.4). A tourniquet should not be used unless there is uncontrolled haemorrhage. The dressings should be removed and the limb cleaned with an aqueous solution of betadine and toweled to exclude the unprepared skin and other surfaces.
5. The extent of contamination of the wound, periosteal stripping, and tissue ischaemia, should be assessed. All visible contaminants should be removed and 2–5 litres of saline used to irrigate the wound and remove blood and contaminants, which should be safely contained (Fig. 26.5). The management of compound wounds is not only associated with the risk of cross-infection to the patient, but also to the surgeon. These operations should therefore be performed by the experienced surgeon used to using universal precautions (Gerberding et al 1990, CDC 1987, CDC 1988). The wound edges should be excised, together with a thin layer of subcutaneous fat (Fig. 26.6). Sufficient fat should be excised, however, to remove the betadine-stained and hence, contaminated layer. The wound may need to be extended for access, so that both bone ends can be inspected and cleaned. Ingrained dirt should be nibbled from the dead bone ends. All small bone fragments devoid of periosteum are dead and should be discarded. Clean periosteum should be preserved at all costs. Segmental bone loss is best dealt with early by planned use of bone transport and bone grafting when necessary (Pennig 1991). The wound should then receive a final 2–5 litre lavage (Fig. 26.7). The wound is not closed but left open for repeat débridement 24–48 hours later. The periosteum should be laid in close proximity to the fractured ends of the bone.
6. Prior to the application of external fixation, the fracture must be reduced and can be held temporarily with bone holding forceps or skeletal traction to achieve anatomical alignment. K-wires and drill holes should be avoided at the fracture site as they produce bone swarf which is dead and can act as a nidus for infection. The best results are obtained by applying an in line fixator to a reduced fracture (Fig. 26.8).
7. Consultation with plastic surgeon colleagues allows planned early coverage of any soft tissue defects (Green 1994). A surgeon should aim to have a wound covered within five days of the fracture. Early bone grafting should be considered if clinical examination and fracture stiffness suggest

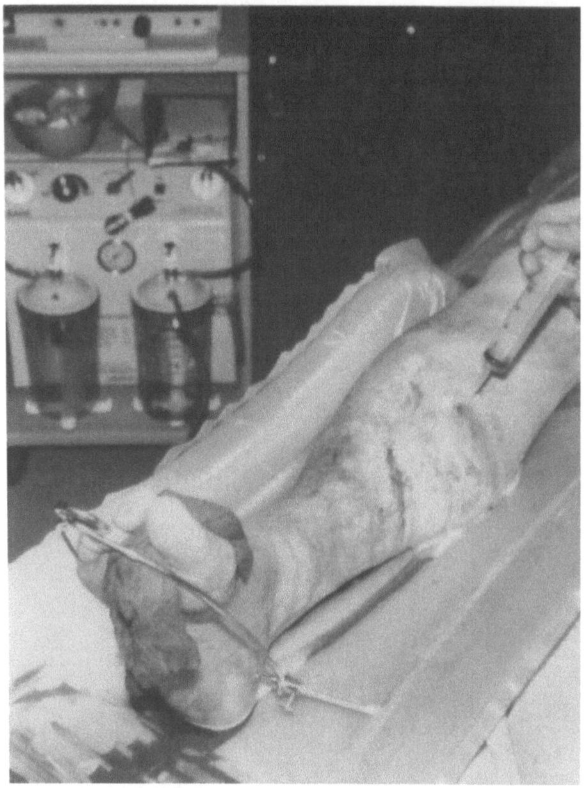

Fig. 26.5 Copius irrigation of the wound with buffered saline can be achieved using a syringe and broken off needle initially, followed by pulsed lavage when the first debridement has been performed.

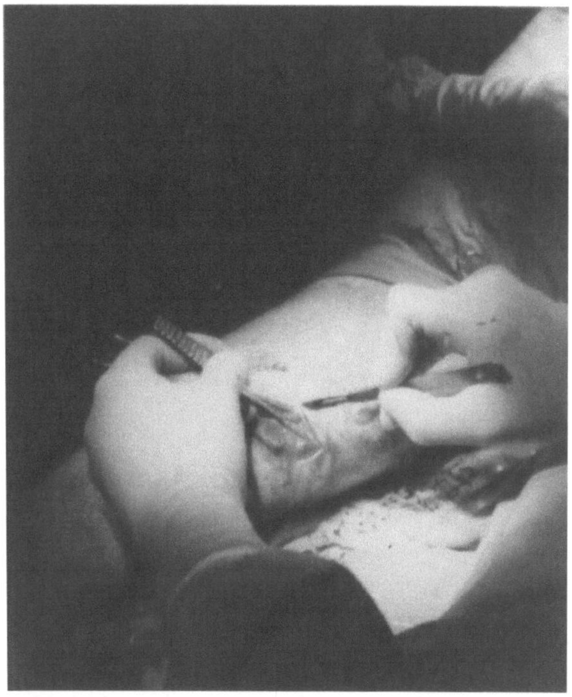

Fig. 26.6 Excision of the wound edges back to healthy bleeding tissues.

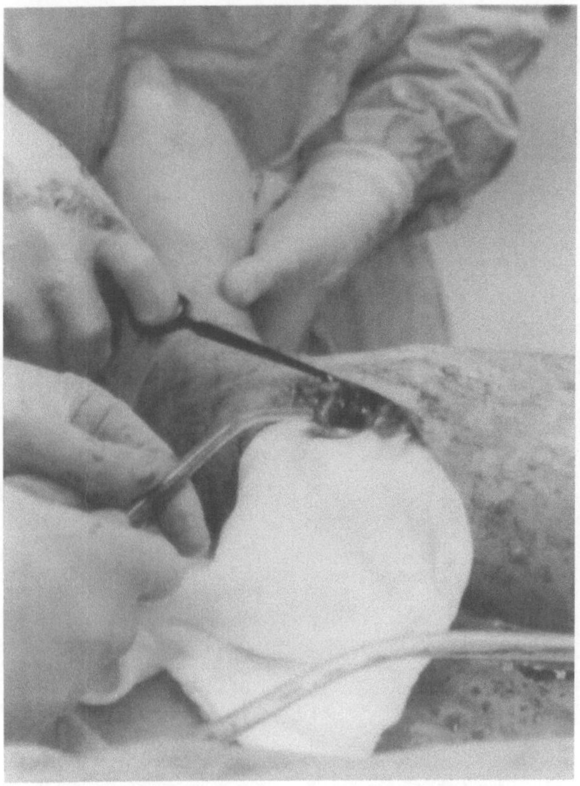

Fig. 26.7 Ensure both ends of bone are brought into the wound for formal inspection and cleaning.

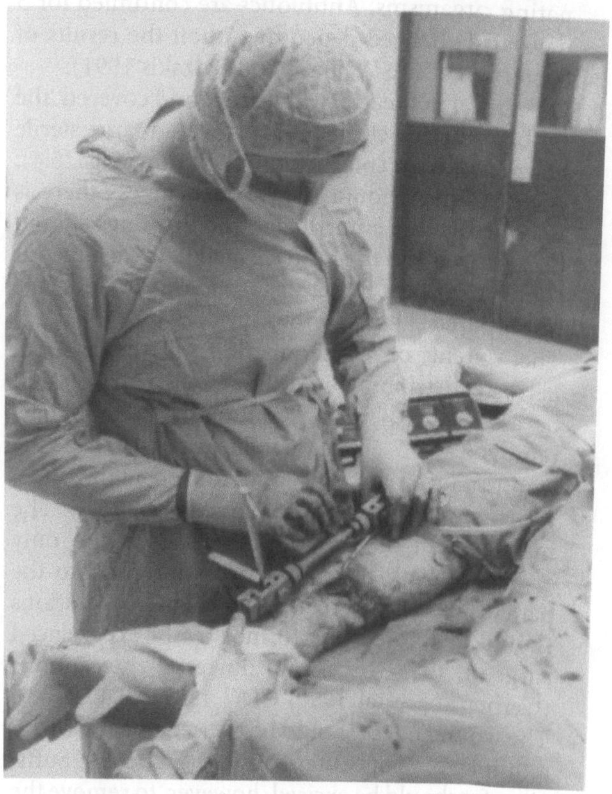

Fig. 26.8 External fixation is performed only after a perfect reduction has been achieved. Here, an Orthofix® template being used to guide pin placement following fracture reduction.

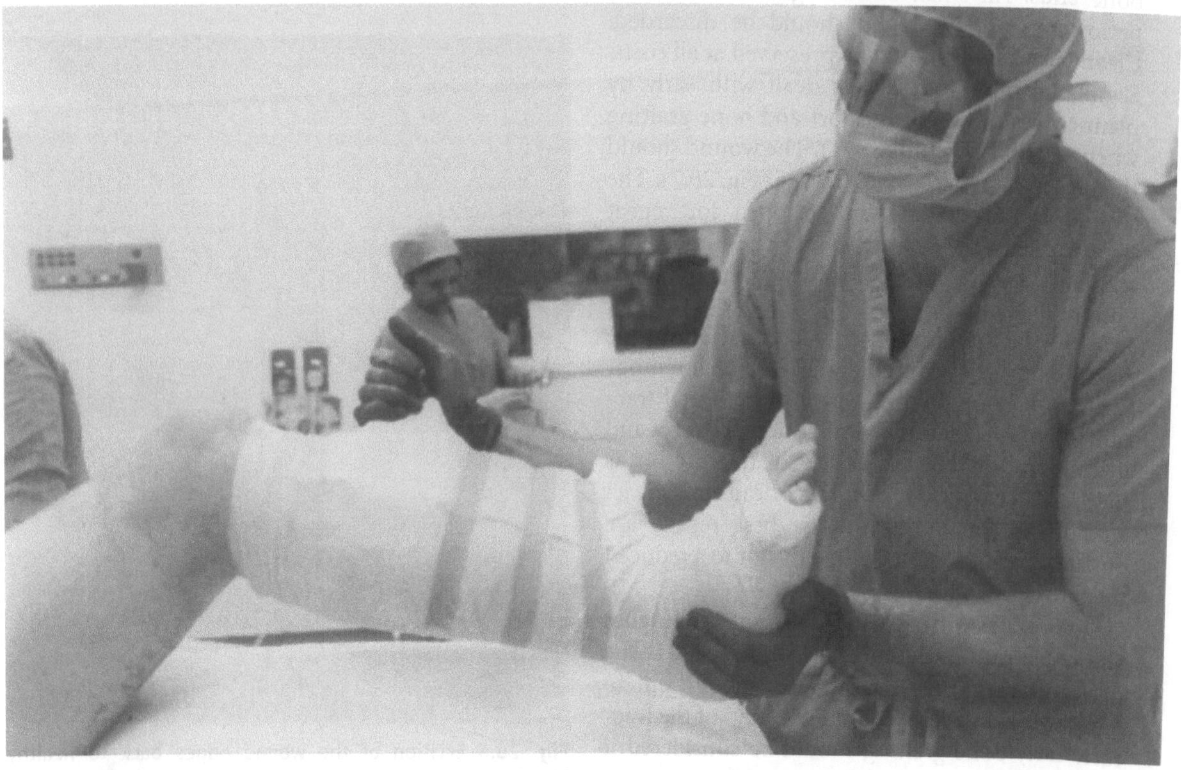

Fig. 26.9 An anti-footdrop orthosis applied beneath bandaging to prevent equinus deformity of the ankle.

an atrophic delay in union. The patient's limb should be elevated in the post-operative period, until the risk of tissue fluid leakage from the wound is minimal. Patients should be encouraged to exercise during this period of elevation, and an equinus deformity of the ankle should be prevented by using a backslab or anti-footdrop orthosis (Fig. 26.9).

8. Early partial weightbearing is important for both closed and compound wounds, although with the latter, the time at which weightbearing is initiated will depend on the condition of the wound.
9. Meticulous pin site care is mandatory in the post-operative period.

External fixation is most commonly used for Types II and III compound wounds. Infection associated with the use of external fixation has been reported in 3–45 per cent of cases in some studies (Gustilo and Gruninger 1987, Behrens and Searls 1986, Court-Brown et al 1985, Court-Brown et al 1990a). The rate seems to depend on the proportion of severe injuries (Caudle and Stern 1978, Checketts et al 1995). There is a trend towards the use of intramedullary nailing for Gustilo types II and III compound fractures with an accepted deep infection rate of 3.2–10 per cent (Court-Brown et al 1990b, Court-Brown et al 1991, Velazco et al 1983, Wiss 1986, Anglen et al 1993, Alho et al 1990, Alho et al 1992, Wu et al 1994, Bone and Johnson 1986). Some of these studies have also demonstrated that deep infections can occur after nailing closed fractures, which emphasises the fact that intramedullary nailing is not always a benign procedure (Wiss et al 1986, Anglen et al 1993, Alho et al 1990, Alho et al 1992, Wu and Zhang 1994, Bone and Johnson 1986). The use of compression plates and screws to immobilize compound fractures has been shown to be detrimental, and most centres now avoid this option (Veliskakis 1959, Bach and Hansen 1989).

All modern treatments carry the risk of complications. Most treatments can be justified as long as the surgeon has the necessary level of competence and expertise to reduce the risks of the procedure (Ribbans and Saleh 1991). A well-prepared surgeon should know whether all the necessary facilities are available for the proposed procedure. It is the surgeon's duty to his patient to obtain informed consent, discussing with the patient all the options and the common complications.

In our own study of 100 patients, treatments were randomly allocated according to prospective studies being undertaken. On admission, fractures were classified according to Gustilo type, displacement on initial radiograph, and finally, according to axial stability after reduction under general anaesthesia. A minimally displaced fracture was defined as a fracture that had no shortening, that had not translated more than 50 per cent of the diameter of the tibia at the level of the fracture and that was not angulated more than 10°.

Following definitive diagnosis, patients were treated according to the algorithm, which separated them into four streams (Hardy et al 1996).

Stream 1 comprised patients whose fractures were either closed and undisplaced or minimally displaced, or were compound Type I undisplaced fractures. These patients were treated with plaster casts. Stream 2 patients had either closed fractures or Type I compound fractures with shortening, which on reduction were stable enough to prevent more than 10mm of shortening. These patients were randomly allocated to plaster cast or external fixation; Stream 3 patients had either closed or Type I compound fractures which were sufficiently unstable to permit more than 10mm of shortening. They were randomly allocated to external fixation or a locked intramedullary nail; Stream 4 patients all had Type II or III compound injuries. All patients allocated to external fixation were treated with an Orthofix monolateral external fixator (Orthofix srl, Verona, Italy).

The commonest cause of injury during the two years of the study was sport (41 per cent) and football accounted for 38 per cent of all fractures.

The average age of the first hundred patients streamed by the algorithm was 29 years (range 16–77 years). There were 89 male and 11 female patients. In 55 patients the right, and in 45 the left tibia was broken. Three patients had fractures in the upper third, 53 in the middle third, and 44 in the lower third of the diaphysis.

Allocation of treatments according to the algorithm and the random allocation process resulted in 50 patients being treated conservatively and the rest by surgery (Table 26.1). Of those treated conservatively only 27 could be treated without resort to general anaesthesia. All patients were treated within 48 hours of admission. Those with compound injuries were all treated within 6 hours of admission.

The average period of follow-up was 29 months (range 20–36 months). Fracture healing, defined by clinical healing, was most rapid in Stream 1 patients and slowest in the Gustilo Type II–III stream (Table 26.2). Up to 86 per cent of this cohort had united fractures within 20 weeks of injury.

Hypertrophic delayed union occurred in 2 patients treated in a plaster cast and in one patient who fatigue-fractured his callus after removal of an external fixator. Hypertrophic callus was treated by reduction of

Algorithm	No. Patients	Plaster cast	External Fixation	I M nail
Stream 1	33	33	0	0
Stream 2	22	17	5	0
Stream 3	29	0	13	16
Stream 4	16	0	16	0
TOTAL	100	50	34	16

Table 26.1 Treatment allocations

Algorithm	No. Patients	Mean IWB (weeks)	Delayed union (>20 weeks)	Non-union (>24 weeks)
Stream 1	33	13	2	0
Stream 2	22	18	3	2
Stream 3	29	14	4	3
Stream 4	16	21	5	3
TOTAL	100		14	8

Table 26.2 Fracture healing as defined in clinical terms. The lower average in Stream 3 is because independent weightbearing (IWB) occurs early in patients with an intramedullary nail, before the fracture has healed.

Algorithm	No. patients	No. patients with hypertrophic callus	No. patients with atrophic non-union	No. patients bone grafted
Stream 1	33	2	0	0
Stream 2	22	0	0	0
Stream 3	29	1	1	1
Stream 4	16	0	2	2
TOTAL	100	3	3	3

Table 26.3 Complications of healing. There were no cases of deep infection.

Shortening (mm)	No. Patients
0–10	95
11–20	4
>20	1

Table 26.4 Shortening

Deformity (degrees)	No. Patients
0–5	83
6–10	2
>10	5

Table 26.5 Deformity at the fracture site.

Complication	Treatment	No. Patients
Sudek's atrophy	Plaster cast	2
DVT	Plaster cast; External fixation	2
Knee pain	Intramedullary nailing	14
Malrotation	External fixation; Intramedullary nailing	2
Refracture	External fixation (2); Intramedullary nailing (1)	3
Excision ring sequestra	External fixation	2
Pin site infection	External fixation	21

Table 26.6 Miscellaneous complications and the treatments with which they were associated

weightbearing through the injured limb in all three cases. Atrophic delayed, or non-union was seen in the streams that included the higher energy injuries and those with excessive periosteal injury. Each of these atrophic cases required bone grafting and has subsequently healed (Table 26.3).

Shortening of more than 2cm occurred in one patient with an unstable, comminuted, compound Type IIIa fracture that went on to atrophic non-union. This degree of shortening was measured after bone grafting and union. Lesser shortening, as measured on final radiographs compared with original radiographs, was not apparent clinically (Table 26.4).

Deformity was minimal (Table 26.5).

Other complications in this cohort of 100 patients are outlined in Table 26.6. Only two patients underwent a change of treatment. The first was a patient who had a short oblique fracture that did not shorten more than 1cm with an axial load under anaesthesia and who was randomly allocated to plaster cast. This patient went on to shorten more than 1cm on weightbearing and so underwent late intramedullary nailing to restore the length of his tibia. The second patient, randomly allocated to a plaster cast, requested to be taken out of the study because of domestic circumstances, and elected for treatment with an intramedullary nail. This patient was subsequently diagnosed as suffering from osteomalacia which caused an apparent non-union, and refracture occurred on nail removal. Both of these tibial fractures eventually healed.

Knee pain is the most common complication following intramedullary nailing, and pin site infection was the most common complication with external fixation (Table 26.6).

Discussion

These results were found to be an improvement on those reported in other studies and justify the use of more than one treatment (Hardy et al 1996). The delayed union rate of 14 per cent was reduced from a previous study in the same hospital in 1988 which found 19 per cent (Oni et al 1988a). Management of a diaphyseal fracture of the tibia should therefore depend on the diagnosis and the nature of the injury as defined by an algorithm.

The time taken for a fracture to heal clinically is almost certainly a reflection of the severity of injury to bone and soft tissue (Ellis 1958a, Court-Brown et al 1990a, Oni et al 1988a, Weissman et al 1966, Nicoll 1964). This seems true in our study, except for those patients treated with an intramedullary nail where clinical healing (i.e. full, pain-free weightbearing through the fractured limb, and no tenderness) does not necessarily represent biological healing. Intramedullary nailing is to be preferred in patients with closed, or Gustilo Type I injuries where healing time is likely to be protracted. These are the patients with a circumferential tear of the periosteum as diagnosed by the ability to distract the fracture gap during examination under anaesthesia.

Hypertrophic delayed union or non-union was related to early excessive use of the limb, usually before removal of the immobilizing device. Atrophic union occurred only in the streams associated with the higher energy injuries or those with significant periosteal damage and stripping. Where external fixation is employed, dynamization should be instituted earlier than the six weeks usually recommended (North et al 1990, Foxworthy and Pringle 1995).

Complications such as infection, shortening, deformity, and malrotation can be accounted for by surgical technique and the type of immobilization chosen. The high incidence of pin track infection in association with external fixation, though easily cured, suggests that external fixation should be avoided in patients with implanted medical devices. None of the closed intramedullary nailings developed infection, which has been reported in larger series of intramedullary nailings. The incidence of knee pain in patients randomly allocated to intramedullary nailing in this series means that this treatment should be avoided in patients with an occupation that requires them to crawl, or rest, on their knees.

One patient, with an oblique fracture, who demonstrated less than 1 cm of shortening under anaesthesia, went on to shorten even further on weightbearing in a plaster cast. Patients with an unstable closed fracture, and an intact periosteal hinge that demonstrates even modest shortening on axial loading under anaesthesia, should therefore be treated with external fixation. Forty-nine of our patients were successfully treated conservatively, which represents a saving in costs. This group had few complications and a good prognosis. The early surgical treatment of axially unstable or compound Type II–III injuries probably saved us the costs of secondary treatment following the failure of treatments inappropriate to the presenting injury. External fixation has a well-defined role in the management of these injuries.

Bibliography

Alho A, Ekeland A, Stromsoe K, Follerås G, Bjørn OT. Locked intramedullary nailing for displaced tibial shaft fractures. *I Bone Joint Surg.* [Br] 1990;72-B:805-9.

Alho A, Benterud JG, Hogevold HE, Ekeland A, Stromsoe K. Comparison of functional bracing and locked intramedullary nailing in the treatment of displaced tibial shaft fractures. *Clin Orthop.* 1992;277:243-50.

Anderson R and Burgess E. 'Delayed union and non-union. *J Bone Joint Surg.* 1943;25:427-32.

Andriole VT, Nagel DA, Southwick WO. A paradigm for human chronic osteomyelitis. *J Bone Joint Sur* [Am] 1973;55-A:1511-15.

Anglen J, Unger D, DiPasquale T, Herscovici JD, Snoke J, Sanders R. The treatment of open tibial shaft fractures using an unreamed interlocked nail – is external fixation obsolete. *J Orthop. Trauma,* 1993;7:163.

Bach AW and Hansen ST. Plates versus external fixation in severe open tibial shaft fractures. *Clin Orthop.* 1989;241:89-94.

Baker JT, McKinney LA, Costa AS, Nepola JV, Marsh LJ, Rodkey WG. Comparison of infection rates in contaminated tibial fractures stabilised with internal vs external fixation in rabbits. *J Orthop, Trauma.* 1992;6:509-10.

Behrens F and Searls K. External fixation of the tibia. Basic concepts and prospective evaluation. *J Bone Joint Surg.* 1986;68-B:246-54.

A report by the BOA/BAPS working party on severe tibial injury. The early management of severe tibial fractures: The need for combined plastic and orthopaedic management. 1993.

Bone LB and Johnson KD The treatment of tibial fractures by reaming and intramedullary nailing. *J Bone Joint Surg.* 1986;68-A:877-87.

Cattermole HR, Hardy JRW, Gregg PJ. The footballer's fracture. *Br J Sports Med* 1996; 30:171-5.

Caudle RJ and Stern PJ. Severe open fractures of the tibia. *J. Bone Joint Surg* 1987;69-A:801-7.

Centres for Disease Coñtrol: Recommendations for Prevention of Human Immunodeficiency Virus (HIV) Transmission in Health Care Settings. *M M W R* 1987; 36(Suppl 2S):1-18.

Centres for Disease Control: Update: Universal Precautions for Prevention of Transmission of Human Immunodeficiency Virus, Hepatitis B Virus, and other Blood-borne Pathogens in Health Care Settings. *M M W R.* 1988;37(24):377-482.

Checketts RG, Moran CG, Jennings AG. 134 tibial shaft fractures managed with the DynamicAxialFixator. *Acta Orthop Scand,*1995;66(3):271-4.

Charnley J. The Closed Treatment of Common Fractures. Churchill Livingstone, London. 3rd Ed. 1961.

Clancey GJ and Hansen ST. Open fractures of the tibia. *Bone Joint Surg.* [Am] 1978;601 A:118-122.

Court-Brown CM, McQueen MM, Quaba AA, Christie J. Hughes external fixator in treatment of tibial fractures. *J Royal Soc Med.* 1985;78:830-7.

Court-Brown CM, Wheelwright EF, Christie J, McQueen MM. External fixation for type III open tibial fractures. *J Bone Joint Sur.* [Br] 1990a; 72-B: 801-4.

Court-Brown CM, Christie J, McQueen MM. Closed intramedullary tibial nailing. *J Bone Joint Sur.* [Br] 1990b; 72-B: 605-11.

Court-Brown CM, McQueen MM, Quaba AA, Christie J. Locked intramedullary nailing of open tibial fractures. *J Bone Joint Surg.* 1991; 73-B: 959-64.

Court-Brown CM, McBirnie J. The epidemiology of tibial fractures. *J Bone Joint Sur.* [Br] 1995; 77-B: 417-21.

Dellinger EP, Caplan ES, Weaver LD, Wertz MJ, Droppert BM, Hoyt N, Brumback R, Burgess A, Poka A, Benirschke SK, Lennard ES, and Lou MA. Duration of preventive antibiotic administration for open extremity fractures. *Arch Surg.* 1988a; 123: 333-9.

Dellinger EP, Miller SD, Wertz MJ, Grympa M, Droppert BM, Anderson PA. Risk of infection after open fracture of the forearm or leg. *Arch Surg* 1988b; 123: 1320-7.

Ellis H. The speed of healing after fracture of the tibial shaft. *J Bone Joint Sur.* 1958a; 40-B: 42-6.

Foxworthy M and Pringle RM. Dynamisation timing and its effect on bone healing when using the Orthofix Dynamic Axial Fixator. *Injury.* 1995;26(2):117-9.

Gerberding JL, Littel C, Tarkington A, Brown A, Schecter WP. Risk of Exposure of Surgical Personnel to Patients Blood During Surgery at San Francisco General Hospital. *New Eng J Med.* 1990; 21: 1788-93.

Green RA. The courage to co-operate: the team approach to open fractures of the lower limb. *Ann R Coll Surg Engl.* 1994; 76: 365-6.

Gustilo RB and Anderson JT. Prevention of infection in the treatment of one thousand and twenty-five fractures of long bones. *Bone Joint Surg* [Br] 1976; 58-A: 453-8.

Gustilo RB, Mendoza RM, Williams DN. Problems in the management of Type III (Severe) open fractures: A new classification of type III open fractures. *The Journal of Trauma.* 1984;24(8):742-6.

Gustilo RB and Gruninger RP. Classification of Type III (Severe) Open fractures relative to treatment and results. *Orthopaedics.* 1987;10:1781-028.

Gustilo RB, Merkow RL, Templeman D. Current Concepts Review - The management of open fractures. *Bone Joint Surg.* [Am] 1990; 72-A: 299-303.

Hardy JRW, Richardson JB, Gregg PJ. Creating an early stable environment for healing by callus: The Leicester algorithm. *International Journal of Orthopaedic Trauma.* 1996; 6(2): 52-61.

Keating JF, Gardner E, Leach WJ, Mcpherson S, Abrami G. Management of tibial fractures with the Orthofix Dynamic External Fixator. *J R Coll Surg Edinb.* 1991; 36: 272-7.

Marsh JL, Nepola JV, Wuest TK, Osteen D, Cox K, Oppenheim W. Unilateral External Fixation until healing with the Dynamic Axial Fixator for severe open tibial fractures: *J Orthop Traumas.* 1991; 5(3): 341-8.

Müller ME, Nazarian S, Koch P,Schatzker, J. The Comprehensive Classification of Fractures of Long Bones. 1990; Springer-Verlag, Berlin-Heidelberg-New York.

Nicoll EA. Fractures of the tibial shaft - A survey of 705 cases. *Bone Joint Surg.* [Br] 1964; 46-B: 373-87.

North AD, Wallace WA, Howard PW, Newton G. Management of tibial diaphyseal fractures with primary dynamic external fixation: a prospective study. *J Bone Joint.* [Br] 1990; 72-B: 531.

Oni OOA, Hui A, Gregg PJ. The healing of closed tibial shaft fractures - The natural history of union rvit c osed treatment. *J Bone Joint Surg.* [Br] 1988a; 70-B: 787-90.

Oni OOA, Gregg PJ, Morrison C, Ponter ARS. An investigation of the fracture characteristics of the tibia of mature rabbits. *Injury.* 1988b; 19: 172-6.

Pennig D. The place of unilateral internal fixation in the treatment of tibial fractures. *International Journal of Orthopaedic Trauma.* 1991;1(3):161-76.

Rang M. Children's Fractures. 2nd Edition. J B Lippincott Company, Philadelphia. 1984.

Ribbans WJ and Saleh M. Orthofix External Fixation for tibial fractures. *J Bone Joint Sur.* [Br] 1991; 73-B [SUPP II]:177.

Robinson D, On E, Hadas N, Hofman S, and Boldur I. Microbiological flora contaminating open fractures: Its significance in the choice of primary antibiotic agents and the likelihood of deep wound infection. *The Journal of Orthopaedic Trauma.* 1989; 3: 283-6.

Tscherne H and Gotzen L. Fractures with soft tissue injuries. Springer-Verlag. New York, Heidelberg and Berlin. 1984.

Veliskakis K P. Primary internal fixation in open fractures of the tibial shaft - the problem of wound healing. *J Bone Joint Surg.* [Br] 1959; 41-B: 342-54.

Velazco A, Whites ides TE, Fleming LL. Open fractures of the tibia treated with the Lottes nail. *J Bone Joint Surg.* [Br] 1983; 65-A: 879-85.

Watson JT. Treatment of unstable fractures of the shaft of the tibia. *j Bone Joint Surg.* [Am] 1994; 76-A: 1575-84.

Weissman SL, Herold HZ, Engleberg M. Fractures of the middle two-thirds of the tibial shaft. *J Bone Joint.* [Am] 1966; 48-A: 257-67.

Wilkins J and Patzakis MJ. Choice and duration of antibiotics in open fractures. *Orthopaedic Clinics of North America.* 1991; 22: 433 7.

Wiss DA. Flexible medullary nailing of acute tibial shaft fractures. *Clin Orthop* 1986; 212: 122-32.

Wu Y-S and Zhang F-B. The treatment of tibial and fibular fractures with the rectangular intramedullary nail. *Orthopaedics.* 1994; 2(5): 437-46.

Distal Tibial and Plafond Fractures 27

J.L. Marsh

Traditionally, fractures of the tibial plafond have been treated by open reduction and internal fixation, with the goals of exact restoration of the articular surface and sufficient stability to allow early motion. Unfortunately, this method of treatment often leads to an unacceptable incidence of complications, many of which are severe. Satisfactory results and a substantial decrease in complications have recently been reported when the metaphyseal portion of the fracture is treated by external fixation. For this reason, the accepted techniques used to treat tibial plafond fractures have changed. The goal is now to preserve the soft tissue envelope by reducing the fracture percutaneously or through limited approaches using stabilization remote from the fracture site by external fixation.

Background

Terminology

What name should we use for high energy fractures of the distal tibia? The terms pilon, pylon, and plafond are all found in the literature. Destot used the term pilon in 1911[5] while likening the distal tibia to a pestle and mortar. However, the word pilon does not appear either in Webster's *Dictionary of the English Language*[21] nor in *Dorland's Illustrated Medical Dictionary*.[8] Pylon, according to Webster, comes from the Greek word pylé and refers to a gate. Dorland's Medical Dictionary defines a pylon as a temporary artificial leg.[8] These definitions of pilon and pylon do not relate generally to the distal tibia or specifically to fractures in this area.

According to Webster,[21] plafond means an elaborate ceiling. Since the articular surface of the bottom of the tibia indeed forms a ceiling over the ankle joint, plafond bears some relationship to the local anatomy in this region. A fracture of the tibial plafond is a fracture of the ceiling of the ankle joint, and this, therefore, should be the preferred terminology.[4]

Mechanism

These fractures can occur from predominantly rotation, predominantly axial loading, or, as is often the case, a combination of the two. Rotation produces lower energy fractures, with less associated soft tissue injury and generally better patient outcomes. These rotational fractures typically disrupt only part of the articular surface of the tibial plafond. They are frequently classified along with ankle fractures and dislocations.

Axial loading fractures occur in motor vehicle accidents or in falls from heights. These rapid loading injuries impart considerable energy to the soft tissues as the distal tibia fails. Typically there is comminution of the articular surface, the metaphyseal region or both. These injuries may involve all or only part of the articular surface, depending on the foot position at the time of impact.

Classification

There is no universally accepted classification. Rüedi and Allgöwer's is important because it is the most commonly used in the literature.[14] It subdivides axial loading injuries into three grades of severity. Type I fractures are cleavage fractures of the joint surface without displacement. Type II fractures have significant displacement of the articular surface without comminution, and Type III fractures are associated with metaphyseal and epiphyseal comminution. Unfortunately, this classification does not provide enough detail to predict outcome accurately. A wide range of fractures with different prognoses lies between the definition of a Type II and a Type III fracture.

Greater anatomical detail is present in the AO Müller Classification of Fractures applied to the distal tibia (Fig. 27.1).[13] Type A are extra-articular distal tibial fractures, Type B are partial articular fractures, and Type C are total articular fractures where the joint surface is completely separated from the tibial shaft. Although non-articular Type A fractures may be high energy and have significant complications after treatment, they are not true fractures of the tibial plafond. Type B1 fractures are more appropriately classified with ankle fractures. Types B2, B3, C1, C2, and C3 are the fractures caused, at least partially, by axial loading. Further anatomical subdivision is based on the location and direction of the major fracture lines. In combination with the classification of malleolar fractures in the same system, the full range of distal tibia injuries can be classified. There is enough detail potentially to define subgroups which require different treatment strategies and/or which have different prognoses, although there are not enough data in the literature to realize this potential at the present time. In addition, this is a complex classification, and the inter- and intra-observer reliability of this fracture classification tool has not been demonstrated.

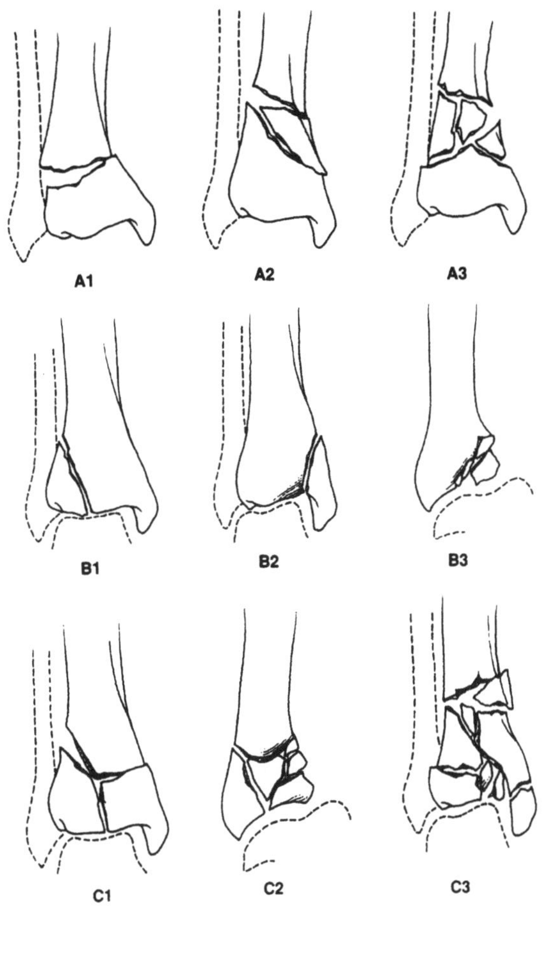

Soft Tissue Injury

For this fracture more than any other extremity injury, the soft tissues must be considered when planning treatment and determining outcome. Open fractures are appropriately classified by the method of Gustilo and Anderson as Type I, Type II and Type III, depending on the size of the open wound.[9] In our experience, the incidence of open wounds associated with tibial plafond fractures is 12 per cent.

Considering only the size of open wounds significantly underestimates the associated soft tissue injury. Tscherne and Goetzen have graded soft tissue injuries associated with closed fractures from Grade 0–Grade III.[19] Closed fractures with no appreciable soft tissue injury are graded as 0. Grade I soft tissue injuries involve abrasion or contusion of skin and subcutaneous tissue. Grade II involve deep abrasion with local contusion of skin and some muscle, and Grade III injuries involve extensive contusion or crush with subcutaneous avulsion and severe muscle damage. Compartment syndrome and arterial rupture are included in Grade III. The at-risk area of the subcutaneous surface of the anteromedial side of the tibia was described by these authors. Unfortunately, this classification does not perfectly apply to tibial plafond fractures, because little muscle is involved, and the fracture occurs from indirect forces, which means that the soft tissue injury is caused by the fracture itself rather than by outside forces. I have found it difficult to apply accurately.

The mechanism of injury, fracture comminution and associated fracture of the fibula provide clues to the amount of soft tissue injury to expect. In each case, however, the surgeon must carefully consider the damage to the soft tissue envelope by examining for tense swelling, contusions, fracture blisters, open wounds and evidence of compartment syndrome.

Fig. 27.1 The AO-Müller classification of long-bone fractures applied to the distal tibia; Type A, nonarticular fractures (A1, nonarticular fracture line; A2, comminuted wedge fracture; A3, complex comminuted metaphyseal fracture); type B, partial articular fractures with a portion of the joint surface intact with the metaphysis and shaft (B1, simple articular fracture line; B2, marginal impaction; B3, comminuted partial articular fracture); type C, complete metaphyseal fractures with articular involvement (C1, non-comminuted; C2, comminuted in the metaphysis with a simple articular fracture; C3, metaphyseal and articular comminution).

Treatment

Internal Fixation

Although the treatment of tibial plafond fractures by internal fixation has been reported to produce good results in the literature, the surgeon should be aware of the possible complications that can occur when using this technique. Major wound complications have been reported in an alarming number of closed fractures treated by open reduction and internal fixation. Teeny and Wiss[16] reported poor results in 50 per cent of their patients, with a 37 per cent infection rate and a 26 per cent fusion rate for Rüedi and Allgöwer Type III fractures. McFerran et al reported on 21 patients who had developed complications following open reduction and internal fixation of a tibial plafond fracture, requiring 77 additional surgical procedures.[12] It is of concern that 50 per cent of the complications in this series occurred in the less severe Rüedi and Allgöwer Type I and II fractures. This indicates that the soft tissue injury can be more severe than the fracture classification implies, which may lead to an underestimation of the risk of wound complications.

The surgeon should take care to prevent these complications. Factors which decrease the incidence of complications include the use of small implants, indirect reduction with minimal stripping, and postponing surgery until soft tissue swelling has decreased. Despite the use of these techniques, cases for internal fixation should be cautiously chosen. The recent favourable experience with external fixation indicates that aggressive techniques of internal fixation for high energy axial loading fractures of the tibial plafond should be considered only by surgeons with considerable experience of these techniques, and even then, only in cases where the soft tissue damage is less severe. I rarely treat any fractures of the tibial plafond by internal fixation, and only consider it in low energy fracture patterns with minimal associated soft tissue injury.

External Fixation

External fixation is becoming increasingly popular for the treatment of severe tibial plafond fractures. The advantage of external fixation is that the metaphyseal portion of the fracture is stabilized without a subcutaneous implant. Clinical reports on the use of a variety of external fixators have shown a substantial decrease in complications, particularly wound breakdown and infection. External fixation screws and wires appear to be well-tolerated about the ankle and the hindfoot. The results and techniques of three methods have been published in the literature. These methods are: (1) use of a hybrid frame and tensioned wires on the tibial side of the joint,[17] (2) use of a non-mobile external fixator to cross the ankle joint,[3] and (3) use of an articulated external fixator to span the joint.[1,10,11,15,18] Further experience is required to determine the advantages and disadvantages and the long-term outcome of each technique.

The hybrid frame technique necessitates obtaining external fixation with wires tensioned on to a ring on the tibial side of the ankle joint. This requires reassembling of the distal tibial articular surface as the first step in the procedure, which is accomplished by an open approach, plate fixation of the fibula and screw fixation of the articular surface. The metaphyseal portion of the fracture is then treated with a hybrid frame. The disadvantage of this technique is that it requires an open approach, which may be difficult when the articular surface is very comminuted.

A second external fixation strategy is to cross the joint with a fixator as the first step in the procedure. Intra-operative distraction with the fixator provides provisional reduction of articular fragments. If necessary, further joint realignment and/or bone grafting can then be accomplished with the use of fluoroscopically guided, minimally invasive or percutaneous techniques. This strategy is easier and less invasive at the distal tibia. Disadvantages include the need to use fixator screws in the hindfoot and ankle joint immobility. Bone et al have reported that in conjunction with spanning external fixation, open reduction and plate fixation can be used safely in some circumstances.[3]

The third approach, which I prefer, uses a hinged articulated external fixator across the ankle (Orthofix srl, Verona, Italy). This fixator combines the advantages of ease of application, cross-ankle intra-operative distraction and early post-operative motion. Fibular fixation is often not necessary. The technique is compatible with either limited or extensive articular repositioning, depending on the surgeon's preference. At the completion of articular reconstruction, the fixator is left in place in the neutralization mode. Post-operatively, limited movements of the ankle are possible through the fixator hinge.

These advantages, combined with the favourable results obtained personally and those reported in the literature, have made this my technique of choice for all high energy fractures of the tibial plafond, including B2, B3, C1, C2, and C3 fractures and all groups of the Rüedi and Allgöwer classification. Occasional non-articular fractures of the distal tibia (Type A fractures,

AO Müller classification) and occasional malleolar fractures where the risks of open techniques have been prohibitively high (pre-existing infection, open venous ulcers, severe open wounds associated with fracture comminution) have also been treated using this technique.

Surgical Technique

Pre-operative Planning

Pre-operative planning requires good antero-posterior, lateral and mortise radiographs. Radiographs after reduction of a dislocated talus reveal more information about the size and location of articular fragments than those taken prior to reduction. If calcaneal traction is required to maintain talar position, radiographs in traction are important for planning because they show the position of the distal tibia that will be achieved after fixator application. If available, a Computerized Tomography (CT) scan of the ankle demonstrates the size and location of the major articular fragments, the direction of fracture lines and the presence of central depressed fragments (Fig. 27.2a). This information is easier to appreciate on an axial CT scan than on plain radiographs. Sagittal and coronal CT reconstructions are less helpful for planning.

With the aid of these radiographs, the surgeon should determine if the fracture is a partial or complete articular fracture. Partial articular fractures leave some of the articular surface intact with the distal tibia. The percentage and location of the intact articular surface and the location and direction of the cleaving fracture line should be determined. This fracture line can be used for visualization of the articular surface through a fracture window if an open approach is chosen (Figs. 27.2a–27.2b).

Complete articular fractures separate the joint surface from the shaft of the tibia. These fractures may involve a single simple articular fracture line or complex unreconstructable comminution of the joint surface. Planning should determine the number, size and location of articular fragments and the presence of a fibular fracture and its location and comminution. Anterolateral and posterolateral articular fragments frequently remain attached to the distal fibula.

Based on these pre-operative investigations, the surgeon should plan which articular fragments will be repositioned, the location for percutaneous application of tenaculum reduction forceps to assist reduction and the entry point and direction of articular fixation screws. The medial location of the external fixator and the location of neurovascular bundles impact on this planning. The amount of metaphyseal comminution

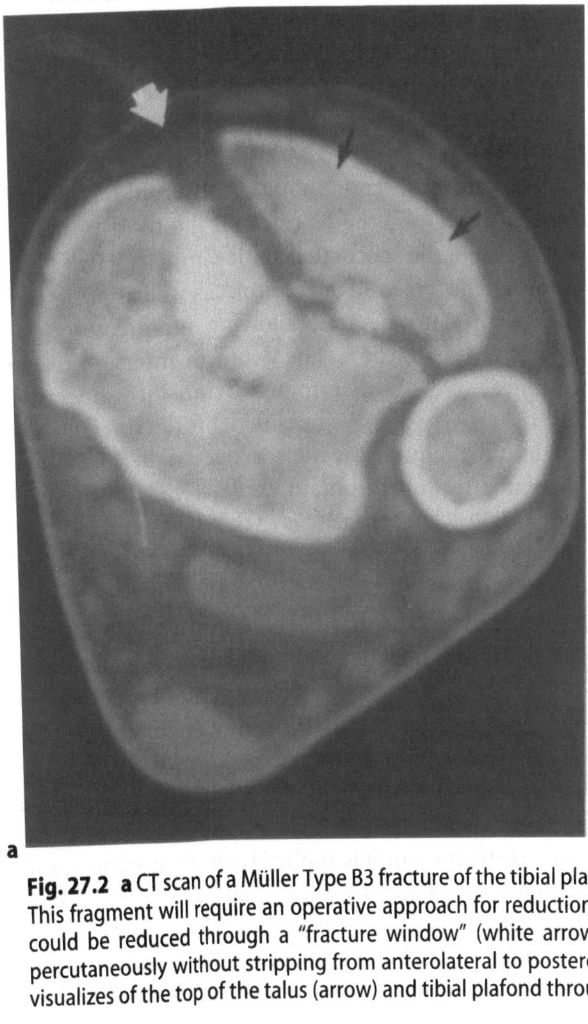

a

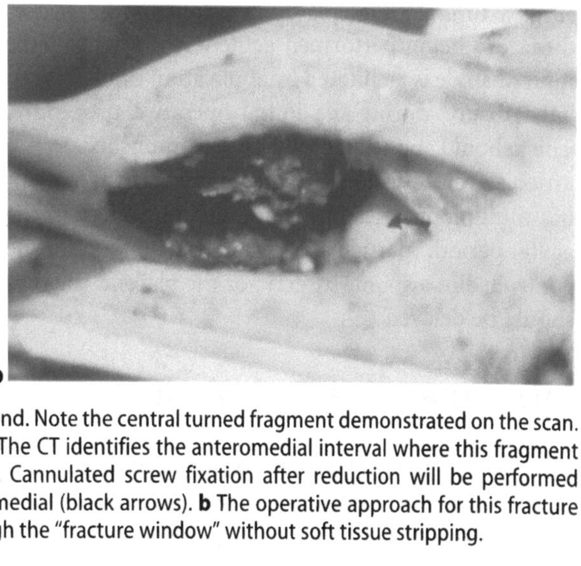

b

Fig. 27.2 **a** CT scan of a Müller Type B3 fracture of the tibial plafond. Note the central turned fragment demonstrated on the scan. This fragment will require an operative approach for reduction. The CT identifies the anteromedial interval where this fragment could be reduced through a "fracture window" (white arrow). Cannulated screw fixation after reduction will be performed percutaneously without stripping from anterolateral to posteromedial (black arrows). **b** The operative approach for this fracture visualizes of the top of the talus (arrow) and tibial plafond through the "fracture window" without soft tissue stripping.

will predict the possible need for a bone graft. In some cases the surgeon may determine pre-operatively that articular repositioning is not possible due to severe comminution.

Timing of Surgery

The timing of surgery is variable at our institution. Factors considered are other systems injuries, the fracture configuration, the condition of the soft tissues, the presence of a communicating open wound, and the availability of an experienced operating team. In patients with isolated fractures of the tibial plafond without open wounds, it is my preference to operate electively under optimal conditions. While awaiting surgery the ankle should be strictly elevated. If the talus will stay centred under the tibia, it should be splinted or casted. If not, longitudinal traction is required through a calcaneal traction pin. Traction obtains a provisional reduction of the articular fragments. In cases where severe soft tissue swelling and fracture blisters develop, definitive surgery is often delayed, depending on the location of the blisters.[20]

When fractures of the tibial plafond are associated with an open wound or compartment syndrome, emergency surgery is indicated to surgically debride the wound and/or release fascial compartments. The fixator should be applied at the time of emergency surgery. This stabilizes the limb, facilitates soft tissue management and realigns the talus. Articular repositioning is not necessary at this initial procedure. At a subsequent procedure for debridement, closure or grafting of fasciotomy wounds, articular reduction and fixation are performed.

In the multiply injured patient, many factors must be taken into account to determine appropriate surgical timing for the plafond fracture. If other procedures are being performed acutely, treatment of the injured ankle is facilitated by application of the articulated fixator during the initial operative procedure. This should be expeditiously accomplished, since articular repositioning is not required. If the patient has multiple injuries but is not having surgery in the acute period, particularly when the ankle can be controlled in a splint, surgery for the plafond fracture should be delayed.

Intra-operative Technique

Fluoroscopy is required for fixator application and articular surface repositioning. Biplane fluoroscopic views are easily obtained by placing the non-operative leg in an elevated stirrup, leaving only the operative leg in extension on the table. Fluoroscopy is performed from the lateral side, which leaves the medial side free for the surgeon. The surgeon should resist the temptation to externally rotate the leg to obtain the lateral view. This position causes rotation through the fracture site and places the subtalar joint in varus. Since the subtalar joint is immobilized in the ankle clamp, this varus position will be maintained during treatment. Lateral views should therefore be obtained by rotating the fluoroscope and not the injured limb.

To begin the procedure, the fluoroscope should first be in position for the lateral view. The skin should be incised over the distal neck of the talus midway between dorsal and plantar aspects. The talar screw is inserted freehand through a sleeve but without the use of the template. I recommend the use of a 3.2mm drill for insertion of a 100/40 Orthofix cancellous screw. Some surgeons utilize cortical screws in this location. The talar screw should be inserted parallel to the dome of the talus. This step is critical, because the rest of the fixator will be assembled in relation to this screw. The depth of insertion of the talar screw is determined on an AP fluoroscopic view of the foot, which is obtained by bending the knee, plantar flexing the foot and slightly obliquing the fluoroscope in a cephalad direction. This view separates the lateral margin of the talus from the calcaneus (Fig. 27.3a).

The calcaneal screw should be inserted high in the posterior angle of the os calcis in the most posterior screw seat of the articulated ankle template. High positioning puts it into stronger bone, as well as presetting the clamp into neutral, allowing for greater post-operative dorsiflexion. The depth of insertion of the calcaneal screw is determined by an intra-operative Harris view, which is obtained by dorsiflexing the ankle and obliquing the fluoroscope axially 40–60° in a plantar direction to obtain an axial view of the heel (Fig. 27.3b). The template is then fully assembled, and the proximal screws are applied in the standard manner.

After the fixator has been applied and the clamps are tightened, the talus should be centred beneath the tibia on both the antero-posterior and lateral fluoroscopic views. If there is any angulation of the distal talar surface, it should be corrected. Once the talus has been positioned, both ball joints should be locked with the torque wrench. A compression–distraction unit is applied to the fixator body, and the talus distracted from the ankle mortise to assist in reduction of the distal tibia (Figs. 27.4a–27.4f).

Based on the intra-operative appearance of the distal tibial articular surface under distraction and on

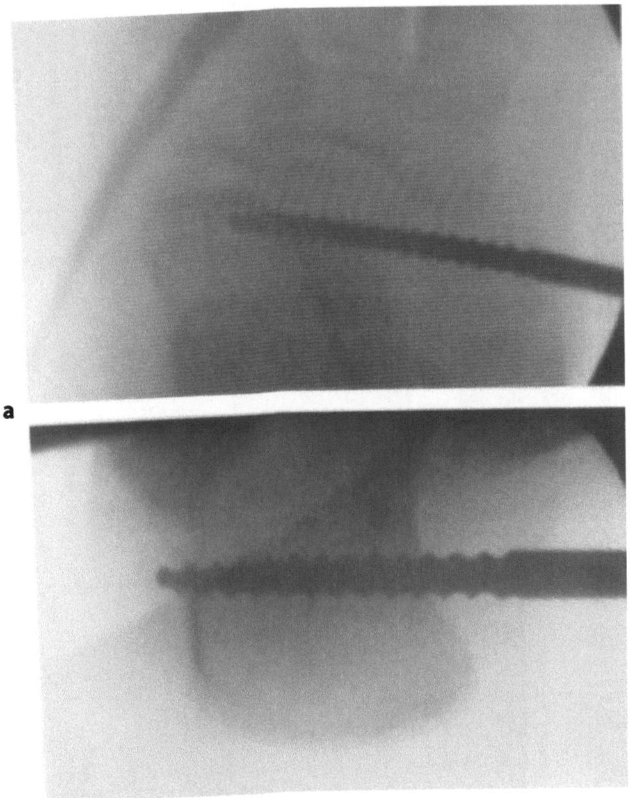

a

b

Fig. 27.3 a The AP fluoroscopic view obtained intra-operatively demonstrates the depth of insertion of the talar screw. This screw should be advanced until two threads protrude through the lateral cortex. **b** An intra-operative fluoroscopic axial view of the heel demonstrates appropriate depth of insertion of the calcaneal screw.

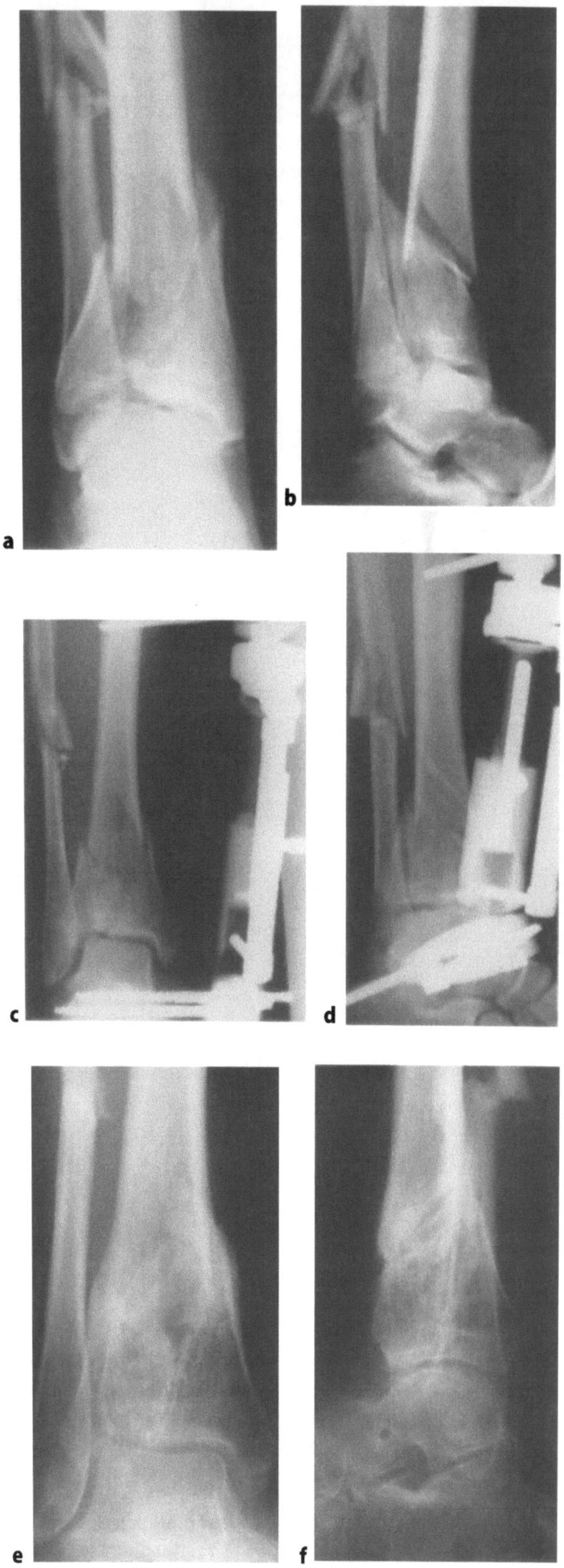

Fig. 27.4 A Müller Type C2 fracture caused by a fall from 10 feet is demonstrated on **a** anteroposterior and **b** lateral radiographs. The position achieved after application of the articulated fixator on **c** AP and **d** lateral radiographs. In this case, articular repositioning was not felt to be necessary. Note that the fibula fracture has not been fixed, and that the ankle is not overdistracted. **e** The healed radiographic appearance on AP and **f** lateral radiographs is demonstrated 8 months after injury and 5 months after fixator removal.

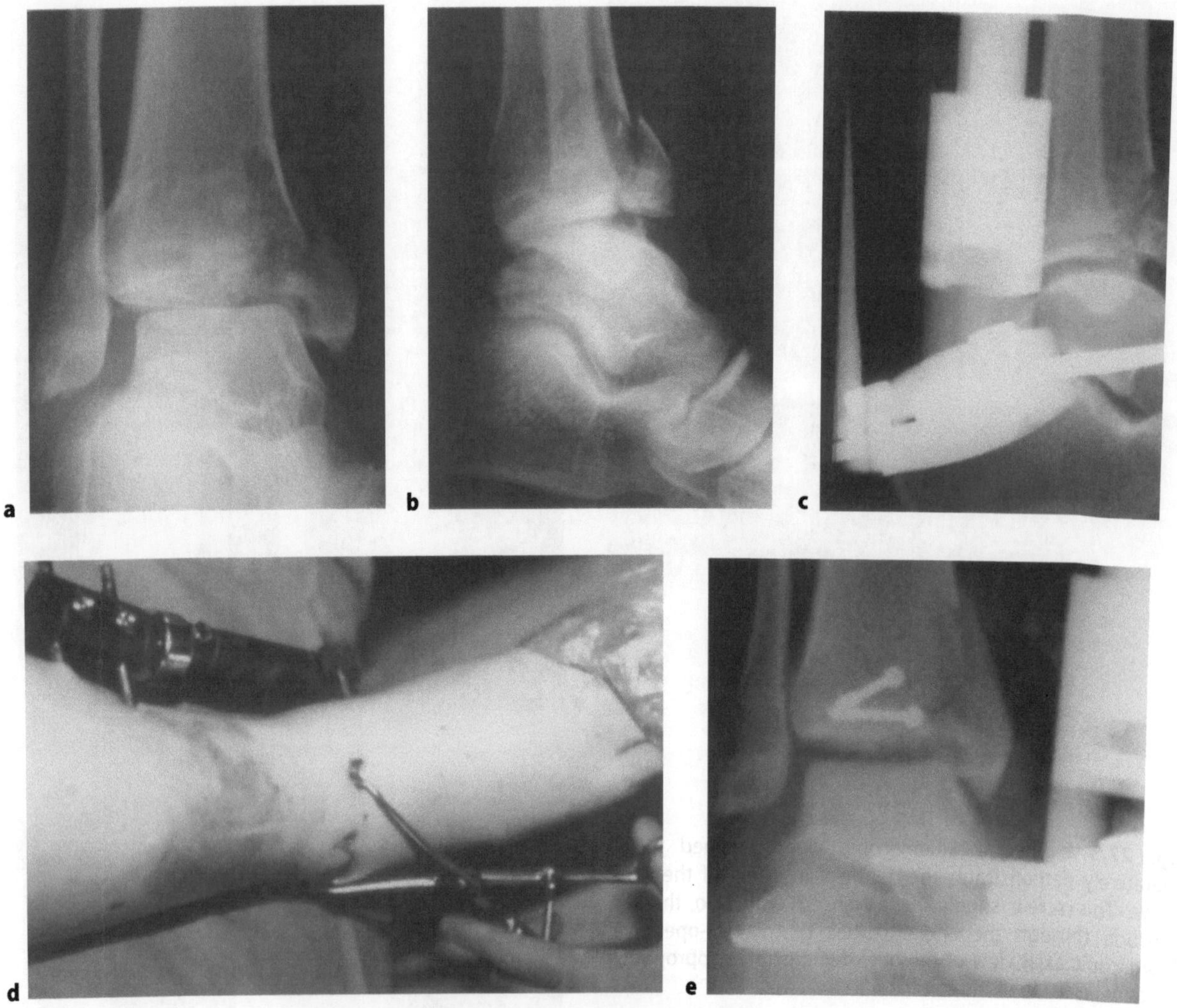

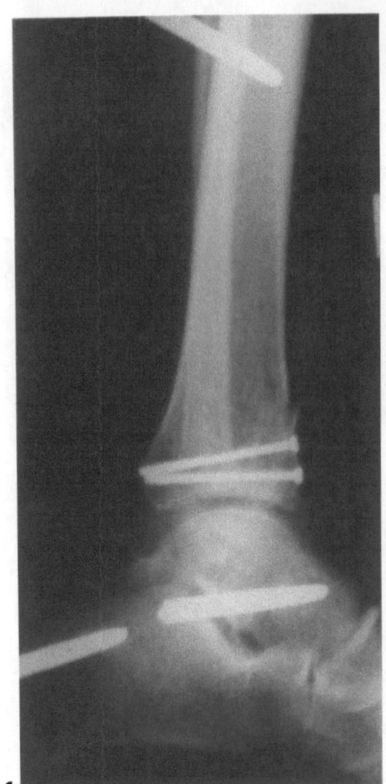

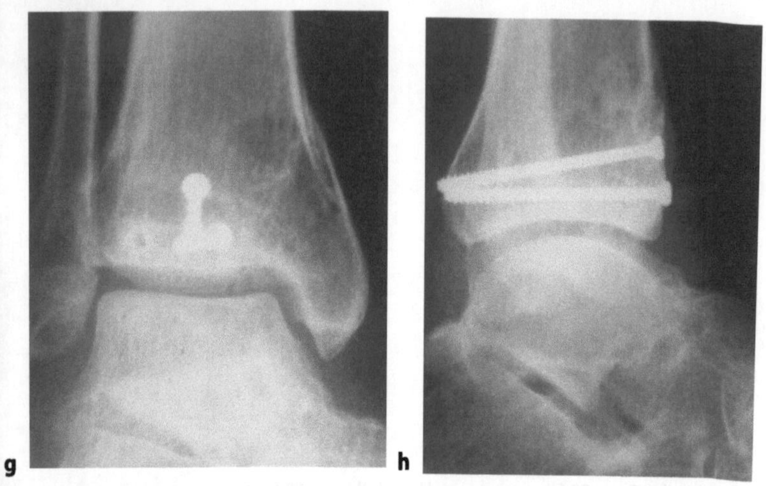

Fig. 27.5 **a** AP and **b** lateral radiographs demonstrate a Müller B3 fracture of the tibial plafond. **c** This lateral radiograph shows the position achieved after articulated fixator application. The anterolateral fragment is not reduced. **d** This intra-operative photograph demonstrates reduction of the anterolateral fragment by percutaneous application of tenaculum forceps placed between the fragment and the posterolateral border of the fibula. **e** The AP and **f** lateral radiographs show fixation of this fragment with 3.5mm cannulated screws. **g** AP and **h** lateral radiographs show the healed appearance 10 months after injury.

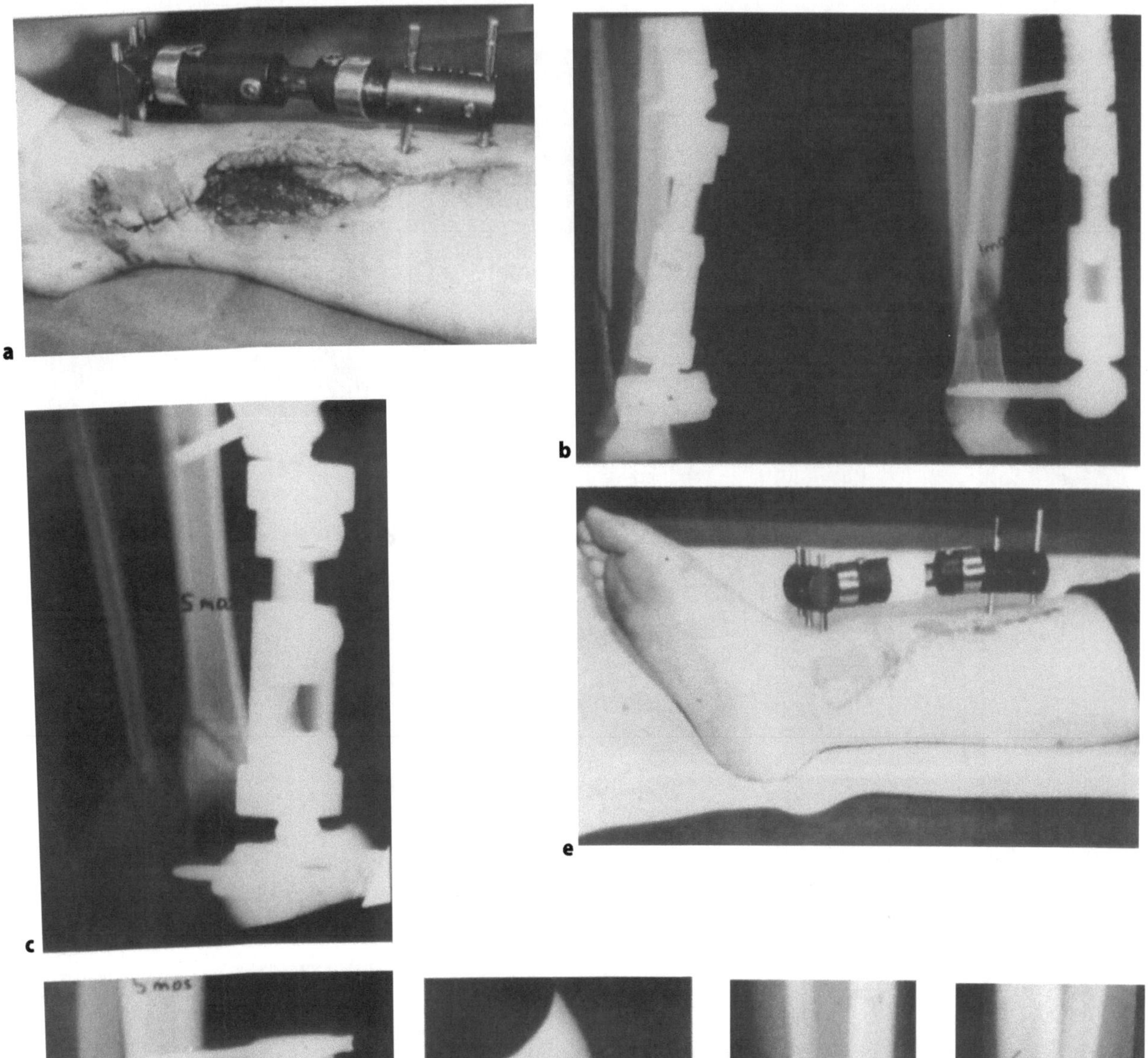

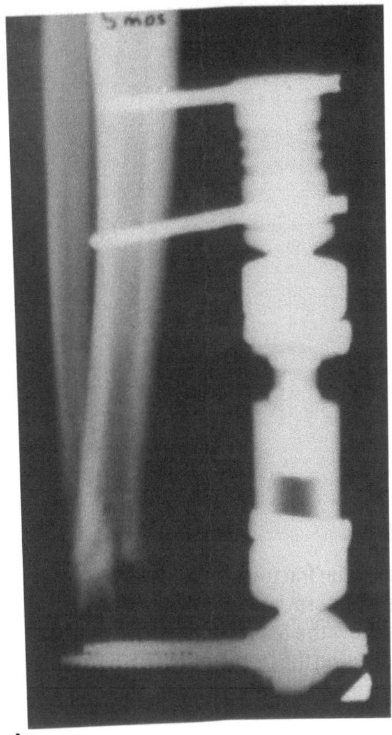

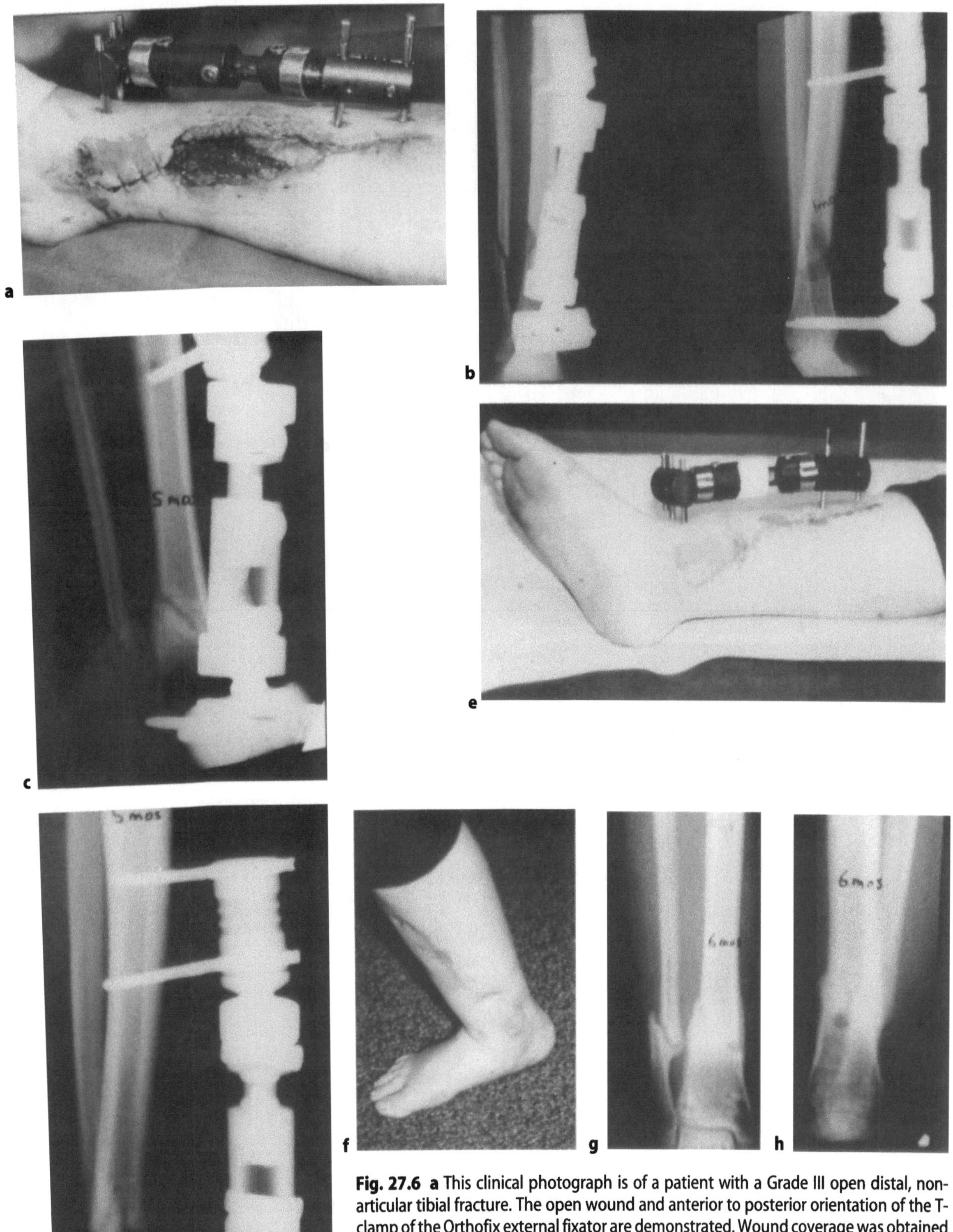

Fig. 27.6 **a** This clinical photograph is of a patient with a Grade III open distal, non-articular tibial fracture. The open wound and anterior to posterior orientation of the T-clamp of the Orthofix external fixator are demonstrated. Wound coverage was obtained by transfer of the muscle belly of the flexor digitorum longus and a split thickness skin graft. **b** AP and lateral radiographs show the reduction and fixation using the Orthofix T-clamp. **c** The appearance on AP and **d** lateral radiographs at 5 months, showing healing with bridging callus. **e** The clinical appearance of the leg at 5 months shows healing of the soft tissue wounds. **f** The final clinical appearance and extent of ankle dorsiflexion. **g** AP and **h** lateral radiographs show sound union at 6 months.

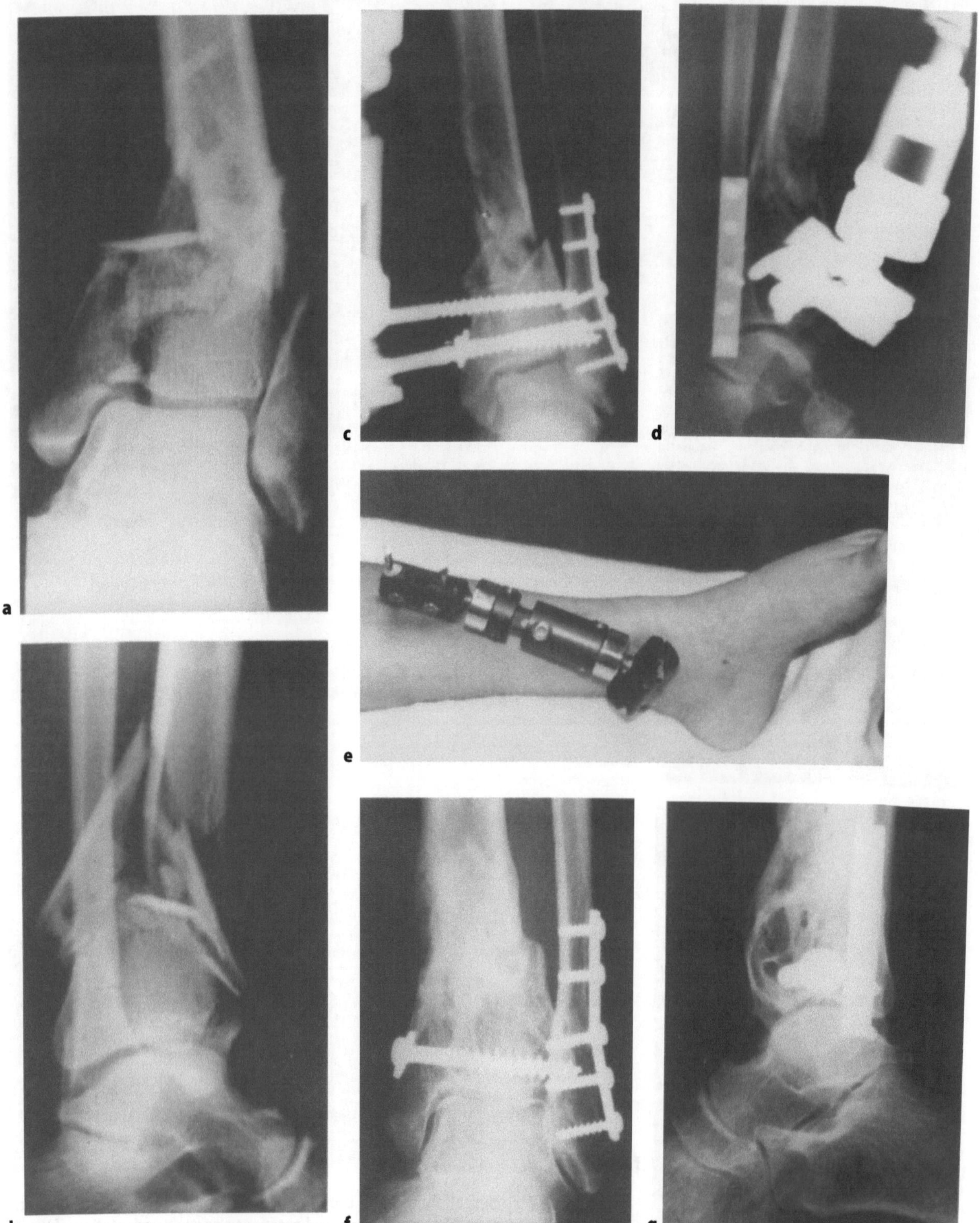

Fig. 27.7 Same side of the joint fixation with the Orthofix T-clamp is possible in distal articular fractures if there is only one simple fracture line. **a** AP and **b** lateral radiographs show a comminuted metaphyseal fracture with associated distal tibia fracture with a fracture through the shoulder of the medial malleolus. **c** AP and **d** lateral radiographs show the reduction obtained after fibular plating and percutaneous screw fixation of the medial malleolus, followed by stabilization using the Orthofix T-clamp. **e** The clinical appearance of the leg. In this case fixator application was antero-medial. **f** AP and **g** lateral radiographs 9 months after injury showing union and good maintenance of joint space.

pre-operative planning, the surgeon may choose to reposition the articular fragments further. Large tenaculum reduction forceps or pelvic reduction forceps are used percutaneously to aid in reducing articular fragments (Figs. 27.5a–27.5h). The size and location of the major articular fragments and the position of the reduction forceps will have been determined during pre-operative planning. Reductions are evaluated fluoroscopically. Open reduction is never done solely for the purposes of visualizing the articular surface. Reduced fragments are fixed with 3.5mm cannulated screws which are percutaneously placed over a wire. Fibular fixation is usually not necessary and is never done before fixator application.

If the articular fragments can not be adequately repositioned using these techniques, open reduction may be required. Articular fragments impacted into the metaphysis and marginal impaction of split fractures defy reduction by indirect techniques. A surgical approach should be planned over a major fracture line, so that access to the articular surface of the tibia is obtained through a "fracture window". This minimizes stripping of the tibia and avoids the necessity of taking down the ankle capsule. Visualization is improved by distraction of the fixator. Impacted fragments can be dislodged and repositioned, and when the major fracture line is closed, the reduced central fragment will be held reduced. Fixation is again accomplished by cannulated screws.

In our experience, bone grafting of the metaphyseal area is necessary in approximately 20 per cent of cases. The less the soft tissues are surgically disrupted, the less frequent will be the need for bone grafting. Grafts of bone are applied to the defect area through limited incisions with the aid of fluoroscopy or through incisions already made for reduction.

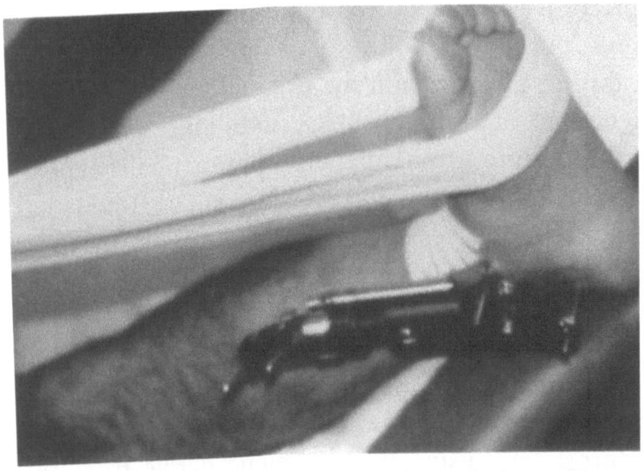

Fig. 27.8 Passive dorsiflexion exercises of the ankle are encouraged. This photograph shows a 3 inch stockinette around the forefoot, which the patient utilized to assist motion.

After articular repositioning and, if necessary, bone grafting, the distraction is reduced until the mortise takes on a symmetrical neutral appearance. During treatment the fixator neutralizes rather than distracts the fracture. Adjunctive screw or plate fixation of the metaphyseal area of the fracture is never used. The articulated hinge is locked in a neutral or slightly dorsiflexed position.

In non-articular distal tibia fractures (Fig. 27.6) and comminuted metaphyseal distal tibia fractures with a simple articular fracture line (Fig. 27.7), the T-clamp module of the Orthofix fixator can be used without crossing the joint. The distal screws will need to be inserted in the 1–3 or the 1–4 positions in the clamp. Pre-operative planning and intra-operative fluoroscopic guidance will ensure good screw positioning and secure fixation in the distal fragment. Bicortical purchase should be obtained with the distal screws. Traditionally, cancellous screws have been used, but some surgeons favour cortical screws. Fixation on the same side of the joint has the advantage of leaving the ankle free and avoiding fixator components in the

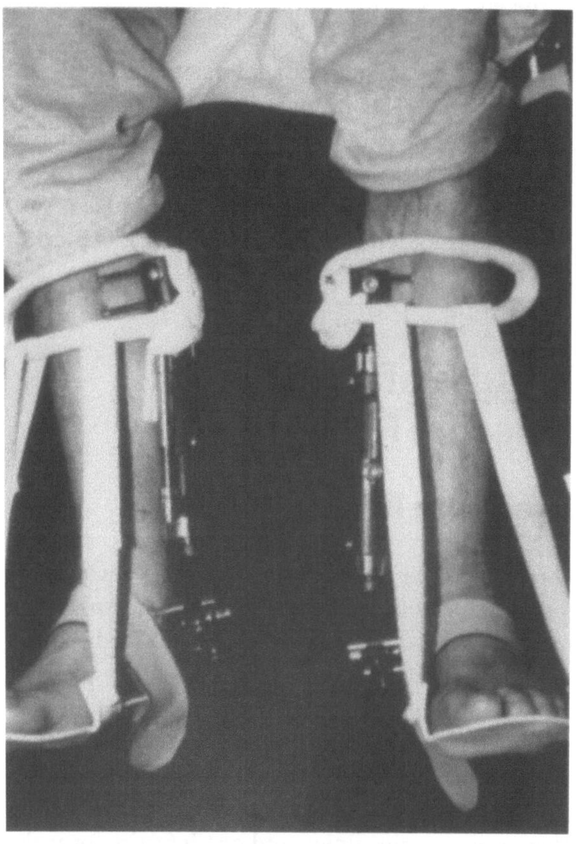

Fig. 27.9 This post-operative photograph of a patient with bilateral fractures of the tibial plafond treated with articulated external fixation shows the use of orthoplast foot plates to control the forefoot and splint the ankle in neutral.

hindfoot bones. This technique is not applicable to high energy, comminuted, intra-articular fractures of the tibial plafond.

There are various other modules of the Orthofix system that may assist in obtaining fixation in this area, such as the metaphyseal clamp, the Orthofix Hybrid Fixator module and the Sheffield Hybrid Fixator Assembly. The author does not have personal experience with any of these devices.

Post-operative Management

Post-operatively, strict elevation is maintained until the soft tissue swelling is controlled. Elastic wraps are used around the fixator to achieve some compression. At approximately 2–3 days, the articular hinge is released and the patient is taught gentle passive and active dorsiflexion and plantar flexion exercises (Fig. 27.8). An orthoplast splint is fashioned for the bottom of the foot and is secured to the fixator through Velcro closures to maintain the foot in a neutral position (Fig. 27.9). Patients are kept non-weightbearing for a period of 4–8 weeks depending on the fracture configuration. At the end of this time the fixator is dynamized, and progressive partial weightbearing is encouraged. Weightbearing dorsiflexion and plantar flexion exercises are begun. The fixator is removed when the fracture is clinically and radiographically healed. The average time in external fixation in our series has been thirteen weeks. After fixator removal the ankle is supported for another 4–8 weeks in a short leg splint or cast.

Results of Articulated External Fixation

Literature Review

Three published reports in the literature describe the use of the Orthofix Articulated Body for the Ankle with a technique similar to that detailed here. Tredwell and Fallot reported successful use in one case. They described the advantages of this technique and noted that precise application was required.[18] Saleh et al reported on twelve patients, five of whom had open plafond fractures.[15] Bone grafts were used in five cases. There was one non-union and one infection over the fibular plate, with no infections over the tibia. They also noted that precise fixator application was required.

Bonar and Marsh reported on their initial experience in twenty-one cases.[1] During this time period, they chose the technique for only the most severe plafond fractures. There were seven open fractures. Articular reconstruction was not possible for five fractures, one resulted in amputation and four in arthrodesis, two of which were performed while the fixator was still in place. The average duration of external fixation in this series was fifteen weeks. There were no tibial wound infections. Eleven of the sixteen patients who had articular repositioning had follow-up X-rays more than one year from injury, and only two of the eleven exhibited significant arthrosis.

Marsh et al studied 42 consecutive patients treated prospectively at three centres.[11] All of these fractures healed. There were no instances of infection, osteomyelitis or wound breakdown over the tibia. There were two infections over fibular plates. At the time of reporting, no patients had required arthrodesis.

Iowa Results

Two surgeons began using variations of this technique in 1987 at the University of Iowa. The technique as described became standardized in 1989 and has been used to treat the vast majority of tibial plafond fractures seen since that time. Currently, 60 cases have been treated. Twelve per cent of these fractures were open. All of them were caused by at least a component of axial loading. The results of this experience have either been reported in previous publications, or involve patients still under follow-up who have not been reported on.

There have been no infections of tibial wounds, either those secondary to open fractures or those surgically created. All soft tissue envelopes over the tibia have healed. There has been one fibular plate infection which required plate removal and antibiotics prior to resolution. There have been five arthrodeses, four from the original series previously described and published, and one subsequent arthrodesis in another patient where articular repositioning was not possible. Additional treatment has been required to obtain fracture union in three patients. The average time of external fixation has been fourteen weeks.

Not all of these patients have had long enough follow-up to determine the rate of arthrosis and functional outcome. The best data available on the arthrosis rate using this technique derive from the prospective study. In this study,[10] thirty-one ankles were followed for a minimum of two years (average 30 months). Radiographs at this follow-up demonstrated mild joint space narrowing in seven and severe joint space narrowing in two.

Function

Despite satisfactory articular reconstructions and successful union, a number of patients still have problems with their ankles many years after their injuries. Mild to moderate pain and ankle stiffness are common complaints. Approximately 75 per cent of patients successfully return to work, but some require changes to lighter jobs. The surgeon should keep in mind that a high energy axial compression fracture of the tibial plafond is a devastating injury that requires a long period of rehabilitation and may leave some permanent symptoms of pain and stiffness. It is my feeling that a majority of these problems have to do with the injury rather than the treatment method employed. It is therefore important for the surgeon to avoid causing additional complications in the treatment of these severe fractures in an unsuccessful attempt to obtain an excellent outcome.

Unresolved Issues

Fibular Fixation

Using AO technique, the fibula is plated as the first step in treating tibial plafond fractures.[14] Fibular plating has been used variably in conjunction with external fixation of the distal tibia. Some investigators have routinely plated the fibula prior to applying an external fixator,[17] while others have felt that this step is often unnecessary.[1] There are several advantages to fibular fixation, which include the restoration of length and alignment, repositioning of the tibial articular fragment attached to the distal fibula and lateral stability.

There are also significant disadvantages to routine fibular plating. In comminuted fractures, fibular plating can be difficult and time consuming, and the incision in this area is at risk for wound complications. In our external fixation series the only wound complications have been over fibular plates. In addition, fibular plating demands reconstruction of the tibia at full length, which in comminuted cases may not be desirable. Some shortening may speed healing, prevent non-union and decrease the need for bone grafting. With the articulated fixator technique fixation is into the talus, which remains attached to the distal fibula through the talofibular ligaments. Fibular fixation is not, therefore, required to restore length and alignment, because the fixator will control the talus and attached fibula in the position the surgeon desires. For this reason, I rarely plate the fibula in conjunction with the articulated technique.

There will probably continue to be advocates of routine fibular fixation for fractures of the tibial plafond. There are currently no data that will resolve this issue and comparative studies will be required.

Hinge Axis

The axis of the ankle closely approximates to a hinge through the majority of the range of motion. The current application technique aligns the fixator hinge along an axis parallel to the dome of the talus. This axis does not reliably approximate to the true ankle axis.[7] With the current fixator design it is not possible to orientate the fixator hinge reliably along the ankle axis because hinge orientation is dependent on screw position in the talus and calcaneus, and the positions of these screws have anatomical constraints and are difficult to place with consistency.

Hinge orientations off the ankle axis could potentially affect fracture healing and talar movements in the fixator, and produce hindfoot pin loosening. One cadaveric study has examined the movements of cadaveric ankles under hinged articulation with different hinge orientations.[7] The hinge positions tested were aligned in the current clinically accepted method in line with the top of the dome of the talus, along an approximate ankle axis, and along a specimen-specific axis determined by a mechanical axis finder. This study demonstrated that near full ankle movements and talar tracking closely approximating unfixated specimens were consistently obtained only with a hinge orientation determined by the specimen-specific axis finder. However, fracture site motion during ankle movements was small for all fixator hinge orientations. This bears out clinical experience that these fractures heal reliably under articulated distraction in spite of off-axis applications. Pin loosening secondary to increased forces from off-axis hinge orientation was not addressed in this study.

Currently, there is enough clinical experience to indicate that articulated movements are safe even with applications off the ankle axis. It is possible that better motion in the frame could be achieved, and the incidence of pin loosening reduced by designing a fixator hinge that could be aligned along the ankle axis. A fixator is currently being tested which would allow this to be achieved clinically.

Factors Which Relate to Outcome

What are the most important factors that predict patient outcome after this difficult fracture and which are under the surgeon's control? Complications of surgical intervention are the single biggest factor that lead to poor outcome and patient morbidity. When these complications are avoided, patient outcome improves.

Even if complications of treatment are avoided, the incidence of poor patient outcome is not insignificant, due to the development of post-traumatic arthrosis. Current literature does not contain enough information to delineate which factors contribute to arthrosis. Articular cartilage damage at the time of injury may be the most significant factor. Although most authors, including myself and others who favour less invasive techniques, recommend articular repositioning, there is no convincing evidence that the quality of reduction alone alters patient outcome. It is not certain whether gaps, steps, angulations or other types of displacement are more significant. Currently, it is logical to reposition fragments in as non-invasive a manner as possible while still avoiding the complications of intervention.

Summary

The treatment of high energy fractures of the tibial plafond by techniques stressing limited soft tissue dissection, articular stabilization with screws only, and external fixation for the major metaphyseal portion of the fracture have recently gained wide acceptance secondary to a decrease in the incidence of complications of treatment.[2] Articulated external fixation offers the advantages of a straightforward application technique, cross-ankle intra-operative distraction and limited ankle mobility in the frame. The talus and calcaneus appear to be safe places for external fixation screws. Excellent results have been reported in several studies. These results have raised the question of whether routine plate fixation of these fractures should be abandoned. Unresolved issues remain, such as those concerning the indications for plate fixation of the fibula, accurate orientation of the articulated hinge along the ankle axis, and which factors correlate with patient outcome.

References

1. Bonar SB, and Marsh JL: 'Unilateral external fixation for severe pilon fractures.' *Foot Ankle* 1993; 14: 57–64.
2. Bonar SB, and Marsh JL: 'Tibial Plafond Fractures: Changing Principles of Treatment.' *Am Academy Orthopaedic Surgeons: A Comprehensive Review* 1994; 2: 297–305.
3. Bone L, Stegemann P, McNamara K, Seibel R: 'External fixation of severely comminuted and open tibial pilon fractures.' *Clin Orthop* 1993; 292: 101–7.
4. DeCoster T.: Personal Communication, 1994.
5. Destot E: *Traumatismes du pied et ryon malleoles, astralage, calcaneus, avant-pied.* Masson: Paris, 1911.
6. Etter C, Ganz R: 'Long-term results of tibial plafond fractures treated with open reduction and internal fixation.' *Arch Orthop Trauma Surg* 1991; 210: 277–83.
7. Fitzpatrick DC, Marsh JL, Brown T.D.: 'Articulated external fixation of pilon fractures: the effects on ankle joint kinematics.' *J Orthop Trauma* 1995; 9: 76–82.
8. Friel JP. *Dorland's Illustrated Medical Dictionary*, 25th ed. WB Saunders, 1974.
9. Gustilo RB, Anderson JT: 'Prevention of infection in the treatment of one thousand and twenty-five open fractures of long bones. Retrospective and prospective analysis.' *J Bone Joint Surg* [Am] 1976; 58A: 453–8.
10. Marsh JL, Bonar S, Nepola JV, Decoster TA, Hurwitz SR. 'Use of an Articulated External Fixator for Fractures of the Tibial Plafond.' *J Bone Joint Surg* [Am] 1995; 77-A: 1498–509.
11. Marsh JL, Bonar S, Nepola, JV, DeCoster T, Hurwitz S, LeClare, W.: 'Tibial plafond fractures – A prospective protocol utilizing articulated external fixation.' *Orthopaedic Transactions*, Vol. 17, No. 4, p. 1038, 1993–1994.
12. McFerran MA, Smith SW, Boulas HJ, Schwartz HS: 'Complications encountered in the treatment of pilon fractures.' *J Orthop Trauma* 1992; 6:195–200.
13. Müller ME, Nazarian S, Koch P, and Schatzker J: *The Comprehensive Classification of Fractures of Long Bones.* Springer-Verlag: Berlin Heidelberg, 1990, pp 170–9.
14. Rüedi TP, Allgöwer M. : 'The operative treatment of intra-articular fractures of the lower end of the tibia.' *Clin Orthop* 1979; 138: 105–10.
15. Saleh M., Shanahan MDG, Fern ED: 'Intra-articular fractures of the distal tibia: surgical management by limited internal fixation and articulated distraction.' *Injury* 1993; 24: 37–40.
16. Teeny SM, Wiss DA: 'Open reduction and internal fixation of tibial plafond fractures: variables contributing to poor results and complications.' *Clin Orthop* 1993; 292: 108–17.
17. Tornetta P, Weiner L, Bergman M, Watnik N, Steuer J, Kelley M, Yang E.: 'Pilon fractures: treatment with combined internal and external fixation.' *J Orthop Trauma* 1993; 7: 489–96.
18. Tredwell JR, Fallat LM: 'Dynamic unilateral distraction fixation: surgical management of tibial pilon fractures.' *J Foot Ankle Surg* 1994; 33: 438–42.
19. Tscherne H, Goetzen L, ed. *Fractures with Soft Tissue Injuries.* Springer-Verlag: Berlin, 1984.
20. Varela CD, Vaughan TK, Carr JB, Slemmons BK: 'Fracture blisters: clinical and pathological aspects.' *J Orthop Trauma* 1993; 7: 417–27.
21. *Webster's Ninth New Collegiate Dictionary*, G and C Merrian Co., 1980.

Hybrid External Fixation in Tibial Trauma 28

M. Saleh and M. El Shazley

Introduction

The third generation monolateral external fixators such as the dynamic axial fixator (Orthofix srl, Verona, Italy) have led to improved patient care and a resurgence of interest in external fixation techniques (Hull et al 1997 Hay et al 1998, Saleh and Rees 1995). Of particular merit is the 6mm tapered screw design and bimodal characteristics of the fixator body which may be converted from rigid to dynamic support. Over a number of years of clinical trials, the 6mm cortical tapered screws have provided strong durable fixation in diaphyseal bone. Osteolysis and infection are rare events, provided that good surgical technique is adhered to and the screws are inserted in the centre of the bone.

By contrast, metaphyseal fixation has been less satisfactory with loosening occuring more frequently. The probable reasons for reduced performance relate to the open "cell like" structure of trabecular bone and cantilever loading. Monolateral external fixators support the bone by cantilever loading (Fig. 28.1a) and this leads to concentrated high stresses on the near cortex. Repeated cyclical loading during gait, is probably the explanation for the loosening which occurs. In one study, cortical screws have been shown to perform better than cancellous screws in metaphyseal bone (Lawes and Goodship, 1997) and in a further study, a zone of poor fixation described as "no man's land" has been defined (Reed et al, 1997).

Circular frames using tensioned Kirschner-wires which cross from one side of the bone to the other, support the bone by beam loading (Saleh et al 1997) and provide variable (multimodal) elastic support to the bone (Ilizarov 1992). Stresses are absorbed by both cortical plates and distributed more evenly across the surface of the bone, an important feature in the support of metaphyseal bone (Fig. 28.1). Clinical experience endorses the improved performance of wires in long term fixation of metaphyseal bone, even where osteoporosis exists. An important prerequisite of stable circular frame fixation is the use of wires with wide crossing angles sited within the central area of the bone. This is certainly possible in the metaphysis, but crossing angles are restricted in the diaphysis due to other soft tissue constraints such as muscles, tendons, nerves and vessels (Faure and Merloz 1987). These narrow crossing angles within the diaphysis lead to instability where all-wire fixation is used.

The combination of wires for fixation of the metaphyseal bone and screws to fix diaphyseal bone is attractive and is reflected by the number of hybrid external fixation frames which are now available. Most of these frames, however, retain their less desirable cantilever loading properties because of the lack of even load transfer between the monolateral and circular frame elements. By using an all-ring construct, a more efficient load transfer system can be achieved, leading to a fixator design whose mechanical characteristics closely match those of the all-wire Ilizarov frame (Fig. 28.1). Unlike other hybrid designs, the use of an all ring design facilitates cross joint fixation and the attachment of hinges for the correction of contracture and deformity (see Ch. 40). Furthermore, the exclusive use of wires in the metaphysis ensures that the device retains its elastic characteristics.

The System Components

The Sheffield Hybrid Fixator Assembly (Orthofix srl, Verona, Italy) consists of reinforced two-thirds rings and one-third rings (arches) capable of supporting up to four 2mm wires, tensioned to 1400

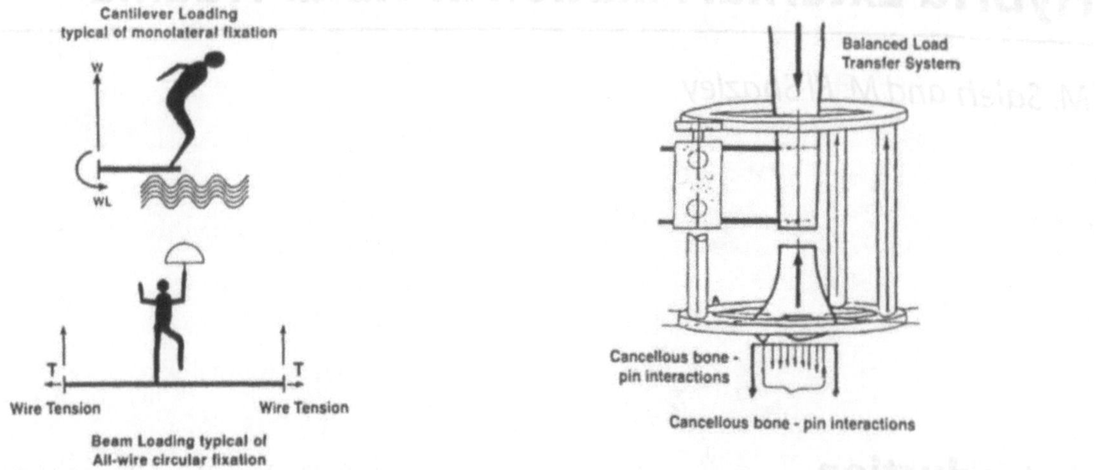

a b

Fig. 28.1 **a** Cantilever and beam loading. **b** Balanced load transfer system.

Newtons. A full ring may be constructed by the attachment of a one-third component to a two-thirds component. These rings are used to support both metaphyseal and diaphyseal segments. In the metaphyseal segment, up to four 2mm wires are attached to the ring using specially designed wire securing pins and wire slider units. The metaphyseal ring may be connected to a diaphyseal ring using three threaded bars or reduction units (Fig. 28.2). Diaphyseal fixation is achieved with the Sheffield clamp. The Sheffield clamp looks similar to the standard DAF clamp (Orthofix srl, Verona, Italy), but has a broad flange connecting it to the ring, and a rotational element to ensure optimal screw placement.

Additional fixation may be achieved by attaching a single screw holder to the ring itself. In this design, the fixator may be used for the treatment of metaphyseal and articular fractures of the proximal and distal tibia. With the addition of hinges and threaded bars, the device may be taken on to the foot or across the knee, and may be used for more complex fracture patterns, as well as for limb reconstruction surgery.

Materials and Methods

Extensive biomechanical and clinical trials were conducted over a four-and-a-half year period, from January 1995 until June 1999. During this period the fatigue characteristics, loading characteristics, and biomechanical properties of the fixator were defined. It has been shown in biomechanical tests, using a materials testing machine, to have the desirable properties of elastic axial fixation, beam loading, and near isotropic bending stiffness. In two-ring form its mechanical properties closely resemble those of the four-ring all-wire Ilizarov frame (Saleh et al 1997, Saleh 1998). As a result of its ease of use, strong mechanical support and comfort, it is indicated for severe tibial trauma situations and, in the majority of instances, it permits early and often immediate weightbearing. More than 200 fixators have been applied for complex trauma and limb reconstruction. Ninety fixators have been applied for acute or delayed complex trauma and the regions treated are shown in Table 28.1.

Results and Conclusions

Satisfactory initial results have been reported for pilon and plateau fractures (Saleh and Hakme 1998), pilon fractures (El Shazley et al 1999) and plateau fractures

Distal Femur	3
Tibial Plateau	17
Proximal Tibia and shaft	23
Distal Tibia	6
Tibial Pilon	41
	90

Table 28.1 Breakdown of the Use of the Sheffield Hybrid Fixator Assembly In Complex Trauma Cases in Sheffield

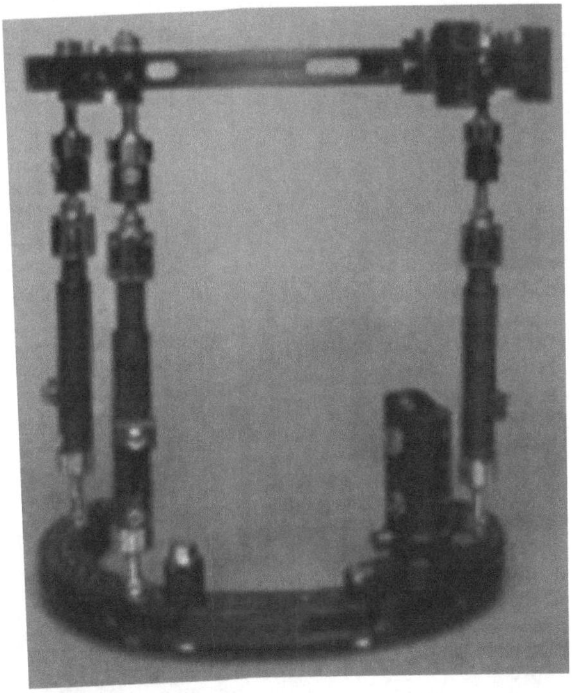

Fig. 28.2 The Sheffield Hybrid Fixator assembled with fracture reduction units.

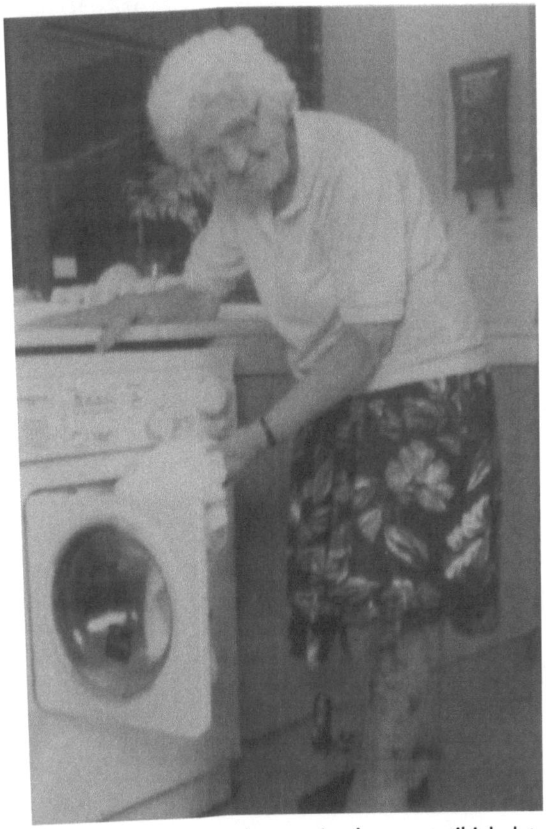

Fig. 28.3 Lady aged 90 who sustained an open tibial plateau fracture mobilizing early post-operatively following the application of a Sheffield Hybrid Fixator. The fixator was removed at 4 months and she regained 135° of motion.

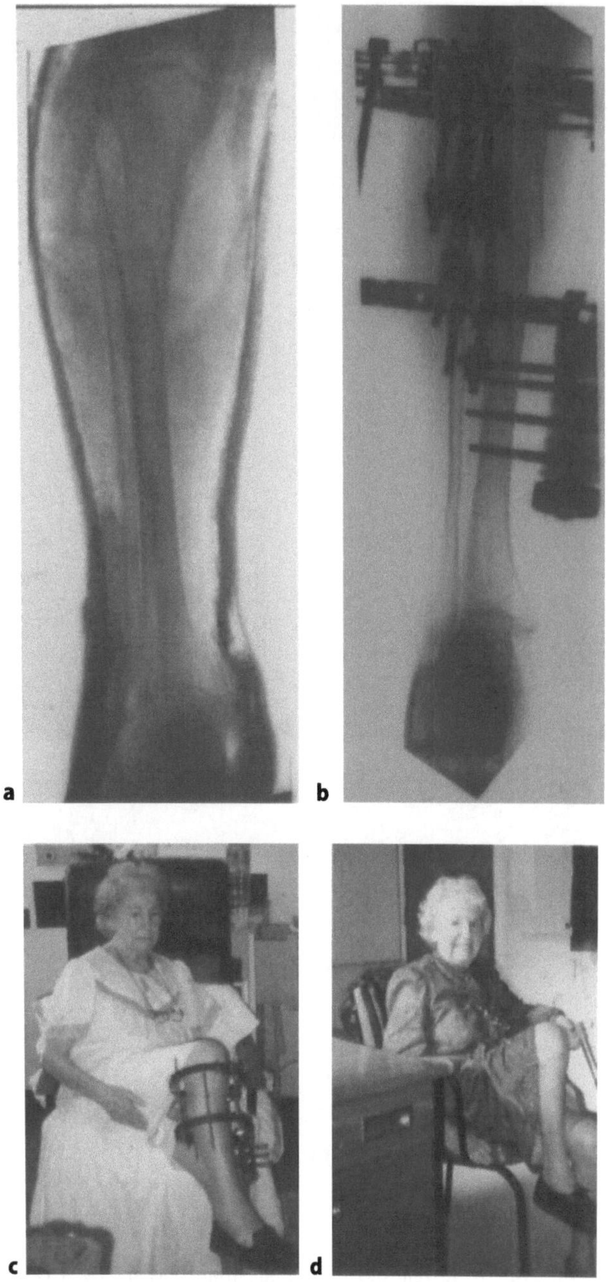

Fig. 28.4 **a** Long spiral, osteoporotic fracture in the proximal tibia in a lady of 78 years of age. Fracture unstable in plaster of Paris. **b** A hybrid fixator was applied. **c** Patient was fully weightbearing at three weeks, and mobilizing her knee. **d** Fixator removed at 5 months.

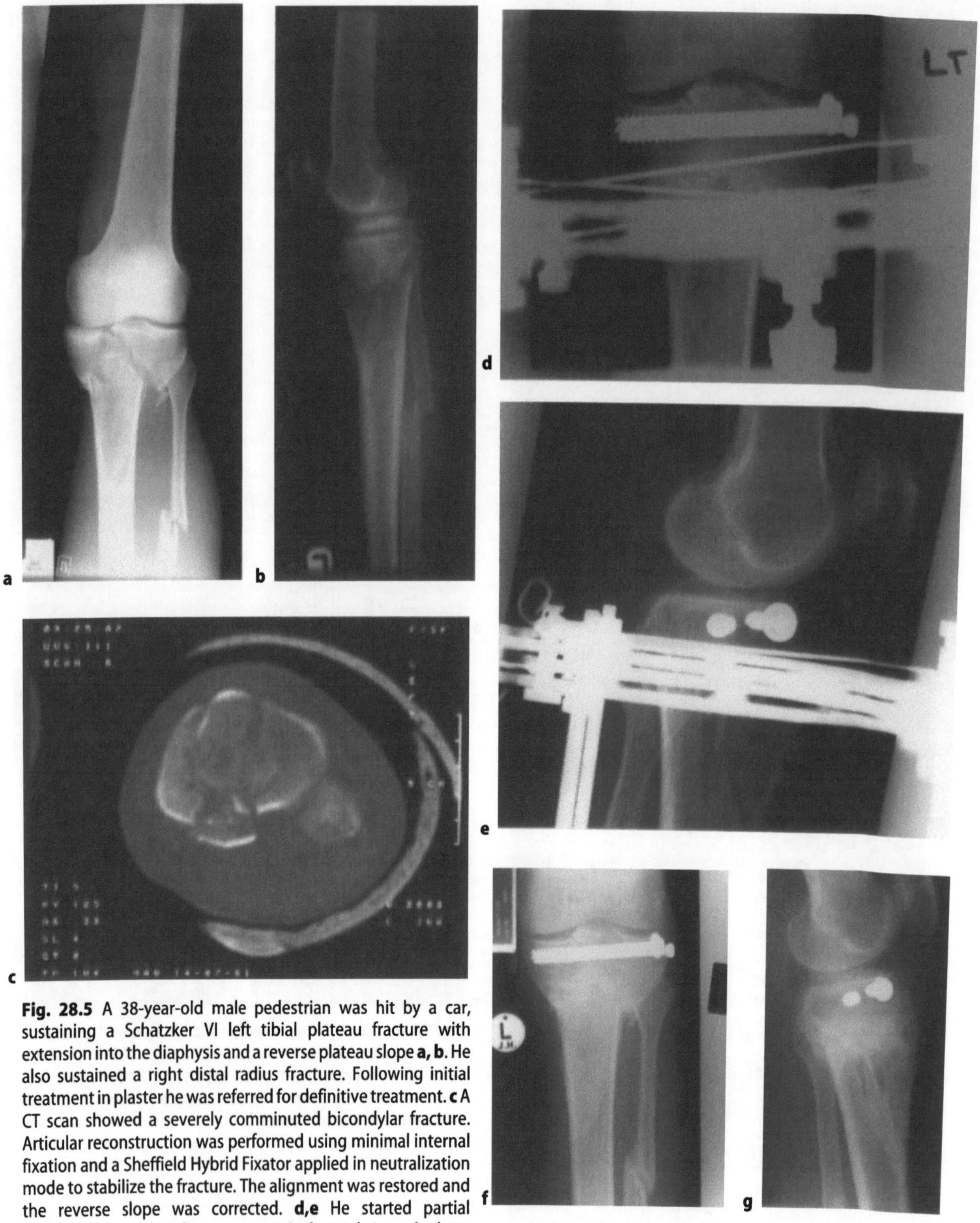

Fig. 28.5 A 38-year-old male pedestrian was hit by a car, sustaining a Schatzker VI left tibial plateau fracture with extension into the diaphysis and a reverse plateau slope **a, b**. He also sustained a right distal radius fracture. Following initial treatment in plaster he was referred for definitive treatment. **c** A CT scan showed a severely comminuted bicondylar fracture. Articular reconstruction was performed using minimal internal fixation and a Sheffield Hybrid Fixator applied in neutralization mode to stabilize the fracture. The alignment was restored and the reverse slope was corrected. **d,e** He started partial weightbearing 2 weeks post-operatively, and 6 weeks later commenced full weightbearing. In view of the diaphyseal extension the frame was left on for 20 weeks and he was dynamized for another 4 weeks after which it was removed **f, g**. He then resumed full activities. At six months following the injury he had no pain and clinical examination showed a full range of movement (5°–135° flexion).

in the elderly (Ali et al 1999). Stable fixation may be achieved in osteoporotic fractures of the tibia in the elderly (Fig. 28.3, Fig. 28.4), as well as in unstable short oblique fractures at the metaphyseal–diaphyseal junction. The device has been used to neutralize articular fractures of the plateau (Fig. 28.5) and pilon (Fig. 28. 6) following percutaneous articular surface reconstruction with cannulated screw fixation, central olive wires or Fragment Fixation System implants (Orthofix srl, Verona, Italy) (Pennig et al 1994). Occasionally, a bone graft may be required to provide further support for the articular surface. The ability of the device to be extended across the knee (Fig. 28.7) and ankle (Fig. 28.8) permits its use in more severely comminuted fractures and those associated with soft tissue injury. At an appropriate stage post-operatively, usually around the sixth week, the transarticular component of the fixation may be disconnected to permit joint mobilization. Schatzker VI tibial plateau fractures are particularly challenging, since in these, a severe articular fracture co-exists with an unstable metaphyseo-diaphyseal fracture. The device provides adequate stability due to the facility it affords to tension four wires on the metaphyseal ring. This is supported by biomechanical studies, where four wires have been demonstrated to be equivalent to medial and lateral buttress plates (Watson, 1996).

In segmental fractures, three rings may be used to provide independent control of each of the fractures (Fig. 28.9). Depending upon the site of the fractures, there may be proximal and distal wire-bearing rings with the middle segment fixed with screws, or one wire-bearing ring and two diaphyseal screw-bearing rings. The fixation at each fracture site is gradually reduced as the fractures heal, thus avoiding the common scenario of one fracture healing and the other progressing to non- or delayed union. Except in the presence of comminuted articular fractures, most patients are able to weightbear, either partially or fully, immediately after fixation. The use of hybrid external fixation in these difficult trauma problems has led to improved results and a reduction in complication rates. As well as ambulating early, patients have been noted to be prepared to exercise, and even run, with the fixator in place; to undergo work retraining, cycling and build-up of muscle bulk (Fig. 28.10).

Dynamization is not usually necessary, but in some cases it may be appropriate to release the telescopic mechanism on the reduction units or to loosen the threaded rods by 3–4mm where they attach to the rings to increase fracture response. This approach is useful where a fracture remains stable but indolent, since no irreversible sacrifice of stability is incurred. As the callus response improves, gradual destabilization may be achieved by removing the supplementary screw and two of the four wires over a period of 6 weeks. The fixator is then removed and the patient advised to build up to full weightbearing. Supplementary cast or orthotic support is rarely required. Satisfactory healing rates and times have been observed, with metaphyseal and articular fractures healing in approximately 13 weeks. Long oblique fractures have occasionally been slow to heal and this may be due to excessive fracture site motion. When fracture site motion was analysed in an in vitro study, more shear motion was recorded with the Sheffield Hybrid Fixator Assembly than with the all-wire Ilizarov fixator (Yang and Saleh 1999). We postulate that this is due to the asymmetrical support provided by wires on one side of the fracture and screws on the other. In another laboratory study we demonstrated increased stability in such fractures when horizontally opposed olive wires were inserted (Koehnlein et al 1999). Since January 1999 we have applied oblique or horizontal olive wires for all fractures with >45° obliquity, with improved results (Fig. 28.11).

The use of hybrid external fixation is a welcome advance over previous external fixation methods. The device chosen, however, should be capable of beam loading support and provide stable long-term fixation.

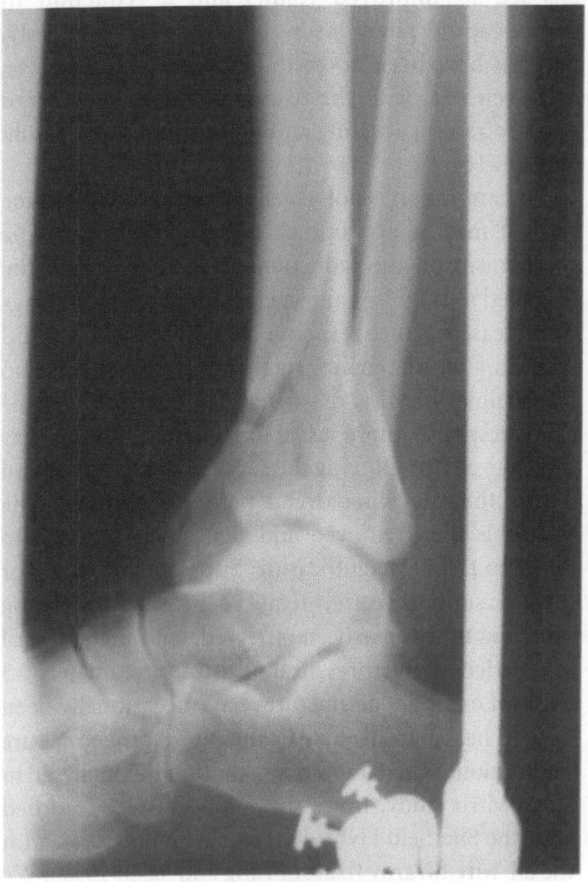

a

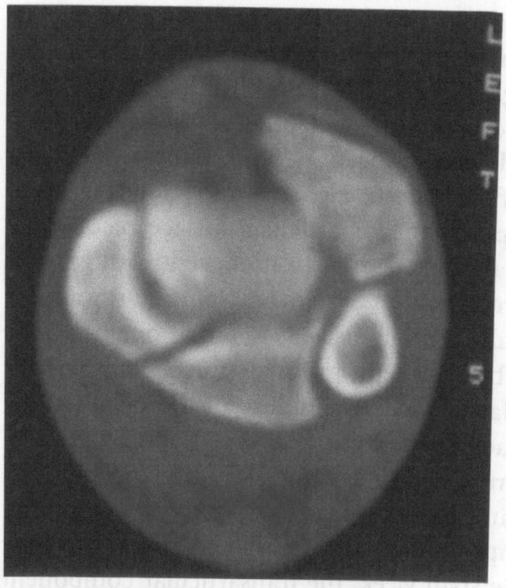

b

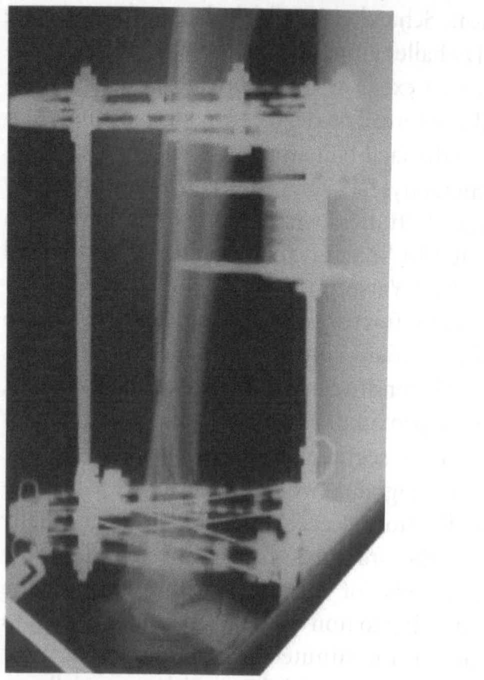

d

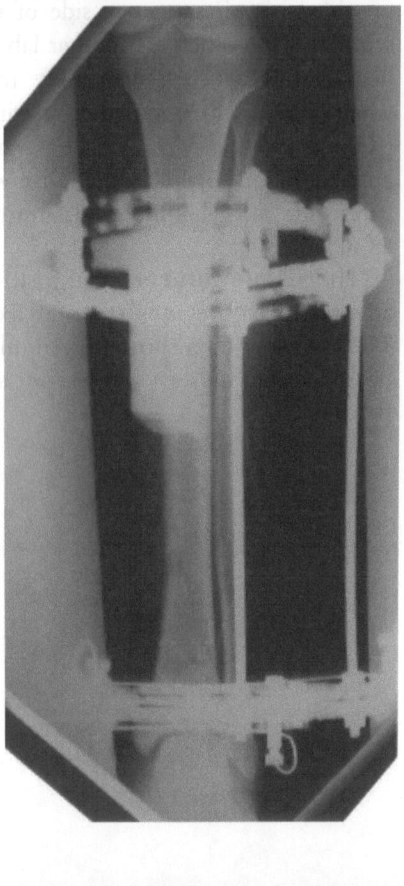

c

Fig. 28.6 **a** A 59-year-old male fell 20 feet from a ladder while cleaning windows, sustaining a closed Rüedi and Allgöwer Type III pilon fracture. The fracture extended into the diaphysis with some comminution. **b** A CT scan of the fracture. **c, d** CT-guided limited open reduction was performed through an anterior incision. The articular surface was restored with a lag screw, K-wires and 2 wires with central olive. The fracture was neutralized using a Sheffield Hybrid Fixator with four wires distally and three screws proximally. The ankle was mobilized immediately post-operatively and these images show the extent of **e** dorsiflexion and **f** plantar flexion. The patient returned to work as a car valeter at 4 weeks, and within two months he was back to full time heavy work which included lifting tyres and washing cars. **g** The X-ray appearances at 6 months and **h** the patient on a ladder again. The fixator was removed at 7 months following healing of the diaphyseal fracture.

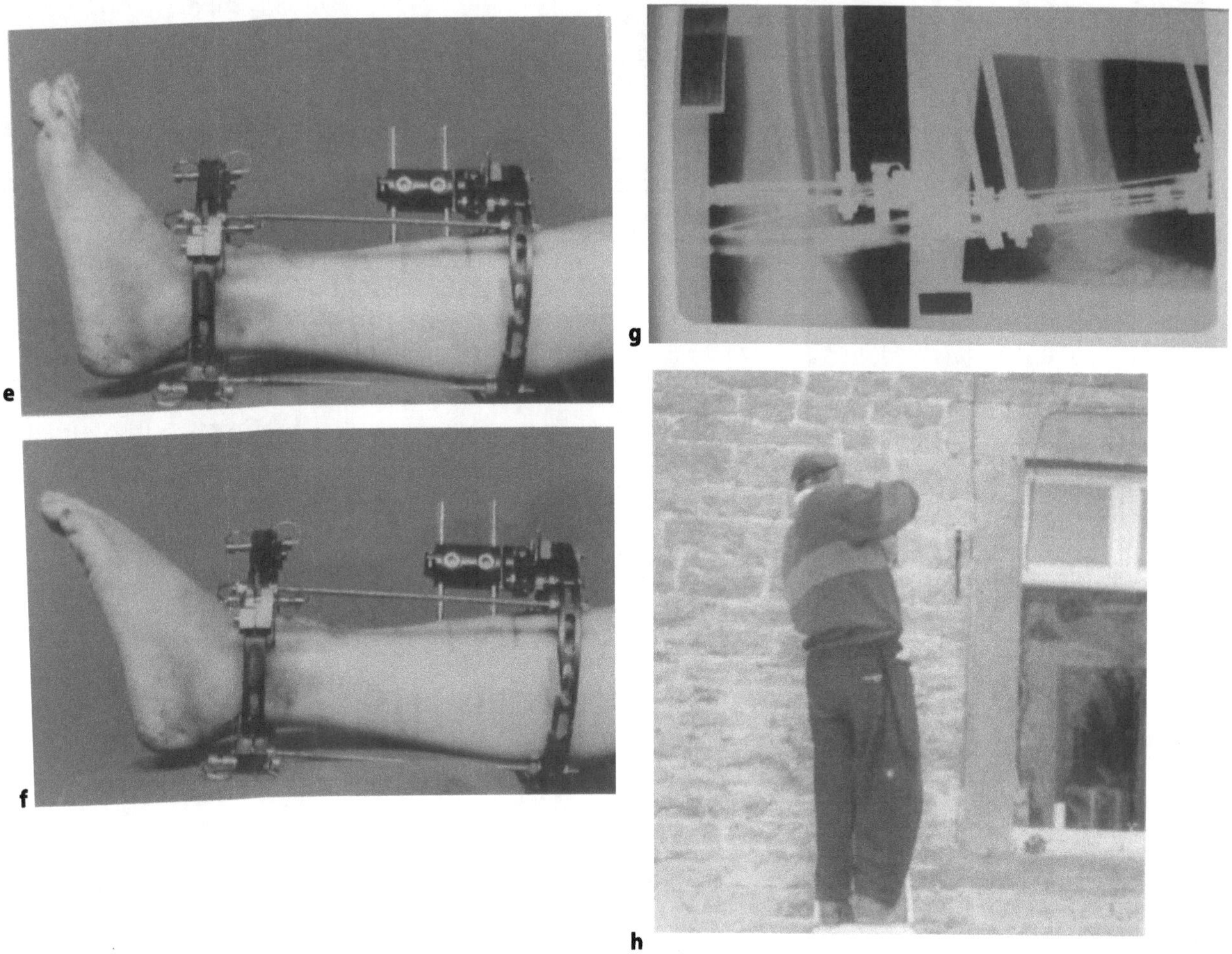

e f g h

Fig. 28.6 (continued)

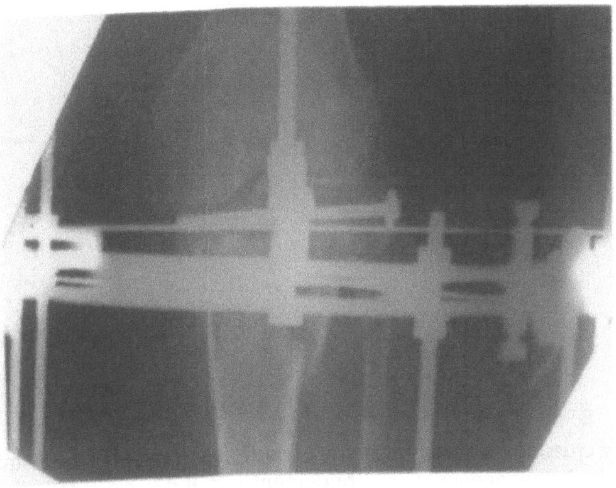

Fig. 28.7 A Schatzker V tibial plateau fracture stabilised using a Sheffield Hybrid Fixator with temporary fixation across the knee with a further ring and Sheffield clamp.

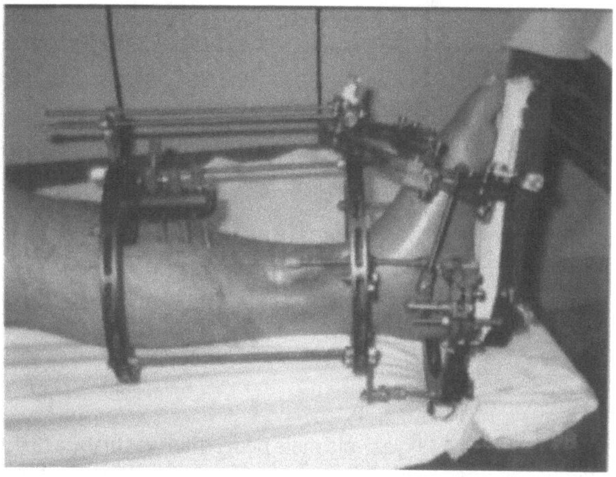

Fig. 28.8 Application of a Sheffield Hybrid Fixator across the ankle with two wires in the hindfoot and two in the forefoot, attached to two-thirds rings.

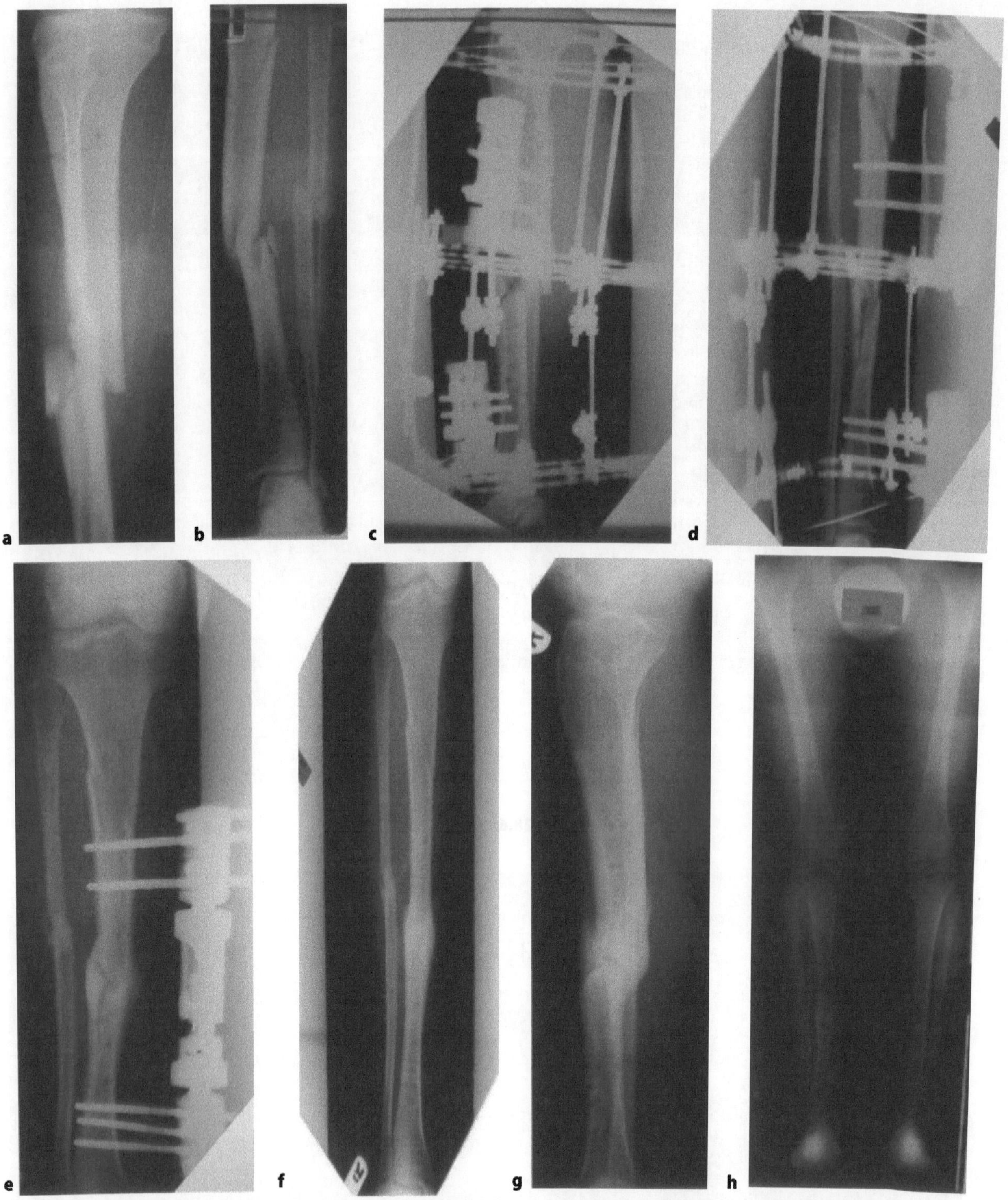

Fig. 28.9 a, b A 31-year-old male pedestrian was hit by a taxi while crossing the road, sustaining a head injury, fracture of the distal radius and open Grade IIIB segmental fracture of tibia and fibula. Initial management with debridement, DAF and fascio-cutaneous flap. **c, d** Two days post-injury a three-ring Sheffield Hybrid Fixator was applied. The proximal metaphyseal ring was fixed with four wires, the middle and distal diaphyseal rings with screws. **e** Following healing of the proximal fracture the hybrid fixator was removed and a DAF applied to support the distal fracture. **f, g** Healing occurred at eleven months. **h** Final limb alignment.

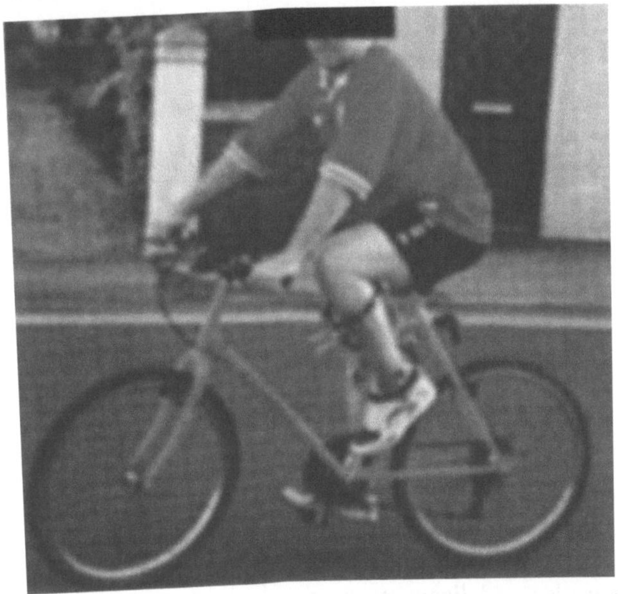

Fig. 28.10 A young patient cycling following the application of a Sheffield Hybrid Fixator. Calf impingement on the proximal ring occurred as a result of exercise induced muscle hypertrophy.

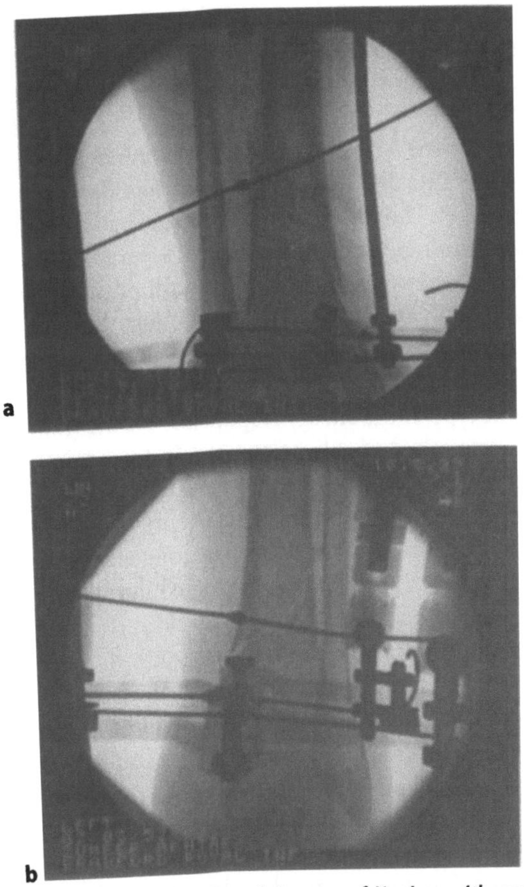

a

b

Fig. 28.11 Two examples of the use of K-wires with central olives used in fractures with an obliquity of greater than 45° to assist approximation and speed healing.

References

Ali A, Hashmi M, Saleh M. 'Treatment of bicondylar tibial fractures in elderly patients with the Sheffield Hybrid Fixator' British Trauma Society Meeting, Stoke-on-Trent 1999; *J Trauma* (in press).

El Shazley M, Dalby-Ball J, Burton M, Saleh M. 'The use of transarticular and extra-articular external fixation for the management of distal tibial intra-articular fractures.' *J Bone Joint Surg* [Br] 1999; Orthop. Proc. III 81B: 275–6.

Faure C, Merloz P. *Transfixation: Atlas of Anatomical Sections for the External Fixation of Limbs.* Springer-Verlag: New York, 1987.

Hay S M, Saleh M, Rickman M. 'Fracture of the tibial diaphysis treated by external fixation and the axial alignment grid. A single surgeon's experience.' *Injury* 1997; 28: 437–43.

Hull JB, Sanderson PL, Rickman M, Bell MJ, Saleh M. 'External Fixation of Children's Fractures: use of the Dynamic Axial Fixator.' *J Pediatr Orthop* 1997; Part B, 6: 203–6.

Ilizarov GA. *Transosseous Osteosynthesis: Theoretical and Clinical Aspects of the Regeneration and Growth of Tissue.* Springer-Verlag: Berlin, Heidelberg, New York, 1992.

Koehnlein W, Yang L, Saleh M. 'The effect of supplementary fixation on fractures of increasing obliquity.' *J Bone Joint Surg* [Br] 1999; Orthop. Proc. III 81B: 341.

Lawes TJ, Goodship AE. 'Cortical profile external fixation screws main torque in the metaphysis.' *J Bone Joint Surg* [Br] 1997; 79B (Suppl 3): 370.

Pennig D, Gausepohl Th, Lukosch R. 'Fragment Fixation for Small Fragment Stabilization in Hand Surgery.' *Handchir Mikrochir Plast Chir* 1994; 26: 270–3.

Reed M, Yang L, Saleh M, Petrone N. 'Metaphyseal "No man's land" - does it really exist?' *J Bone Joint Surg* [Br] 1997; Suppl IV p. 462.

Saleh M, Rees A. 'Bifocal surgery for deformity and bone loss after lower-limb fractures. Comparison of bone-transport and compression-distraction methods.' *J Bone Joint Surg* [Br] 1995; 77(3): 429–34.

Saleh M, Yang L, Nayagam S, 'Can a Hybrid Fixator perform as well as the Ilizarov Fixator?' *J Bone Joint Surg* [Br] 1997; Suppl IV p. 462

Saleh M. 'The Sheffield Hybrid Fixator: design considerations and clinical experience.' *Orthopaedic Product News* 1998; May/June: 33–6.

Saleh M, Hakme A, 'Fixation of intra-articular fractures of the tibia using hybrid external fixation – a prelimininary report.' *Injury* 1998; 29: 155.

Watson JT. *Biomechanical stability of Schatzker 6 fractures treated with fine wire external fixation.* ASAMI North America: Atlanta, 1996.

Yang L, Saleh M. 'Fracture site motion with external fixators.' *J Bone Joint Surg* [Br] 1999; Orthop. Proc. III 81B: 330.

Os Calcis Fractures

29

L. Nogarin, A. Rebeccato and B. Magnan

Introduction

The description of calcaneal fractures as extra-articular or intra-articular (thalamic) is universally accepted. Thalamic fractures are a controversial issue in traumatology, particularly in terms of treatment. Although the current trend is towards surgery, which offers a wide range of options, conservative treatment also has its advocates.

External fixation can be considered an option which lies somewhere between radical surgery and conservative treatment, and incorporates the best features of both. It involves closed reduction and synthesis, requiring thorough knowledge of the morphology of the lesion in this anatomically complex site. It is essential both to understand the causative mechanism of the injury, and to have access to a comprehensive imaging system. Computerised tomography (CT) fulfils the latter requirement.

Biomechanics

Despite the complexity of the forces involved, calcaneal fractures are essentially the result of shear forces followed by compression forces. Shear forces cause the so-called primary fracture line of Palmer.[34] According to Essex Lopresti,[16] this fracture line starts laterally. At the moment of impact with the ground, the weight of the body is transferred to the os calcis through the lateral process of the talus. This impinges on the os calcis at the angle of Gisanne and the external cortex, resulting in a vertical fracture line immediately in front of the posterior articular facet. The fracture then extends medially, separating the os calcis into two fragments: an anteromedial or sustentacular fragment and a posterolateral or tuberosity fragment.

If the shear force is completely spent in the production of the primary fracture line, the result is a compound fracture. If the shear force is not confined to this initial fracture line, the result is a displaced fracture with two fragments, the posterolateral fragment being dislocated superolaterally and distally, while the sustentacular is almost invariably maintained by the capsular and ligamentous structures by which it is attached to the talus.

When the energy responsible for the trauma is not limited to the initial shear force, a compression force is also exerted by the violent impingement of the talus on the posterolateral fragment. While the sustentacular fragment slips downwards and medially along the medial cortex, the posterolateral fragment is impacted by the talus. This results in a further, or secondary, fracture line[33] and a third, thalamic fragment. According to the direction of this secondary fracture line, Essex Lopresti[16] distinguishes between joint depression type and tongue type fractures. The main difference between these is the length of the thalamic fragment,[40-41] which extends only just beyond the posterior articular facet in the joint depression type but as far as the posterior wall of the tuberosity in the tongue type. If the energy responsible for the trauma is sufficient, the articular fragment is forced into the calcaneal cancellous bone and the lateral wall of the os calcis is pushed outwards. This occurs more often in the joint depression type than the tongue type, where the fragment is too large to be forced into the underlying cancellous bone to any major degree.

In the opinion of Essex Lopresti,[16] only four per cent of calcaneal fractures are so grossly comminuted that they cannot be assigned to either the depression type or tongue type. True blow-out fractures should therefore be considered rare.

The three main fragments (sustentacular, tuberosity, thalamic) created by the shear and compression forces can thus be identified as fairly consistent morphological features of heel fractures.

Diagnostic Imaging

While traditional X-rays often fail to provide optimal information, the CT scan, as a source of imaging not subject to overlap, has come to play a decisive role in the diagnosis, and hence the treatment, of thalamic calcaneal fractures.[11,14,20,21,29,30,38,43]

Traditional X-ray imaging of calcaneal fractures can still provide useful information if the following three standard views[8,23,38] are obtained:

mediolateral: to identify "depressed" and "tongue" fractures, blow-out fractures and the type of disruption (vertical and/or horizontal);

axial (descending retrotibial): to visualise the posterior subtalar joint, the posterior tuberosity and the body of the os calcis, the sustentaculum tali and lesions to these sites;

dorsoplantar view of the foot: to determine whether the fracture lines extend to the large apophysis, whether or not the calcaneo-cuboid joint is involved and whether other bones of the foot are damaged.

The CT scan is indispensable in the evaluation of thalamic fractures. It identifies the number of fracture lines, their exact morphology, the number and volume of fragments, the position of each fragment in relation to the others, and the extent to which the joint surfaces are involved.

The *coronal view* identifies the course of the fracture lines, both primary and secondary. The primary fracture line is responsible for the separation of the posterolateral and anteromedial fragments. The secondary fracture line isolates the thalamic fragment. It is also vital for the displacement of each fragment to be evaluated. Downward, medial displacement of the *sustentacular fragment* produces a "spike" on the profile of the medial cortex. The position of this fragment in relation to the talus is in most cases normal, but internal rotation with asymmetrical widening of the joint line is occasionally present.

The *tuberosity fragment* is the most mobile of all. It tends to move in a superolateral direction, lowering and widening the os calcis. The increase in transverse calcaneal diameter thus depends not only on the fracture of the external cortex, but primarily on the superolateral dislocation of the tuberosity which in most cases is rotated into a varus position.

The *thalamic fragment* varies in size according to the position of the primary and secondary fracture lines. It penetrates more deeply into the cancellous tissue of the tuberosity in joint depression than in tongue type fractures. In most cases, the thalamic fragment is externally rotated, with asymmetrical widening of the joint line.

The *axial view* can identify the course of the primary (pre-, trans- and retrothalamic) and secondary fracture lines; the lateral and distal dislocation of the tuberosity with widening and shortening of the bone and the involvement of the large apophysis and calcaneo-cuboid joint.

Pre-operative planning requires a thorough evaluation of this information, in terms of the number and volume of fragments and the position of each fragment in relation to the others.

Technique

The usual position for the frame is on the lateral face of the os calcis. The patient is placed in the lateral decubitus position on the uninjured side, with the thigh flexed at 45° and the knee at 90°. Under image intensification, two self-tapping, self-drilling 90mm pins are placed in the thalamic fragment first, parallel to the joint surface. Since the thalamic fragment is externally rotated in most cases, the pins must be slightly oblique from top to bottom. These pins are used to lift or derotate the thalamic fragment in order to reduce it, depending upon whether horizontal or vertical disruption is involved. The pins are then advanced manually into the medial calcaneus.

Two further pins are placed in the os calcis, in a suitable position to provide a counter force for reduction and stability. If the fracture involves vertical disruption and the need for derotation, the preferred position for the fixator will be on the anterior apophysis (Fig. 29.1). If the fracture line extends to the large apophysis and calcaneo-cuboid joint, an anterior assembly on the os calcis alone is impossible. In such cases, one pin must be placed in the cuboid. When the fracture involves horizontal or mixed disruption and elevation of the fragments is required, the preferred site is the posterior tuberosity (Fig. 29.2).

Once the mini-fixator (Orthofix srl, Verona, Italy) has been assembled, the ball jointed clamp is used to perform further reduction, locking the ball joint once this is complete and applying distraction or compression as required.

The sural nerve, which passes close to the lateral malleolus and on the lateral face of the os calcis, must be carefully avoided, to prevent any superficial paresthesia. It is particularly important to avoid the tendons of the peroneal muscles, to prevent any tension when the thalamic fragment is further reduced. Difficult reduction of depressed fractures can be aided by an incision at the site of the sinus tarsi,

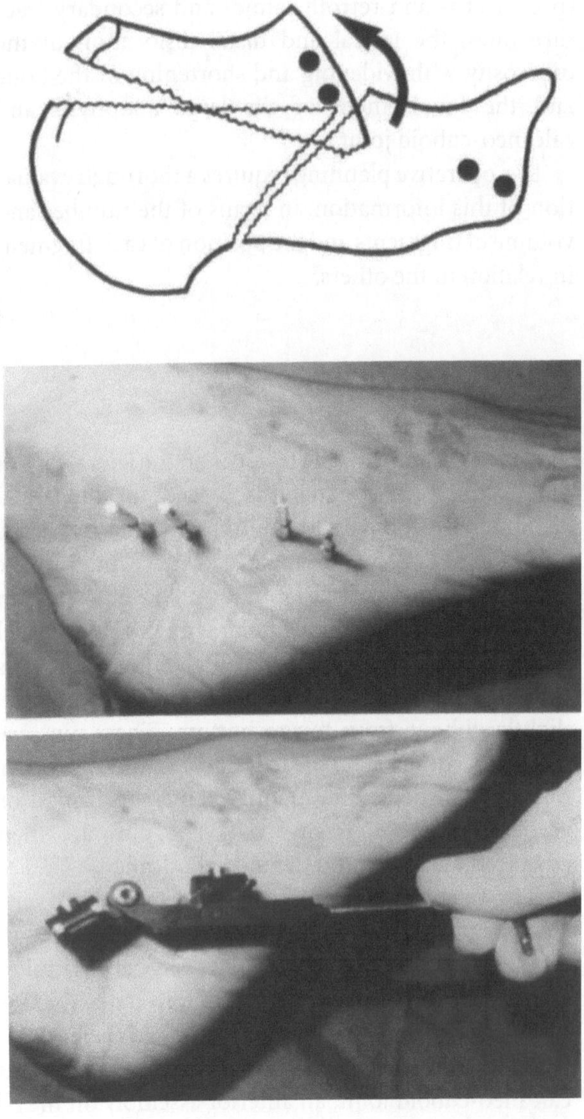

a b c

Fig. 29.1 a Schematic drawing of a B3.1 heel fracture (AO classification) showing vertical depression; the "tongue" type fracture according to Essex Lopresti. **b** and **c** Positioning of the screws and mounting of the assembly anteriorly for derotation of the thalamic fragment.

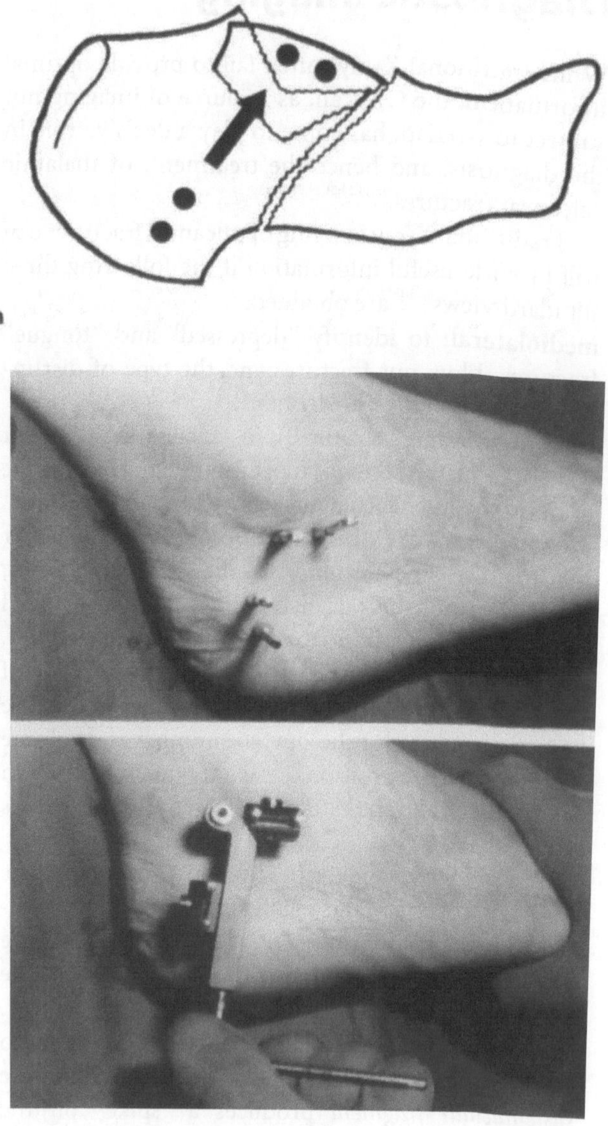

a b c

Fig. 29.2 a Schematic drawing of a B3.2 fracture (horizontal or mixed depression); the "depression" type fracture according to Essex Lopresti. **b** and **c** Positioning of the screws and mounting of the assembly posteriorly for elevation of the thalamic fragment.

through which a blunt instrument can be inserted into the fractured lateral cortex to raise the thalamic fragment (Fig. 29.3).

The superolateral and distal dislocation of the tuberosity fragment, which is the main cause of altered calcaneal length, width and height, may require medial application of the fixator. This makes it possible to restore the normal juxtaposition of the sustentacular and tuberosity fragments, and thus the morphology of the os calcis. For this additional manoeuvre, the patient must be moved from the lateral to the supine decubitus position, with the knee flexed at 80°. An intraoperative axial view is thus facilitated.

The distal pins, which are the first to be inserted, are positioned immediately below and distal to the sustentaculum. This position avoids damage to the posterior tibial neurovascular bundle. The two proximal pins are placed in the posterior tuberosity of the os calcis, perpendicular to its medial wall (Fig. 29.4). Taking account of the usual displacement of this fragment, the direction of the pins must be from distal to proximal, from top to bottom and, of course, from medial to lateral.

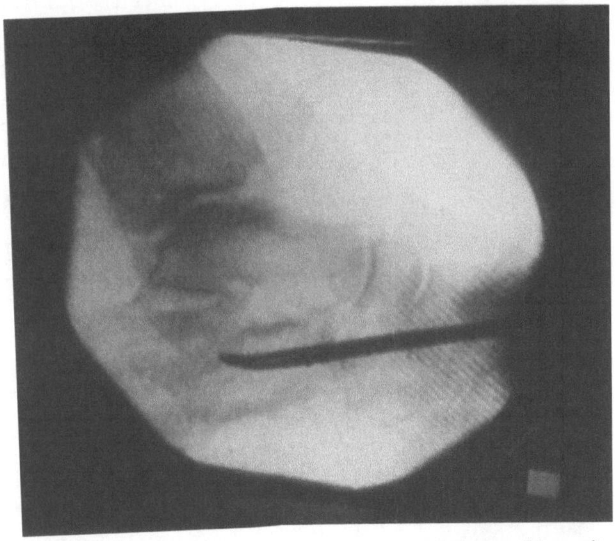

Fig. 29.3 Shows use of a blunt instrument inserted into the fractured lateral cortex to raise a depressed thalamic fragment.

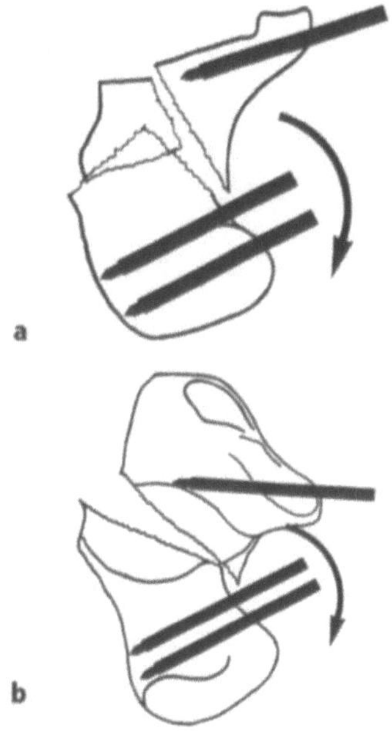

Fig. 29.4 Schematic representation of the position of the pins for a medial assembly: **a** Coronal view; **b** Axial view. The pins in the tuberosity must be perpendicular to the medial wall cortex and must transfix the bone for effective correction.

To realign the posterior tuberosity with the sustentacular fragment, the proximal pins must completely transfix the posterior tuberosity as far as the lateral face of the os calcis. This ensures that none of the distraction force is lost as a result of the screws moving within the cancellous bone of the os calcis. The pin positions must also be as far plantar as possible, to ensure that they do not engage the thalamic fragment still embedded in the cancellous calcaneal bone. The distal pins do not have to transfix the bone, since the sustentacular site is made up of thick bone and affords good purchase. A second fixator is then applied to the lateral face, in an anterior or posterior position according to the type of thalamic disruption.

The rationale for using both a medial and a lateral frame is the need for correction of both the articular and the non-articular components of the fracture. The articular component, comprising the thalamic disruption, is treated by the lateral frame; the medial fixator reduces and stabilizes the non-articular component, restoring the overall morphology of the os calcis. This means in practice the displacement of the posterolateral fragment, since the CT scan in most cases shows that the position of the sustentacular fragment in relation to the talus remains normal.

Post-Operative Management

Reduction can be improved in the first few post-operative days, by adjustment of the fixator clamps and body. This allows derotation and compression–distraction.

Since the application of the fixator differs from most others in the literature in that it is generally monosegmental, active and passive post-operative mobilization of the peritalar joint complex is possible as early as the first few days following operation. This accelerates the resolution of any post-traumatic haematoma and limits any risk of secondary stiffness as a result of periarticular fibrosis. Gradual weightbearing is usually introduced only after two months, often with the minifixator in situ. X-rays after the first two months no longer show the gap at the centre of the calcaneal body just below the reduced thalamic fragment. This gap is conspicuous in the immediate post-operative views, especially with depressed fractures. The os calcis is well vascularized and damage to its cancellous tissue heals rapidly, without the need for a bone graft.[40,41]

As regards to dressings and removal of the fixator, the same considerations apply as for any fixator applications.

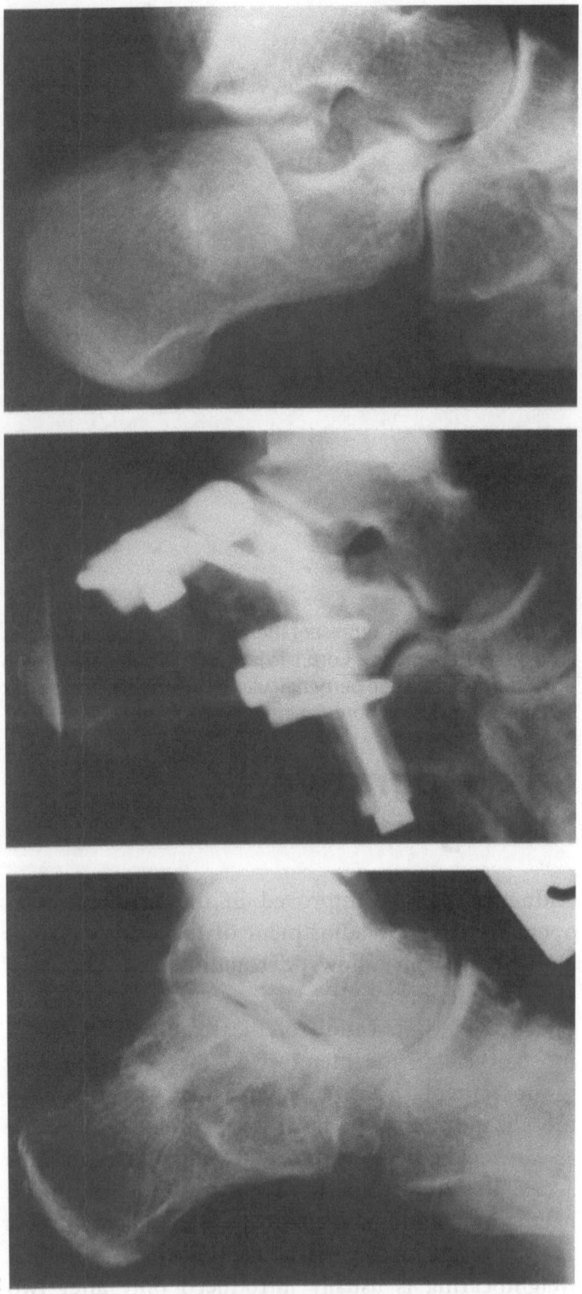

a b c

Fig. 29.5 Case 1: **a** A B3.1 fracture of the calcaneus. **b** Anterior positioning of the fixator assembly. **c** Final result.

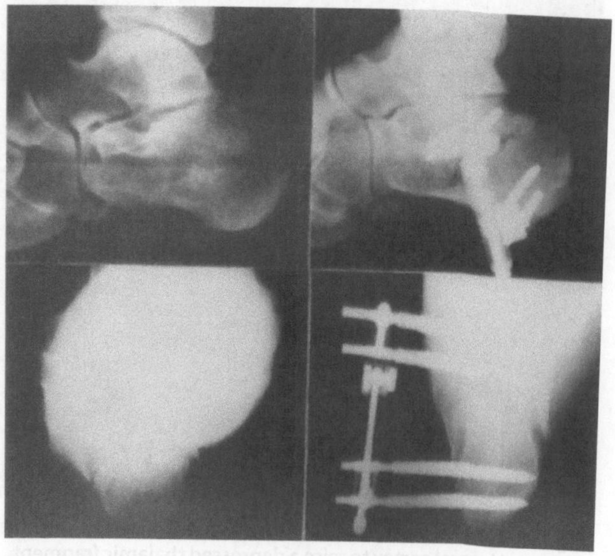

Fig. 29.6 Case 2: Posterior positioning of fixator assembly; reduction of the thalamic fragment and recovery of calcaneal height.

Patients

The present series includes 38 thalamic calcaneal fractures, in 37 patients (age range 20–70 years) treated in the Departments of Orthopedics of the Vicenza and Verona Hospitals. Two fractures were open, and the remainder closed. The fixator was applied 1–19 days following injury (mean 6 days).

Twenty-nine patients, with a total of 30 calcaneal fractures, were reviewed. The right and left sides were involved in 18 (60 per cent) and 12 (40 per cent) cases, respectively. One case was bilateral.

Twenty-seven fractures were treated with a simple assembly on the lateral face of the os calcis. In two cases, two fixators were applied using three pin groups, again on the lateral aspect of the os calcis. In only one case was a combined medial and lateral non-monosegmental assembly used. This procedure has recently become far more common practice in the two departments concerned, but most cases have been excluded because of insufficient follow-up.

Follow-up ranged from 5 to 61 months (mean 24 months). The AO classification was used, with division of thalamic fractures of the os calcis into three types:

B3.1: vertical thalamic disruption
B3.2: horizontal or mixed thalamic disruption
B3.3: "blow-out" (total destruction of joint surface).

The advantage of this classification is that it provides a ready guide to the external fixation technique to be used: anterior derotational configuration for B3.1, posterior assembly to raise depressed fragments in type B3.2, and combined medial/lateral application for B3.3.

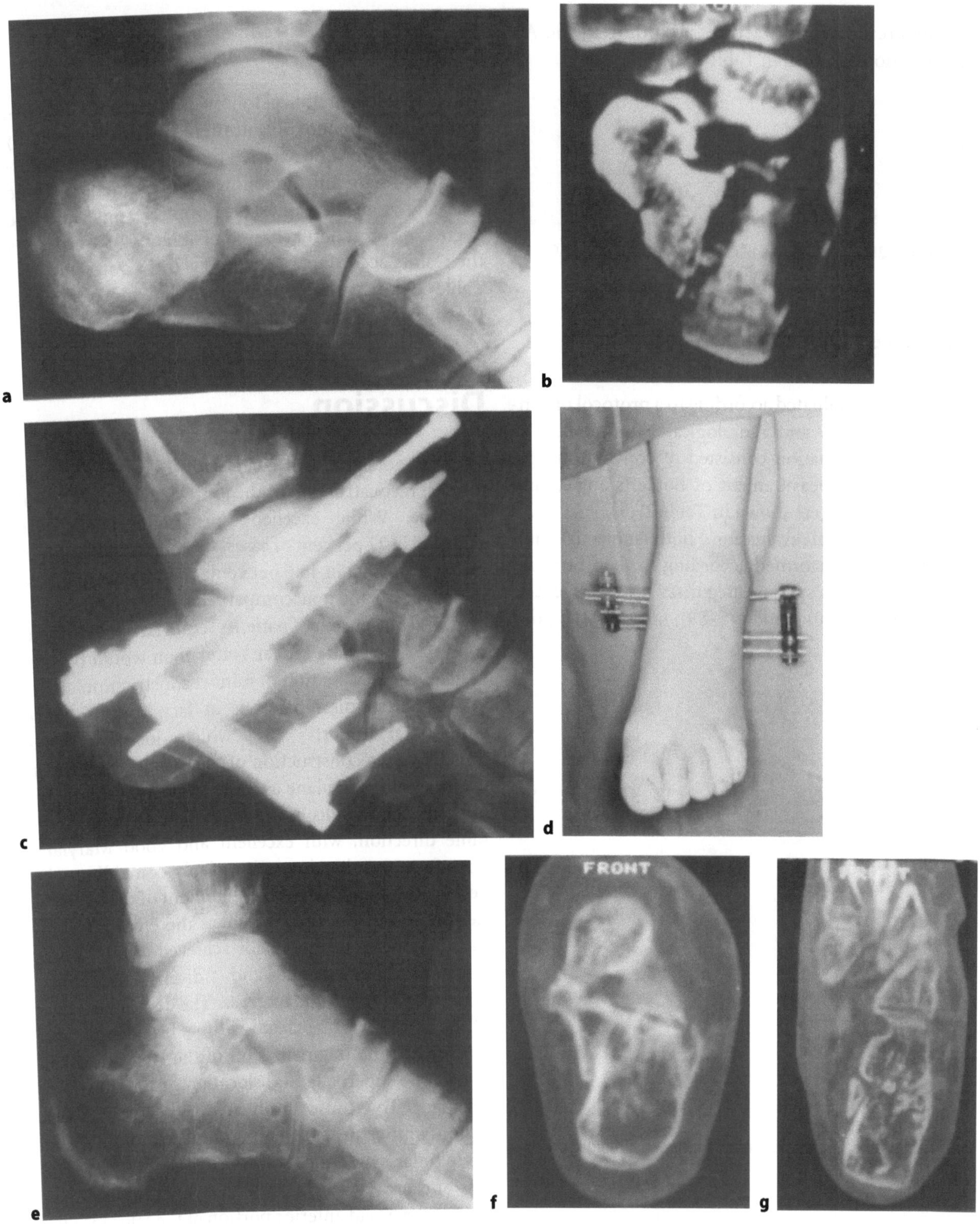

Fig. 29.7 Case 3: **a** B3.3 fracture. **b** CT scan showing extent of comminution. **c** Radiographic view and **d** clinical view of the medial and lateral fixators in place. **e** lateral X-ray and **f** and **g** CT scans of the healed fracture.

The breakdown of fractures according to the AO classification is shown in Table 29.1.

B 3.1	12	40%
B 3.2	14	47%
B 3.3	4	13%

Table 29.1 Breakdown of cases according to the AO classification.

Evaluation Protocol

Patients were evaluated according to a protocol of clinical (Table 29.2) and radiological assessment. The radiological evaluation consisted of conventional X-rays, including measurement of Böhler's angle,[4] and CT scan (parameters shown in Table 29.3).[28]

Overall clinical evaluation, both subjective and objective, was performed according to the Maryland Foot Score.[37] This system categorises results as: excellent (score 90–100); good (75–89); fair (50–74); poor (<50).

Hindfoot appearance
Forefoot appearance
Talo-navicular prominence
Plantar arch (podogram)
Subtalar joint mobility
Metatarsalgia
Pain at rest
Walking
Pain on walking
Orthoses

Table 29.2 Clinical parameters assessed at follow-up

Joint congruence
Sustentaculum tali
Sagittal axis
Longitudinal axis
Calcaneal height

Table 29.3 CT scan evaluation at follow-up

Results

Table 29.4 details clinical follow-up on the 29 patients, comprising a total of 30 calcaneal fractures treated by closed reduction and external fixation. Table 29.5 presents post-treatment and follow-up CT scan data. Table 29.6 shows mean values of Böhler's angle and the degree of correction achieved. Table 29.7 summarises the results according to the Maryland Foot Score and Table 29.8 lists the complications during treatment. Illustrative cases are shown in Figs. 29.5, 29.6 and 29.7.

Discussion

There is no significant correlation between the anatomical reconstruction of the joint surface and clinical outcome. While excellent joint congruence was achieved in 27 per cent of cases, subtalar articular function was normal in 46.6 per cent; walking was painless in 57 per cent and unaccompanied by limping in 76 per cent, and 80 per cent of patients required no additional support. These data are far better than would be suggested by CT evaluation of joint reconstruction alone. This apparent discrepancy is in fact in consonance with other reports[5,20,21,27,30] which identify three-dimensional reconstruction of the os calcis in relation to the supporting plane as more important than joint integrity. The results of the present study point in the same direction, with excellent and good Maryland Foot Score results almost invariably coinciding with better frontal and transverse alignment of the os calcis. Restoration of calcaneal height is therefore a significant parameter. If this is not achieved, symptoms of fibular impingement and distal tibiofibular syndesmosis syndrome increase. The decreased height of the os calcis is associated with its broadening, due not only to the fragmentation of the lateral wall but also to the superolateral dislocation of the tuberosity fragment. This causes problems in the submalleolar region with respect to the peroneal tendons.[38] Distal tibiofibular syndesmosis syndrome is also related to loss of calcaneal height, leading to continuous intrusion of the broad anterior portion of the talus into the tibio-fibular mortice.[35]

X-ray data provide a solid rationale for the use of external fixation in thalamic calcaneal fractures. The objective of the technique in these fractures is the restoration of bone morphology, regardless of perfect joint congruence. Closed reduction of the thalamic surface by a minifixator restores Böhler's angle adequately, even in the presence of major corrections

Hindfoot appearance	normal 25 (83%)	valgus 3 (10%)	varus 2 (7%)
Forefoot appearance	normal 28 (94%)	adducted 1 (3%)	abducted 1 (3%)
Talo-navicular prominence	absent 30 (100%)		present 0 (0%)
Plantar arch (podogram)	normal 20 (67%)	flat 8 (26%)	cavus 2 (7%)
Subtalar joint mobility	normal 14 (46.6%)	Reduced <50% 14 (46.6%)	Reduced >50% 2 (7%)
Metatarsalgia	absent 30 (100%)	present 0 (0%)	
Pain at rest	absent 22 (73%)	present 8 (27%)	
Walking	normal 23 (76%)	limp 7 (24%)	
Pain on walking	absent 17 (57%)	present 13 (43%)	
Orthoses	no 24 (80%)	yes 6 (20%)	

Table 29.4 Clinical results (mean duration of follow-up 23.6 months).

Joint Congruence	good 8 (27%)	fair 13 (43%)	poor 9 (30%)
Restoration of sagittal and longitudinal axes		yes 18 (60%)	no 12 (40%)
Calcaneal height		maintained 17 (57%)	reduced 13 (43%)

Table 29.5 Results from CT scan

Mean value of angle	pre-operative 0° (±15°)	follow-up 18° (±11°)
Resoration of angle >20°	yes 18 (60%)	no 12 (40%)

Table 29.6 Radiographic measurement of Böhler's angle

Excellent (90–100)	10 (33.3%)
Good (75–89)	15 (50%)
Fair (50–74)	4 (13.3%)
Poor (<50)	1 (3.3%)

Table 29.7 Results according to the Maryland Foot Score

Superficial Pin Track infection	2 (6.7%)
Algodystrophy	8 (26.7%)
Secondary thalamic perforation due to premature weightbearing	2 (6.7%)

Table 29.8 Complications

(mean 26° in fractures with an originally negative angle (range –30° to –10°) and 12° in those with a reduced angle (range 0° to +24°)). An angle of more than 20° was achieved in 18 cases (60 per cent).

Excellent and good results according to the Maryland Foot Score together accounted for 83 per cent of cases. In addition to confirming that the high initial expectations of the technique were justified, this statistic bears out the known principle that the functional outcome of thalamic calcaneal fractures is always better than the corresponding clinical and X-ray outcomes.

Two cases of superficial pin track infection were treated by early removal of the frame, with no major effect on final outcome. The incidence of algodystrophy, frequent with fixation in distraction of the wrist and tibial pilon, was minimal, and where it was observed, the condition resolved gradually with resumption of weightbearing.

Conclusion

Thalamic calcaneal fractures involve an articular component, the subtalar joint; they also have an equally important extra-articular component, the overall shape of the os calcis and the alignment of the hindfoot. The treatment method described offers the known advantages of external fixation (minimal invasiveness, no internal synthesis, the possibility of further post-operative reduction and early mobilization). It restores thalamic anatomy, albeit not always optimally, and achieves three-dimensional calcaneal reconstruction. The latter provides significant benefit in terms of its effect on final functional outcome.

References and Additional Bibliography

1. Andreasi A. 'Trattamento chirurgico delle fratture del calcagno.' *Chir Piede* 1992; 16: 273–6.
2. Baumgaertel FR, Gotzen L. 'Two-stage operative treatment of comminuted os calcis fractures; primary indirect reduction with medial external fixation and delayed lateral plate fixation.' *Clin Orthop Rel Res* 1993; 290: 132–41.
3. Bezes H, Massart P, Delvaux D, Fourquet JP, Tazi F. 'The operative treatment of intraarticular calcaneal fractures; indication, technique and results in 257 cases.' *Clin Orthop Rel Res* 1993; 290: 55–9.
4. Böhler L. 'Diagnosis, pathology and treatment of fractures of the os calcis.' *J Bone Joint Surg* 1931; 13: 75–89.
5. Bradley SA, Davies AM. Computed tomographic assessment of old calcaneal fractures. *Brit J Radiol* 1990; 63: 926–33.
6. Burdeaux BD.'Reduction of calcaneal fractures by the McReynolds medial approach technique and its experimental basis.' *Clin Orthop Rel Res* 1983; 177: 87–103.
7. Burdeaux BD. 'The medial approach for calcaneal fractures.' *Clin Orthop Rel Res* 1993; 290: 96–107.
8. Burghele N, Luppino T, Caroli A. *Le fratture del calcagno* Piccin Ed.: Padova, 1972.
9. Carr JB. 'Mechanism and pathoanatomy of the intraarticular calcaneal fracture.' *Clin Orthop Rel Res* 1993; 290: 36–40.
10. Carr JB, Hamilton JJ, Bear LS. 'Experimental intraarticular calcaneal fractures: anatomic basis for a new classification.' *Foot Ankle* 1989; 10: 81–7.
11. Crosby LA, Fitzgibbons T. 'Computerized tomography scanning of acute intraarticular fractures of the calcaneus; a new classification system.' *J Bone Joint Surg* [Am] 1990; 72–A: 852–9.
12. De Marchi F, Treccani PG, Boreatti V. 'Inquadramento anatomo-patologico delle fratture talamiche di calcagno.' *Chir Piede* 1992; 16: 259–62.
13. Duparc J, de la Caffiniere JY. 'Mechanisme, anatomo-pathologie, classification des fractures du calcaneum.' *Ann Chir* 1970; 24: 289–301.
14. Eastwood DM, Gregg PJ, Atkins RM. 'Intraarticular fractures of the calcaneum. Part I: pathological anatomy and classification.' *J Bone Joint Surg* [Br] 1993; 75-B: 183–8.
15. Eastwood DM, Langkamer VG, Atkins RM. 'Intraarticular fractures of the calcaneum. Part II: open reduction and internal fixation by the extended lateral transcalcaneal approach.' *J Bone Joint Surg* [Br] 1993; 75-B: 189–95.
16. Essex Lopresti P. 'The mechanism, reduction technique and results in fractures of the os calcis.' *Brit Surg* 1952; 39: 395–419.
17. Giachino AA, Uhthoff HK. 'Current concept review: intraarticular fractures of the calcaneus.' *J Bone Joint Surg* [Am] 1989; 71-A: 784–7.
18. Gui L. *Fratture e lussazioni.*Aulo Gaggi Ed.: Bologna, 1952.
19. Hammesfahr Rick JF. 'Surgical treatment of calcaneal fractures.' *Orthop Clinics North America* 1989; 20: 679–89.
20. Heger L, Wulff K. 'Computed tomography of the calcaneus: normal anatomy.' *Am J Radiol* 1985; 145: 123–9.
21. Heger L, Wulff K, Seddiqui MSA. 'Computed tomography of calcaneal fractures.' *Am J Radiol* 1985; 145: 131–7.
22. Johnson EE, Gebhardt JS. 'Surgical management of calcaneal fractures using bilateral incision and minimal internal fixation.' *Clin Orthop Rel Res* 1993; 290: 117–24.
23. Koval KJ, Sanders R. 'The radiologic evaluation of calcaneal fractures.' *Clin Orthop Rel Res* 1993; 290: 41–6.
24. Lanfranco G. Gnemmi G, Bertuzzi B. 'Fratture del calcagno; quando e come operare.' *G.I.O.T.* 1987; vol. XIII; fasc. 3: 346–56.
25. Lanzetta A. *Le fratture del calcagno* Verducci Ed.: Roma, 1975.
26. Letournel E. 'Open treatment of acute calcaneal fractures.' *Clin Orthop Rel Res* 1993; 290: 60–7.

27. Magnan B, Caudana R, Campacci A, Barzoi A, Molinaroli F, Ricci M. 'Follow-up clinico e radiografico mediante T.C. delle fratture di calcagno trattate con Mini-Fea.' *Chir Piede* 1992; 16: 145–50.
28. Magnan B, Montanari M, Bragantini A, Bartolozzi P. 'A system for prognostic evaluation of CT imaging of heel fractures: the Score Analysis Verona (SAVE).' *Foot Disease* 1995; II (1): 19–27.
29. Magnan B, Nogarin L, Bragantini A, Molinaroli F, Ricci M. 'L'impiego di mini-fissatori esterni nell'ortopedia e nella traumatologia del calcagno.' *Chir Piede* 1990; 14: 57–64.
30. Neri M, Grandi A, Querin F. 'L'indagine T.C. nelle fratture del calcagno.' *Chir Piede* 1992; 16: 263–8.
31. Neri M, Querin F. 'La T.C. del piede: quadri patologici.' *Chir Piede* 1989; 13: 363–9.
32. Olmeda A, Turra S, Bonaga S. 'Risultati a distanza del trattamento incruento delle fratture talamiche di calcagno' *Chir Org Mov* 1989; LXXIV: 35–43.
33. Paley D, Fischgrund J. 'Open reduction and circular external fixation of intraarticular calcaneal fractures.' *Clin Orthop Rel Res* 1993; 290: 125–31.
34. Palmer I. 'The mechanism and treatment of fractures of the calcaneus. Open reduction with the use of cancellous grafts.' *J Bone Joint Surg* [Am] 1948; 30-A: 2–8.
35. Pescatori G, Fioriti M. 'Il trattamento delle fratture talamiche di calcagno mediante apparato di Ilizarov.' *G.I.O.T.* 1989; 15: 327–38.
36. Pisani G. 'La talizzazioni dell'astralago negli esiti di frattura di calcagno.' *Chir Piede* 1992; 16: 289–93.
37. Ross Steven DK, Sowerby Maren RR. 'The operative treatment of fractures of the os calcis.' *Clin Orthop Rel Res* 1985; 199: 132–43.
38. Sanders R, Fortin P, DiPasquale T, Walling A. 'Operative treatment in 120 displaced intraarticular calcaneal fractures. Results using a prognostic computed tomography scan classification.' *Clin Orthop Rel Res* 1993; 290: 87–95.
39. Societa Italiana di Medicina e Chirurgia del Piede: *Fratture del Calcagno.* Aulo Gaggi Ed.: Bologna, 1994.
40. Souer R, Remy R. 'Fractures of the calcaneus with displacement of the thalamic portion.' *J Bone Joint Surg* [Br] 1975; 57–B: 413–21.
41. Stephenson JR. 'Treatment of displaced intraarticular fractures of the calcaneus using medial and lateral approaches, internal fixation and early motion.' *J Bone Joint Surg* [Am] 1987; 69-A: 115–30.
42. Stephenson JR. 'Surgical treatment of displaced intraarticular fractures of the calcaneus, a combined lateral and medial approach.' *Clin Orthop Rel Res* 1993; 290: 68–75.
43. Utheza U, Flurin PH, Colombier JA, Chiron Ph, Tricoire JL, Potel JF, Puget J. 'Les fractures thalamiques du calcaneum: description anatomo-pathologique. Apport de la densitometrie.' *Rev Chir Orthop* 1993; 79: 49–57.
44. Warrick CK, Bremner AE. 'Fractures of the calcaneum. With an atlas illustrating the various types of fractures.' *J Bone Joint Surg* [Br] 1953; 35-B: 33–45.
45. Zwipp H, Tscherne H, Thermann H, Weber T. 'Osteosynthesis of displaced intraarticular fractures of the calcaneus; results in 123 cases.' *Clin Orthop Rel Res* 1993; 290: 76–86.

Metatarsal Fractures, Phalangeal Fractures and Reconstructive Procedures: the Pennig MiniFixator in the Foot

30

D. Pennig and K. Mader

Introduction

Injury to the foot producing skeletal instability in combination with soft tissue injury presents a difficult problem. A compromised soft tissue envelope in the foot does not lend itself to further exposure for the use of internal fixation. The combination of joint dislocation and fractures of the metatarsals requires not only stabilization of the fracture but also reduction and retention of the joint. External fixation being a minimally invasive procedure seems advantageous in the management of difficult foot injuries because of its wide range of applications coupled with the flexibility provided by modern systems. External fixation allows easy monitoring of the soft tissue situation.

In reconstructive procedures, minimally invasive techniques which respect the soft tissues and especially the periosteum, permit lengthening as well as the treatment of contractures.

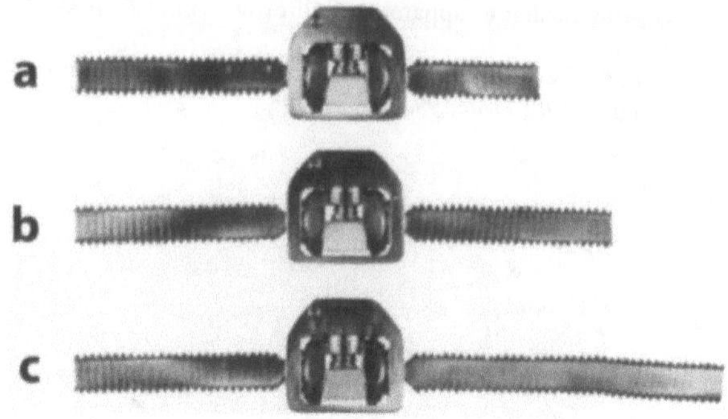

Fig. 30.1 The central element of the MiniFixator is a double ball joint with a single screw locking mechanism embedded in a module 15.5 × 15mm square. The central element connects two threaded bars to constitute **a** short (bars 28.1mm and 18.1mm), **b** standard (both bars 28.1mm) and **c** long (bars 28.1mm and 43.1mm) MiniFixators.

Design of the MiniFixator

Fracture Fixator

The central element of the Pennig MiniFixator is a double ball joint with a single screw locking mechanism embedded in a module 15.5 × 15mm square. The central element connects two threaded bars to constitute (a) short (bars 28.1mm and 18.1mm), (b) standard (both bars 28.1mm) and (c) long (bars 28.1mm and 43.1mm) MiniFixators (Fig. 30.1).

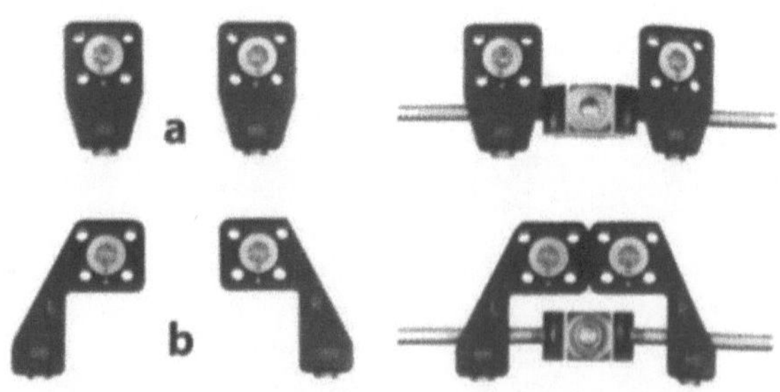

Fig. 30.2 Clamp modules:(a) standard clamp; (b) L-clamp. The L-clamp is designed to be used when the distance between the bone fixation points is too small to accommodate two standard clamps. There is a left and a right L-clamp.

The threaded bars are attached in turn to the clamp modules, of which there are two types: a standard clamp and an L-clamp (Fig. 30.2). The L-clamp is designed to be used when the distance between the bone fixation points is too small to accommodate two standard clamps. Two L-clamps facing one another, as shown in Fig. 30.2 will permit the insertion of two pairs of wires as little as 6mm apart. In view of this and because the hexagonal locking screw must always face the surgeon, the L-clamp is available in two models, left (L) and right (R). The standard clamp is normally used for metacarpal or metatarsal bones and the L-clamp for the phalanges.

Compression and distraction are possible using supplementary nuts in association with the threaded bars to move the clamps in the desired direction. The nuts are turned using the 3mm Allen wrench and one full turn of the nut through 360° will compress or distract respectively by one millimetre (Fig. 30.3). The nuts are not generally used in association with fresh fractures.

The clamp modules can each accommodate threaded wires in four different positions. Two wires are sufficient in most circumstances. The wires are specifically designed for use with the MiniFixator to ensure good bone purchase. Standard Kirschner-wires are inadequate for the purchase and should not be used. The threaded wires are supplied in two combinations of diameter and length: 2.0mm diameter and 100mm long, or 1.6mm diameter and 70mm long (Fig. 30.4). In both sizes the threaded portion is 15mm long. The wires are trimmed to length following insertion, increasing the versatility of the system and reducing the inventory required.

Before the threaded wires are inserted into the clamp, the dot on the surface of the cam must be aligned with the white dot on the surface of the clamp. This opens up the holes in the clamp, allowing easy passage of the wires. When the wires are inserted into the clamp in a plane along the axis of the bone, they emerge parallel; when they are inserted in a plane at right angles to the diaphyseal axis, they converge (Figs. 30.5a, 30.5b). This is particularly useful when it is necessary to insert wires close to the joint, or into very small fragments. The wires are locked into the clamp by tightening the cam. When wires are inserted into the bone, the clamp will always be stable provided the cam is securely tightened.

Reduction can be carried out with the fixator in situ, using manipulation forceps and the maintenance of reduction is facilitated by the small number of locking screws requiring only one size of Allen wrench.

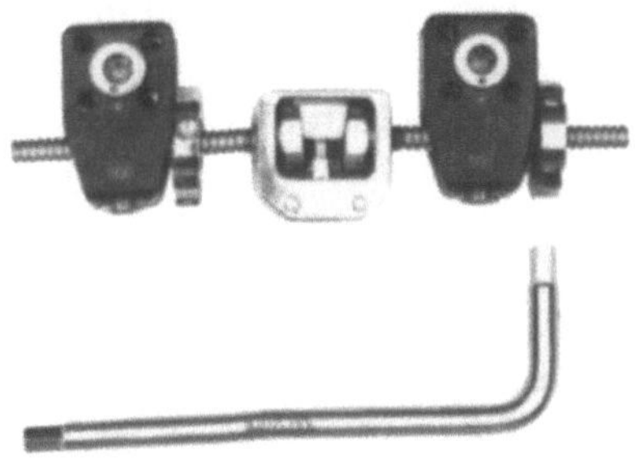

Fig. 30.3 Compression and distraction with the MiniFixator. With the nut outside the clamp compression is performed; with the nut between clamp and ball joint housing distraction is possible.

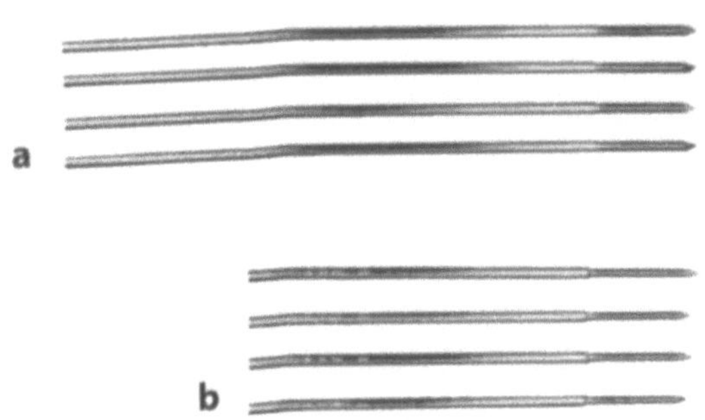

Fig. 30.4 Threaded wires: **a** 2mm thread diameter and 100mm long; **b** 1.6mm thread diameter and 70mm long.

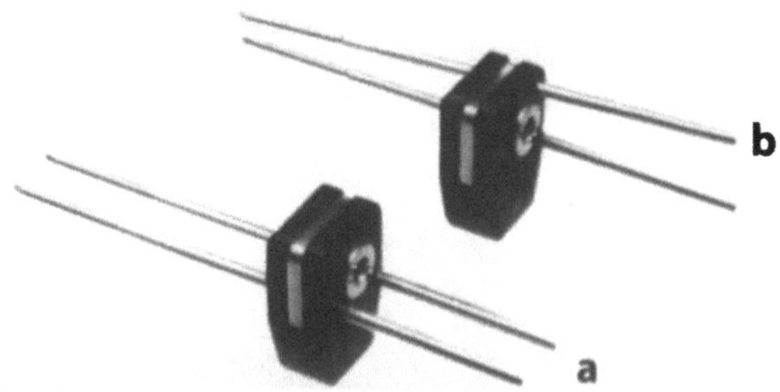

a

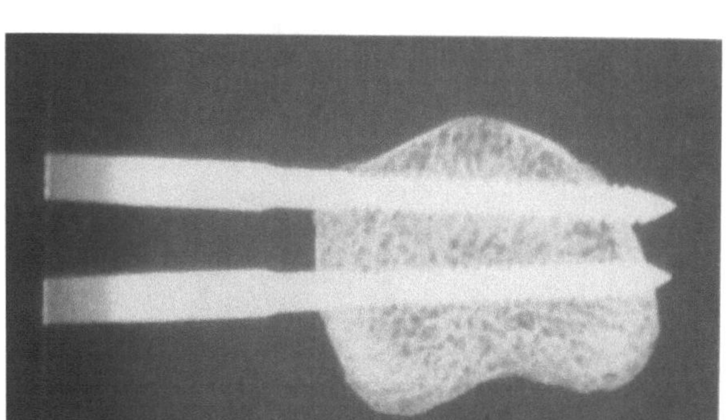

b

Fig. 30.5 **a** The wires emerge parallel (a) when inserted along the axis of the bone; (b) wires inserted at right angles to the diaphyseal axis converge. **b** Cross section of the proximal metaphysis in the proximal phalanx illustrating the convergence of the wires to allow secure fixation of small fragments.

Lengthening and Reconstructive Device

For lengthening or bone transport the ball jointed MiniFixator body is replaced by a lengthening bar. These are supplied in three sizes: (a) short (80mm), (b) standard (100mm) and (c) long (120mm) and are used in association with either standard or L-clamps and 2mm wires, compression–distraction nuts and spacers (Figs. 30.6, 30.7). A third wire may be added in each clamp to improve stability especially in osteoporotic bone and metatarsals.

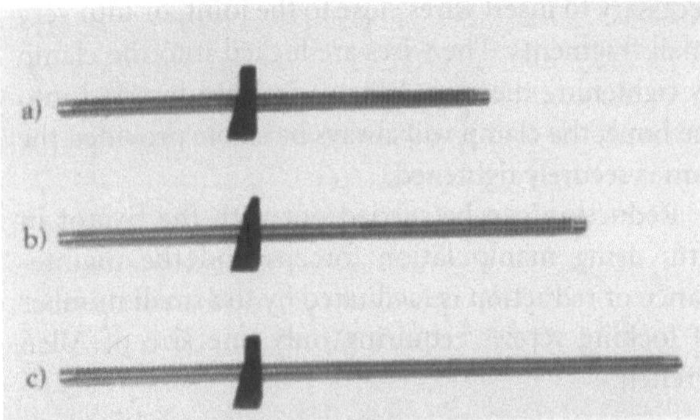

Fig. 30.6 For lengthening or bone transport the ball jointed Pennig MiniFixator body is replaced by a lengthening bar with spacer. Short: 80mm; standard: 100mm; long: 120mm.

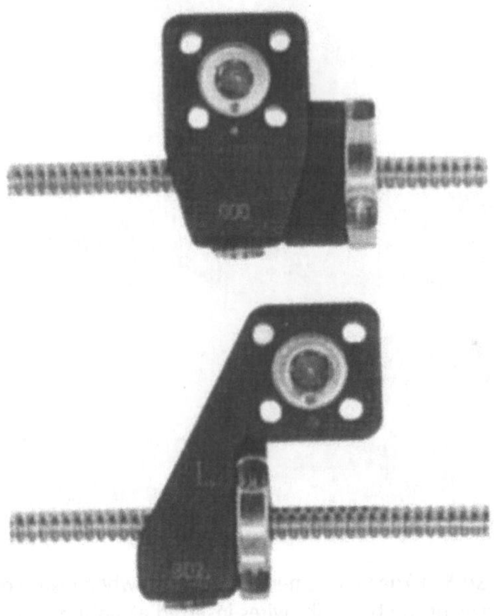

Fig. 30.7 A spacer is used in conjunction with the standard clamp (top) whereas the L-clamp does not require a spacer (bottom) for proper use of the nut.

Operative Technique

Anatomical Landmarks

With the exception of the sole of the foot, external fixation may be used from the dorsal, the medial or the lateral sides. In general the skin on the dorsal side is without much fat and the subcutaneous soft tissue very flexible. This may, however, be a disadvantage since oedema formation on the dorsal side can be pronounced. In the subcutaneous tissue the terminal branches of the superficial peroneal nerve spread out. On the lateral side the terminal branch of the sural nerve can be found. The tendons are covered by the superficial fascia. From the retinaculum extensorum in about the midline of the foot the tendons to toes II–V spread out like a fan (Fig. 30.8). The space between the extensor hallucis longus tendon and the adjacent tendon of the second toe is rather wide. The extensor digitorum brevis muscle lies beneath the tendons. The dorsalis pedis artery is situated between the tibialis anterior muscle and the extensor hallucis longus muscle. This vessel must be avoided when using external fixation in the tarsal bones. The dorsalis pedis profunda fascia separates the muscles, tendons and vessels from the metatarsal bones and the interosseous muscles. Considering the anatomy of the foot, metatarsal I is best approached from the medial or dorso-medial side, metatarsal II from the dorso-medial side and metatarsal V from the dorso-lateral side. Metatarsals III and IV may be approached from either side but open insertion of the fixator pins may be advisable (Figs. 30.9–30.11). The phalanges are approached from the same sides.

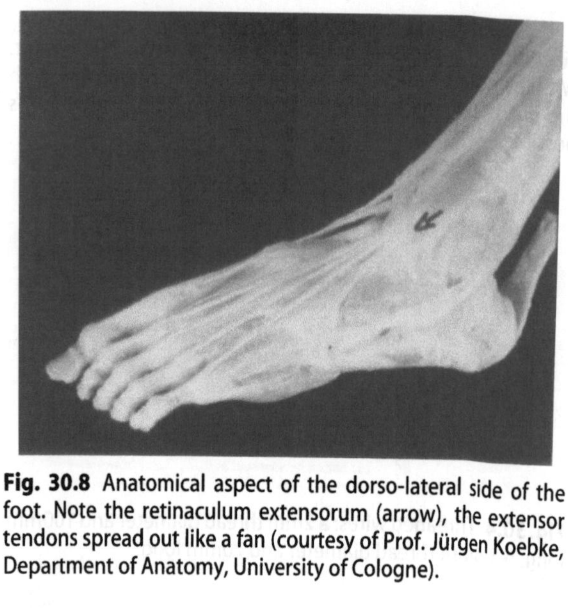

Fig. 30.8 Anatomical aspect of the dorso-lateral side of the foot. Note the retinaculum extensorum (arrow), the extensor tendons spread out like a fan (courtesy of Prof. Jürgen Koebke, Department of Anatomy, University of Cologne).

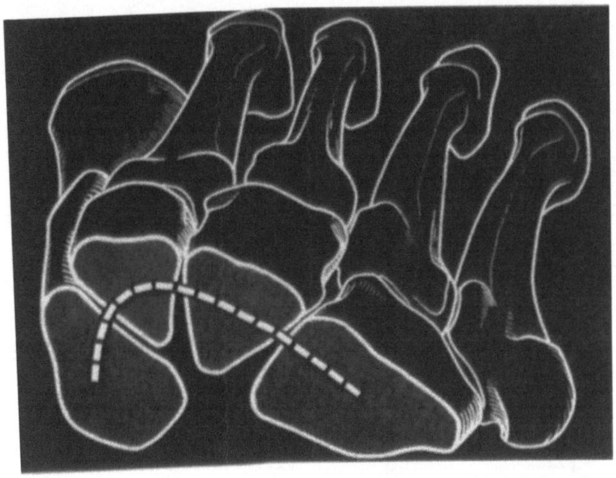

Fig. 30.9 Cross-section of the foot at the tarsal level showing metatarsals II and III as the most dorsal bones while metatarsals I and V form the plantar frame. This illustration clarifies why the approach to metatarsal II is easier from the medial side whereas metatarsals III, IV and V are best approached from the lateral side (courtesy of Prof. Jürgen Koebke, Department of Anatomy University of Cologne).

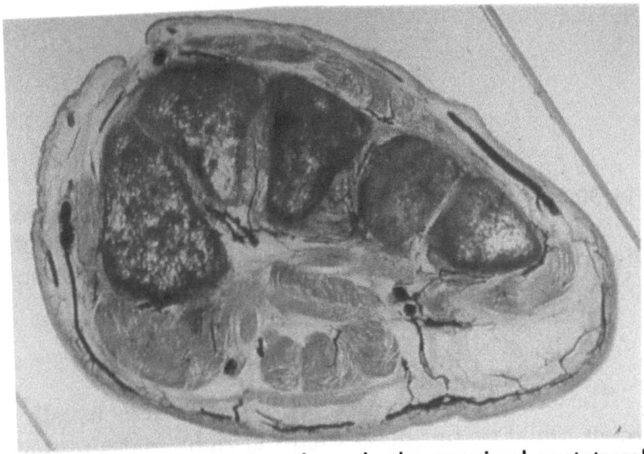

Fig. 30.10 Cross-section through the proximal metatarsal metaphysis (courtesy of Prof. Jürgen Koebke, Department of Anatomy, University of Cologne).

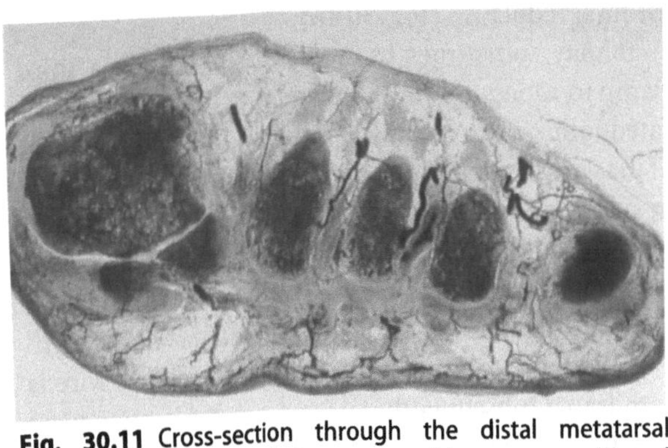

Fig. 30.11 Cross-section through the distal metatarsal metaphysis. On this level the metatarsal bones are positioned side by side (courtesy of Prof. Jürgen Koebke, Department of Anatomy University of Cologne).

Fixator Application in Metatarsals and Phalanges

Most commonly the fixator will be applied in metatarsal I and V injuries as well as fracture dislocations of the adjacent joints.

In the first and fifth metatarsals the fixator is applied in the frontal (coronal) plane whereas in the second, third and fourth metatarsals, the wires are placed 45° dorsal to that plane. Again careful attention should be paid to avoid injury to the extensor tendons, and neurovascular structures on the plantar aspect of the metatarsal bones. In fractures of the toes, the principles are the same as those described for the fingers (Ch. 19).

Shaft Fractures of the First Metatarsal

For metatarsals, the 2mm threaded wires are used. A decision must be made, based on the X-rays, as to whether the wires can be inserted in an axial plane or whether they will need to be introduced in a plane transverse to the bone axis. If there is one small fragment, transverse placement of the wires in this fragment is advisable. The minimum distance between a wire and the fracture should not be less than 3mm.

The first wire to be inserted is the one closest to the joint. It is introduced in the frontal plane using power instrumentation and since its thread is not conical it can be backed out if it has been advanced too far. With all applications of the MiniFixator, the wires should just penetrate the far cortex, protruding no more than one millimeter beyond it, to avoid damage to adjacent structures. This should be confirmed using image intensification (Fig. 30.12).

A standard clamp is inserted over the wire, ensuring that the dot on the surface of the cam is in line with the dot on the clamp surface. The clamp must be posi-

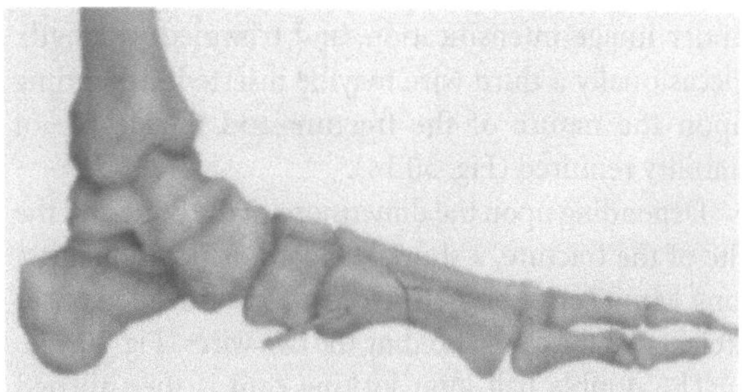

Fig. 30.12 Placement of threaded wires in metatarsal shaft fracture: First wire. 2mm wires only should be used.

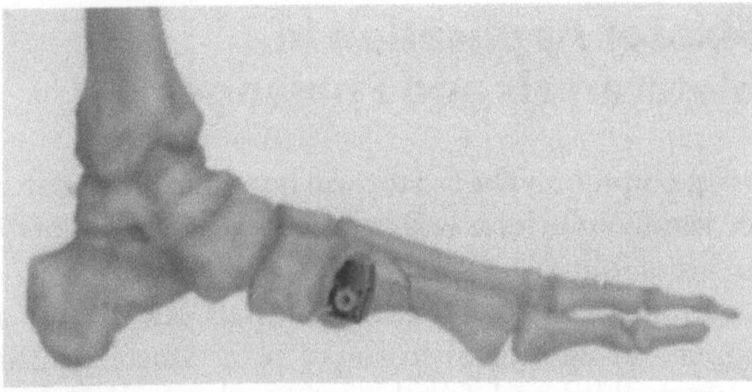

Fig. 30.13 Standard clamp is inserted over the wire and the wire trimmed.

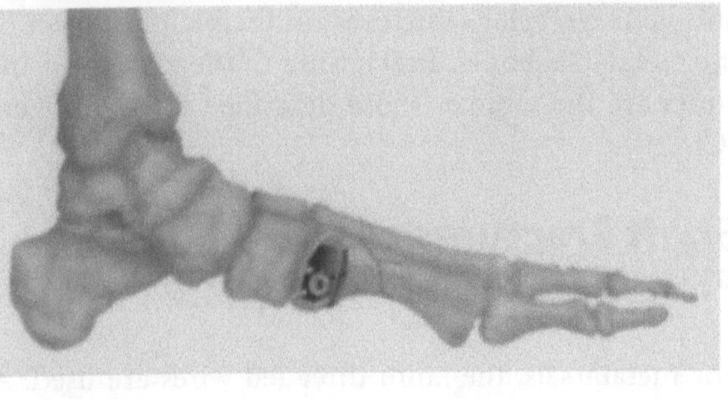

Fig. 30.14 The second and third wires are inserted and trimmed.

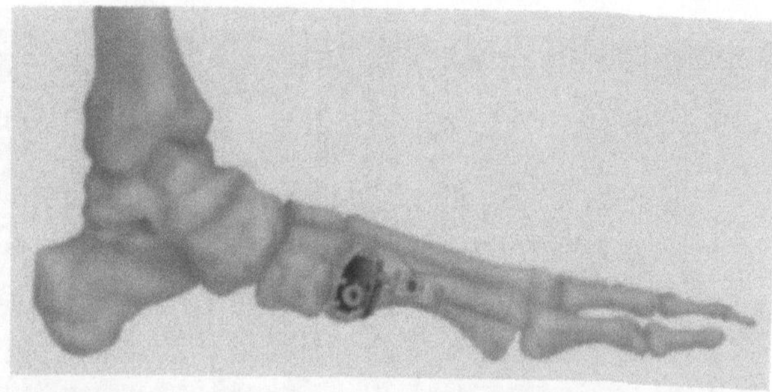

Fig. 30.15 Insertion of a standard MiniFixator body into the clamp.

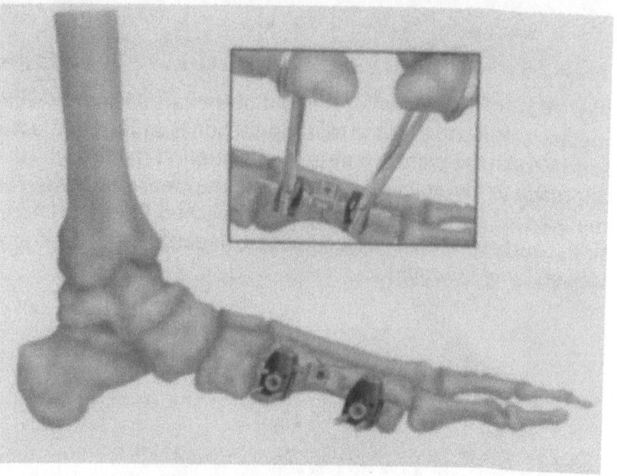

Fig. 30.16 Application of second clamp and placement of two (if required, three) threaded wires. The insert shows the use of the reduction forceps with the double ball joint and one clamp locking screw unlocked.

tioned so that the head of the cam faces away from the bone, to allow for subsequent locking of the wires (Fig. 30.13).

As a general rule, the clamp should be positioned about 5–10mm from the skin, to allow for some post-operative swelling. The first wire is then trimmed so that about 5mm projects beyond its margin. It should be noted that each wire must be trimmed after insertion, to avoid obstructing the drill during insertion of the next wire.

The second wire is inserted either axially or transversely with respect to the first, according to the length of the fragment. When inserted in a transverse plane the wires converge, so that they can be inserted into very small fragments. The second wire is now inserted under image intensification, and trimmed to length. Occasionally a third wire may be inserted, depending upon the nature of the fracture and the degree of stability required (Fig. 30.14).

Depending upon the dimensions of the bone and the site of the fracture, a short, standard or occasionally, a long MiniFixator body is selected. One threaded bar is attached to the clamp holding the two wires (Fig. 30.15).

The double ball joint locking cam is then turned clockwise a little, so that ball joint movement becomes slightly stiff. The long axis of the fixator can now be aligned with the long axis of the metatarsal, which should be reduced clinically. The second clamp is now attached to the other threaded bar.

The second set of wires is now inserted, usually longitudinal to, but occasionally at right angles to the diaphyseal axis. When choosing the position for these wires, care should be taken to ensure that the clamps have sufficient room on their respective bars to allow for final reduction (Fig. 30.16).

It may sometimes be necessary to attach a third clamp to a long module allowing one to bridge a dislocated joint which has to be reduced prior to insertion of the wire in the extra clamp. This would be applicable in cases with a fracture of metatarsal I in association with a dislocation of the metatarso-phalangeal joint I. It is important to reduce the joint anatomically and temporary K-wire fixation may be advisable prior to insertion of two 2mm threaded wires. The K-wire is withdrawn subsequently.

Once all the wires have been inserted, the clamps are locked to them, by turning the cam on each firmly. Before final reduction, one of the clamps can be locked to its bar with the clamp locking screw, checking that the other clamp has room to move along its bar during the reduction procedure.

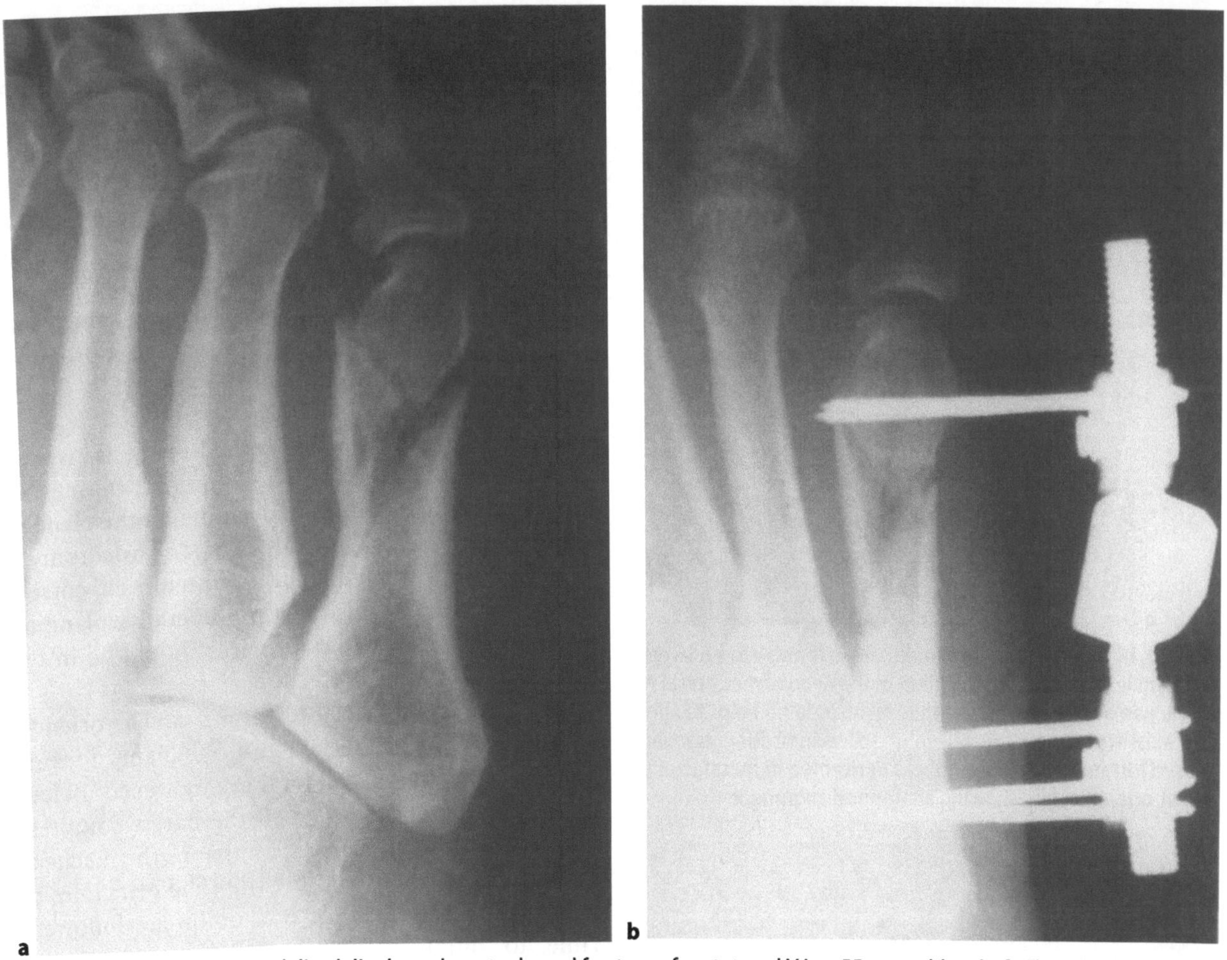

a b

Fig. 30.17 **a** Comminuted distal diaphyseal–metaphyseal fracture of metatarsal V in a 55-year-old male. **b** Closed reduction with restoration of length and axis.

The fracture is now reduced using traction and counter-traction, taking particular care to avoid any rotational deformities and bearing in mind that in flexion, all toes converge on the topographic location of the navicular. The reduction forceps are provided to distance the surgeon's hands from the radiation source. For additional protection, radiation gloves are available and may be worn for this manoeuvre. The forceps grip the clamps to permit manipulation and, after reduction, tightening of the necessary screws without loss of position (Fig. 30.16 inset).

While the reduction is held the second clamp is locked to the bar, maintaining the length of the bone. Following this, the double ball joint of the MiniFixator body is locked to control angulation, by turning the cam in the centre of the MiniFixator body, clockwise.

At the end of the operation, a check should be made to ensure that sufficient space has been left between the skin and the fixator (minimum 5mm). The wires are finally trimmed such that 2mm of wire protrudes from each clamp. This helps to prevent the sharp ends of the wires catching in the patient's clothes. A dressing is applied in such a way that the MiniFixator is fully covered. No circumferential dressing is necessary.

The patient is encouraged to move toes and adjacent joints from the day of operation. Partial weightbearing is allowed after the swelling has subsided and a plaster sole may be applied until then. Special shoes are available to allow mobilization of the patient. Illustrative cases are shown in Figs. 30.17–30.20.

Correction of Deformity, Lengthening and Bone Transport

In post-traumatic malunion and congenital deformity, the fixator can be used to correct metatarsal or phalangeal malalignment. This is particularly valuable in rotational deformities of the phalanges. As a general

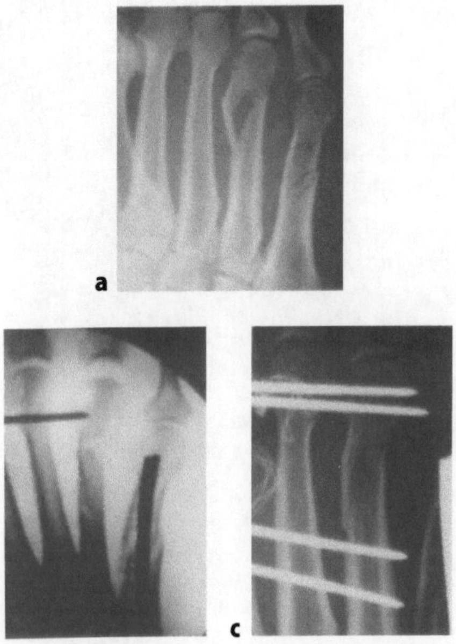

Fig. 30.18 **a** Serial fracture of metatarsals IV and V in a 66-year-old female. Note the displacement of the head of metatarsal IV. **b** Traction on the fourth toe applied with a clamp helps to align the axis. Note the wide MP joint space indicating traction. Closed intramedullary nailing was performed in metatarsal V. **c** Post-operative film showing anatomical alignment.

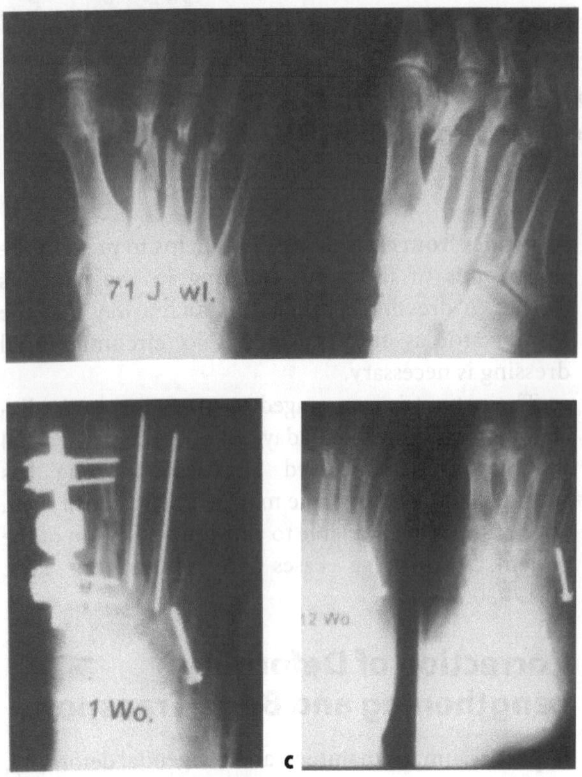

Fig. 30.19 **a** Serial fracture of metatarsals II, III and IV and proximal fracture of metatarsal V in a 71-year-old female. **b** Closed reduction using the MiniFixator in metatarsal II, K-wire fixation in metatarsals III and IV and screw fixation in metatarsal V allowed early mobilization of the patient. **c** Final results 12 weeks post-operatively; the fixator was removed at six weeks.

rule correction should be carried out at the site of the original injury in post-traumatic cases. Bone healing usually proceeds faster at the metaphyseo-diaphyseal junction, and this site should be preferentially selected whenever possible. The application technique for corrective osteotomies is similar to that for metatarsal fractures, but one set of wires is applied at such an angle to the second pair that will result in correction of the deformity when they are reduced to the same plane following osteotomy. A typical example is a proximal metatarsal I osteotomy in hallux valgus (Fig. 30.23a and b).

The first pair of wires is applied in the transverse plane close to the joint. The required amount of correction is estimated when deciding on the plane of insertion of the second pair of wires. The osteotomy is then carried out preserving the periosteum and correction performed. Provided that pre-operative planning was correct, the two pairs of wires should be in the same plane following correction.

The clamps are locked to the wires. The orientation of the bone is checked and one clamp locking screw and the double ball joint are tightened. Before the second clamp is locked to the bar, a compression–distraction nut is used to enhance the mechanical stability of the osteotomy site. The principles of compression described for non-union are followed. Time to union is usually longer in corrective osteotomies than in fractures and healing times of 9–12 weeks may be expected. During this period, physiotherapy plays an important role.

In principle it is possible to lengthen both phalanges and metatarsal bones. The most common indication, however, is likely to be lengthening of the fourth metatarsal in congenital shortening. A lengthening bar with standard clamps is applied with the wires in the axial plane. A proximal osteotomy is normally performed to permit good fixation in each fragment. A compression–distraction nut and a spacer should be placed on the lengthening bar before the second clamp is applied (Fig. 30.21a).

A delay of two weeks before commencing distraction is advisable. Distraction is then performed at a rate of 0.5mm per day (one-quarter turn of the nut twice a day). Callus formation should be carefully monitored with standard radiographs weekly.

For the treatment of bone loss, the technique of bone transport can be employed. A lengthening bar with three clamps is used (Fig 30.21b). Two clamps are applied to the larger segment and the osteotomy performed between them. The segments must be aligned before wire insertion and fixator application.

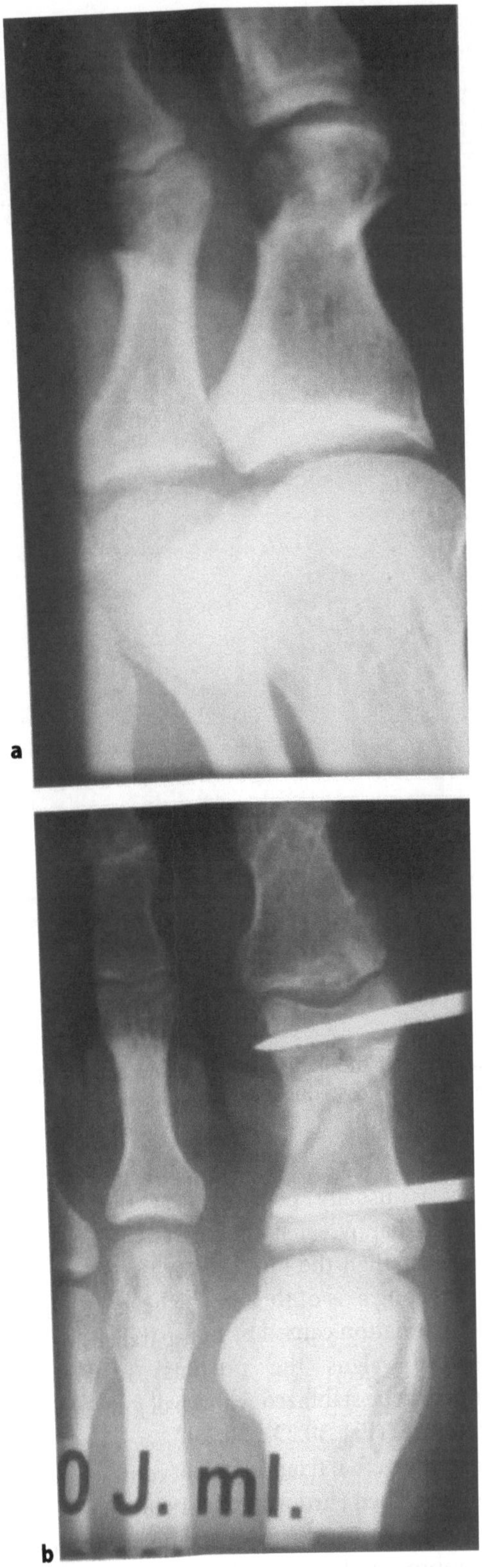

a

b

Fig. 30.20 **a** Comminuted and displaced fracture of the proximal phalanx in D I with severe soft tissue injury in a 30-year-old male. **b** Closed reduction and fixation with two convergent 2mm threaded wires in the distal and the proximal metaphysis.

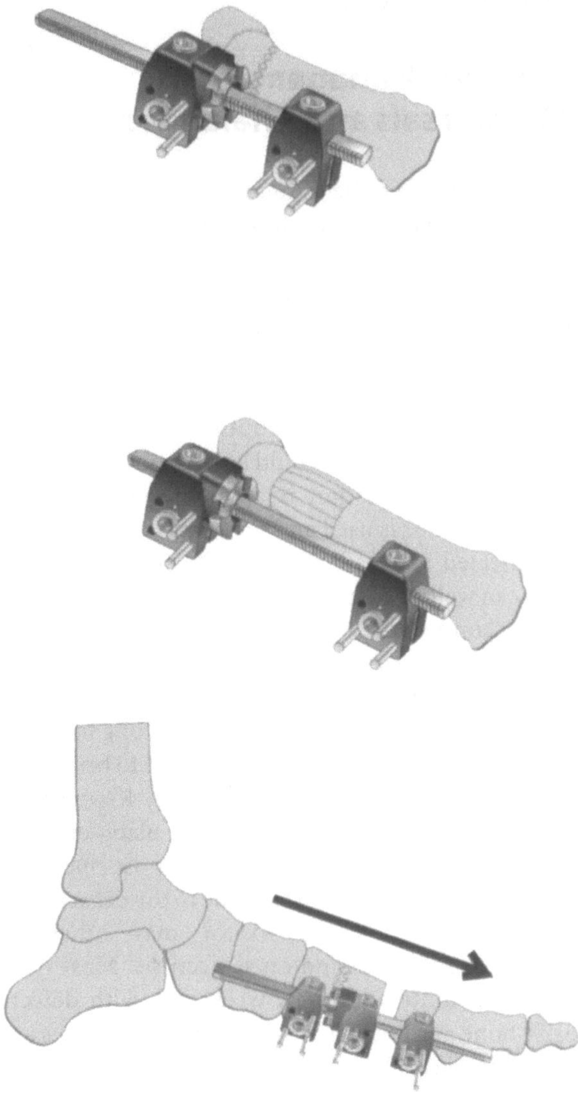

a

b

Fig. 30.21 **a** Use of the lengthening bar and compression-distraction nut for lengthening of a metatarsal; proximal osteotomy. Note that where a midshaft osteotomy is performed three wires per clamp are used. **b** Assembly for bone transport to fill a defect in the first metatarsal. Middle clamp is moved in the direction of the arrow.

Indications

Fracture Management in Metatarsals and Phalanges

Few reports are to be found in the literature on the use of external fixation in foot injuries. Most authors agree that the compromised soft tissue envelope in closed and certainly in open injuries is an indication. In 22 fresh fractures there were 14 open and eight closed injuries with six fracture dislocations of the Lisfranc joint. Closed midfoot fracture dislocations with significant joint disruption merit consideration. Joint reduction should be performed and temporary K-wire fixation is advisable. The shortest possible fixator is used and preferably no more than the affected joint is bridged (de Coster et al 1986). This can well be achieved with either the standard or the L-clamp of the MiniFixator. In cases with fracture of a metatarsal and dislocation in the adjacent joint, the joint will have to be reduced after reduction of the metatarsal fracture. Once a long fixator is applied a third clamp may be employed to bridge the joint after reduction. Again temporary K-wire fixation of the joint is advisable. When using external fixation on the dorsal side of the foot post-operative swelling has to be allowed for. Due to the capacity for oedema formation the fixator may otherwise impinge on the skin and cause necrosis. Most fractures will unite within six weeks but with defects early bone grafting is advisable. Illustrative cases are shown in Figs. 30.17–30.20.

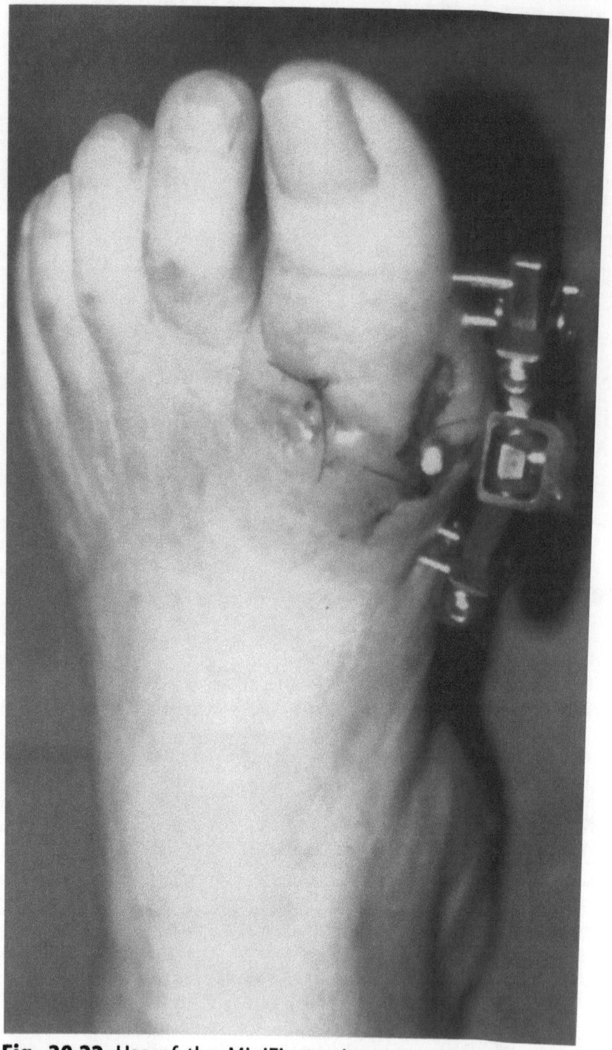

Fig. 30.22 Use of the MiniFixator in treatment of MP-joint empyema after corticosteriod injection.

Osteomyelitis

Osteomyelitis, infected non-unions and joint infections are classical indications for external fixation (Fig. 30.22). When using external fixation in these cases the bone may be osteoporotic and a longer application time than in fractures may be expected. A third or even a fourth 2mm wire may be used per clamp to provide additional stabilization. It is also possible to use two fixators on one bone in a V-shaped manner. External fixation will not cure osteomyelitis by itself and additional procedures should be followed.

Reconstructive Procedures

The lengthening bar of the MiniFixator may be used for callus distraction of metatarsal bones. One of the more common sites is metatarsal IV and the osteotomy is usually performed at the proximal metaphyseal–diaphyseal junction. It is of particular importance to align the long axis of the lengthening bar with the long axis of the bone to be lengthened to avoid axial deviation caused by non-parallelism.

In hallux valgus the proximal metatarsal I osteotomy may be stabilized with a ball jointed fixator in selected cases (Fig. 30.23a, 30.23b).

The use of external fixation in foot contractures has also been described (Erdogan et al 1996). Burns are a common cause of contractures and open procedures in the compromised skin are not advisable. External fixation allows slow distraction of the soft tissues and the distraction rate is 1–2mm per day. Application of the fixator depends on the site of the problem and careful pre-operative planning is mandatory.

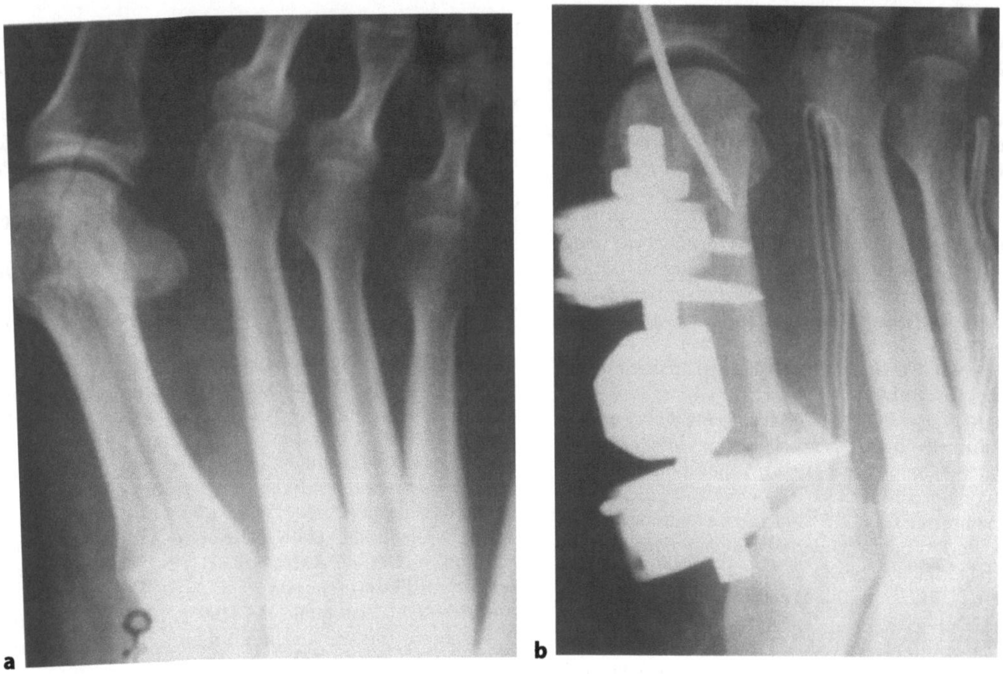

Fig. 30.23 a Painful bunion in a 57-year-old female. b Proximal metatarsal osteotomy stabilized with a MiniFixator.

Contraindications

Contraindications to the use of the MiniFixator in the foot are similar to those for external fixation in general. These include severe osteoporosis, patients who are HIV positive and patients with severe, poorly controlled diabetes mellitus. In addition, in uncooperative or predictably difficult patients, external fixation is not advisable. Careful patient selection will therefore avoid problems at a later stage.

Post-operative Management

Post-operatively the leg should be elevated. A cast sole is usually applied and the AV Impulse System may be used to reduce swelling (Pennig and Gladbach 1999). Partial weightbearing is allowed once the soft tissues have healed and full weightbearing commences after radiological fracture healing. The cast sole may be replaced by a special orthosis available for foot surgery (Fig. 30.24).

Routine review of the wire entry sites twice weekly is advisable. In general, dressings are not necessary after two weeks. The patient should not be allowed to use soap on the wires, but tap water is permitted.

Physiotherapy is advisable and this applies to the operations described in this chapter. The MiniFixator is removed when in the opinion of the attending surgeon, bony union has occurred.

Removal of the fixator is carried out by unlocking all the fixator screws and sliding the fixator clamps off the threaded wires. The wires are then removed using the threaded wire extractor since, because of their threaded ends, they cannot be simply pulled out. The protruding end of the wire is inserted into the threaded wire extractor with the locking screw open. After tightening the locking screw with the 3mm Allen wrench, the wire is removed from the bone by turning the threaded wire extractor in a anticlockwise direction. Removal of the wires can normally be done in the outpatient clinic without analgesics.

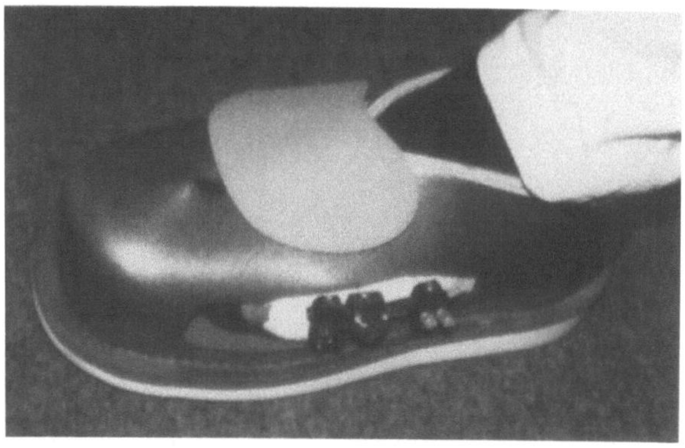

Fig. 30.24 Special orthosis accommodating the MiniFixator allows early mobilization of the patient.

Bibliography

Ahmed A, Espley A (1988) 'Fractures of the metatarsals: Management of complicated injuries with a simple traction technique.' *Injury* 19: 345—59.

Andersen LD (1977) 'Injuries to the forefoot.' *Clin Orthop* 122:18–27.

Armanek DL, Juda EL, Oloff LM et al (1986) 'Opening base wedge osteotomy of the first metatarsal utilizing rigid external fixation.' *J Foot Surg* 25:321–6.

Bellacosa RA, Pollak RA (1991) 'Complications of lesser metatarsal surgery.' *Clin Podiatr Med Surg* 8.

De Coster T, Alvarez R, Trevino S (1986) 'External fixation of the foot and ankle.' *Foot Ankle* 7:40–8.

Eastaugh-Waring SJ, Saleh M (1994) 'The management of a complex midfoot fracture with circular external fixation.' *Injury* 25:61–3.

Erdogan B, Görgü M, Girgin O et al (1998) 'Application of external fixation in major foot contractures.' *J Foot Ankle Surg* 35:218-21.

Giannestras NJ, Sammarco GL (1975) 'Fractures and dislocations in the foot.' in: Rockwood CA, Green DP (eds.) *Fractures.* J B Lippincott: Philadelphia: p 1400.

Gudas CJ, Cann JE (1991) 'Non-unions and related disorders.' *Clin Pod Med Surg* 2:321–39.

Johnson VS, Batemann JE (1976) (eds.) 'Treatment of fractures of the forefoot in industry.' in: *Foot Science,* WB Saunders: Philadelphia: p 257.

Kenzora JE, Edwards CC, Browner BD et al (1981) 'Acute management of major trauma involving the foot and ankle with Hoffmann external fixation.' *Foot Ankle* 1: 348–61.

Kortmann HR, Wolter D, Bisgwa F et al (1992) 'Die Frakturbehandlung des Kalkaneus und des Mittelfuáes mittels geschlossener Reposition und Fixation im Ilisarow-Fixateur.' *Unfallchirurg* 95 (8): 541–6.

Laughlin RT, Calhoun JH (1995) 'Ring fixators for reconstruction of traumatic disorders of the foot and ankle.' *Orth Clin North Am* 26: 287–94.

Mooney JF, DeFranzo A, Marks MW (1998) 'Use of cross-extremity flaps stabilized with external fixation in severe pediatric foot and ankle trauma: An alternative to free tiusse transfer.' *J Ped Orthop* 18: 26–30.

Müller KH, Müller-Färber J (1982) 'Der Fixateur externe - seltene Indikationen, Kombination von internen und externen Osteosynthesetechniken, Sekundäreingriffe.' *Langenbecks Arch Chir* 358: 133–40.

Myerson MS (1993a) 'Crush injuries and compartment syndromes of the foot.' in: Myerson M (ed.) *Current therapy: Foot and ankle surgery.* MosbyYear Book: St. Louis.

Myerson MS (1993b) 'Management of fractures and dislocations of the forefoot.' in: Jahss M (ed.) *The foot* (ed. 2) WB Saunders: Philadelphia.

Pennig D (1998) *Treatment of Fractures and Deformities in Small Bones. The Pennig Minifixator. Operative Technique.* Orthofix srl., Bussolengo, Italy.

Pennig D, Gladbach B (1999) 'Use of the AV Impulse System in the Hand.' in: Gardner AMN, Fox RH (eds.) *The return of blood to the heart* (3rd Ed) (in press).

Sammarco GJ, Carrasquillo HA (1995) 'Intramedullary fixation of metatarsal fracture and non-union.' *Orth Clin North Am* 26: 265–72.

Smith GH, Green AL (1983) 'Cerclage wiring of metatarsal fractures: A case report.' *J Am Pod Assoc* 73: 25–6.

Spector FC, Karlin JM, Scurran BL et al (1984) 'Lesser metatarsal fractures: Incidence, management and review.' *J Am Pod Assoc* 74: 259–64

Walter JH (1985) 'External fixation: Its use in podiatric surgery.' *Clin Pod* 2: 3–26.

Wilson PD (1933) 'Fractures and dislocations of the tarsal bones.' *South Med J* 26: 833.

Fracture Management in Children

31

J. Bennek

Introduction

Fracture treatment in children differs from that in adults, since the special problems of the growing skeleton and delayed deformities must be taken into consideration. In addition, there are some fractures that do not occur in adults and certain peculiarities of fracture healing.

Callus begins to form very rapidly, and after only a few days many residual deformities can no longer be corrected. To a certain extent, functional transformation may take place during growth, but bone remodelling takes place in a different way in different parts of the body and in the individual planes. The most favourable tendency to compensation occurs in fractures of the newborn; with increasing age this tendency is reduced and virtually disappears between the tenth year and skeletal maturity. Impaction fractures occur frequently in infants and greenstick fractures are also encountered, due to the elasticity of the periosteum. In the case of epiphyseal injuries, immediate, exact repositioning with maintenance of the appropriate position is always required to prevent later growth disorders with deformities of the articular planes.

In view of the peculiarities of fracture healing in children, conservative treatment was favoured until relatively recently, but a change in attitude is now becoming apparent. There is a trend away from purely static, rigid forms of therapy towards a more functional and dynamic approach. The aim should always be a form of treatment which takes the child's needs into account and which is accepted by the child (Table 31.1). Rigid, conservative fracture management cannot readily be reconciled with this philosophy. Today the mission statement should be: "Less plaster means an enhanced quality of life for the child".

The growing tendency, therefore, is to employ operative or semi-operative forms of management. In addition to Kirschner-wires and screws and tension wires especially for intra-articular and periarticular fractures, flexible fixation is gaining importance in the treatment of diaphyseal and metaphyseal fractures. Plate osteosynthesis has been largely abandoned. For fracture healing, so-called flexible fixation adopts the biological principle of callus induction and bone remodelling through movement, in order to reconstruct the bone to match the appropriate function.

External fixation and intramedullary stable elastic splinting have both proved to be useful methods. In 1984, De Bastiani et al [13] presented the results with an axial dynamic unilateral fixator, which ensures stable fracture fixation even in children and at the same time facilitates the application of dynamic stress through the fracture. Intramedullary stable elastic splinting relies on the insertion of pre-bent nails into the straight

Fracture treatment in line with needs of child
Acceptable to child
Maintenance of quality of life, with early mobilization and loadbearing
Short hospital stay
Minimal complications
Optimal long-term results

Table 31.1 Aims of Treatment

medullary cavity; this provides adequate stabilization of the fracture without preventing axial micromovement.[17,24,31–34,47,52,53] With these methods, the thrust and shear forces that prejudice fracture healing are converted to tractional and compressive forces.

External fixation and intramedullary stable elastic splinting have distinct advantages for fracture management in children (Table 31.2). Both methods, however, also have disadvantages which must be taken into consideration (Table 31.3). External fixation and intramedullary stable elastic splinting are not rival methods of treatment, but are procedures that may complement each other. They therefore allow fracture-specific adaptation. The present chapter reports exclusively on external fixation as a method of treatment.

Simple, low risk surgical technique
Minimal surgical trauma
Rapid, definitive stabilization
Minimal trauma to the soft tissues
Fracture haematoma undisturbed
Callus induction through micromovement
Maintenance of quality of life with early mobilization and loadbearing

Table 31.2 Advantages of flexible fixation

External fixation
Pin-track infection
Some discomfort
Transfixion of the iliotibial tract during pin insertion into the femur
Intramedullary stable elastic splinting
Contraindicated in open fractures and where there are major soft tissue defects
No secondary correction of position possible
Rotational instability
Full weightbearing only possible after 3–4 weeks
Second surgical intervention necessary to remove hardware

Table 31.3 Disadvantages of flexible fixation

Indications For External Fixation

At the present time, the indications for the use of external fixation in childhood fractures are those shown in Table 31.4. The classical indications[9,10,16,25,26,35] may be supplemented by diaphyseal and metaphyseal fractures of the lower extremity.[1–6,12,14,23,25,27–29,36,39,41,42,44–46,48,50,51]. Fractures in the trochanteric region and transcervical fractures are also indications. In diaphyseal fractures of the upper extremity conservative management is still the mainstay of treatment and external fixation is a treatment of second choice. In irreducible fractures, intramedullary stable elastic splinting is the predominant form of treatment.

Primary indications for external fixation
Fractures in multiply injured patents
Grade (I)/II/III open fractures (Gustilo)
Closed fractures associated with severe soft tissue trauma
Fractures of the proximal femur (trochanteric, transcervical)
Proximal tibial fractures
Extra-articular complex fractures (spiral, segmental, irregular) of the tibia and femur
Wedge fracturės of the tibia and femur
Transverse and oblique fractures of the medial zone in the tibia and femur
Distal fractures of the femur and tibia
Secondary indications for external fixation
Diaphyseal fractures of the humérus
Fractures of the radius/ulna
Pathological fractures

Table 31.4 Indications for external fixation

Surgical Technique

Pre-operative Planning

Stabilization of the fracture with external fixation should be carried out as early as possible; this applies especially to open fractures. In children with multiple injuries, the treatment of injured body cavities and intensive-care measures to restore organic functions have priority. The timing of fracture management, however, must not be neglected (Fig. 31.1). Mobile fractures increase the risk of secondary pulmonary damage and haemodynamic disorders during the course of intensive therapy. Trauma-induced alterations of the immune system may also occur with severe soft tissue injuries.[10,38]

Because of the modular nature of the system, the unilateral Dynamic Axial Fixator (Orthofix srl, Verona, Italy) is readily adaptable to childhood fractures from about the 3rd to 4th year of life onwards

Orthofix Model	Age group (years)
Femur	
Standard body	8–15
Short body	6–9
Small body	3–8
Tibia	
Standard body	10–16
Short body	8–11

Table 31.5 Size of Orthofix Fixator in relation to age

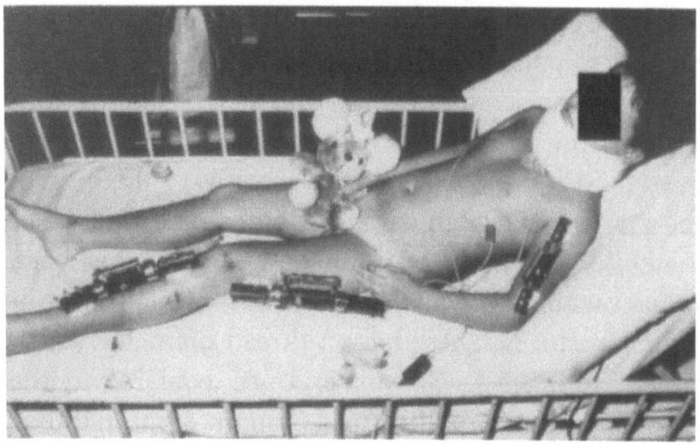

Fig. 31.1 A 9-year-old boy with multiple injuries including three long bone fractures stabilized with Orthofix external fixators.

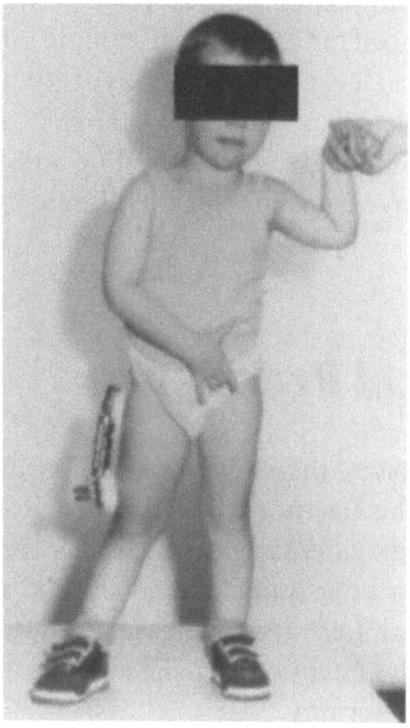

Fig. 31.2 A boy aged 3 years and 4 months, with a spiral fracture of the right femur stabilized with small Orthofix fixator.

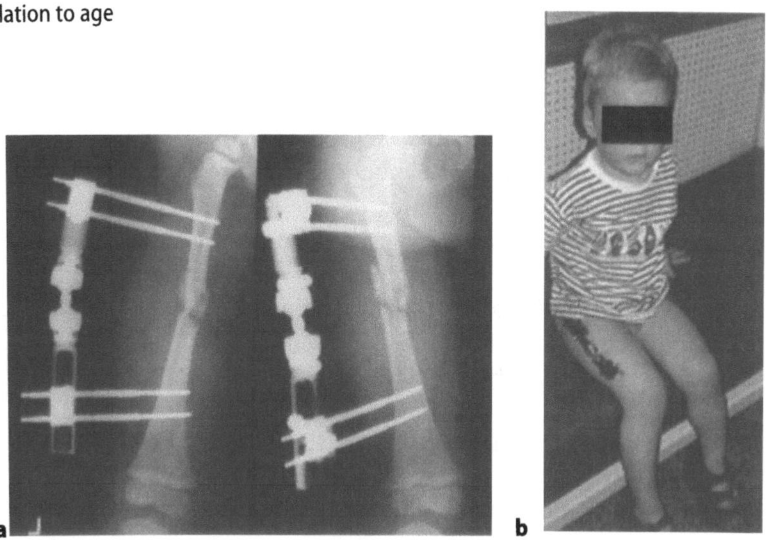

a b

Fig. 31.3 a Open diaphyseal spiral fracture of the right femur (first degree) in a boy aged 2 years and 4 months, treated by means of a special paediatric Orthofix fixator. **b** Clinical view.

(Fig. 31.2). A survey of the application of the system in relation to patient age is shown in Table 31.5.

Pin (bone screw) position and size of pin are estimated from the X-ray, using a special transparent overlay. It is important to take account of the bulk of the soft tissues, which will vary according to the age of the child. The standard adult range of pins has been supplemented by special pins for the treatment of children's fractures. These have a thread diameter which tapers from 4.5 to 3.5mm and are available in the following total length/thread length combinations: 120/30, 100/30, 100/20, 90/20. Drill guides with lengths of 90mm and 55mm and a special pertrochanteric clamp for the small fixator body are also available. For the treatment of children from the 2nd to the 4th year of life, a special external fixator has been developed for use with self-drilling pins with total length/thread length combinations of 60/20, 70/30 and 100/30. This infant fixator (Orthofix®) requires no modification; the design is appealing and the application is convenient in small children (Figs. 31.3a, 31.3b).

Surgical Procedure

Where possible, the child is placed on an extension table and the fracture reduced approximately. In all but a very few cases the external fixator can be applied on a standard operating table. It is important that an assistant maintains reduction via traction at the foot and also pays attention to axial alignment to prevent rotational deformity.

Pin insertion is carried out according to the standard procedure, using image intensification. In fractures of the femur and humerus, the external fixator is applied from the lateral side; in tibial fractures, just posterior to the anterior tibial edge (Fig. 31.4). Application from medial side at an angle of 30° from the sagittal plane hampers walking. Anatomical and clinical studies have confirmed that ventral tibial pin placement does not endanger anatomical structures. The tendon of the tibialis anterior deviates distally towards lateral side, because it is not fixed by the retinacula.[43]

Stab incisions in the skin at the entry points of the pins should correspond to the diameter of the drill guides; this is cosmetically beneficial. It is followed by blunt dissection of the soft tissues to the greatest circumference of the bone. In the thigh, the iliotibial tract is slit where the pin passes through, to limit the risk of transfixion. The pins that are furthest away from

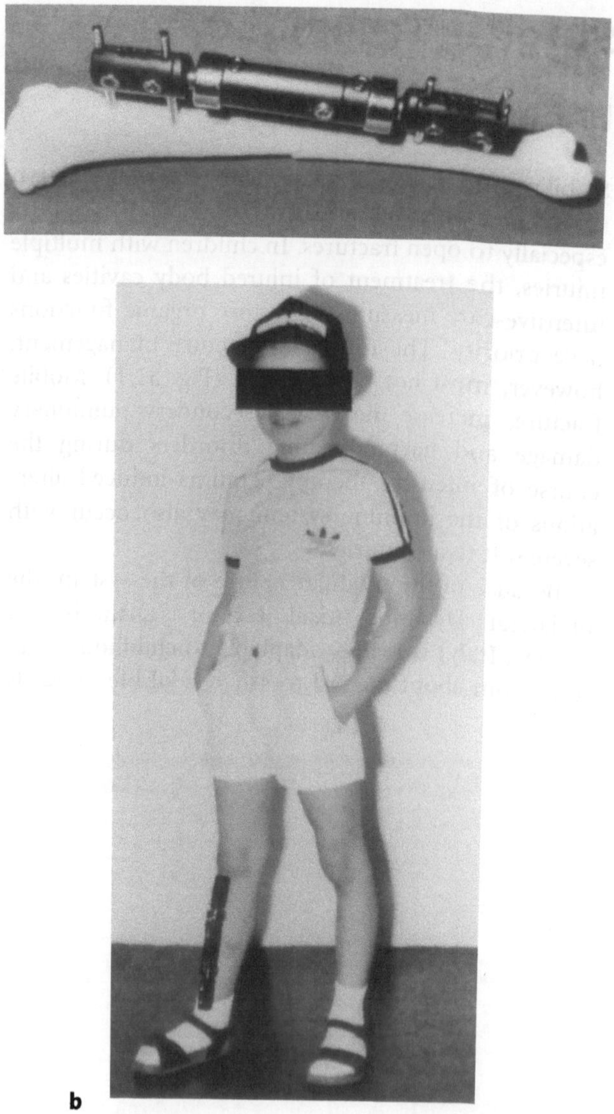

a

b

Fig. 31.4 **a** Application of the external fixator in the tibia, just posterior to the anterior tibial border (sawbone application). **b** Clinical view.

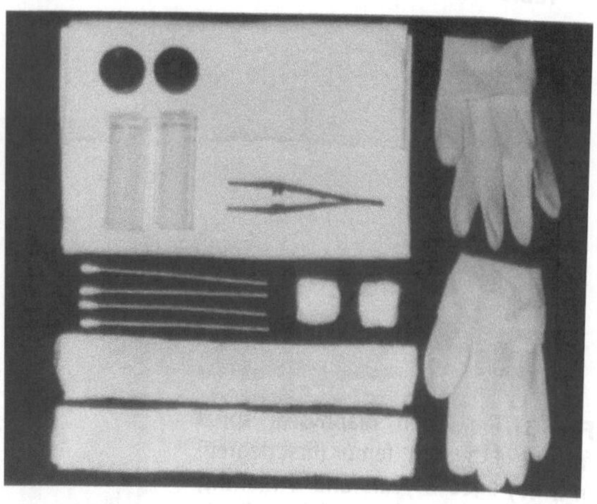

Fig. 31.5 Special child pack for unaided pin site care at home.

the fracture are generally inserted first. The body template should be open approximately 0.5cm and fixed in this position; if it is not applied open in this way, subsequent dynamization will not be possible. In children, four pins generally suffice to stabilize the fracture. T-clamps and, less frequently, a ring fixator are used in metaphyseal fractures.

Following application of the external fixator, final reduction is carried out. Here, reduction forceps have proved extremely useful. Even in children, adequate fracture reduction should always be the primary aim despite the tendency for alignment to correct spontaneously. Long bone remodelling accompanied by excessive callus formation frequently leads to increased longitudinal growth. Sometimes the fracture must be reduced anatomically before the fixator body is applied. Subsequent reduction causing lesions of soft tissue and entailing the risk of a pin-track infection should be avoided. Deliberate overriding to avoid increased longitudinal growth is not acceptable.[2,4,5,6,8,18,30,31]

Immediately after the application of the external fixator and while the patient is still anaesthetised, the adjacent joints should be mobilized fully. This is especially important at the knee joint when the iliotibial tract has been transfixed by pins. Any tautness of skin around the pins requires incision.

Post-operative Management

The main features of post-operative management are pin site care; early mobilization and load-bearing according to a defined programme of physiotherapy; the timing of dynamization and the removal of the external fixator after fracture healing.

Pin site care involves an assessment of the entry points of the pins and pin care itself (Table 31.6). In general, the children learn to look after their own pin sites and do this alone, daily and very conscientiously, even at home (see Ch.11). From a psychological point of view, encouragement to assume responsibility for pin care plays an important role. The child must understand that the external fixator is, for a time at least, a part of his or her own body.[40] We produce a special pin care pack for our patients (Fig. 31.5).

In addition to pin care, physiotherapy plays an important role in treatment and must not be neglected. A step-by-step programme of physiotherapy corresponding to the phases of treatment (Table 31.7) has proved invaluable. It facilitates efficient exercising until sufficient movement has been achieved.[11] Immediately following surgical intervention, exercises on a movement rail (motor rail) are carried out. Mobility of the knee joint soon becomes pain-free and the children require very few analgesics (Fig. 31.6).

Despite full mobility of the knee-joint under anaesthesia, if pins have been inserted in the femur, there is restricted mobility post-operatively, with a maximal

Stage 1	No irritation
Stage 2	Secretion
Stage 3	Granulation
Stage 4	Pin-track infection with osteolysis
Stage 5	Loose pins with osteolysis
Stage 6	Osteomyelitis with sequestrum

Table 31.6 Assessment of Pin Sites and Pin-track Infection

1. At Operation
Mobilization of adjacent joints under anaesthesia after application of external fixator
2. Post-operative Phase (days 1–6)
A) start of motorised rail exercises immediately after the operation
B) isometric tension exercises and electro-myostimulation in bed from day 2 onwards
C) active and active-passive exercises in bed from day 3 onwards
2. Load-bearing phase (from day 7 onwards)
A) partial weightbearing
B) use of special aids and devices for movement exercises under static and later dynamic conditions
C) walking exercises, climbing steps
3. Physiotherapy at follow-up appointments
A) walking exercises
B) specific exercises
C) correction of pathological movement patterns

Table 31.7 Graded Programme of Physiotherapy

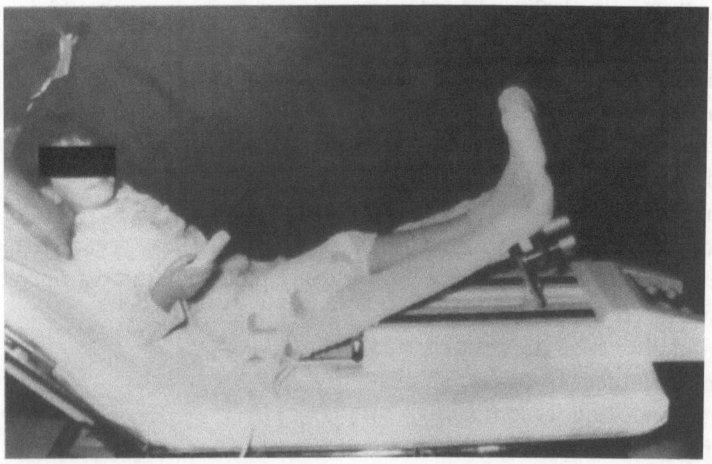

Fig. 31.6 Exercise treatment on a motorised rail.

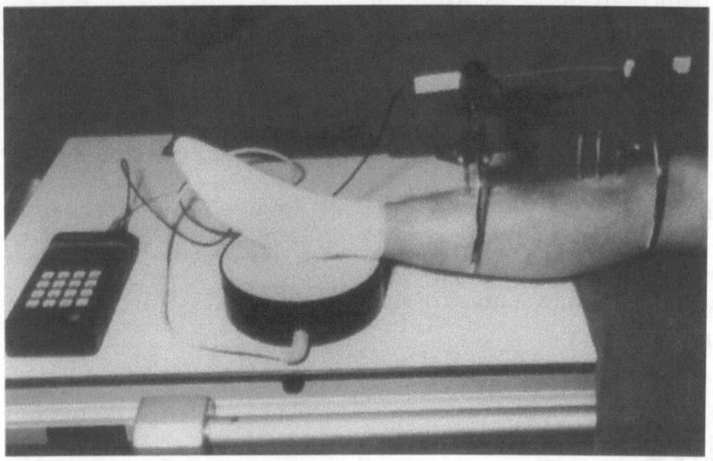

Fig. 31.7 Testing fracture stiffness with the aid of an Orthometer (Orthofix).

degree of movement between 0/0/20° and 0/0/90°. Transfixion of the iliotibial tract by pins is thought to be the reason for this. Clinical studies of the anatomy have shown that the iliotibial tract cannot relax sufficiently for full flexion. The children tolerate this restriction of movement without problems, and as soon as the pins have been removed on the completion of treatment, they regain full mobility. The load-bearing phase on the locked fixator starts in the second week. With single injuries, hospitalization lasts for 2–3 weeks.

The timing of dynamization depends on the length of the fracture gap. In transverse and oblique fractures, axial dynamization starts as early as the second week. If interfragmentary collapse occurs following release of the central body locking nut of the fixator, dynamization must be abandoned, or a Dyna-Ring used to control the extent of dynamization. Even with a locked fixator, micromovement due to minimal flexion of the screws will initiate callus formation. The effect of dynamization on callus production has been verified scientifically. There are no studies on the duration of fracture healing in conjunction with dynamization in children, however. The problem lies in the age-dependent duration of fracture healing and in fracture-specific peculiarities.

Full weightbearing in hospital means that the children can go to kindergarten or school after being discharged. Out-patient follow-up takes place once a week at a special clinic. The course of fracture healing can be monitored with the aid of an Orthometer (Orthofix) (Fig. 31.7). This measures the stiffness of the fracture and according to initial results, tibial fractures in children may be considered as healed when values in excess of 14 Nm/° are achieved. In infants, fracture healing takes about 6 weeks and in older children, around 10 to 12 weeks. The children remove the pins themselves in the out-patient clinic without the need for anaesthesia or analgesia (Fig. 31.8). The entry points of the pins heal within one week. Sometimes keloid or extensive scars remain after excessive skin incisions for pin insertion.

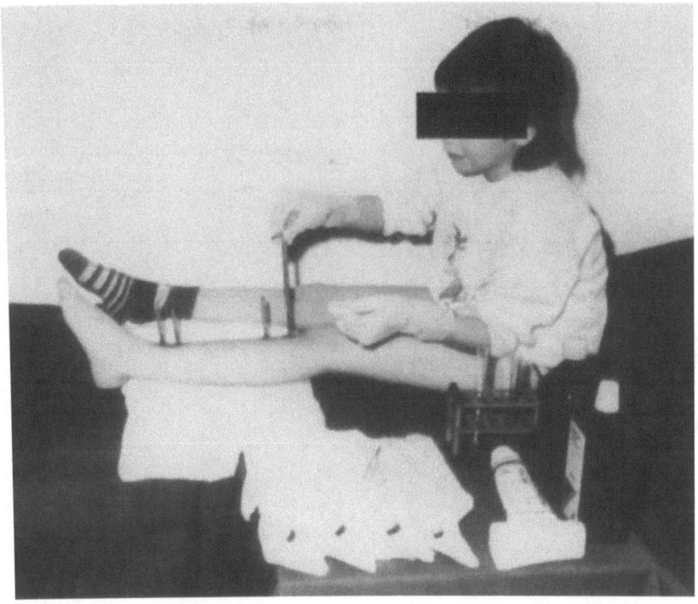

Fig. 31.8 A 9-year-old boy removing his pins by himself in the out- patient department following healing of a fracture of the left tibia.

406 Fractures in 389 Patients	
200 femoral fractures (3/I, 4/II, 5/III)	
15 fractures of humerus	
183 tibia/fibula fractures (15/I, 16/II, 15/III)	
8 radius/ulna fractures (3/I, 2/II, 1/III)	
Single injuries	292
Multiple injuries	87
Without trauma	10

Table 31.8 Experience with Orthofix External Fixation in the clinic for paediatric surgery of the University of Leipzig June 1990–December 1998 (Distribution of open fractures, Grades I–III shown in brackets)

skull	+	+	+	+	+	+		
thorax			+	+				
abdomen		+	+					
extremity	+	+	+	+	+	+	+	+
extremity					+	+	+	+
extremity					+		+	
n =	39	10	1	8	5	4	3	17
Craniocerebral injury (GCS 8–12)						39		
Blunt abdominal trauma						10		
Critically injured children in shock suffering other Organ damage						19		

Table 31.9 Distribution of trauma pattern in multiple injuries (n = 87)

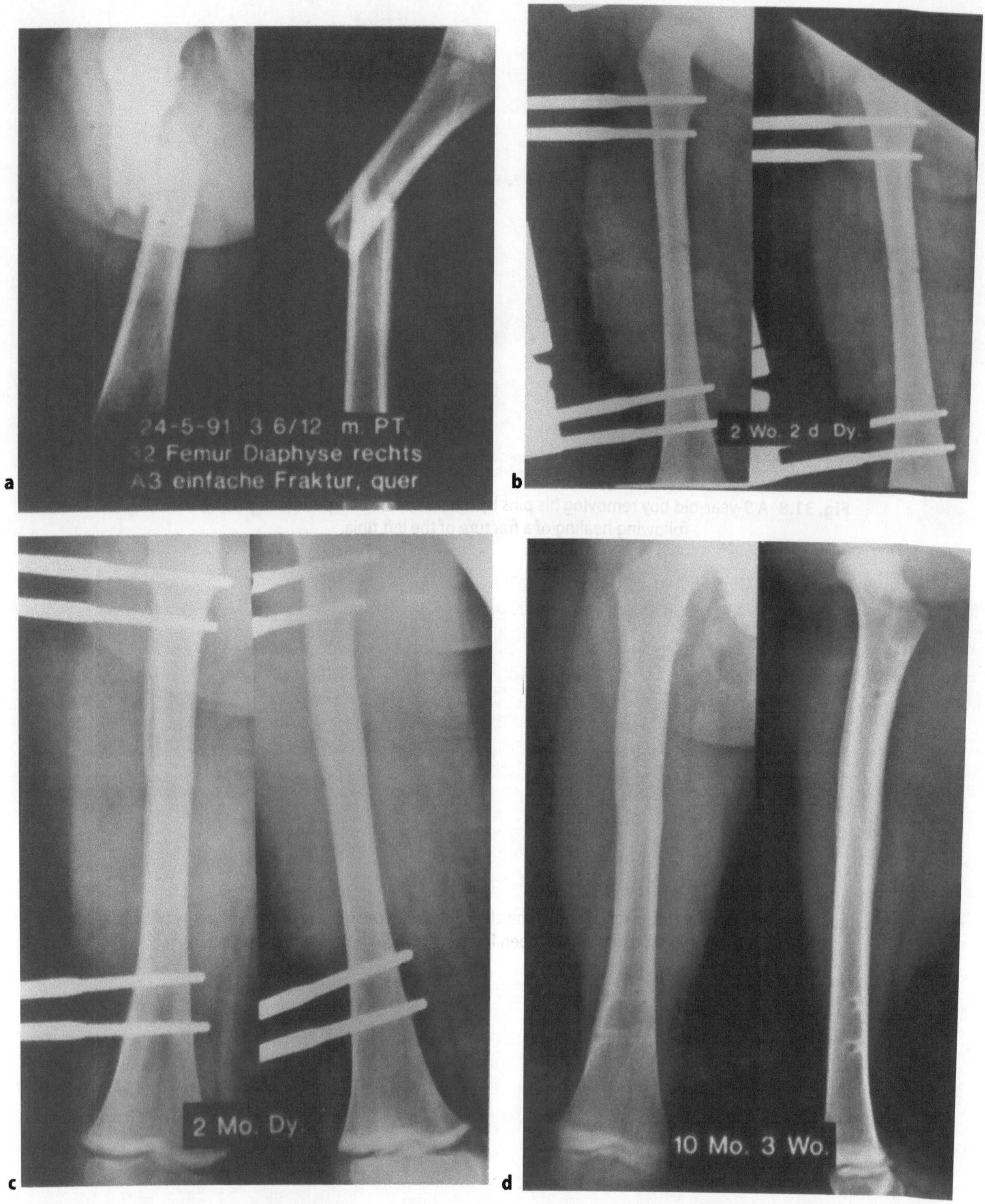

Fig. 31.9 **a** A 3½-year-old boy with multiple injuries, including this transverse fracture of the right femoral diaphysis. **b** Follow-up 2 weeks after application of the fixator. **c** Follow-up at 2 months; this fracture was dynamized. **d** Follow-up at 10 months 3 weeks; fracture healed, fixator removed.

Results

During the period between June 1990 and December 1998, 406 fractures in 389 children were treated in our clinic with external fixation. A fracture-related summary is shown in Table 31.8. Of these fractures, 342 were closed and 64 open. In this group, 292 had a single injury and 87 had multiple injuries. In 10 children without trauma, a disorder of bone maturity was observed. The injury patterns of the multiply injured children are shown in Table 31.9. In 39 cases, extremity injuries were combined with craniocerebral injury (Glasgow Coma Scale 8–12). Nineteen critically ill children were in shock and had other injuries; 17 children had a double extremity injury and 3 patients had a triple extremity injury. Age at accident ranged from 1 year and 3 months to 16 years and 6 months, with an average age of 9 years and 8 months. Road traffic accidents were the most common cause of injury (>50 per cent). The sex ratio was 2.3:1 with boys predominating.

As a basis for a comparative assessment, the AO classification was used.[37] The external fixator was applied on the femoral shaft in 139 simple fractures (32 A1–A3), in 37 wedge fractures (32 B1–B3) and in 8 complex fractures (32 C1–C3); 3 fractures were third degree open, 3 were second degree and 3 were first degree. In the proximal femur, 4 intertrochanteric and 2 transcervical fractures (31 A3/B2) were treated. Distally, external fixation was performed in 7 metaphyseal fractures (33 A1/A3) with one third degree. One partial articular fracture (33 B1) and 2 complete articular fractures, second and third degree open, Aitken classification 3 (33 C2–3) occurred (Table 31.10). Figs. 31.9–31.15 show selected examples of the use of external fixators on the femur. In shaft fractures, external fixation may be used to obtain definitive stabilization regardless of fracture type.

Special fractures of the proximal and distal zone are of some interest. Intertrochanteric, pertrochanteric and transcervical fractures can be treated by inserting the pins into the femoral neck or into the fracture region, using an angled clamp attached to the external fixator. Metaphyseal fractures are fixed by inserting the pins either crosswise or obliquely in conjunction with either a straight or T-clamp, depending upon location. Here, external fixation is superior to intramedullary stable elastic splinting, because faulty axial or rotational positions can be safely avoided. In meta-epiphyseal fractures, external fixation is applied only in exceptional cases, e.g. in multi-planar fractures accompanied by articular injuries. Segmental fragments are fixed with additional pins. Isolated meta-epiphyseal fractures always require exact reconstruction with the aid of screws and are not an indication for external fixation.

In the tibial shaft, 123 simple fractures (42 A1–A3), 24 wedge fractures (42 B1–B3) and 7 complex fractures (C1–C3) were treated; 12 fractures were third degree open, 13 were second degree and 12 first degree. In the proximal tibia, external fixation was applied to 5

31 Proximal Femur	
A3 fracture of trochanteric region, intertrochanteric	4
B2 cervical fracture, transcervical	2
32 Femoral Diaphysis	
A1 simple fracture, spiral	50
A2 simple fracture, oblique	26
A3 simple fracture, transverse (2/I, 2/II, 1/III)	63
B1 wedge fracture, spiral wedge (1/I)	14
B2 wedge fracture, bending wedge(1/II)	17
B3 wedge fracture, fragmental wedge (2/III)	6
C1 complex fracture, spiral	5
C2 complex fracture, segmental	2
C3 complex fracture, irregular	1
33 Distal Femur	
A1 extra-articular fracture, simple (1/III)	5
A3 extra-articular fracture, metaphyseal complex	2
B1 partial articular fracture, metaphyseal, simple	1
C2 complete articular fracture, simple (1/II)	2
C3 complete articular fracture, multiple-fragmental (Aitken classification 3) (1/III)	2

Table 31.10 Femoral fractures: fracture type according to the AO classification

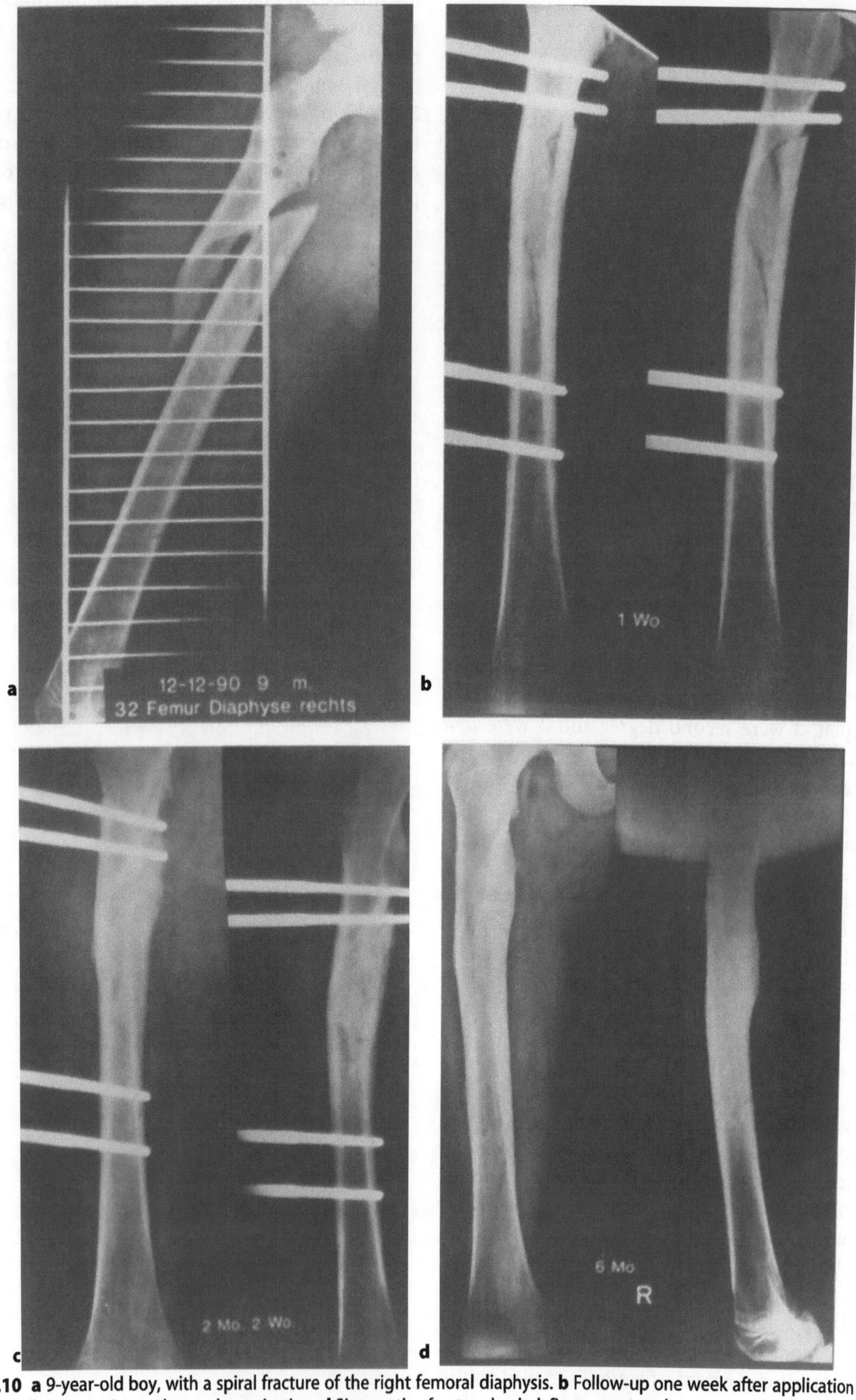

Fig. 31.10 **a** 9-year-old boy, with a spiral fracture of the right femoral diaphysis. **b** Follow-up one week after application of the fixator. **c** Follow-up at 2 months; no dynamization. **d** Six months; fracture healed, fixator removed.

metaphyseal fractures (41 A2–A3); 23 metaphyseal fractures of the distal tibia (43 A1–A3) were treated. Distally, 3 fractures were third degree open, 3 were second degree and 3 first degree. One partial articular fracture (43 B1) occurred (Table 31.11). Figs. 31.16–31.20 show typical examples of the use of external fixation in the tibia.

In the tibia, external fixation is also suitable for the definitive treatment of diaphyseal and metaphyseal fractures. Children with closed fractures of the lower extremity generally achieve full weightbearing in the first week. The advantages of external fixation in open tibia/fibula fractures deserve special emphasis. In the presence of major soft tissue defects, this method allows soft tissue reconstruction under stabilization via shortening, with secondary callus distraction.[19] Even combined injuries of the lower extremity and foot can be fixed externally via temporary arthrodesis using a special module (Orthofix®). The same treatment is also available for open meta-epiphyseal fractures.

In the humeral shaft, 14 simple fractures (12 A1–A3) and one wedge fracture (12 B2) were stabilized externally, as were 7 simple fractures (22 A1/A3) of the radius/ulna shaft and one distal fracture (23 A2). In the forearm, one fracture was a third degree open fracture, 2 second degree and 3 first degree (Table 31.12). In children, external fixation is, for the most part, an indication of second choice in fractures of the upper extremity (Fig. 31.21), and intramedullary stable elastic splinting is favoured; open fractures, however, are an exception (Fig. 31.22).

41 Proximal Tibia/Fibula	
A2 extra-articular fracture, metaphyseal simple	4
A3 extra-articular fracture, metaphyseal, multi-fragmental	1
42 Tibia/Fibula Diaphysis	
A1 simple fracture, spiral (1/I, 3/II, 2/III)	54
A2 simple fracture, oblique (3/I, 3/II, 2/III)	39
A3 simple fracture, transverse (4/I,3/II)	30
B1 wedge fracture, spiral wedge (2/III)	6
B2 wedge fracture, bending wedge (1/I, 2/II, 3/III)	12
B3 wedge fracture, fragmental wedge (3/I, 1/II)	6
C1 complex fracture, spiral (1/III)	4
C2 complex fracture, segmental (1/II)	1
C3 complex fracture, irregular (2/III)	2
43 Distal Tibia/Fibula	
A1 extra-articular fracture, metaphyseal simple (3/I, 1/III)	18
A2 extra-articular fracture, metaphyseal wedge (Aitken classification 1) (2/II, 2/III)	4
A3 extra-articular fracture, metaphyseal complex (1/II)	1
B1 partial articular fracture, metaphyseal, simple	1

Table 31.11 Tibia/fibula fractures: fracture type according to the AO classification

Open Fractures

In open fractures in children, the same philosophy as that for adult fractures applies. Interest focuses on stabilization of the fracture via external fixation. The

12 Humeral Diaphysis	
A1 simple fracture, spiral	7
A2 simple fracture, oblique	2
A3 simple fracture, transverse	5
B2 wedge fracture, bending wedge	1
22 Radius/Ulna Diaphysis	
A1 simple fracture of ulna, Monteggia fracture (1/I)	1
A3 simple fracture, complete (2/I, 2/II)	6
23 Radius/Ulna Distal	
A2 extra-articular fracture, simple (1/III)	1

Table 31.12 Upper limb fractures: fracture type according to the AO classification

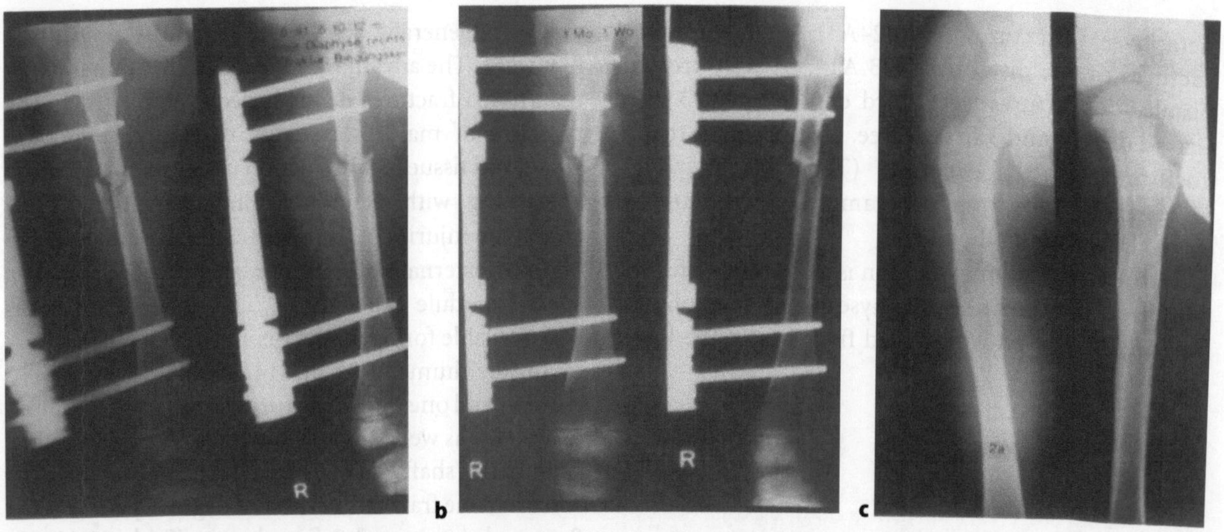

a b c

Fig. 31.11 **a** Boy aged 5 years and 10 months with a wedge fracture of the right femoral diaphysis stabilized with an Orthofix. **b** Follow-up after one month without dynamization. **c** Healed.

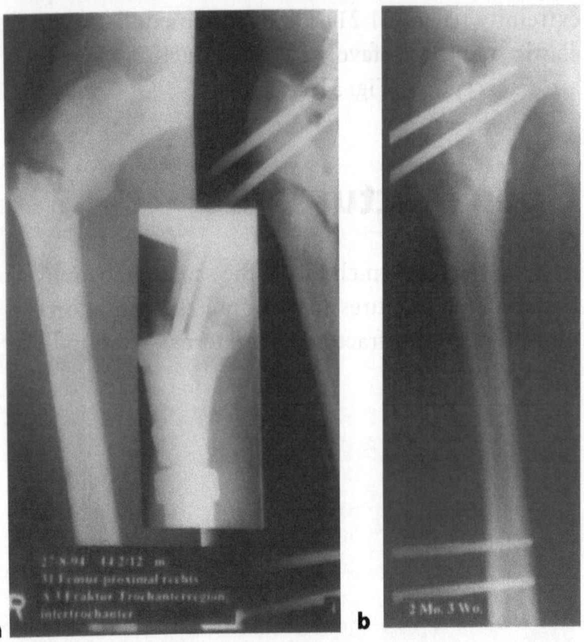

a b

Fig. 31.12 **a** Intertrochanteric fracture of the right femur in a 14-year-old boy treated with an Orthofix fixator with angled clamp for insertion of screws along the femoral neck. **b** Healing after 2 months and 3 weeks.

extent of surgical debridement necessary depends on the extent of the bone and soft tissue injury. In general, systemic antibiotics are given for 3–5 days, and in second or third degree open fractures, local antibiotic treatment is also administered.

We treated 64 open fractures with external fixation. Of these, 21 fractures were first degree fractures, 22 second degree and 21 third degree. Four children also had a severe soft tissue injury of the lower leg with or without involvement of the foot. In one case, soft tissue reconstruction of the lower leg was performed, with stabilization via shortening. Secondary callus distraction to compensate for the limb length discrepancy followed. In two cases, the skin defect was treated first with a synthetic skin substitute and finally covered by multiple skin grafts (Fig. 31.23). In one instance, bone and soft tissue defects later required a free flap skin graft with microvascular connection in addition to secondary callus distraction. In these cases, temporary post-operative post-traumatic osteitis occurred.

All open fractures healed within a period of not more than 8 months. For definitive stabilization, the external fixator alone was used and a change of procedure was never required. Open fractures were not dynamized. Our own treatment regime so far has proved its worth, especially with regard to the possibility of secondary callus distraction. Autologous cancellous bone grafts and segmental transfer are exceptional procedures in the treatment of childhood fractures.

Complications

In children, pin-track infections are common and prejudice treatment with external fixation. According to the literature, the reported frequency of pin track infection varies considerably (Table 31.13). This can be explained by differing definitions of pin-track infection. Secretion from the pin sites and granulation around them must be differentiated from a true pin-

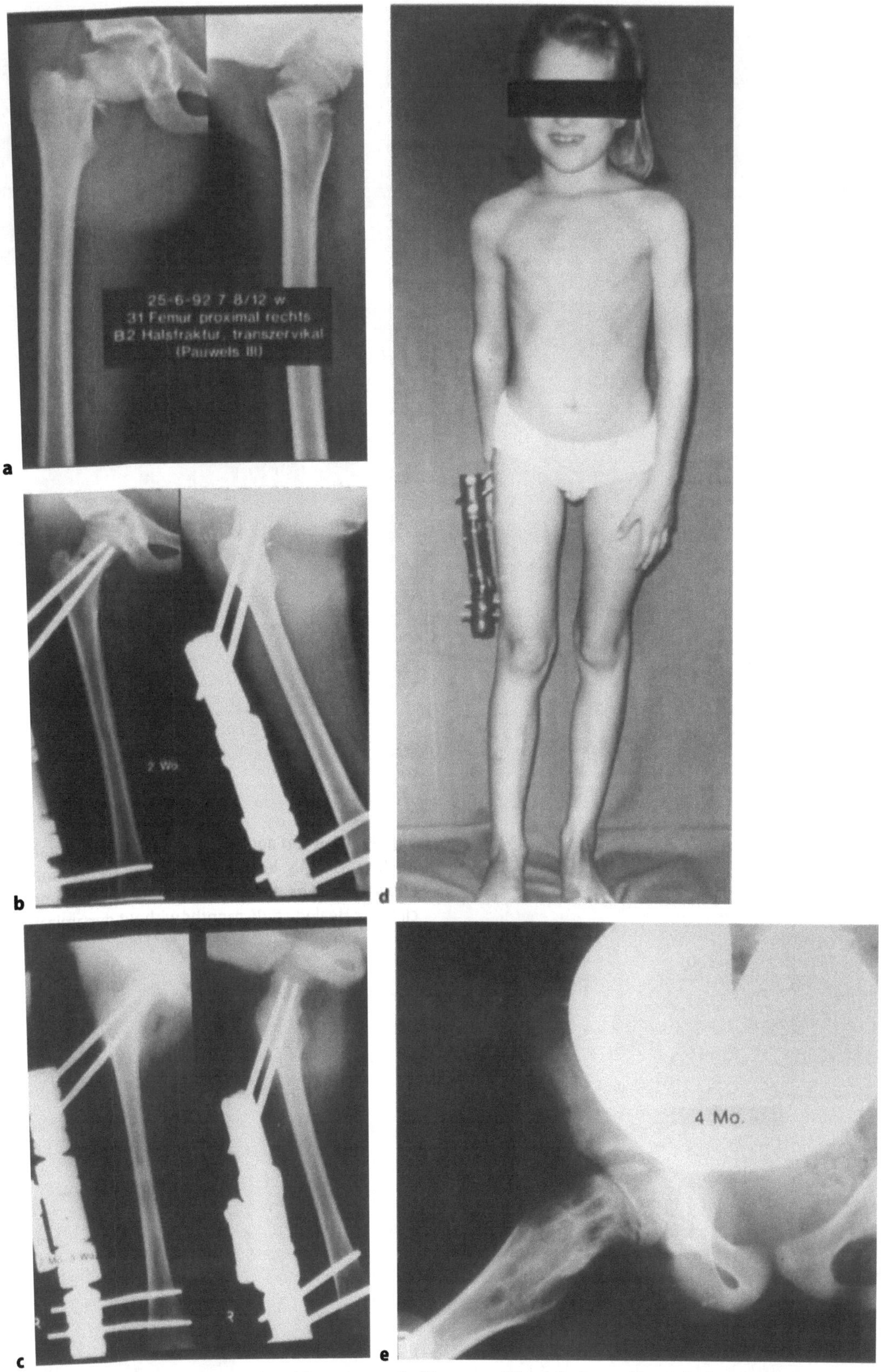

Fig. 31.13 **a** Girl aged 7 years and 8 months with a transcervical fracture of the right femur (Pauwels classification 3). **b** Follow-up at 2 weeks following application of Orthofix fixator with angled clamp. **c** Follow-up at 2 months. **d** Clinical picture. **e** Healing at 4 months.

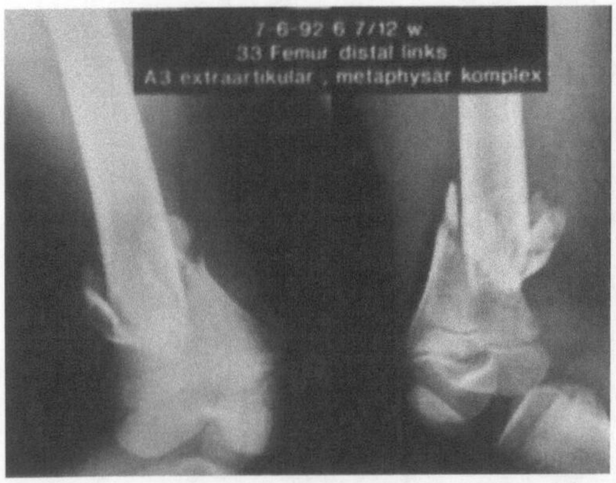

a

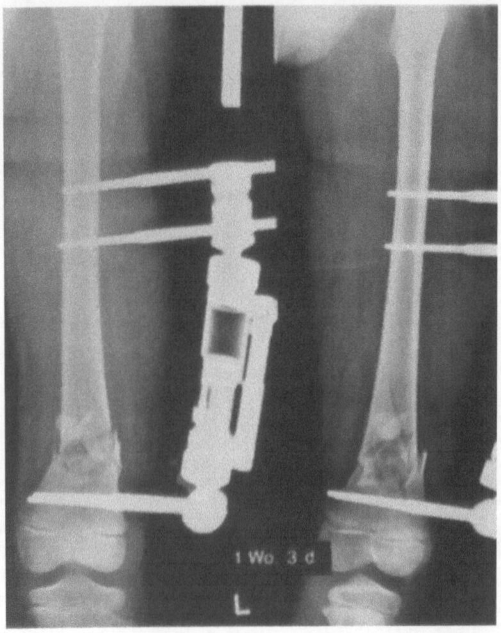

b

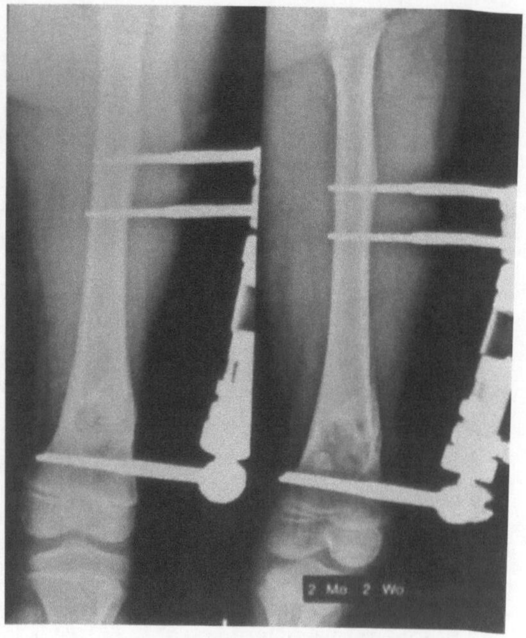

c

Fig. 31.14 **a** Girl aged 6½ with a complex distal metaphyseal fracture of the left femur. **b** Follow-up one week after application of fixator with proximal straight clamp and distal T-clamp. **c** Healed at 2½ months without dynamization.

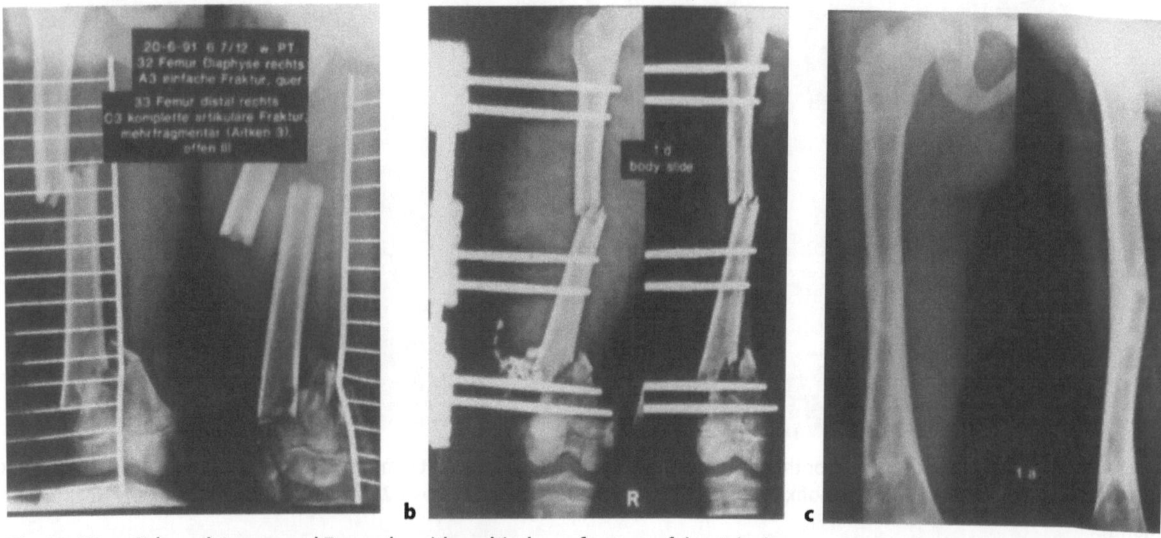

a b c

Fig. 31.15 **a** Girl aged 6 years and 7 months with multi-planar fracture of the right femur accompanied by an open third degree meta-epiphyseal fracture (Aitken classification 3). **b** External fixation with an Orthofix Limb Reconstruction System; temporary septopal bead chain implantation. **c** Healed appearance.

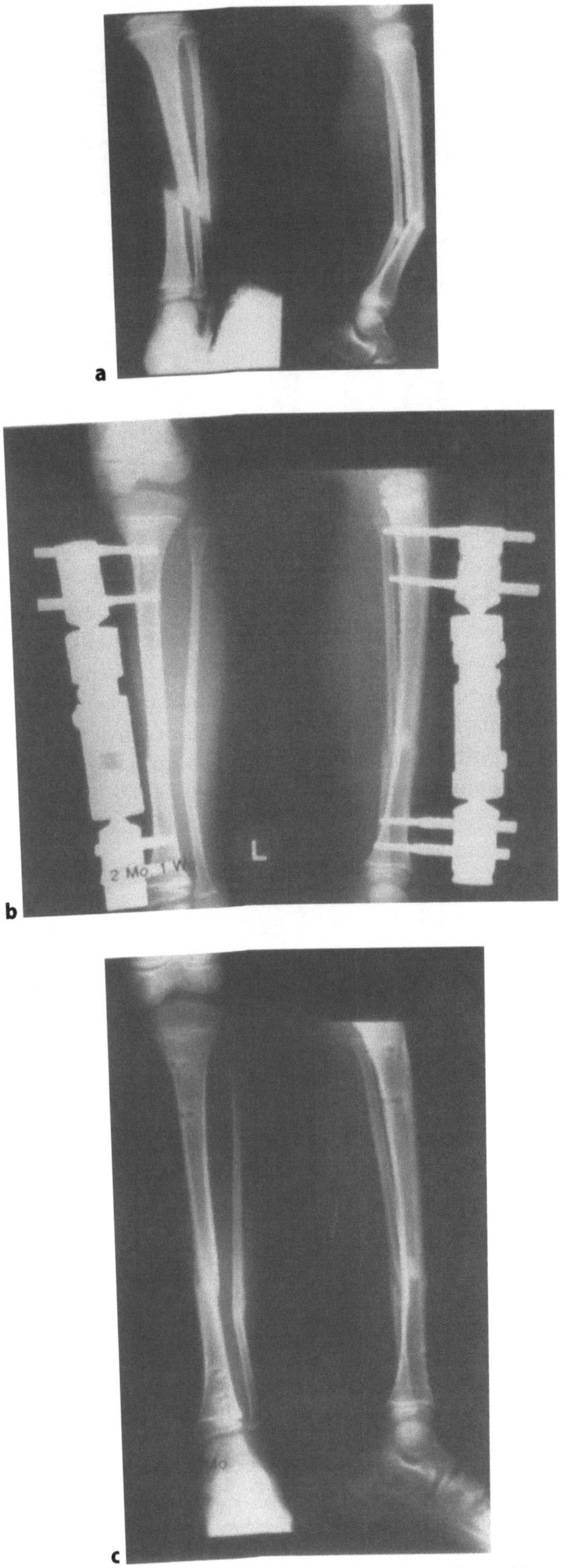

a b c

Fig. 31.16 **a** Girl aged 4 years and 7 months with an oblique diaphyseal fracture of the left tibia/fibula. **b** Follow-up after two months, with dynamization. **c** Healed appearance.

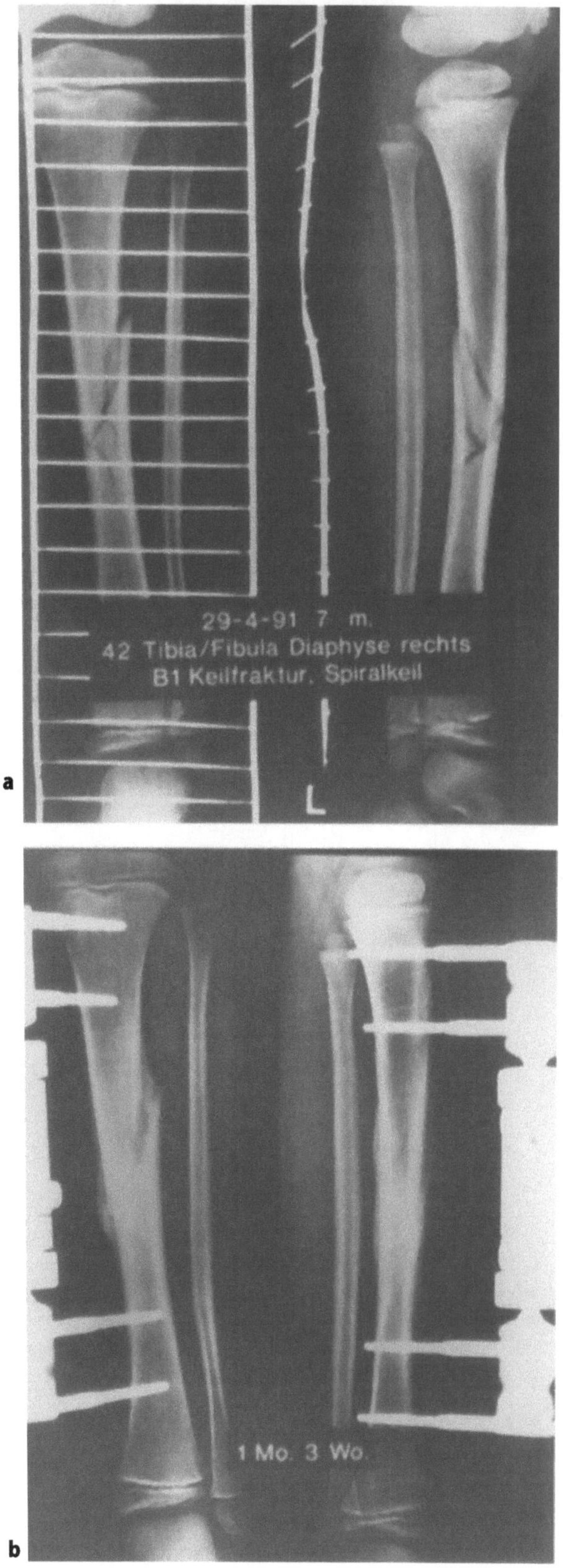

a b

Fig. 31.17 **a** Diaphyseal wedge fracture of the tibia/fibula in a 7-year-old boy. **b** Follow-up after 2 months, with dynamization; healed.

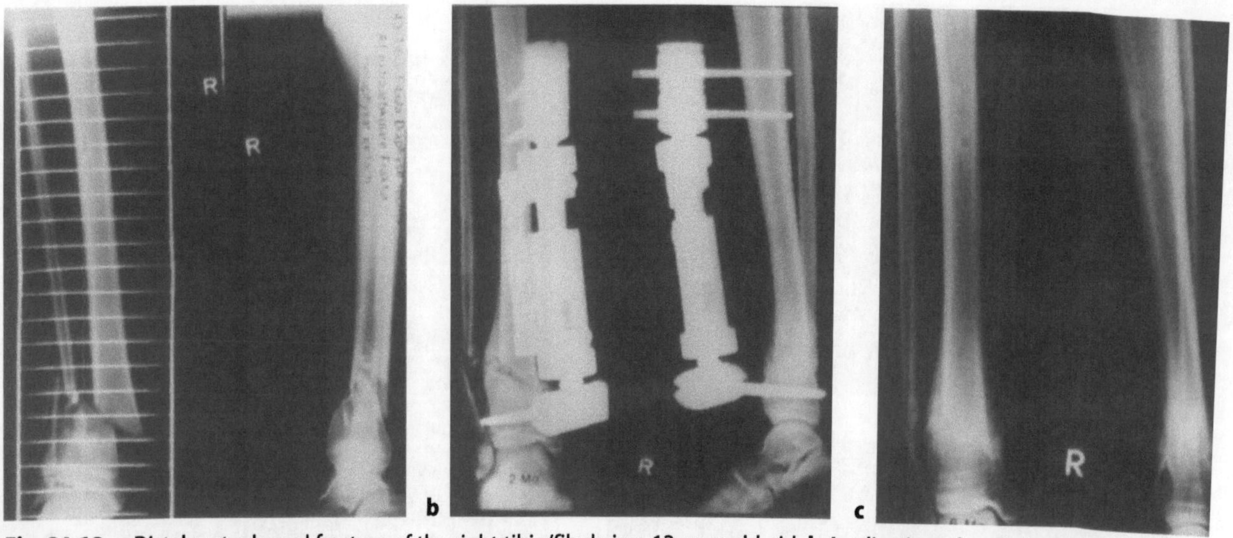

Fig. 31.18 **a** Distal metaphyseal fracture of the right tibia/fibula in a 12-year-old girl. **b** Application of an Orthofix fixator with a straight clamp proximally and a T-clamp distally; follow-up at 2 months. **c** Healed result at 6 months, following fixator removal.

track infection which consists of a fistula accompanied by bacterial contamination and radiological evidence of osteolysis (Fig. 31.24).

In our patients, 16 pin-track infections were observed in 389 children (4.1 per cent). A summary of the organisms involved is shown in Table 31.14. Pin-track infections occur almost exclusively in association with femoral pins and proximal pins are especially affected. Here, the bulk of the soft tissue and its movement around the pins is responsible. Except for an increased sedimentation rate, laboratory values were unremarkable. Leukocytes and C-reactive protein were within normal limits. Blood cultures were always sterile and no septic shock was observed.[49]

	n	infection	%
Asche (1989)	111	1	0.9
Krettek, Haas, Tscherne (1989)	16	4	25
Shih et al (1989)	22	0	0
Kirchenbaum et al (1990)	10	3	30
Keating et al 1991)	100	30	30
Aronson, Tursky (1992)	44	15	34
Dietz, Rösch (1992)	6	4	67
Laer von (1992)	33	14	42
Schranz, Gultekin, Colton (1992)	20	2	10
Van Tets, van der Werken (1992)	15	6	40
Bennek et al (1993)	125	7	5.6
Mittmann, Klein, Brug (1993)	19	2	10.5
Scavenius et al (1993)	18	1	6
Weinberg et al (1994)	89	4	4.5
De Sanctis et al (1996)	82	7	8.6
Blasier et al (1997)	132	6	4.5
Kapukaya et al (1997)	57	3	5.3

Table 31.13 Survey of Pin-Track Infections in the Literature

Period of Study: June 1990–December 1998 Total 16 pin-track infections (4.1 %)			
Femur n = 14		Tibia n = 2	
12	*Staphylococcus aureus*	2	*Staphylococcus aureus*
1	*Staphylococcus aureus* *E. Coli* *Klebsiella*		
1	*Staphylococcus aureus* *E. Coli* *Proteus*		

Table 31.14 Pin-Track Infections: Organisms Isolated

Children with pin-track infections are generally treated in hospital with systemic antibiotics. In contrast to the situation in adults, pin-track infections in children do not normally require surgical intervention. Pin loosening was not considered an indication and resiting of pins was performed only in exceptional cases. Tightening pins which are loose as a result of infection is risky and should not, therefore, be performed. In our patients, the external fixator was not removed prematurely in any case of pin-track infection. These infections healed, and subsequent radiographs revealed the development of a periosteal edge around the entry points of the pins. In 6 children, pins were found to be loose on removal of the external fixator after fracture healing.

In 2.0 per cent of patients refractures occurred after removal of the external fixator. This is no different from the frequency encountered with other methods of treatment.[18,21] To date, pseudarthrosis has not been observed. In our patients, 3 femoral refractures after 10, 12 and 16 weeks and 3 tibial refractures after 10, 11 and 12 weeks were found. In 2 cases, femoral refracture occurred after 11 and 12 weeks respectively, accompanying a disorder of bone maturity; in one case, it was associated with infantile cerebral palsy.

Long Term Follow-up

We have followed up 383 fractures in 367 children for periods ranging from 4 months to 8 years and 2 months. Differences in leg length and rotational malalignment were determined clinically, and axial malalignment radiologically. Computerised tomography and sonography studies of the femoral necks were not carried out.

Of 190 femoral fractures, 170 (89.5 per cent) had healed in axial alignment and without any length discrepancy; 6.8 per cent remained axially malaligned. There were 6 cases of antecurvatum of 10–15°, 2 cases of recurvatum of 10°, 4 cases of valgus deformity of 10 and 15° respectively, and one case of varus deformity of 10°. Pathological rotational deformities did not occur. In 3.7 per cent, measurable length discrepancies occurred; in 6 children, a lengthening of ≥ 2 cm was observed, and in one a lengthening of ≥ 3 cm. A breakdown of these results is shown in Table 31.15.

Of 179 tibial-fibular fractures, 171 (95.5 per cent) healed in axial alignment and without length discrepancy. In 3.4 per cent, axial malalignment, remained. There were two instances of antecurvatum of 15°, one case of recurvatum of 10°, 2 valgus deformities of 10° and one varus deformity of 10°. In 1.1 per cent a length discrepancy occurred: 2 children showed a lengthening of ≥ 2 cm (Table 31.16). 14 fractures of the humerus healed axially aligned and without length discrepancies.

Overall, our follow-up showed that 355 fractures healed in an anatomical position. In 28 fractures (7.3 per cent), axial malalignment and/or limb length discrepancies remained (Table 31.17). Restricted mobility was not observed. The maximum limb length discrepancy (3cm) observed in our patients corresponds to the findings of other authors who used external fixators.[1,18,23,25,39,41] It should be stated that a primary idiopathic difference of leg length cannot be excluded[20] and the accuracy of the clinical measurement has an error of 1cm which must also be taken into consideration. With intramedullary stable elastic splinting and plate osteosynthesis, the reported rate of additional longitudinal growth is smaller, but a statistically significant difference could not be demonstrated.[18]

Discussion

The aims of fracture treatment in children have changed. Hitherto conservative therapy was favoured, but a tendency towards surgical or semi-operative treatment has become apparent. In addition to the minimal osteosynthesis (Kirschner-wire fixation, screws, tension banding) required in intra-articular and periarticular fractures, flexible fixation in diaphyseal and metaphyseal fractures is being used with increasing frequency. Here, external fixation and intramedullary stable elastic splinting have proved

	AO Classification	Number of follow-ups (n = 190)
31	A3	4
	B2	1
32	A1	46
		1 AC 10°
		1 VR 10°
	A2	25
	A3	50
		1 AC 10°/L + 2.0cm
		2 AC 15°
		1 AC 10°
		2 RC 10°
		1 VG 10°
		2 L + 2.0cm
		1 L + 3.0cm
32	B1	12
		2 L + 2.0cm
	B2	11
		1 AC 15°
		2 VG 10°
	B3	5
		1 VG 15°
	C1	5
	C2	1
	C3	1
33	A1	4
	A3	2
	B1	1
	C	1
		1 L + 2.0cm
	C3	1

Number of Follow-up Visits free of complications = 170 (89.5%)
Key: AC = antecurvatum; RC = recurvatum; VR = varus deformity;
VG = valgus deformity; L = length discrepancy

Table 31.15 Follow-Up in Patients with Femoral Fractures Treated with External Fixation

	AO Classification	Number of Follow-ups (n = 179)
41	A2	4
	A3	1
42	A1	52
		1 VR 10°
	A2	36
		1 AC 15°
		1 VG 10°
	A3	28
		1RC 10°
		1L + 2.0cm
	B1	6
	B2	11
		1 VG 10°
	B3	4
	C1	4
	C2	1
	C3	1
		1 L + 2.0cm
43	A1	18
	A2	3
		1 AC 15°
	A3	1
	B1	1

Number of Follow-up Visits free of complications = 171 (95.5%)
Key: AC = antecurvatum; RC = recurvatum; VR = varus deformity; VG = valgus deformity; L = length discrepancy

Table 31.16 Follow-Up in Patients with Tibial Fractures Treated with External Fixation

	No Abnormality at Follow-Up	Deformity (axis/length)
	n	n
femur	170	20
tibia	171	8
humerus	14	0
Totals	355	28 (7.3%)

Table 31.17 Overall Results at Follow-Up

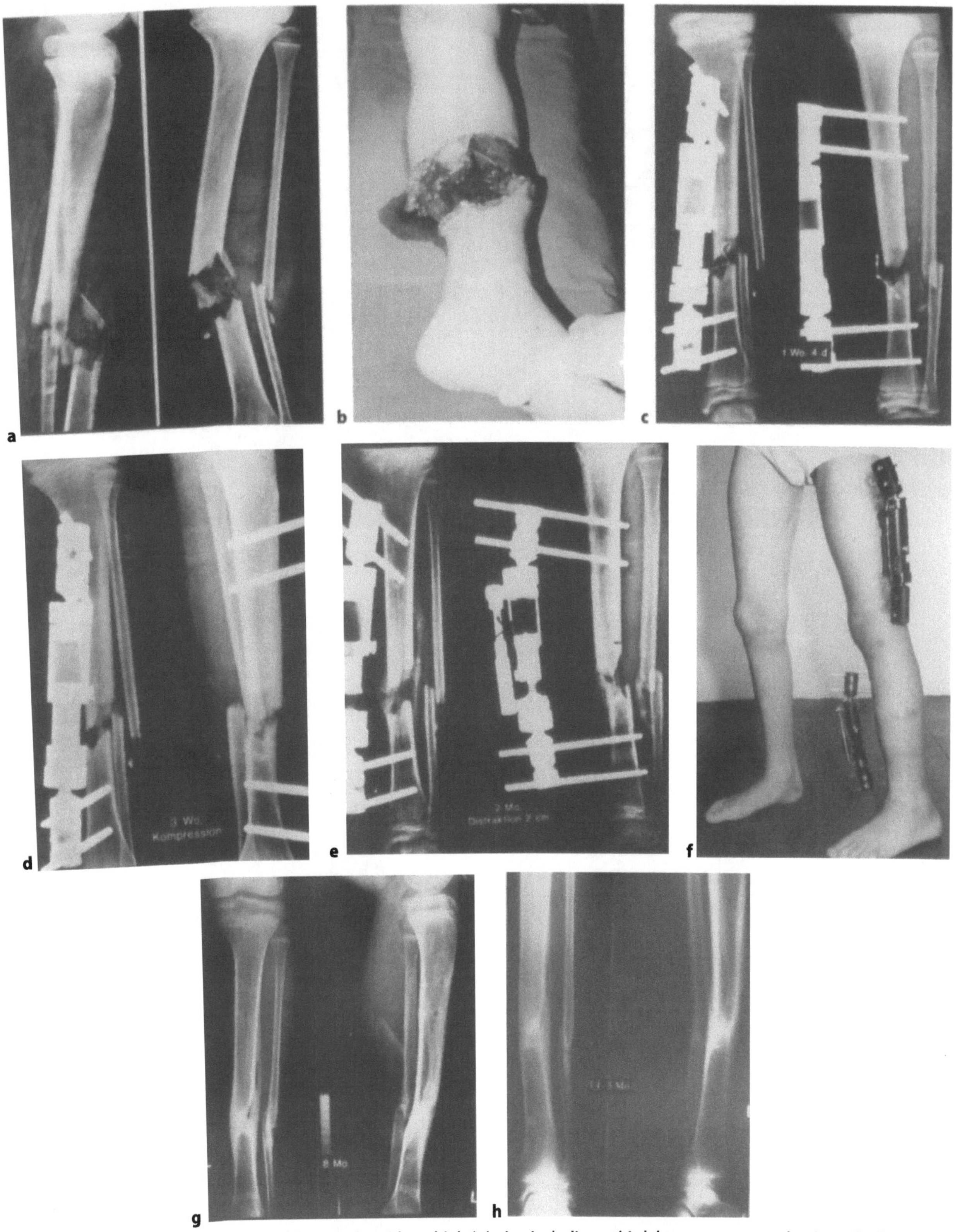

Fig. 31.19 **a** Boy aged 12 years and 7 months with multiple injuries, including a third degree open, complex, irregular fracture of the left tibia/fibula. **b** Clinical appearance. **c** Reconstruction with stabilization via shortening; temporary implantation of septopal bead chain. **d** Follow-up at 3 weeks with fracture under compression. **e** Follow-up at 2 months, after 2cm of callus distraction. **f** Clinical picture showing additional fixator on ipsilateral femur for stabilization of a wedge fracture. **g** Follow-up at 8 months showing healed result. **h** Long-term follow-up at 3 years and 3 months, showing remodelling.

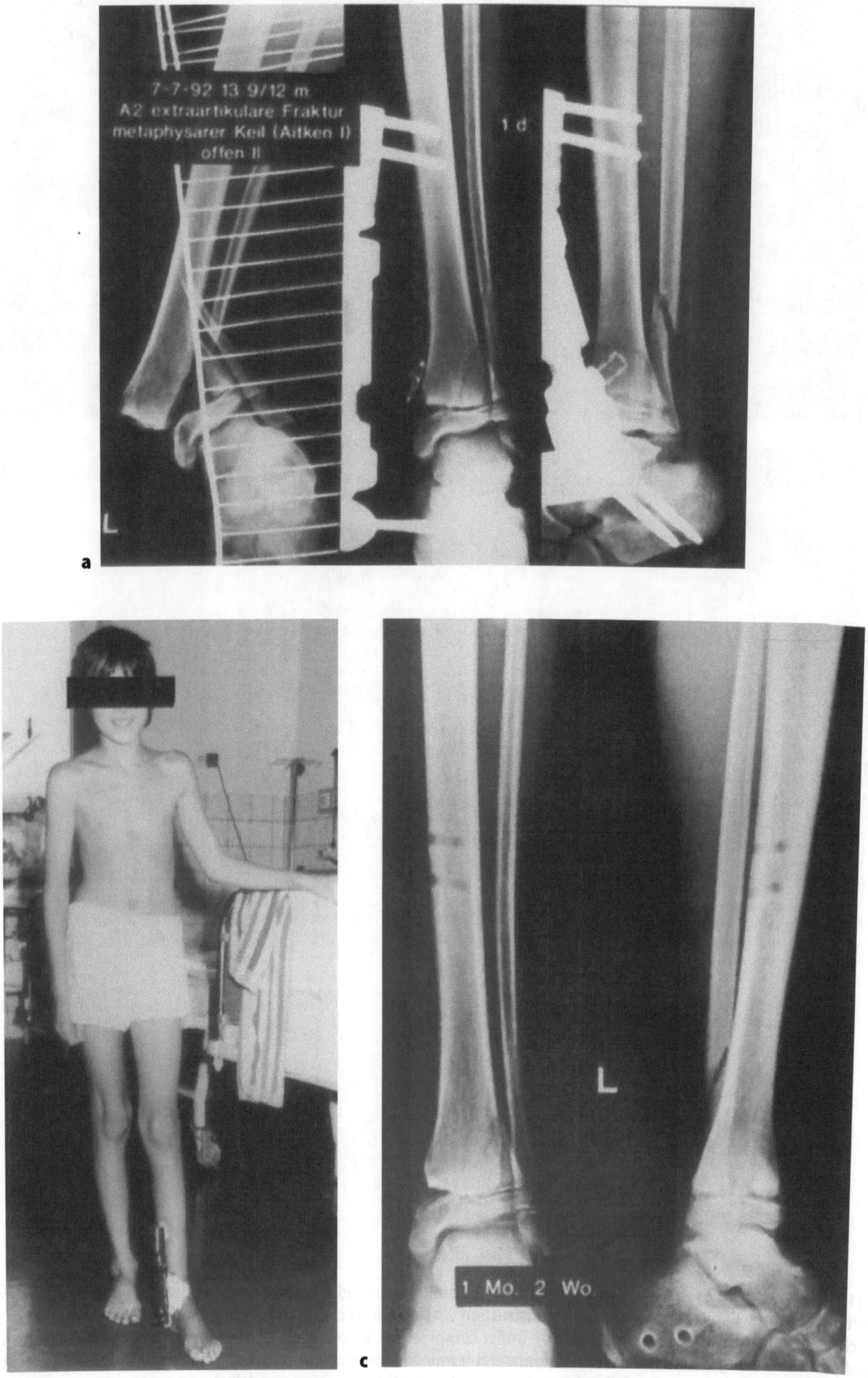

Fig. 31.20 a Boy aged 13 years and 9 months with a second degree, open, meta-epiphyseal fracture of the left tibia/fibula (Aitken classification 1); reconstruction with temporary ankle arthrodesis. **b** Clinical picture with fixator in situ. **c** Healed result at 6 weeks, following fixator removal.

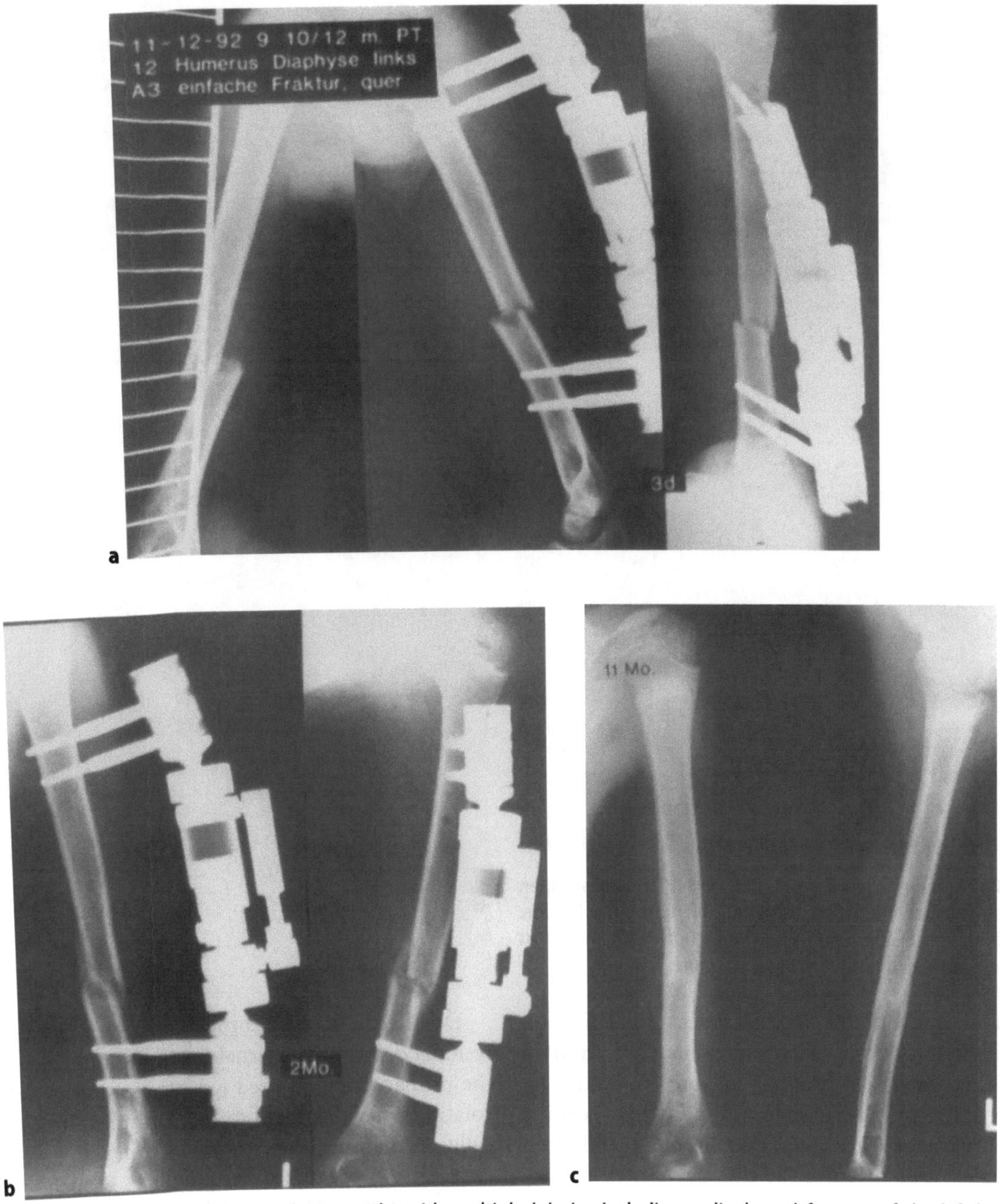

Fig. 31.21 **a** Boy aged 9 years and 10 months with multiple injuries including a diaphyseal fracture of the left humerus; stabilization with Orthofix fixator. **b** Follow-up at 2 months; no dynamization. **c** Follow-up at 11 months showing healed result with remodelling.

useful. In open fractures with or without severe soft tissue injury and in children who have sustained multiple injuries and fractures, external fixation is a treatment of first choice. Even fractures in the intertrochanteric and transcervical regions can be treated with external fixation. In diaphyseal and metaphyseal fractures of the lower extremity, both methods can be used for stabilization.

In our patients, the external fixator is favoured. In the upper extremity, however, external fixation is rarely used and intramedullary stable elastic splinting is preferable in irreducible fractures.

The modular nature of the Orthofix Dynamic Axial Fixation System means that it can be adapted to treat a variety of fracture types from about the 3rd or 4th year onwards. The availability of additional inventory, specific to paediatric applications coupled with the development of an infant fixator (Orthofix®) have now made it possible to provide adequate fracture treatment from the second year of life onwards.

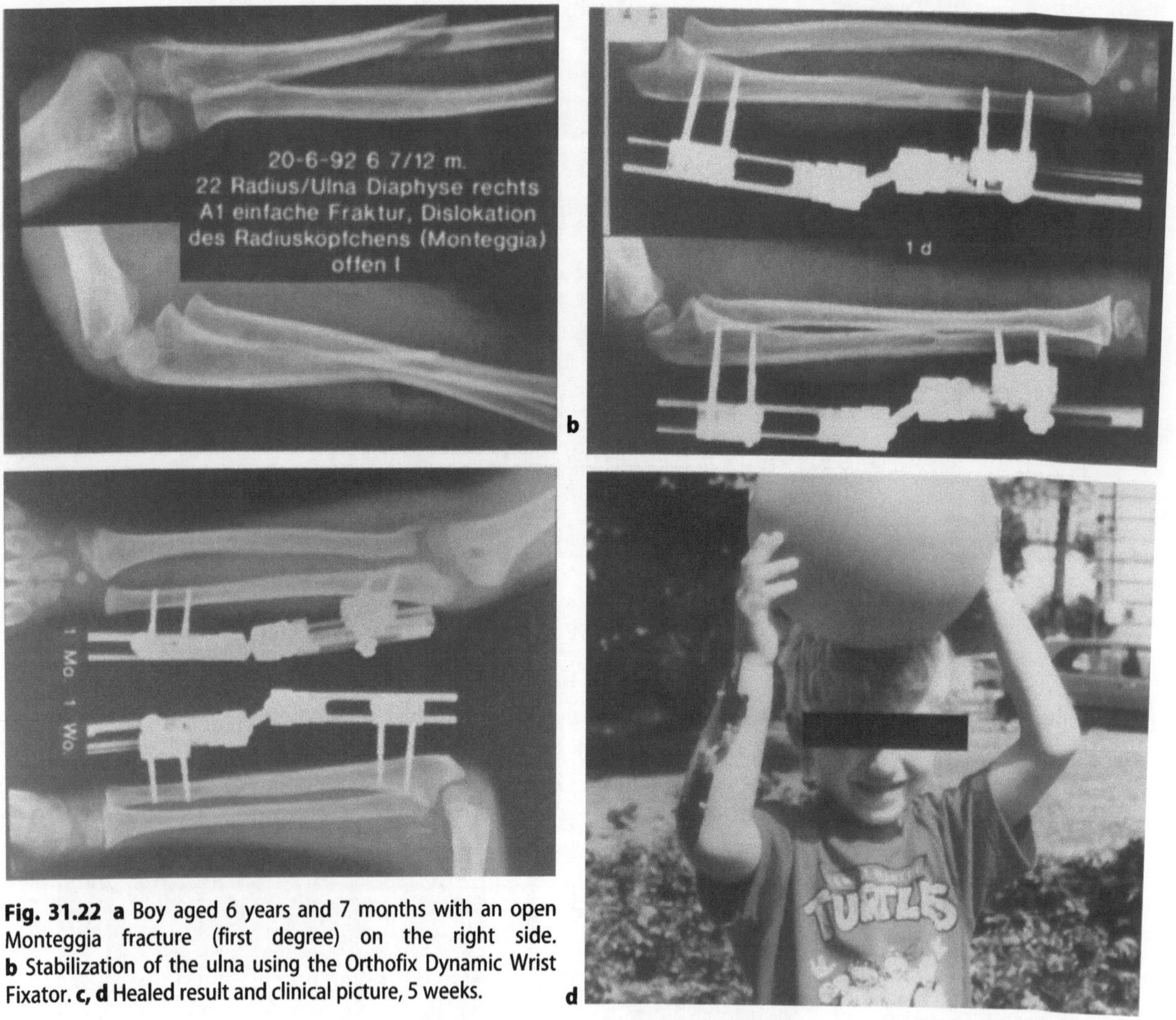

a b c d

Fig. 31.22 a Boy aged 6 years and 7 months with an open Monteggia fracture (first degree) on the right side. **b** Stabilization of the ulna using the Orthofix Dynamic Wrist Fixator. **c, d** Healed result and clinical picture, 5 weeks.

Stabilization of the fracture by external fixation should be initiated as early as possible. The reported problems which can occur if fractures in adults are allowed to remain in a mobile state, particularly during intensive therapy, are equally applicable to children's fractures. Application of the external fixator directly adjacent to the anterior tibial edge in tibial fractures has distinct advantages in terms of the child's ability to walk easily.

Our anatomical and clinical studies have shown that the recommended corridors for pin insertion do not endanger any vital structures. Scarring is minimal with clearly circumscribed skin incisions at the entry points of the pins, and the technique has no cosmetic disadvantages in comparison to other methods. Incising the iliotibial tract at the entry points of the pins in femoral fractures coupled with mobilization of the adjacent joints under anaesthesia does not wholly avoid restricted mobility of the knee-joint in femoral fractures while the fixator is in situ.

Despite the known compensating tendencies of a residual deformity, external fixation should always be the primary method used for stabilization. Axial and rotational malalignment must be avoided. If excessive callus formation occurs in conjunction with long bone remodelling, increased longitudinal growth occurs almost automatically, but deliberate overriding is not acceptable. The duration of surgery and fluoroscopy is similar to that reported for intramedullary stable elastic splinting. Here, the advantages of using the template for pin insertion are particularly apparent.

In open fractures, systemic and local antibiotic treatment have proved a useful adjunct to surgical debridement in second and third degree fractures. For definitive fracture healing, external fixation has always been suitable, and a change of method has never been required during the course of treatment. The technique of secondary callus distraction in association with major bone and soft tissue loss can also be applied to children's fractures.

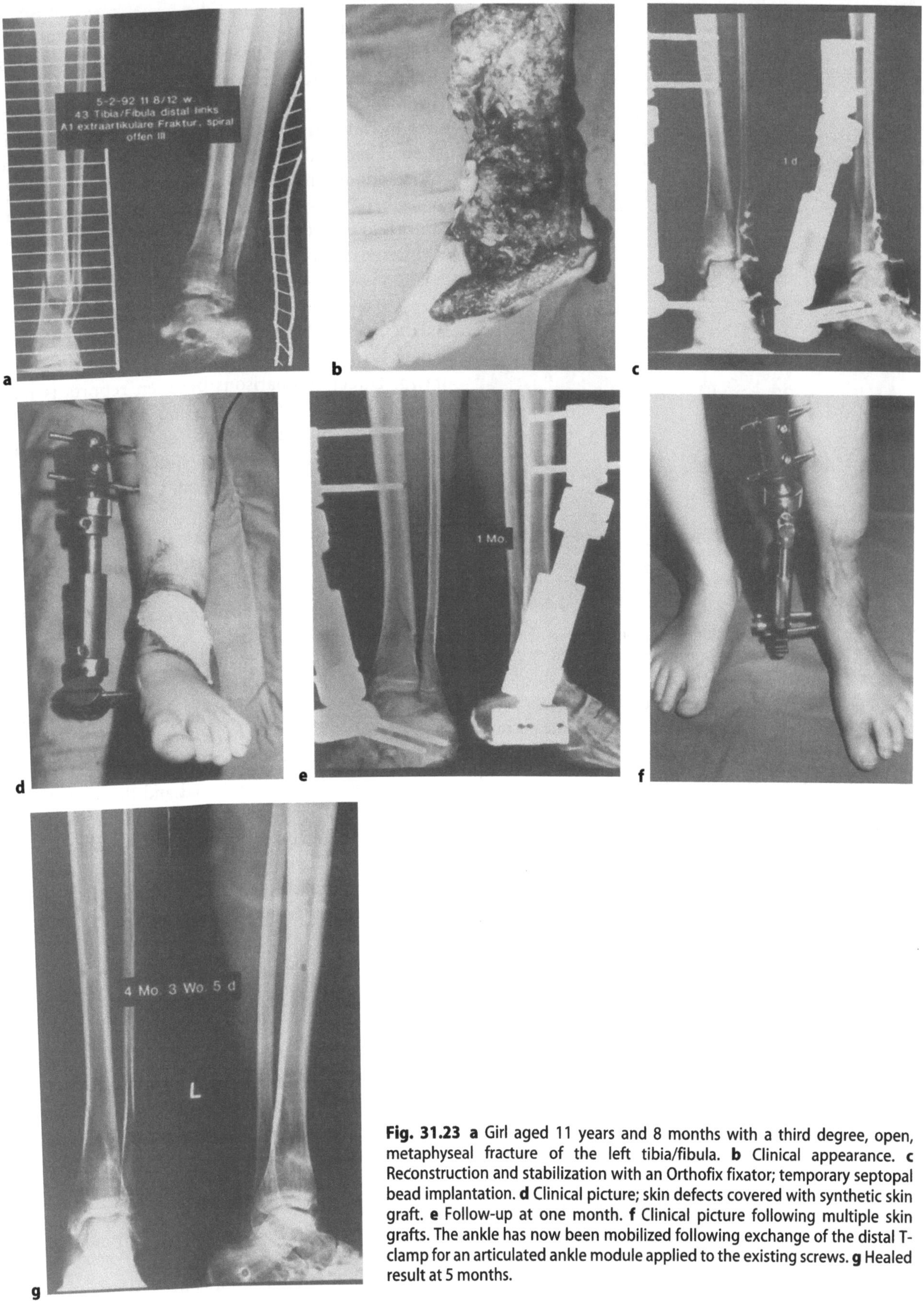

Fig. 31.23 **a** Girl aged 11 years and 8 months with a third degree, open, metaphyseal fracture of the left tibia/fibula. **b** Clinical appearance. **c** Reconstruction and stabilization with an Orthofix fixator; temporary septopal bead implantation. **d** Clinical picture; skin defects covered with synthetic skin graft. **e** Follow-up at one month. **f** Clinical picture following multiple skin grafts. The ankle has now been mobilized following exchange of the distal T-clamp for an articulated ankle module applied to the existing screws. **g** Healed result at 5 months.

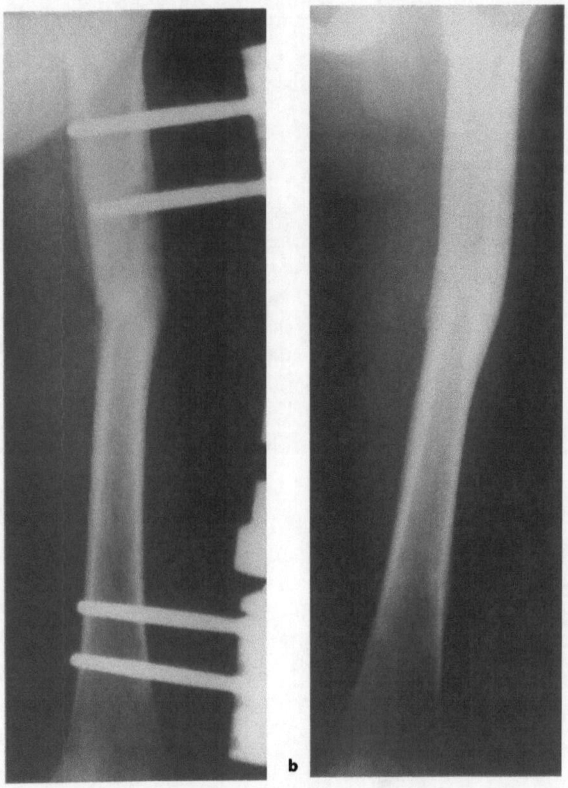

Fig. 31.24 a Pin track infection with radiological evidence of osteolysis in the region of the proximal pins. **b** Healed result.

In post-operative management, physiotherapy has a special part to play. A step-by-step programme permits children with single injuries to return to full weightbearing as early as the second week. With intramedullary stable elastic splinting, on the other hand, full weightbearing is possible after 3–4 weeks at the earliest. Generally, the children treated with external fixation stay in hospital until full weightbearing has been achieved. After discharge, in the second to third week, they can attend school or kindergarten.

Axial dynamization for childhood fractures remains controversial. Even when the fixator is locked, micromovement is sufficient to initiate callus formation. There are no published studies on the duration of fracture healing in children where dynamization has been employed. Fracture-specific peculiarities and the variable, age-dependent duration of fracture healing do not permit us to draw reliable conclusions at this stage. It is our impression, however, that even where axial dynamization is instituted, the duration of fracture healing is unlikely to be markedly shortened.

The conical thread of the pins permits their unaided removal in the out-patient department without anaesthesia or analgesia, once the fracture has healed. A second surgical intervention under anaesthetic is not necessary.

Refractures are rare and generally occur after premature removal of the external fixator. These must be regarded as treatment errors.

Pin-track infections prejudice the treatment of fractures in children by external fixation, and this fact is often quoted by those who use other methods. Despite conscientious pin care, the frequency in our patients is somewhere between 4 and 5 per cent. However, in contrast to the situation in adults, pin-track infections in children do not require surgical intervention.

Follow-up results refer to limb length discrepancies as well as residual axial and rotational malalignment. The reports published in the literature to date, do not permit any definitive conclusions to be drawn. Direct comparisons between reports is not possible, because there is as yet no uniform fracture classification or standardized series of follow-up criteria. It has been shown, however, that post-traumatic alterations in leg length generally remain during the growth period.[1,7,12,14,22,29,30,31,42,51] In our patients, maximum discrepancies in leg length of 3cm were found. This does not differ significantly from the values reported for other methods, but information on primary idiopathic differences in limb length remain unknown.

In our patients, residual axial malalignment was observed in 6.8 per cent of femoral fractures. Our overall figure for axial malalignment of 5.0 per cent is relatively low in comparison to other studies. The idea that any remaining axial malalignment fully corrects itself has not yet been confirmed and the long-term results after full bone remodelling should be awaited, since in most of our cases, growth is still in progress. To avoid axial malalignment, the primary aim should always be stabilization of the fracture using an external fixator. Rotational errors did not occur.

Summary

Our experience, which is confirmed by other reports, indicates that fractures in children may be treated adequately with unilateral dynamic axial fixators (Orthofix®). In addition to the classical indications, diaphyseal and metaphyseal fractures of the lower extremity and fractures of the trochanteric and transcervical regions can be treated. In the upper extremity, however, external fixation is only indicated in exceptional circumstances.

The versatile, modular Orthofix System can be adapted to treat fractures from the second year of life onwards, and the advantages for the child are:

1. definitive fracture management over a short period of time without traumatizing the soft tissues
2. early mobilization and full weightbearing, permitting early return to school or kindergarten
3. stabilization of open fractures whether or not accompanied by excessive soft tissue injury
4. the possibility of secondary callus distraction
5. no need for a second surgical intervention to remove hardware
6. no prolonged period of physiotherapy
7. fracture treatment in line with children's needs, maintaining their quality of life.

The application of external fixation is simple and does not involve high risks. The primary aim when using it is always stabilization of the fracture. Complications are rare. Temporary pin-track infections are a method-induced disadvantage. The follow-up results are comparable to those of competing methods.

References

1. Aronson J, Tursky EH (1992) 'External fixation of femur fractures in children.' *J Pediatr Orthop* 12: 157–63.
2. Asche G (1986) 'Die Anwendung des Fixateur externe bei kindlichen Frakturen.' *Zentbl Chir* 111: 391–7.
3. Asche G (1990) 'Erfahrungen mit dem Fixateur externe bei der Behandlung kindlicher Frakturen.' in: Asche G (Hrsg.): *Wege der Osteosynthese mit dem Fixateur externe.* Howmedica: Schönkirchen, S. 69–74
4. Bennek J, Brock D, Rothe K, Bühligen U (1993) 'Versorgung kindlicher Schaftfrakturen mit dem Fixateur externe.' *Langenbecks Arch Chir Suppl* (Kongreßbericht): 901–4.
5. Bennek J (1993) 'Die Versorgung kindlicher Frakturen.' in: Neumann HS, Klein W, Brug E (Hrsg.): *Die dynamisch-axiale externe Fixation.* Marseille: München, S. 125–37.
6. Bennek J, Müller W, Brock D, Bühligen U (1995) 'Versorgung kindlicher Femurschaftfrakturen mit dem Fixateur externe.' *Langenbecks Arch Chir* Suppl II (Kongreßbericht): 1290–5.
7. Blasier RD, Aronson J, Tursky EA (1997) 'External Fixation of Pediatric Femur Fractures.' *J Pediatr Orthop* 17, 342–6.
8. Breitfuß H, Muhr G (1988) 'Läßt sich vermehrtes Längenwachstum nach kindlichen Oberschenkelfrakturen vermeiden?' *Unfallchirurg* 91: 189–94.
9. Brug E, Klein W, Grünert J (1987) 'Die Behandlung der offenen Frakturen mit dem Fixateur externe – mit Berücksichtigung der dynamisch-axialen Fixation "Orthofix".' *Chirurg* 58: 699–705.
10. Brug E, Pennig D, Gähler R, Haeske-Seeberg H (1988) 'Polytrauma und Femurfraktur.' *Akt Traumatol* 18: 125–8.
11. Bühligen U, Herpisch D (1993) 'Das physiotherapeutische Stufenprogramm von Kindern mit Orthofix-Versorgung.' in: Neumann HS, Klein W, Brug E (Hrsg.): *Die dynamisch-axiale externe Fixation.* Marseille: München, S. 237–40.
12. Canale ST, Tolo VT (1995) 'Fractures of the Femur in Children.' *J Bone Joint Surg* [Am] 77 A: 294–315.
13. De Bastiani G, Aldegheri G, Renzi-Brivio L (1984) 'Treatment of fractures with a dynamic axial fixator.' *J Bone Joint Surg* [Br] 66B: 538–45.
14. De Sanctis N, Gambardella A, Pempinello C, Mallano P, Della Corte S (1996) 'The use of external fixation in femur fractures in children'. *J Pediatr Orthop* 16, 613–20.
15. Dietz HG, Rösch B (1992) 'Infektionen nach Osteosynthesen im Kindesalter.' *Unfallchirurg* 95: 160–2.
16. Engert J (1982) 'Indikation und Anwendung des Fixateur externe im Kindesalter.' *Z Kinderchir* 36: 133–7.
17. Erikson E, Hovelius L (1979) 'Internal nailing in fractures of the diaphysis of the femur.' *J Bone Joint Surg* [Am] 61A: 1178–81.
18. Feld C, Gotzen L, Hannich T (1993) 'Die kindliche Femurschaftfraktur in der Altersgruppe 6–14 Jahre. Ein retrospektiver Therapievergleich zwischen konservativer Behandlung, Plattenosteosynthese und externer Stabilisierung.' *Unfallchirurg* 96: 169–74.
19. Giebel G (1992) *Callus Distraction: Clinical Applications.* Thieme: Stuttgart New York.
20. Guichet JM, Spivak JM, Trouilloud P, Grammont PM (1991) 'Lower limb-length discrepancy. An epidemiologic study.' *Clin Orthop* (US) 272: 235–41.
21. Hehl G, Kiefer H, Bauer G, Völck C (1993) 'Posttraumatische Beinlängendifferenzen nach konservativer und operativer Therapie kindlicher Oberschenkelschaftfrakturen.' *Unfallchirurg* 96: 651–5.
22. Kapukaya A, Subasi M, Necmioglu S, Arslan H, Kesemenli C, Yildirim K 1998) 'Treatment of closed femoral diaphyseal fractures with external fixators in children.' *Arch Orthop Trauma Surg* 117, 387–9.
23. Keating JF, Gardner E, Leach WJ, Macpherson S, Abrami G (1991) 'Management of tibial fractures with the orthofix dynamic extemal fixator.' *J R Coll Surg Edinb* (Scotland) 36: 272–7.
24. Kirby EM, Winquist RA, Hansen ST (1981) 'Femoral shaft fractures in adolescents: a comparsion between traction plus cast treatment and closed intramedullary nailing.' *J Pediatr Orthop* 1: 193–7.
25. Kirschenbaum D, Albert MC, Robertson WW, Davidson RS (1990) 'Complex femur fractures in children: treatment with external fixation.' *J Pediatr Orthop* 10: 588–91.
26. Klein W, Pennig D, Brug E (1989) 'Die Anwendung eines unilateralen Fixateur externe bei der kindlichen Femurfraktur im Rahmen des Polytraumas.' *Unfallchirurg* 92: 282–6.
27. Klein W, Pennig D, Brug E (1990) 'Dynamic axial fixation for femoral fractures in children.' in: Vidal JG, Dossa JG (Hrsg.): *Evolution de la fixation externe... et l'orthofix! ... Du statique au dynamique... Traitement déxception? Traitement de routine?* Université de Montpellier.
28. Klein W, Pennig D, Grünert J, Brug E (1990) 'Die Behandlung kindlicher Femurschaftfrakturen mit einem unilateralen Fixateur externe.' *Hefte Unfallheilk* 212: 50–1.
29. Krettek C, Haas N, Tscherne H (1989) 'Versorgung der Femurschaftfrakturen im Wachstumsalter mit dem Fixateur externe.' *Akt Traumatol* 19: 255–61.
30. Laer von L (1977) 'Beinlängendifferenzen und Rotationsfehler nach Oberschenkelfrakturen im Kindesalter.' *Arch Orthop Unfallchir* 89: 121–37.
31. Laer von L (1991) *Frakturen und Luxationen im Wachstumsalter.* Thieme: Stuttgart New York
32. Ligier JN, Metaizeau A, Prevot J, Lascombes P (1985) 'Elastic stable intramedullary pinning of long bone shaft fractures in children.' *Z Kinderchir* 10: 209–12.
33. Linhart WE, Spendel S, Mayr H, Schwendenwein E (1992) 'Die elastisch stabile intramedulläre Schienung kindlicher Schaftfrakturen.' *Zent bl Kinderchir* 1: 215–20.
34. Mann DC, Weddington J, Davenport K (1986) 'Closed internal nailing of femoral shaft fractures in adolescents.' *J Pediatr Orthop* 6: 651–5.
35. Melendez EM, Colon C (1989) 'Treatment of open tibial fractures with the Orthofix fixator.' *Clin Orthop* (US) 241: 224–30.
36. Mittmann CH, Klein W, Brug E (1993) 'Die Indikation für die dynamisch-axiale Fixation bei Frakturen im Kindesalter.' in: Neumann HS, Klein W, Brug E (Hrsg.): *Die dynamisch-axiale externe Fixation.* Marseille: München, S. 119–24.

37. Müller ME, Nazarian S, Koch P (1989) *AO-Klassifikation der Frakturen.* Springer: Berlin Heidelberg New York.
38. Nast-Kolb DC, Jochum M, Waydhas CH, Schweiberer L (1991) *Die klinische Wertigkeit biochemischer Faktoren beim Polytrauma.* Springer: Berlin Heidelberg New York.
39. Neugebauer R, Becker U, Stinner A (1990) 'Die Behandlung der kindlichen Oberschenkelfraktur mit dem lateralen Klammerfixateur (Technik, Nachsorge, Ergebnisse).' *Hefte Unfallheilkd* 212: 363.
40. Purschke CH, Bühligen U (1993) 'Akzeptanz des Gerätes "Orthofix" beim Kind.' in: Neumann HS, Klein W, Brug E (Hrsg.): *Die dynamisch-axiale externe Fixation.* Marseille: München, S. 241–7.
41. Saleh M (1992) 'External fixation of long bone fractures in children.' *J Bone Joint Surg* [Br] 74B 2: 152.
42. Scavenius M, Ebskov LB, Sloth C, Torholm C (1993) 'External Fixation with the Orthofix System in Dislocated Fractures of the Lower Extremities in Children.' *J Pediatr Orthop* Part B 2: 161–9.
43. Schmidt W, Rolle U, Bennek J (1994) 'Klinisch-anatomische Studien zur Pin-Implantation bei "äußerer" Osteosynthese von Schaftfrakturen mit dem Fixateur externe.' *Osteologie Suppl* 13: 43.
44. Schranz PJ, Gultekin C, Colton CL (1992) 'External fixation of fractures in children.' *Injury* 23: 80–2.
45. Shih HN, Chen LM, Lee ZL, Shih CH (1989) 'Treatment of femoral shaft fractures with the Hoffmann external fixator in prepuberty.' *J Trauma* 29: 498–501.
46. Siegmeth A, Wruhs O, Vécsei V (1998) 'External fixation of lower limb fractures in children.' *Eur J Pediatr Surg* 8, 35–41.
47. Sim E, Schaden W (1990) 'Indikation und Technik der operativen Behandlung von Schienbeinschaftbrüchen bei offenen Epiphysenfugen.' *Unfallchir* 93: 262–9.
48. Stedtfeld HW, Taruttis H, Schneider M (1993) 'Die Oberschenkelfraktur des (Schul-) Kindes.' in: Neumann HS, Klein W, Brug E (Hrsg.): *Die dynamisch-axiale externe Fixation.* Marseille: München, S. 139–48.
49. Turker R, Lubicky JP, Vogel LC (1992) 'Toxic Shock Syndrome in Patients with External Fixators.' *J Pediatr Orthop* 12: 658–62.
50. van Tets WF, van der Werken C (1992) 'External fixation for diaphyseal femoral fractures: a benefit to the young child?' *Injury* 23: 162–4.
51. Weinberg AM, Reilmann H, Lampert C, Laer von L (1994) 'Erfahrungen mit dem Fixateur externe bei der Behandlung von Schaftfrakturen im Kindesalter.' *Unfallchirurg* 97: 107–13.
52. Winquist RA, Hansen ST, Clawson DK (1984) 'Closed intramedullary nailing of femoral shaft: a report of five hundred and twenty cases.' *J Bone Joint Surg* [Am] 66A: 529–39.
53. Ziv I, Blackburn N, Rang M (1984) 'Femoral intramedullary nailing in the growing child.' *J Trauma* 24: 432–4.

The Management of Acute Bone Loss Following Trauma

32

M. Saleh

In recent years orthopaedic surgeons have been increasingly faced with the problem of bone loss following open tibial fractures. Advances in fracture fixation techniques and in the handling of soft tissues have meant that many more limbs are now saved. In previous years severe open tibial fractures associated with bone loss were frequently treated by primary or secondary amputation. Recently, however, the incidence of infection following open tibial fracture has dropped dramatically and the problem of how to manage large bone defects is now the most challenging problem that orthopaedic traumatologists encounter.

Occasionally patients will present with a missing bone segment but more commonly it becomes clear at the time of the initial debridement that there is extensive bone damage and periosteal stripping. Consequently the surgeon has to resect bone, thereby creating a bone defect. If this defect is left, a malunion or a non-union will inevitably ensue. Occasionally the orthopaedic surgeon will be faced with a bone defect that has followed bone resection carried out for infected non-union, osteomyelitis or malignancy. The treatment of these secondary defects is the same as for a primary defect that has occurred following a severe open tibial fracture.

In this chapter the various options for treating tibial bone loss are discussed with particular reference to limited bone grafting and the use of callus distraction. Bifocal techniques are described for simultaneous osteosynthesis and bone lengthening. In addition, the technique of primary bone shortening to facilitate union followed by secondary bone lengthening using callus distraction will be described.

Classification

Any classification of bone loss should make the distinction between partial and complete bone loss and any comprehensive description of the problem should include the volume of bone loss or the length of the bone defect. The classification of the Orthopaedic Trauma Association is in widespread use (Fig. 32.1) In this classification the type 1 lesion involves less than 50 per cent of the diameter; type II bone loss is present when there is more than 50 per cent of the diameter missing; in type III bone loss there is complete bone loss involving a circumferential segment (Gustilo, 1991).

In the AO classification (Müller et al, 1990) of tibial diaphyseal fractures the C3 group consists of irregular complex fractures and the C3.3 subgroup is composed of diaphyseal fractures which are associated with significant comminution. Thus many of the tibial fractures that present with bone loss will be C3.3 in severity. Although the degree of bone loss is not selectively defined by the AO classification, an extensive description of the soft tissue and bony damage may be compiled using the various descriptors that are allied to the main AO classification. The Gustilo classification of open fractures (Gustilo and Anderson, 1976; Gustilo et al, 1984) does not address the problem of bone loss but obviously only IIIB and IIIC fractures will be associated with bone loss. There is no current classification for bone shortening but shortening should be described in terms of its location within the bone and its extent, the latter being expressed as a percentage of the current segment length.

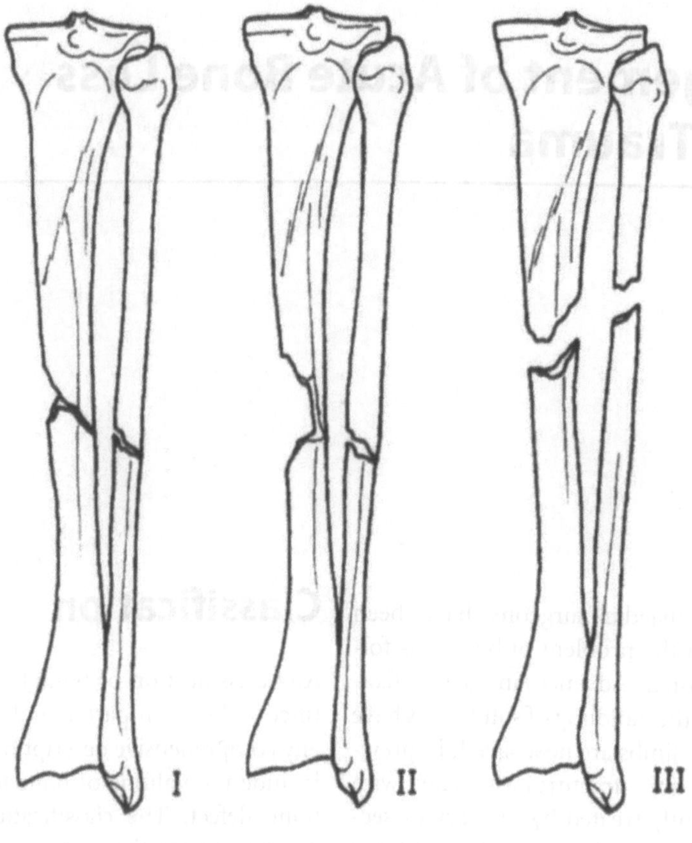

Fig. 32.1 The OTA classification of bone loss.

Management Principles for Fractures with Bone Loss

Analysis of data from the Edinburgh Orthopaedic Trauma Unit concerning open tibial diaphyseal fractures (Court-Brown and Rose, 1995) has shown that 27 per cent of patients who present with a Gustilo IIIB open tibial fracture are multiply injured and that 70 per cent of these patients have other orthopaedic injuries. It is therefore obvious that many patients who present with tibial bone loss will be seriously injured. It is therefore vital that a surgeon carefully evaluates the overall condition of the patient as well as carrying out an adequate assessment of the injured limb.

Primary examination of the injured limb should involve a careful evaluation of the state of the soft tissues and the bone. If possible, the surgeon should ask about the pre-operative physical state of the patient and ascertain whether he or she may have had peripheral vascular disease, diabetes or any other condition that might have affected the viability of the limb. These and other factors such as the amount of muscle damage and the presence of posterior tibial nerve damage may suggest to the surgeon that primary amputation is the treatment of choice.

Initial treatment should aim to restore the circulation to the limb by volume replacement, fracture reduction and vascular repair if this is required. It is mandatory that a thorough debridement be undertaken and that the surgeon should interally or externally fix the diaphyseal fracture and any related adjacent articular fractures. Keating et al (1994) have shown that 5 per cent of tibial diaphyseal fractures are associated with intra-articular fractures of either the knee or ankle. Failure to treat these adequately will lead to severe disability. Early mobilization of the knee, ankle and subtalar joints is essential and fracture fixation, must aim to allow this as soon as possible after surgery. The goal of fracture treatment is not merely to achieve union but to achieve the best possible mobility for the limb and the patient. The surgeon must be particularly aware of the problems of leaving untreated foot fractures. These are frequently ignored and lead to crippling disabilities. It is advised that compartment pressure monitoring should be carried out where possible, but if this is not available for the surgeon he or she must have a low threshold for fasciotomy. The effects of compartment syndrome occur rapidly and last for the patient's lifetime.

Initial Fracture Surgery

The most important part of the initial operation is debridement. It is vital that all devitalized soft tissue and bone are removed at the time of the initial wound exploration. Care must be taken to assess the state of the skin around the open wound and the extent of any associated degloving. The viability of the local musculature must be assessed and all devitalized muscle removed. Failure to do this will greatly increase the risk of infection. Gentle lavage is recommended, together with appropriate use of intravenous antibiotic prophylaxis. The open wounds should not be closed under any circumstances and can be treated by secondary closure, split-skin grafting or flap cover at a later time.

All Gustilo type III fractures should be treated by a secondary debridement 24–36 hours after the initial wound inspection. If the wound remains dirty at this time a third debridement must be performed. If by the third debridement the wound still contains devitalized tissues the surgeon must consider whether there has been significant muscle crushing and that it may not be possible to save the limb.

Bone grafting should only be undertaken after good soft tissue healing has been achieved. If bone grafting is undertaken at the time of skin closure or flap cover there is a risk of infection and the bone graft will be lost. The Papineau technique (Papineau et al, 1979) involves packing areas of bone loss with graft and allowing the skin to granulate. With the introduction of improved plastic surgery techniques this technique has now been superseded by either flap cover and corticocancellous grafting or by bone transport. Following initial debridement the treatment principles are bone realignment and stabilization followed by fracture stimulation to secure union (Ribbans et al, 1992; Saleh and Scott, 1992).

Fracture Realignment and Stabilization

At the time of the initial debridement it may not seem important to realign the bone adequately. However, there is no better time to achieve correct bony alignment. The bone will almost invariably be easily visible in the wound and the surgeon must undertake adequate fracture stabilization with correct alignment.

In the management of severe open tibial fractures associated with bone loss there is no place for the use of casts or braces. Such methods of managing severe open tibial fractures are outdated and should not be used. Three major fixation methods are available to the surgeon. These are bone plating, intramedullary nailing, using either a reamed or unreamed nail, and external skeletal fixation.

The AO group were responsible for revolutionary new ideas in the management of open tibial fractures. They advocated the use of rigid bone plates but it became clear that there were a number of problems associated with this technique. Bone plating is the most difficult of the three techniques to do well, as the soft tissues must be stripped away from the bone to allow the plate to be inserted. If this is not done carefully there can be significant bone avascularity and infection and non-union will ensue. Even if done carefully, the use of bone plates in the presence of bone loss means that a very large plate must be applied and considerable soft tissue dissection undertaken.

Other disadvantages of plating were that surgeons often left devitalized bone segments in position to provide structural "stability". Bone healing using rigid plate fixation was slow with callus formation being significantly lessened by the rigid nature of the implant. Thus there was a high incidence of non-union and infection with Clifford et al (1988) quoting an infection rate of 7.8 per cent in Gustilo type II fractures and 44.4 per cent in type III open fractures.

Plate fixation of open tibial fractures has now largely been superseded by either intramedullary nailing or external skeletal fixation. There is still debate about the relative merits of intramedullary nailing and external fixation and about whether surgeons should use reamed or unreamed nails if intramedullary nailing is selected. Court-Brown and his co-workers have reported on the use of reamed intramedullary nails in Gustilo type III open fractures over the past four years (Court-Brown et al, 1991; Court-Brown and Rose, 1995). In the initial paper they reported the incidence of infection in Gustilo type III fractures to be 11.1 per cent with the infection rate in the IIIB subgroup being 23 per cent. A later analysis undertaken by Court-Brown and Rose (1995) of intramedullary nailing of open tibial fractures over a 7-year period showed that the overall infection rate in Gustilo type III open tibial fractures had dropped to 5.5 per cent with a 10.7 per cent incidence in the IIIB subgroup. Despite these excellent results the use of nailing in more severe cases is still viewed with caution by many surgeons as they feel that retained devitalized tissue may lead to intramedullary infection which is perceived to be difficult to treat. With careful surgery, however, and adherence to the strict surgical principles of treating infection, it is possible to treat sepsis associated with intramedullary nailing (Court-Brown et al, 1992). Unreamed nails have been investigated by a number of authors (Whittle et al, 1992; Fairbank et al, 1995). The literature concerning the advantages of reamed or unreamed nails is confusing, but at this time clinical studies have not indicated that unreamed nails are superior to reamed nails and they are certainly mechanically weaker and associated with higher breakage rates.

The third method of bone fixation is external skeletal fixation. This is viewed by many surgeons as the safest method of treatment as the screws remain at a distance from the fracture site and this is thought to reduce the incidence of deep infection. In recent years there have been considerable advances in the philosophy and design of external skeletal fixators. Older external fixators tended to produce rigid fixation and often lead to unacceptably high pin site infection rates as well as delayed and non-union (Edge and Denham, 1981; Court-Brown et al, 1990), although Edwards et al (1988) achieved excellent results in grade III open fractures using primary external fixation but changing later to plaster cast management. As a result of the relatively poor results obtained using earlier external fixators some surgeons investigated the role of initial external fixation followed by secondary intramedullary nailing (McGraw and Lim, 1988; Maurer et al, 1989; Blachut et al, 1990). There was debate about the use of this technique but some of the investigators had a high incidence of post-traumatic osteomyelitis which was thought to be due to seeding from pin sites and this technique is probably best reserved for the management of failed cases (Marshall et al, 1991).

In recent years third generation fixators have been devised. These are bimodal external fixation devices which allow the mechanical environment to be switched from rigid to elastic (De Bastiani et al, 1984). Marsh et al (1991) showed that high union rates and a low infection rate could be achieved using the third generation Orthofix fixator (Orthofix srl, Verona, Italy), although malunion rates tended to be somewhat higher than with intramedullary nailing. External fixation is particularly indicated when there is doubt about tissue viability, overt infection or established shortening or significant bone loss. Ideally, external fixation should be applied in such a way that it can be used for definitive fracture treatment. With the Orthofix external fixation device two or three 6mm screws are inserted into each of two clamps, one on each side of the fracture. If the fracture is eccentric in the limb a supplementary screw may be placed in the longer bone segment for additional stability (Fig. 32.2). For maximum stability the inner screw should be no more than 6cm from the fracture site. If obese or osteoporotic patients are being treated it is recommended that three screws are inserted into each clamp. As with all external fixation devices the exact placement of the screws should be discussed with the plastic surgeon if there is a large area of soft tissue loss. Recommendations have been made for safe screw placement (BOA/BAPS, 1993) but the exact positioning of individual pins will depend on the area of soft tissue loss and the proposed reconstructive technique. The anterior mounting, although technically demanding, is safe for all soft tissue reconstructive procedures (Fig. 32.3). In some circumstances circular or hybrid constructs may be preferred since tensioned wires appear to produce superior holding power in soft and metaphyseal bone and the constructs are easily adapted to cross joints.

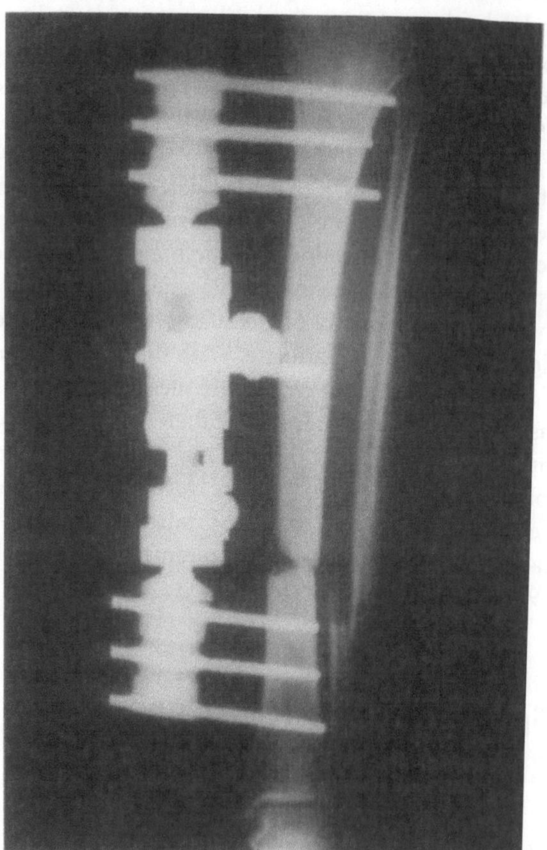

Fig. 32.2 An open fracture of the distal third of the tibia with grade II bone loss. A supplementary external fixator screw has been used to provide enhanced stability.

Fracture Stimulation

Fractures require stability and bone contact for healing. Contact areas may be improved by square osteotomy or bone grafting. Cancellous bone grafting remains the mainstay of this aspect of treatment. Smaller bone defects should be filled with cancellous autograft. If structural support is required a corticocancellous graft may be used. The iliac crest donor site is the source of significant and often understated morbidity. The incidence of donor site complications in one series was 9.4 per cent and included chronic wound pain and hypersensitivity, buttock anaesthesia, muscle herniation, meralgia paraesthetica and even subluxation of the hip (Cockin, 1971). Meralgia paraesthetica was also described by Weikel and Habal (1977). In another series chronic donor site pain was reported in 25 per cent of patients but this was associated particularly with tricortical grafts (Summers and Eisenstein, 1989). A limited percutaneous approach for harvesting grafts using a trephine is preferred to open techniques (Saleh, 1991) and is associated with reduced donor site morbidity (Kreibich et al, 1994).

If a fracture fails to progress to union this may be due to biomechanical or vascular reasons. Biomechanically the fracture may be excessively mobile or too stable. Fractures with biomechanical instability tend to produce hypertrophic non-unions and these can be treated either by exchange nailing (Court-Brown et al, 1995), plating (Müller and Thomas, 1978) or by altering the configuration of the external fixator. An unstable external fixator may be due to inadequate screws, loose screws or soft bone, and stability may be increased by adding extra screws or a supplementary cast. A tight Achilles tendon should be released as this is a potent stress point. If the fixation is producing stress protection, reducing the level of fracture support may be achieved with a fibular osteotomy, dynamization or progressive destabilization. Other means of stimulation include increasing vascularity and loading with exercise, weightbearing and flap surgery.

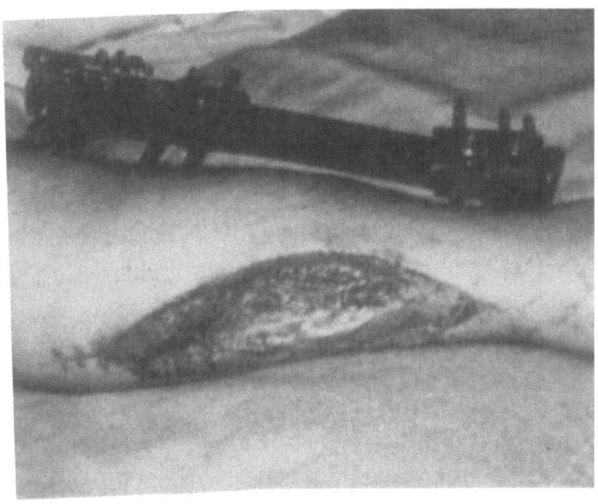

Fig. 32.3 An anteriorly mounted unilateral external fixator allows good access to most soft tissue defects.

Type I Bone Loss

Type I bone loss represents less than 50 per cent of the diameter of the bone (see Fig. 32.1). In this situation the fracture should be reduced accurately and stabilized using either an intramedullary nail or an external fixation device. Depending on the degree of comminution, the length should be easily maintained and bone contact will contribute to overall stability. Usually the nail or external fixator is not unduly stressed because of the degree of shared loading with the bone. The limb is initially elevated to allow the soft tissues to rest, and monitored carefully for signs of compartment syndrome. Non-weightbearing or partial weightbearing mobilization is then commenced depending on the degree of stability achieved with the fixation system. The soft tissues are allowed to heal and autogenous cancellous bone grafting performed at 6 weeks. The surgical approach is dictated by the location of the defect and is usually mid-lateral or posteromedial. A direct anteromedial approach should be avoided since this could result in a wound problem. If flap cover has been performed, the surgical approach must be carefully planned to avoid the base or pedicle of the flap. Mobilization of a flap may require a large skin incision as the tissues are often firm and difficult to mobilize. If a fixator has been used it is recommended that the leg be elevated for 24 hours before bone grafting and that the pin sites are as clean as possible.

Surgical Technique For Type I Bone Loss

If a fixator has been used the fixator and pin sites are isolated from the operative site. The skin is prepared with an aqueous antiseptic, as are the pin sites. The convenient way of covering the fixator is with a bowel bag which has a drawstring tie at its opening. The bag ties around the screws adjacent to the skin and is covered by a 5cm crepe bandage. The limb is covered with stockinette or a plastic leg bag and the wound area exposed by cutting into the bag and applying a clear adhesive wound dressing. A tourniquet is not usually necessary. The levels of the defect are carefully marked on the skin either by transfer of a radiological measurement or X-ray screening. The approach is chosen according to soft tissue constraints and the site of the bone defect.

If the posteromedial. approach is used, a 5cm incision provides direct access to the bone. Using a mid-lateral approach a 7cm incision is usually required. The deep fascia is incised and the extensor muscles are displaced posteriorly to gain access to the lateral side of the tibia. The incision is marked on the skin and the approach continued down to the bone. The approach should permit direct access to the fracture on one surface only. Bone levers should not be used since these strip the tissues unnecessarily. Whenever possible a subperiosteal approach is made to the bone. Occasionally, when working in a submuscular region, the Judet technique of decortication (Judet and Patel, 1972) may be used, although in general this technique is more useful in the femur than the tibia. Even at 6 weeks the defect may be filled with fibrous tissue and the bone should be palpated with a dissector until a soft area is entered or a break in continuity is detected. Sharp dissection is then used followed by curettage with a Volkmann's spoon to expose the defect. A high speed dental burr may be used to denude the bone ends of fibrous tissue. The bed is correctly prepared when the bone edges are exposed and bleeding and the surrounding tissue is shown to be vascular. It is recommended that if a tourniquet has been used it is deflated at this stage.

Fine cancellous autograft is packed into the defect and the author's preference is to harvest this using a percutaneous approach (Saleh, 1991). Grafts may also be laid in the submuscular plane adjacent to the presenting cortex. If the presenting cortex looks avascular it may be petalled using an osteotome. The wound is then closed in layers and a drain placed in a separate layer from the graft. If, following this procedure, the bone gap is eliminated but the fracture line persists, dynamization or fibular osteotomy may be required. Occasionally, a second bone graft is required for a persistent defect. The aim of this early active intervention is to ensure that shared loading is achieved as rapidly as possible and fracture healing occurs well before fixation failure.

Type II Bone Loss

In type II bone loss there is a loss of more than 50 per cent of the bone diameter (see Fig. 32.1). These injuries may be complicated by vascular damage and soft tissue loss. Realignment and stabilization are carried out rapidly with a view to restoring the circulation and permitting vascular repair. Since there may be little in the way of shared loading, fixation stability is much more critical than for type I injuries. If there is an extensive soft tissue defect the fixator screws should be placed well away from the fracture site providing adequate temporary support whilst the patient is on supervised bed rest. Fasciotomies are not infrequently required. Supplementary external fixator screws may be added within one or two weeks, if necessary, through the site of the flap, taking care not to damage its vascular pedicle. Good quality soft tissue cover is vital to healing since at least two bone grafts will be required. Occasionally, and particularly in the elderly where soft tissue is poor, acute shortening may be used to convert the fracture line to a more stable configuration with well vascularized bone ends (Edwards, 1983). Grafting should be performed at around 6 weeks, adhering to the same careful surgical principles used in type I injuries. Often, however, the most appropriate approach is posterolateral. At 12 weeks an anterior graft is inserted using a mid-lateral or posteromedial approach (Fig. 32.4). Cancellous autograft is preferred, although corticocancellous grafting may occasionally be considered where stability is a problem. This technique is less than ideal since there remain two fracture surfaces to be incorporated and typically one heals preferentially. Where there is major pelvic damage, a poor quality iliac crest or a large defect, morcellized allograft mixed with the patient's own marrow has proved useful in the author's experience. In very resistant cases a repeat posterolateral approach may be used for tibiofibular grafting (Vidal et al, 1982).

Surgical Technique For Type II Bone Loss

The posterolateral approach is contraindicated if the posterior tibial artery is the only blood supply to the leg. This is, however, rare and a posterolateral approach will commonly be used for type II bone loss. The procedure is best performed with the patient in the prone position, although if the patient has respiratory problems the lateral position may be chosen. Depending on the quality of the tissue a 10-15cm incision may be required. This is sited just posterior to the

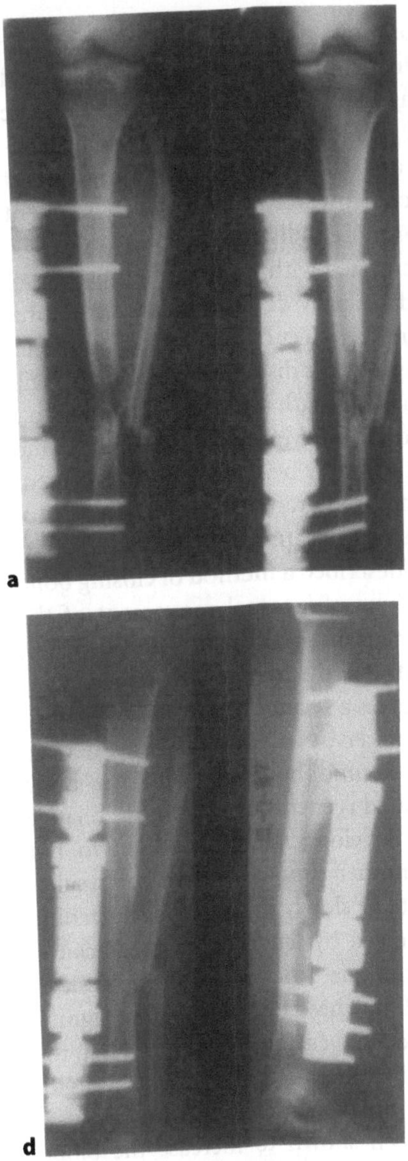

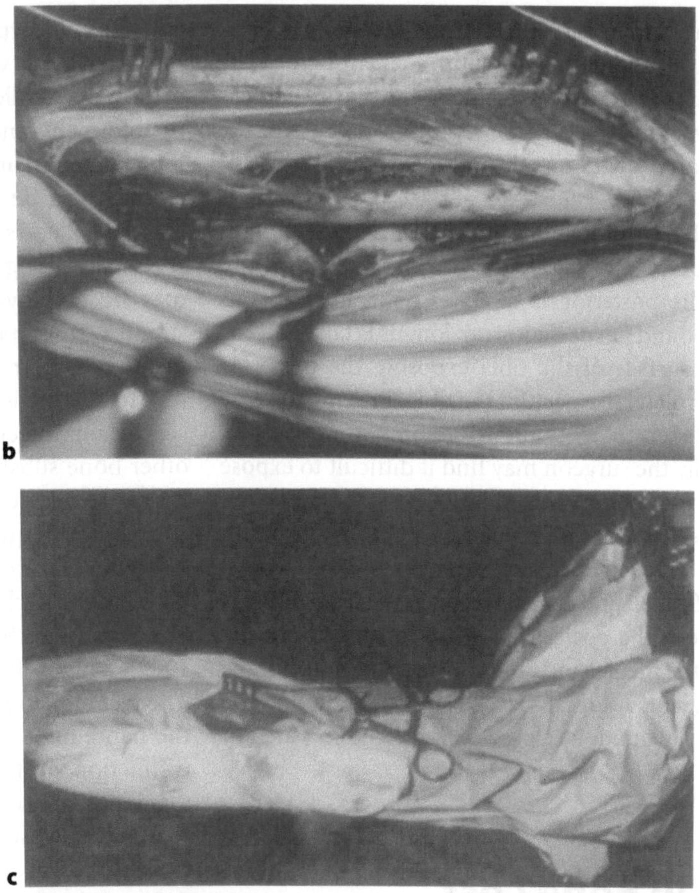

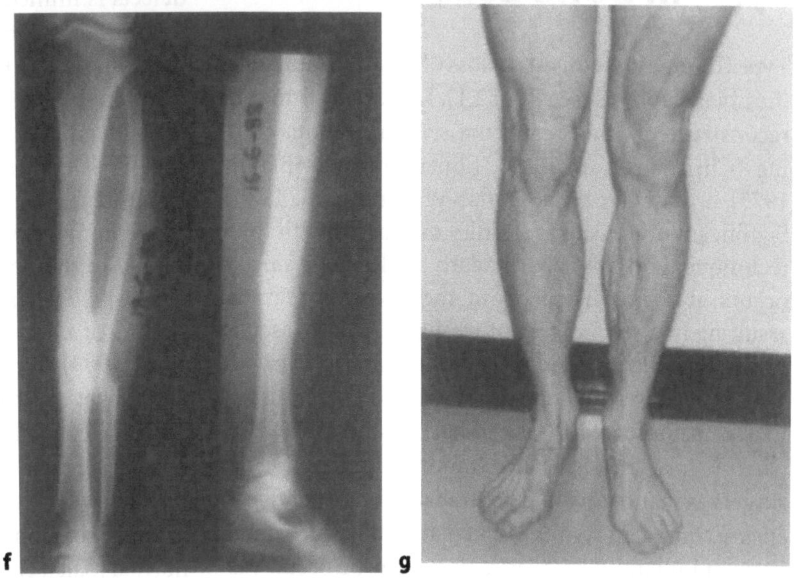

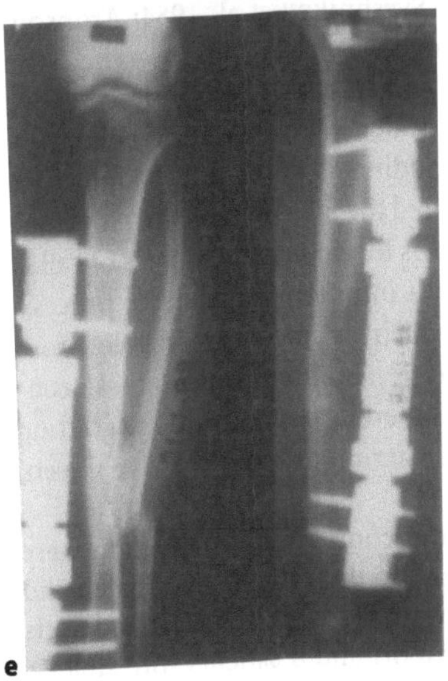

Fig. 32.4 The management of a Gustilo IIIC open tibial fracture. **a** A unilateral external fixator has been used to stabilize the fracture. **b** Posterolateral bone grafting was undertaken at 6 weeks; the operative approach is shown. **c** Anterolateral bone grafting was undertaken at 14 weeks; the operative approach is illustrated. Note how the external fixator has been isolated. **d** Radiological appearance of graft incorporation at 13 weeks. **e** Radiological appearances of graft incorporation at 22 weeks. **f** Radiological appearances of bone healing at one year. **g** Clinical appearance of leg at one year after fracture. Note the satisfactory cosmesis.

fibula. The deep fascia is divided and the thin posterior peroneal intermuscular septum identified. The peronei are separated from soleus and flexor hallucis longus by splitting along the septum. Branches of the peroneal artery winding around the fibula are identified and divided. The flexor surface of the fibula is exposed by stripping off the flexor hallucis longus which protects and carries the peroneal artery with it. The tibialis posterior is swept off the interosseous membrane and flexor digitorum longus is taken off the posterior surface of the tibia exposing the posterior and posterolateral aspects of the tibia. Proximally, care must be taken to avoid the common peroneal nerve, and distally the surgeon may find it difficult to expose the lower quarter of the tibia. Bone is laid into the defect after appropriate preparation of the non-union site as described in the management of type I bone loss. For tibiofibular grafting more bone is harvested and laid between the posterior and lateral surfaces of the tibia and the medial and anterior surfaces of the fibula. If insufficient autograft is present allograft may be used. The wound is closed in layers over suction drains.

Type III Bone Loss

Type III bone loss consists of loss of the full diameter of the tibial diaphysis (see Fig. 32.1). Large defects may be reconstructed with repeated massive autogenous grafting (Christian et al, 1989), fibular transfer (Blauth, 1973) or vascular bone grafts (Weiland et al, 1983). Significant donor site morbidity may occur with these techniques and this is particularly undesirable since it occurs at a site distant from the involved segment resulting in a second area of weakness. Microvascular procedures have a good record of reliability. They are long procedures but may be expedited by the use of two teams of surgeons, one to harvest and one to prepare the host area. Specialist training in microvascular surgery is mandatory and centralization is desirable to ensure consistent results. Particular caution is required in the traumatized limb since there may be occult vascular injury. The choice remains between transfer of the ipsilateral or contralateral fibula where a composite flap based on the deep circumflex iliac artery may be used. Such flaps may be raised with a soft tissue and skin component. In some tibial defects the ipsilateral fibula may be mobilized on its vascular pedicle and transplanted medially. Whether vascular or nonvascularized grafts are used, bone must be protected from stress for a considerable period to encourage full incorporation and hypertrophy of the imported bone. Close cooperation between plastic and orthopaedic colleagues is essential to ensure adequate re-alignment and stabilization. Microvascular techniques remain an attractive option, providing instant closure of a defect. However, the replaced segment may take 2 years or more to hypertrophy.

Cortical allograft fixed with an intramedullary nail may be employed to provide immediate structural support. Incorporation occurs by local junctional fusion. Vascular ingrowth is discouraged since this will lead to a reduction in strength and is associated with a significant infection risk. Morcellized allograft and other bone substitutes may be used as a replacement for autogenous cancellous graft but clinical experience of these techniques remains limited.

In 1969 Ilizarov described a method of closing bone defects by a technique of internal movement of the bone known as bone transport (Ilizarov and Ledyaev, 1969). This is illustrated diagramatically in Fig. 32.5. The technique involves a second bone division, hence the name bifocal surgery. New bone is generated by distraction at the second bone cut and the bone segment that is created is encouraged to move relative to the soft tissue envelope maintaining length but closing the gap. Another similar strategy for smaller defects is immediate or slowly progressive shortening to close a gap followed by lengthening at a healthy metaphysis, a technique known as compression-distraction (Fig. 32.5). These techniques have significant advantages over conventional methods. First, the surgery is confined to the affected segment. Second, using technetium uptake studies the metaphyseal corticotomy has been shown to increase the blood supply to the bone (Sveshnikov et al, 1984; Aronson, 1994). This has important implications when the healing of a non-union of the tibia is considered. Paley et al (1989) demonstrated the value of this clinically and believed that adding a corticotomy improved union rates and lowered the incidence of atrophic non-union. The new bone is formed by the process of callus distraction, a slow but infinitely controllable process, leading to bone which is indistinguishable from normal (Saleh et al, 1993). In three studies bifocal techniques have proved superior to repeated bone grafting (Marsh et al, 1994; Cierny and Zorn, 1994; Green, 1994).

Bone transport and compression-distraction were compared in one series in the author's unit (Saleh and Rees, 1995). There were 8 patients with large defects treated by bone transport and 8 patients with smaller defects or deformity treated by compression-distraction. There were 5 femoral and 11 tibial cases. At

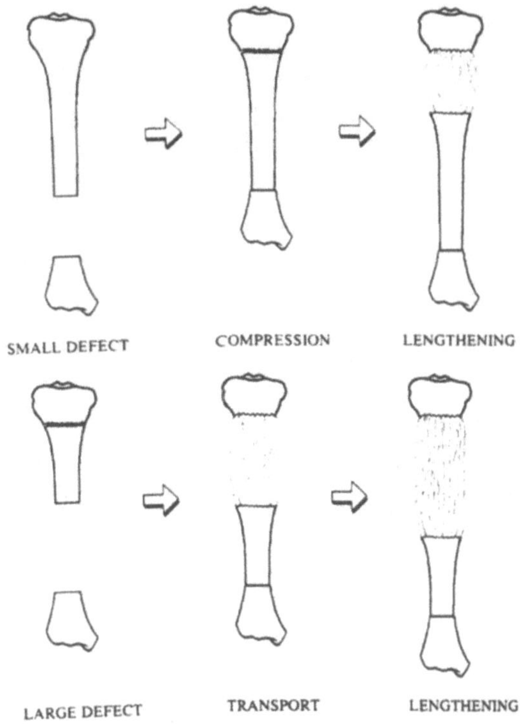

a

b

Fig. 32.5 A management scheme for bone loss. **a** Compression–distraction: for small defects (<3cm tibia or <5cm femur) compression of the defect is followed by osteotomy and lengthening at the other end of the bone. **b** Bone transport: in larger defects, lengthening and compression occur simultaneously so the middle segment of bone is transported to fill the defect. Once the defect has been closed, further lengthening can be carried out as required (from the *British Journal of Bone and Joint Surgery*, with permission).

a mean follow-up of 24 months all 16 patients had excellent or good results with union of the fracture, correction of deformity and restoration or near restoration of leg length without major complications. Treatment times were longer (mean 16 months) for bone transport compared with compression-distraction (mean 9.8 months) and the procedure was more complicated, requiring on average 2.2 additional operative procedures compared to only one for compression–distraction. Femoral cases had shorter treatment indices than tibial cases but were associated with a less favourable outcome.

In general, surgeons can choose between two types of external fixator. We have used the Orthofix monolateral fixator since it is a simple system with excellent rigidity. It is preferred to circular frames as it is less cumbersome, quicker to apply and better tolerated by the patient. However, circular frames are useful in certain situations. Their use should be considered where the fracture is adjacent to a joint, the bone is osteoporotic, or gradual correction of angulation or a soft tissue contracture is necessary. Where previous microvascular free flaps have been performed it may not be safe to use transfixion wires in the transported segment because of the risk of pedicle transection.

Surgical Technique For Type III Bone Loss

Circular frames are built pre-operatively from radiographs, plans and plaster casts. They are checked on the patient prior to surgery and then sterilized. Monolateral frames need little prior planning except to select the correct size and length and ensure that any special clamps that may be required are available. Final detailed planning is performed in the operating theatre and screw lengths are selected and osteotomy sites rehearsed. When the patient is asleep, joint ranges are checked. The image intensifier is used to identify bony landmarks and the anatomical and mechanical axes and these are then marked on the skin. Scars are also marked out and the pre-operative plan is then transferred to the skin to show screw positions and osteotomy sites.

Circular frames are designed to contour to the tibial deformity and appropriately placed hinges facilitate progressive post-operative correction whereas monolateral frames are usually applied with immediate deformity correction. Three fixation points are required. Three clamps are used in the case of a monolateral frame and three paired rings, or their equivalent, with a circular device. An alignment grid may be used in combination with an image intensifier to allow accurate immediate angular corrections (Saleh et al, 1991). An example of the use of a circular frame in the management of a 15cm length of bone loss is shown in Fig. 32.6. Here the proximity of the missing segment to the knee joint necessitates the use of a circular frame.

Once the fixator is applied, a bone cut is made between two of the fixation points with minimal thermal and vascular damage to avoid inhibiting the callus response. Although a medulla-sparing osteotomy (corticotomy) was initially described by Ilizarov, there has been increasing evidence of early recovery of the medullary blood supply and there is no particular advantage in this technique provided a sufficient delay is allowed before lengthening (White and Kenwright, 1990). We recommend an osteotomy under tension (Saleh, 1992a), which allows precise division of the bone. The distractor unit is applied to

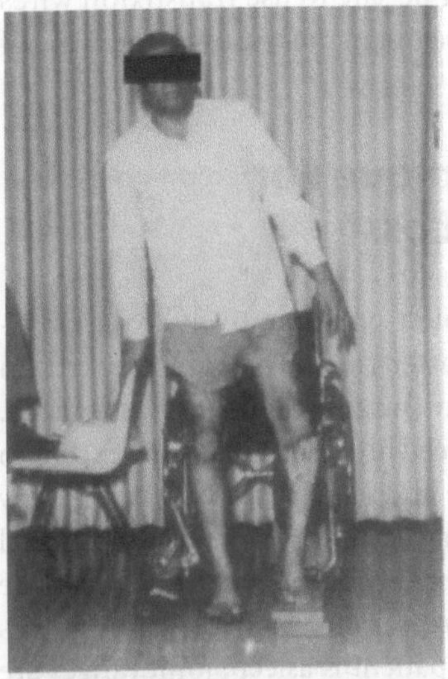
a
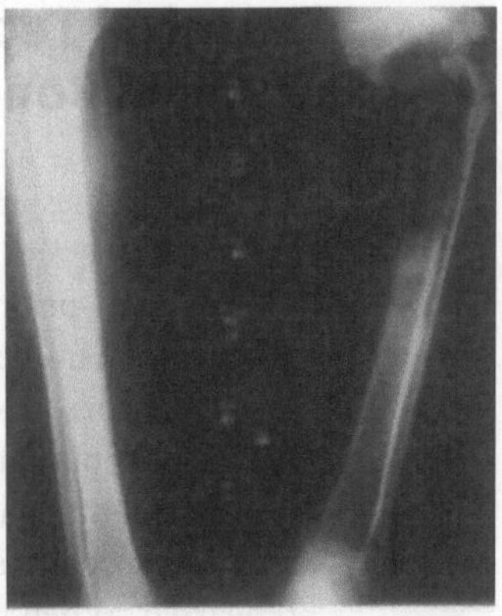
b
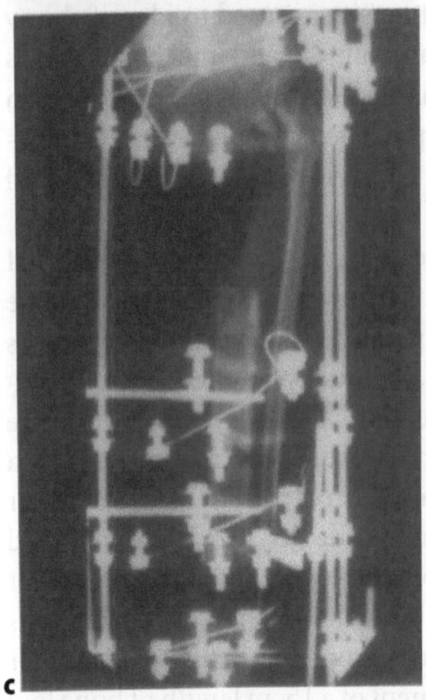
c
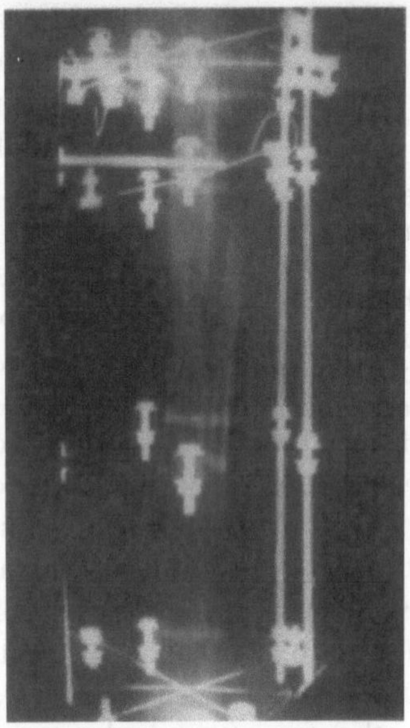
d
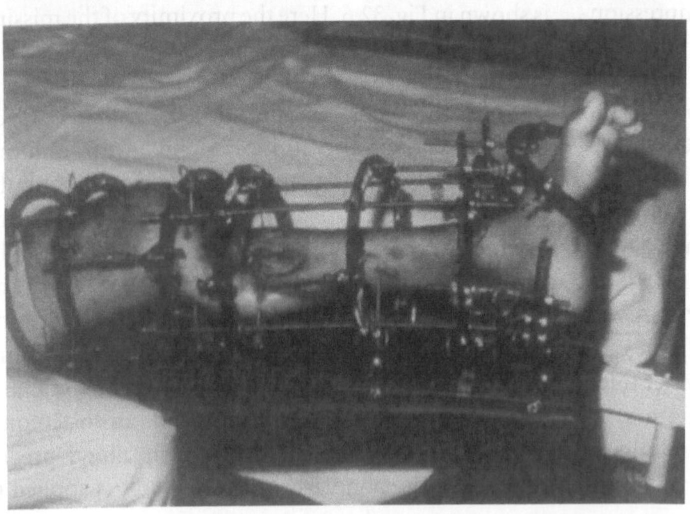
e
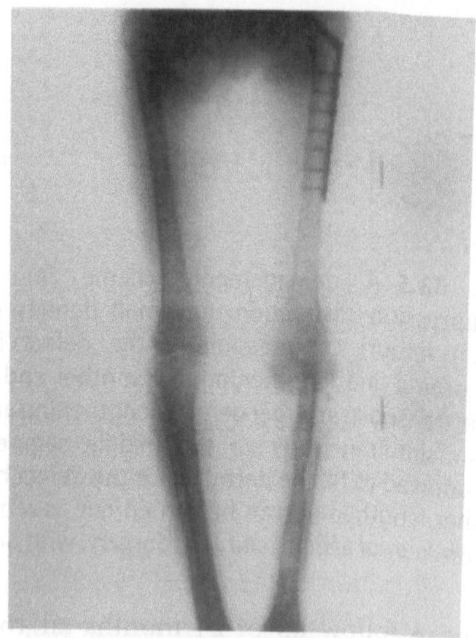
f
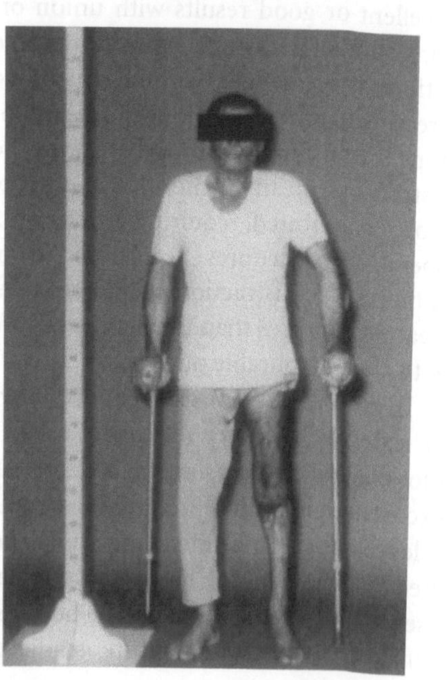
g

Fig. 32.6 A 15cm bone defect in the proximal tibia treated by bifocal transport using an Ilizarov frame. **a** The clinical appearance of the patient before surgery. Note the varus knee, the short leg and the equinus foot deformity. **b** The pre-operative radiological appearance showing a large segment of bone loss. **c** The radiological appearance after application of the Ilizarov device. **d** The proximal tibia has been straightened and bone transport undertaken. **e** The clinical appearance of the Ilizarov frame. It has been applied across the ankle and knee joints. The pre-operative equinus deformity has been corrected. **f** The radiological appearance after bone union and cessation of treatment. **g** The final clinical appearance.

the fixator and 3-5mm of distraction applied. The bone is approached in a normal way through an anteromedial longitudinal incision and the periosteum is reflected with stay stitches. A 3.2mm drill is used to drill through the whole diameter of the bone at three or four sites. The drill holes are connected with an osteotome, paying particular attention to division of the posteromedial and posterolateral corners. Once the cortex is sufficiently broken down, the osteotomy will gradually drift open under the applied tension force. Having confirmed that the osteotomy is complete, it should be closed down since contact between the bone ends is essential for callus generation. A drain should be inserted but left clamped to preserve fracture haematoma and only opened if there is significant haematoma or wound tension. A fibular osteotomy may be required if angular correction or further lengthening is planned. The bone defect or site of resection may be closed immediately (compression-distraction) or held apart for internal transport. For immediate closure appropriate fibular resection may be necessary. Lengthening is commenced on the seventh post-operative day at a rate of 0.25mm four times per day and thereafter varied according to the rate of new bone formation. Follow-up must be meticulous in order to avoid complications (Paley, 1990; Saleh and Scott, 1992). In compression-distraction the defect site is often healed before the lengthening site. In bone transport, however, docking is a much more complicated and delayed process. The fixation system is gradually destabilized once the bone is mature.

Docking

When bone transport is used, soft tissue obstruction, docking site mismatch or limited contact and non-union may occur. Bone grafting, manipulation and realignment and resection may be required. Although Ilizarov originally described the procedure without bone graft or resection, and in some cases this has been adhered to (Morandi et al, 1989; Paley et al, 1989; Dagher and Roukoz, 1991), other authors have recommended routinely resecting bone to achieve a satisfactory docking configuration (Cattaneo et al,

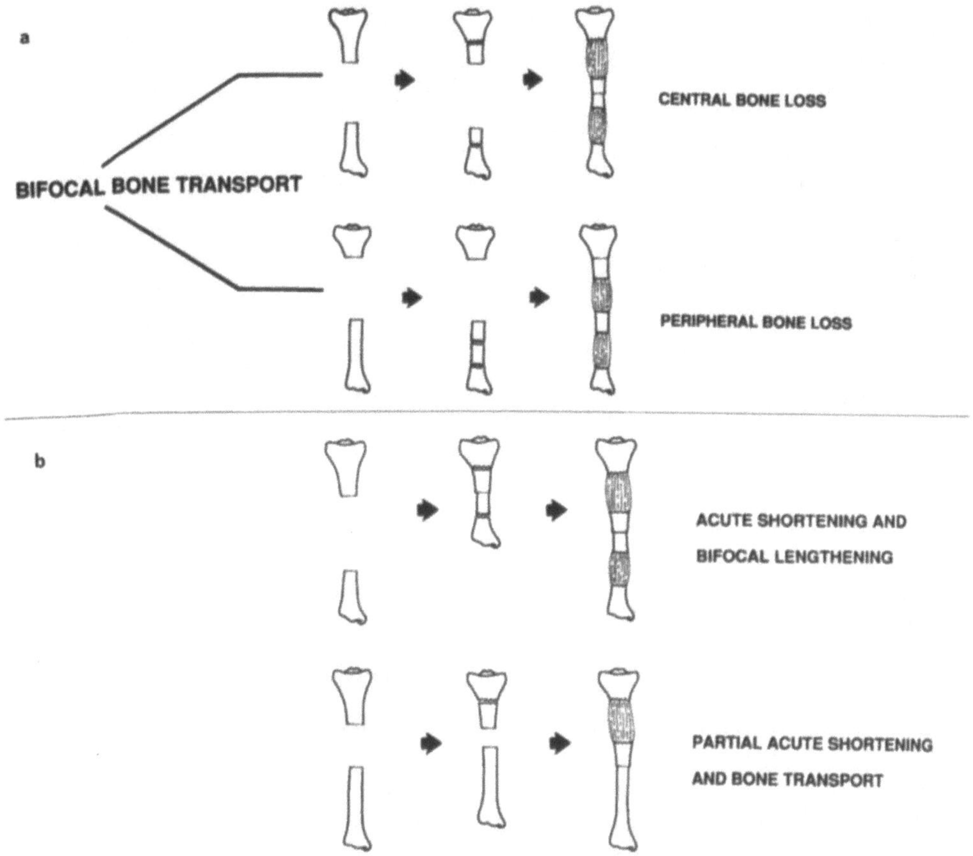

Fig. 32.7 A management scheme for extensive bone loss. **a** Normal bone. **b** Where there is poor bone stock and early shared loading between the fixator and bone is desirable.

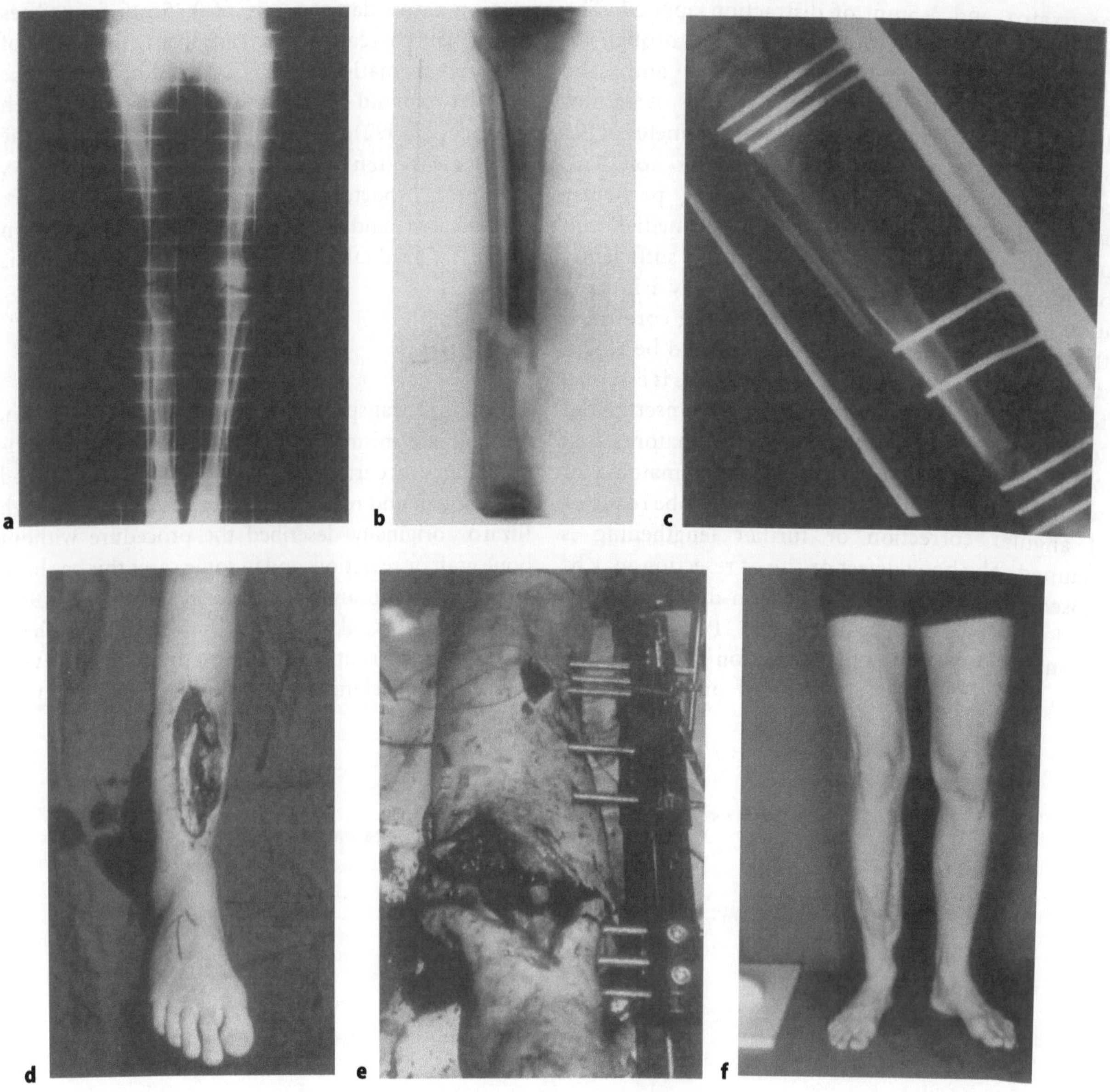

Fig. 32.8 The management of a combined soft tissue and bone defect. An open tibial diaphyseal fracture was initially treated by plating and soft tissue closure. Infection ensued. After debridement there was a 10cm bone defect. **a, b, c** Radiographs before, during and after fixation. **d, e, f** Clinical appearance before, during and after treatment.

1992; Green et al, 1992). Green also found bone grafting necessary on occasion, and biopsies taken at the time of grafting showed empty lacunae at the forward end of the transported segment indicating avascular bone. Routine bone grafting does not seem to be necessary, although it is indicated when the contact area is small. Many authors have reported high complication rates and the need for further procedures with bone transport (Paley et al, 1989: Cattaneo et al, 1992; Green et al, 1992; Marsh et al, 1994). In our series further operations were necessary at a rate consistent with the intrinsic complexity of the procedure, and although minor complications occurred, none was serious or persisted following the end of treatment. In part this may be due to careful patient selection and preparation prior to surgery.

Surgical Treatment of Defects of 6–10cm

A number of options are available to the surgeon in addition to microvascular bone transfer. These are summarized in Fig. 32.7. The choice of management method will, to a certain extent, depend on the quality of the bone stock that is left. A clinical example of the

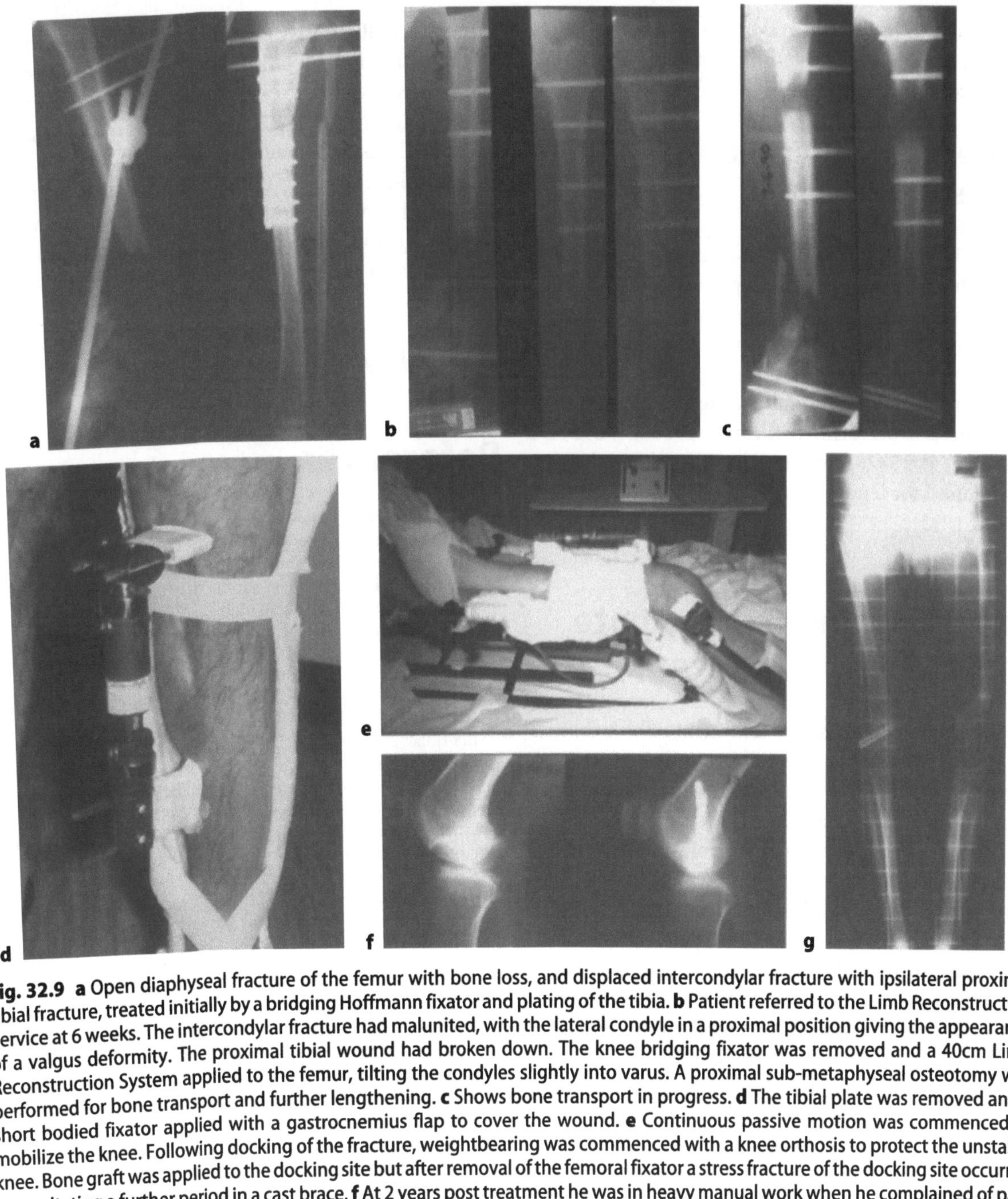

Fig. 32.9 **a** Open diaphyseal fracture of the femur with bone loss, and displaced intercondylar fracture with ipsilateral proximal tibial fracture, treated initially by a bridging Hoffmann fixator and plating of the tibia. **b** Patient referred to the Limb Reconstruction Service at 6 weeks. The intercondylar fracture had malunited, with the lateral condyle in a proximal position giving the appearance of a valgus deformity. The proximal tibial wound had broken down. The knee bridging fixator was removed and a 40cm Limb Reconstruction System applied to the femur, tilting the condyles slightly into varus. A proximal sub-metaphyseal osteotomy was performed for bone transport and further lengthening. **c** Shows bone transport in progress. **d** The tibial plate was removed and a short bodied fixator applied with a gastrocnemius flap to cover the wound. **e** Continuous passive motion was commenced to mobilize the knee. Following docking of the fracture, weightbearing was commenced with a knee orthosis to protect the unstable knee. Bone graft was applied to the docking site but after removal of the femoral fixator a stress fracture of the docking site occurred necessitating a further period in a cast brace. **f** At 2 years post treatment he was in heavy manual work when he complained of pain in the contralateral knee, where a large osteochondral fracture was identified and fixed. **g** At 7 years post-injury he remains in full-time employment in a shipbuilder's yard.

treatment of a 10cm tibial defect is shown in Fig. 32.8. It must be remembered that this type of surgery is difficult and it is suggested that patients who have large bone defects should be transferred to surgeons experienced in these techniques. No matter which method is used, the treatment time is long and the morbidity is not inconsiderable.

Management of Bone and Soft Tissue Loss

Acute shortening of extensive bone defects has been recommended by Giebel (1991) in order to close soft tissue and bone defects whilst length is restored by simultaneous metaphyseal osteotomy and lengthening. Using this technique major plastic surgery may be avoided. However, the safe limits of acute shortening are not yet fully understood.

Acute Shortening and Staged Lengthening

If acute shortening is performed in the interests of rapid rehabilitation, lengthening by callotasis may be offered one year to 18 months after completion of treatment. The patient should use a temporary shoe raise. When the bone is sufficiently strong to support an external fixator, lengthening by distraction osteogenesis is performed (Ilizarov, 1989a, 1989b; De Bastiani et al, 1987; Saleh, 1992b). Bifocal lengthening may be used for lengthenings of over 6 cm (Saleh and Hamer, 1993).

Some Comments on Acute Bone Loss in the Femur

The principles governing the treatment of bone loss in the femur are essentially similar to those described above for the tibia, but some aspects merit additional comment. The femur has a more extensive and continuous soft tissue envelope than the tibia and devitalised bone is much less common, although it may still be encountered, particularly in the distal third of the bone. Fractures of the femur are relatively common and include segmental fractures, intertrochanteric cervical fractures and supracondylar and intercondylar fractures. They often occur in combination. A pattern which occurs frequently in motorcyclists includes a Gustilo IIIB distal diaphyseal fracture with bone loss and an associated intercondylar fracture.

The femur requires much stronger external support because of the increased fixator bone distance and greater applied muscle forces. Re-construction may be achieved with screw fixation of the metaphyseal and articular fragments and neutralization using the Limb Reconstruction System with three clamps. The most efficient distal fixation is a metaphyseal clamp, with two straight clamps proximally to permit lengthening or bone transport. Fixation of the lateral soft tissues, particularly in association with the metaphyseal screws, may lead to knee stiffness; in the case of an articular fracture, therefore, fixation may be taken across the knee initially, using the Sheffield Hybrid Fixator and hinged to facilitate exercise (see Ch. 23 on supracondylar and intercondylar fractures of the femur). An illustrative case study is shown in Fig. 32.9. Because the distal fixation is critical to the success of the procedure, hydroxyapatite-coated screws may be used (Magyar et al 1997; Moroni, Heikkila et al 1998; Moroni, Toksvig-Larsen et al 1998).

Techniques based on callus distraction provide salvage of more difficult bone loss problems without significant donor site morbidity. They require careful planning and patient preparation and surgeons should be well versed in callus distraction techniques. Post-operative care is fairly labour intensive and treatment times are long.

References

Aronson, J. (1994) 'Temporal and spatial increases in blood flow during distraction osteogenesis.' *Clin Orthop*, 301, 124-31.

Blachut, P.A., Meek, R.N. and O'Brien, P.J. (1990) 'External fixation and delayed intramedullary nailing of open fractures of the tibial shaft.' *J Bone Joint Surg* 72A, 729-35.

British Orthopaedic Association and the British Association of Plastic Surgeons (1993). *A report by the BOA/BAPS working party on severe tibial injuries.* BOA/BAPS

Blauth, W. and Von Tome, O. (1978) 'Die fibula-pro-tibiafusion (hahn-brandes-plastik) in der behandlung von knochendefekten der tibia.' *Z Orthop*, 116, 20-6.

Cattaneo, A., Catagni, M. and Johnson, E.E. (1992) 'The treatment of infected non-unions and segmental defects of the tibia by the methods of Ilizarov.' *Clin Orthop*, 280, 143-52.

Christian, E.P., Bosse, M.J. and Robb, G. (1989) 'Reconstruction of large diaphyseal defects, without free fibular transfer, in grade IIIB tibial fractures.' *J Bone Joint Surg*, 71A, 994-1004.

Cierny, G. and Zorn, K.E. (1994) 'Segmential tibial defects: comparing conventional and Ilizarov methodologies.' *Clin Orthop*, 301, 118-23.

Clifford, R.P., Beauchamp, C., Kellum, J.F., Webb, J.K. and Tile, M. (1988) 'Plate fixation of open fractures of the tibia.' *J Bone Joint Surg*, 70B, 644-8.

Cockin, J. (1971) 'Autologous bone grafting: complications at the donor site.' *J Bone Joint Surg*, 53B, 153.

Court-Brown, C.M., Wheelwright, E.F., Christie, J. and McQueen, M.M. (1990) 'External fixation for type III open tibial fractures.' *J Bone Joint Surg*, 72B, 801-4.

Court-Brown, C.M., McQueen, M.M., Quaba, A.A. and Christie, J. (1991) 'Locked intramedullary nailing of open tibial fractures.' *J Bone Joint Surg*, 73B, 959–4.

Court-Brown, C.M., Keating, J.F. and McQueen, M.M. (1992) 'Infection after intramedullary nailing of the tibia: incidence and protocol for management.' *J Bone Joint Surg*, 74B, 770-4.

Court-Brown, C.M. and Rose, C. (1995) 'Reamed nailing of open tibial fractures.' *Osteo Int*, 3, 178-82.

Court-Brown, C.N.M., Keating, J.F., Christie, J. and McQueen, M.M. (1995) 'Exchange intramedullary nailing. Its use in aseptic tibial non-union.' *J Bone Joint Surg*, 77B, 407-11.

Dagher, F. and Roukoz, S. (1991) 'Compound tibial fractures with bone loss treated by Ilizarov technique.' *J Bone Joint Surg*, 7313, 316-21.

De Bastiani, G., Aldegheri, R. and Brivio, L.R. (1984) 'The treatment of fractures with a dynamic axial fixator.' J Bone Joint Surg, 66B, 538-45.

De Bastiani, G., Aldegheri, R., Renzi Brivio, L. and Trivella, G. (1987) 'Limb lengthening by callus distraction (callotasis)' *J Paed Orthop*, 7, 129-34.

Edge, A.J. and Denham, R.A. (1981) 'External fixation for complicated tibial fractures.' *J Bone Joint Surg*, 63B, 92-7.

Edwards, C.C. (1983) 'Staged reconstruction of complex open tibial fractures using Hoffmann external fixation: clinical decisions and dilemmas.' *Clin Orthop*, 178, 130-61.

Edwards, C.C., Simmons, S.C., Browner, B.D. and Weigel, M.C. (1988) 'Severe open tibial fractures. Results treating 202 injuries with extent fixation.' *Clin Orthop*, 230, 98-115.

Fairbank, A.C., Thomas, D., Cunningham, B., Curtis, M. and Jinnah, R.H. (1995) 'Stability of reamed and unreamed intramedullary tibial nails: a biomechanical study.' *Injury*, 26, 483-5.

Giebel, G. (1991) 'Resektions debridement mit kompensatorischer kallusdistraktion.' *Unfallchirurg*, 94, 401-8.

Green, S.A., Jackson, J.M., Wall, D.M., Marinow, H. and Ishkanian, J. (1992) 'Management of segmental defects by the Ilizarov intercalary bone transport method.' *Clin Orthop*, 280, 138-42.

Green, S. (1994) 'Skeletal defects: a comparison of bone grafting and bone transport for segmental defects.' *Clin Orthop*, 301, 111-17.

Gustilo, R.B. and Anderson, J.T. (1976) 'Prevention of infection in the treatment of one thousand and twenty-five open fractures of long bones: retrospective and prospective analysis.' *J Bone Joint Surg*, 58A, 453-8.

Gustilo, R.B., Mendoza, R.M. and Williams, D.N. (1984) 'Problems in the management of type III (severe) open fractures: a new classification of type III open fractures.' *J Trauma*, 24, 742-6.

Gustilo, R.B. (1991) *The Fracture Classification Manual*, Mosby Year Book, St Louis.

Ilizarov, G.A. (1989a) 'The tension-stress effect on the genesis and growth of tissues. Part 1: the influence of stability of fixation and soft tissue preservation.' *Clin Orthop*, 238, 249-81.

Ilizarov, G.A. (1989b) 'The tension-stress effect on the genesis and growth of tissues. Part 2: the influence of the rate and frequency of distraction.' *Clin Orthop*, 239, 263-85.

Ilizarov, G.A. and Ledyaev, V.I. (1992) 'The replacement of long tubular bone defects by lengthening by distraction osteotomy of one of the fragments.' Reproduced in *Clin Orthop*, 280 7-10 (Original in Russian, *Vestn Khir*, 1969; 102: 77).

Judet, R. and Patel, A. (1972) 'Muscle pedicle bone grafting of long bones by osteoperiosteal decortication.' *Clin Orthop*, 87, 74-80.

Keating, J.F., Kuo, R.S. and Court-Brown, C.M. (1994) 'Bifocal fractures of the tibia and fibula.' *J Bone Joint Surg*, 76B, 395-400.

Kreibich, D.N., Wells, J., Scott, I.R. and Saleh, M. (1994) 'Donor site morbidity at the iliac crest: comparison of percutaneous and open methods.' *J Bone Joint Surg*, 76B, 847-8.

McGraw, J.M. and Lim, E.V.A. (1988) 'Treatment of open tibial shaft fractures. External fixation and secondary intramedullary nailing.' *J Bone Joint Surg*, 70A, 900-11.

Magyar G, Toksvig-Larsen S, Moroni A. (1997) 'Hydroxyapatite-coating of threaded pins enhances fixation.' *J Bone Joint Surg* (Br) 79B: 487–9.

Marsh, J.L., Nepola, J.V., Wuest, T.K. et al (1991) 'Unilateral external fixation until healing with the dynamic axial fixator for severe open tibial fractures.' *J.Orthop Trauma*, 5, 341-8.

Marsh, J.L., Prokuski, L. and Biermann, S. (1994) 'Chronic infected tibial non-unions with bone loss: conventional techniques versus bone transport.' *Clin Orthop*, 301, 139-46.

Marshall, P., Saleh, M. and Douglas, D.L. (1991) 'Intramedullary nailing following the use of external fixators: the risk of deep infection.' *J R Coll Surg Edinb*, 36, 268-71.

Maurer, D.J., Merkow, R.L. and Gustilo, R.B. (1989) 'Infection after intramedullary nailing of severe open tibial fractures initially treated with external fixation.' *J Bone Joint Surg*, 71A, 835-8.

Morandi, M., Zembo, M.M. and Ciotti, M. (1989) 'Infected tibial pseudarthosis: a 2-year follow-up on patients treated by the Ilizarov technique.' *Orthopaedics*, 12, 497-508.

Moroni A, Heikkila J, Toksvig-Larsen S, Stea S, Giannini S. 'Hydroxyapatite-Coated Tapered Pins Are Better Fixed; A Multi-Center Prospective, Randomized Clinical Study.' Presented at the AAOS 1998.

Moroni A, Toksvig-Larsen S, Maltarello MC, Orienti L, Stea S, Giannini S. (1998) 'A Comparison of Hydroxyapatite-Coated, Titanium-Coated and Uncoated Tapered External Fixation Pins.' *J Bone Joint Surg* 80A: 547–54.

Müller, M.E. and Thomas, R.J. (1979) 'Treatment of non-union in fractures of long bones.' *Clin Orthop*, 138, 141-53.

Müller, M.E., Nazarian, S., Koch, P. and Schatzker, J. (1990) *The Comprehensive Classification of Fractures of Long Bones.*, Springer-Verlag: Berlin.

Paley, D. Catagni, M.A., Argnani, F. et al (1989) 'Ilizarov treatment of fibial non-unions with bone loss.' *Clin Orthop*, 241, 146-65.

Paley, D. (1990) 'Problems, obstacles and complications of limb lengthening by the Ilizarov technique.' *Clin Orthop*, 250, 81-104.

Papineau, L.J., Alfageme, A., Dalcourt, J.P. et al (1979) 'Chronic osteomyelitis: excision and open cancellous bone grafting after extensive saucerisation'. *Int Orthop*, 3, 165-76.

Ribbans, W.J., Stubbs, D.A. and Saleh, M. (1992) 'Non-union surgery. Part 11: the Sheffield experience – 100 consecutive cases, results and lessons.' *Int J Orthop Trauma*, 2, 19-24.

Saleh, M., Harriman, P. and Edwards, D.J. (1991) 'A radiological method for producing precise limb alignment.' *J Bone Joint Surg*, 73B, 515-16.

Saleh, M. (1991) 'Bone graft harvesting. A percutaneous technique.' *J Bone Joint Surg*, 73B, 867-8.

Saleh, M. (1992a) 'Technique selection in limb lengthening: the Sheffield practice.' *Semin Orthop*, 7, 137-51.

Saleh, M. and Scott, B. (1992) 'Pitfalls and complications in leg lengthening: the Sheffield experience.' *Semin Orthop*, 7, 207-22

Saleh, M. (1992b) 'Non-union surgery. Part 1: Basic principles of management.' *Int J Orthop Trauma*, 2, 4-18.

Saleh, M. and Hamer, A. (1993) 'Bifocal lengthening – preliminary results.' *J Paed Orthop*, 2, 42-8.

Saleh, M., Stubbs, D.A., Street, R.J., Lang, D.M. and Harris, S.C. (1993) 'Histologic analysis of human lengthened bone.' *J Paed Orthop*, 2, 16-21.

Saleh, M. and Rees, A.R. (1995) 'Bifocal surgery for deformity and bone loss – bone transport and compression–distraction compared.' *J Bone Joint Surg*, 77B, 429-34.

Summers, B.N. and Eisenstein, S.M. (1989) 'Donor site pain from the ileum.' *J Bone Joint Surg*, 71B, 677-80.

Sveshnikov, A.A., Barabash, A.P., Chepelenko, T.A., Smotrova, L.A. and Larionov, A.A. (1984) 'Radionuclide studies of osteogenesis and circulation in substitution of large defects of the leg bones.' *Exp Ortop Traumatol Protex*, 11, 33-7.

Vidal, J. Buscayret, C., Finzi, M. and Melka, J. (1982) 'Les greffes inter-tibio-perionières dans le traitement des retards de consolidation jambier.' *Rev Chir Orthop*, 68, 123

Weikal, A.M. and Habal, M.B. (1977) 'Meralgia paraesthetica: a complication of iliac bone procurement.' *Plast Reconstr Surg*, 60, 572-4.

Weiland, A.J., Moore, JR. and Daniel, R.K. (1983) 'Vascularised bone grafts. Experience with 41 cases.' *Clin Orthop*, 174, 87-95.

White, S.H. and Kenwright, J. (1990) 'The timing of distraction of an osteotomy.' *J Bone Joint Surg*, 69A, 356-61.

Whittle, A.P., Russell, T.A., Taylor, J.C. and Lavelle, D.G. (1992) 'Treatment of open fractures of the fibial shaft with the use of interlocking nailing without reaming.' *J Bone Joint Surg*, 74A, 1162-71.

SECTION 7 ANCILLARY EQUIPMENT

Ancillary Equipment for Fracture Management

33

S. Salvagno

The Orthofix range includes a number of additional items which are of value in the treatment of certain diaphyseal fractures. These items are described in this chapter.

Supplementary Screw Holder

Where there is a large, unstable third fragment, one or two supplementary screws may be used. The fragment may be reduced either via a closed procedure (sometimes involving the use of K-wires with olive) or an open procedure.

The supplementary screw or screws are inserted, at a suitable angle, using the standard technique and taking care to avoid damage to the neurovascular structures. The supplementary screw holder is designed to be attached either to the body of the fixator (Fig. 33.1) or to an existing screw (Fig. 33.2) according to circumstances. It comprises a bar 150mm long and 6mm in diameter, two clamps and a modular attachment for the body of the fixator. Each clamp contains one attachment point for the bar, and a second attachment point for either the modular attachment for the body, or an existing screw shaft.

Any supplementary screws should be removed prior to the institution of dynamization.

Alignment Grid

This is a perspex sheet (Figs. 33.3a–d) with metal rods embedded in it, which is designed to be used in

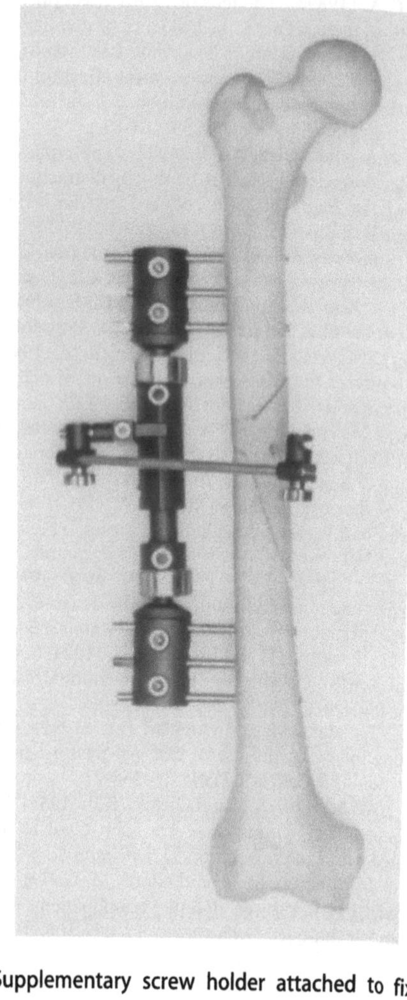

Fig. 33.1 Supplementary screw holder attached to fixator body.

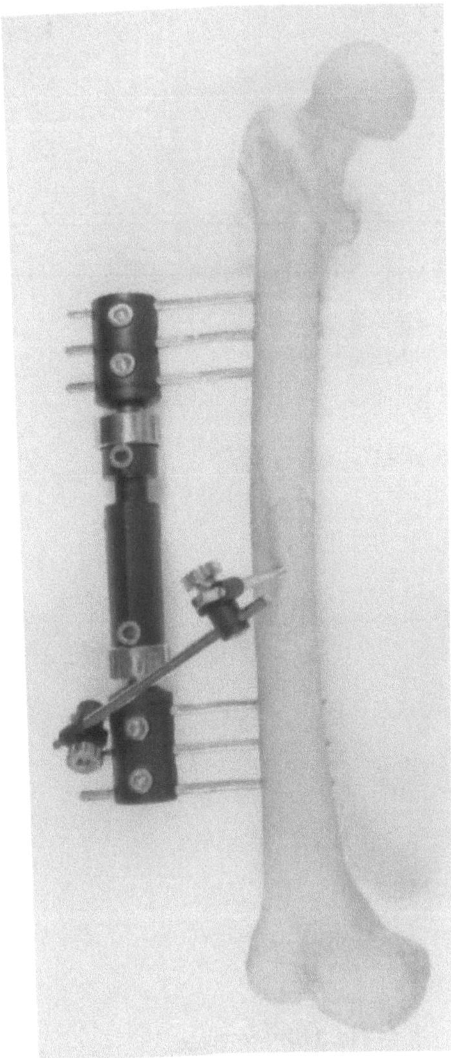

Fig. 33.2 Screw holder attached to an existing screw.

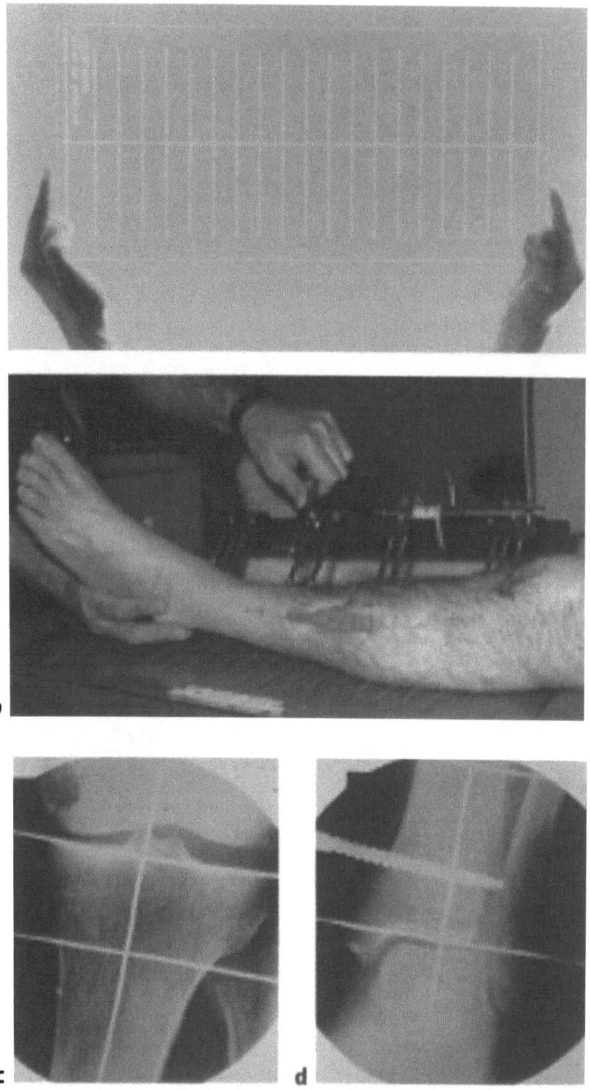

a b c d

Fig. 33.3 a Alignment grid. **b** Grid placed under limb. **c** The image intensifier is used to align the grid with the knee. **d** If the alignment is correct the grid lines will align with the ankle.

conjunction with a mobile image intensifier before fixator application, to enable the surgeon to identify and correct angulation and to detect any translation of the joint above and below the deformity, with a mean accuracy of 2.5°.[1]

Reduction System

This device may be used intra-operatively in conjunction with the fixator once the latter has been applied, to maintain the reduction achieved in one plane while correcting in another (Fig. 33.4).

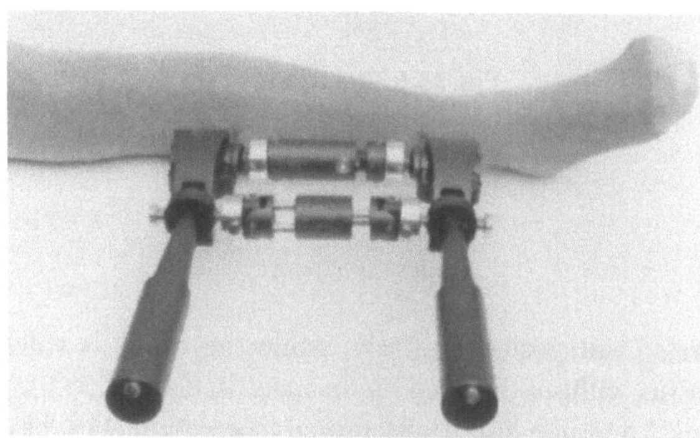

Fig. 33.4 Reduction system.

Micrometric Correction Device

This device, which is designed to be attached to the fixator clamps, allows fine-tuning of reduction to be

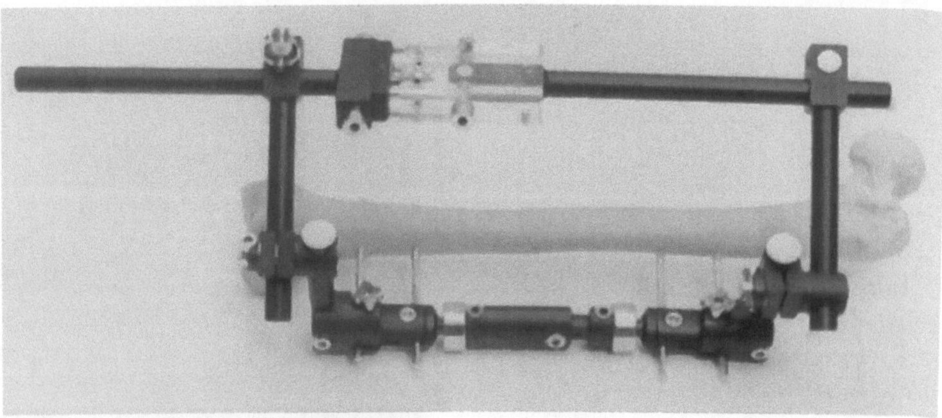

Fig. 33.5 Micrometric correction device.

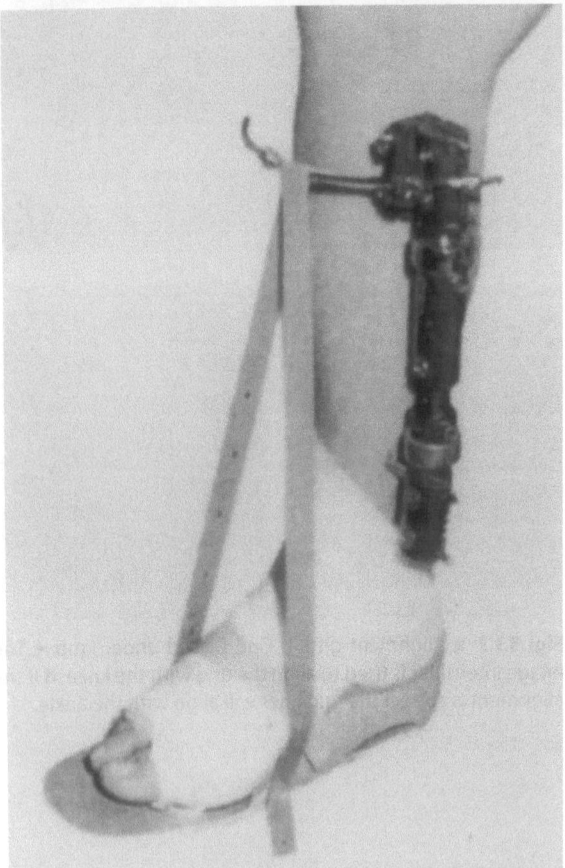

Fig. 33.6 Dyna-Foot.

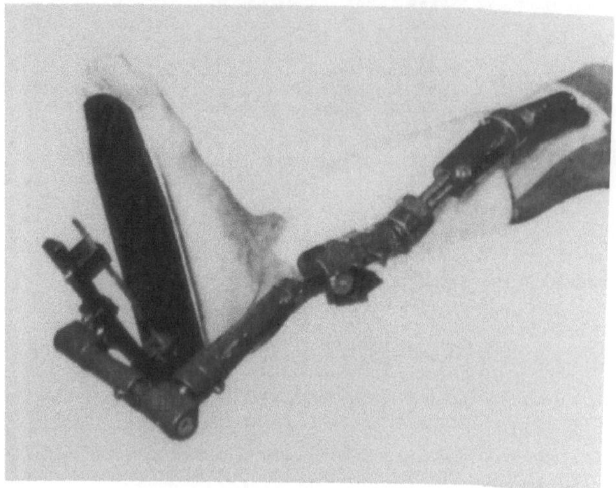

Fig. 33.7 Foot plate.

carried out post-operatively, while the callus is still plastic, without the need for an anaesthetic (Fig. 33.5). Axial, angular and translational correction can be made in any given plane at the fracture site itself.

Dyna-Foot and Foot Plate

These are two specially designed, adjustable devices (Figs. 33.6, 33.7) for attachment to a tibial fixator to prevent the development of equinus position of the foot due to muscle contracture.

Exchange Unit

This device helps to maintain reduction if the fixator is temporarily removed to allow easier access to soft tissues or the fracture site, to enable plastic surgery or bone grafting procedures to be carried out. It is also used to replace a fixator or lengthener with a larger model without losing reduction (Figs. 33.8a, 33.8b).

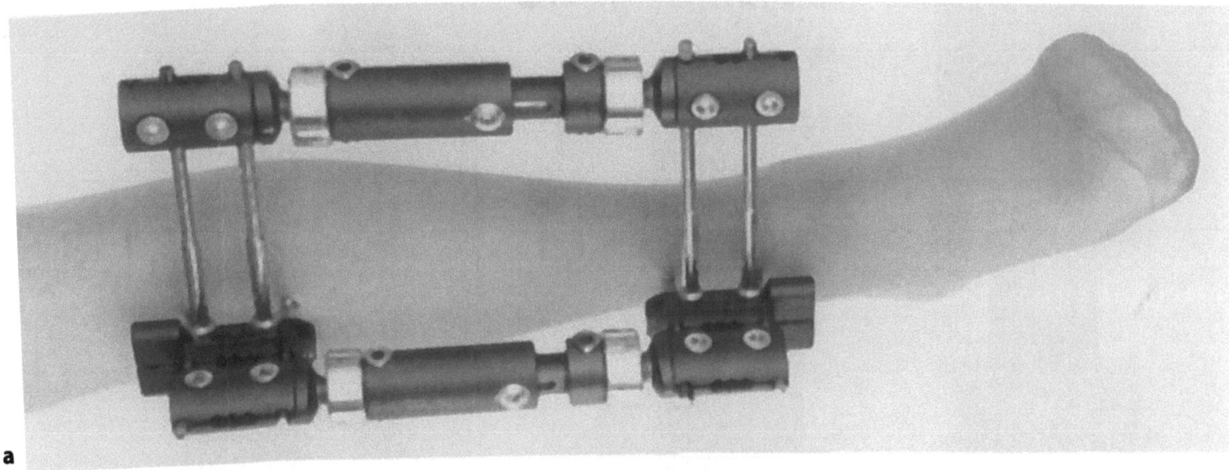

a

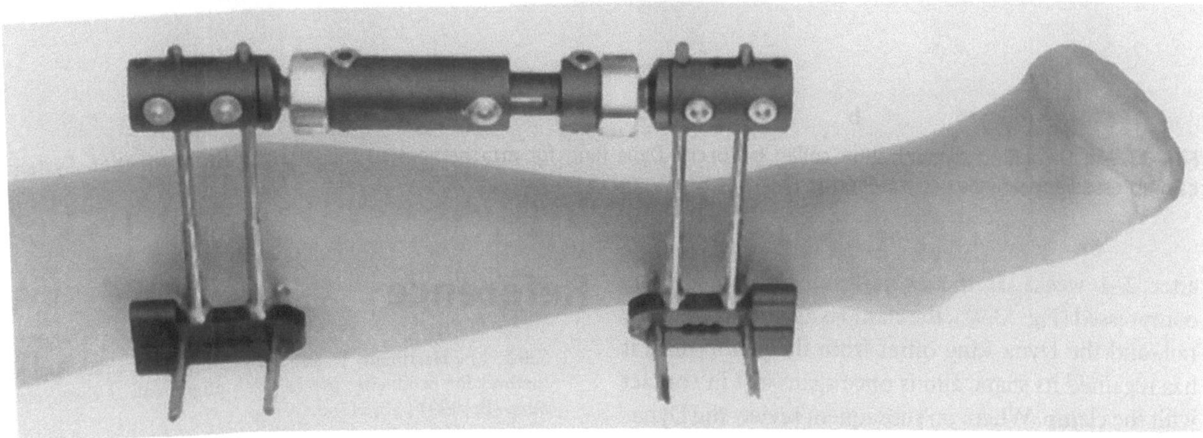

b

Fig. 33.8 **a** Exchange unit in place; **b** Reduction maintained while fixator has been temporarily removed.

The Dyna-Ring

Fractures

A Dyna-Ring dynamization collar is available for early, controlled dynamization. This device incorporates a silicone cushion and is attached to the stem of the male part of the fixator. It is designed to prevent collapse of the fracture, and at the same time to permit limited micromovement of up to 2mm on weightbearing.

A guide to its use is as follows: on the second postoperative day, the fracture site is distracted by 2mm if the two bone segments are perfectly in contact. The Dyna-Ring is then attached with its silicone cushion facing the rim of the female part of the fixator, and just in contact with it (Fig. 33.9a). The central body locking nut is now loosened. Weightbearing may now commence immediately, regardless of the type of fracture.

As a general rule, the Dyna-Ring may be removed after 3 weeks in stable fractures and after 6–8 weeks in unstable and comminuted fractures, at which time full dynamization is permitted.

Lengthening, Bone Transport

This special module (Fig. 33.9b) is locked to the rail of the Limb Reconstruction System with the silicone cushion facing the clamp which has been unlocked for dynamization, and just in contact with it. When attached in this way, it permits only limited dynamization of the segment concerned and thus acts as a safeguard against collapse. The Dyna-Ring therefore allows earlier conversion from a rigid to a dynamic mode, and a corresponding reduction in the neutralization period.

A guide to its use is as follows: when, after a variable period in neutralization, the callus shows evidence of early corticalization, the Dyna-Ring is attached to the rail as described above. The patient is then reviewed

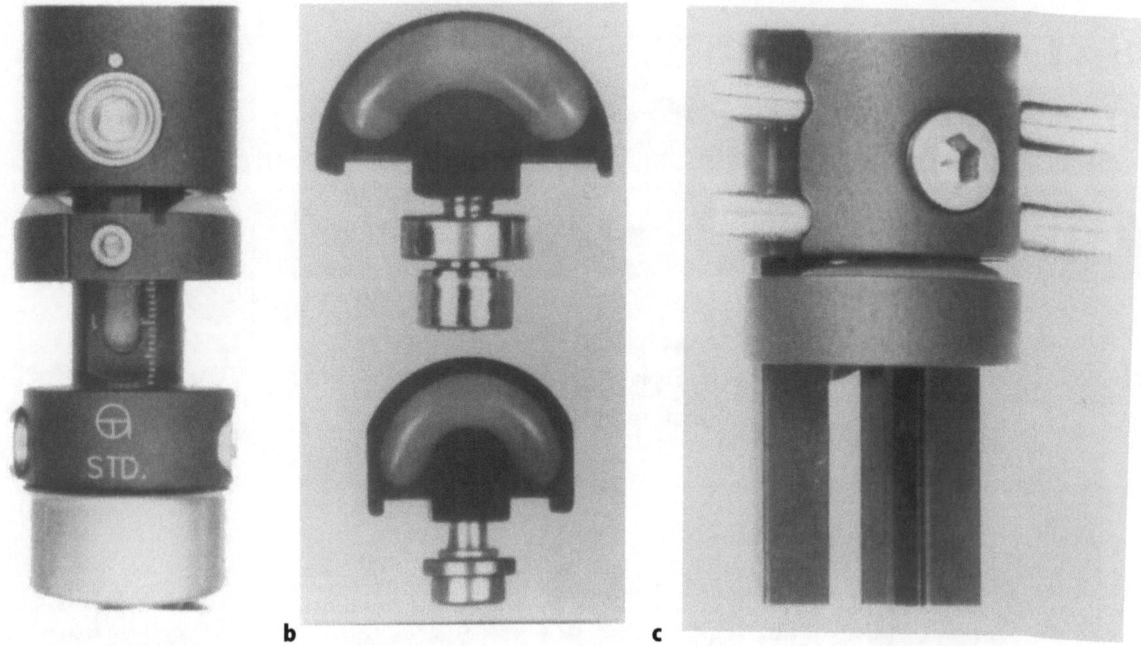

a b c

Fig. 33.9 **a** Dyna-Ring dynamization collar; **b** Special Dyna-Ring for attachement to rail of Limb Reconstruction System; **c** Compressed appearance of Dyna-Ring on rail.

after 2–4 weeks. If the Dyna-Ring cushion appears compressed (Fig. 33.9c), the clamp is again locked to the rail, and the Dyna-Ring offset from the clamp until it has regained its shape and is once again just in contact with the clamp. When, on subsequent review the Dyna-Ring no longer appears compressed, it may be left in this position until full corticalization is evident.

Reference

1 Saleh, M., Harriman, P. and Edwards, D.J. 'A radiological method for producing precise limb alignment.' *J Bone Joint Surg*, [Br] 1991 73B, 515–6.

The Fragment Fixation System in Intra-articular and Periarticular Fractures

34

T. Gausepohl and D. Pennig

History

In 1969 a group of well-known surgeons, all members of the AO, produced a manual of osteosynthetic techniques (Müller et al 1969). For the first time they attempted to standardize fragment fixation based on biomechanical information derived from cadaver and animal experiments as well as clinical data. In the preceding century various techniques had been used and every surgeon had his preferred method – many of which worked very successfully. Nevertheless, it is to the credit of the AO group that they collected a great deal of information on fracture treatment and healing and then summarized their experiences in a technical manual. Even today, however, secure fixation of bony fragments remains a point of discussion. The reason for that is the fact that no single method of fixation can solve every problem and many different methods are available to solve the same problem, each having their own advantages and disadvantages in a given fracture situation. With this in mind, and taking account of the development of new materials over the past three decades, we are obliged to revisit and reappraise existing techniques and strategies and to compare them with newer methods for dealing with these problems.

But the basic requirements defined in their book are still, however, the guiding principles in fracture care:

1. Stable anatomical reduction
2. Early active mobilization.

The AO group is particularly noted for its work on screw and plate fixation. Catchwords like "interfragmentary compression" seemed to provide the key to a secure fixation for a long period of time. To achieve this, emphasis was placed on a special thread design and a meticulous protocol was established on exactly how to predrill and pretap an adequate screw hole. Engineers were engaged to optimize the screw–bone interface and different screws for cortical and cancellous bone were developed.

Although the benefits of this work are undeniable, we cannot stop at this point. Surveying more than a century of trauma surgery we are faced with the fact that the most simple techniques have survived all the innovations. There is one tool in the armamentarium of every surgeon, whatever philosophy he follows, which is never overlooked: the K-wire. If we ask ourselves why this simple instrument has never fallen from grace the answer is easy: its tempting simplicity. When developing new materials and techniques we should never lose sight of this fact.

Technical Aspects of Conventional Screw Design

In the early days surgeons borrowed established principles from other handicrafts. As bone appears to be comparable to wood the screw design was at first similar to that of wood screws. But as early as 1912 Sherman wrote in his article about plate and screw design: "There is no mechanical reason why a wood screw should be used when the self tapping machine screw answers all requirements. It has a much greater holding power and is much more readily inserted." (Fig. 34.1). The difference between a wood screw and a machine screw is mainly the conical shape of the core in the wood screw and the constant core diameter in the machine screw. In addition, the wood screw normally has a greater pitch than the machine screw (Fig. 34.2). The standard cortical screw developed by the

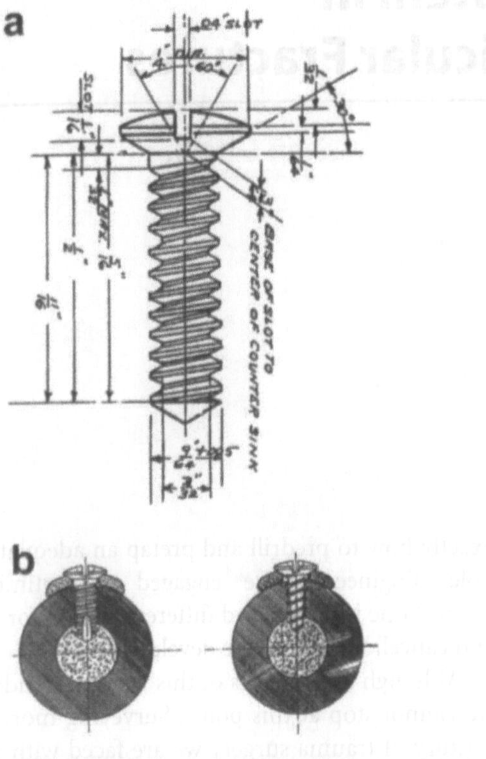

Fig. 34.1 Drawing for the original article of Sherman 1912. **a** Technical drawing of the machine screw design. **b** Difference between a machine screw and a wood screw.

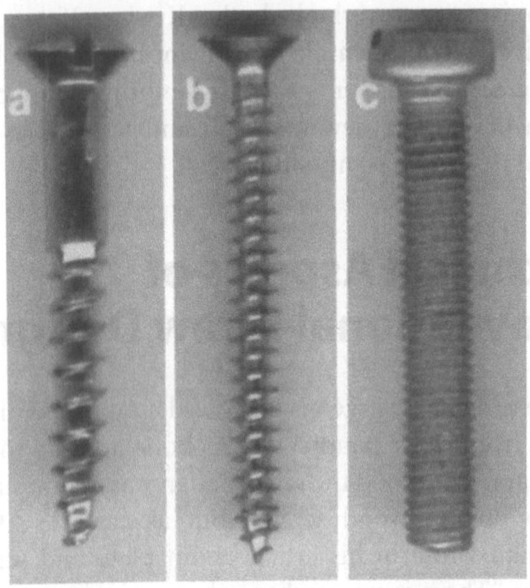

Fig. 34.2 Different screw types. **a** Typical shape of a wood screw; **b** Self drilling wood screw; **c** Machine screw.

AO group has a constant core diameter but a pitch similar to that used for wood screws (Figs. 34.3, 34.4). This kind of pitch needs a well prepared hole and pretapping, especially in cortical applications. According to the industrial standard the pitch design has been improved to allow for more interfragmentary compression (Fig. 34.5).

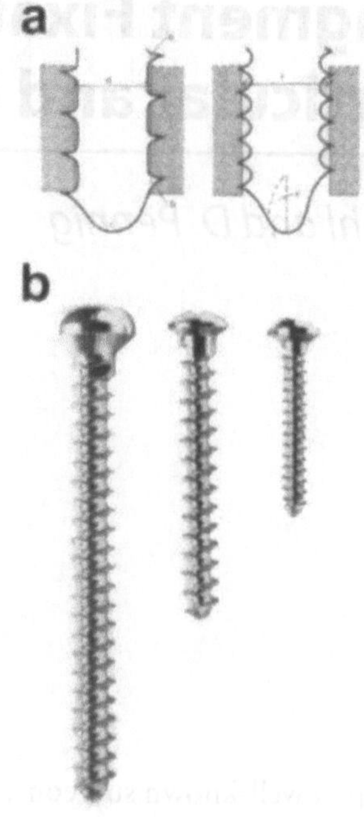

Fig. 34.3 Improved screw design for cortical screws. **a** Improvement of the bone-screw interface as developed by the AO group; **b** Different cortical screw sizes.

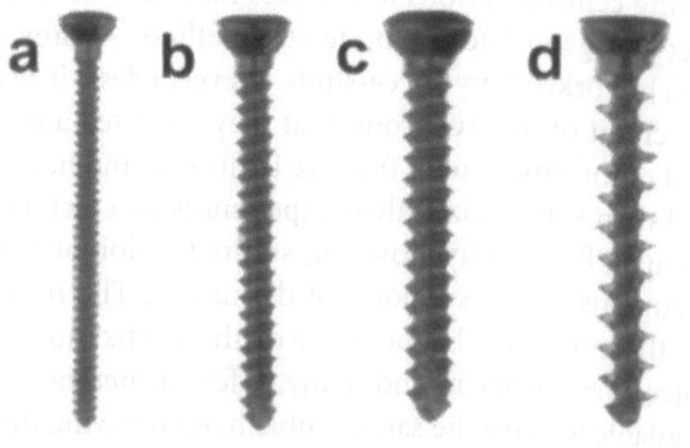

Fig. 34.4 Screw types available on the market. **a, b, c** Different screw diameters. The pitch increases with the core diameter. **d** Design for cancellous screws. Typical small core diameter and large pitch.

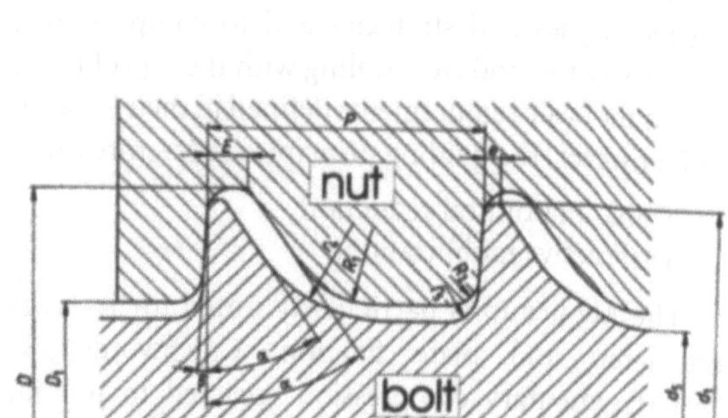

Fig. 34.5 Technical construction of bone screws (German Industrial Standard, DIN).

Principles of the Fragment Fixation System (FFS)

We return to the simplicity principle. In developing fragment fixation from the simple – but in terms of purchase insecure – K-wire to the sophisticated AO technique with improved purchase in the bone, handling for the surgeon became increasingly complicated. The limits of the AO screw technique are related to the size of the fragments which have to be secured. In hand surgery particularly, there is frequently the need to stabilize extremely small bone fragments, for example, bony avulsed extensor tendons in the third phalanx (bush fracture), bony collateral ligament disruptures, avulsion of the palmar plate with bone fragments or comminuted fractures of the base of the phalanges which typically display a pattern of multiple small fragments. While we are reluctant to sacrifice the advantages of screw fixation, for the lack of anything better the K-wire comes into prominence again.

The newly developed Fragment Fixation System (FFS, Orthofix srl, Verona, Italy, Fig. 34.6) provides the missing link between K-wire and screw. Each implant has a three–edged tip similar to that of the K-wire and a fine machined thread followed by a polished shaft. Because the shaft has an increased diameter compared to the threaded portion a "shoulder" appears at the connection between thread and shaft similar to that of a screw head (Fig. 34.7a, 34.7c). If there is any need to increase the size of the "shoulder" a washer can be used (Fig. 34.7b). The washers are stored in slots in front of the boxes. They are available only for the medium sized and large sized FFS implants. They can be taken out of the slot by simply spearing the washer with the FFS implant and can easily be replaced as shown in Fig. 34.6c.

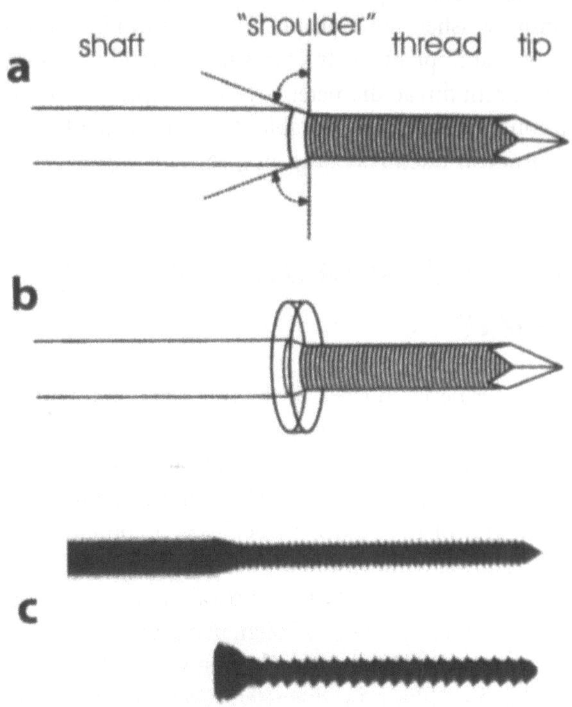

Fig. 34.7 **a** Schematic drawing of the technical features of the FFS system. **b** A washer can be used. **c** Comparison between a conventional cortical screw and the FFS implant.

Like a conventional screw the threaded portion of the FFS is available in different lengths, and in three different diameters. The smallest thread diameter is 1.2mm and is only used for extremely small fragments in hand surgery. Washers are not available for this small size. If a washer could be used with a 1.2mm implant it would be possible to use a larger FFS implant. The

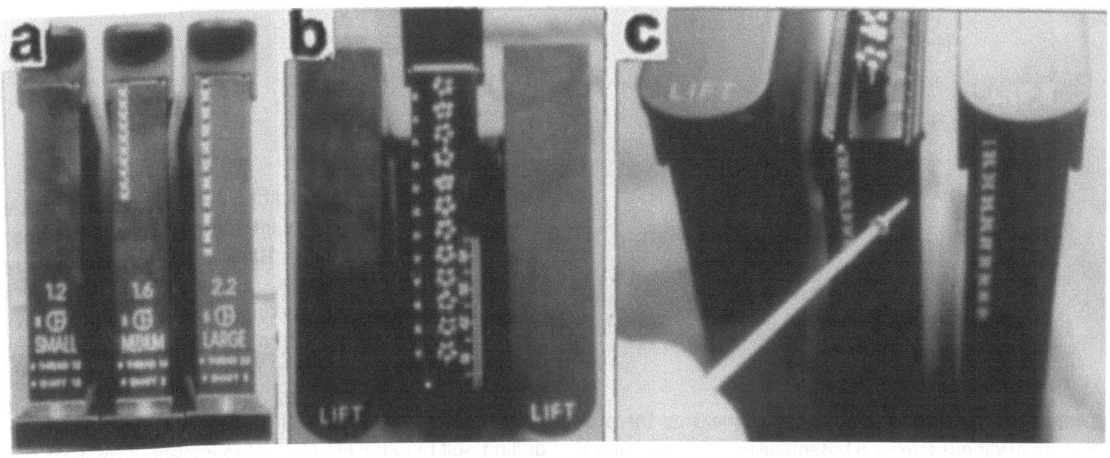

Fig. 34.6 The Fragment Fixation System. **a** Front view of the boxes. Three different diameters of implant are available. **b** View from top. Every box provides different lengths. **c** Slots in front of the medium and large sized implants house washers.

medium sized implants have a thread diameter of 1.6mm. Washers are available. This medium implant is the typical implant for fractures in the hand and foot. The 2.2mm thread diameter large FFS implants with or without washers are suitable for intra-articular or periarticular fractures of the long bones.

Screw Design and Holding Power

Previous experiments (Rovinsky et al 1997) comparing 4.0mm cancellous screws with 2.2mm FFS implants have demonstrated a significant pull-out strength and an equivalent resistance to axial load in the stabilization of fractures of the medial malleolus. To compare the holding power of the fine machine thread with the holding power of conventional cortical and cancellous screws we designed an experiment using a homogenous testing material (Baydur™). The test material was cut into blocks 13mm in diameter. Cortical screws of 3.5mm and 2.7mm diameter both pretapped and self tapping, were inserted into the test blocks as were 4.0mm predrilled and pretapped cancellous screws (Fig. 34.8a–34.8c). The blocks were mounted in a biomechanical testing machine (Losenhausen™) and the screws pulled out of the test block at a constant speed of 0.1mm/sec). The maximum holding power was registered. At least twenty screws of each type were tested and the results compared with the holding power of the FFS implants with diameters of 1.2, 1.6 and 2.2mm. The mean values and standard deviations of the holding powers for the tested screws is shown in Fig. 34.9. There was no statistical difference between the 4.0mm cancellous screw and the 3.5mm cortical self tapping screw in spite of the clear difference in screw diameters. A similar situation exists between the 2.7mm cortical screw and the 2.2mm FFS implant. The holding power of the FFS implant was as good as the holding power of the cortical screw but the diameter of the FFS implant was 0.5mm less than that of the cortical screw.

In a second experiment the holding power was tested in cancellous bone. Bone blocks of 13mm diameter were cut out of bovine humeral heads. X-rays were taken from every bone block to identify non-homogeneous material. As in the previous experiment the different screws and FFS implants were inserted and mounted in the testing machine. The holding

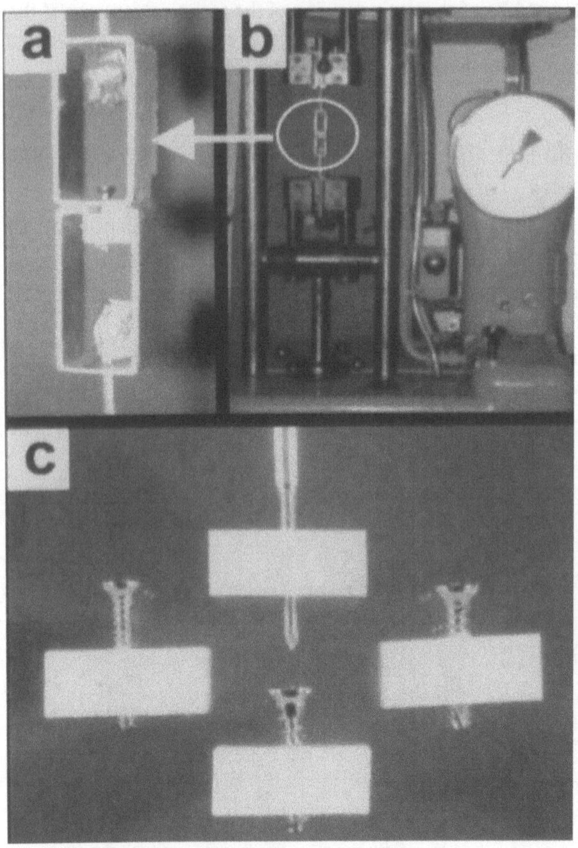

Fig. 34.8 **a** Testing apparatus designed to measure the pull-out strength of various screws. **b** Losenhausen™ biomechanical testing machine. **c** Screws inserted into testing material with a constant screw bone interface.

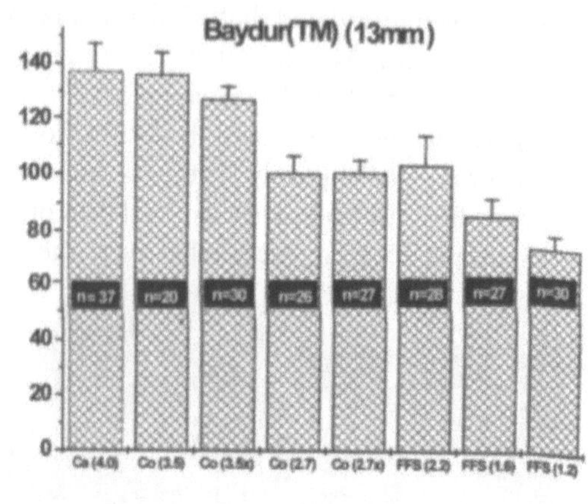

Fig. 34.9 Holding power of different screws in testing material (Baydur™). The screw–bone interface is 13mm. The value on the y-axis is given in kp (1kp = 10nN).Ca(4.0) = cancellous screw, diameter 4.0mm, predrilled, pretapped; Co(3.5) = cortical screw, diameter 3.5mm, predrilled, self tapping; Co(3.5x) = cortical screw, diameter 3.5mm, predrilled, pretapped; Co(2.7) = cortical screw, diameter 2.7mm, predrilled, self tapping; Co(2.7x) = cortical screw, diameter 2.7mm, predrilled, pretapped; FFS (2.2) = FFS implant, diameter 2.2mm, self drilling, self tapping; FFS (1.6) = FFS implant, diameter 1.6mm, self drilling, self tapping; FFS (1.2) = FFS implant, diameter 1.2mm, self drilling, self tapping.

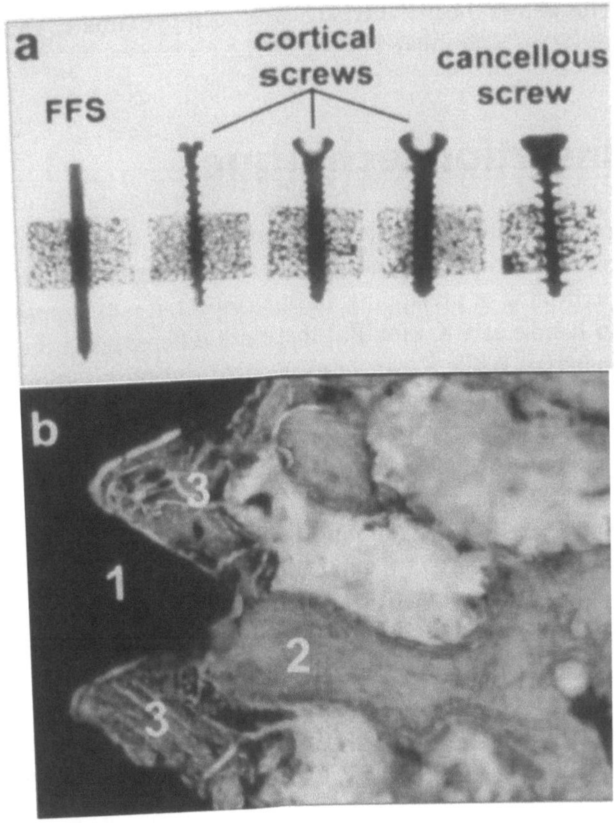

Fig. 34.10 a Histological slices of 1mm thickness through screw and bone. The bone is stained with silver nitrate. **b** Close-up demonstrating the impacted drill flour. 1 = thread of the FFS implant; 2 = cancellous trabecula; 3 = drill flour.

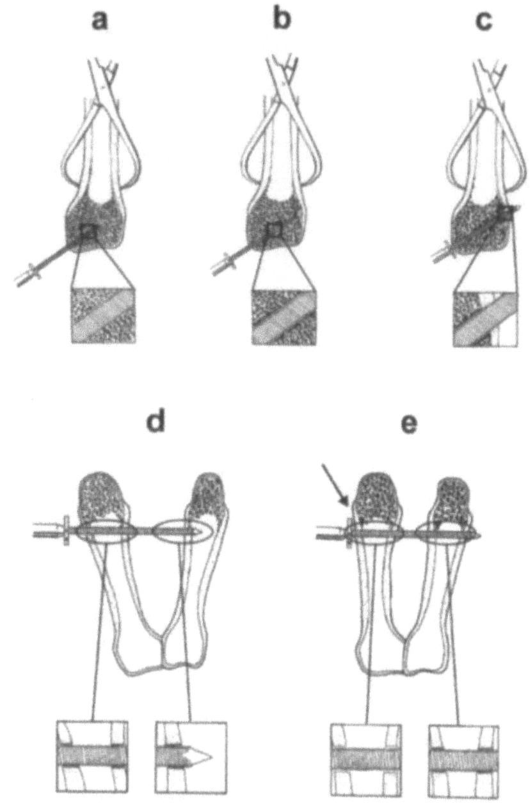

Fig. 34.11 Schematic drawing to explain the "compression effect".

power of the FFS implants was strikingly superior to that of the cortical screws with conventional screw design. There was no statistically significant difference between the pretapped cortical screw of 3.5mm diameter and the self drilling and self tapping 2.2mm FFS implant (unpublished data).

To explain this remarkable result we need to look more closely at the bone–screw interface. Fig. 34.10 shows slices of 1mm thickness through screw and cancellous bone. In Fig. 34.10a a dense zone can be seen around the thread of the FFS implant. This dense zone can be interpreted as impacted drill flour which is pushed aside and pressed into the cancellous caverns while the implant is inserted (Fig. 34.10b) (The Orthofix Fragment Fixation System: Technical Monograph). The other examples in Fig. 34.10a show conventional predrilled screws where the drill flour is removed by the drill. There is less impaction around the thread. It can be concluded that the improved holding power of the FFS implants is at least partially due to the non-predrilled design. Another aspect is the decreased pitch of the FFS implants compared to the conventional screws. The improved holding power of screws with a decreased pitch has previously been studied by Asnis (Asnis et al 1996).

Compression Effect

It is self evident that a screw with a continuous thread cannot exert a compression effect under normal conditions. Connecting two pieces of bone these screws work like adjusting screws. In some clinical situations, however, a certain compression effect was observed with the FFS implants. Looking more closely at this phenomenon the explanation is simple. There are two situations where a compression effect can be exerted. If, for example, a bone fragment at the base of a phalanx has to be reattached, the FFS implant is inserted in an oblique direction starting at the cancellous base of the bone with the tip directed towards the contralateral cortex (Fig. 34.11a). In Fig. 34.11a the fragment is reduced with Weber forceps. When the implant enters the bone it produces a thread. The implant is then pro-

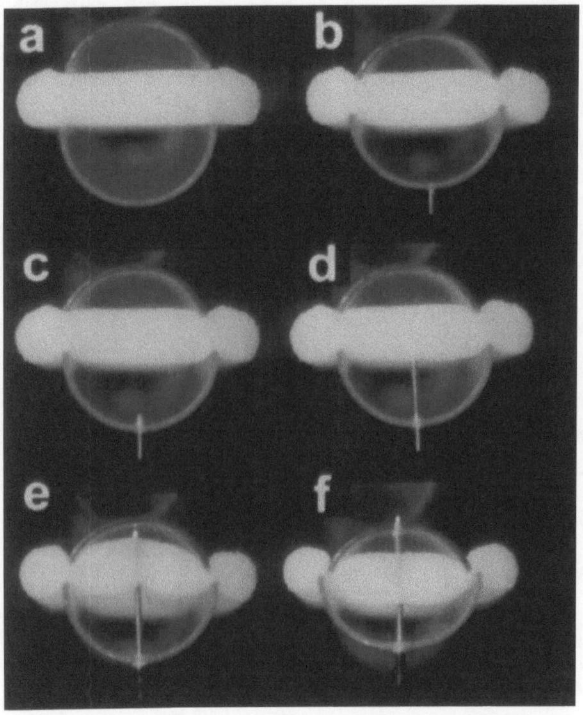

Fig 34.12 Model to explain the compression effect. **a** Two plastic half rings are mounted in front of each other with a soft sponge in between. **b** The tip of the FFS implant is placed on the near "cortex". With a slight pressure against the near cortex the sponge shows some compression. **c** The FFS implant is drilled into the near cortex producing a thread. **d** The implant is advanced towards the far cortex. **e** When the tip of the FFS implant reaches the far cortex it makes a number of revolutions before the tip enters the cortex. At this point the thread in the near cortex is stripped with the washer abutting against the near cortex. **f** The threaded portion of the FFS implant has entered the far cortex. The sponge now shows considerable compression.

gressively inserted until its tip meets the contralateral cortex (Fig. 34.11b). At this point the implant meets the resistance of the hard cortical bone. The thread makes several revolutions without advancing initially, leading to a stripping of the thread in the cancellous bone. The result is a gliding hole proximally and a threaded hole distally (Fig. 34.11c). A similar situation occurs if the near cortex of the fragment reaches the washer at the end of the FFS implant before the fracture gap is firmly closed (Fig. 34.11d, 34.11e, 34.12). In the example shown (Fig. 34.11d) a ruptured intermetacarpal ligament resulted in a wide gap between adjacent metacarpal heads. The fully threaded FFS implant is first drilled into the near metacarpal producing a threaded hole. On reaching the far metacarpal it also produces a threaded hole. At the moment the washer reaches the near metacarpal cortex (Fig. 34.11e) the FFS implant revolves without advancing thus producing a gliding hole in the near metacarpal. This allows the metacarpal heads to approximate. The situation is simulated in Fig. 34.12.

Insertion techniques

Just as with a simple K-wire, the FFS implant is mounted in a drill. It is designed to be inserted without predrilling or pretapping. In this respect, it is as simple to handle as a K-wire. But there are differences in the material. While K-wires can be bent during insertion into the bone, the steel used for FFS implants is comparable to screw material. Bending is not intended and not possible. As with a screw, it would lead to deformity and breakage. This means, therefore, that the intended position of the FFS implant must be determined before it is inserted. Fig. 34.13 demonstrates the operative technique. The first step is reduction of the fracture. A Weber forceps is used to achieve interfragmentary compression in an intra-articular fracture of the proximal phalanx of the big toe (Fig. 34.13a). The joint line should be perfectly reconstructed. It is of the utmost importance to turn either the extremity or the image

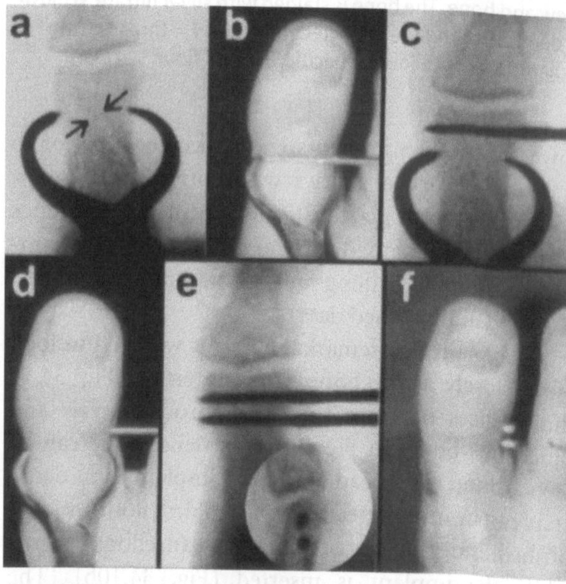

Fig. 34.13 Basic technique of fracture fixation in a fracture of the proximal phalanx of the big toe. **a** The extremity is turned until the X-ray beam is aligned with the fracture gap. A forceps is used for reduction and interfragmentary compression. **b,c** The length of the implant is determined by overlaying the bone with an implant of adequate size. **d** The implant is inserted perpendicular to the X-ray beam until the shoulder meets the near cortex. **e** A second implant ensures rotational stability (inset shows a lateral view to confirm correct placement). **f** Implants cut with pliers.

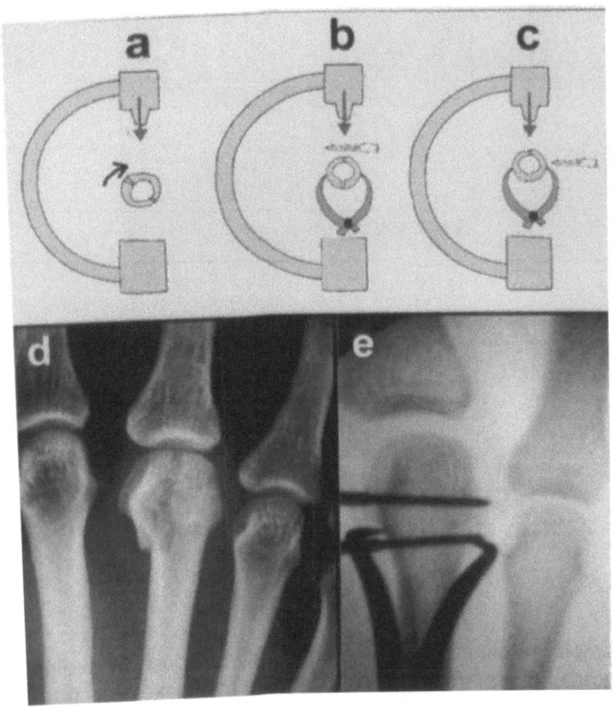

Fig. 34.14 Operative technique. **a** The extremity is turned until the X-ray beam is aligned with the fracture gap. **b** A forceps is used for reduction and interfragmentary compression. The length of the implant is determined by overlaying the bone with an implant of adequate size. **c** The implant in then inserted percutaneously. **d, e** Example of a fracture in the metacarpal head.

intensifier to obtain a perfect view of the fracture gap (Figs. 34.14a, 34.14b). The second step is to estimate the required length of the implant. The length can be measured in the pre-operative X-ray but it is easier to use the image intensifier overlaying the bone with an implant of adequate size as demonstrated in Figs. 34.13b, 34.13c and 34.14b. The implant is then inserted perpendicular to the X-ray beam. In this case a percutaneous technique is used. The skin is penetrated by the FFS implant and the tip of the implant is securely placed on the bone. It is then drilled in until the shoulder meets the near cortex (Fig. 34.13d). A second implant is used to achieve rotational stability and an exact side view is taken to make sure that both implants are inserted correctly (Fig. 34.13e). The last step is to shorten the implant with pliers. Whenever the subcutaneous layer is deep enough the sharp end of the implant should be covered with skin. In the fingers and toes this is sometimes not possible as in the example in Fig. 34.13f. In such cases the ends of the implants are draped with a sterile dressing. The implants are left in place until fracture healing, normally for 6 weeks, and removed in the ambulatory stage. If FFS implants must be left in place for a longer period of time, where for example, they are used for arthrodesis of a PIP joint, they should always be cut short enough to be covered with skin to minimize the risk of infection.

Clinical Use of the Fragment Fixation System

Use in the Upper Extremity

FFS Implants in the Hand

Fig. 34.15a shows a bony avulsion of the extensor tendon at the base of the third phalanx. There are various techniques described to refix the small fragment, most of them considerably time consuming. The FFS implant can solve the problem in a simple percutaneous way. After piercing the skin the tip of the implant (1.6mm) is placed on the fragment and with a slight pressure it is pushed back to its anatomical position (Fig. 34.15b). The correct positioning of the fragment is controlled with the aid of an image intensifier. The fine machine thread is then slowly advanced into the fragment and the base of the phalanx until the "shoulder" of the implant abuts against the cortex of the fragment (Fig. 34.15c). The implant is cut leaving 2mm of the shaft outside for easy removal as demonstrated in Figs. 34.15d and 34.15e. As an additional stabilizer for the first three weeks in these cases a "Stack" splint is used to immobilize the DIP joint. In Figs. 34.15d and 34.15e the final result after 6 weeks at the time of removal of the implant is demonstrated. Instead of one medium sized implant it is sometimes advantageous to use two small implants (1.2mm). Reduction of the fragment can be assisted with forceps as demonstrated in Fig. 34.16a. Ideal stability is achieved if the implants are inserted in a converging fashion (Fig. 34.16b) as sliding of the fragment under the pull of the extensor tendon is thus prevented.

Figs. 34.17a, 34.17b shows an osteotomy at the base of the first phalanx which was produced by a kitchen knife. The base fragment was anatomically reduced under direct vision (Fig. 34.17c). The shafts of the implants after shortening should be long enough to allow easy removal (at least 2mm, Fig. 34.17d). In this position they can be completely covered with skin. Figs. 34.17e and 34.17f demonstrate the function of the MCP joint after removal of the implants.

Fig. 34.18a shows an unusual case of a carpometacarpal dislocation. To reduce the dislocation a

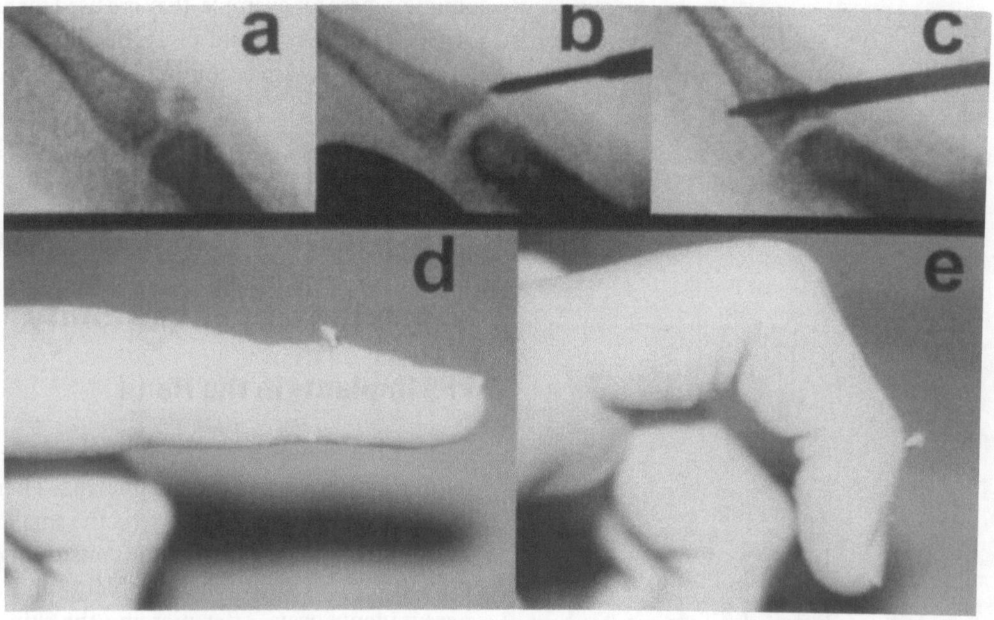

Fig. 34.15 **a** Lateral view of a "bush fracture". **b** The tip of the FFS implant is placed on the fragment percutaneously. With slight pressure the fracture gap disappears. **c** The implant is slowly advanced until the "shoulder" of the implant meets the near cortex. **d, e** Function shortly before removal of the implant at six weeks.

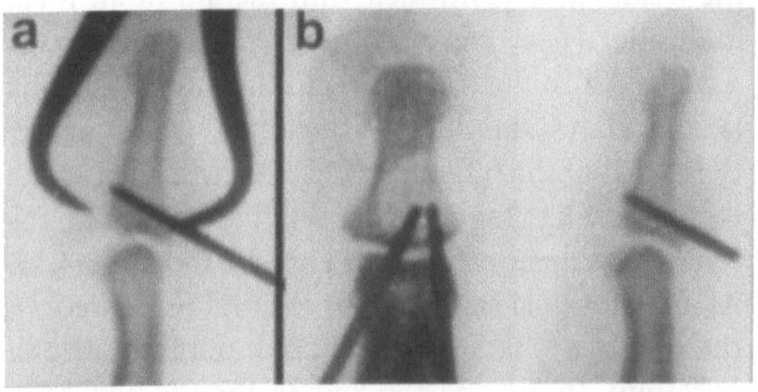

Fig. 34.16 **a** Lateral view of a "bush-fracture". The reduction was performed with a Weber forceps. The first FFS implant (small size) is inserted. **b** AP and lateral views after insertion of two small sized implants in a slightly converging fashion.

FFS implant was drilled into the proximal third of the metacarpal shaft (Fig. 34.18b). Using the FFS implant like a joystick it was now possible to perform a closed reduction under image intensification. Fig. 34.18b shows an anatomically aligned carpo-metacarpal joint. To maintain the anatomical position a medium sized FFS implant armed with a washer was drilled through the base of the fifth metacarpal into the fourth metacarpal (Fig. 34.18c). Compression between the metacarpals was not intended with this implant. While the proximal dislocation was anatomically aligned the broad gap between the fifth and fourth metacarpal heads indicated rupture of the distal intermetacarpal ligaments (Fig. 34.18d). To solve the problem a medium sized FFS implant with a washer was inserted

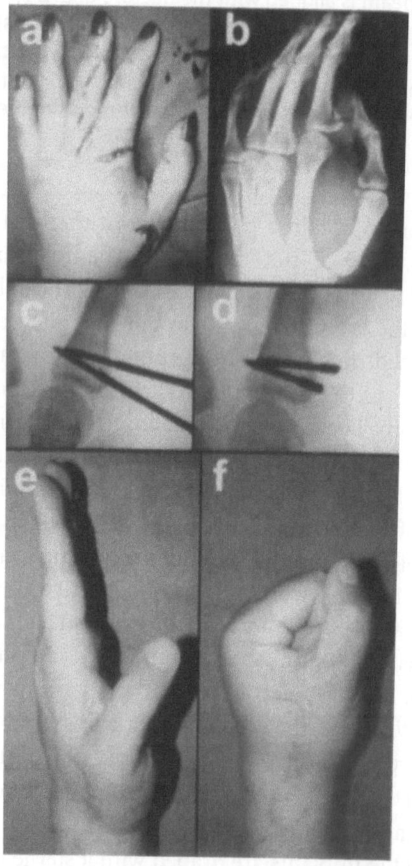

Fig. 34.17 **a, b** Fracture at the base of the first phalanx. c, d Two medium sized FFS implants are inserted after open reduction and cut close to the "shoulder" leaving 2–3mm outside the bone. **e, f** Function after removal of the implants.

into the subcapital region of the fifth metacarpal (Fig. 34.18d). As the tip of the implant approached the near cortex of the fourth metacarpal the washer reached the near cortex of the fifth metacarpal (Fig. 34.18d). With the washer firmly pressed against the cortex of the bone, the thread in the fifth metacarpal previously produced by the implant was stripped and thus converted into a gliding hole. With a thread in the fourth metacarpal and a gliding hole in the fifth metacarpal the FFS implant was slowly advanced into the fourth metacarpal until the distance between the metacarpal heads was corrected (Fig. 34.18e, theoretical explanation in Figs. 34.11d, 34.11e). The post-operative X-ray is shown in Fig. 34.18f ; the healing after implant removal is demonstrated in Fig. 34.18g.

FFS Implants in the Wrist Joint and Distal Radius

There are many indications for the use of threaded wires in fractures of the upper extremity. Whenever screws and K-wires are alternative methods the Fragment Fixation System (FFS) is appropriate.

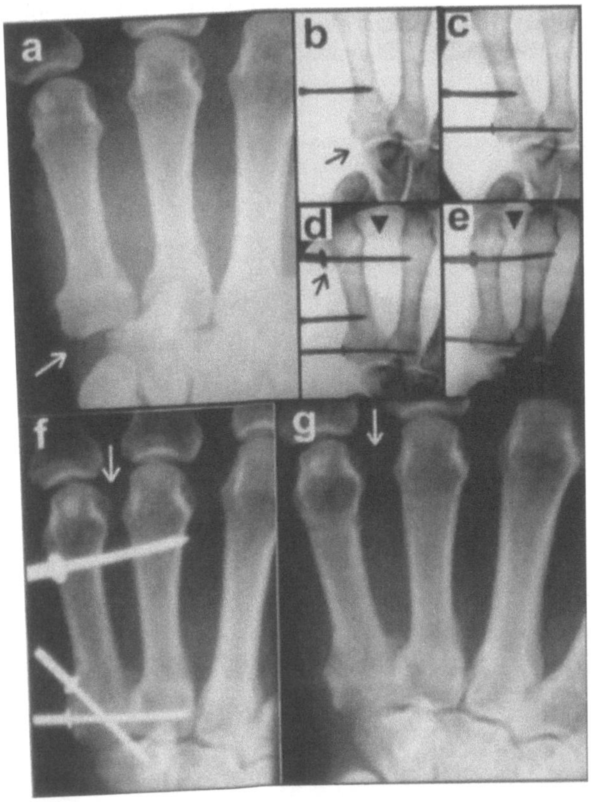

Fig. 34.18 The use of FFS implants in a carpo-metacarpal dislocation. **a** Dislocation; **b** "Joystick" function; **c** Fixation of the base; **d, e** Reduction and maintenance of the corrected intermetacarpal "gap". **f** Post-operative X-ray; **g** X-ray after implant removal.

For example, in comminuted fractures of the distal end of the radius many surgeons use K-wires to stabilize the fragments. As an alternative, the fragment fixation system can be used. The threaded portion provides much more purchase in the cancellous bone, especially in elderly people with osteoporosis. As with K-wires the FFS implants can be used percutaneously. Fig. 34.19 shows a distal radius fracture where the FFS implants have been used as an adjunct to external fixation to stabilize the fracture. They are used in a crossed fashion to prevent secondary loss of radial length. The concomitant ulnar fracture is treated with a single medium sized FFS implant. In intra-articular fractures the implants are inserted parallel to the radio-carpal joint line after reduction of the fracture (Fig. 34.20).

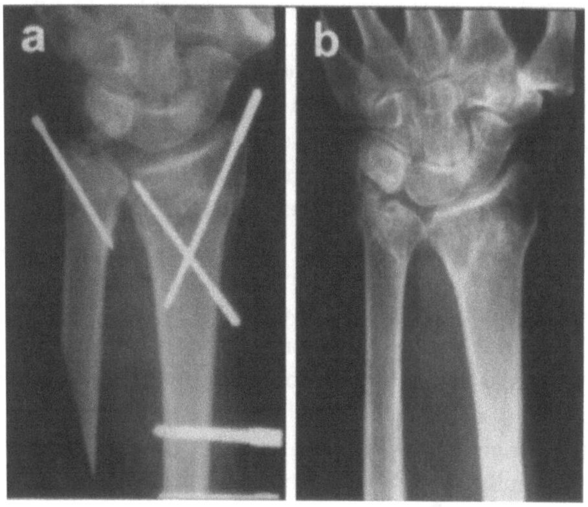

Fig. 34.19 a Distal radius fracture treated with external fixation. As an additional measure two FFS medium implants are inserted in a crossed fashion to prevent a secondary loss of radial length and angulation. The concomitant ulnar fracture was treated with a single FFS implant. **b** No loss of length or angle occurred after removal of the implant.

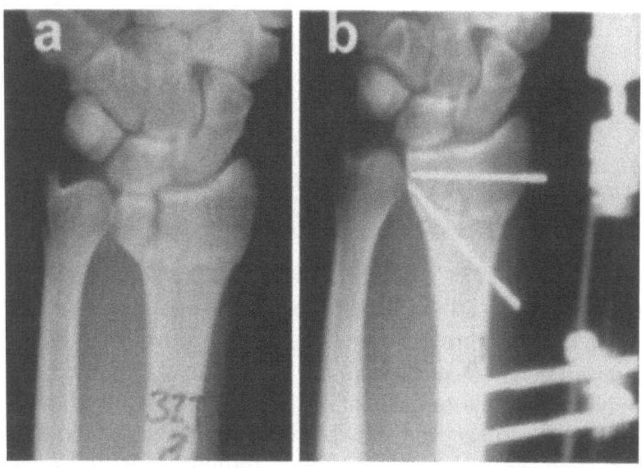

Fig. 34.20 a Intra-articular fracture of the distal radius. **b** Instead of K-wires FFS implants are used percutaneously after closed reduction of the radio-carpal joint line.

Bony avulsions of the radio-ulnar ligament at the ulnar side of the radius can be refixed under direct vision following a minimally invasive approach. In these cases the use of a washer with a medium sized implant is recommended.

As a general rule fractures with a dorsal instability can usually be treated with a minimally invasive technique. The FFS implants are inserted either percutaneously from the radial side or, with a small incision, from the dorsal side between the extensor tendon compartments (Figs. 34.21a, 34.21b). In some cases, however, especially in comminuted fractures and osteoporotic bone, a dorso-radial bone graft as an additional technique is advisable. Regardless of this, fractures displaying palmar instability should be treated from the palmar side. The surgical approach to the palmar distal radius is much more extensive since the fracture elements must be stabilized under direct vision. Plates are commonly used for these fractures. As an alternative method we recommend a limited surgical approach and the use of mini-plates combined with medium sized FFS implants and washers. The malleable mini-plate can be perfectly adapted to the palmar shape of the distal radius and is fixed after reduction using medium FFS implants with washers. The FFS implants can be inserted through the holes of the plate in various directions in accordance with the individual fracture situation (Fig. 34.22) and the polished shaft is cut with pliers close to the shoulder after implantation. The sharp ends of the shortened FFS implants are then covered by the pronator muscle. This Minimally Invasive Osteosynthesis Technique (MIOT) provides sufficient stability to prevent a secondary palmar displacement. We frequently use this technique as an additional measure in combination with a joint bridging wrist fixator (Figs. 34.22,

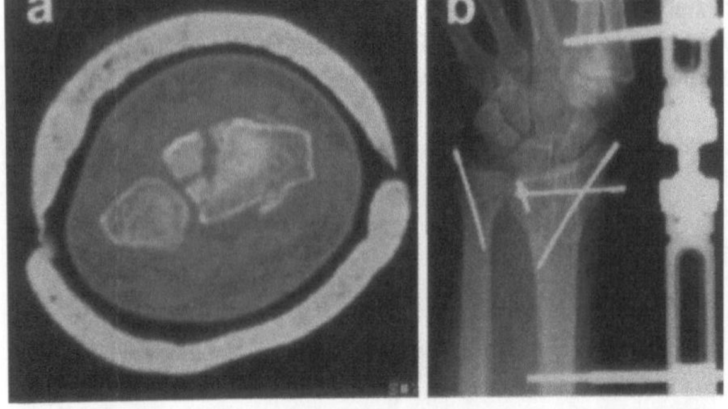

Fig. 34.21 **a** CT-scan of a distal radius fracture at the level of Lister's tubercle. The scan helps to plan the operative strategy. **b** The fracture is treated with an external fixator. FFS implants inserted percutaneously from the radial side are employed to stabilize the radio-carpal joint line and to prevent loss of radial length. The ulnar "die punch" fragment is held, following reduction, by a single FFS implant through a limited open approach between the fourth and fifth extensor tendon compartments. A concomitant ulnar fracture is stabilized by a medium sized FFS implant.

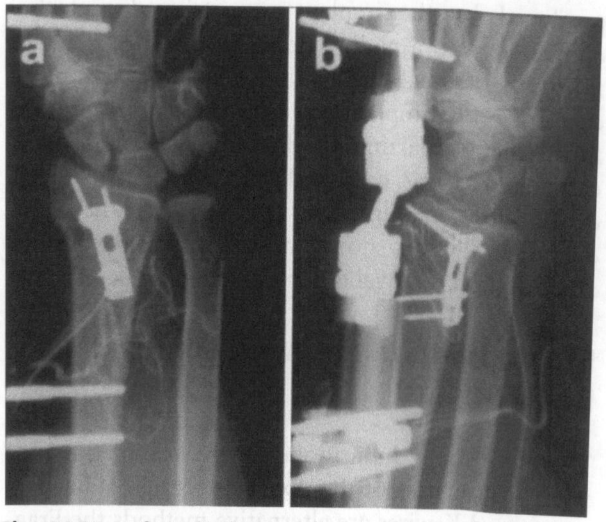

Fig. 34.22 **a, b** A displaced radius fracture is treated with external fixation. Through a limited palmar approach a small plate is used to stabilize the main fragment. The plate is fixed to the distal radius using medium sized FFS implants with washers. This technique allows independent choice of the direction of the FFS implants according to the fracture situation.

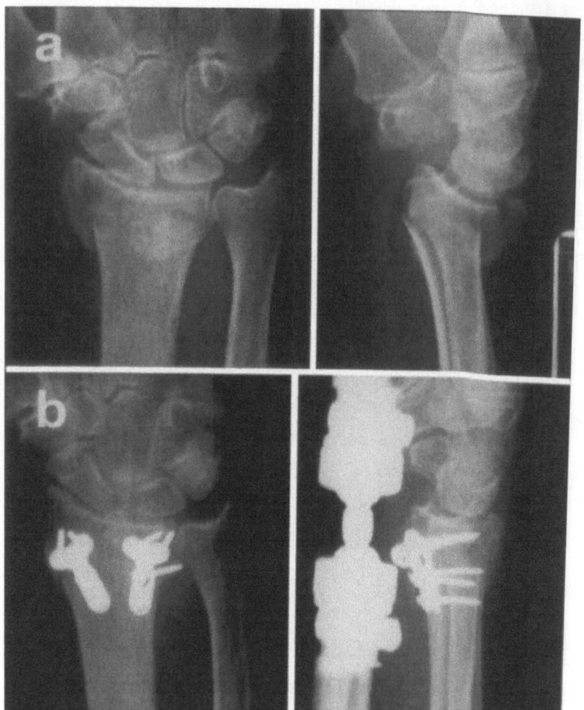

Fig. 34.23 Intra-articular radius fracture. Two mini-plates are used to stabilize the radial "pilon" on the ulnar and radial sides.

34.23). If necessary, two of these mini-plates can be combined to counteract instability on both the ulnar and radial sides of the distal radius: for example, to reattach a ligament-bearing fragment at the radio-ulnar joint and at the same time to treat a fractured radial styloid which tends to dislocate under the pull of the brachioradialis muscle (Fig. 34.23).

FFS Implants in the Elbow

FFS implants can be used for any kind of bony disruption at the distal end of the humerus. As an example, Figs. 34.24a, 34.24b show a radial condyle fracture. Either medium or large sized implants each with a washer can be employed (Figs. 34.24c, 34.24d). The free elbow function is demonstrated in Figs. 34.24e, 34.24f. In disruption of collateral ligaments which must be reattached to the bone, the FFS implants are used in combination with plastic washers as illustrated in Fig. 34.25. This technique allows secure and broad contact of the disrupted ligament with the bone. The technique is demonstrated in Fig. 34.26. The ligament is held firmly in place with two pincers or forceps as demonstrated in Fig. 34.26b. The FFS implant is then slowly drilled into the bone until the plastic washer presses the ligament against the bone. The same technique is used for the reattachment of ligaments in other sites, for example, reattachment of a collateral ligament at the base of the thumb.

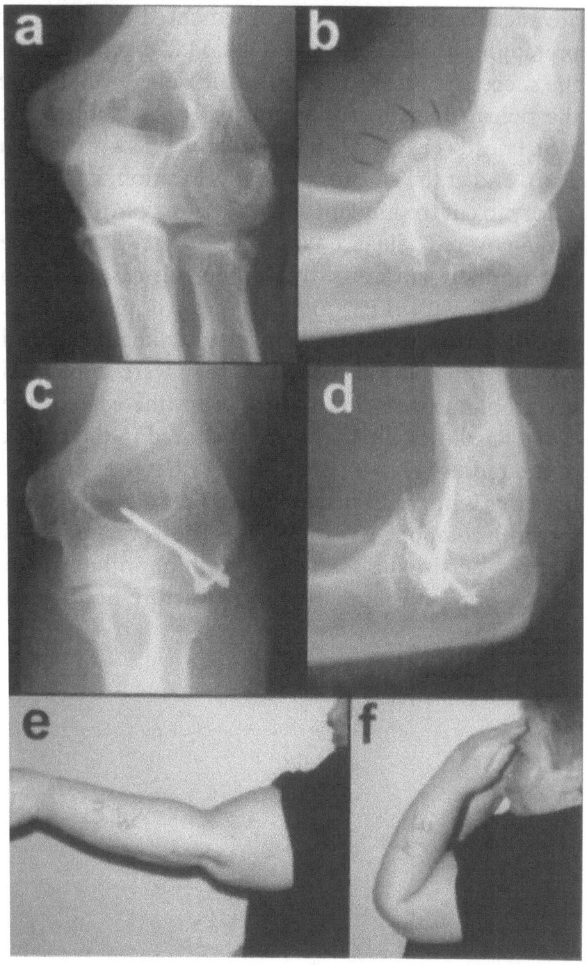

Fig. 34.24 **a, b** Fracture of the radial condyle. **c, d** A large size and a medium size FFS implant both bearing washers were inserted after open reduction. **e, f** Function after 3 weeks.

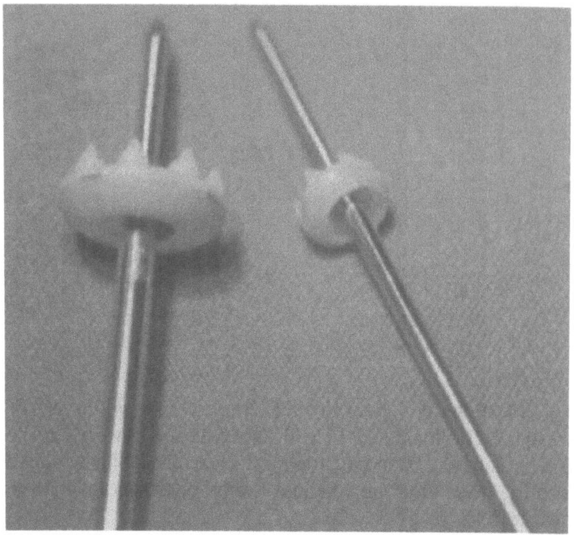

Fig. 34.25 The use of plastic washers. Medium and large size FFS implants fit to plastic washers. This allows secure refixation of ligamentous disruptions.

Radial Head Fractures

Radial head fractures are either intracapital "chisel" fractures or subcapital fractures. Not infrequently, however, both fracture types are combined. These combined intra- and subcapital fractures indicate an extremely unstable situation and frequently lead to resection of the radial head. As a late sequel to radial head resection persistent pain in distal radio-ulnar and radio-carpal joint has been described. This is due to proximal movement of the radius leading to a relative overlength of the distal ulna. For this reason reconstruction of the radial head should be attempted whenever possible. The medium sized FFS implants are most helpful especially in the reconstitution of multiple fragment radial head fractures. The scenario is illustrated in Figs. 34.27a–b which show a three part intracapital fracture combined with a subcapital fracture. As demonstrated in Fig. 34.27c–e the first step is the reconstruction of the radial head. Use of FFS implants (medium size without washer) simplifies the operative technique. The implant is drilled into the fragment and then used as a joystick to manipulate the fragment into its anatomical position. Once the anatomical position is attained the implant is slowly advanced into the adjacent fragment. Predrilling or pretapping is not necessary. Figs. 34.27e, 34.27f show the successful reconstruction of the radial head before the polished shaft of the implant is cut close to the radial head (Fig. 34.27g). Because the pliers produce a sharp end at the cut surface in this location, it is mandatory to cut the implant as close as possible to the cartilage-covered surface of the radial head. The concomitant subcapital fracture in this case was also stabilized with FFS medium size implants (Fig. 34.27h). After reconstruction of the radial head and adequate anatomical reduction, they were implanted in an oblique direction starting from the edge of the radial head. Distally they were anchored in the cortex of the radius (Figs. 34.27h, 34.27i). Removal of these implants is not indicated as long as they do not disturb forearm rotation. In some cases, however, patients report a persistent "scratching" with or without pain during pro- and supination after fracture healing. In these cases removal of the FFS implants is indicated if ultrasound discloses a chronic intra-articular effusion. This was diagnosed in the case illustrated and the FFS implants were subsequently removed. Fig. 34.28c shows the healed situation after removal of the implants and clinically free and painless function is demonstrated in Fig. 34.29.

Fractures of the Olecranon

Various techniques are available to stabilize olecranon fractures. As the most common technique, tension band wiring provides enough stability for early active mobilization. As an alternative to K-wires inserted from the tip of the olecranon in an oblique direction and anchoring in the ventral cortex of the ulna, FFS implants can be used. We use large implants of ade-

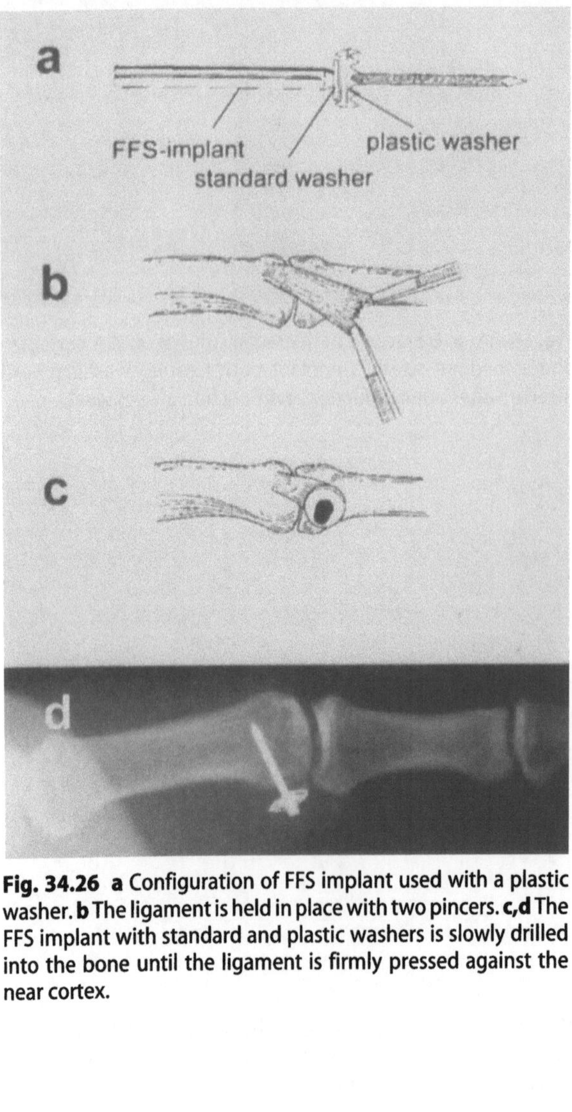

Fig. 34.26 **a** Configuration of FFS implant used with a plastic washer. **b** The ligament is held in place with two pincers. **c,d** The FFS implant with standard and plastic washers is slowly drilled into the bone until the ligament is firmly pressed against the near cortex.

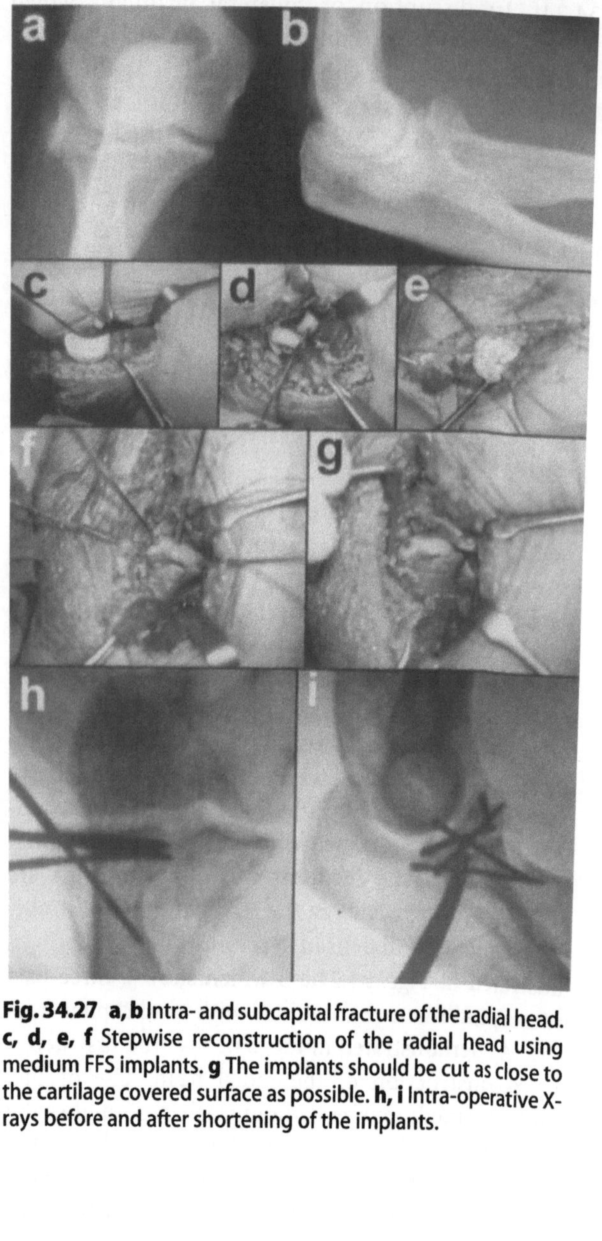

Fig. 34.27 **a, b** Intra- and subcapital fracture of the radial head. **c, d, e, f** Stepwise reconstruction of the radial head using medium FFS implants. **g** The implants should be cut as close to the cartilage covered surface as possible. **h, i** Intra-operative X-rays before and after shortening of the implants.

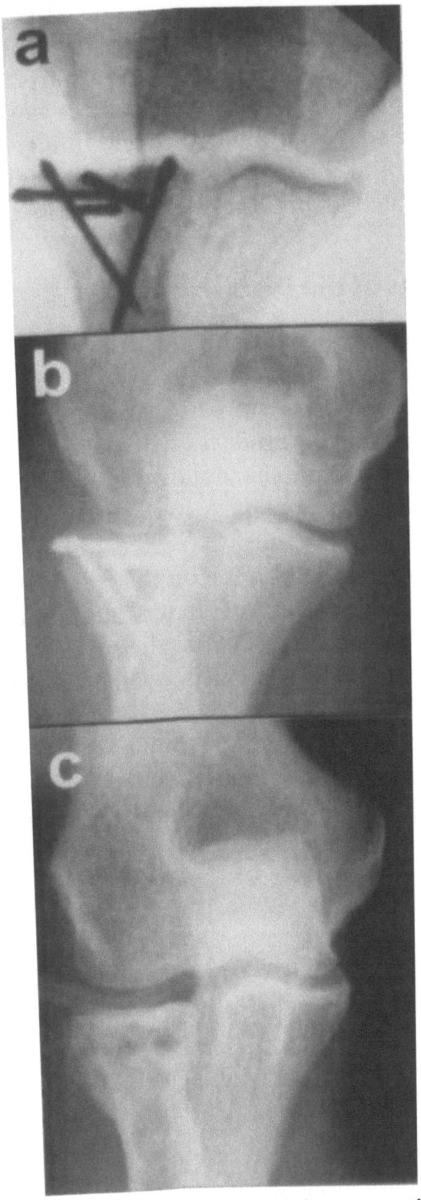

Fig. 34.28 Same case as in Fig. 34.27. **a** Intra-operative X-ray; **b** post-operative X-ray; **c** X-ray after removal of the implants.

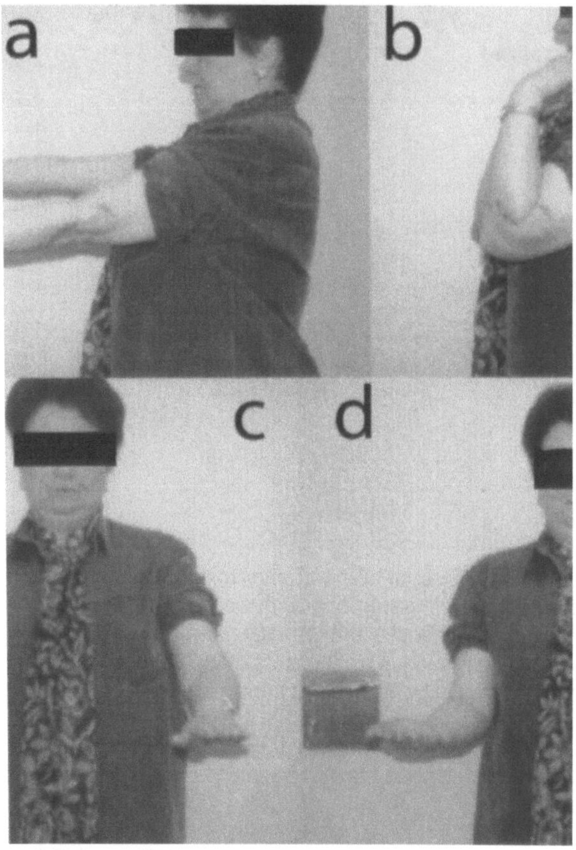

Fig. 34.29 a, b, c, d Free function of the elbow joint after removal of the implants.

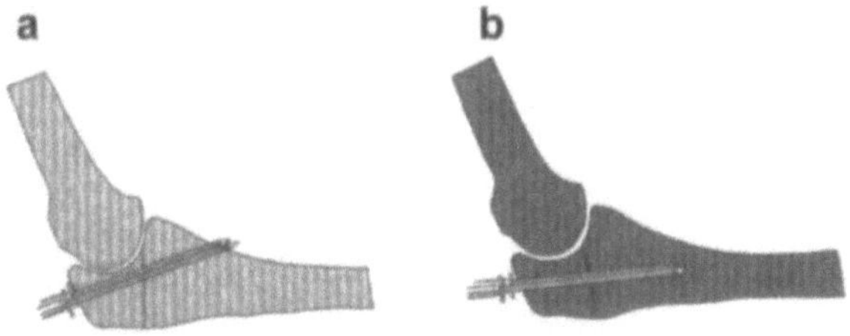

Fig. 34.30 a Stabilization of an olecranon fracture in an elderly patient. Both implants should be anchored in the contralateral cortex. **b** Stabilization of an olecranon fracture in a young patient. The FFS implants (large size) can be securely anchored in the cancellous bone; penetration of the contralateral cortex is not necessary.

quate length with washers. The fracture site is exposed through a dorsal approach and the elbow joint cleaned of blood clots. Starting at the tip of the olecranon, two FFS implants are inserted parallel to one another or in a slightly v-shaped configuration across the fracture line. In younger patients with dense cancellous bone it is sufficient to anchor the threaded portion of the implants in the cancellous bone (Fig. 34.30b). In elderly patients with considerable osteoporosis, however, the threaded portion should be anchored in the ventral cortex of the ulna (Fig. 34.30a). In younger patients the purchase of the fine machine thread is normally good enough so that additional tension band wiring is not necessary. In severe osteoporosis, or if there is any doubt about the purchase of the FFS implant, a tension band wire should be used in addition to the FFS implant. Fig. 34.31a shows a simple olecranon fracture which was anatomically stabilized with two large FFS implants. Tension band wiring with two FFS implants replacing K-wires is shown in Fig. 34.31b. In this case an additional fragment was fixed with two medium FFS implants. In both cases immobilization of the elbow joint is necessary only in

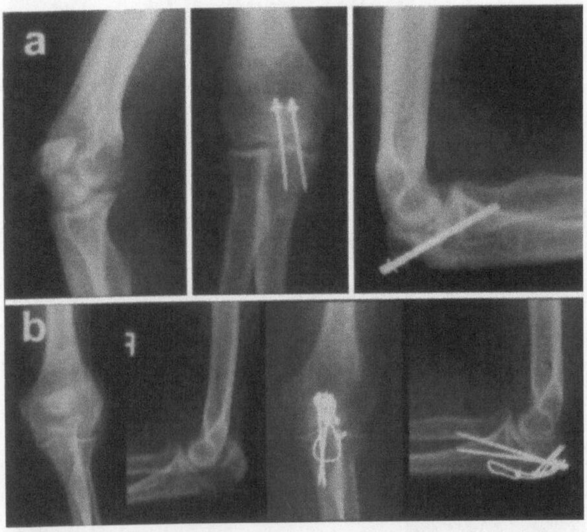

Fig. 34.31 **a** Example of an olecranon fracture treated with two large sized FFS implants, each with washer. The thread of the implants is anchored in the contralateral cortex. **b** Example of an olecranon fracture in an osteoporotic patient. Two large implants were used, anchored in the contralateral cortex. In this case the situation was not stable enough, so an additional tension band wire was employed. Two medium sized implants were used to stabilize a smaller fragment.

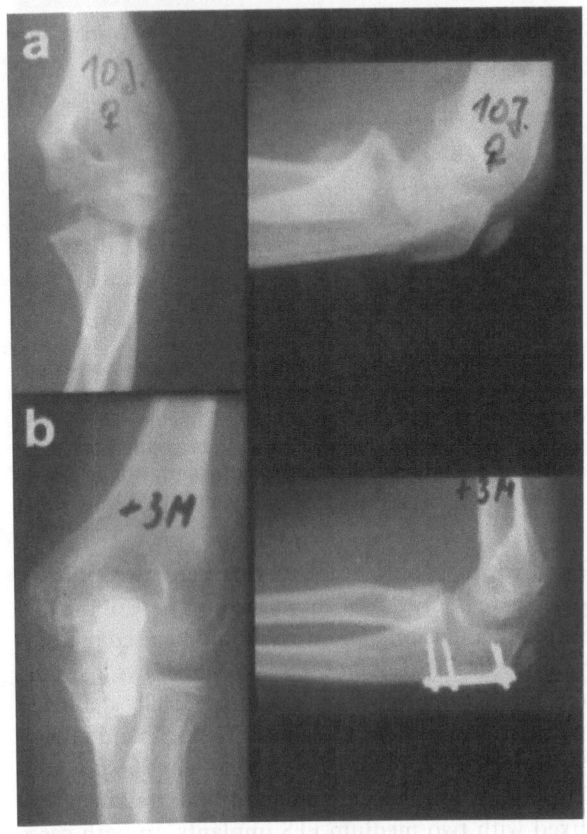

Fig. 34.32 a, b Olecranon fracture in a 10-year old girl stabilized with a mini plate and medium FFS implants with washers (MIOT technique).

the early post-operative period until uneventful wound healing occurs. Mobilization starts with passive physiotherapy during the first three weeks. Later, increasing active motion is allowed. In Fig. 34.32 the use of a mini-plate with FFS medium implants is demonstrated in an olecranon fracture in a 10-year-old girl.

Fractures of the Distal Humerus

Intra-articular fractures of the distal humerus frequently require open reduction and internal fixation. The main objectives are perfect realignment of the joint surface and the production of a stable enough situation at the fracture site to allow early passive mobilization of the elbow joint. A frequently observed late sequel in these fractures is severe loss of motion. Screws and plates are typical implants for the internal osteosynthesis technique. FFS implants of medium or large size can help to minimize the surgical approach instead of, or combined with, conventional osteosynthesis techniques. Fig. 34.33a shows a distal intra-articular fracture of the humerus with multiple fragments and displacement. As seen in Fig. 34.33b FFS implants were used to reduce the fracture. The operative technique was completed with the applica-

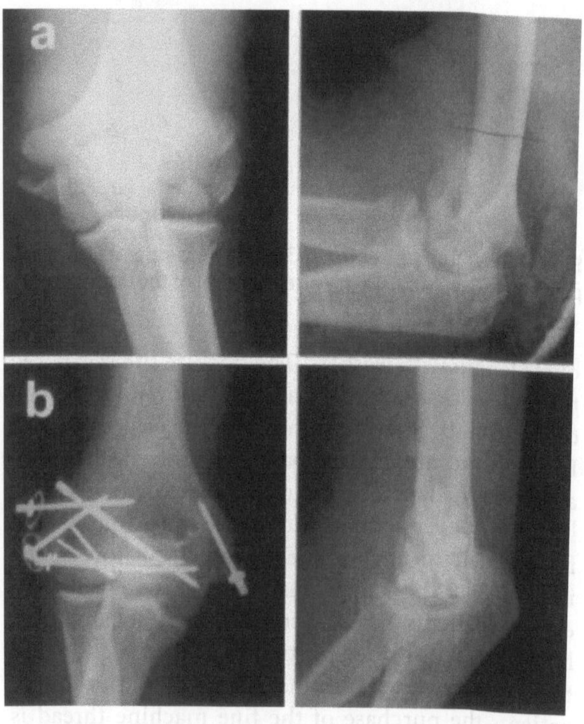

Fig. 34.33 **a** Comminuted intra-articular fracture of the distal humerus. **b** FFS implants are used instead of screws and K-wires for the stabilization of small fragments. The technique was completed with a joint-bridging hinged fixator.

tion of a unilateral joint bridging elbow fixator with motion capacity to allow early active mobilization.

Fractures of the Proximal Humerus and Scapula

Isolated fractures of the greater tuberosity are securely fixed by two large FFS implants with washers (Fig. 34.34). They can also be used as an additional technique in multi-fragment proximal humerus fractures where the greater cartilage-bearing fragment is stabilized with a T-plate and smaller fragments with attachments of the rotatory cuff are secured with FFS implants. Due to the large soft tissue envelope composed mainly of the deltoid muscle, and the course of the axillary nerve, an open technique is most advisable. The same is true for fractures of the glenoid, which require reduction. Fig. 34.35 shows a scapula fracture where the dorsal fragments of the glenoid were reattached with medium FFS implants through a dorsal approach. Removal of these implants is not indicated. As in the use of FFS implants for radial head fractures, therefore, it is most advisable to cut the ends of the implants as short as possible.

FFS implants are not suitable for "Tossy" injuries. The relative movement between the acromion and the clavicle needs flexible implants. The temporary transfixion of the AC-joint is best performed, therefore, with K-wires and an additional tension band wire. The use of FFS implants would inevitably lead to early breakage.

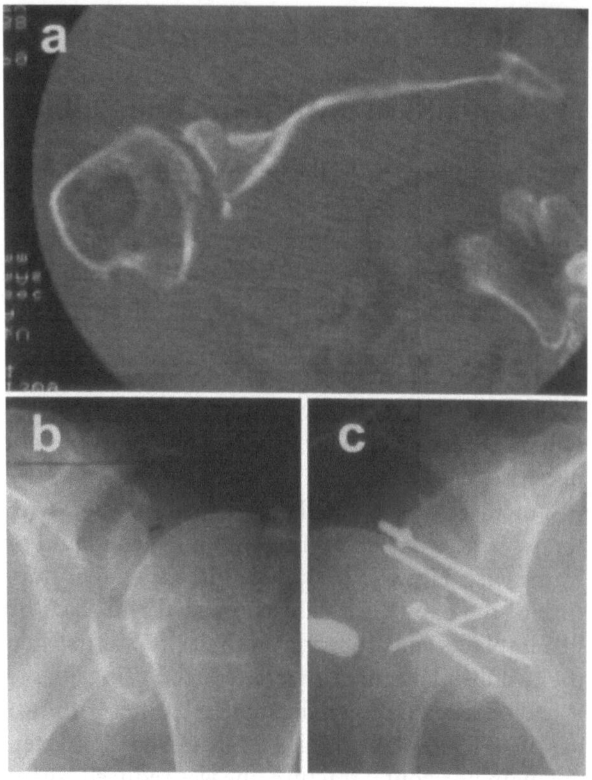

Fig. 34.35 Fracture of the glenoid. **a** CT-scan showing a displaced major fragment. **b** Pre-operative AP view. **c** Post-operative view.

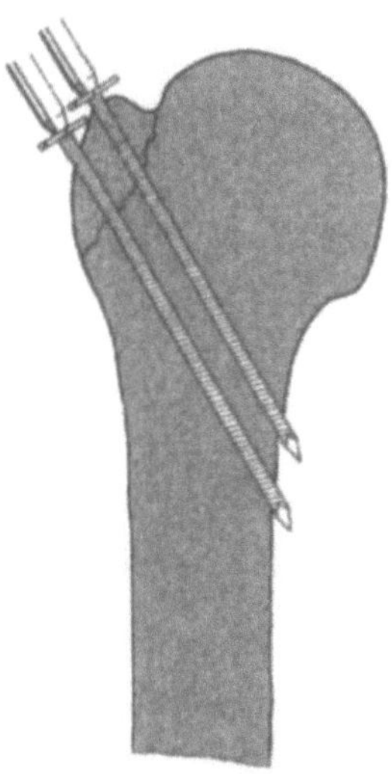

Fig. 34.34 Schematic drawing to demonstrate the stabilization of a fracture of the greater tuberosity of the humerus.

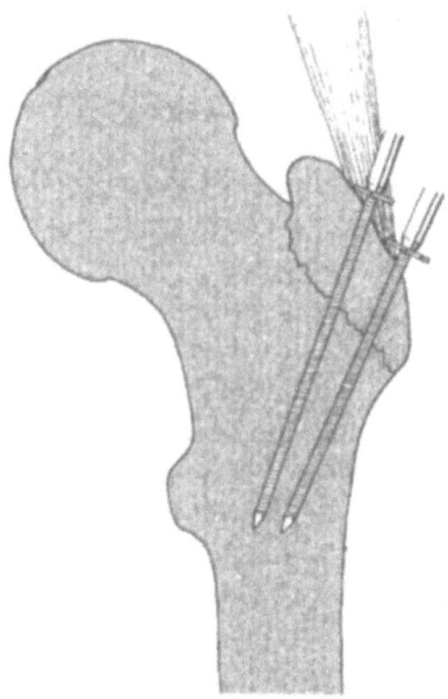

Fig. 34.36 Schematic drawing to demonstrate reattachment of the greater trochanter. In younger patients additional tension band wiring is not necessary.

Use in the Lower Extremity

FFS Implants in the Hip and Knee Joints

As discussed previously, the fine machine thread of FFS implants is best suited for cancellous bone. Except in the presence of severe osteoporosis, reattachment of the greater trochanter can easily be performed using large FFS implants. As described in the treatment of olecranon fractures the implants used for securing the greater trochanter should be armed with washers (Fig. 34.36). A tension band wire as an additional technique is only necessary if the bone quality would lead to poor purchase.

Fractures of the patella are usually treated with screws or K-wires combined with a tension band or frame wire. Fig. 34.37a shows a three fragment fracture of the patella which was reduced and fixed by FFS implants (medium and large size). As a first step the two distal fragments were reduced using a large Weber forceps and then fixed to each other with two parallel FFS implants (Fig. 34.37b). In a second step the main horizontal fracture line was reduced, again with a Weber forceps, and two FFS implants inserted vertically parallel to one another (Fig. 34.37c). To increase stability in this case a frame wire was used as shown in Fig. 34.37d. Long term post-operative immobilization is not necessary. After wound healing, early passive physiotherapy is employed to achieve a minimum knee flexion of at least 90°. In simple vertical and horizontal fractures in younger patients with good bone substance, the use of FFS implants (medium or large size) alone would be sufficient (Fig. 34.38). This technique can be performed percutaneously thus minimizing iatrogenic trauma.

Fig. 34.39 shows disruption of a tibial tuberosity which was reduced and reattached using three large FFS implants with washers. Simple monocondylar fractures of the proximal tibia can be treated percutaneously with two FFS implants of adequate length (large size). Prior to FFS implantation, forceps can be used to reduce the fracture. The FFS implants are introduced under image intensification parallel to the tibial joint line. In more comminuted tibial plateau fractures, open reduction and internal fixation is advisable. T- or L-shaped plates are in common use to stabilize the condyles and bone grafting is frequently unavoidable. In many of these cases FFS implants can function as an additional measure to reattach smaller joint-building bone fragments to achieve the maximum joint congruence.

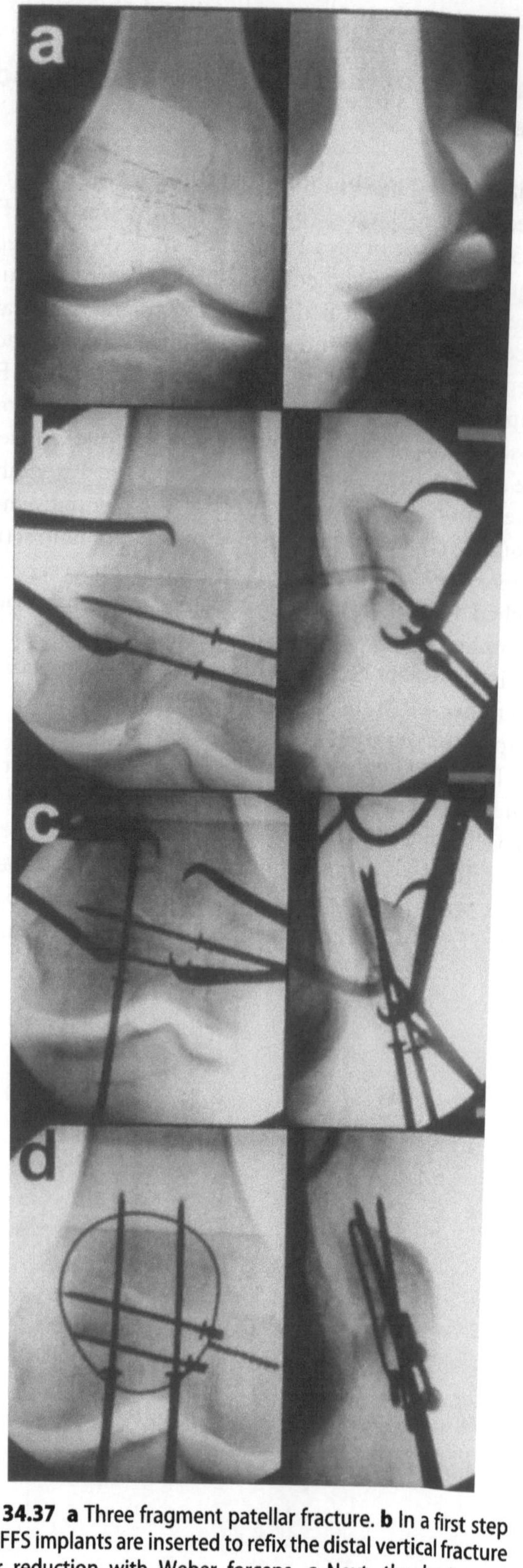

Fig. 34.37 **a** Three fragment patellar fracture. **b** In a first step two FFS implants are inserted to refix the distal vertical fracture after reduction with Weber forceps. **c** Next, the horizontal fracture is stabilized with two vertically inserted FFS implants. **d** In this case an additional "frame-wire" was used to secure the fracture.

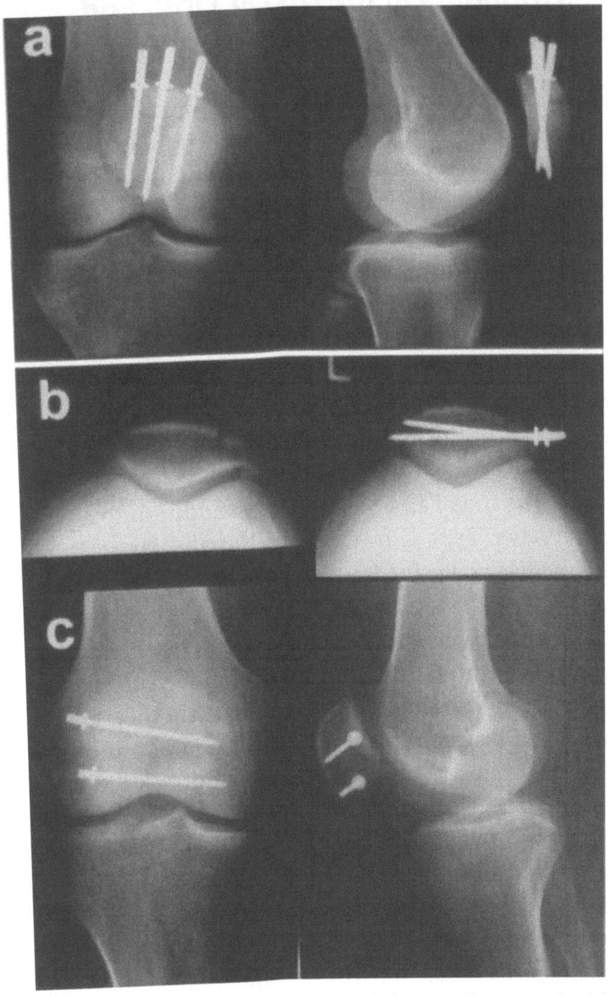

Fig. 34.38 a Horizontal fracture of the patella treated with three large sized FFS implants. **b,c** Vertical fracture fixed with two medium sized implants.

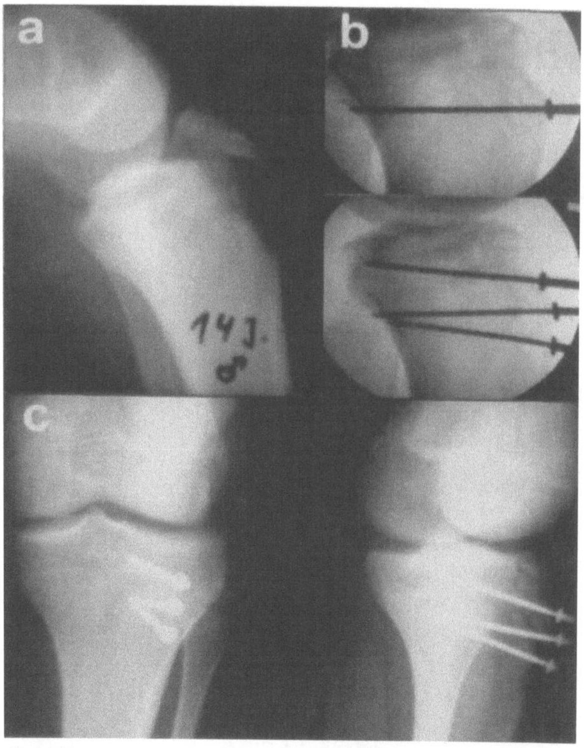

Fig. 34.39 a Disruption of the tibial tuberosity. **b** FFS implants are inserted using the compression effect. **c** Post-operative X-rays.

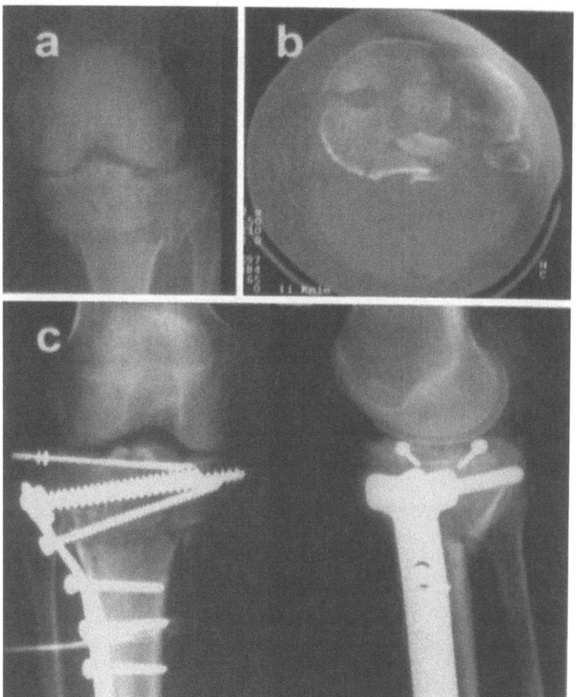

Fig. 34.40 a AP view of a severely comminuted tibial head fracture. **b** The CT scan shows multiple fragmentation and gross displacement. **c** Post-operative views. The FFS implants are introduced into the subchondral bone layer as an additional measure.

Here, medium and/or large sized implants can sometimes be inserted into the subchondral bone under direct vision (Fig. 34.40). These implants are not intended to be removed as long as they do not disturb knee function. They are cut close to the bone surface. In an extremely comminuted distal femur fracture as demonstrated in Fig. 34.41a the primary stabilizer is a retrograde nail. In addition to this the smaller fragments are reconstituted with FFS implants. In Fig. 34.41b the post-operative X-ray shows multiple use of the FFS system in the distal femur. The patella was partially reconstructed and also fixed with FFS implants. The X-ray in Fig. 34.41c shows the fracture site at 4 months with healing in progress. The patient was allowed full weightbearing at that time. The FFS implants did not move during the entire treatment period.

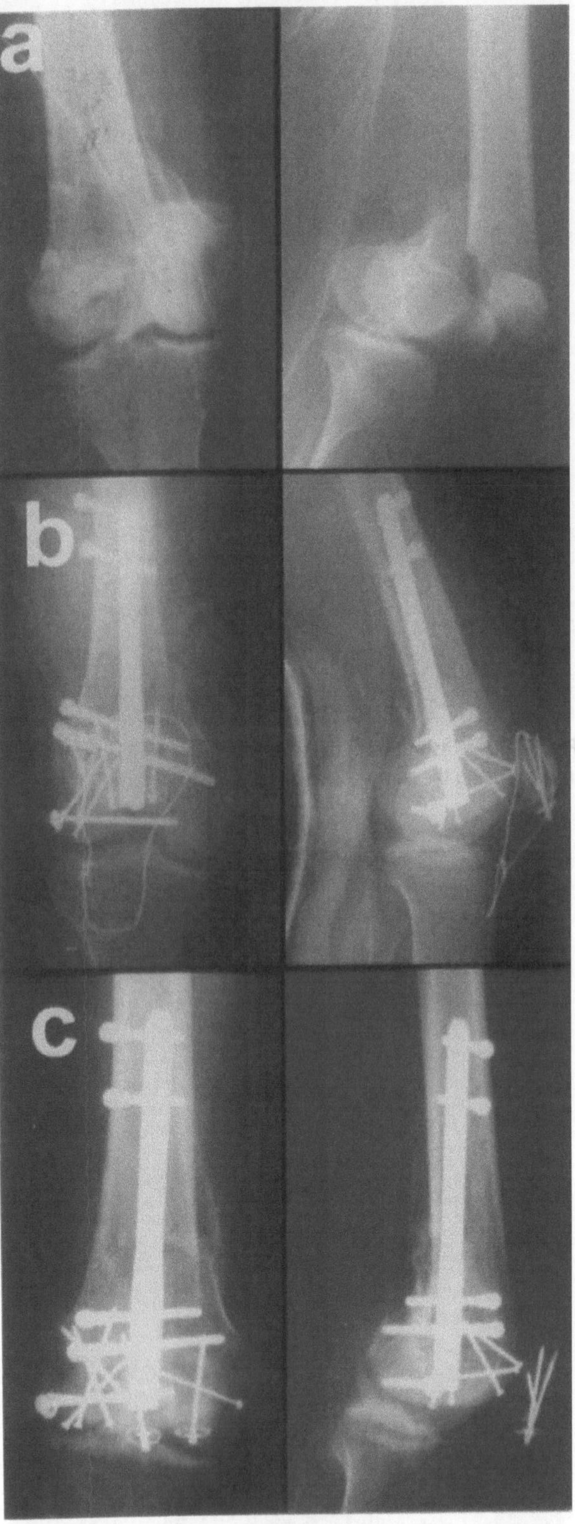

Fig. 34.41 **a** Comminuted fracture of the distal femur. **b** A retrograde nail serves as the primary stabilizer. Multiple FFS implants with and without washers are used to fix small fragments. **c** X-ray at 4 months.

FFS Implants in the Distal Tibia and Ankle Joint

Fractures of the distal fibula are commonly treated with open reduction and a lag screw for interfragmentary compression. A lateral plate secures the fracture site. In Weber Type C fractures, bony disruptions, especially of the ventral tibio-fibular ligament, are frequently encountered. Reattachment of these fragments is desirable, but due to the small size of the fragments the use of a conventional screw can be complicated. The FFS technique allows simple refixing of the fragment and the ligament in a single step procedure. The use of plastic washers as demonstrated in Figs. 34.25, 34.26 is recommended. Fig. 34.42 demonstrates the use of an FFS implant in addition to a plate in a Weber Type C fracture. In bimalleolar fractures the medial malleolus frequently requires open reduction due to the interposed periosteum. After cleaning the fracture site an FFS osteosynthesis with two large implants with washers is a simple and secure procedure. After insertion into the fragment they enable reduction of the fracture under image intensification or direct vision (joystick) and after anatomical repositioning is achieved they are simply advanced through the fracture line into the tibia until the washer abuts securely against the near cortex (Fig. 34.42b). The joystick function is most helpful in severely comminuted tibial pilon fractures (Fig. 34.43a, 34.43b). The main problem in these fractures is the poor soft tissue envelope which does not permit an extensive surgical approach. Reduction is assisted with use of a joint-bridging fixator with proximal screws in the tibia and distal screws either in the calcaneus or in the talus and calcaneus (Fig. 34.44). Slight distraction exerted by the fixator helps to reduce the fracture. The FFS implants (large size) can then be inserted percutaneously into the fragments. The joystick function subsequently allows one to move and to align the joint-bearing fragments as demonstrated in Figs. 34.43c–e. Once a satisfactory position is achieved they are simply advanced into the adjacent fragment as shown in Figs. 34.43f–h or another FFS implant can be inserted parallel to the joint line while the anatomical position of the fragments is maintained by holding the shafts of the previously inserted FFS implants.

FFS Implants in the Foot

It is self-evident that the use of FFS implants in fractures of the foot is as useful as in the hand. Here they provide valuable assistance for the surgeon in a wide

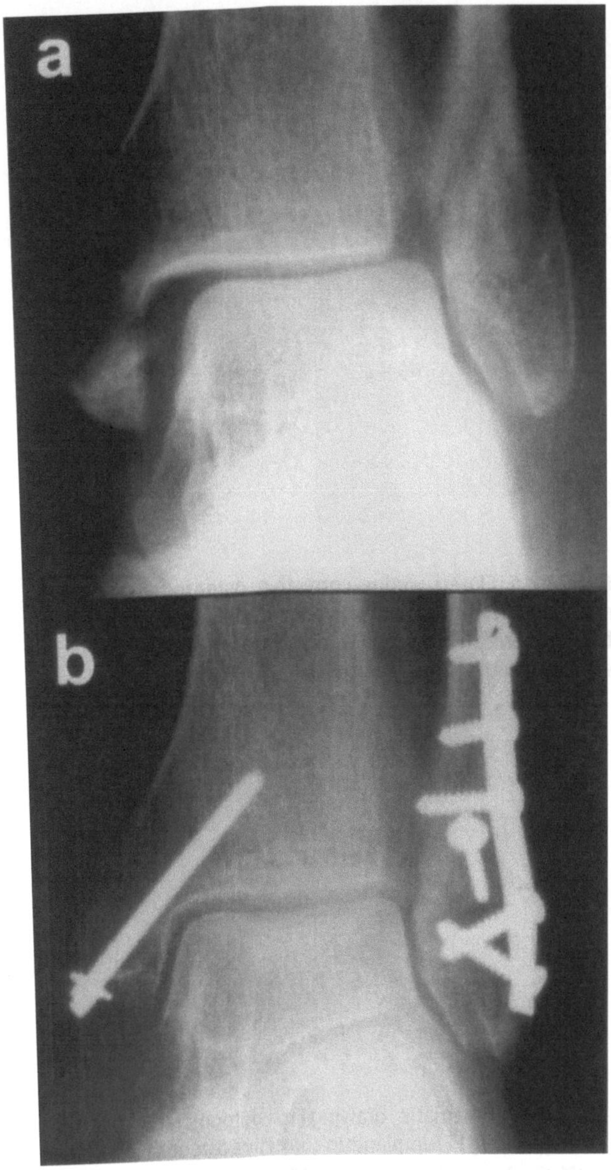

Fig. 34.42 **a** Bimalleolar fracture of the ankle joint. **b** Plate fixation of the fibula. The disrupted syndesmosis is fixed with an FFS implant. The fracture of the medial malleolus is treated with two large sized implants.

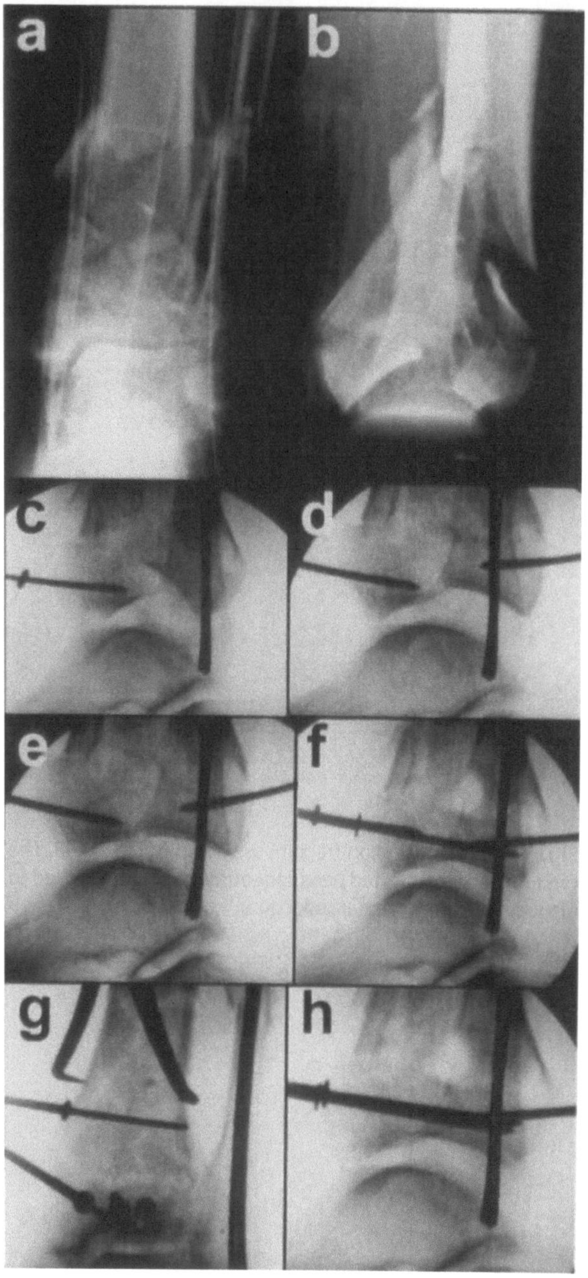

Fig. 34.43 **a, b** Tibial pilon fracture with poor soft tissue envelope. **c, d, e** The percutaneously inserted large FFS implants are used as "joysticks" to reduce the main joint-building fragments. **f, g, h** After achieving an anatomical reduction the FFS implants are inserted fully.

range of indications. Fractures at the base of the fifth metatarsal are easily treated with FFS implants (Fig. 34.45). An open reduction in displaced fractures is necessary.

In Fig. 34.46a a closed wedge corrective osteotomy of the fifth metatarsal bone is illustrated. The technique is demonstrated in the schematic drawing in Fig. 34.47. The FFS implant is first inserted into the distal fragment. The direction of the implant represents the angle of correction as demonstrated in Fig. 34.47a. According to the pre-operative plan a bone wedge is removed. The FFS implant is then swung round (joystick) until the gap is closed (Figs. 34.47b,c). The wedge is closed and the FFS implant is slowly drilled into the far cortex (Fig. 34.47c,d, Fig. 34.46b). If necessary, a second implant can be inserted to provide rotational stability. A similar technique can be used to perform corrective osteotomies at the base of the first metatarsal in order to correct hallux valgus.

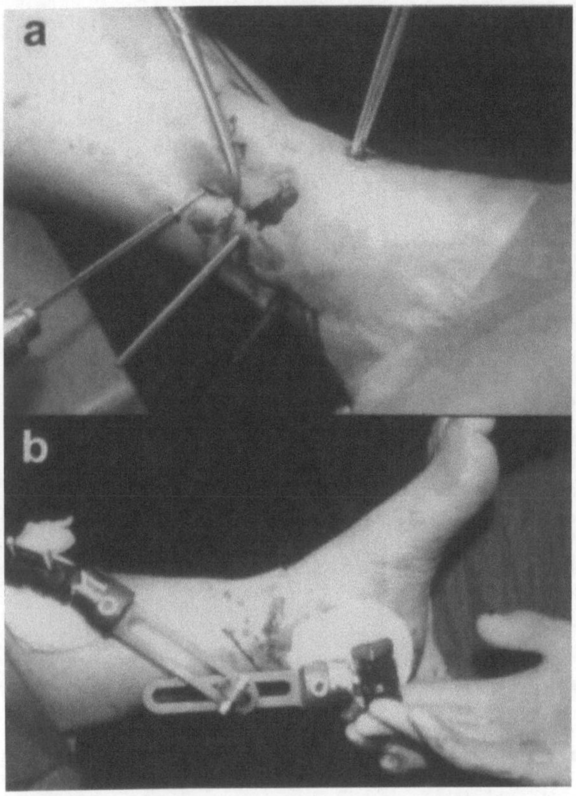

Fig. 34.44 **a** Tibial pilon fracture as shown in Fig. 34.43. The FFS implants are inserted percutaneously. **b** A fixator is used to distract the joint for easier reduction.

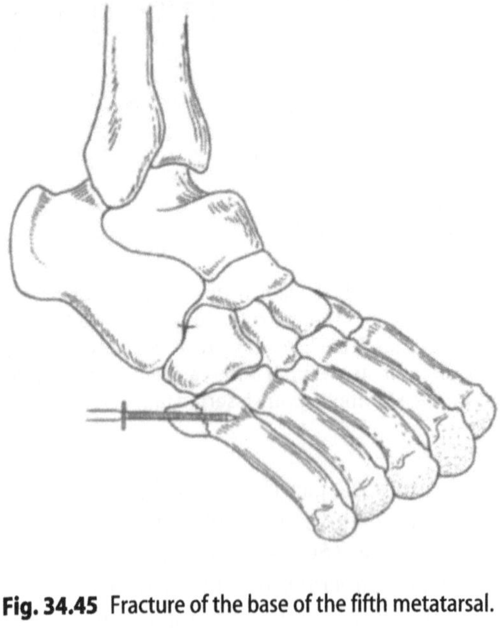

Fig. 34.45 Fracture of the base of the fifth metatarsal.

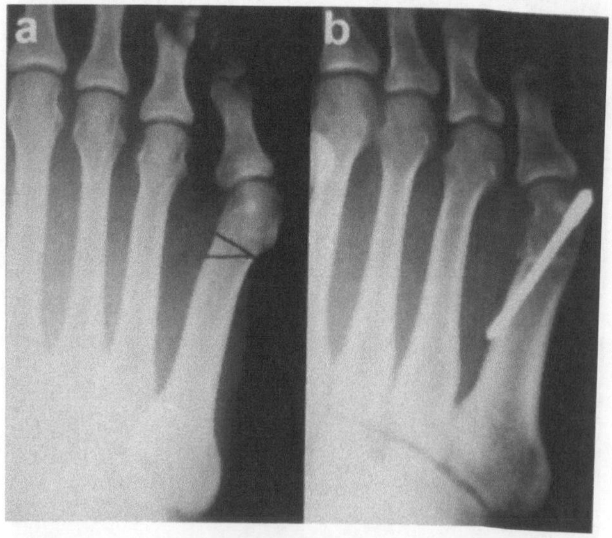

Fig. 34.46 Closed wedge corrective osteotomy of the fifth metatarsal. **a** Planning of the wedge in the pre-operative X-ray. **b** Post-operative X-ray. The wedge is closed and the osteotomy stabilized with a large FFS implant.

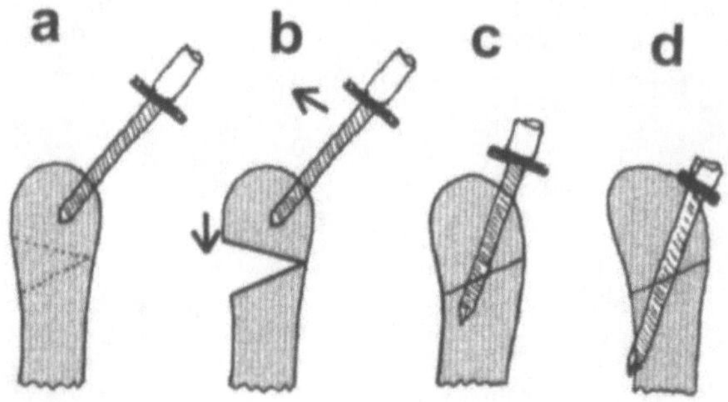

Fig. 34.47 Schematic drawing to demonstrate the basic technique using FFS implants in corrective osteotomies of small bones. **a** The FFS implant is drilled into the head of the bone before the osteotomy is performed. **b** The wedge is removed and the FFS implant used as a lever is swung round to close the wedge. **c, d** After closure of the wedge the FFS implant is advanced into the far cortex.

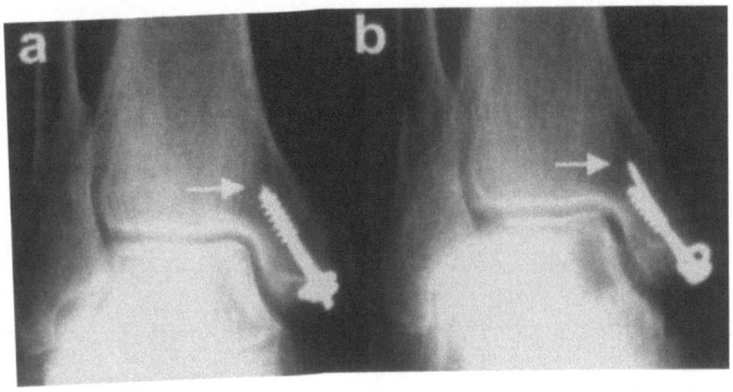

Fig. 34.48 **a** Fracture of the inner malleolus treated with a partially threaded cancellous screw and an addition FFS implant. **b** Watch the displacement of the cancellous screw while the FFS implant is still in place.

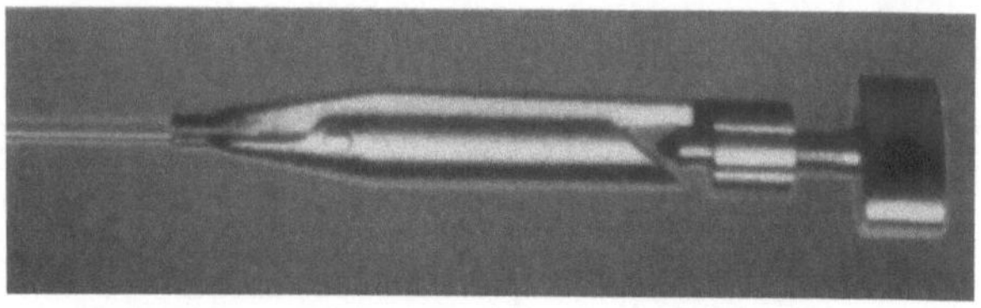

Fig. 34.49 Extractor for FFS implants. Two sizes are available (for small/medium implants and large implants). The screw at the end of the extractor is turned counterclockwise to lock the end of the FFS implant to the extractor. By further turning counterclockwise the implant is then unscrewed.

Implant Removal Technique and Timing

Removal of the FFS implants can be an exacting task. When we first began to use the Fragment Fixation System we left the implants in place as long as other conventional screws. Many of them were removed a year or more after implantation. But we noticed that the torque necessary to unscrew these implants is much greater than that associated with cortical screws. It seems that the fine machine thread design provokes a wall especially in cancellous bone substance. Another phenomenon probably related to this wall in effect is the fact that we rarely see displacement of the FFS implants once they are inserted. Fig. 34.48a shows a fracture of the medial malleolus fixed with a cancellous screw and an additional FFS implant. Weeks later we observed slow displacement of the screw, but the FFS implant as seen in Fig. 34.48b was still in place. For this reason we now tend to remove these implants much earlier at around 3–6 months. To facilitate removal of the implants an extractor shown in Fig. 34.49 is available.

The manifold advantages of this technique cannot be described comprehensively in a single article. The examples provided should, however, give some idea of the scope and benefits of this technique.

Bibliography

Asnis S.E., Ernberg J.J., Bostrom M.P., Wright T.M., Harrington R.M., Tencer A., Peterson M. 'Cancellous Bone Screw Thread Design and Holding Power.' *J Orthop Trauma* 1996 10(7): 462–9.

Müller M.E., M. Allgöwer, H. Willenegger: *Manual Der Osteosynthese.* Springer Verlag: Berlin, Heidelberg, New York, 1969

Pennig D., Gausepohl T., Lukosch R. 'Der Einsatz von Fixationsstiften zur Fragmentstabilierung in der Handchirurgie.' *Handshirurgie-Mikrochirurgie-Plastische Chirurgie* 1994 26: 270–4.

Rovinsky D., Q.Liu, G. Patement, S. Robinovitch: *Evaluation of a New Method of Small Fragment Fracture Fixation.* In press

Sherman W.O. 'Vanadium Steel Bone Plates and Screws.' *Surgery, Gynecology and Obstetrics*, 1912 Vol. XIV: 629–34.

The Orthofix Fragment Fixation System. Technical Monograph.

Part III Orthofix External Fixation in Orthopaedics

Orthofix External Fixation in Orthopaedics

Introduction

M. Saleh

In parallel with the development of the ball-jointed Dynamic Axial Fixator, a telescopic lengthener was developed. A derivative of the standard Orthofix fixator, this model did not have ball joints at either end, and the clamps for the bone screws were integral with the body of the device. This model proved its value in association with the technique of callotasis as a stable device for limb lengthening procedures. It could be dynamized in the same way as the ball jointed fixator, to encourage bone maturation. Additional modular attachments for both systems widened the scope of application to include progressive angular correction, lengthening with angular correction and articulated distraction.

The Limb Reconstruction System (LRS), which is a monolateral clamp and rail system, was developed in order to perform multisegmental surgery, such as bone transport and bifocal lengthening. The design of this device enabled screws to be placed very close to an osteotomy site, and the additional stability this confers has also led to its use in monofocal lengthening procedures. Used in conjunction with an acute correction template, the system may be used for the correction of deformities at multiple sites. The template is applied to the segment in such a way that, following osteotomy, the desired correction is achieved once the LRS is in place. The importance of the LRS is its ability to achieve complex deformity correction and lengthening in a simpler manner than with the Ilizarov device and with a higher degree of patient acceptability.

Some features of circular fixation are desirable, however, in certain situations. These include: long-term fixation in metaphyseal bone; progressive deformity correction and cross-joint fixation. This has led to the development of a hybrid fixation system which combines the use of wire fixation in the metaphysis with screw fixation in the diaphysis. This may be used as a stand-alone system for trauma and reconstructive procedures. In addition, since the diaphyseal fixation elements are compatible with the clamp design of the LRS, the two systems may be coupled together for more complex procedures.

Many of the above systems are also available in sizes suitable for paediatric use.

This part of the book will concentrate in the main on the lower limb, since lengthening and reconstructive procedures are less commonly performed in the upper limb. Reconstructive procedures specific to the upper limb are, however, discussed in several of the chapters in Part II of this volume.

The Scope of Orthofix External Fixation in Lower Limb Reconstruction

35

M. Saleh

Limb reconstruction is rapidly becoming a significant and expanding subspecialty of orthopaedics. It may be defined as the use of biomechanical and biological principles to restore a limb to its optimal alignment surgically, avoiding arthroplasty or amputation. Presenting problems include lower limb bony deformity, joint contracture, non-union, bone loss and shortening with or without infection. Patients may come to limb reconstruction following trauma, with congenital deformity or as a result of disease or surgery. It has evolved as surgeons have become aware of the biology of fracture healing, and in particular that of distraction neogenesis. Ilizarov noted that gradual distraction of living tissues created stresses that stimulated and maintained active regeneration in certain tissue structures. This concept is perhaps a more specialised statement of Wolff's law (Wolff, 1892)[1] and has been termed the Tension Stress Effect (Ilizarov 1989a;[2] 1989b,[3] 1990[4]). This had a major impact on the approach to the treatment of such diverse conditions as post-traumatic malunion, non-union, congenital fibula hemimelia, Blount's disease, congenital pseudarthrosis of the tibia, club foot and radial club hand.

Bony stabilization may be achieved with internal fixation techniques, such as plating or closed locked intramedullary nailing. The former requires extensive soft tissue dissection, but may still be an important option for periarticular osteotomies. The latter produces less soft tissue damage, and may be used to correct diaphyseal deformities. Metaphyseal deformities may be similarly corrected; however, the use of an external fixator to maintain the correction prior to reaming may improve both the fixation and the accuracy of the correction (Fig. 35.1).

External fixation is the most widely used form of stabilization in limb reconstruction since it causes minimal surgical trauma and is safer to use in previously infected tissues. It is, furthermore, the only technique which can be used to lengthen and correct deformity progressively. The ability to operate at multiple levels and to cross joints, permits extensive corrections to be achieved following a single surgical intervention.

Classification of Limb Reconstruction Procedures

Limb reconstruction techniques increase in complexity as the aims of treatment become more complex: from deformity (non-union, malunion) correction alone, to deformity correction plus lengthening, to deformity correction plus lengthening plus correction of contracture.

A classification system has been designed which can serve as the basis for treatment, prognosis, and the comparative evaluation of results (Ali and Saleh 1999).[5] The Sheffield Classification is used to describe the major primary operative intervention. It is an alpha-numeric classification with five descriptors. The first and second descriptors detail the overall aims and procedure; the third and fourth descriptors describe the precise aim and procedure at a single site, while the fifth descriptor indicates the location, both side and site. The first descriptor is unifocal (u), bifocal (b), or multi-focal (m) and relates to the number of operative sites in the limb. The second descriptor is simple or complex, and this relates to whether one or more aims was effected at a single site. The third descriptor is the surgical aim and the fourth descriptor qualifies the third by an (a) or a (b) (Table 35.1).

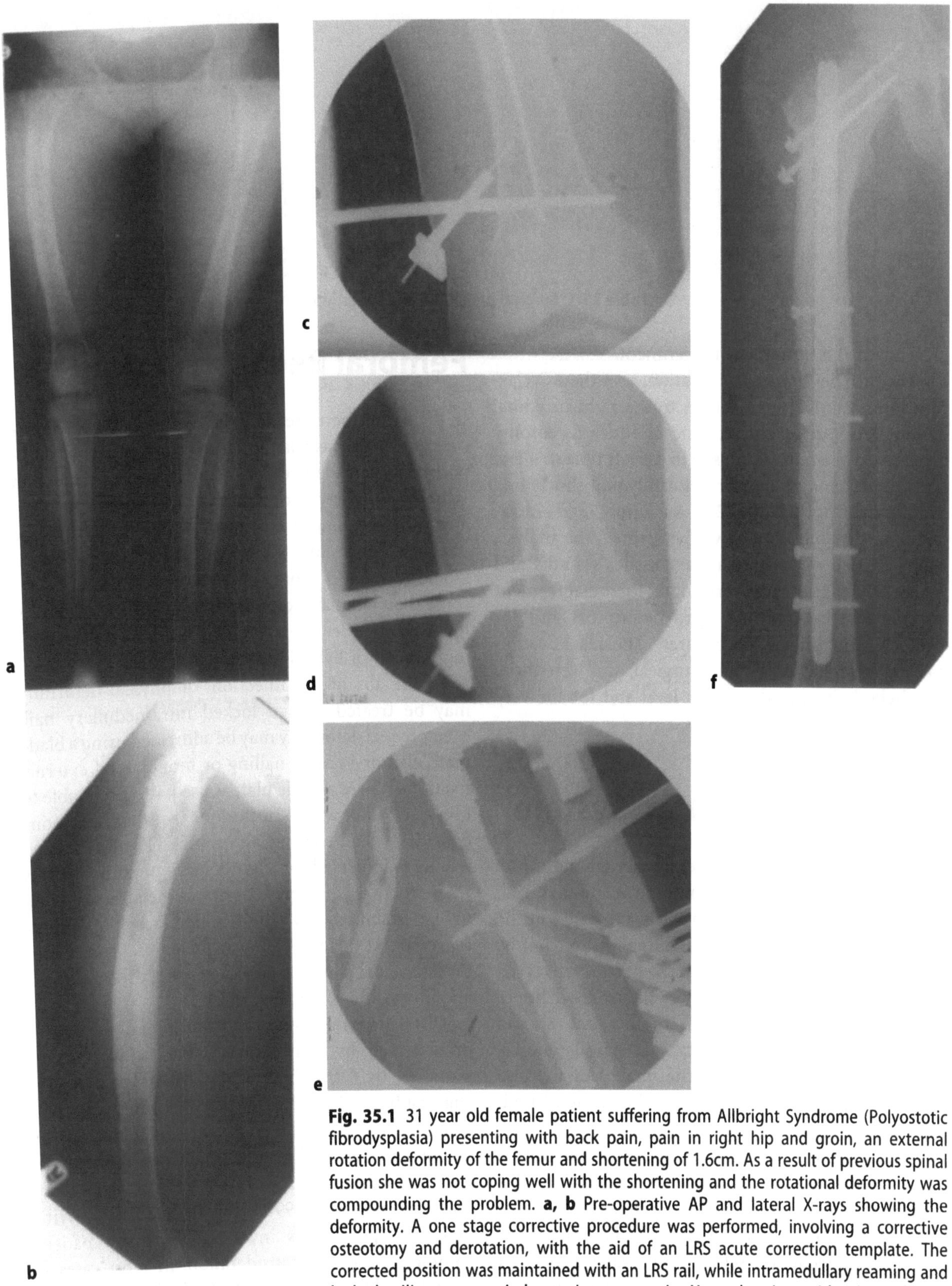

Fig. 35.1 31 year old female patient suffering from Allbright Syndrome (Polyostotic fibrodysplasia) presenting with back pain, pain in right hip and groin, an external rotation deformity of the femur and shortening of 1.6cm. As a result of previous spinal fusion she was not coping well with the shortening and the rotational deformity was compounding the problem. **a, b** Pre-operative AP and lateral X-rays showing the deformity. A one stage corrective procedure was performed, involving a corrective osteotomy and derotation, with the aid of an LRS acute correction template. The corrected position was maintained with an LRS rail, while intramedullary reaming and locked nailing were carried out. **c** Intra-operative X-ray showing guide wire and vent. **d** Reaming in progress, LRS in situ. **e** Insertion of proximal locking screws. **f** The locked intramedullary nail. Post-operatively she achieved a normal gait and normal foot progression angle, full pain relief and a good cosmetic result.

1	realignment osteotomy:	a =immediate	b = progressive
2	arthrodesis:	a = good bone stock	b = poor bone stock
3	limb equalization:	a = lengthening	b = shortening
4	osteosynthesis:	a = acute (6 months)	b = non-union
5	soft tissue correction:	a = closed	b = open
6	articulated distraction:	a = acute	b = elective
7	bony debridement:	a = minor	b = major

Table 35.1 Surgical procedure and subgroup.

Thus 1(a) is immediate realignment.

The fifth descriptor, the location, uses the AO classification; e.g. R31 would refer to the right proximal femur. As an example, an oblique osteotomy performed at a non-union site in the left tibia to allow acute correction of angular deformity and shortening would be "uc1(a)3(a)L42". An inter- and intra-observer variability study was performed, the analysis being carried out with Kappa statistics (Landis and Koch 1977).[6] There was very good or good agreement for the first, second and third descriptors and for unifocal and bifocal procedures. The classification proved less reliable when the surgical aims were more precisely defined at the fourth level and for the very complex multifocal procedures.

Selecting a Fixation System

The choice of fixation system will depend upon patient-related factors, the anatomical site involved, and the surgical aims. It is important to assess at the outset the patients' ability and willingness to comply. Do they appreciate the long treatment times involved and can they cope with these? What are their hopes and expectations? Assessment of the limb should include the tissue quality, infection status, neurovascular integrity and the quality of the end organ as a prerequisite to any consideration of limb reconstruction.

The pre-operative planning of correction will be based upon the mechanical axis and anatomical features of the limb, with reference to the malalignment test described by Paley and Tetsworth.[7] The surgical technique selected must take account of the available muscle cover, the neurovascular structures in the region, the constraints imposed by the deep compartments and whether the site is diaphyseal (cortical), or metaphyseal (cancellous).

Femoral Reconstruction

In the femur there are large strong muscles, lax soft tissues and neurovascular structures, and generous compartments. For these reasons acute deformity correction is preferred. Many reconstructive procedures are associated with prolonged treatment times, and from the patient's perspective, therefore, monolateral external fixation, which is more comfortable and less cumbersome than circular fixation, is the treatment of choice, followed, in order of preference, by intramedullary nailing, circular or hybrid fixators, and plates.

In the absence of infection, diaphyseal deformity may be treated with a locked intramedullary nail. Metaphyseal deformity may be addressed using a blade plate, fixator-assisted nailing or monolateral external fixation. Where a blade plate is used, it is preferable to use a closing wedge technique so that the bone provides load-sharing support. Fixator-assisted nailing is indicated for slightly more proximal lesions where there is sufficient diaphyseal/metaphyseal bone to be stabilised by the locking screws without toggeling. At the end of any acute femoral correction, the alignment should be checked using the bovie cord and image intensifier (Fig. 35.2).

Distal femoral valgus deformities may be treated progressively by hemicallotasis using a monolateral frame, e.g the Orthofix ProCallus fixator with the self-aligning body (Fig. 35.3). Where deformity and limb length discrepancy co-exist, and the deformity is diaphyseal, a gradual lengthening nail system may be used in combination with a corrective osteotomy (Guichet and Caser, 1997;[8] Cole JD et al, 1998[9]). With long-term procedures involving the thigh, patient comfort is a major consideration. In most cases, a monolateral fixator such as the Orthofix Limb Reconstruction System, in conjunction with an Acute Correction Template is the treatment of choice, providing stable fixation for both diaphyseal and metaphyseal deformity. This system enables lengthening to be performed with a very strong monolateral construct (Fig. 35.4). A range of modular attachments has been developed for enhanced fixation and progressive deformity correction (see Ch. 40).

Where deformity, shortening and contracture coexist, strong fixation systems are required. The addition of rings to the monolateral system in such situations provides a stable construct for joint neutralization (for limb lengthening), compression (for arthrodesis) and distraction (for contractures). The Limb Reconstruction System may still be used in the femur and the Sheffield Hybrid Fixator Assembly (SHF) with two rings and two Sheffield clamps provides a simple means of bridging and supporting the knee. One Sheffield clamp is fixed to the diaphyseal screws of the Limb Reconstruction System and the other is attached via screws inserted directly into the diaphysis of the proximal tibia (Fig. 35.5).

Knee stiffness may occur as a result of the restriction of normal soft tissue movement, and this is more likely to occur with wires than with screws, since the former transfix the tissues on both sides of the knee. Residual stiffness in the joint may resolve spontaneously, or with soft tissue release around the external fixation tracks or arthroscopic arthrolysis. Occasionally quadricepsplasty is required and the Judet technique (Judet 1959[10]) used.

Tibial Reconstruction

In the tibia, external fixation is possible without transfixing muscle because there is a subcutaneous bony surface. Diaphyseal deformities of the tibia in varus may be corrected acutely using the Limb Reconstruction System, or an intramedullary nail, but in the case of valgus deformities, correction must be effected slowly, to avoid compartment syndrome and damage to the peroneal nerve which is very sensitive to stretching. In general, therefore, progressive corrections are safer in the tibia, and for this reason hybrid external fixation is preferred in most instances, followed, in order of preference, by monolateral fixation and intramedullary nailing. Unlike the situation in the femur, ring-wire systems are well tolerated. A number of the problems associated with circular frames have been addressed successfully in the Sheffield Hybrid Assembly, where wires are used exclusively in the metaphysis and screws in the diaphysis. With this construct, metaphyseal fixation is particularly strong, since four wires may be tensioned on a single ring.

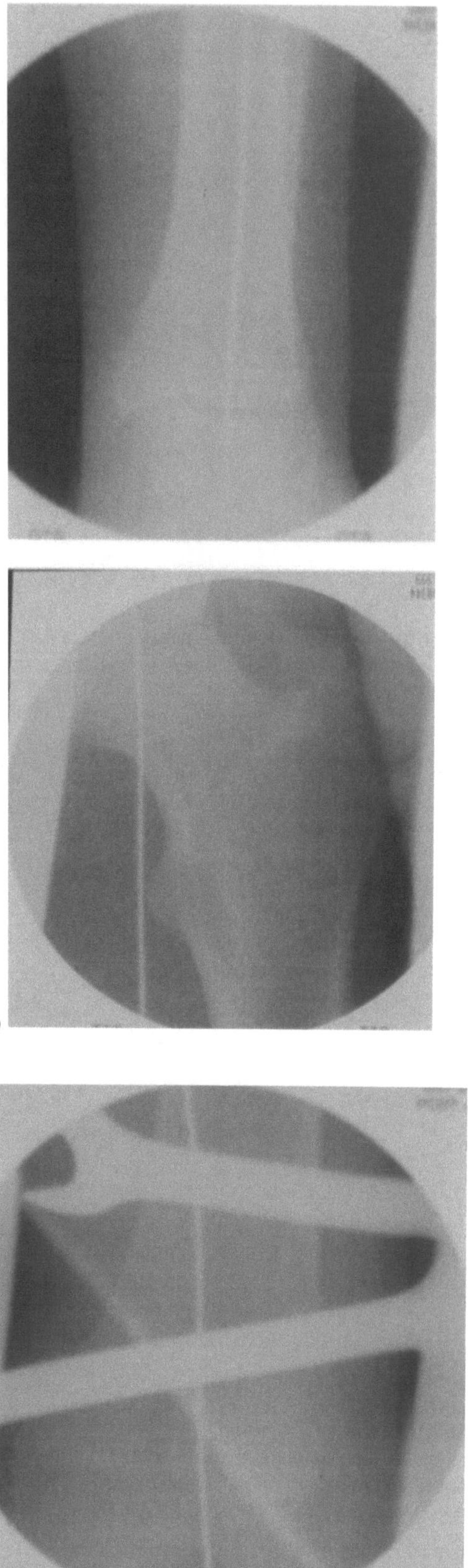

a b c

Fig. 35.2 a, b, c Following the acute correction of a femoral deformity, alignment of ankle, hip and knee should be checked using the Bovie (diathermy) cord and Image Intensifier.

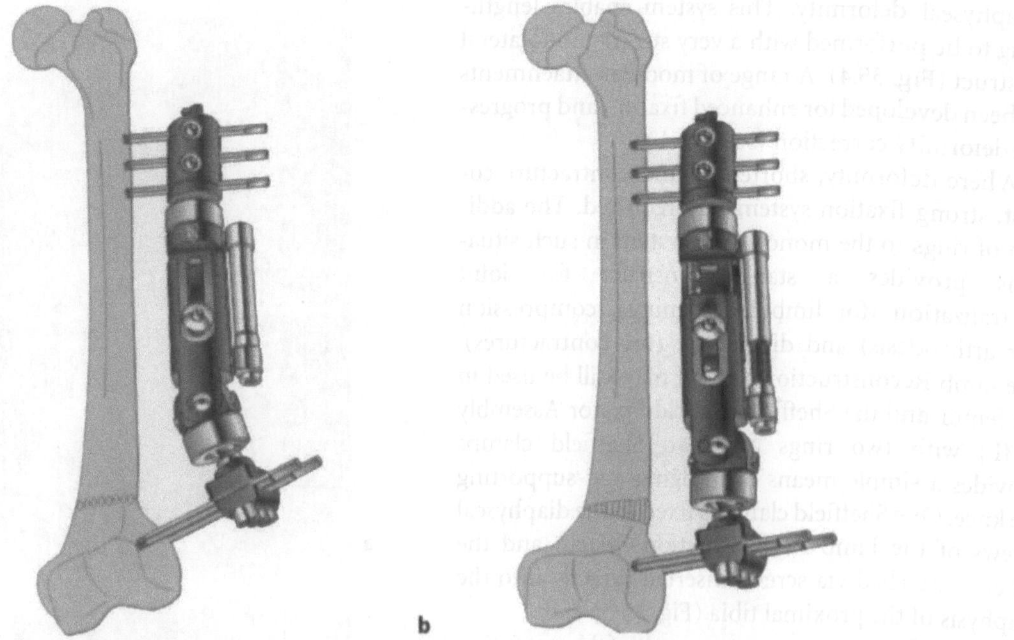

Fig. 35.3 Valgus deformity of the distal femur. **a** ProCallus fixator in place with a self-aligning body and Torbay-Garches clamp distally. A distal metaphyseal osteotomy has been performed. **b** Progressive correction of the deformity by hemicallotasis.

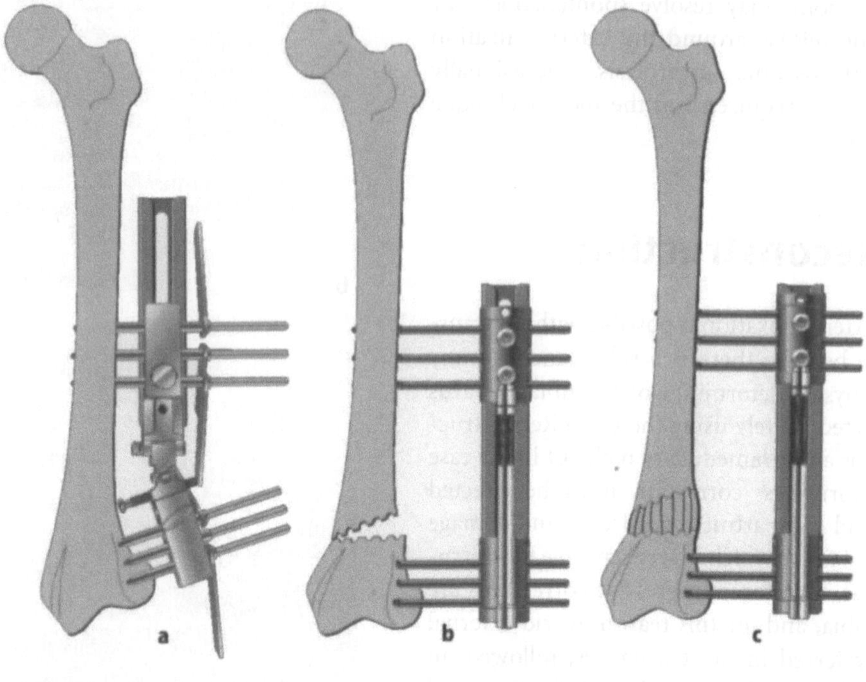

Fig 35.4 Distal valgus deformity in a short femur; correction using the Limb Reconstruction System. **a** LRS being applied; note Acute Correction Template at distal end of rail. **b** Osteotomy performed and deformity corrected; definitive fixator in place. **c** Lengthening to restore original bone length.

Monolateral external fixation remains a valuable technique in the tibia and progressive metaphyseal deformity correction may be achieved by means of hemicallotasis. Fig. 35.6 shows the use of a ProCallus fixator applied medially in conjunction with a self-aligning body and Torbay-Garches clamp, and Fig. 35.7 the LRS applied anteriorly in conjunction with an OF-Garches T-clamp. Intramedullary nails may be used to correct varus or translational diaphyseal malunions, but despite their convenience, problems

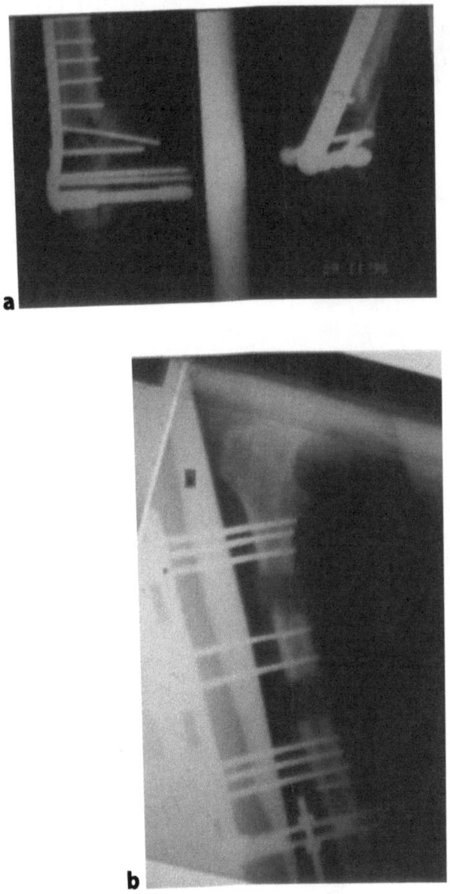

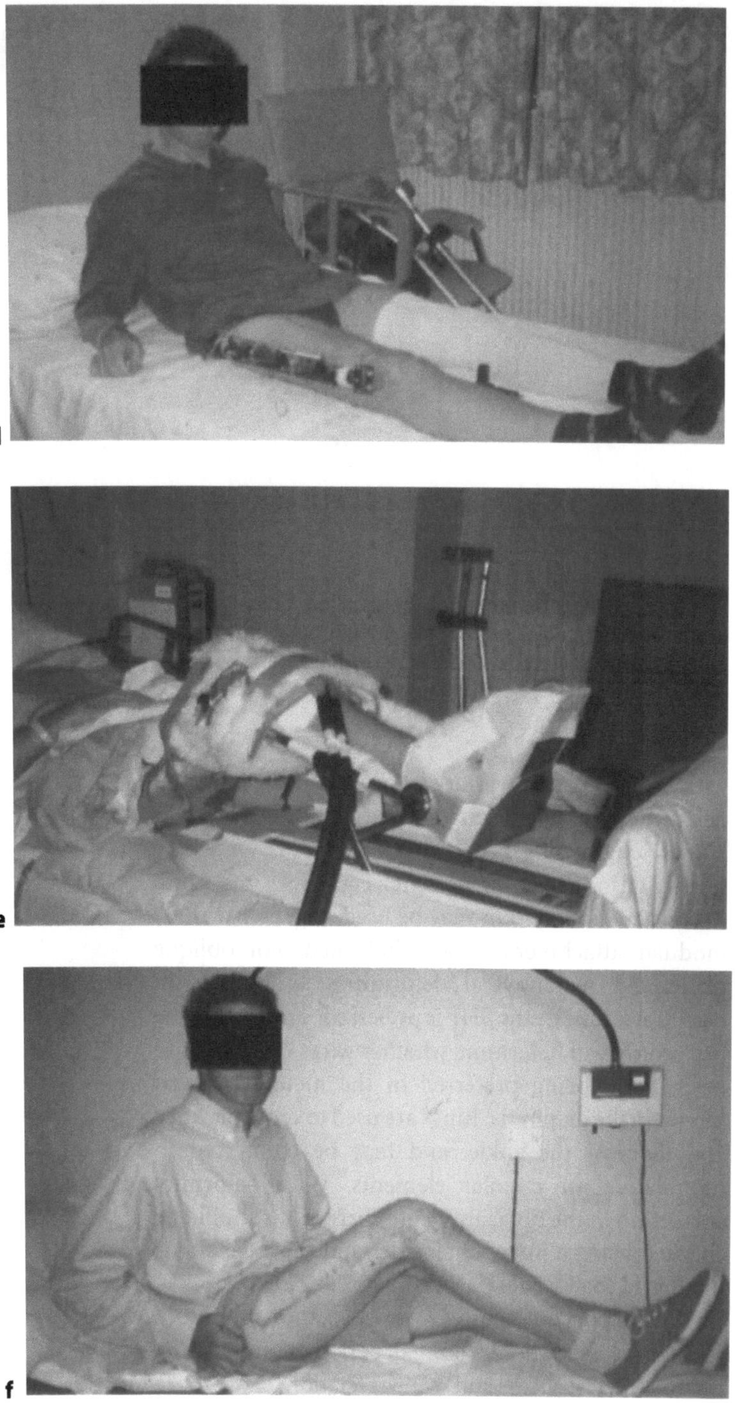

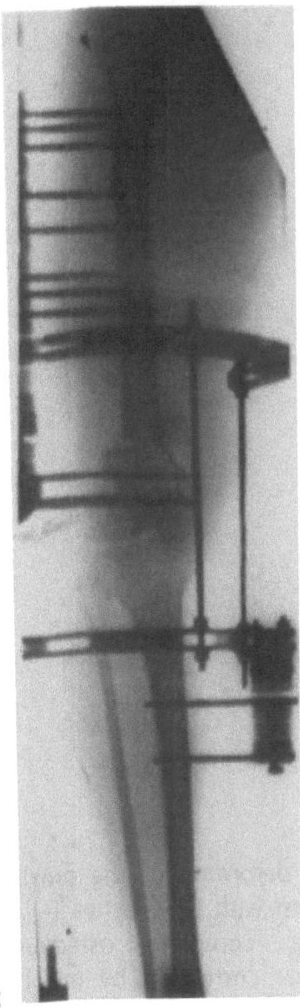

Fig. 35.5 **a** Non-union of the distal femur following a motorcycle accident. Patient treated with internal fixation, resulting in medial translation, varus deformity, 8cm of shortening and a stiff knee. Referred to author's centre. **b** Following removal of the blade plate, an osteotomy was performed through the malunion for realignment, and lengthening performed with an LRS at mid-diaphyseal and proximal osteotomies. No attempt was made to lengthen through the distal femoral osteotomy due to the relatively poor bone quality and limited condylar fixation due to previous surgery. **c** Support was provided by an LRS with a metaphyseal clamp in the distal femur and a Sheffield Hybrid Fixator Assembly taken across the knee to protect the relatively weak distal femoral fixation and neutralize the lower limb lever arm and stiff knee. **d** The SHF was removed at the end of lengthening. **e** CPM following a quadricepsplasty performed 6 months after fixator removal. **f** The final result.

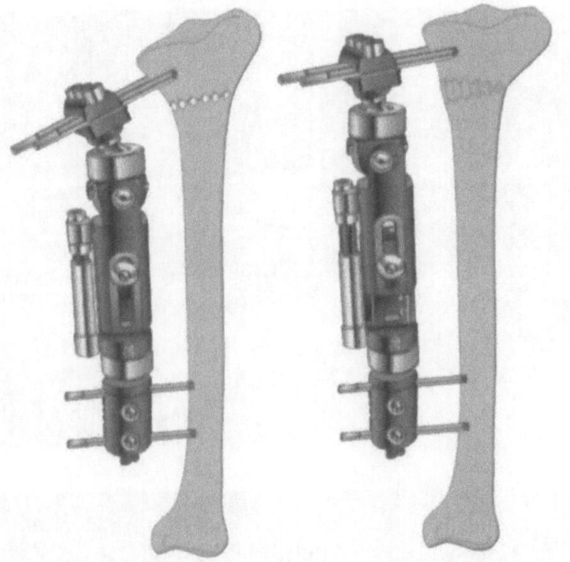

Fig. 35.6 **a** Varus deformity of the proximal tibia; ProCallus fixator applied medially, with self-aligning body and Torbay-Garches clamp; osteotomy performed with fixator in place. **b** Gradual correction by hemicallotasis.

with knee pain, nerve injury from acute correction and delayed union may occur.

For lengthening procedures (Fig. 35.8), or where segmental bone loss is present (Fig. 35.9), the Limb Reconstruction System may be used, together with its modular attachments where indicated. For oblique plane and metaphyseal deformities as well as in osteoporotic bone the SHF is preferred. The level of the osteotomy will determine whether wires or screws are used, wires being preferred in the metaphysis and screws in the diaphysis. Rings are used to cross the knee and to cross the ankle, and may be connected to monolateral or circular elements. With deformity correction in the tibia, any acute corrections should be checked using a image intensifier and the axial alignment grid (Saleh et al)[11]. (See Ch. 36.)

Where foot contractures co-exist, fixation in the foot may be achieved for a limited period of time using monolateral devices and screw fixation. For more concentric support and long-term fixation, the LRS or SHF may be extended on to the foot using a two-thirds ring attached to the hindfoot, or the hindfoot and midfoot (Fig. 35.10). For control of the forefoot a further two-thirds ring is applied with wires passing through the metatarsal necks. Such techniques may also be used to protect the foot during tibial lengthening.

In summary, monolateral frames and acute corrections are preferred in the femur. Hybrid frames and progressive corrections in the tibia. Rings are used to cross the knee and ankle/foot.

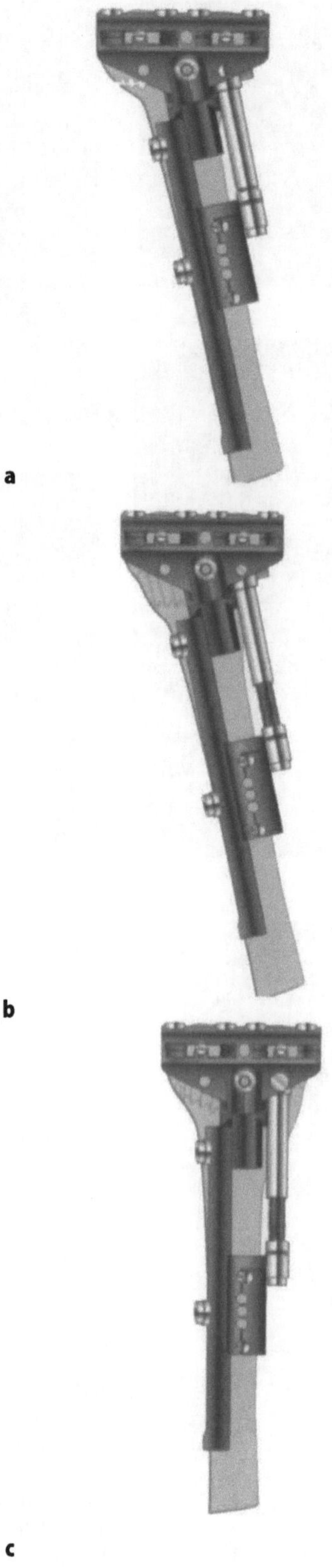

Fig. 35.7 **a** Valgus deformity of the proximal tibia; Limb Reconstruction System with OF-Garches T-clamp proximally, mounted anteriorly; complete osteotomy performed. **b** Progressive angular correction by initial lengthening – **c** Followed by hemicallotasis.

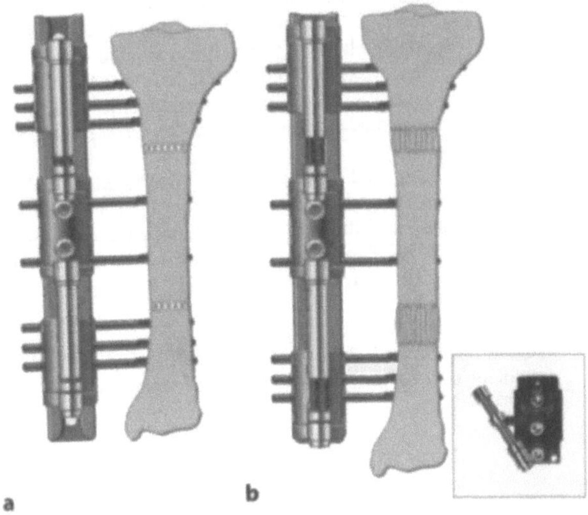

a b

Fig. 35.8 a Very short tibia, LRS mounted medially; proximal and distal osteotomies performed. b Simultaneous lengthening at each osteotomy site. Inset shows a micrometric swivelling clamp which can be attached at either end of the adult rail to correct any varus or valgus occurring during lengthening. See also case report in Fig. 35.5.

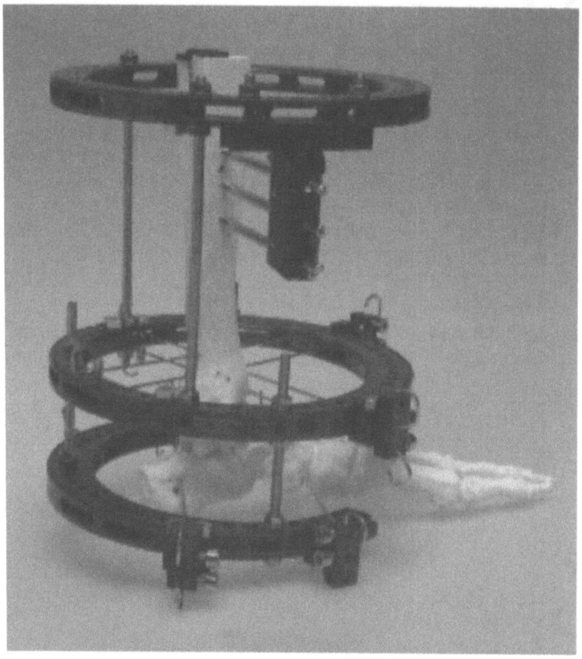

Fig. 35.10 Shows SHF extended on to the foot using a two-thirds ring attached to the hindfoot and mid-foot. The forefoot may be protected with a simple orthosis.

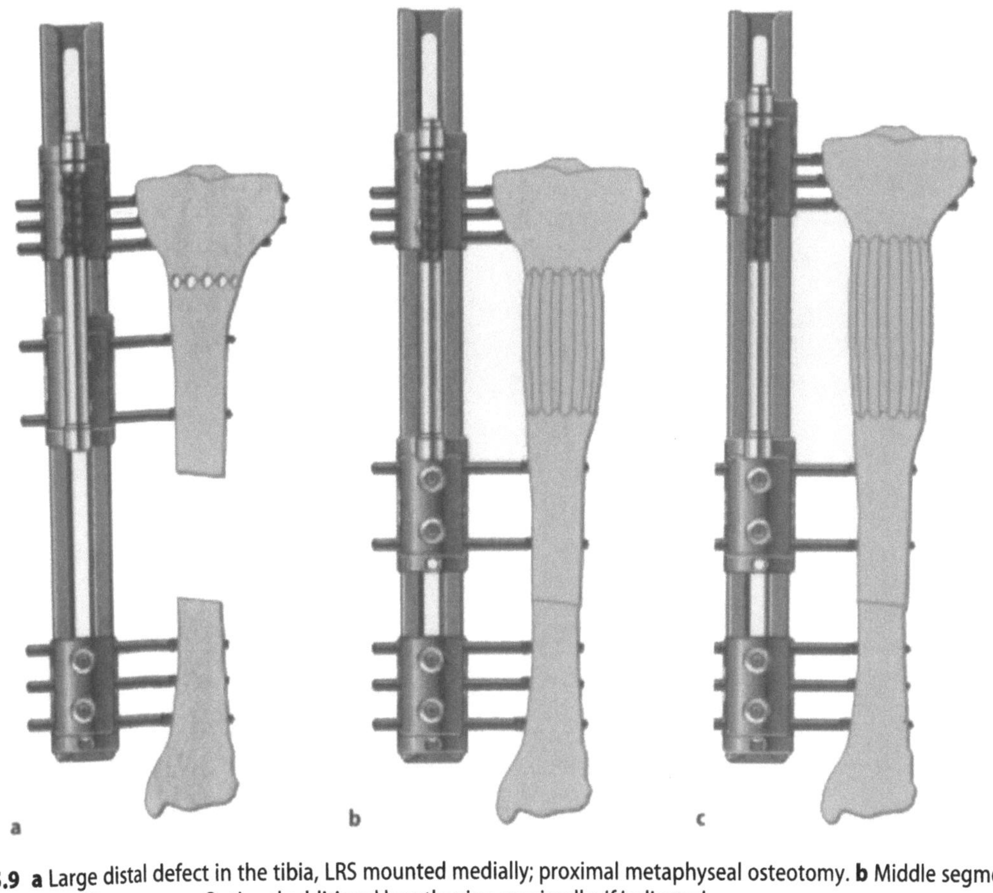

a b c

Fig. 35.9 a Large distal defect in the tibia, LRS mounted medially; proximal metaphyseal osteotomy. b Middle segment moved distally until docking occurs. c Optional additional lengthening proximally, if indicated.

References

1. Wolff J. *Das Gesetz der Transformation der knochen.* A.Hirschwald: Berlin, 1892.
2. Ilizarov GA. 'The tension–stress effect on the genesis and growth of tissues. Part 1: The influence of stability of fixation and soft tissue preservation.' *Clin Orthop* 1989; 238: 249–81.
3. Ilizarov GA. 'The tension–stress effect on the genesis and growth of tissues. Part 2: The influence of the rate and frequency of distraction.' *Clin Orthop* 1989; 239: 263–85.
4. Ilizarov GA. 'Clinical application of the tension–stress effect for limb lengthening.' *Clin Orthop* 1990; 250: 8.
5. Ali F, Saleh M. 'The development, validation and clinical usage of a new classification for limb reconstruction surgery.' *J Bone Joint Surg* [Br] 1999; *Orthop Proc* III; 81-B: 279.
6. Landis JR, Koch GG. 'The measurement of observer agreement for categorical data'. *Biometrics* 1977; 33: 159–74.
7. Paley D, Tetsworth K. 'Mechanical axis deviation of the lower limbs; pre-operative planning of uniapical angular deformities of the tibia or femur.' *Clin Orthop* 1992; 280: 48–64.
8. Guichet JM, Casar RS. 'Mechanical characterisitics of a totally intramedullary gradual elongation nail.' *Clin Orthop* 1997; 337: 281–90.
9. Cole JD, Justin DF, Kasparis T, DeVlught D. 'The Intramedullary Skeletal Kinetic Distractor (ISKD): First Clinical Results of a New Intramedullary Nail for Lengthening of the Femur and Tibia' Paper No. 51, presented at the German Trauma Association Meeting 1998.
10. Judet R, 'Mobilisation of the stiff knee.' *J Bone Joint Surg* [Br] 1959; 41B: 856–7.
11. Saleh M, Harriman P, Edwards DJ. 'A radiological method for producing precise limb alignment.' *J Bone Joint Surg* [Br] 1991; 73B: 515–6.

SECTION 1 THE CORRECTION OF BONY AND SOFT TISSUE DEFORMITY

The Acute Correction of Deformity by Means of Monolateral External Fixation 36

M. Saleh and S. Nayagam

Introduction

In its simplest form, the monolateral fixator can be used to stabilize the skeleton following the acute correction of a diaphyseal deformity. This will often be encountered in the form of a uniplanar or multiplanar deformity in the lower limb. The type of procedures which will be described can be effected with minimal interference to the soft tissues and healing can be accelerated by weightbearing and dynamization.

Since deformities of the skeleton are frequently associated with either real or apparent shortening of the limb, a device which will enable the smooth transition from correction of deformity to lengthening procedure is integral to a successful outcome. The Limb Reconstruction System (LRS) which is a strong monolateral rail to which a variety of modular clamps can be attached, is specifically designed to accomplish this transition. Even where the problem is primarily one of deformity, without any overt shortening, acute correction of the deformity may of itself result in some minor degree of lengthening, shortening (with a closed wedge osteotomy) or translation at the osteotomy site at the end of the procedure, as will be seen below, and this can readily be compensated for using the LRS.

The Use of Acute Correction Templates

Where the LRS is used to stabilize a bone following an osteotomy made for the purpose of correcting a deformity, the screws in each of the bone fragments must end up parallel to each other and in the plane of the rail, to enable them to be secured by the clamps on the rail. The screw clusters must therefore be introduced in such a way that they will reflect the plane of the deformity. The planning of screw positions is not always straightforward, however, and to facilitate the procedure a series of Acute Correction Templates is available for attachment to either the adult or the paediatric models of the Limb Reconstruction System. Use of these articulated templates allows the fixator to be applied accurately to reflect the bony deformity. Now, following a properly executed osteotomy, the bone screws are brought into alignment with the rail clamps to correct the deformity, and lengthening can subsequently be performed, if need be. These templates can be used to correct antero-posterior/ medio-lateral angulation, or internal/external rotation respectively. Where angular and rotational deformities co-exist, the impact of the angular deformities on the perceived degree of rotation should be carefully assessed. The limits of such corrections depend on the site, quality of the bone and the tension generated in tissues, especially nerves. As a general rule, correction in any one plane should not exceed 20° if lengthening at the same site is proposed. In a series of cases, those patients who underwent a >30° angular correction were 7.7 times more likely to have a Bone Healing Index in excess of 45 days/cm. (Donnan et al 1999).[1] These procedures are particularly useful in the femur and may be used for smaller corrections in the tibia. In a monofocal deformity both angulation and rotation may be corrected simultaneously (Donnan and Saleh, 1998).[2]

The acute correction templates for angular deformity (varus/valgus, procurvatum/recurvatum) attach to the end of the rail of the Limb Reconstruction System and three are available, corresponding to the straight clamp, the T-clamp and the OF-Garches T-clamp (Fig. 36.1). To use the straight clamp, for example, the medio-lateral plane (coronal plane) and antero-posterior plane (sagittal plane) deformities are first measured from full length radiographs. These angles are then set into the clamp by adjusting the two locking screws which control the coronal and sagittal plane hinges respectively. This enables precise bone screw placement so that once the osteotomy has been performed, the two screw clusters can be manually manipulated into the same plane ready for the attachment of the definitive clamp-rail assembly. Figs. 36.2a–36.2g illustrate the use of the straight clamp template for the acute correction of a varus deformity of the distal femur.

Where a monolateral fixator is used to correct a deformity, the surgeon must be aware of the axis around which the correction is occurring. The centre of rotation for the correction may not always be at the apex of the deformity and this may result in an undesirable shortening, lengthening or translational effect which will necessitate an appropriate compensatory manoeuvre. Fig. 36.3 shows the centre of rotation of angulation (CORA)[3] of the deformity, which is the point at which the proximal and distal anatomical axes of the bone cross. Ideally, this is the point at which the osteotomy and the angular correction should be made.

In theory, where the centre of rotation of the actual correction coincides exactly with the CORA within the bone, angular correction alone will occur, without any associated translation; where it is situated outside the bone somewhere along the bisector of the angle, e.g. at C2 on the convex side of the bone, or C3 on the concave side, angular correction will be associated with some degree of lengthening or shortening. A hinge placed above or below the osteotomy level will increase the amount of translation between the proximal and distal axes.

In practice, when an angular correction is being performed with a monolateral system, the centre of

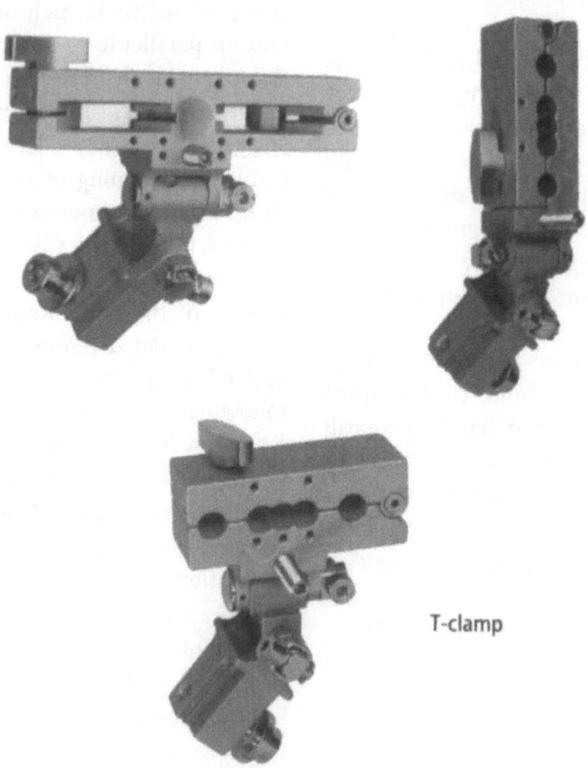

Fig. 36.1 The Acute Correction Templates for angular deformity.

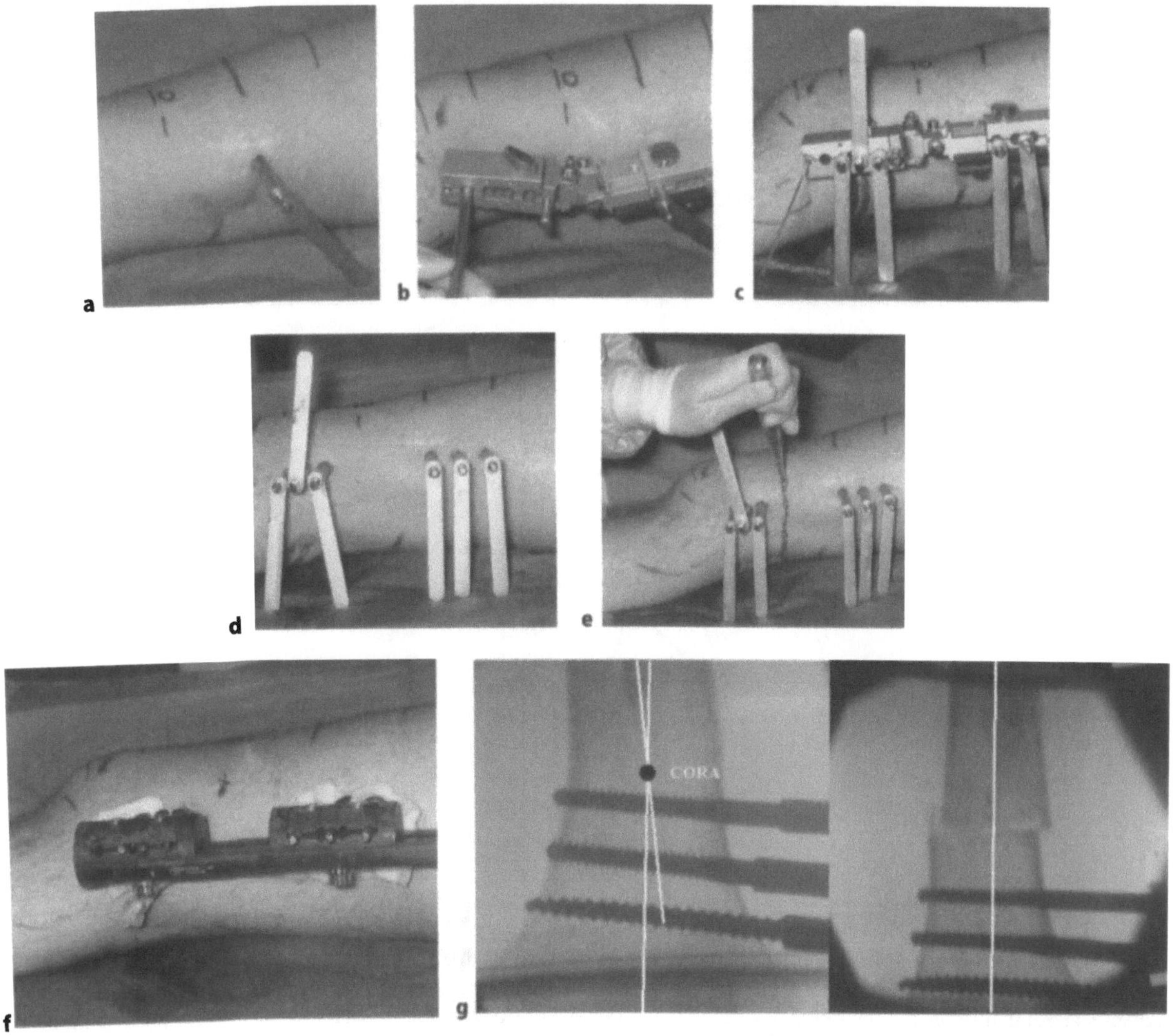

Fig. 36.2 Use of the straight clamp Acute Correction Template to correct a varus deformity of the distal femur. **a** First (most distal of proximal set) screw inserted at right angles to the bone. **b** Acute Correction Template applied at an angle corresponding to the deformity of the bone and second screw inserted through standard clamp template on the rail. **c** All screws inserted. **d** Template removed. **e** Osteotomy performed. **f** Correction performed by manipulating the pin groups; definitive rail and clamps applied. **g** Radiological appearance prior to and following correction of deformity.

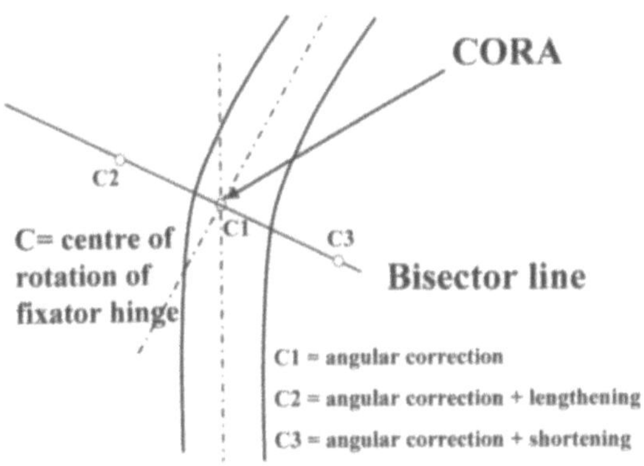

Fig. 36.3 The centre of rotation of angulation (CORA) is the point at which the proximal and distal anatomical axes of the bone cross (C1); the bisector is the line dividing the angle formed by the two axes. Ideally, the centre of rotation of the actual correction should coincide with C1. Where it is outside the bone but on the bisector line, e.g. at C2 or C3, angular correction will be associated with some degree of shortening or lengthening.

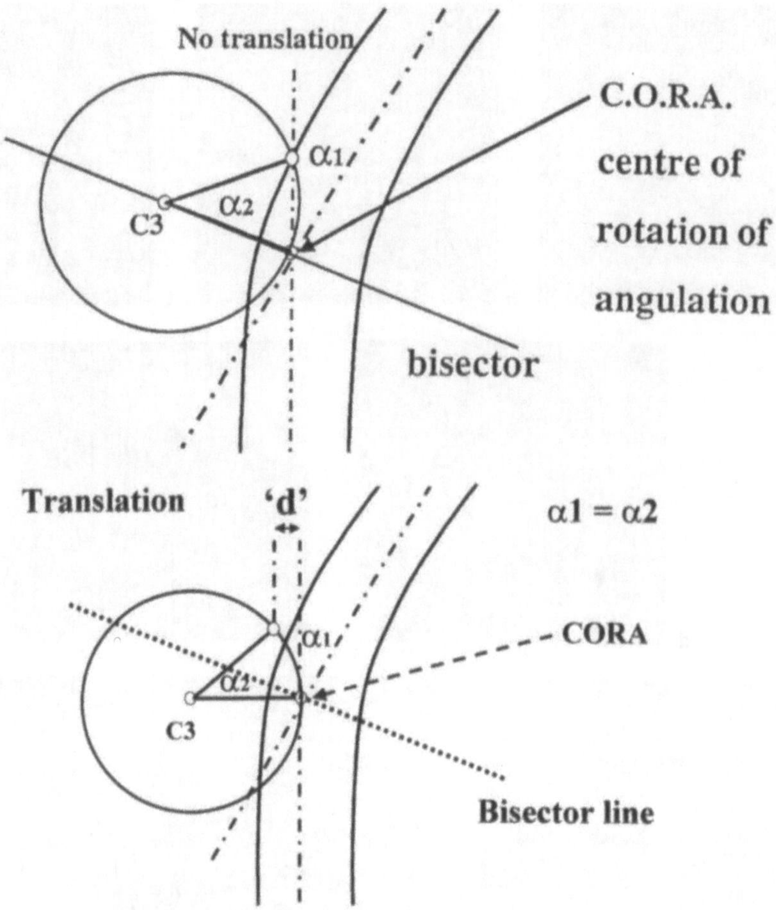

b **Translation 'd' if hinge not on bisector line**

Fig. 36.4 **a** Where the centre of rotation of the clamp (C3) is placed in line with the osteotomy either at its centre (CORA) or at some point along the bisector, the amount of correction (α2) will equal the amount of deformity (α1) and the bone ends should align with minimal translation. **b** If the centre of rotation of the clamp is not on the bisector line, this will increase the amount of translation ('d') between the proximal and distal axes.

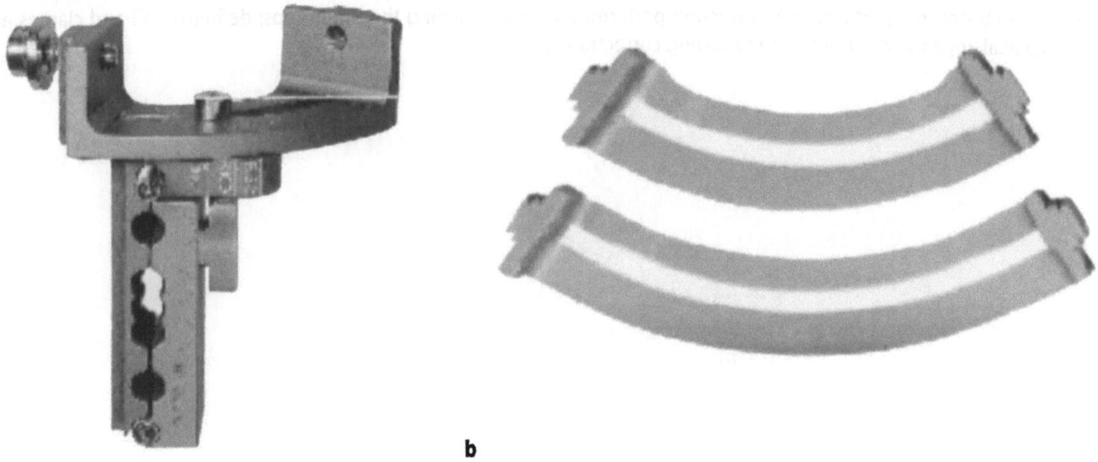

a **b**

Fig. 36.5 The Acute Correction Template for rotational deformity.

rotation of the clamp of the fixator will normally be situated at a distance from the CORA (unless it can be placed directly over it as in the case of the OF-Garches T-clamp). It therefore follows that angular correction will usually be accompanied by some degree of lengthening or shortening at the site of the osteotomy, and the precise amount of this will depend upon the diameter of the bone.

Where the centre of rotation of the clamp (C3 in Fig. 36.4) is placed in line with the osteotomy either at its centre (CORA) or at some point along the bisector, the amount of correction ($\alpha 2$) will equal the amount of deformity ($\alpha 1$) and the bone ends should align with minimal translation (Fig. 36.4a). A small amount of translation is bound to occur with monolateral fixation, however, since the screw lengths in the proximal and distal screw clamps will not be identical. If the centre of rotation of the clamp is not on the bisector line, this will increase the amount of translation ('d') between the proximal and distal axes (Fig. 36.4b). With ring fixation, where the distance of the fixation to the central axis of the bone is equal in both segments, the bone ends will align without translation.

Following angular correction, therefore, it is important to determine whether any translation has occurred at the site of the osteotomy. Where this is observed, it can be corrected by loosening the appropriate clamp cover screws and moving the screw cluster further into, or out of the clamp as necessary.

There is another Acute Correction template for rotational deformities (Fig. 36.5). This template is free to slide along the length of the rail, and three sizes of arc are available to accommodate varying bulks of soft tissues. The correct arc radius to use is calculated by adding together the radius of the bone, the bulk of the soft tissues and the fixator-skin distance in millimetres (Fig. 36.6a). Use of the correct size of arc is particularly important since if too large or too small an arc is used the rotational correction will be accompanied by some degree of translation (Fig. 36.6b). When using the device, the degree of rotation is determined clinically or by CT scan. The template arc should curve around the limb and its straight clamp template component is preset to reflect the number of degrees required for rotational correction. Once the template frame has been prepared to mimic the deformity, and the screws in each clamp have been inserted, the osteotomy is performed and the proximal and distal screw clusters rotated into the same plane. The definitive clamp rail assembly is then applied. A clinical example of the correction of a rotational deformity of the femur is illustrated in Figs. 36.7a–36.7d.

It is perfectly possible to correct a co-existing angular and rotational deformity using a single assembly, by attaching one of the angular correction templates to one end of the rail, and the rotational template at an appropriate site along the rail, as illustrated in Fig. 36.8a.

In the example cited a 20° varus and a 45° internal rotation deformity in the midshaft of the left femur is to be corrected acutely. The screws must be placed in such a way that after the correction has been achieved they lie parallel in two planes ready for attachment to the rail using two straight clamps. A pre-operative plan is made using an overlay tracing of the radiograph. Screw insertion positions may be referenced to the anatomical axis or joint plane. In this case the proximal clamp template has been adjusted to reflect the varus

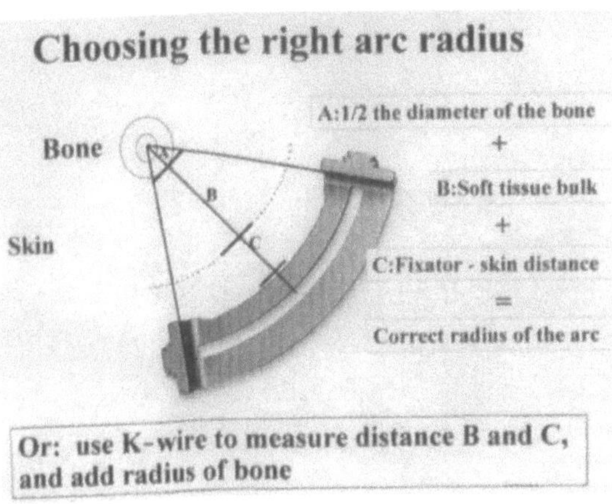

a

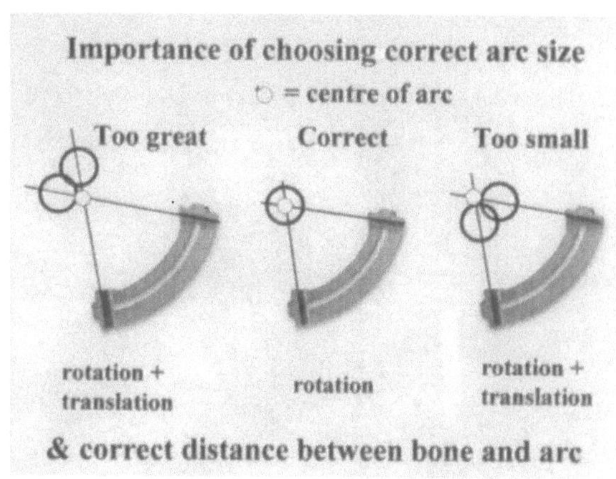

b

Fig 36.6 **a** Selecting the right diameter of arc to use with the Acute Correction Template for rotational deformity. **b** Translation will occur if the size of arc and its distance from the centre of the bone are incorrect.

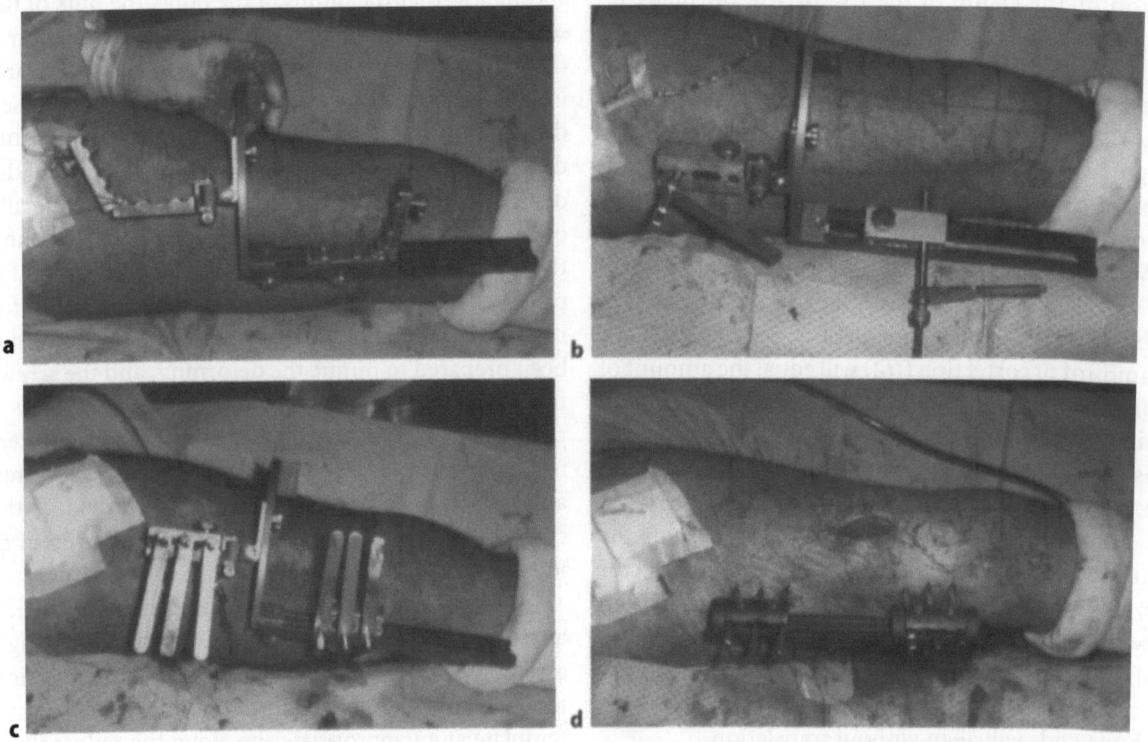

Fig. 36.7 Using the Acute Correction Template to correct a rotational deformity in the femur (clamp shown is a prototype; see Fig. 36.8 for the current version of this clamp). **a** First (most proximal) screw inserted through the straight clamp template attached to the arc of the rotational correction template, which has been preset to reflect the amount of rotational correction needed. **b** Second (most distal) screw inserted in the clamp on the rail. The assembly is now stabilized. **c** All the screws have been inserted. **d** Following osteotomy and removal of the templates the segments are rotated into alignment and the definitive rail and clamps applied.

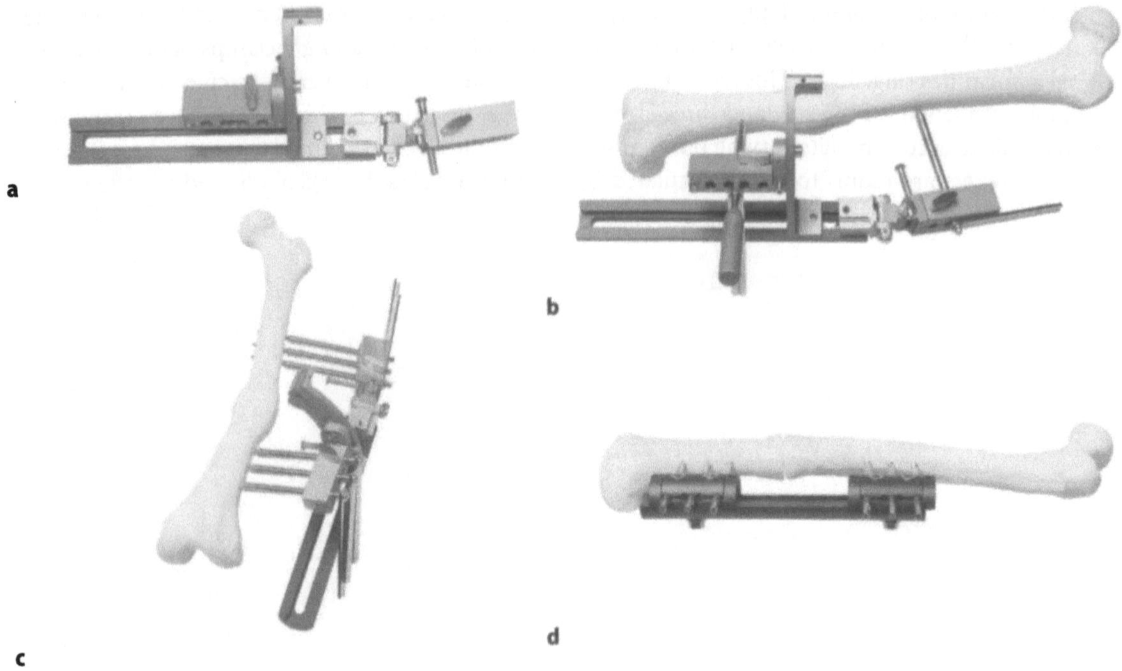

Fig. 36.8 Use of the Acute Correction Templates to correct a co-existing angular and rotational deformity. **a** A rotational template used distally and a straight clamp template proximally, preset to reflect the rotational and angular deformities, respectively. **b** Proximal screw inserted at 90° to bone segment; distal screw guide and trocar inserted to confirm that bone screw will be in the centre of the bone. **c** All screws are now inserted, 3 in each clamp. **d** Template assembly removed, osteotomy performed; correction implemented and definitive rail with straight clamps applied.

deformity and the distal clamp the rotational deformity.

The limb is now positioned with the patella facing anteriorly. The rail with templates attached is placed so that the hinge in the angular correction template is opposite the apex of the deformed bone. A screw is inserted at right angles to the axis of the proximal femoral segment, just proximal to this apex. The rail is held 3–4cm from the skin, and the spacing screws in both clamp templates advanced until they touch the skin. The distance between the rail and the centre of the bone is now checked and confirmed to be equal to the radius of the arc. It is important that this is checked at this time as later correction will not be possible. A trocar is now inserted down to the distal segment through the clamp template mounted on the arc. If the template has been set up correctly, the trocar will point towards the centre of the bone, perpendicular to the axis of the distal femur (Fig. 36.8b). If it is not at 90° to the axis of the distal segment or does not point to the centre of the bone, the settings of the angulation template and the distance of the rail from the bone should be reviewed. Once it has been confirmed that the trocar is in the correct position, the second screw is inserted.

With the template held in a fixed relation to the limb, screws are inserted in seats 1 and 5 of each clamp (seats 1and 3 where the paediatric LRS is used). Three screws may be used in each clamp (Fig. 36.8c). The bone is now cut at the planned level with a 3.2mm drill and osteotomes. The template is now replaced with the definitive straight clamps on the rail which are compressed together to close the gap (Fig. 36.8d). At the end of the procedure the Bovie (diathermy) cord is placed on the centre of the femoral head and run down the limb to the centre of the talus to confirm the correction and the mechanical alignment.

Other Modules For Acute Correction

In addition to the acute correction templates described above, several other accessory modules are available which attach to the rail of the Limb Reconstruction System and enable acute corrections to be carried out. Their use is described below.

The Ball-Joint Coupling

This is a fixed module (Fig. 36.9) which can be sited at either end of the rail, but cannot slide along it. It has a bayonet fitting which will accept an Orthofix straight clamp or T-clamp with ball-joint. When unlocked, it allows free rotation, and up to 36° of angular movement in any plane. It is applied with a dedicated template. It is used to perform precise, immediate correction at an osteotomy or deformity site corresponding to the axis of the ball joint. Once the desired position has been achieved, final locking of the ball joint is performed using the torque wrench.

The Micrometric Swivelling Clamp

This clamp (Fig. 36.10) is usually sited at one or other end of the LRS rail and allows free movement of up to 50° in the plane of the screws. It can be used for a planned acute corrective osteotomy, e.g. a pre-existing varus or valgus deformity in the femur; a corrective osteotomy combined with lengthening, or correction of an axial deviation occurring during lengthening or transport. There are five screw seats in this clamp, corresponding to the five seats in a standard adult LRS straight clamp with which it is interchangeable.

Where an immediate on-table correction is planned, screws are inserted as close to the plane of the deformity as possible, using the dedicated template for this module attached to the rail. The centre of articulation of the template (and hence of the clamp itself) should be placed at the level of the planned osteotomy (Fig. 36.11a). Since correction of a valgus deformity of the distal femur in this way may actually cause the distal fragment to impact and bind on the proximal fragment

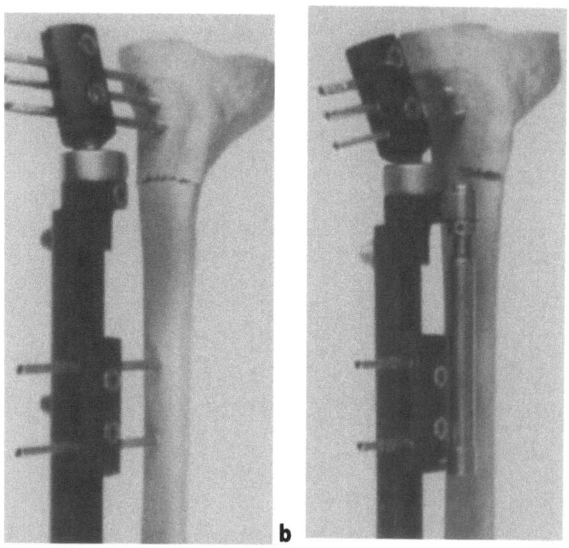

a b

Fig. 36.9 Use of the Ball-Joint Coupling to correct a deformity of the proximal tibia. **a** LRS applied with straight clamp with ball-joint proximally; osteotomy performed. **b** Manipulation of ball-joint to correct deformity.

before full correction has been achieved, it is always necessary to distract the bone ends slightly prior to commencing the corrective manoeuvre. Then, with the definitive clamp in place, free to slide on the rail, turning the screw of the distractor unit of the clamp in the appropriate direction will correct the deformity (Fig. 36.11b). Translation is not unusual and can easily be corrected at the end of the procedure by sliding the screws in the clamp manually. If the soft tissue tension involved in correction becomes great, so that the distractor is difficult to turn, it is better to use the standard compression–distraction unit to stretch the soft tissues, shorten, and only then make the correction.

If minimal additional length is required following the correction of deformity this can be achieved by a further small amount of distraction between the bone ends. Where any major increment in length is required, lengthening can be effected by callotasis (see Ch. 42).

The Multiplanar Clamp

In some instances it is very difficult to predict the exact amount of correction which will be needed. This is particularly so where there is angulation at a single level on both AP and lateral X-rays. In these cases a clamp that can take account of such oblique plane deformities and which allows fine tuning of angulation and translation at the end of the procedure can be used. The Multiplanar Clamp (Fig. 36.12) attaches to either end of the LRS rail and can be used to correct angular deformities in any plane. It has five screw seats

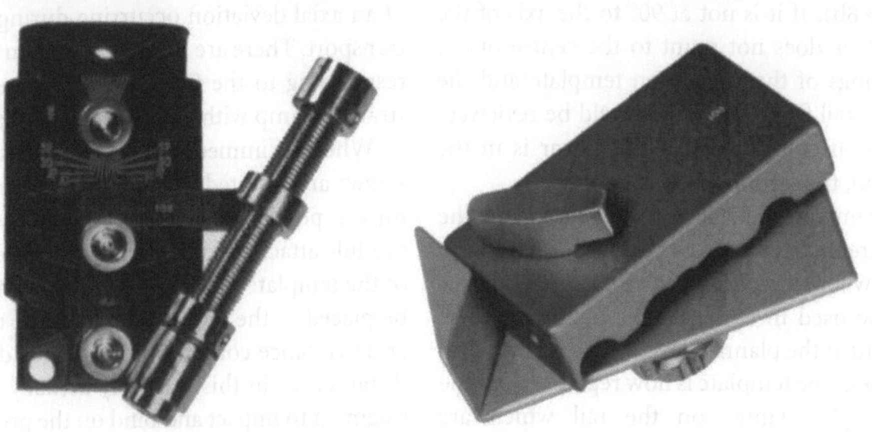

Fig. 36.10 The Micrometric Swivelling Clamp and its template.

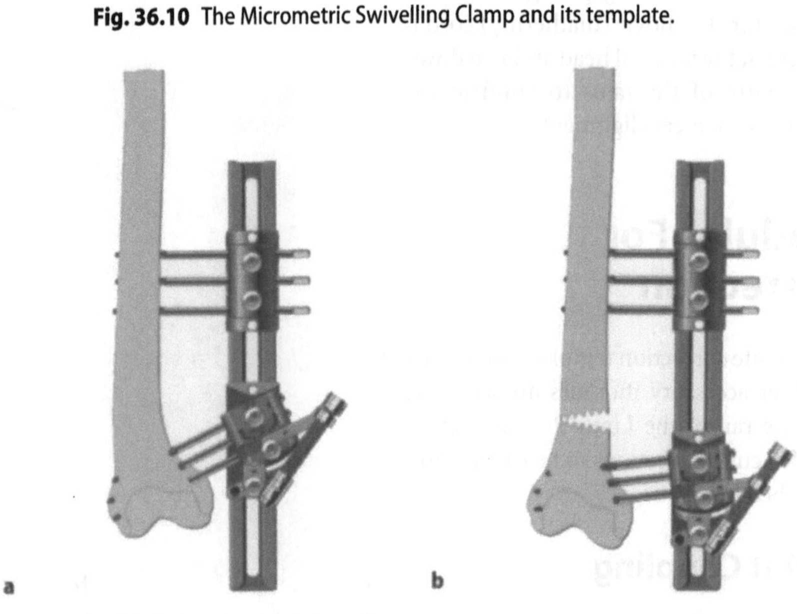

Fig. 36.11 Use of the Micrometric Swivelling Clamp for the immediate correction of a valgus deformity of the distal femur. **a** Distal screws inserted in the plane of the deformity; the osteotomy is at the level of the articulation of the clamp, which is free to slide on the rail. **b** Correction of the deformity by turning the screw of the distractor unit on the clamp in the appropriate direction (see text for a full description of the technique).

corresponding to those of a standard adult straight clamp, and a translation screw which can correct up to 12mm of translation. The central part of the clamp is termed the angulator. This part can rotate through 360°, can be locked in any desired position and determines the plane of angular correction independently of the bone screw positions. The centre of rotation of the clamp is indicated in Fig. 36.12. Application of the clamp requires the use of a dedicated template.

When the fixator is on the convex side of the bone (e.g. varus or anterior angulation in the femur, or valgus or anterior angulation in the tibia), correction will tend to *open* the osteotomy, whereas when the fixator is on the concave side of the deformity (e.g. valgus or posterior angulation in the femur, or varus or posterior angulation in the tibia), correction will tend to *close* the osteotomy. When the fixator is being used to make an acute correction, the adjacent straight clamp must move on the rail to compensate for the opening or closing of the osteotomy gap during this correction. This can be achieved with a standard compression–distraction unit between the two clamps. Initial separation of the osteotomy by 2–3mm will prevent the bone ends from binding. Correction is then made acutely with the distractor, while the osteotomy gap of 2–3mm is simultaneously maintained by shortening or lengthening between the clamps. After correction is complete, the osteotomy is closed.

In either circumstance, the design of the clamp is such that it can be used to correct, at the same time, deformities with components in two planes. Fig. 36.13 shows a femur with 15° of procurvatum in the sagittal plane and 20° of varus in the coronal plane. The anatomical axes of the bone have been drawn to determine the CORA. The plane in which the angulator of the clamp should be mounted can then be determined from the diagram illustrated in Fig.. 36.14. The parameters of the deformity are entered on the appropriate axes as shown. Perpendiculars are then dropped from these points, and the resultant indicates the plane in which the angulator should be placed. Fig. 36.15 shows the application of the Multiplanar Clamp to the above deformity.

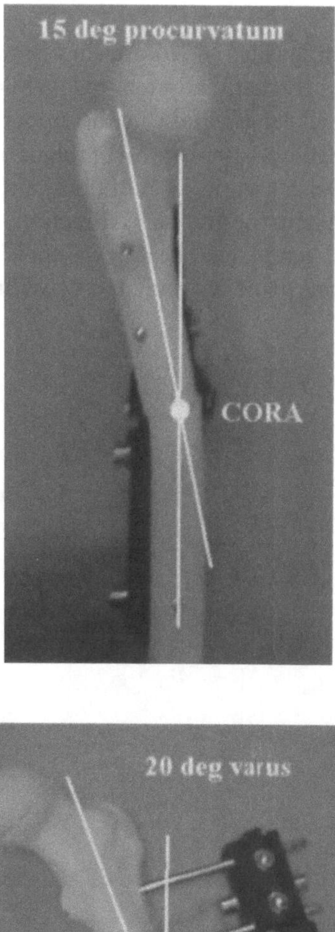

a

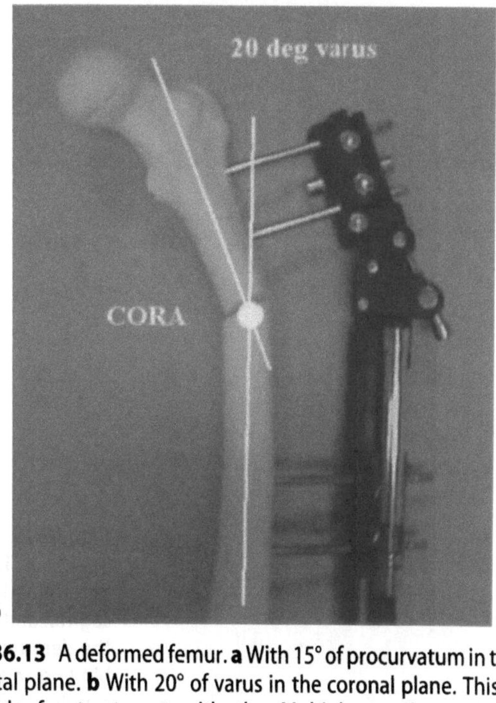

b

Fig. 36.13 A deformed femur. **a** With 15° of procurvatum in the sagittal plane. **b** With 20° of varus in the coronal plane. This is suitable for treatment with the Multiplanar Clamp. Note position of the CORA.

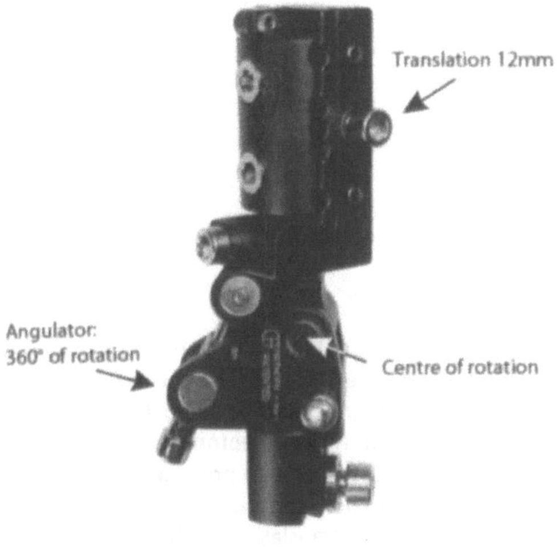

Fig. 36.12 The Multiplanar Clamp.

In addition to its use in the acute correction of deformity, this clamp can also be used to treat deformities occurring during a lengthening procedure or for a lengthening in the presence of a pre-existing deformity which also requires to be corrected. Both of these situations involve callus manipulation and are dealt with in Chs. 40, 42).

The OF-Garches T-Clamp

This module (Fig. 36.16) attaches to one end of the Limb Reconstruction System rail. While its main use is for tibial lengthening in the upper metaphyseal region to allow better control of valgus or varus deviation, it is also used in cases of tibia vara or tibia valga for immediate (or gradual) correction. It has its own dedicated template. The OF-Garches T-Clamp can move in one plane only, and has swivelling screw seats

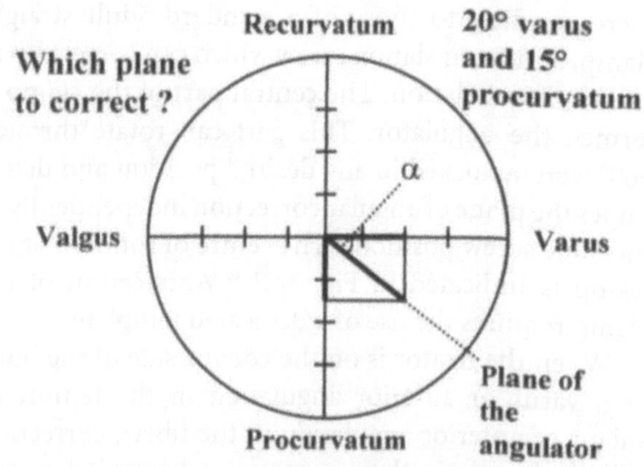

Fig. 36.14 Determination of the plane in which the angulator of the multiplanar clamp should be applied for a femur with 15° of procurvatum and 20° of varus. The co-ordinates are plotted on the diagram and the resultant is the plane to which the angulator should be aligned. In this case α = 37° from the frontal plane.

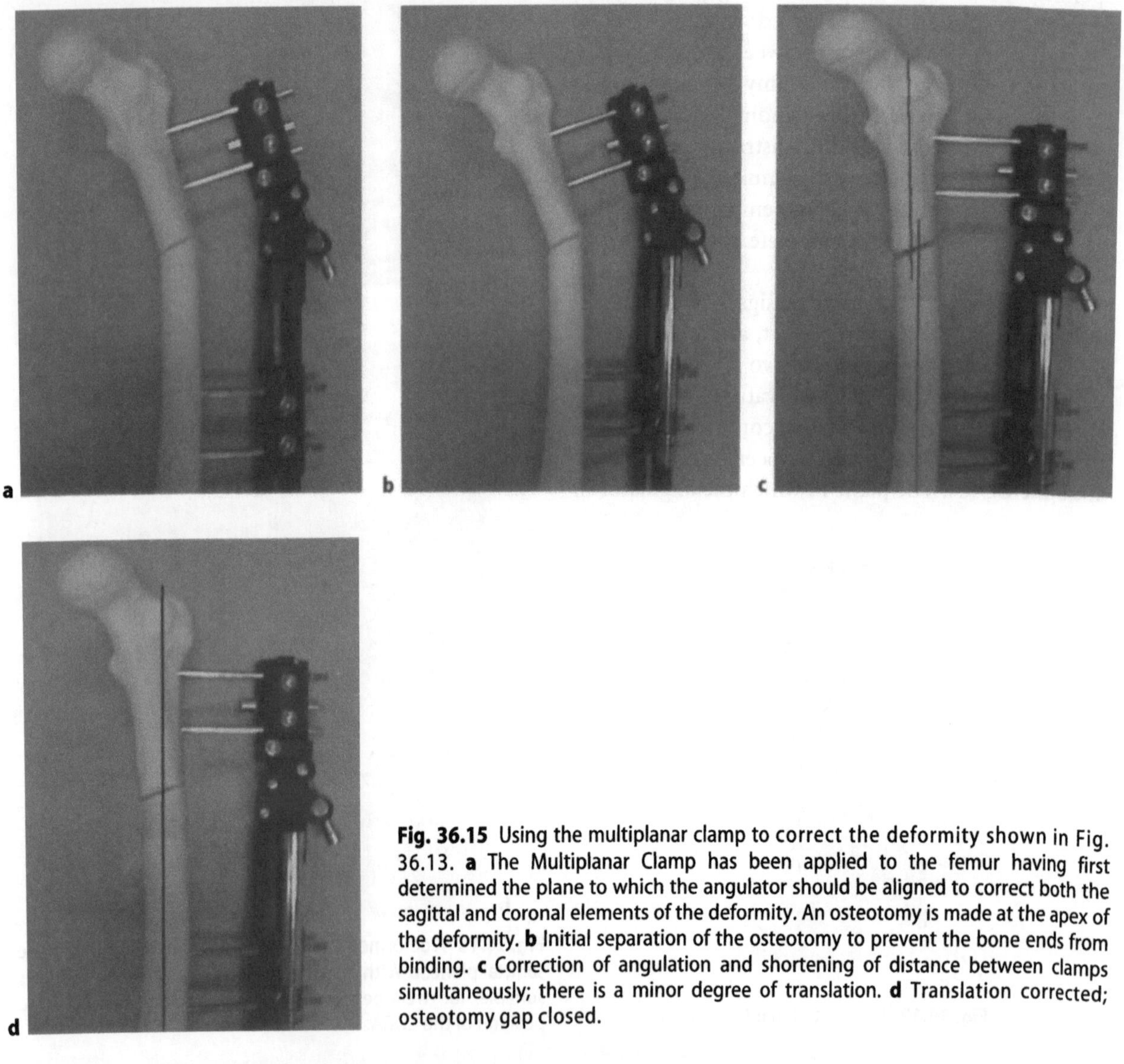
a b c d

Fig. 36.15 Using the multiplanar clamp to correct the deformity shown in Fig. 36.13. **a** The Multiplanar Clamp has been applied to the femur having first determined the plane to which the angulator should be aligned to correct both the sagittal and coronal elements of the deformity. An osteotomy is made at the apex of the deformity. **b** Initial separation of the osteotomy to prevent the bone ends from binding. **c** Correction of angulation and shortening of distance between clamps simultaneously; there is a minor degree of translation. **d** Translation corrected; osteotomy gap closed.

which allow convergent siting of the upper screws. Its compression–distraction unit can be attached in one of two ways, depending upon whether lengthening or angular correction is desired (Fig. 36.19). A paediatric version is also available.

Where used for immediate correction of, for example, a varus tibia, a fibular osteotomy with distal fixation of the fibula is performed. The clamp is applied parallel to the upper surface of the tibia in the coronal plane such that the clamp axis locking nut is at the same level as the upper border of the proposed osteotomy. It is important to bear in mind that the bone screws should be sited below the growth plate in children (Fig. 36.17). With the clamp and rail assembly in place (Fig. 36.18), a subtraction or dome osteotomy is performed, 1cm below the upper screws.

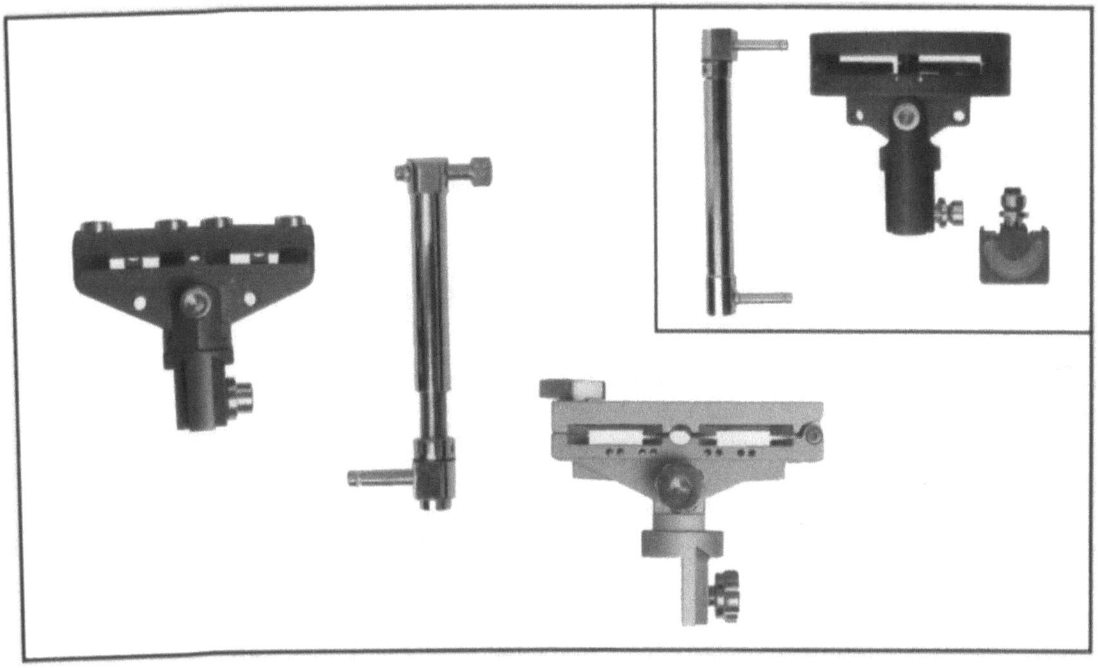

Fig. 36.16 The OF-Garches T-Clamp and its template; the paediatric version is shown in the inset. Because the axis of rotation of the T-clamp passes throught the centre of the osteotomy, translation should not occur during its use.

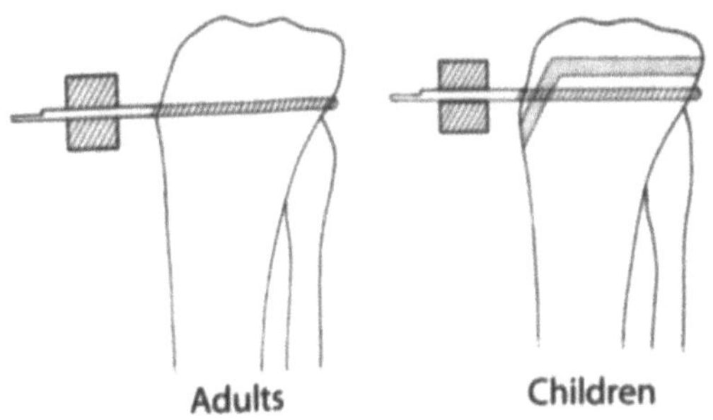

Fig. 36.17 The correct position for the proximal screws for the OF-Garches T-Clamp in adults and children. In the latter the screws are sited below the growth plate.

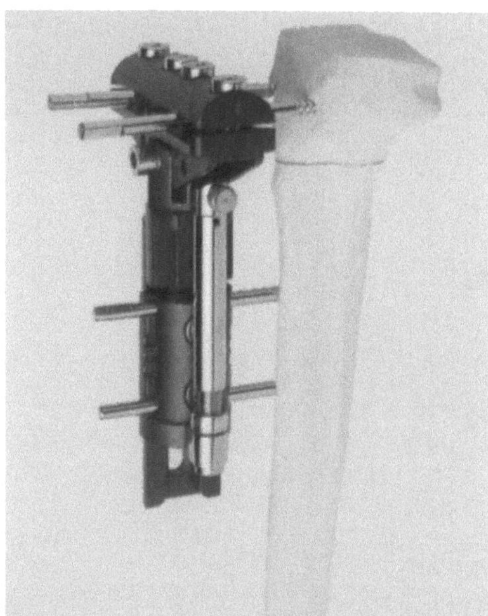

Fig. 36.18 The OF-Garches T-Clamp attached to the LRS for proximal tibial procedures.

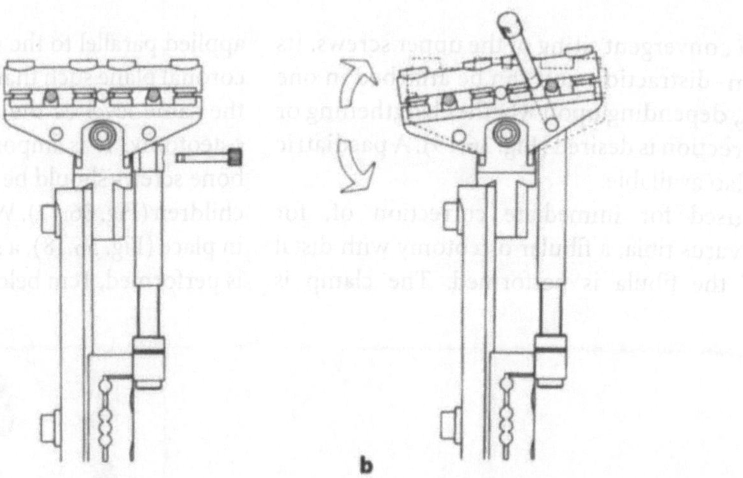

Fig. 36.19 The OF-Garches Clamp: Position of the removable locking pin **a** for lengthening, **b** for angular correction.

Correction is by manipulation, and the fixator is locked with the osteotomy closed. Optimal alignment is best judged post-operatively by means of an AP X-ray of the entire lower limb with the patient standing. Any additional correction may be achieved, where necessary, using the compression–distraction unit, connected as shown in Fig. 36.19b.

Use of this module for lengthening coupled with angular correction is described in Ch. 42.

References

1. Donnan LT, Rigby AS, Saleh M. 'Acute correction of bony deformity and simultaneous lengthening by callotasis.' *J Bone Joint Surg* [Br] 1999; Orthop Proc III; 81-B: 278.
2. Donnan LT, Saleh M. 'Monolateral External Fixation in Paediatric Limb Reconstruction.' *Current Orthopaedics* 1998; 12: 159–66.
3. Paley D, Tetsworth K. 'Mechanical axis deviation of the lower limbs; pre-operative planning of uniapical angular deformities of the tibia or femur.' *Clin Orthop* 1992; 280: 48–64.

Upper Tibial Osteotomy: A Critical Review 37

A.G. MacEachern and A.E. Weale

Bone may be deformed as a consequence of fracture, abnormal growth or disease, such as osteoarthritis. Correction of deformity can be achieved immediately, at operation, by means of a step cut osteotomy, by dome osteotomy, or by removing or adding a wedge of bone; the position must then be held until the osteotomy has united.

Correction may also be achieved by means of a partial osteotomy followed by gradual asymmetrical distraction of the callus. This method, known as hemicallotasis, will be described in this chapter. The advent of modern external fixation has made hemicallotasis an exciting possibility, although external fixation and osteotomy can also be used in the conventional manner, as suggested by Aldegheri et al.[1] The area which will be focused upon is upper tibial osteotomy in the osteoarthritic knee, but the principles of the technique can be related to other conditions and other sites.

Jackson[2] first described the use of tibial osteotomy for osteoarthritis of the knee in 1958, and later reported results with Waugh and Green[3]. The latter authors described a series of 70 dome osteotomies, for varus and valgus deformity, fixed by a variety of methods including staples, pins and plates. There were several cases of delayed union, three of which required bone grafting, eight cases of peroneal nerve palsy, four wound infections and 13 pin track infections. Harris and Kostuik[4] reported on four laterally-based closing wedge osteotomies, fixed with staples. There were two cases of peroneal nerve palsy, three wound infections, one intra-articular fracture and one delayed union.

The name of Coventry[5] has been closely associated with upper tibial osteotomy for many years. He stated "the results of upper tibial osteotomy have been uniformly good if the proper correction has been obtained and no technical complications have ensued." He cited a number of potential complications. These included intra-articular fracture through the proximal fragment, avascular necrosis, delayed union and non-union. He suggested that peroneal nerve palsy may be due to one of several causes. Pressure on the nerve from a cast or a tight bandage was probably the most common cause, but proximal fibular osteotomy was also implicated.

Gibson, Barnes, Allen and Chan[6] monitored compartment pressures and peroneal nerve palsy. They described 20 closing-wedge osteotomies, with concomitant fibular osteotomy, and noted raised compartment pressures over 50mm Hg in 7 of 10 cases in which no drain was inserted. Of these, 5 had transient signs of peroneal nerve palsy. Even in the drained group some pressure rise was noted. Curley, Eyres, Brezinova et al[7] further examined peroneal nerve dysfunction after high tibial osteotomy. They concluded that proximal fibula division is an important factor in common peroneal nerve palsy after osteotomy.

Correction

The correction required for osteotomy is generally estimated from standing radiographs, preferably including the hip and ankle. Measurements may then be made of the tibiofemoral angle, and of the mechanical axis. Coventry stated that the tibiofemoral angle should not only be corrected to normal, i.e. 5 to 7° of anatomical valgus, but overcorrected to 10° of anatomical valgus. This represents a mechanical axis angulation of 3–5° (see Fig. 37.1).

Insall[8] reviewed 95 knees at a mean of 8.5 years after operation. Although still suggesting that 5–14° of valgus correction is appropriate, he believed that the passage of time (since the operation) was the most important factor in determining outcome. He noted that recurrence of pain was associated with under-correction.

Tjórnstand et al[9] reported a 7-year follow-up of 89 osteotomies. They described adequate correction as a normal post-operative mechanical axis. Of 24 patients adequately corrected, 22 had no progression of osteoarthritis. Two-thirds of the 65 patients in whom satisfactory correction was not achieved, showed some evidence of osteoarthritic progression.

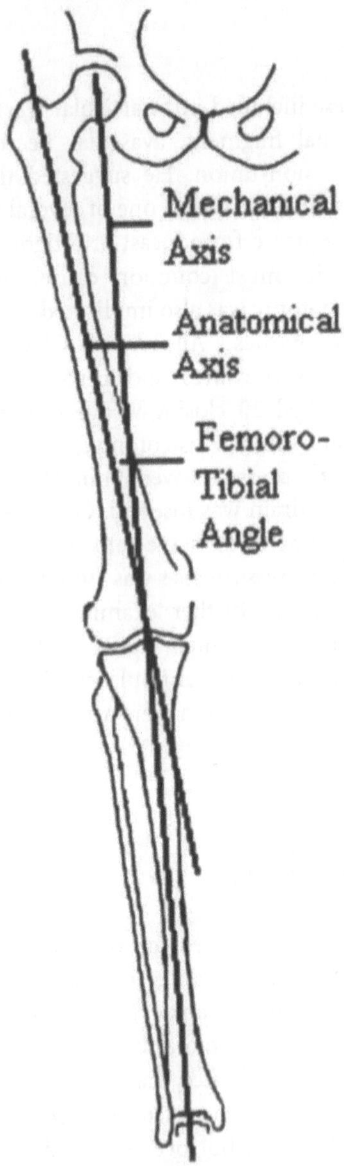

Fig. 37.1 The mechanical axis is a straight line passing through the head of the femur, the centre of the knee joint, and the centre of the ankle joint; it should also be at right angles to the articular surfaces of the knee and ankle joints. The femoro-tibial angle is the angle between the diaphyseal axes of the femur and the tibia, and varies from 5° to 7° of valgus.

Hernigou[10] reported a 10–13 year follow-up of 93 knees treated with a medial opening wedge osteotomy and bone grafting. In this group, 20 patients were corrected to 3–6° of valgus, with a good result; 68 were "under-corrected", with less satisfactory results. Five knees were overcorrected and developed progressive lateral compartment osteoarthritis. He concluded that "exact post-operative alignment is the prerequisite for the largest possible relief of symptoms."

Thus, although the precise degree of correction may still be a matter for discussion, it is largely accepted that under-correction is to be avoided, and that the results deteriorate with time.

Patient Selection

Coventry has stressed the importance of patient selection. He suggested that the knee should be mobile, but that a flexion deformity of up to 15° was acceptable. The patient's age, weight and activity level are also important. Those under the age of 65 years with high activity levels are more suited to osteotomy than those over 65 with low demands, in whom total knee replacement may be more appropriate.

Prodromos et al[11] provided a vital clue as to why some patients appear to do better than others after upper tibial osteotomy. Pre-operative gait analysis showed that patients could be divided into two groups – those with a high adduction moment, and those with a low adduction moment who had developed a compensatory short-stride, toe out gait. At a mean of 3.2 years post-operatively the low adduction moment group had 100 per cent excellent or good results, compared with 50 per cent in the high adduction moment group. Andriacchi[12] confirmed the value of gait analysis. Correction may be better assessed dynamically, by reduction of the adduction moment and the transfer of force to the lateral compartment. This method has now, in fact, been studied and a preliminary report by Thomas et al[13] on three cases appears encouraging.

Knee Replacement

It is important to remember that patients treated by osteotomy may later become candidates for total knee replacement. The latter procedure is more difficult and the results less satisfactory after conventional proximal tibial osteotomy (Windsor et al).[14]

Hemicallotasis

It seems clear, therefore, that conventional methods, involving either dome or wedge osteotomy, have the potential for serious complications. An alternative method of correcting malalignment is hemicallotasis. In 1983, De Bastiani[15] explained this procedure and its advantages in high tibial osteotomy. It avoids the need for fibular osteotomy, committed on-table geometry, immobilization in a cast, compartment syndrome, non-union and subsequent loss of position.

Original Technique

Initially, two cancellous screws, parallel to the articular surface of the tibia, were applied to the medial tibial border and held with a T-clamp. This was attached to an articulated hinge, connected to a standard fixator, with two distal cortical screws. A hemicorticotomy was performed through the medial half of the tibia, proximal to the tibial tuberosity. Distraction was tested at operation, and commenced, after a period of 10–14 days, at 4 × ¼ turns of the compression-distraction unit screw per day, until the desired correction was achieved. A neutralization phase followed until the new bone appeared sufficiently strong to allow dynamization of the frame, which continued until union of the osteotomy.

Recently, a revised T-clamp (the Torbay Garches clamp) has become available, allowing the surgeon to angle the pins slightly and thus accommodate them more easily within the narrow upper tibia. The original simple hinge permitted lateral translation of the proximal fragment. A self-aligning body with a hinge incorporating a slot was therefore designed. With this module, the pivot moves within the slot during distraction, and translation of the tibia is avoided (Fig. 37.2).

Current Technique

Image intensification is required. Using appropriate templates, two cancellous screws are inserted into the upper tibia, from the medial side, and two distal cortical screws are inserted into the diaphysis. Through an anteromedial incision, placed so as not to compromise a subsequent incision for total knee replacement, the periosteum is carefully reflected.

The osteotomy line is drilled with a 3.2mm drill bit, extending over the medial two-thirds of the upper tibia, in an anterior and posterior direction. The osteotomy may be sited proximal to the insertion of the patellar tendon, or more distally, according to the patient's anatomy and pathology, and the surgeon's preference. The osteotomy is completed with an osteotome; this can be done with the fixator in place, as distraction is applied. As the osteotomy proceeds from medial to lateral, it begins to open under tension, indicating that sufficient bony division has occurred. It is then opened widely to ensure that satisfactory correction can be achieved and a note is made of the opening distance on the telescopic scale. The osteotomy is then allowed to close, the periosteum is carefully resutured and the wound closed. Early weightbearing and knee movement are encouraged in the early post-operative phase.

After 7–10 days, distraction is commenced at a rate of 6 × ¼ turns per day (or 3 × ½ turns, if more convenient) until adequate correction is achieved. Distraction is then discontinued and a Dyna-Ring applied. Further weightbearing is encouraged. The fixator and pins are removed once union has been achieved.

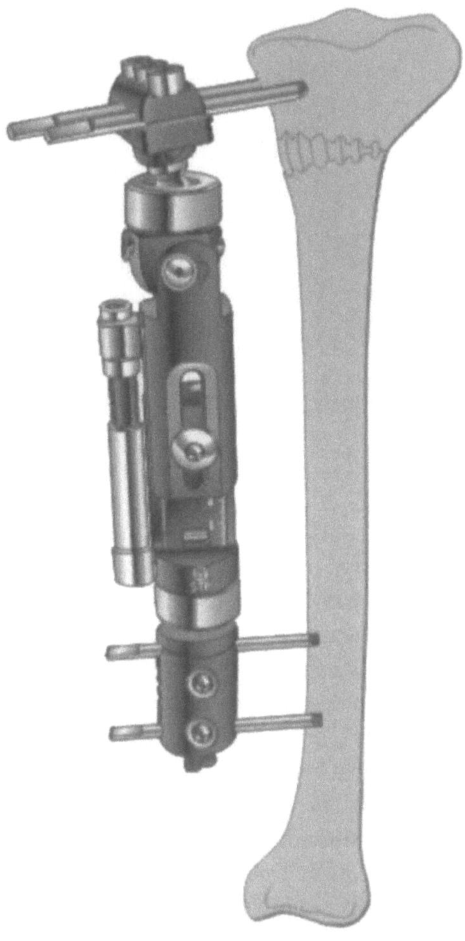

Fig. 37.2 Upper tibial hemicallotasis; the 90.000 fixator with Torbay Garches clamp and self-aligning articulated body.

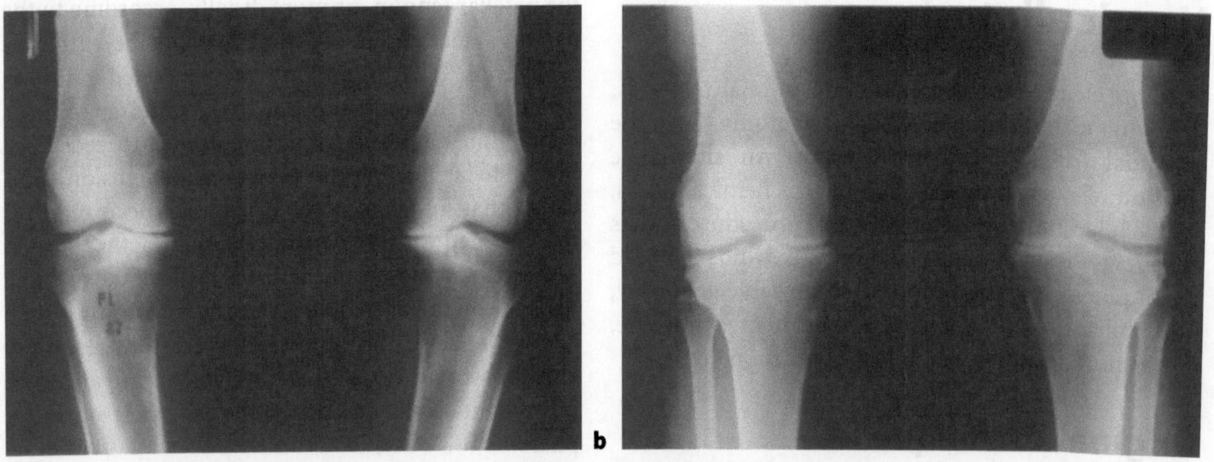

a b

Fig. 37.3 The treatment of bilateral varus tibiae in a man with medial osteoarthritis of both knees. **a** Pre-operative films. **b** Post-operative films; right knee: 5½ years post-operatively; left knee: 7 years post-operatively.

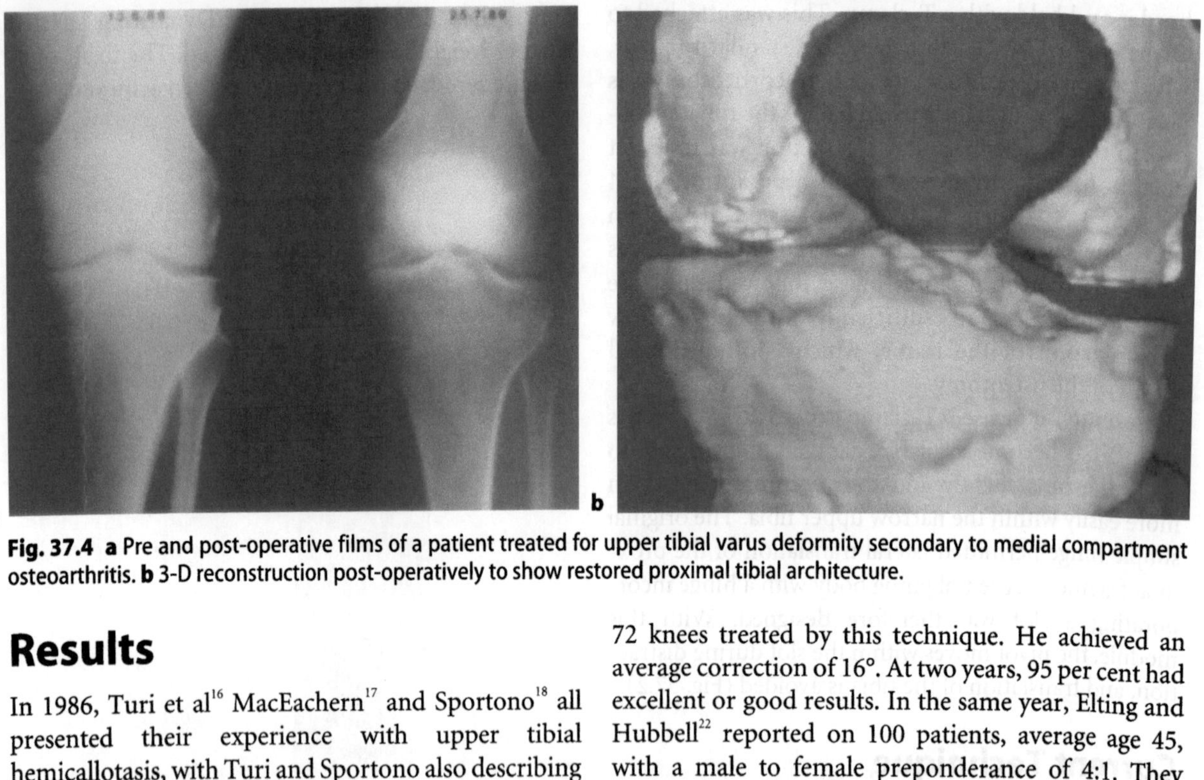

a b

Fig. 37.4 **a** Pre and post-operative films of a patient treated for upper tibial varus deformity secondary to medial compartment osteoarthritis. **b** 3-D reconstruction post-operatively to show restored proximal tibial architecture.

Results

In 1986, Turi et al[16] MacEachern[17] and Sportono[18] all presented their experience with upper tibial hemicallotasis, with Turi and Sportono also describing distal femoral hemicallotasis for the valgus knee. Turi et al[19] reported their findings in 1987. Fowler et al[20] were the first to describe the technique in the English language in 1991, on an initial series of 21 patients. It was observed that the method allows limb alignment to be controlled precisely by post-operative adjustment, and that since the proximal tibial architecture is restored, subsequent total knee replacement may be easier than after conventional osteotomy. Post-operative compartment pressures were monitored and no rise above 30mm Hg was recorded.

In 1992, Oppenheim[21] described his experience with 72 knees treated by this technique. He achieved an average correction of 16°. At two years, 95 per cent had excellent or good results. In the same year, Elting and Hubbell[22] reported on 100 patients, average age 45, with a male to female preponderance of 4:1. They noted 98 per cent good or excellent results at two years, and expressed satisfaction with the advantages of this technique over conventional wedge osteotomy.

In 1994, MacEachern and Fowler[23] reported on 36 cases, (follow-up 44–123 months, mean 83 months.) Two patients had died of unrelated causes; one had left the area and had been reviewed by a colleague; that patient had developed sepsis of the upper tibia, requiring curettage and bone grafting, which appeared to have been curative. Of the remaining 33 knees, good and fair results were reported in 79 per cent and poor results in 21 per cent.

Prospective studies from Sweden have shown that the outcome following osteotomy in conjunction with the hemicallotasis technique is equivalent to that following closing-wedge osteotomy, and that complications are infrequent and rarely serious.[24,25] At 5 and 10 years following upper tibial hemicallotasis using external fixation, the results were still good in 89 and 63 per cent of cases respectively.[26]

Hemicallotasis can also be used to correct other deformities, e.g. recurvatum of the knee, using an anterior application, as reported by O'Dwyer et al.[27] It can also be used for realignment of the distal femur to treat a valgus knee, and in the distal tibia for a varus ankle.

Summary

Orthofix External Fixation has proved itself capable of a wide variety of uses in the correction of limb malalignment, both in uniplanar and multiplanar deformities as described elsewhere in this book. With respect to the use of hemicallotasis in upper tibial osteotomy, there appear to be certain clear advantages over conventional methods. These include the ability to adjust the position of the knee post-operatively, to the satisfaction of surgeon and patient (Fig. 37.3). An excessively valgus position may be cosmetically unacceptable, particularly if the other knee is somewhat varus – the windswept deformity. The absence of a fibular osteotomy is associated with a reduction in the incidence of both compartment syndrome and peroneal nerve palsy. The knee remains mobile throughout treatment, avoiding the problems associated with cast immobilization. Non-union has not been observed. Proximal tibial architecture is restored (Fig. 37.4) facilitating subsequent total knee replacement.

The potential disadvantages of hemicallotasis include the need for patient compliance through the period to union – approximately three months. The greatest worry, however, is the possibility of pin site sepsis. Of the 208 patients reported in the English language, there has been only one case of significant sepsis. It may be that routine pin site curettage at pin removal should be considered, to reduce problems further.

The consensus view appears to be that the advantages of hemicallotasis far outweigh the disadvantages. Moreover, careful patient selection and gait analysis studies should help us to achieve better long-term results for our patients.

References

1. Aldegheri R, Renzi Brivio L, Spagnol G. 'L'osteotomia di Ginocchio con il Fissatore Esterno. Assiale.' *La Chirurgia degli Organi di Movimento*. Vol. LXVIII.II, 207–211.
2. Jackson J P. 'Osteotomy for osteo-arthritis of the knee.' *J Bone Joint Surg* [Br] 1958; 40-B: 826.
3. Jackson J P, Waugh W, Green J P. 'High tibial osteotomy for osteo-arthritis of the knee.' *J Bone Joint Surg* [Br] 1969; 51-B: 88–94.
4. Harris W R, Kostuik JP. 'High tibial osteotomy for osteo-arthritis of the knee.' *J Bone Joint Surg* [Am] 1970; 52-A: 330–336.
5. Coventry M B. 'Upper tibial osteotomy for osteo-arthritis.' J *Bone Joint Surg* [Am] 1985; 67-A: 1136–1140.
6. Gibson M J, Barnes M R, Allen M J, Chan R M W. 'Weakness of foot dorsiflexion and changes in compartment pressures after tibial osteotomy.' *J Bone Joint Surg* [Br] 1986; 68-B: 471–475.
7. Curley P, Eyres K, Brezinova V, Allen M, Chan R, Barnes M. 'Common peroneal nerve dysfunction after high tibial osteotomy.' *J Bone Joint Surg* [Br] 1990; 72-B: 405–408.
8. Insall J N, Joseph D M, Miska C. 'High tibial osteotomy for varus gonarthrosis. A long term follow up study.' *J Bone Joint Surg* [Am] 1984; 66-A: 1040–1048.
9. Tjórnstrand B, Egund N, Hagstedt B. 'High tibial osteotomy: A seven year clinical and radiographic follow up.' *Clin Orthop* 1981; 160: 124–136.
10. Hernigou P H, Medevielle D, Debeyre J, Goutallier P 'Proximal tibial osteotomy for osteo-arthritis with varus deformity. A ten to thirteen year follow-up study.' *J Bone Joint Surg* [Am] 1987; 69-A: 332–354.
11. Prodromos C C, Andriacchi T P, Galante J. 'A relationship between gait and clinical change following high tibial osteotomy.' *J Bone Joint Surg* [Am] 1985; 67-A: 1188–1194.
12. Andriacchi T P. Personal Communication. 1987.
13. Thomas P B M, Wooton J R, Patrick J H. 'Preliminary report of a novel use of gait analysis in proximal tibial callotasis for medial compartment osteo-arthritis of the knee.' *J Bone Joint Surg* [Br] 1994; 76-B: suppl. p.47.
14. Windsor R E, Insall J N, Vince K G. 'Technical considerations of total knee arthroplasty after proximal tibial osteotomy.' *J Bone Joint Surg* [Am] 1988; 70-A: 547–555.
15. De Bastiani G. Personal Communication. 1983.
16. Turi G, Tomasi P S, Armotti P A, Cassini A. 'The dynamic axial fixator in directional osteotomy of the knee.' in *Proceedings of Recent Advances in External Fixation* Riva del Garda, 1986, p.138.
17. MacEachern A G. 'Valgus osteotomy of the upper tibia for osteo-arthrosis of the knee.' in *Proceedings Recent Advances in External Fixation*, Riva del Garda, 1986, p 139.
18. Sportono L. 'A new method for the correction of femoral tibial axial deviations.' in *Proceedings of Recent Advances in External Fixation.* Riva del Garda, 1986.
19. Turi G, Cassini M, Tomasi P S, Atmotti P, Lavini F. 'L'osteotomia Direzionale di ginocchio mediante La 'emicallostasi'.' *Chir Organi Movimenti* 1987; 72: 250–209.
20. Fowler J L, Gie G A, MacEachern A G. 'Upper tibial valgus osteotomy using a dynamic external fixator.' *J Bone Joint Surg* [Br] 1991; 73-B: 690–691.
21. Oppenheim W S, Jaffe L, Rosa R. 'Upper tibial osteotomy utilizing hemicallotasis.' Paper No. 220, 59th AAOS meeting, Washington DC, 1992.
22. Elting J, Hubbell J. 'Unilateral frame distraction. Proximal tibial valgus osteotomy for medial gonarthritis.' *Contemp Orthop* 1993; 27: 435–444.
23. MacEachern A G, Fowler J L. 'Upper tibial osteotomy by hemicallotasis with the dynamic external fixator.' *J Bone Joint Surg* [Br] 1994; 76-B: 49.

24. Magyar G, Ahl TL, Vibe P, Toksvig-Larsen S, Lindstrand A. 'Open-wedge osteotomy by hemicallotasis or the closed-wedge technique for osteoarthritis of the knee. A randomised study of 50 operations.' *J Bone Joint Surg* 1999; 81B: 444–448.
25. Magyar G, Toksvig-Larsen S, Lindstrand A. 'Hemicallotasis open-wedge osteotomy for osteoarthritis of the knee. Complications in 308 operations.' *J Bone Joint Surg* 1999; 81B: 449–451.
26. Weale AE, Lee AS, MacEachern AG. 'High tibial osteotomy using a dynamic external fixator.' *Clin Orthop*: in press.
27. O'Dwyer K J, MacEachern A G, Pennig D. 'Osteotomia tibiale corretiva perginocchio recurvato con distrazione del callo mediante fissatore esterno.' *La Chirurgia degli Organi di Movimento* 1991; 70: 355–358.

Upper Tibial Hemicallotasis Using a Self-Aligning Articulated Body

38

J.J. Elting

Introduction

There has emerged in recent years a distinct group of patients who pose a difficult problem for the orthopaedic surgeon. These are the patients with medial compartment degenerative disease who are young and active, who may have had multiple arthroscopic procedures and who have been advised to "take it easy and wait until the time is right for a total knee replacement". This may not, however, be an acceptable option for an individual in a full-time occupation.

If the knee is in varus, we would advocate unilateral frame distraction upper tibial corticotomy. Turi et al[9] of the School of De Bastiani in Verona suggested in 1987 that the technique of hemicallotasis, or asymmetric distraction of the developing callus following a corticotomy, might be used to achieve a valgus tibia and described a method in which a unilateral dynamic external fixator is applied to the medial aspect of the limb and gradually distracted until the appropriate degree of valgus is attained. Fowler et al[4] reported their experience with the technique in 1991 and in 1992 Oppenheim et al[8] reported on a series of 75 patients treated by this method.

We have performed upper tibial corticotomy in conjunction with unilateral frame distraction over time as a treatment for symptomatic medial osteoarthritis of the knee since 1988. Our early experience prompted us to demonstrate this technique at the American Academy of Orthopaedic Surgeons' annual meeting in 1992 and to report our initial results.[2,3] Further favourable communications have followed as realignment of the tibia by this method has gained acceptance in North America.[7] The present chapter will document our own experience in terms of patient selection, surgical technique and management of the hemicallotasis, and will describe clinical outcomes.

Materials and Methods

The patient will typically present as a hard working male in his forties (male: female 3:1; mean age 48 years) who may, some years previously, have sustained a medial compartment injury and had transarthroscopic or open meniscectomy or other surgical intervention (average 1.7 previous operations). While the patient may have remained active over the period of time following the initial injury, the pain has become symptomatic to the point where it is difficult to function at work, much less in any recreational activities. Many of our patients are farmers or outdoor workers who are on their feet and moving about during the working day. The single leg X-ray mimics stance phase and depicts a 'kissing' lesion as described by Coventry.[1] In addition, there seems to be a varus angulation or medial cortical collapse in the metaphyseal portion of the proximal tibia.

We first ensure that the patient has carried out a rehabilitation programme either under the direct supervision of a member of the rehabilitation staff, or adequately at home. It is preferable that the range of movement of the affected knee is comparable to that on the unaffected side or, if both knees are symptomatic, that the range of motion is deemed adequate and full. There should be no synovitis present, and on occasion we will perform arthroscopy to treat synovitis or remove a meniscal remnant which is blocking full extension. The patient must be able to carry out a standard protocol which includes distraction of the frame and pin site care, and must have a bodily configuration that will accept the assembly. The individual need not be thin or small, but massive obesity may be associated with a higher incidence of pin track complications or inability to distract the frame.

Surgical Technique

As in any operative procedure, it is helpful for all involved to be aware of the proposed sequence of events as well as having a familiarity with the Orthofix equipment. The patient is supine on the operating table, with the affected extremity draped free and elevated on folded linen so that the surgeon, who is standing across the table, will not be hindered by the near leg.

Two tapered cancellous screws are placed, under fluoroscopic control, in what was once the proximal tibial epiphyseal line. Image intensification is essential in order to avoid perforating the subchondral plate and entering the joint, and to ensure that the screws are inserted parallel to one another. Two cortical screws are introduced distally in the tibial shaft, the guide to their position being the closed frame. The frame we used (Orthofix Srl, Verona, Italy) consisted of (1) a horizontal T-clamp for the proximal cancellous screws, with ball-joint attachment to (2) a self-aligning articulating body with a male stem which fits into (3) the female component of a standard or small dynamic axial fixator which in turn is attached by a ball joint to (4) a straight clamp for the distal screws. It is best applied in the closed position to the medial surface of the tibia.

Using the axis of rotation of the self-aligning articulating body as a guide, a medial corticotomy is now performed at this level (Fig. 38.1). This corticotomy encompasses approximately five-sixths of the circumference of the tibia. Following minimal disturbance of the periosteum, multiple drill holes are placed in the anterior, medial and posteromedial cortices, leaving the lateral cortex intact. The drill holes are now connected via cortical perforation with a small short osteotome and the frame, having been applied, is distracted to ensure that the corticotomy opens unilaterally (Fig. 38.2). The intact lateral cortex along with its periosteum, attendant soft tissues, and the proximal fibula, serves as a hinge. The small medial incision is closed loosely with interrupted nylon skin sutures. Neither a drain nor a tourniquet is used. The frame is locked in its closed position, and the patient admitted to hospital overnight. Pin site care is taught on the day following surgery and the patient encouraged to bear weight to tolerance with a crutch.

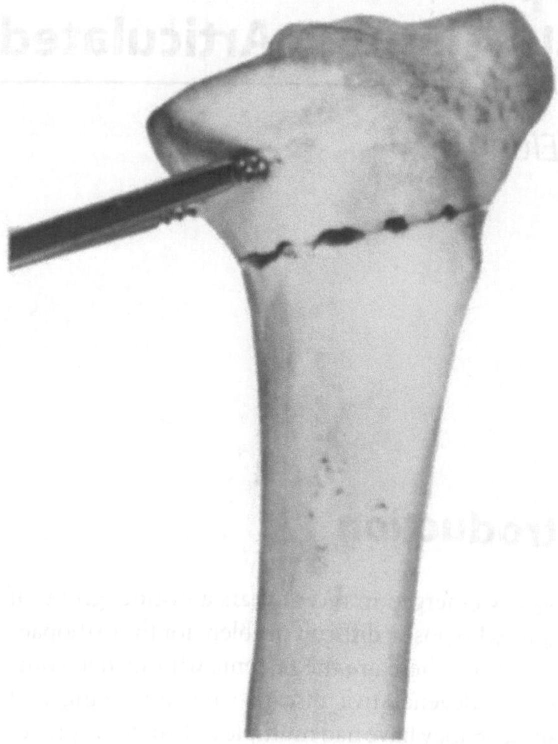

Fig. 38.1 Proximal screws in position; medial osteotomy performed. The lateral cortex remains intact and acts as a hinge.

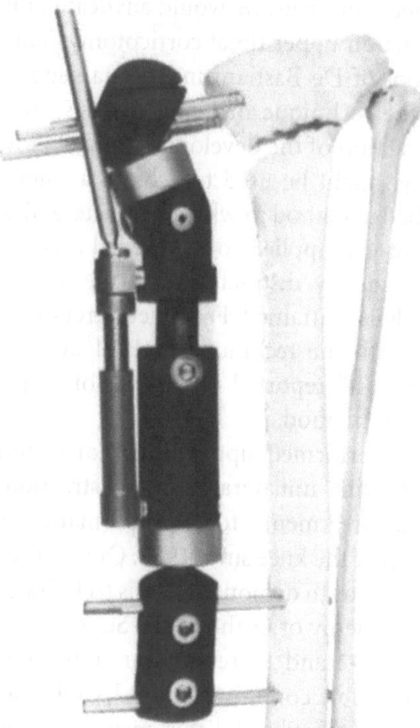

Fig. 38.2 With the fixator in place the compression-distraction unit is used to ensure that the osteotomy opens unilaterally, and that correction is achievable, before bringing the segments back into contact.

Management of Hemicallotasis

At 10 days, when early callus formation has begun, distraction is commenced at the rate of 1mm per day at the medial cortex (2mm per day at the frame). Distraction and alignment are checked every few days and, at a certain point in time, the patient will state that the medial knee pain which had provoked the need to seek treatment has disappeared. We stop the distraction when it is judged to be sufficient roentgenographically, symptomatically, and aesthetically. This will usually take place when more than 10° of valgus is achieved.

The frame is then locked, careful follow-up continued, and some 3–4 weeks thereafter, or at 7–10 weeks post surgery, the frame is dynamized. This allows axial loading of the corticotomy site which now becomes progressively mineralized and corticalized. A dynamization collar incorporating a silicone cushion is attached to the male stem as it enters the female component of the frame, thus preventing collapse of more than 2mm at the osteotomy site. The frame is usually removed at 12–14 weeks. The patient has been bearing full weight, usually with a cane, and is allowed to walk about for an hour or two without the frame before the screws are finally removed. The X-rays are taken antero-posterior, with the patient standing. A useful method of comparison is to overlay the images obtained at successive visits.

The patient and family participate in this intensive exercise in bone physiology. They are guided by our staff in pin site care and operation of the frame. We schedule several of these patients in the clinic at the same time, so that they may observe the X-rays, compare experiences, and encourage each other. Where callotasis is not progressing, as reflected in several X-rays or by collapse of the corticotomy on dynamization, the frame may be used in compression for a few days and then redistracted. It is important that patients bear weight on the operated extremity, to transmit axial load and to provide micromotion at the site of the corticotomy and callus distraction.

We anticipate that the patient will return to a full range of activities within six months of surgery.

Results

We have now treated 150 patients using this technique over the past 10 years. The results have been rewarding, and over the entire period, only 10 patients (11 knees) have progressed to total knee arthroplasty 2–7 years (mean 4.1 years) following the procedure. All have fared well. The total knee arthroplasty was performed in a routine manner and presented no technical surprises in any instance. Follow-up clinical and roentgenographic ratings in the 10 patients who eventually received a total knee replacement in our series have compared favourably with our population of "virgin knees" (Table 38.1). In the past four years, no patient who has undergone upper tibial hemicallotasis has developed symptoms requiring total knee replacement.

Iliac marrow aspirate was instilled for one individual whose distraction hemicallotasis had not been stable at 12 weeks. She had had a non-union of a "conventional" upper tibial osteotomy in the same area many years before. By 17 weeks, she had stabilized after redistraction. Two anterior cruciate reconstructions were performed in two individuals six and nine months following the distraction upper tibial osteotomy respectively.

There have been no neurovascular complications and no deep infections in our series, and as our experience has increased, our incidence of skin and pin track problems has fallen from an initial 25 per cent to less than 10 per cent who require oral antibiotics. Overall satisfaction with the procedure is high, with 90 per cent of our patients reporting that they are pleased with the outcome following unilateral frame distraction upper tibial valgus osteotomy.

A typical case history is illustrated in Fig. 38.3. A male college professor and football referee presented at age 41 with bilateral knee pain, more severe on the left. The pain was particularly associated with the medial joint interval on weightbearing. As a teenager he had played in the English premier league, but had no history of severe knee injury, or any previous surgery. Examination demonstrated a relative quadriceps insufficiency and a shortening on both sides. A single leg standing film showed a varus deformity of the left knee with medial compartment narrowing (Fig. 38.3a). He was introduced into a rehabilitation programme aimed primarily at lengthening his quadriceps, and received intra-articular injections. Under this regime he was able to continue as a referee for a further season.

During the following winter the patient underwent upper tibial osteotomy with medial application of a standard Orthofix fixator with self-aligning body and T-clamp. The fixator was initially locked for 10 days, after which distraction began, and was continued for 2 weeks (Figs. 38.3b, 38.33c). He achieved symptomatic shift of force plate, excellent cosmesis and an X-ray

Fig. 38.3 41-year-old male referee with severe left knee pain in the medial joint interval on weightbearing. **a** Single leg standing X-ray showing varus deformity of the left knee with medial compartment narrowing. **b** 10 days after upper tibial osteotomy; distraction phase about to commence. **c** After 10 days distraction; callus visible within the opening osteotomy gap. **d** 7 weeks post-operation; dynamization collar in place, and dynamization phase about to commence. **e** 5 months post-operation; deformity corrected; patient fully functional. **f** 6 months post-operation; refereeing at an international tournament.

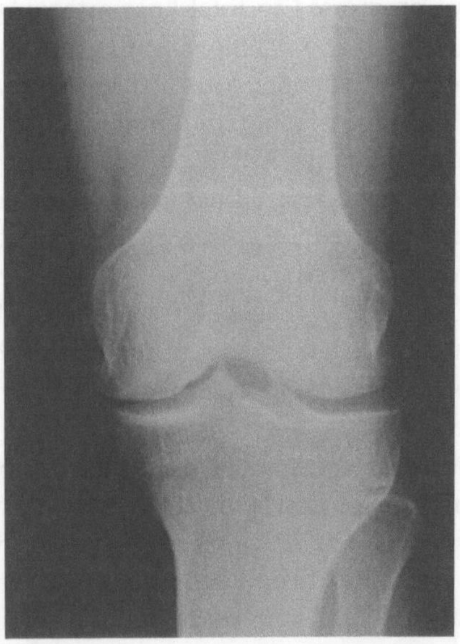

a

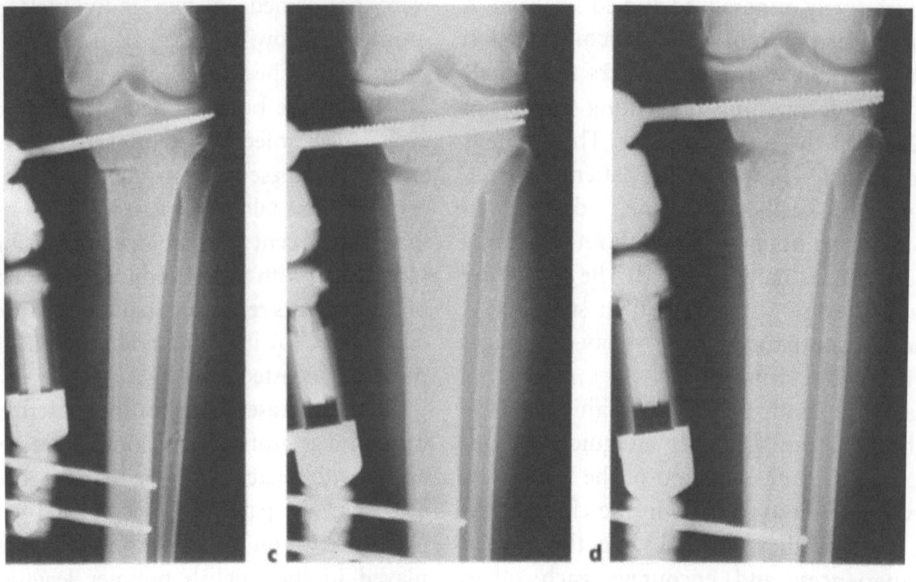

b c d

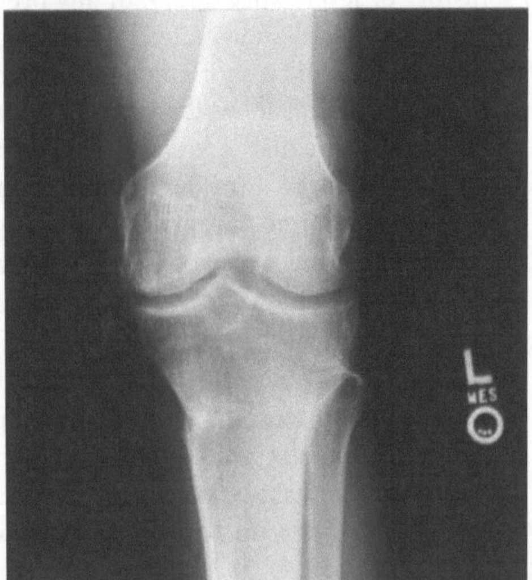

e

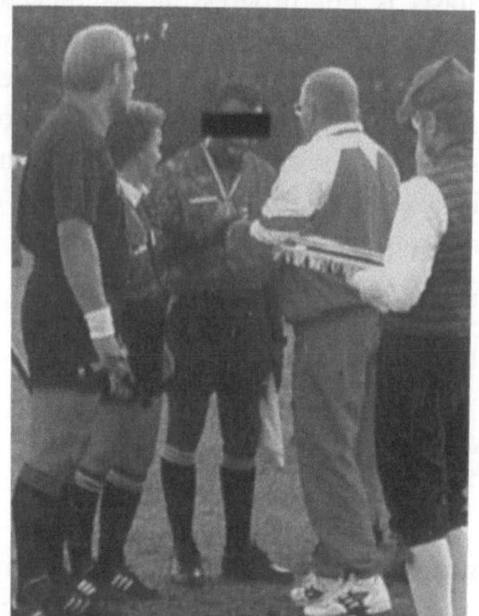

f

reflecting acceptable valgus. The frame was then locked, and the patient participated in an active exercise programme, gaining full extension of the knee. At 7 weeks post-osteotomy a dynamization collar was applied to the fixator, and dynamization commenced (Fig. 38.3d). The frame was removed at 12 weeks. At 5 months post-operation (Fig. 38.3e) the patient was fully functional and had returned to refereeing. Six months after surgery he participated in an international tournament in Denmark (Fig. 38.3f), officiating at 21 matches in 6 days.

Discussion

Unilateral frame distraction proximal tibial valgus osteotomy is a relatively new technique for medial osteoarthritis of the knee. The procedure is straightforward, as is the clinical follow-up. It has particular application in the younger age group for whom joint resurfacing is not a rational alternative and who have been largely neglected by the orthopaedic fraternity.

Post HTO TKR (6 months–7 years)		
	10 patients	11 TKR
	Age	59.7 yrs (58–72)
Follow-up	4.1 yrs (2–7)	
	Pre –	Post –
Flexion	89.2° (70–105)	108° (95–120)
Extension	13.7° (0–25)	1.2° (0–5)
Knee Score	63 (35–90)	90.7 (85–95)
Function Score	67.5 (55–80)	95 (90–100)
Virgin TKR		
	110 patients	150 TKR
	Age	66.2 yrs (57–84)
Follow-up	5.2 yrs (3–7)	
	Pre –	Post –
Flexion	87.2° (70–107)	110° (95–125)
Extension	15.2° (0–30)	1° (0–5)
Knee Score	66 (40–94)	91 (84–96)
Function Score	64 (50–85)	96 (88–100)

Table 38.1 Clinical and functional ratings in patients who have come to total knee replacement (TKR) at some time following upper tibial osteotomy (HTO), and in patients who have had primary total knee replacement ("Virgin TKR").

Fowler et al,[4] Oppenheim et al[8] and Kelikian et al[7] have all reported good results in the short term, and our own results have been excellent. The overall anatomical and physiological result is superior to that obtained with traditional high tibial osteotomy and the incidence of complications minimal.

While Coventry[1] has maintained that a valgus overcorrection is essential for pain relief in tibial valgus osteotomy, other authors, notably Insall et al,[5] have seen no correlation between either pain-relief or longevity of the procedure and the degree of angular over-correction.

We have deliberately not placed our patients in extreme valgus, as the knee mechanics resulting from this manoeuvre are often as unsatisfactory as those with which the patient presented. In our series, the amount of angular correction has been dictated more by symptomatic and aesthetic considerations than by X-ray appearance. It must be said, however, that the present method permits the angle of varus correction to be determined with a precision hitherto impossible with traditional closing wedge high tibial valgus osteotomy.

Shortening of the tibia due to loss of bone stock is an unavoidable consequence of the closing wedge osteotomy and this, together with the extreme realignment of forces, accounts for the frequently observed ankle pain in patients undergoing this procedure. Tibial shortening does not occur in the present technique, which in fact preserves and enhances bone stock. Ankle pain is thus avoided and complementary procedures or eventual total knee replacement are facilitated. Follow-up in the small group of patients who eventually received a total knee replacement in our series has shown that there is no difference in outcome in cases where total knee replacement was performed after hemicallotasis and those in whom it was the primary treatment. Our experience is in marked contrast to that of Windsor, Insall, and Vince[10] who concluded that the results of total knee arthroplasty after "conventional" high tibial osteotomy are similar to those for revision total knee arthroplasty.

There have been no neurovascular complications and no deep infections in our series. This contrasts with the closing wedge high tibial valgus osteotomy, where dissection around the fibular head jeopardizes the peroneal nerve.[1,5,6] Similarly, compartment syndrome does not appear to be a potential problem, as the dissection is limited and the correction gradual.

As in any innovative surgical procedure and orthopaedic management, we have made errors in patient selection, both in terms of severity of disease as an indicator, and ability of some patients to carry out the treatment protocol properly. These errors accounted for one early (one year post-corticotomy) total knee replacement and two instances of late loss of correction. These circumstances have not recurred as we have become more experienced in the procedure.

Longer term follow up is necessary, particularly in view of the young age of our patients. Even if the surgeon is not optimistic about the long-term pain relief, and predicts that the eventual outcome will be a total knee arthroplasty, this method, by which bone stock is actually enhanced, length maintained and ligamentous structures about the knee undamaged, is superior to methods previously described.

References

1. Coventry MB: 'Current concepts review. Upper tibial osteotomy for osteoarthritis.' *J Bone Joint Surg* [Am] 1985; 67A: 1136–40.
2. Elting J: 'Hemicallotatic upper tibial osteotomy.' *Orthopaedics Today* 1992; 26: 7.
3. Elting J et al: 'Proximal tibial osteotomy and unilateral frame distraction for osteoarthritis of the knee.' *Int J Orthop Trauma* 1993; Suppl (3), 89–91.
4. Fowler JL, Gie GA, MacEachern AG: 'Upper tibial valgus osteotomy using a dynamic external fixator.' *J Bone Joint Surg* [Br] 1991; 73B: 690–1.
5. Insall JN, Joseph DM, Msika C: 'High tibial osteotomy for varus gonarthrosis. A long-term follow-up study.' *J Bone Joint Surg* [Am] 1984; 66A: 1040–8.
6. Jackson JP: 'Osteotomy for osteoarthritis of the knee' in: Proceedings of the Sheffield Regional Orthopaedic Club. *J Bone Joint Surg* [Br] 1958; 40B: 826.
7. Kelikian A, Robb W et al: 'Hemicallotatic high tibial osteotomy.' Scientific Exhibit AAOS meeting 1997
8. Oppenheim WC, Jaffe L, Rosa R: 'High tibial osteotomy utilizing hemicallotasis.' AAOS Proceedings Final Program: 142, 1992
9. Turi G, Cassini M, Tomasi, PS, Arrmotti P, Lavini F: 'L'osteotomia direzionale di ginocchio mediante la 'emicallotasi'.' *Chir Organi Mov* 1987; 72(3): 205–9.
10. Windsor RE, Insall JN, Vince KG: 'Technical considerations of total knee arthroplasty after proximal tibial osteotomy.' *J Bone Joint Surg* [Am] 1988; 70A: 547–55.

Upper Tibial Hemicallotasis Using the OF-Garches

39

S. Toksvig-Larsen

Introduction

The rationale for performing a proximal tibial osteotomy is to correct abnormal loading of the arthrotic knee caused by deviation of the mechanical axis.[3,14] Medial osteoarthrosis is the most common, but lateral arthrosis, which comprises about 5 per cent of cases,[3] requires special consideration in terms of whether the corrective osteotomy should be performed in the tibia or the femur.[6]

The closing wedge osteotomy developed by Bauer,[3] Coventry[7] and Koshino[11] is the most widely used method, with good results reported in several studies, but the dome osteotomy also has its advocates[13], and should be considered, especially, where large deformities associated with more advanced cases of osteoarthrosis are encountered. Long-term results are closely linked to the accuracy of the correction achieved,[5,19,24] which should correspond to an overccorrection to 3–8° of valgus from the mechanical axis. The recurrence of symptoms is most common in cases where the initial arthrotic changes were severe and the final result an excessive under- or overcorrection. The achieved correction reported in the literature is highly variable (Table 39.1). Major complications include a 4 per cent incidence of pseudarthrosis and peroneal palsy in up to 10 per cent of cases, which tends to recover in most cases over the first post-operative year, but loss of correction and clinical deterioration with time must also be taken into account.

Indications for Osteotomy

The indication for an osteotomy for unicompartmental osteoarthrosis of the knee is Albacks Classification grade 1–3[1] in the younger (aged less than 60–65 years), active patient. Osteotomy can also be considered in the very active older patient with the disease, where we know that the risk of failure of a prosthesis is quite high. In most cases, the arthrosis is in the medial compartment and this is treated with a proximal valgus osteotomy. Involvement of the lateral compartment alone, which is much less common, can be treated by a proximal varus tibial osteotomy or a distal valgus femoral osteotomy, depending on the deformity and the "inclination" of the knee. Once the indication for surgical treatment of the osteoarthrosis has been confirmed, the operative technique employed – conventional osteotomy or a distraction technique – is a matter of surgeon preference. There are virtually no contraindications to the technique of asymmetric callus distraction as compared to the more conventional osteotomy techniques.

Acceptable correction	n	Per cent
Veinionpaa (1981)	46/95	50
Tjornstrand (1981)	44/52	85
Matthews (1988)	30/40	75
Hernigou (1987)	20/93	22
Koshino (1989)	96/176	54
Odenbring (1991)	51/52	98

Table 39.1 Upper Tibial Osteotomy with Immediate Correction; a Summary of Published Data

Why Change from an Established and Proven Technique?

We are aware, and it has been stated by others[21], that even experienced surgeons find the closed wedge or the dome osteotomy difficult to perform and often choose instead to use a uni- or a bi/tri-compartmental knee prosthesis in these patients. These surgeons consider the results unpredictable and this fact, coupled with the relatively high risk of complications, has tended to deter them from using these osteotomy techniques. Patients have a long period of sick leave and rehabilitation, often lasting for 6 to 12 months. The ability to re-operate on a failed osteotomy by performing a second proximal tibial osteotomy is very limited, and conversion to a knee prosthesis is the more appropriate procedure. Technically, subsequent prosthetic surgery is more demanding; it is often difficult to get good access (especially laterally), and balance during the operation.

The Theoretical Advantage of Hemicallotasis

The hemicallotasis technique, which involves asymmetric distraction of callus to produce a progressive opening-wedge osteotomy, has the advantage that it is relatively simple to perform, and in theory, it should be easy to achieve optimal correction. Patients maintain a high activity level with a good range of knee movement during the treatment and can probably recognize when correction is adequate. The method can be repeated if correction is lost for any reason, and it is probably easier to perform a knee prosthesis at a later date, should this become necessary.

A drawback of the technique is the possibility of pin track infection, at a site close to the knee. The risk of septic arthritis should be considered, since it could jeopardize the success of a knee prosthesis in the future. Even a local infection around a pin can create a focus for future infection when performing surgery on the lower extremity.

Methods

Most of our patients with osteoarthrosis of the knee are participating in a major, ongoing research programme involving different protocols, scoring systems and radiological techniques during the follow-up period. Since our experience suggests that patients with grade 1–3 osteoarthrosis (Ahlback Classification) form a homogeneous group, these were the patients used in our evaluation of the hemicallotasis technique. We chose to use the Orthofix OF-Garches fixator (Orthofix srl, Verona, Italy) for the procedure, primarily because we believed that an anteriorly placed device would be more comfortable for the patient than a medially placed one, despite the fact that X-ray control during follow-up was likely to be more difficult.

The line of the knee joint must be located carefully, both in the frontal and the sagittal planes, and the template should be attached using K-wires, such that the upper limit of the T-clamp will be about 1cm below, and parallel to the articular surface of the tibia. It is particularly important to avoid malrotation of the T-clamp.

We find this the most difficult part of the operation and it should not be rushed. It is important to use the template, the screw guides and the drill guides on every occasion. To minimize the risk of pin track infection, we routinely use only 2 screws proximally, and 2 screws distally in the tibial shaft.

The bone screws are inserted under fluoroscopic control, starting with the proximal (epiphyseal) screws. These are inserted in a convergent mode, with an angle of convergence of 30°. It is important that these screws are not sited at the outermost margins of the T-clamp template, as this may make it difficult to apply the distractor later. K-wires drills and pins (screws) should not be permitted to penetrate more than a short distance beyond the second cortex, and when positioned, the bone screws should penetrate it by only a few threads. This will avoid the risk of damage to the popliteal vessels which do not always move away from the posterior aspect of the tibia when the knee is flexed[26].

After an initial trial period we decided to use cortical screws in the epiphysis as opposed to cancellous ones, but we pre-drill using the 3.2mm drill rather than the 4.8mm drill and find that this enables the screws to get a good hold in the bone. Technically, it can be a little more difficult to insert the lateral screw, which may show a tendency to slip during insertion, but this has not proven to be a major problem. We insert two cortical pins in the tibial diaphysis after predrilling with the 4.8mm drill in the normal way.

A 5cm longitudinal skin incision for the osteotomy is made over the anterior aspect of the proximal tibia. This is done to reduce the likelihood of wound problems should it later become necessary to convert the osteotomy to an arthroplasty. The osteotomy/

corticotomy is performed with a slightly oblique inclination at the medio-distal end of the tibial tuberosity, such that it engages the most distal part of the insertion of the patellar ligament. Following sharp incision of the periosteum, the latter is gently separated from the bone over a length of 3–5mm in the region where the osteotomy is planned. This is done in order to preserve as much of the periosteum as possible.

Initially, the osteotomy was performed using special chisels following predrilling around the cortex. In one instance, however, an unplanned fracture developed in the posterior cortex and extended proximally, narrowly avoiding the exit hole of the lateral screw. Distraction was possible in this case, but following it, the technique was modified. Current practice involves the use of a reciprocal saw, sawing from the inside out, and trying to preserve as much of the bone marrow as possible. A retractor is always used to protect the soft tissues posteriorly. The osteotomy is monitored fluoroscopically, and extends from the medial aspect of the tibia to involve approximately three-quarters of the circumference of the bone. In this way, the lateral cortex acts as a hinge. It has not proved necessary as yet, to perform a fibular osteotomy, even in association with large corrections.

At this point we confirm that there is slight elasticity so that the osteotomy can be opened some 3–4mm. The periosteum is then sutured back and the wound closed without drainage. The patient is then draped and the OF-Garches mounted (Fig. 39.1). Finally, a test is made to ensure that the device can distract slightly. The distractor is then locked with no tension applied to the bone. The patient is allowed to weightbear immediately (Fig. 39.2) and asked to return to the outpatient clinic 7–10 days later to start distraction. At this visit the clamp axis locking nut (the proximal locking nut) and the lengthener body locking nut (the distal locking nut) are both loosened. Distraction is then performed, ideally at a rate of a quarter turn of the compression–distraction unit screw 4 times per day (1mm), but the patient can reduce the rate if pain is experienced on distraction.

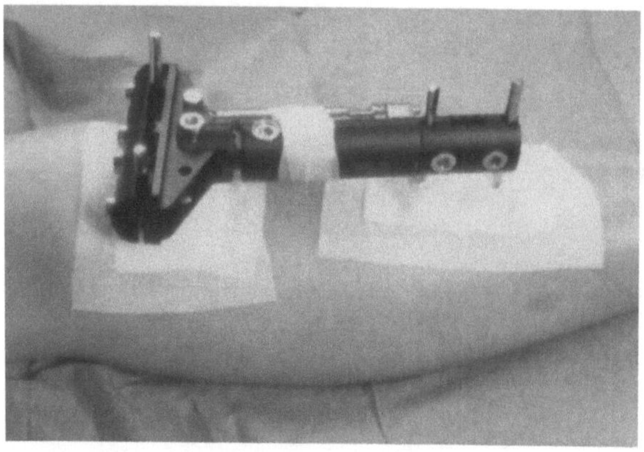

Fig. 39.1 The Orthofix OF-Garches device positioned ventrally at operation. Note attachement of the proximal pole of the compression–distration unit to the wing of the clamp.

Patients receive prophylactic antibiotics during the first week and are instructed to take additional antibiotics if even the slightest symptoms of pin track infection are experienced. Initially, pin care is performed daily by the nursing staff, but subsequently, by the

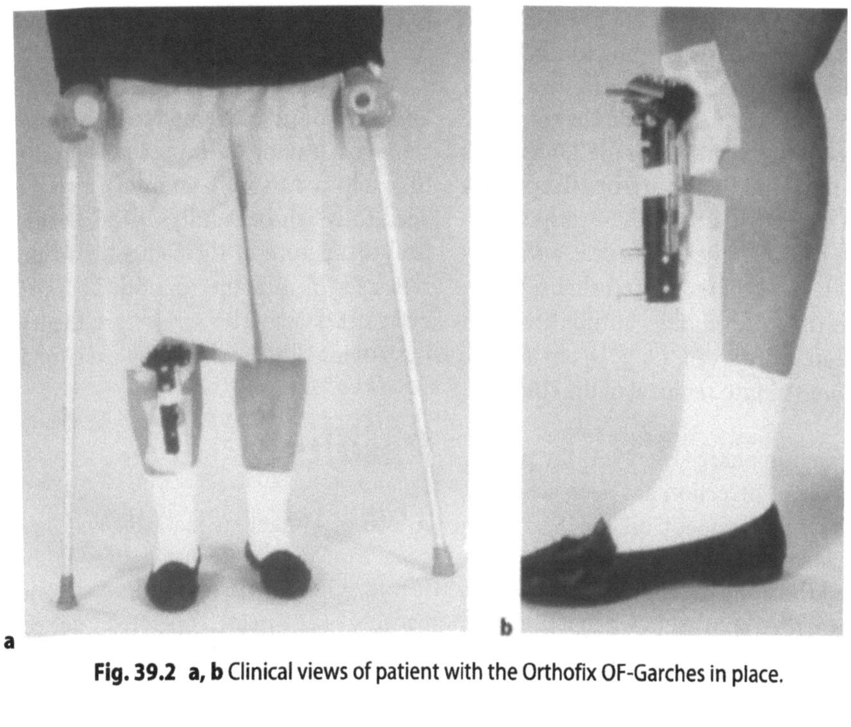

Fig. 39.2 a, b Clinical views of patient with the Orthofix OF-Garches in place.

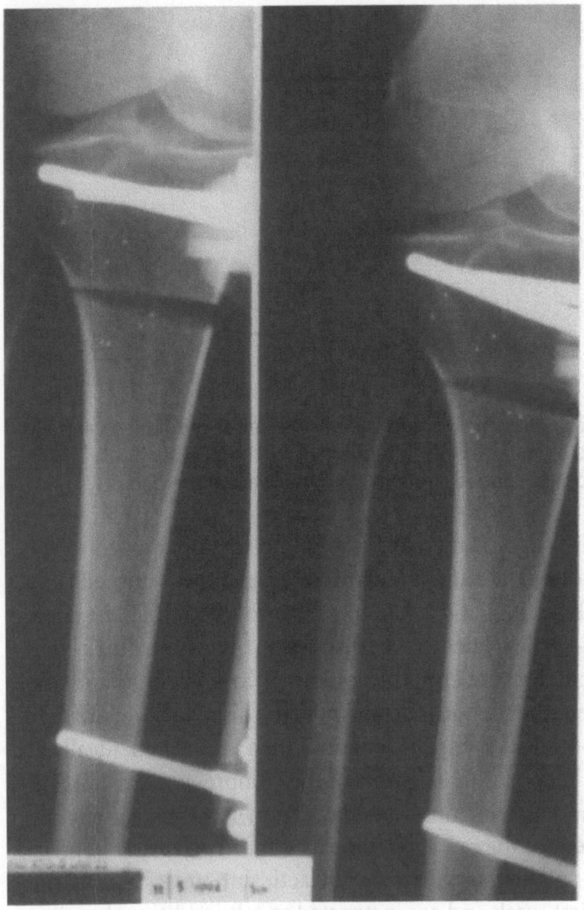

Fig. 39.3 The osteotomy.

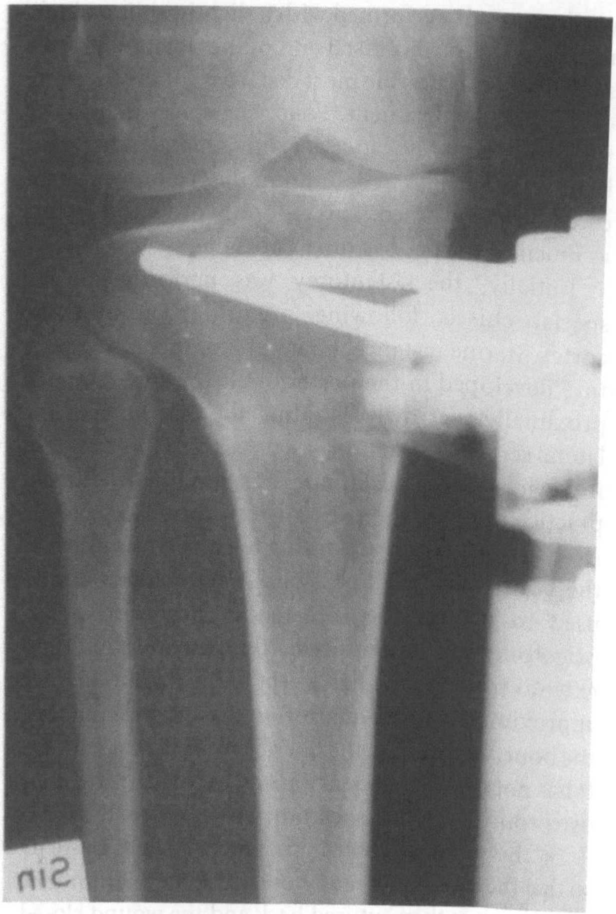

Fig. 39.4 The healed osteotomy.

patients themselves. The pins and the skin should be cleaned daily with sterile water and the skin around the pins should be massaged gently.

Pin track infection is graded according to Checketts et al[22]. Grade 1 infections are characterised by a slight redness around the pins with a little discharge; these settle with improved pin site care. In Grade 2 infections there is redness of the skin, discharge from the pin site and tenderness in the soft tissues. These respond to improved pin site care together with oral and local antibiotics. In Grades 3–6 there is increasing severity, which may require intravenous antibiotics and surgical intervention which can range from simple resiting of one or more pins to removal of the complete fixator assembly.

During the distraction phase (Fig. 39.3) the patient is seen weekly, and once correction has been achieved, as demonstrated by measurement on the X-rays, in terms of both the calculated hip–knee angle (mechanical correction) and the bony correction, the device is locked. The patient is then seen again when it is judged that healing will have occurred, usually at about 10 weeks, and further follow up is planned according to the clinical healing, the healing on X-ray (Fig. 39.4) and ultrasound investigation. To facilitate the taking of X-rays we often remove the OF-Garches during this investigation.

When the quality of the callus as judged by X-ray and ultrasound is deemed to be adequate, the fixator is removed, leaving the bone screws in situ. The patient is then allowed to walk about for two days and encouraged to weightbear fully. If this should cause pain or lead to fracture of the callus the fixator can easily be replaced for a further period. To date, this has never been necessary. The screws are then removed in the outpatient clinic without the need for any analgesia.

Results

A total of 45 patients requiring angular correction have been treated to date using the Orthofix OF-Garches fixator. Our initial results in this series comprise 30 patients (22 men) operated on for Grade 1–3 osteoarthrosis of the knee (Ahlback Classification).[1] The mean age was 52 (range 33–63) years; mean weight 68kg (range 64–113kg) and mean height 175cm (range 155–194cm). The mean pre-operative Hip–Knee–Ankle angle (HKA) was 172° (range 161–179°) (varus = <180°).

The mean correction achieved using the device was 12° (5–24°), and the mean alignment when the device was locked was 184° (4° of valgus), (range 178–187°). The mean distraction time was 14 days (range 7–35 days) with a correction of 1.33° (range 0.5–2.4°)/turn. Mean change in correction of the HKA angle during healing was 2°.

Patients remained in hospital for a mean of 1.4 days (range 1–4) days and the fixator was in situ for a mean of 89 days (range 61–146) days. Mean duration of sick leave was 99 days (range 11–257) days.

Pin track infection Grade 1 and 2 (Checketts et al Classification) [22] was recorded in about 25 per cent of pins. No severe infections (Grades 3–6) were encountered. No knee joint infections or effusions were seen.

There were three complications, all of which occurred in our pilot study. These were: one complete corticotomy, one per-operative fracture and one late, deep venous thrombosis. There were no knee joint problems or neurovascular complications in our entire series of patients treated by the hemicallotasis technique.

The security of pin fixation was assessed by measurement of insertion and removal torque. In a pilot series, pins with a hydroxyapatite coating were tested (n = 5 patients; 20 pins), and in all cases pin fixation was enhanced (Table 39.2).

Discussion

We chose to use a ventrally applied device despite the fact that some mechanical and practical considerations tended to favour use of a medially applied fixator. We felt that patient comfort, which is quite difficult to measure, would be better, and our experience to date has confirmed this. We are, nonetheless, aware that similar results can be achieved with a medially-placed device.

We produced a slight overcorrection with the Orthofix OF-Garches device, which is recommended by several authors.[3,7,11,17] It was interesting to note that many patients were themselves able to state when they felt that the correction was optimal. The change in correction during healing was comparable to that seen with the closing wedge technique.[9,20,23] The accuracy and reproducibility of measurement of the HKA angle is 2°,[18] and the high degree of correlation noted between the magnitude of the correction as calculated from the HKA radiographs and that derived using the high precision RSA technique (Roentgen Stereophotogrammetric Analysis) indicates that measurements from HKA radiographs are reliable and accurate in assessing the amount of surgical correction achieved.[25] However, the degree of correction may be difficult to assess by means of the mechanical (HKA) axis alone, as some patients cannot

Standard Pins				
	Insertion torque (Ncm)		Extraction torque (Ncm)	
	mean	range	mean	range
PM	213	90–350	10	0–50
PL	158	50–250	8	0–50
DP	430	400–>440	254	25–>440
DD	428	380–>440	185	15–>440
Hydroxyapatite-Coated Pins				
	Insertion torque (Ncm)		Extraction torque (Ncm)	
	mean	range	mean	range
PM	189	140–230	538	250–780
PL	177	90–325	477	300–700
DP	430	420–>440	553	250–750
DD	430	400–>440	450	300–800

Key: PM = Proximal medial pin; PL = Proximal lateral pin; DP = Diaphyseal proximal pin; DD = Diaphyseal distal pin

Table 39.2 Security of pin fixation (Standard vs Hydroxyapatite-Coated)

weightbear fully in the early stages. For this reason we used both the HKA angle and the osseous correction measured as the angle between the tibial condyles and the longitudinal axis of the tibia to assess the extent of correction.

The monitoring of callus quality and the progress of healing using a combination of radiography and ultrasound was valuable. In the future, digital radiographs, ultrasound, Dexa (Dual Energy X-ray Absorptiometry), MRI or CT, single or dual photon absorptiometry and mechanical measurements with devices such as the Orthometer may all contribute to our ability to assess the rate of callus production and maturation.

The preliminary results from a randomized study currently in progress, comparing the closing wedge and hemicallotasis techniques, have shown that sick leave time is significantly reduced from 5 months to 3 months in patients treated by hemicallotasis. These values for the hemicallotasis technique and the closing wedge technique were both less than those quoted in earlier reports on the dome osteotomy technique.[2] Hospital stay with hemicallotasis was also reduced in comparison to the closing wedge technique, from 5 days to 1.4 days. We believe that in the future it will be possible to perform most hemicallotasis operations as an outpatient procedure. Clinical scores, the HSS, the Lysholm and the Tegner scores and the NHP (Nottingham Health Profile) as might be expected, have not so far shown any differences between the groups.

Pin track infection is always worrying, but the figure of 25 per cent of pins in our patients probably represents a slight overestimation, since it is debatable whether a Grade 1 infection should be defined as such. It is not unusual for a mild serous discharge to occur, especially in association with the proximal pins. This should not be regarded as an infection and responds to improved hygiene. Our results are in fact comparable with, or better than those reported by others.[10, 12, 22]

The better pin purchase and improved fixation strength for screws with a ceramic coating, looks promising and is in accord with other pin studies.[4,15] We found a tendency, (which did not attain statistical significance), for the HA pins to be associated with less pin track infection and less pain during treatment (as judged using a visual analogue scale). More pin studies and improved drilling techniques[8,16] will undoubtedly enhance the appeal of hemicallotasis.

In comparison with the more usual closing wedge osteotomy, patients treated by hemicallotasis seemed to experience rather more pain. We have not performed a fibular osteotomy in any instance, although some would advocate doing this, particularly where corrections in excess of 15° are contemplated. The largest angular correction in our patient group to date, has been 24°.

The three complications we encountered were all at the beginning of our pilot study. In one patient, a complete corticotomy with lateral translation half the bone width occurred following a fall during the first week (Fig. 39.5). We did not reoperate, but the patient had the frame on for a very long period (146 days) and had the longest sick leave of any patient (257 days). In addition to this, correction was lost over the first year. He was, however, pain free. In one patient a per-operative fracture of the posterior cortex occurred while the corticotomy was being performed with a chisel. The fracture was close to a proximal pin, but had no influence on outcome. We decided, however, following this, to change our technique and to perform the corticotomy with a saw, since we felt that such a fracture had the potential to jeopardize pin fixation and with it the technique itself. Since changing, no complications or disadvantages, such as delayed healing, have been observed. The third complication we encountered was a deep venous thrombosis 6 weeks post-operatively in a very active man, who experienced this on a return flight from abroad where he had been participating in a

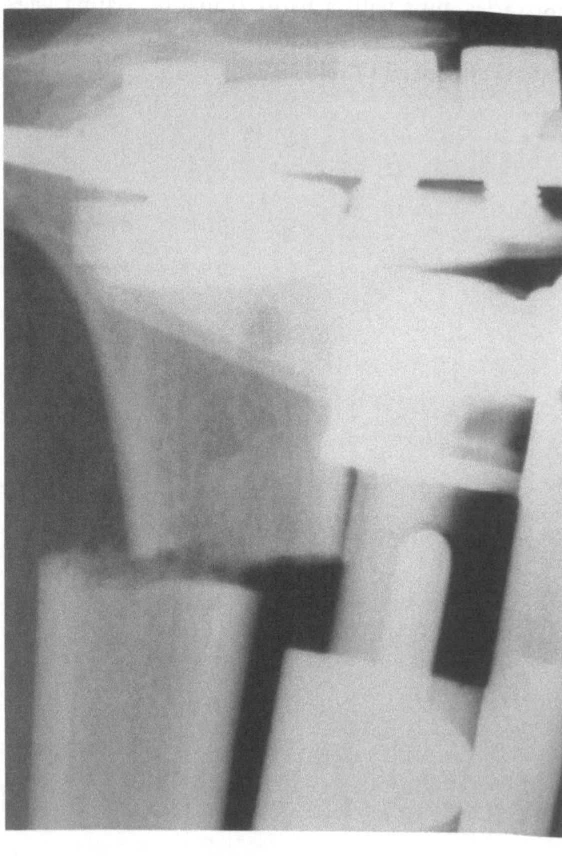

Fig. 39.5 Complication with lateral translation.

showjumping competition.

We feel that the Orthofix OF-Garches is well tolerated, even by older patients and that the progressive opening-wedge osteotomy using the hemicallotasis technique is a valid alternative to conventional forms of osteotomy. It does, however, place certain demands on the surgeon. Frequent outpatient appointments are required and it is mandatory for the patient to have ready access to the team. The economic advantages of the technique are substantial, however, with a dramatic reduction in both hospitalization time and the overall duration of sick leave.

Conclusion

Longer term follow-up is essential for full evaluation of the hemicallotasis technique in the treatment of unicompartmental osteoarthrosis of the knee. The more conventional closing wedge osteotomy remains the reference operation, and can still be regarded as a safe technique when performed carefully.[17] Eventual loss of correction with time must be carefully assessed on long-term review. Even if we believe that all osteotomies will eventually fail and require total knee replacement, the technique of hemicallotasis, which enhances bone stock, maintains bone length and preserves the ligaments around the knee joint, will probably prove superior to earlier techniques. Pin track infection is still, however, a problem which could jeopardize a future knee arthroplasty. Further improvements in surgical technique, instrumentation and especially, pin fixation, are predicted.

Acknowledgements

I would like to thank my co-workers, Goran Magyar M.D. and Associate Professor Anders Lindstrand for their enthusiasm and their contribution to these studies.

References

1. Ahlback S. 'Osteoarthritis of the knee. A radiographic investigation.' *Acta Radiol* 1968; (Suppl. 277.): 1–72.
2. Alnehill H, Dolk T. 'Complications after proximal tibial dome osteotomy.' 51:SOF (Swedish Orthopedic Society) meeting : 1995; 53.
3. Bauer GCH, Insall JN, Koshino T. 'Tibial osteotomy in gonarthrosis (osteo-arthritis of the knee).' *J Bone Joint Surg* 1969; 51: 1545–63.
4. Caja V, Ruiz J, Aliaga F. 'Clinical trial of hydroxyapatite-coated external fixation pins for external fixation.' *J Bone Joint Surg* 1995; 77-B (supplement II): 227.
5. Coventry MB, Ilstrup D, SL. W. 'Proximal tibial osteotomy. A critical long-term study of eighty-seven cases.' *J Bone Joint Surg* [Am] 1993; 75-A: 196–201.
6. Coventry MB. 'Osteotomy about the knee for degenerative and rheumatoid arthritis.' *J Bone Joint Surg* [Am] 1973; 55-A : 23–48.
7. Coventry MB. 'Upper tibial osteotomy for gonarthrosis; the evolution of the operation in the last 18 years and long-term results. *Orthop Clin N Am* 1979; 10: 191–210.
8. Eriksson AR, Adell R. 'Temperatures during drilling for the placement of implants using the osseointegration technique.' *Journal of Oral Maxillofac Surgery* 1986; 44 (1): 4–7.
9. Hagstedt B, Norman O, Ohlsson H, Tjórnstrand B. 'Technical accuracy in high tibial osteotomy for gonarthrosis.' *Acta Orthop Scand* 1980; 51 : 963–70.
10. Haugegaard M, Albrecht-Olesen P, Torholm C. 'Occurrence of infection when using Orthofix.' *Acta Orthop Scand* 1993; 64 (Suppl 253): 41.
11. Koshino T, Morii T, Wada J, Saito H, Ozawa N, Noyori K. 'High tibial osteotomy with fixation by a blade plate for medial compartment osteoarthritis of the knee.' *Orthop Clin N Am* 1989; 20 (2): 227–43.
12. Mahan J, Seligson D, Henry S, Hynes P, Dobbins J. 'Factors in pin tract infections.' *Orthopaedics* 1991; 14 (3): 305–8.
13. Maquet P. 'The treatment of choice in osteoarthritis of the knee.' *Clin Orthop* 1985; 192: 108–12.
14. Maquet P, Simonet J, de Marchin P. 'Biomechanique du genou et gonarthrose.' *Rev Chir Orthop* 1967; 53 : 111-38
15. Moroni A, Caja VL, Maltarello C, Nicoli Aldini N, Stea S, Visentin M. 'Enhancement of the bone external fixation pin interface: a biomechanical and morphological in vivo experimental study.' *Bioceramics* 1994; 7: 229–34.
16. Moyes S, Debastini M, Williams L. 'Thermally efficient bone drilling.' *J Bone Joint Surg* [Br] 1995; 77-B (Suppl II): 227.
17. Odenbring S. 'Osteotomy for medial gonarthrosis.' Thesis, 1991; Lund University, Sweden
18. Odenbring S, Berggren A-M, Peil L. 'Roentgenographic assessment of the Hip–Knee–Ankle axis in medial gonarthrosis: A study of reproducibility.' *Clin Orthop* 1993; 289 : 195–6.
19. Odenbring S, Egund N, Knutsson K, Lindstrand A, Toksvig-Larsen S. 'Revision after osteotomy for gonarthrosis: A 10–19 year follow-up of 314 cases.' *Acta Orthop Scand* 1990; 61 (2): 128–30.
20. Odenbring S, Egund N, Lindstrand A, Tjórnstrand B. 'A guide instrument for high tibial osteotomy.' *Acta Orthop Scand* 1989; 60 (4): 449–51.
21. Port J, DiGioia A, Kwoh C, Harner C. 'A technique for valgus high tibial osteotomy.' *Am J Knee Surg* 1993; 6 (4): 135-44
22. Checketts RG, Otterburn M, MacEachern G. 'Pin track infection: definition, incidence and prevention.' Suppl to *Int J Orthop Trauma* 1993; 3 (3): 16–8.
23. Tjórnstrand B, Egund N, Hagstedt B, Lindstrand A. 'Tibial osteotomy in medial gonarthrosis. The importance of overcorrection of varus deformity.' *Arch Orthop Trauma Surg* 1981; 99: 83–9.
24. Valenti JR, Calvo R, Lopez R, Canadell J. 'Long term evaluation of high tibial valgus osteotomy.' *Int Orthop* 1990; 14: 347–9.
25. Weidenhielm L, Wykman A, Lundberg A, Brostrom L. 'Knee motion after tibial osteotomy for arthrosis. Kinematic analysis of 7 patients.' *Acta Orthop Scand* 1993; 64 (3): 317–9.
26. Zaidi SHA, Cobb AG, Bentley B. 'Danger to the popliteal artery in high tibial osteotomy.' *J Bone Joint Surg* [Br] 1995; 77-B (3): 384–6.

Progressive Correction in Bone and Soft Tissue Deformity Using Monolateral Fixation or the Sheffield Hybrid System

40

M. Saleh and M. Hashmi

Introduction

Progressive deformity correction is indicated where acute correction might lead to nerve or vessel injury or to compartment syndrome. In the thigh, acute corrections are well tolerated, but in the lower leg such corrections are associated with an increased risk. This is due in part to the fact that the muscle compartments are tighter, predisposing to compartment syndrome, and in part to the sensitivity of the peroneal nerve to acute stretching. Progressive deformity correction relies on the use of hinges around which the bone rotates. Specially adapted monolateral fixators such as the ProCallus fixator in conjunction with the self-aligning articulated body, or the Limb Reconstruction System in conjunction with the OF-Garches, have a hinge whose position is fixed in relation to the adjacent screws. Such devices may be used for progressive deformity correction provided that the osteotomy is sited at the same level and is in the same plane as the hinge. Unwanted translational effects may occur if the osteotomy is either too high or too low (see Ch. 36).

Proximal or Distal Tibial Varus Deformity

Progressive correction of a proximal or distal tibial varus deformity can be carried out using the self-aligning articulated body attachment with the ProCallus fixator. Fig. 40.1 shows the fixator assembly applied to the medial aspect of the tibia. The proximal screws, shown here in a Torbay-Garches clamp, are inserted parallel to the tibial plateau, reflecting the deformity, and the hinge in the self-aligning articulated body positioned at the end of the slot closest to the bone. A metaphyseal partial osteotomy is performed with the fixator in situ. Once callus has started to form, the osteotomy is opened unilaterally at a rate of 1mm per day (0.25mm four times a day), thus correcting the deformity by hemicallotasis. As distraction proceeds, the hinge in the self-aligning body moves towards the end of the slot furthest from the bone, thus correcting any translational effect.

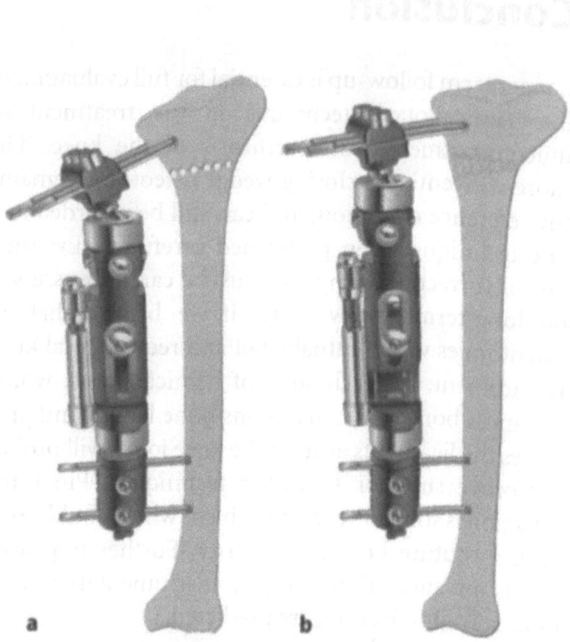

Fig. 40.1 Upper tibial hemicallotasis using the ProCallus fixator in conjunction with the self-aligning articulated body and Torbay-Garches clamp proximally. **a** Fixator in situ; osteotomy performed. **b** Gradual correction by hemicallotasis.

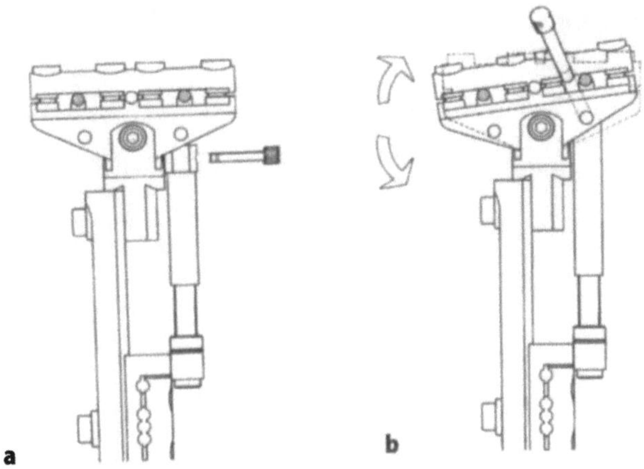

a b

Fig. 40.2 The OF-Garches clamp. Position of the removable locking pin: a For lengthening. b For angular correction.

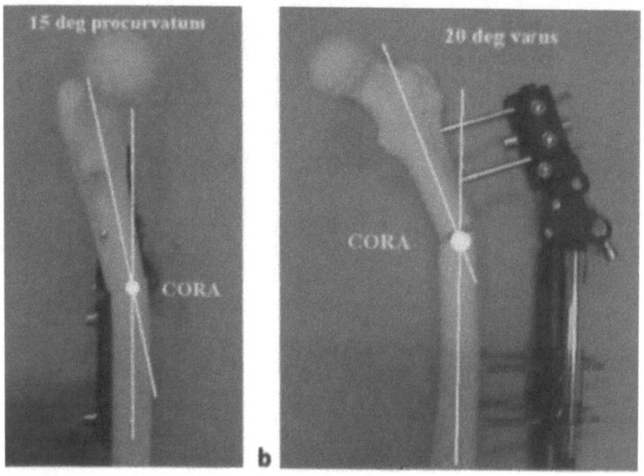

a b

Fig. 40.3 Identification of the CORA, the centre of rotation of angulation.

Upper Tibial Valgus or Varus Deformity

Progressive correction of an upper tibial valgus or varus deformity can be carried out using the OF-Garches clamp in association with the Limb Reconstruction System. Where there is angular deviation together with a discrepancy of more than 2cm, the following technique may be used. Following osteotomy, and after a waiting period of 10 days to allow initial callus formation, the compression–distraction unit is placed in the concavity of the deviation with the removable locking pin connected in the "lengthening mode" (Fig. 40.2a). It is preferable in these circumstances to achieve some lengthening prior to angular correction, in order to ensure that the bone ends do not bind together at the osteotomy site. The callus is therefore distracted by 1–2cm at a rate of 1mm per day (0.25mm four times a day) with the clamp axis locking nut tightened and the straight clamp locking screw loosened. After 1–2cm of distraction, the straight clamp locking screw is tightened, the removable locking pin connected in the "angular correction mode" (Fig. 40.2b), and the clamp axis locking nut loosened. Correction is then implemented at a rate of 0.25mm four times a day by stretching the callus on one side and compressing it on the other side. After correction, further lengthening may be implemented as necessary.

Centre of Rotation of Angulation (CORA)

Mechanical axis and lateral radiographs are used to identify the apex of deformity known as the CORA (Centre Of Rotation of Angulation) (Paley and Tetsworth 1992)[1] as shown in Fig. 40.3. For a fuller description of the CORA and its importance, see Ch. 36.

The Multiplanar Clamp

Progressive correction of deformity may be carried out using the multiplanar clamp in association with the Limb Reconstruction System. The multiplanar clamp can be used when lengthening a bone with an oblique plane deformity, as illustrated in Fig. 40.4. If, for example, the femur shown requires lengthening, and has in addition a varus deformity coupled with anterior angulation, the correct plane in which to apply this clamp can be worked out by plotting the amount of deformity in each plane, in degrees, on a diagram similar to that in Fig. 40.8. When the resultant is constructed, this corresponds to the plane into which the angulator of the multiplanar clamp is turned following its application.

The tendency will be to lengthen the segment during correction of the deformity, because the fixator is on its convex side. This would create soft tissue tension too great for the distractor unit on the clamp. Lengthening at the osteotomy site between the

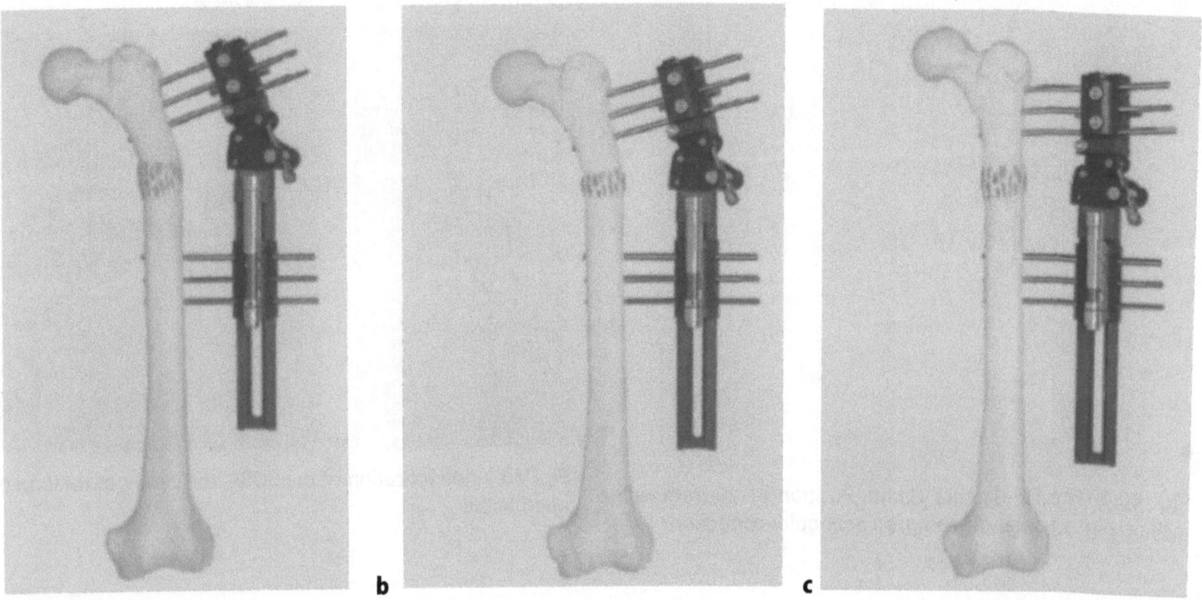

Fig. 40.4 Use of the Multiplanar Clamp to correct a varus deformity coupled with anterior angulation in a short femur. **a** Initial lengthening to stretch the soft tissues. **b** Shortening at the osteotomy site by compression of the callus using the compression-distraction unit; this reduces soft tissue tension prior to correcting angulation. **c** Correction of the deformity using the micrometric screw on the angulator; further lengthening as required.

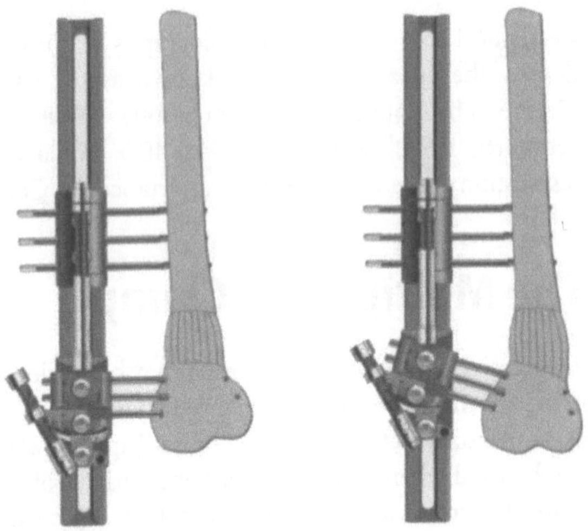

Fig. 40.5 Use of the micrometric swivelling clamp to correct a distal varus deformity in the femur. As in Fig. 40.4 after initial lengthening, the callus is shortened to reduce tension in the soft tissues prior to correction of the deformity.

multiplanar clamp and the distal clamp as illustrated is therefore carried out first (Fig. 40.4a). The callus thus produced can now be manipulated in two stages, both of which can be performed progressively in a single session. The osteotomy site is shortened as shown in Fig. 40.4b with the compression–distraction unit. Correction of the deformity is now carried out by turning the micrometric screw on the angulator. Fig. 40.4c shows that as angular correction proceeds, the callus is lengthened again. If translation occurs, this is readily corrected by turning the appropriate screw on the clamp. Lengthening can now be continued as needed by further distraction of the callus between the multiplanar and distal clamps.

If the fixator is on the concave side of the deformity, initial lengthening is again necessary, to avoid binding of the bone ends during correction. After lengthening, progressive correction can again be made in a single session by shortening the lengthened callus.

Use of the Micrometric Swivelling Clamp

The use of this clamp (see Fig. 36.10 on p. 416) in the acute correction of deformity is described in Ch. 36. Where it is possible to insert the bone screws in the plane of the deformity, e.g medial to anterior in the tibia, and lateral to anterolateral in the femur, this can be used for the progressive correction of deformity in a single session by callus manipulation, in conjunction with the protocol described for the multiplanar clamp above (Fig. 40.5).

The Sheffield Hybrid Fixation System

Progressive correction of deformity can be carried out using the Sheffield Hybrid Fixation System. Circular frames have a three-dimensional external scaffold and hinges may be placed at any level or orientation. This permits both oblique plane corrections (Fig. 40.6) and planned translational effects where the osteotomy cannot be placed at the level of the deformity (Fig. 40.7).

Unlike other hybrid designs the Sheffield Hybrid Fixator was designed as a full ring system capable of crossing joints to permit correction of bony deformity and joint contracture (Saleh et al, 1999).[2] The ability to achieve strong metaphyseal bone fixation is particularly important since large soft tissue forces are generated during such corrections.

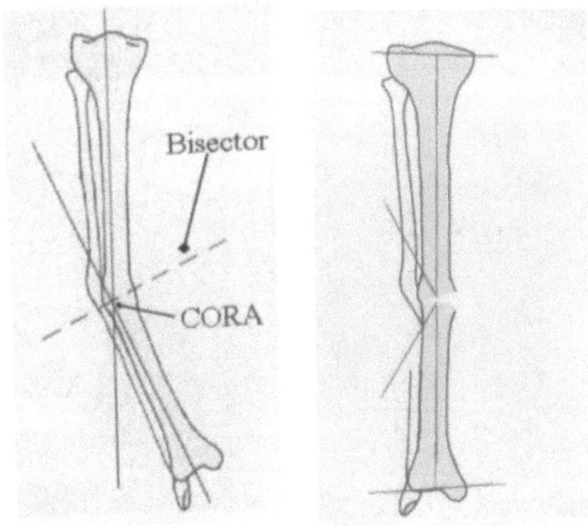

a

Fig. 40.6 Oblique plane correction. **a** Oblique plane deformity; determination of the CORA (Centre of Rotation of Angulation) by the mechanical axis method. **b** Osteotomy and corrected tibia.

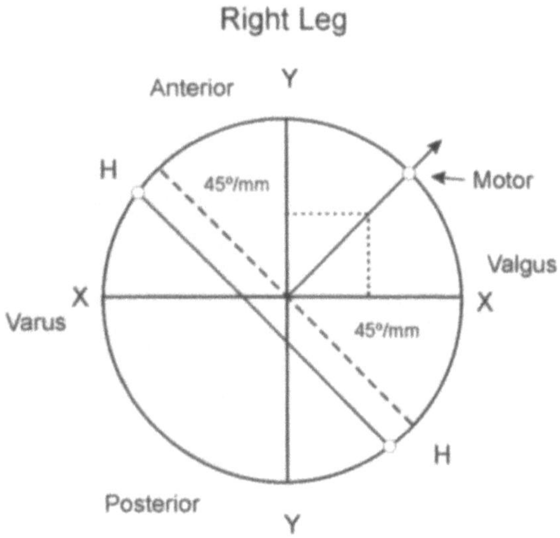

Fig. 40.8 Calculation of the magnitude of correction in the oblique plane, and hinge and motor placement. Motor: at angle where oblique plane vector crosses the circle; Hinges (H): at right angles to the base of the oblique plane vector.

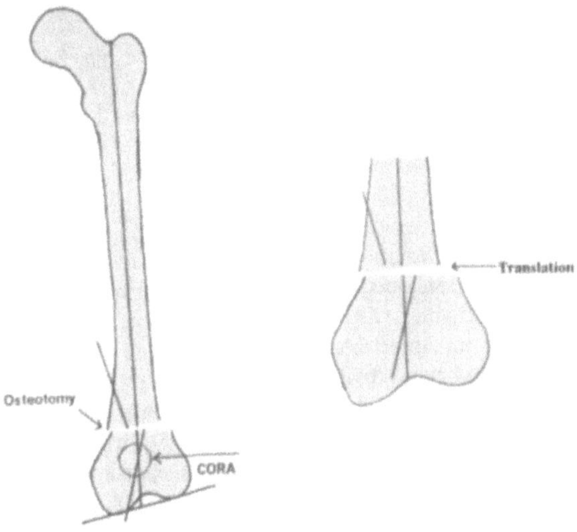

a b

Fig. 40.7 Planned translational effect where osteotomy is not placed at the level of the deformity.

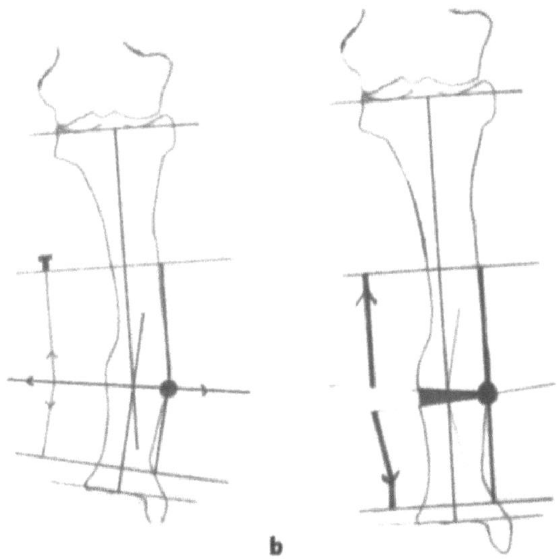

a b

Fig. 40.9 a The deformity and CORA; note hinge placement on convex side of deformity. **b** Opening wedge effect of correction by hinges on convex side.

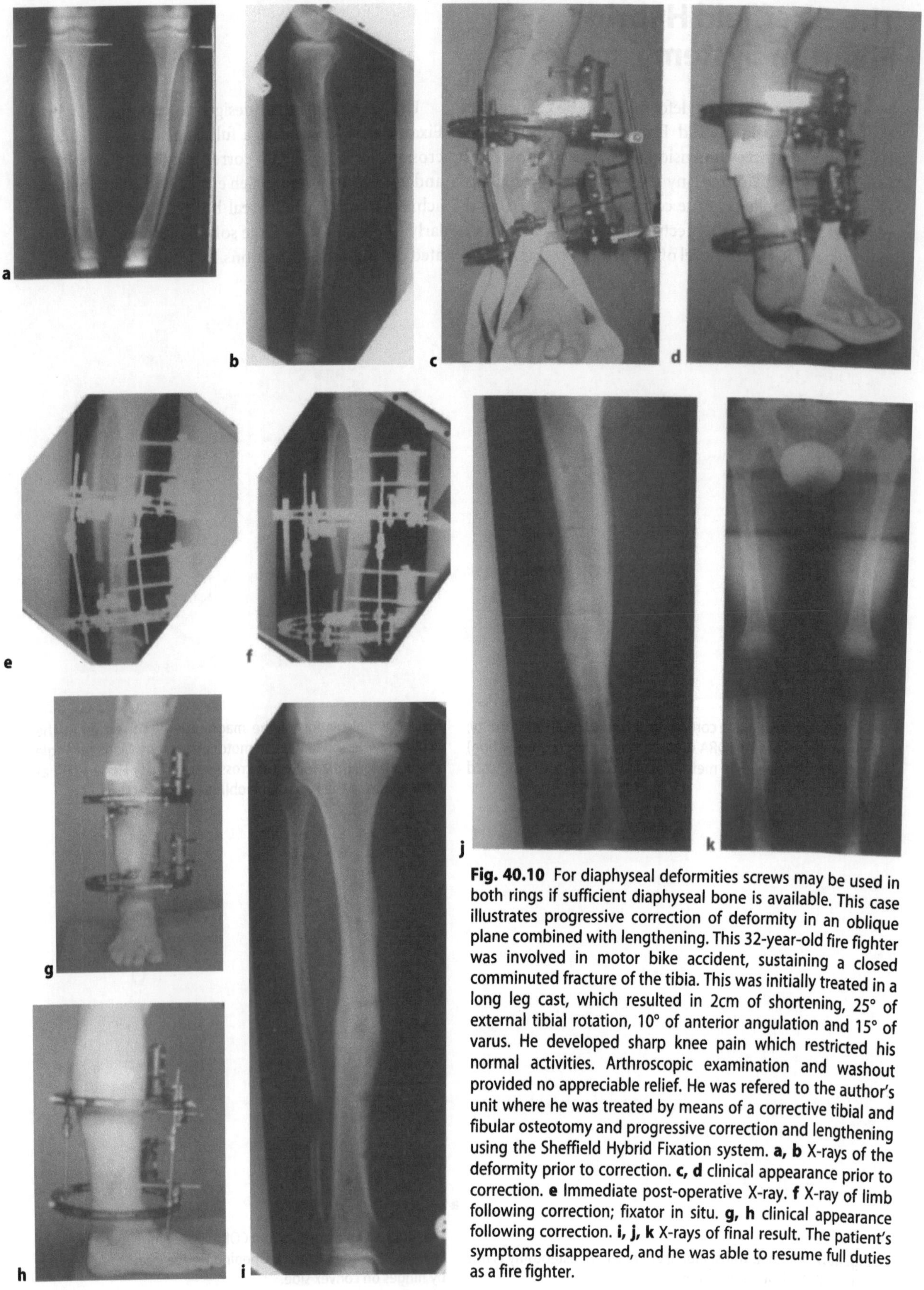

Fig. 40.10 For diaphyseal deformities screws may be used in both rings if sufficient diaphyseal bone is available. This case illustrates progressive correction of deformity in an oblique plane combined with lengthening. This 32-year-old fire fighter was involved in motor bike accident, sustaining a closed comminuted fracture of the tibia. This was initially treated in a long leg cast, which resulted in 2cm of shortening, 25° of external tibial rotation, 10° of anterior angulation and 15° of varus. He developed sharp knee pain which restricted his normal activities. Arthroscopic examination and washout provided no appreciable relief. He was refered to the author's unit where he was treated by means of a corrective tibial and fibular osteotomy and progressive correction and lengthening using the Sheffield Hybrid Fixation system. **a, b** X-rays of the deformity prior to correction. **c, d** clinical appearance prior to correction. **e** Immediate post-operative X-ray. **f** X-ray of limb following correction; fixator in situ. **g, h** clinical appearance following correction. **i, j, k** X-rays of final result. The patient's symptoms disappeared, and he was able to resume full duties as a fire fighter.

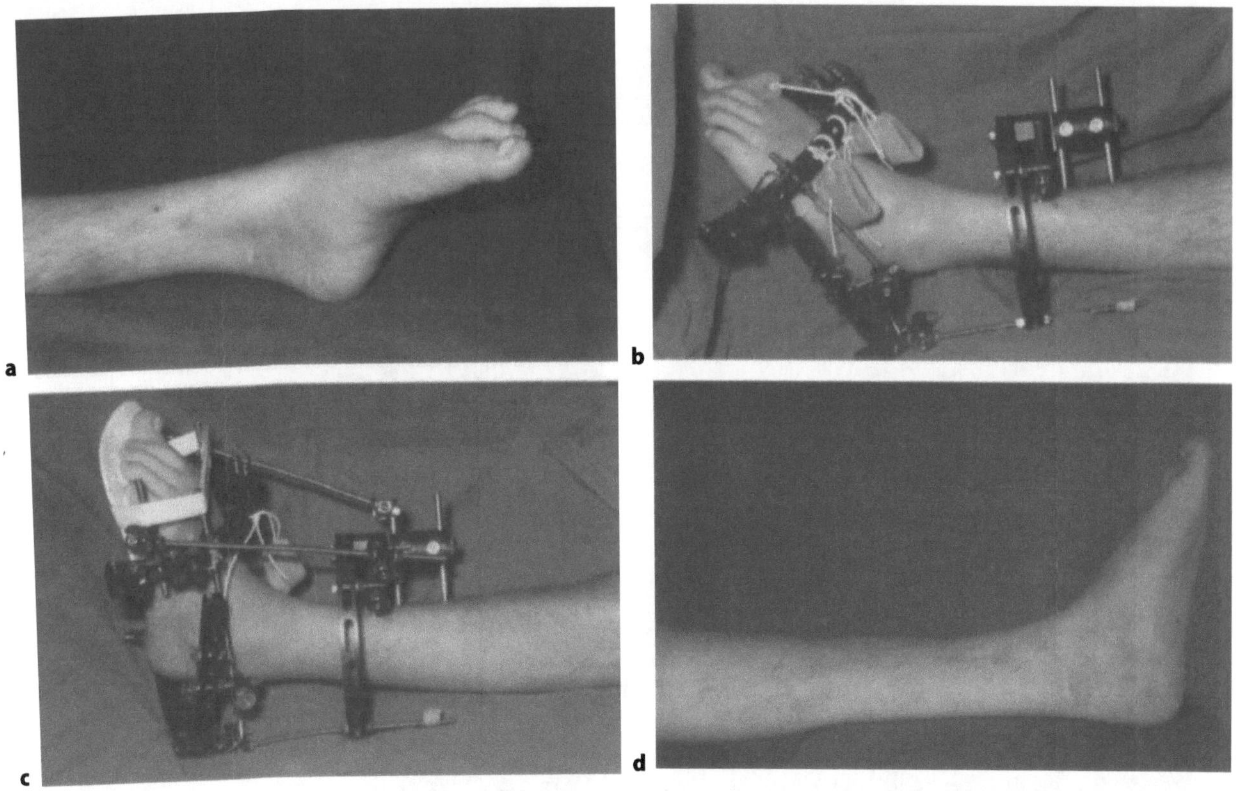

Fig. 40.11 Soft tissue correction. **a** Equinovarus deformity. **b** A pushing system between the tibia and hindfoot and hindfoot and forefoot is used to distract the joints and achieve part of the correction. **c** The motors and hinges are now changed to pull up on the foot. **d** Final correction.

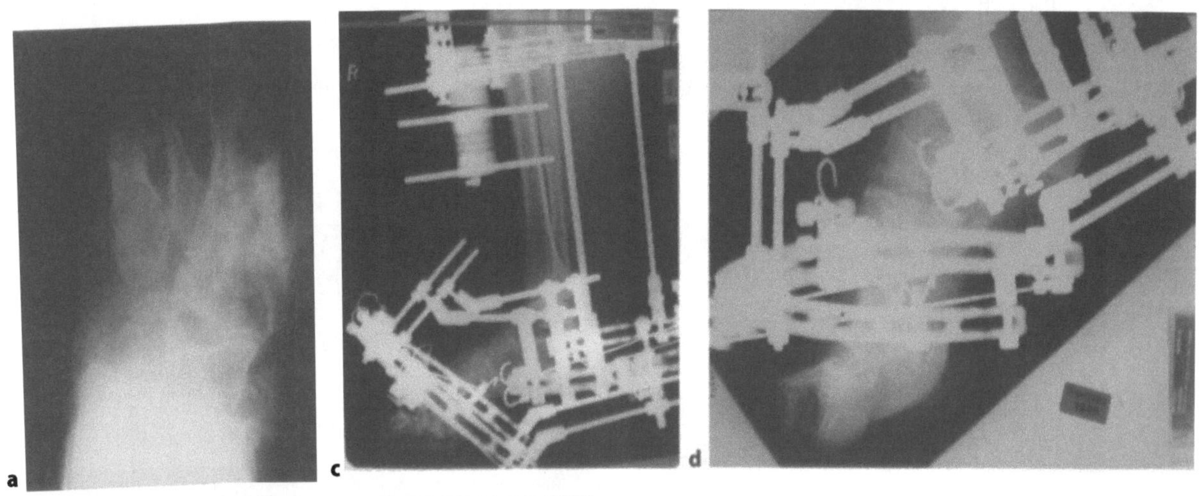

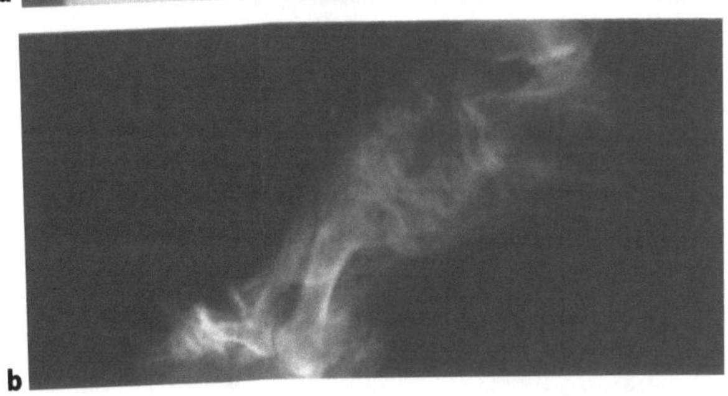

Fig. 40.12 A mid foot bony correction is used to correct this severe congenital cavus deformity. A powerful frame has been devised with 4 wires in the hindfoot and 4 in the forefoot. **a, b** AP and lateral views of initial deformity. **c** Hybrid construct with Sheffield clamp supporting a diaphyseal ring, connected to hind foot ring by threaded rods. **d** Mid foot osteotomy and strong hybrid construct. **e** Hybrid rings with 4 wire fixation for forefoot and hindfoot. **f, g** X-ray showing correction in progress through osteotomy. **h** X-ray of completed correction. **i, j** X-rays of foot after fixator removal. (**e, f, g, h, i, j** on next page.)

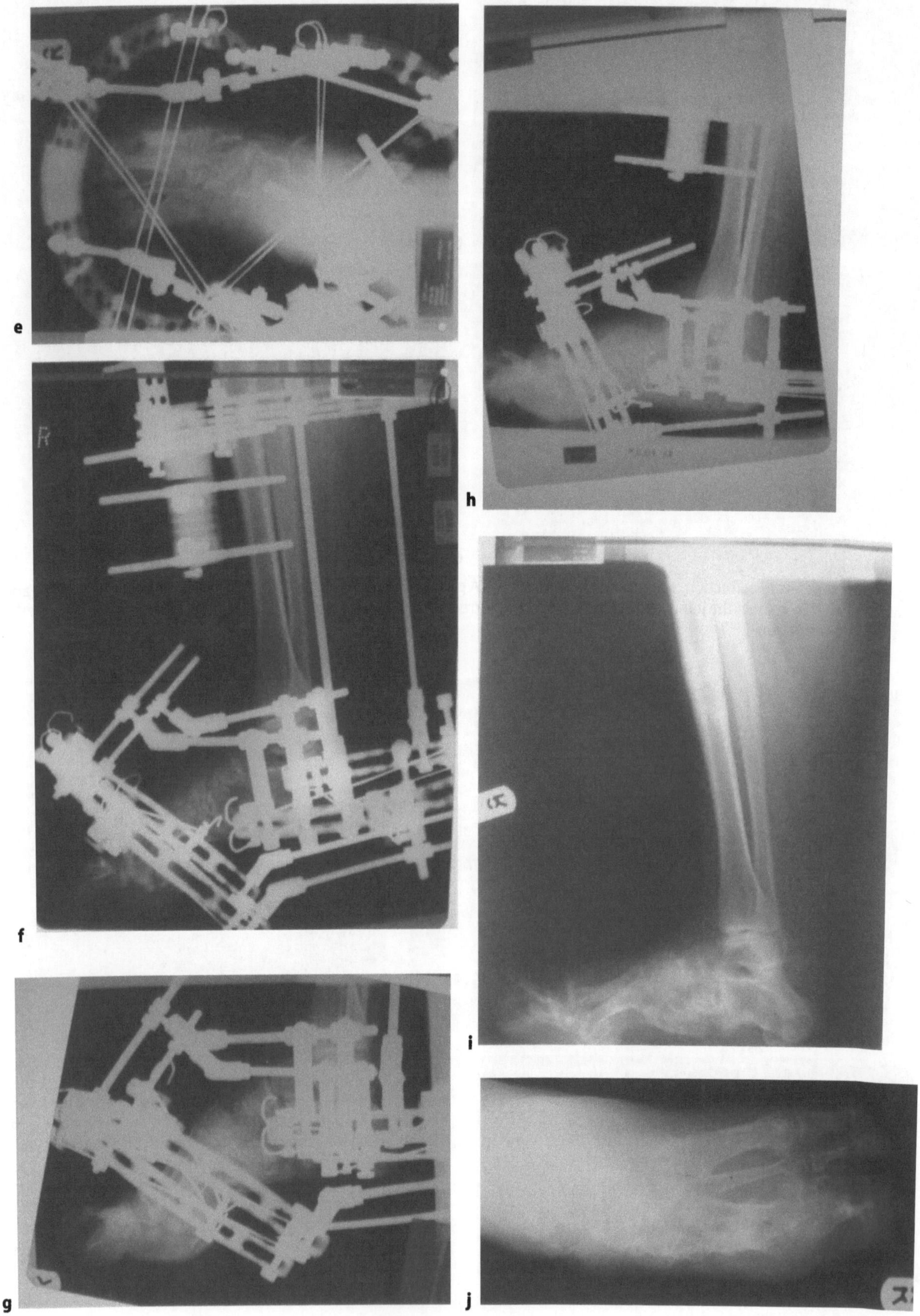

Fig. 40.12 (continued)

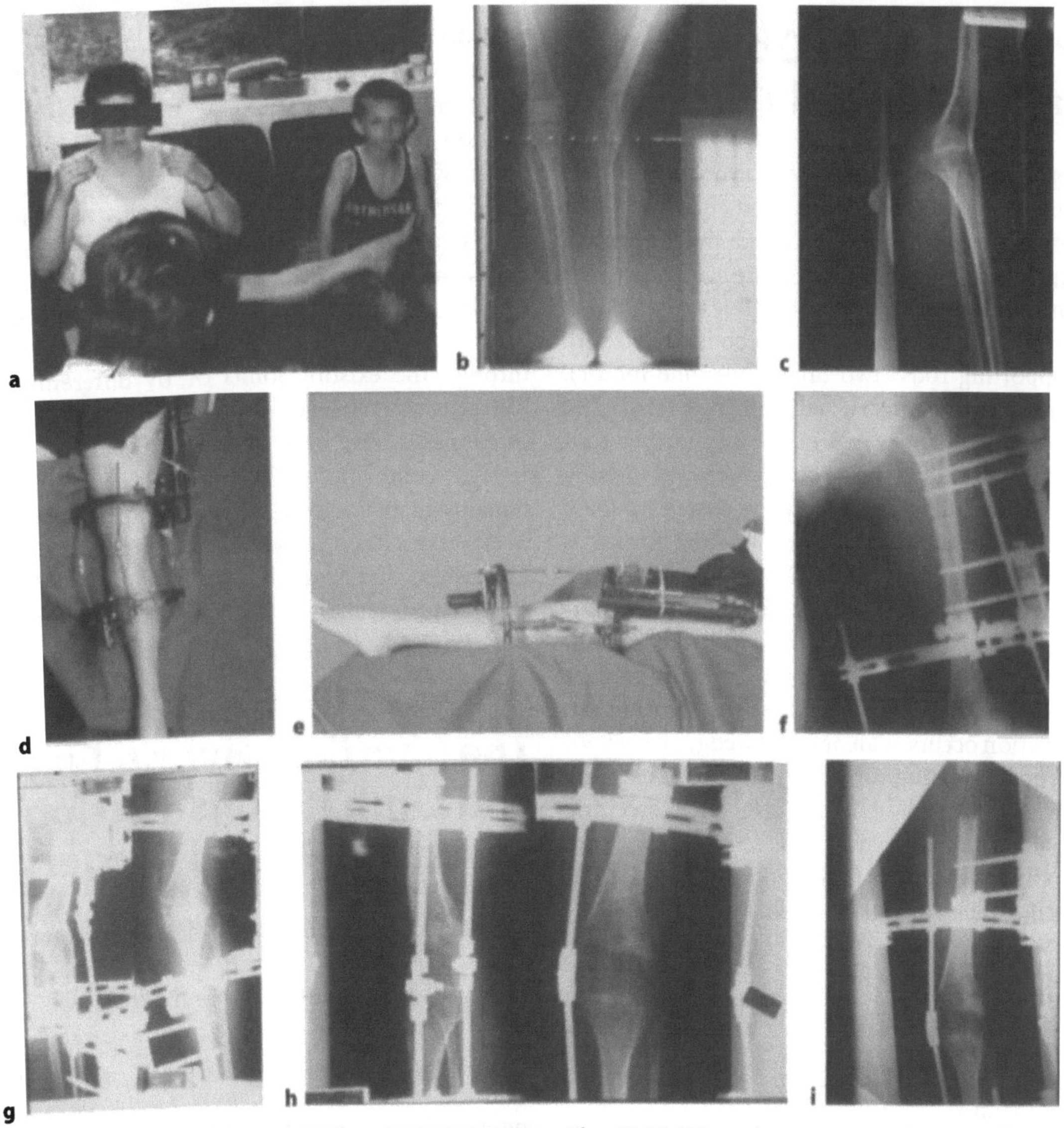

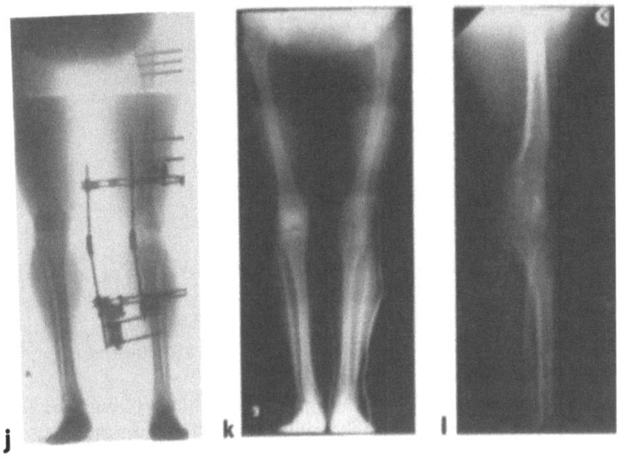

Fig. 40.13 This patient was run over at age 3, sustaining a degloving injury to the left knee, followed by distal femoral growth arrest. At age 14 she underwent patellectomy and knee arthrodesis. She presented at age 26 with a functionally limited leg with an unsightly appearance. **a** Clinical examination revealed extensive skin grafts, structural scoliosis concave to the left, 8cm of shortening, a stiff knee and mobile ankle, subtalar joint and midfoot. **b, c** Radiographs showed 78mm shortening; 44mm lateral mechanical axis deviation; 25° anterior bowing and 25° valgus at the knee. Bifocal surgery was indicated because length required was >6cm. **d, e, f, g** A Sheffield Hybrid Fixator with oblique plane hinges was attached across the knee with screw fixation only. Osteotomy was performed through the arthrodesis area for lengthening and deformity correction. Using the screws already in situ in the distal femur an LRS was applied to the femur and a mid-diaphyseal osteotomy performed for lengthening. **h, i** Callus formation increased in the metaphyseal bone of the knee as compared to that in the diaphyseal bone in the femur. **j** Alignment and length were restored 3 months post-surgery. Note that only 9 screws were used for the entire construct. **k, l** Final result.

Correction of an Oblique Plane Deformity In the Tibia

The magnitude of the correction in the oblique plane is calculated using the graphical method (Fig. 40.8). The plane of the hinges and motor are derived from the graph and the hinge level from plane radiographs by measuring the distance from the joint line to the CORA.

A two-ring Hybrid frame is then constructed with three supporting rods (two hinges and one motor). Complete rings are constructed from two-thirds and one-third components. Two of the supporting rods contain hinges and the third rod is placed off the ring with rotational supports to apply the corrective force (motor). For metaphyseal deformities the fixator is attached in the usual way with wires in the metaphysis and screws in the diaphysis. For diaphyseal deformities, screws may be used in both rings if sufficient diaphyseal bone is available. It is good practice to align the hinges with the convex surface of the deformity so that correction occurs as an opening wedge (Fig. 40.9). A case report involving correction of an oblique plane deformity is detailed in Fig. 40.10. Such eccentric distraction techniques may be used to realign and heal hypertrophic non-unions (Saleh and Royston, 1996).[3] A case is illustrated in Fig. 49.4 (Ch. 49).

Correction of a Joint Contracture

Preconstructed hybrid frames may be used to correct joint contractures of the knee and foot. Large forces are generated during such corrections and stable fixation is required with additional soft tissue releases where necessary.

For knee flexion contractures, stable mid-diaphyseal ring fixation in the femur and tibia is achieved with two screws in the Sheffield clamp and one offset screw. Hinges are placed slightly anterior to the centre of rotation of the knee to protect the joint from compressive forces. Correction is achieved with a posterior motor after 3–5mm of initial joint distraction. In severe cases a hamstring release may be required.

The most common indication for such corrections is in the foot for equinovarus and cavo-varus deformities (O'Doherty et al 1992).[4] Again the surgery may be combined with conventional soft tissue releases. The mid-diaphyseal tibial fixation must be sufficiently stable to act as a fulcrum around which the hindfoot and forefoot corrections may be achieved. Hindfoot fixation is achieved with a two-thirds ring and 2–4 2mm wires tensioned to 800N and crossing at 45°. Forefoot fixation is achieved with a two-thirds ring fixed to the foot with one wire in the medial metatarsal necks and one in the lateral metatarsal necks. Further stability and directional control may be achieved using central olive wires. Correction may be achieved through the existing joints or by differential callus distraction. Various hindfoot and midfoot osteotomies have been described (Saleh and Jackson 1994).[5] Following slight overcorrection the frame remains in place for a neutralization period of 6–8 weeks and is then removed and replaced by a plaster for 4 weeks and an ankle foot orthosis for a further 6 months to a year. Two illustrative cases are shown in Figs. 40.11 and 40.12.

The Sheffield Hybrid Fixator and Limb Reconstruction System in Bifocal Surgery

The Sheffield Hybrid Fixator may be combined with the LRS for bifocal surgery. In this case (Fig. 40.13) the SHF has been mounted across the knee with screws only, to permit an oblique plane correction and lengthening following osteotomy through an arthrodesis. Further lengthening is achieved by attaching an LRS to the femur using the same screws for distal fixation of the LRS and proximal fixation for the hybrid.

References

1. Paley D, Tetsworth K. 'Mechanical axis deviation of the lower limbs; pre-operative planning of uniapical angular deformities of the tibia or femur.' *Clin Orthop* 1992; 280: 48–64.
2. Saleh M, Yang L Simms M. 'Limb reconstruction after high energy trauma.' *Brit Med Bull* 1999; 55: 870–84.
3. Saleh M, Royston S 'Management of non-union of fractures by distraction with correction of angulation and shortening.' *J Bone Joint Surg* [Br] 1996; 78B:105–9.
4. O'Doherty D, Street R, Saleh M. 'The Use of Circular External Fixators in the Management of Complex Disorders of the Foot and Ankle.' *The Foot* 1992; 2:135–42.
5. Saleh M, Jackson A 1994, 'The Ilizarov Technique.' in *Children's Orthopaedics and Fractures.*(ed) Benson M, Fixsen J, MacNicol M. Churchill Livingstone: Edinburgh.

An Historical Perspective Prior to Callotasis

41

M. T. Dahl

Introduction: A Difficult Course of Events

Indications for limb lengthening have changed considerably over time. While devices and technologies have experienced a slow progression in history, the enthusiasm to correct these deformities has remained.

In the early history of limb lengthening, the majority of treatments were applied for post-traumatic aetiologies. This phase was followed by a phase of lengthening for post-infectious aetiologies (e.g. poliomyelitis and tuberculosis). Lengthening for congenital anisomelia, physeal infection or fracture, and fracture malunion or non-union are more common today. Even lengthening for stature, rarely considered in the past, has been performed by some surgeons in the last twenty years.

Trial and error was frequently the fundamental mode of discovery during the early years of limb lengthening surgery. Events leading to contemporary methods of bone lengthening, specifically callotasis, did not always follow an orderly progression. There are many reasons for this slow evolution, for example:

1. Much of what early surgeons discovered about bone lengthening was lost on the surgeons' assistants who were immediately exposed to their work. First assistants who did not possess the attention to detail that was necessary could become discouraged and give up on bone lengthenings for their patients.
2. Physicians working in relative isolation may not have had the scientific discipline, knowledge, or the time and resources to perfect an idea or test an hypothesis. Results of their work in leg lengthening were often not recorded in the medical literature.
3. The sharing of information between surgeons doing similar work was often limited by geography, nationality, language, costs and cultural differences.
4. Metal material improvements occurred in slow steps.
5. Communication technology slowed the transfer of knowledge during the first half of the century.

Achieving success in limb lengthening has always been difficult. Generations of orthopaedists have come to learn a similar lesson, namely, that complications are a recurring theme of limb lengthening. Pin track infections, loosening, fracture, axis deviation, malunion, non-union, and soft tissue contractures continue to plague patients and their surgeons. Despite improved materials and techniques, these complications continue.[1-6]

Alternatives to Bone Lengthening

Surgical attempts at bone growth stimulation have included: periosteal stripping,[7] drilling of the metaphysis,[8] foreign body implantation near the physes,[9] arteriovenous fistula,[10] and lumbar sympathectomy. None of these became predictable treatment for leg length discrepancy.

Contralateral shortening by physeal arrest in the growing child was popularized by Phemister.[11] Resectional osteotomy with internal fixation was developed by Kuntscher in the 1930s for use in the mature patient.[27] The decision to lengthen a bone as opposed to contralateral shortening, orthotic support, amputation or prosthetic management, has always been dependent on the diagnosis and available treatment options, as well as the patient's expectations and the surgeon's bias. The magnitude of the discrepancy necessary to consider limb lengthening has consistently been 5cm or greater. But as techniques have improved, lesser magnitudes are considered for lengthening surgery.

Technical Developments

As early as 1775, iron wires were used for internal fixation, but soft-tissue reactions around these wires and other implants caused concern. Biocompatible materials that allowed mutual tolerance between host and implant were sought for years. The concept of biocompatibility meant the host should not react to the implant and that the implant should not corrode, decay or break. The developments of antisepsis by Lister, followed later by antibiosis, allowed surgeons to use and develop biocompatible materials. Iron, cobalt chrome, stainless steel, titanium, and other alloys were tried and tested in order to improve biocompatibility while maintaining strength.[15]

With the exception of acute lengthening, and limited efforts at internally implanted lengtheners,[12] bone lengthenings have relied on an external distraction force, maintained with either a cast, traction pins, external fixator or internal fixator (plate), to support the limb. It is evident, therefore, that technical developments in limb lengthening parallel the evolution of external fixation.

The rigidity of the external frame presented challenges for limb length surgeons.[3,18] Some researchers felt that early problems with pin track infection and loosening were associated with an inappropriate degree of rigidity. To create greater stability, modifications in fixator design continued.

The Story of Ignacio de Loyola

It is unknown when the very first bone lengthening occurred. The story of Ignacio Lopez de Loyola (translated from Spanish to French and now to English) may be one of the very first. The following is an excerpt from *The Testament and Spiritual Exercises*, a description of events occurring in 1521.

> On the day of the artillery attack on May 20, 1521, Ignacio Lopez de Loyola confided his thoughts to one of his colleagues. After quite a long struggle, artillery fire hit his leg and broke it completely, and since the cannonball passed between his two legs, the other was also badly injured. Because he could not fight any more, the defenders surrendered him immediately to the French, who, having secured the citadel, dealt civilly with him and were very polite and kind. After a stay of 12 to 15 days at Pamplona, the French moved Ignacio to his family home... At Loyola, Ignacio began to feel very badly and all the doctors and surgeons who were called to examine him agreed that his leg should be reduced a second time. They thought it looked as if the bones had been improperly adjusted the first time, or that they had moved during the voyage home. Healing seemed impossible under the circumstances. Ignacio's condition was worsening. He could not feed himself and other symptoms announcing death were already appearing. The bones were fusing, but under the knee a bone superimposed itself on to another and resulted in a shortening of the leg. So obvious was the prominence of this condition. This displeased Ignacio greatly but he would not accept it. He thought that the deformity would not allow him to live his life as he wished, so he asked the surgeons if they could re-cut the bone. They told him that this could probably be done but the pain would be worse than anything he had ever endured. Also, since the fracture was already healed, the operation would be long and difficult. He decided nevertheless to suffer through the procedure. The incision was made and the bone was cut. Many various attempts were made trying to lengthen the leg. They applied ointments, they lengthened the leg non-stop using instruments - stretching it and supporting it so that Ignacio could not move at all. Ignacio endured great pain but the Lord was going to give him back his health. There was such an improvement that his general state was diagnosed as excellent with the exception that he could not steadily stand on that limb which forced Ignacio to stay in his bed.... After.... happy end.[13]

Although this story is very old and short on technical details, it underscores the difficulties encountered by surgeons who have attempted bone lengthening by any method. The story also shows how the process of limb

1905	***Codivilla combined external pins and plaster of Paris to perform limb lengthenings after an osteotomy. The traction was applied to the cast, which transferred the distraction to the patient's bone via the skin.***
1907	***Lambotte's "bone clamp" required the reduction of the focus of the fracture before setting the fixator. His apparatus marked the beginning of external fixation.***
1913	***Magnuson reported his initial clinical experience lengthening the femur. Another early report of Hopkins, in 1889 (cited by Magnuson in 1913), describes lengthening legs with acute distractional osteotomies maintained by a bone spacer.***
1921	***Putti published his experience using a technique of skeletal traction to lengthen femurs at a time when most others were restricting lengthenings to tibias. He was the first to use Kirschner wires and traction bows during distraction.***
1927	***Abbott improved the concepts of Codivilla and Putti by creating an apparatus with two pins in each of the fragments to improve stability.***
1932	***Haboush and Finkelstein designed an apparatus that rested on a flat surface, eliminating the need for traction. Subperiosteal osteotomies, latency period, as well as functional use of the limb, were recommended.***
1938	***Hoffmann designed the first external fixator with threaded pins, 3mm in diameter, which engaged both cortices. This unilateral frame was equipped with a system of overlaying bars which allowed external adjustments to reduce the fragments.***
1948	***Allan introduced "positive elongation."***
1949	***Anderson designed a transfixed system with four pins to lengthen the tibia.***
1950	***Wittmoser publishes a report on a circular fixator for treatment of fractures of the tibia.***
1953	***Ilizarov introduced a circular fixator, made up of many mechanical elements that allow different frame positions. He and coworkers focused their attentions for decades before their methods became known to the west.***
1956	***Bost and Larsen compared oblique, Z, and transverse osteotomies and concluded there was no difference in healing.***
1968	***Kawamura and coworkers combined extensive laboratory experiments with clinical experience to determine the maximum safe lengthening limit of 10-15%.***
1969	***Judet designed a new external lengthening device with a slotted rail mounted parallel to a distraction rod.***
1971	***Wagner introduced an external fixator consisting of a solid telescopic body with 6 mm pins that would allow both elongation and compression. Along with his portable fixator design, Wagner proposed a method involving an open osteotomy followed by distraction as soon as possible. A special lengthening plate and bone graft were used in a secondary operation.***
1976	***Vidal promotes the use of fixators transfixed in one or two planes for fracture applications.***
1979	***De Bastiani introduced his first rigid external fixator with dynamic capabilities.***
1980	***Ilizarov's fixator and methods are introduced to the west by surgeons in Italy.***
1984	***De Bastiani introduced a dynamic, axial, unilateral aluminum alloy fixator with a covering to improve resistance. The linear design was simple, comfortable, rigid and not transfixed.***
1986	***Canadel published his modifications to Wagner's unilateral external fixator, making it a dynamic system.***
1990s	***Hybrid (variations on circular and monolateral frames) fixators to treat large length discrepancies and more complex deformities become popular.***

Fig. 41.1 The evolution of limb lengthening: time scale.

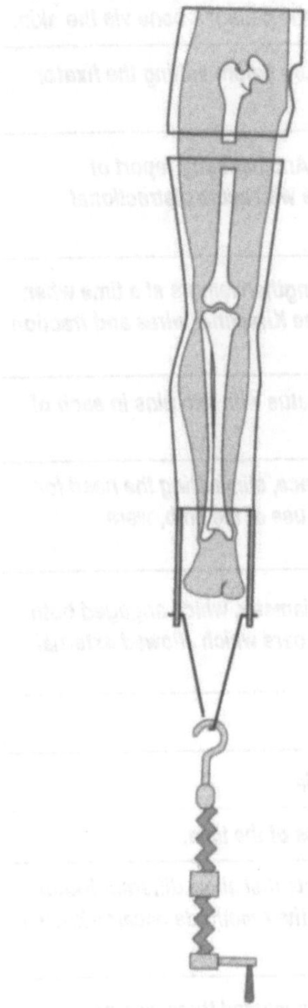

Fig. 41.2 Codivilla's technique of traction by plaster against skin was later modified to include a distal calcaneal pin.

lengthening is endured with sometimes significant morbidity and poor outcome. A condition that requires an intervention as dramatic as bone lengthening is complex and high risk. Patient expectations are significant, especially when a return to near normal function is expected. Any surgeon intent on pleasing the patient and achieving success undertakes a difficult task when surgically lengthening a bone.

Bone Lengthening From 1889 To Callotasis

The evolution of limb lengthening (Fig. 41.1) has occurred out of a desire to treat patients who could not be helped by conventional methods of orthopaedics. Even today, after years of refinement, limb lengthening is still placed in a category of last resort, used most often after less complicated methods to help the patient have been exhausted.

The concept of external fixation (using percutaneous pins to join the bone to a rigid frame) was conceived by Joseph Malgaigne in 1847, but it was not until 1907 when Albin Lambotte published his work on a system for securing the femur and other long bones to a rigid frame, that external fixators became useful.

The first known medical publication on the subject of limb lengthening was by the Italian surgeon, A. Codivilla in 1905.[1] He performed a transverse osteotomy, through which an abrupt intra-operative distraction was performed. The gap was maintained by applying traction against the skin with a plaster cast. Every few days the plaster was cut circumferentially, new traction applied, and the gap re-plastered (Fig. 41.2). This led to an incidence of skin and soft tissue necrosis, which Codivilla referred to as "inconveniences". He later modified the technique by incorporating a calcaneal pin in the plaster distally, with proximal counter-traction against the skin. Even with this early publication, Codivilla emphasized that attention should be focused on soft tissue resistance and the maintenance of articular function.

In 1913, Magnuson reported his initial clinical experience of lengthening the femur.[14] Like Codivilla, Magnuson performed acute distraction at the time of surgery, attempting to gain several inches. He did so using a long Z-shaped osteotomy fixed with ivory screws and maintained in position with a plaster cast.

In 1921, Vittorio Putti published eleven years of experience using piano wires and skeletal traction to lengthen the femur.[2] He was the first to use transverse wires and traction bows, one placed sagittally through the proximal femur and fixed to the head of the bed, and one inserted transversely through the distal femur and fixed to applied weights which controlled distraction. After completing distraction, a plaster cast was applied, incorporating the pins.

Putti emphasized the importance of overcoming resistant soft tissue forces with a gradual and continuous traction of the limb. This system of traction, consisting of a telescopic tube with a screw and spring attached to two traction pins, became known as an "osteoton". Considerable lengthening activity followed Putti's publication and presentations. One surgeon who gained insight from Putti's experience was LeRoy C. Abbott.

Abbott considered the delayed unions seen in Putti's work to be secondary to malignment of the fragments in the osteoton. He improved the osteoton by using one lengthener on each side of the limb and incorporating

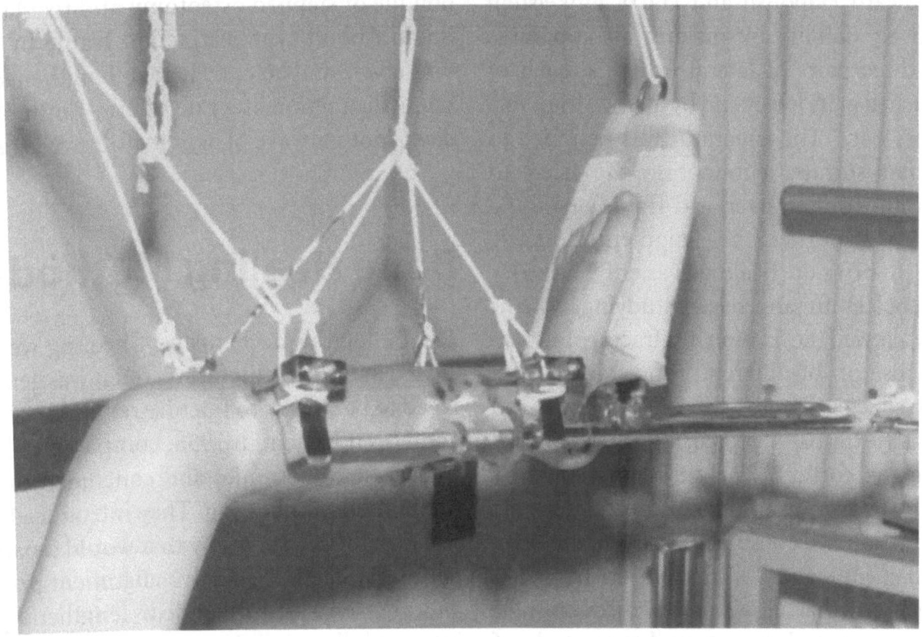

Fig. 41.3 This device, used by Dr. Wallace Cole, was known as the Princess Margaret fixator. The patient was confined to bed in traction. The similarities to Abbott's device are remarkable. Photo courtesy of Steven E. Koop, M.D., Gillette Children's Hospital.

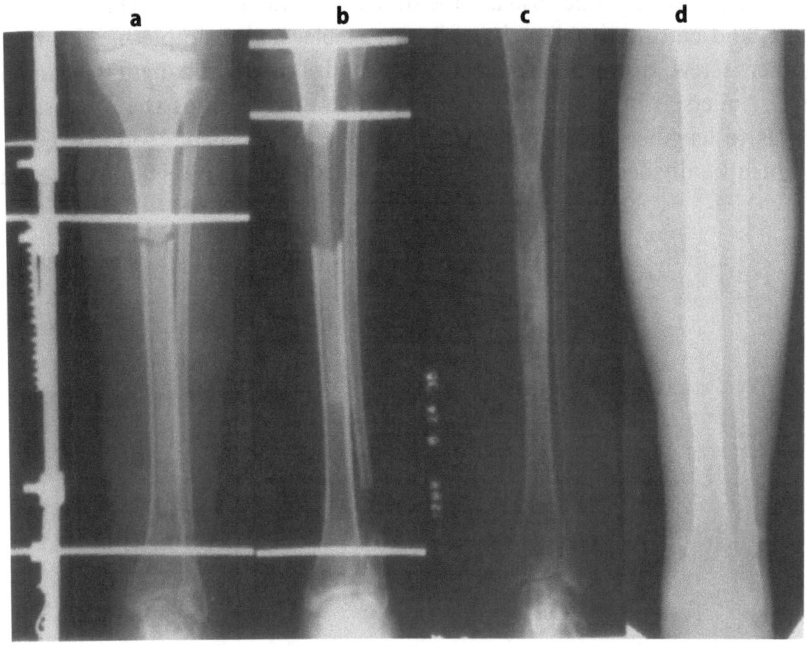

Fig. 41.4 This lengthening, performed by Dr. Wallace Cole in 1935, involved distracting the tibia of a patient with poliomyelitis. A long-slotted osteotomy was performed. **a** Two pins above the osteotomy and a pin in the distal tibia with a further pin in the calcaneum provided stability. **b** Double level fibular osteotomies show abundant intramembraneous new bone, with less abundant new bone at the tibial distraction site. **c** Follow-up X-rays two years post-lengthening. **d** 57 years post-lengthening.

an external supporting sleeve to improve control of the bone segments.[3] He later further improved stability by applying two pins to each bone segment. Abbott emphasized the osteogenic value of periosteal preservation and a 7–10 day waiting period before distracting the osteotomy. The Abbott method took 8 to 12 weeks to complete distraction, during which time the patient was confined to bed and immobilized. Due to substantial difficulties (his longest lengthening was 4.76cm) and complications with skin necrosis and osteomyelitis, Abbott recommended limb lengthening be used as a method of last resort.

In 1932, Edward Haboush and Harry Finkelstein further improved stability by making an apparatus consisting of three pairs of lateral uprights, each of which was attached at its lower end by a hinge joint to a horizontal cross-bar.[16] The apparatus was designed to rest on any flat surface, eliminating the need to suspend the limb from an overhead frame or tie the patient to a bed during the lengthening. Early weightbearing, to promote healing, was emphasized.

In 1938, Raoul Hoffmann began studying systems which not only allowed the fixation of a fracture but also modified the position of different bone fragments, a concept referred to as "osteotaxis"[17]. Hoffmann designed the first external fixator using threaded pins which engaged the cortices. This new pin geometry, combined with stacking bars, offered greater support for fracture reduction and eventually, limb lengthening.

In 1948, Allan introduced a mechanism he called "positive elongation" that allowed screw distraction of bone fragments to control the rate and magnitude of lengthening.[18] He emphasized the need to minimize soft tissue dissection, sparing local blood supply. The osteotomy was performed within a periosteal tube by predrilling the site, and cutting it obliquely with an osteotome. Another screw distraction system was designed by Roger Anderson in 1949.[19] The method Anderson used was to lengthen the Achilles tendon first, following which he divided the tibia by a long oblique or stepped osteotomy and fixed the fragments on an Abbott type distraction frame by double fixed pins above and below. He then lengthened the limb by screw distraction at a rate of one-ninth of an inch per day. Another wave of activity followed these reports.

Bone Healing Methods

The biological mechanism of healing was briefly discussed in the early literature, but it was generally recognized to be similar to fracture repair.[3,18,20] Frederic Bost and Loren Larsen, in 1956, compared oblique, Z, and transverse osteotomies and concluded that there was no difference in healing. They introduced the concept of a transverse osteotomy that would separate within a periosteal sleeve.[22] To solve alignment problems, Bost and Larsen recommended lengthening over an intramedullary rod. Bone grafts were often necessary, however, and complications were frequent.

In the late 1960s, Heinz Wagner introduced a monolateral fixator (Fig. 41.5) that was sufficiently stable, had a simple hand-turned distracting motor, and allowed the patient to be mobilized.[23] Three operative interventions were necessary. The first involved generous, open, soft tissue releases, diaphyseal osteotomy with section of the periosteum, and slight

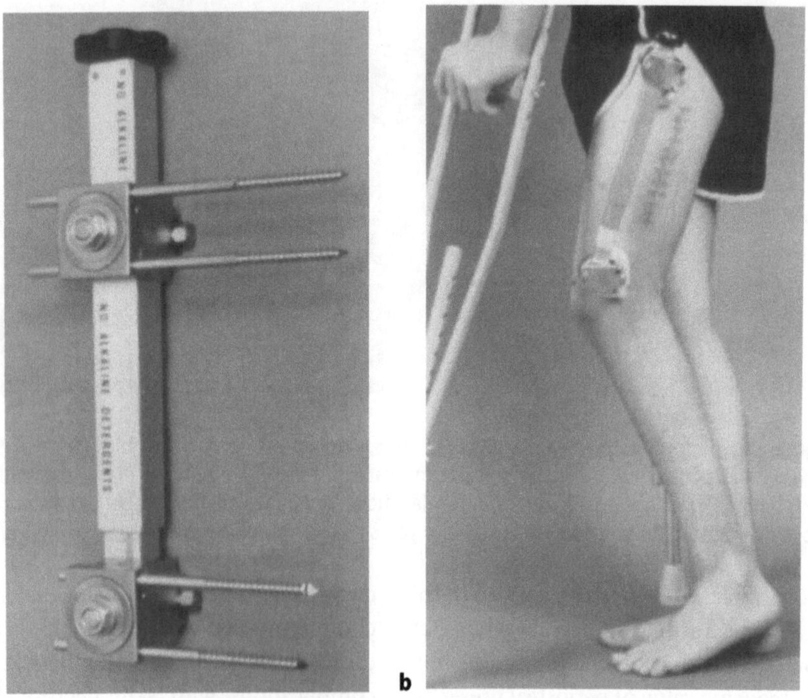

a b

Fig. 41.5 a, b Wagner's device is a low profile, monolateral fixator that allows the patient to be out of bed during distraction. Author's case.

immediate distraction. Subsequent distraction was relatively rapid, at a rate of 1.5mm per day. The second operation involved inserting cancellous bone graft and a special lengthening plate. Lengthening site healing occurred by creeping substitution, requiring prolonged protection and limited weightbearing. The third operation involved plate removal when remedullarization was evident. Patient mobility improved and external fixation time was shortened. This method was widely adopted by surgeons, but after 10 to 15 years of follow-up, it became evident that complications of fracture, infection and soft tissue contracture were still high.

B. Kawamura and co-workers performed extensive laboratory experiments, including microscopy, microangiography, histochemistry, electromyography, and plethysmography.[20,21] Their lengthenings involved subperiosteal osteotomies, separated in small increments under three or four anaesthetics. They combined their experimental work with results of their clinical experience, proposing a lengthening limit of 10–15 per cent of the original bone length.

Robert Judet and his brother Jean began performing femoral lengthenings over intramedullary rods in 1965[12]. They applied a plate and iliac bone graft to promote bone formation (Fig. 41.6). This technique, however, was promptly abandoned because of the frequent occurrence of axis deviation, infection and joint subluxation. In 1969, Judet introduced a new external lengthening device which consisted of a slotted rail mounted parallel to a distraction rod.

In 1975 and 1981, Jean-Claude Pouliquen reported results using the Judet technique, including a description of the prevention of axis deviation by careful alignment of the fixator along the mechanical axis and the inclusion of 3–4 pins in each cluster.[25,26] Foot equinus was prevented in high risk cases (e.g. congenital aetiologies) by the use of calcaneal pins incorporated in a plaster bandage or by orthotically suspending the foot and knee. Pouliquen's reports detail how late subluxation, soft tissue tension, and further bone growth contributed to the occurrence of complications. Pouliquen further modified the Judet technique by performing low-energy transverse subperiosteal osteotomies.

The Siberian surgeon, Gavriil Ilizarov, began developing methods of distraction osteogenesis in the early 1950s but due to political restraints his work was unknown to western surgeons until 1981.[24] Ilizarov developed his concepts of circular external fixation, utilizing tensioned multiplanar wires in conjunction with the biological principles of distraction

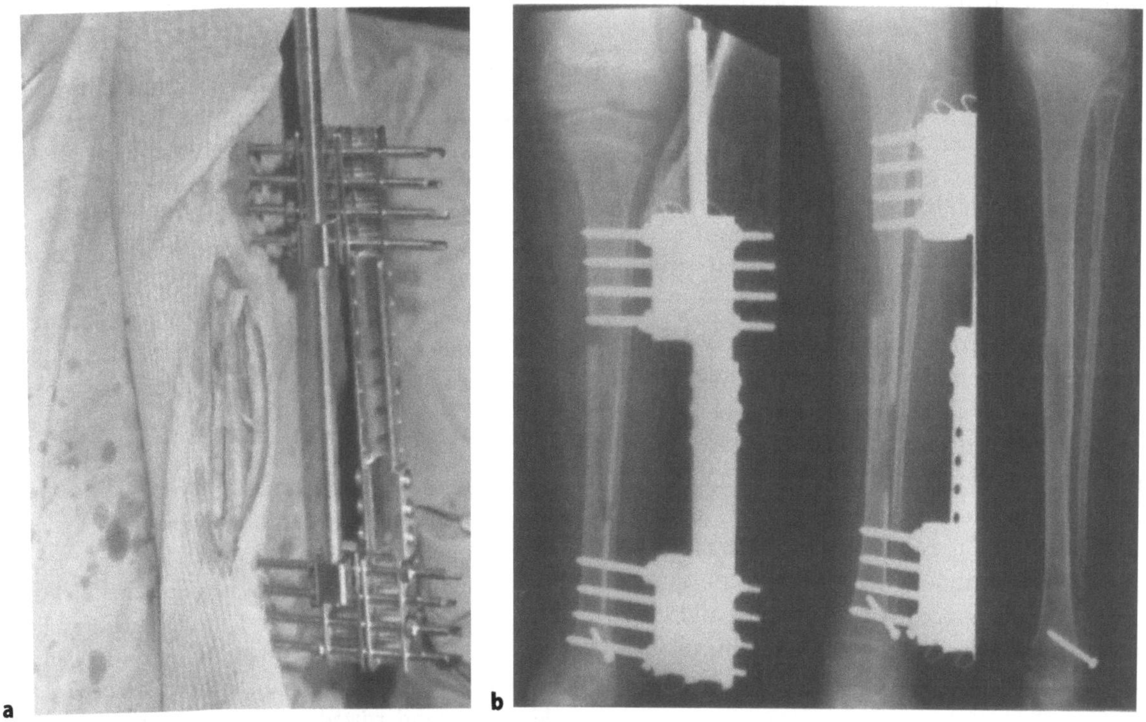

Fig. 41.6 Judet's technique incorporated a long oblique osteotomy with a monolateral fixator and distraction rod. **a** Osteotomy performed through drill holes. **b** Distraction of the osteotomy site. Note the screw transfixion of the fibula to the tibia. Four-year follow-up X-ray. Photo and X-rays courtesy of J.C. Pouliquen, M.D.

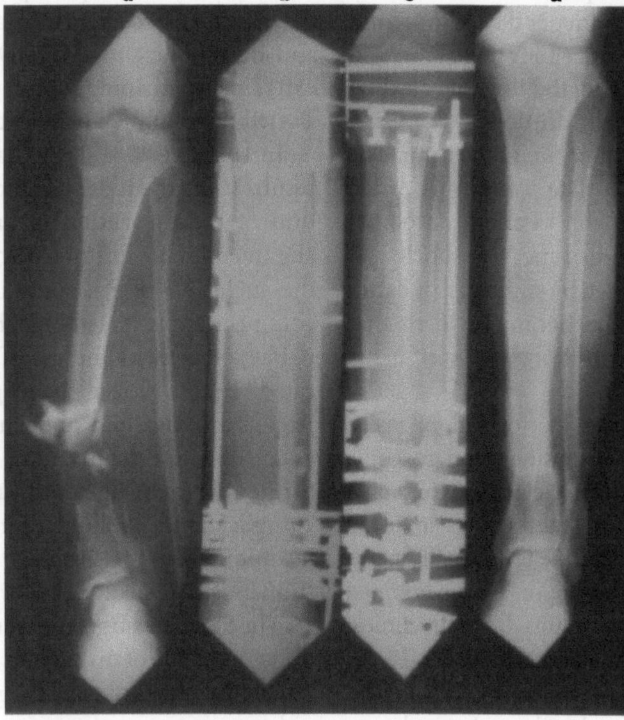

Fig. 41.7 **a** Ilizarov's circular fixator was applied to a patient with segmental bone loss from open trauma. **b, c** The case involved myocutanous soft-tissue coverage followed by circular fixation and bone transport of 11 cm. **d** Healing at 3-year follow-up. Author's case.

osteogenesis (Fig. 41.7). These principles were studied in laboratories at his institute and widely applied clinically.

The principles refined by Ilizarov include:

1. Stable external fixation
2. Low energy corticotomy
3. A latency period before initiating distraction
4. A lengthening rate and rhythm that allowed direct intramembranous new bone formation
5. Functional use of the limb with weightbearing and physiotherapy.

These concepts were developed in relative isolation but with a commitment and focus not previously seen in limb lengthening. Ilizarov also recognized the importance of allowing the bone to mature before removing the frame, thus avoiding many of the complications of fracture and subsequent deformity commonly encountered with previous methods. The multiplanar nature of ring fixation allowed the surgeon to correct axis deviation as it occurred. The patient and surgeon paid a price for this advantage, however, in bulkiness of frame and tedium of treatment.

Summary

The evolution of limb lengthening has clearly undergone many changes since Codivilla's first limb lengthening publication on bedridden patients treated without antibiotics. Advances in limb lengthening devices, surgical techniques, and an appreciation of the principles involved in preserving the blood supply, have been important steps forward. Many of the problems we still face today (e.g. soft tissue resistance) are identical with those encountered by our predecessors.

It is evident that a lack of communication between investigators has been responsible for repeated mistakes and has slowed the acceptance and advancement of limb lengthening considerably. When the history of limb lengthening is reviewed again 30 or 40 years from now, it is this author's hope that the greatest contribution of the present generation will be seen to have been that of communication. To benefit all those interested in limb lengthening, we need to establish a deformity classification and stratification as well as a systems approach to limb lengthening. We need also to develop a standardized means of measuring complications, and the way in which they are recorded and reported, to help diminish their incidence and severity.

Methodologies of bone lengthening continue to evolve, allowing safer, quicker, and more comfortable applications for our patients. These contributions have led to the development of the principles and technique of callotasis.

Acknowledgements

Special thanks to Professor Jean-Claude Pouliquen, Hopital Raymond Poincare, Garches, France, for his historical contributions to this chapter.

References

1. Codivilla, A. 'On the means of lengthening, in the lower limbs the muscle and tissue shortened through deformity.' *Am J Orthop Surg* 1905; 2:353.
2. Putti, V. 'The operative lengthening of the femur.' *J Am Med Assn* 1921; 77–934.
3. Abbott, L.C. 'The operative lengthening of the tibia and fibula.' *J Bone Joint Surg* 1927; 9:128–52.
4. De Bastiani, G., Aldegheri, R., Renzi-Brivio, L., Trivella, G. 'Limb lengthening by callus distraction (callotasis).' *J Pediatr Orthop* 1987; 7: 129–34.
5. Dahl, M.T., Gulli, B., Berg, T. 'Complications of limb lengthening: A Learning Curve.' *Clin Orthop.* 1994; 301:10–8.
6. Moseley, C., Mosca, V. 'Complications of Wagner Leg Lengthening.' in: *Behavior of the Growth Plate.* edited by Hans K. Uhthoff and James J. Wiley. Raven Press: New York, 1988.
7. Wu, Y.K., Miltner, L.J. 'A procedure for stimulation of longitudinal growth of bone.' *J Bone Joint Surg* 1937; 19:909–21.
8. Ferguson, A.B. 'Surgical stimulation of bone growth by a new procedure.' *J Am Med Assn* 1933; 100:26–7.
9. Bohlman, H.R. 'Experiments with foreign materials in the region of the epiphyseal cartilage plate of growing bones to increase their longitudinal growth.' *J Bone Joint Surg* 1929; 11: 365–84.
10. McCarroll, H.R. 'Trials and tribulations in attempted femoral lengthening.' *J Bone Joint Surg* [Am] 1950; 32-A: 132–42.
11. Phemister, D. 'Operative arrestment of longitudinal growth of bones in the treatment of deformities.' *J Bone Joint Surg* 1933; 15: 1–15.
12. Judet, R., Judet, J. 'Allongements Femoraux.' in: *Actualities Orthopedidues De Garches.* Masson Ed: Paris. 37–47, 1969.
13. *The Testament and Spiritual Exercises*
14. Magnuson, P. 'Lengthening of shortened bones of the leg by operation. Ivory screws with removable heads as a means of holding the two bone fragments.' *Surg Gynecol Obstet* 1913; 16: 63–71.
15. Laing, P.G. *Clinical experience with prosthetic materials: Historical perspectives, current problems, and future directions. Corrosion and Degradation of Implant Materials.* ASTM STP 684. B.C. Syrett and A. Acharya, Eds., American Society for Testing and Materials 199–211, 1979.
16. Haboush, E., Finkelstein, H. 'Leg lengthening with new stabilizing apparatus.' *J Bone Joint Surg* 1932; 14: 807.
17. Hoffman, R.' "Rotules a os" pur la "reduction dirigee", non sanglante, des fractures ("osteotaxis").' *Helv Med Acta* 1938; 5: 844–50.
18. Allan, F.G. 'Bone lengthening.' *J Bone Joint Surg* [Br] 1948; 30B: 490.
19. Anderson, W.V. 'Leg lengthening.' *J Bone Joint Surg* [Br] 1952 34B: 150.
20. Kawamura, B., Hosono, S., Takahashi, T. 'The principles and technique of limb lengthening.' *International Orthopaedics* (SICOT) 1981; 5: 69–83.
21. Kawamura, B., et al 'Limb lengthening by means of subcutaneous osteotomy.' *J Bone Joint Surg* [Am] 1968; 50A(5): 851–77.
22. Bost, F.C., Larson, L.J. 'Experiences with lengthening of the femur over an intramedullary rod.' *J Bone Joint Surg* [Am] 1956; 38A: 567–84.
23. Wagner, H. 'Operative lengthening of the femur.' *Clin Orthop* 1978; 136: 125–42.
24. Ilizarov, G. 'The tension–stress effect on the genesis and growth of tissues: Part I., The influence of stability of fixation and soft-tissue preservation.' *Clin Orthop* 1989; 238: 249–81.
25. Pouliquen, J.C., Beneux, J., Verneret, C., Hardy, J., Mener, G. 'Allongement de tibia selon la methode de Judet: A propos de 108 cas chez l'enfant.' *Revue de Chirurgie Orthopedique* 1984; 70: 29–39.
26. Pouliquen, J.C., Gorodischer, S., Verneret, C., Richard, L. 'Allongement de femur chez l'enfant et l'adolescent. Etude comparative d'une serie de 82 cas.' *Revue de Chirurgie Orthopedique* 1989; 75: 239–51.
27. Kuntscher G: *Practice of Intramedullary Nailing.* Charles C. Thomas. pp. 279–84, 1967.

The Technique of Callotasis and its Application to Monofocal Limb Lengthening

42

M. Saleh and L. Donnan

Introduction

Monolateral fixators have been used in limb lengthening since the late 1970s. Wagner[1] employed a technique for femoral lengthening which utilised a mid-diaphyseal osteotomy and a process of progressive lengthening at a rate of 1–2mm per day. This was continued until the desired increase in limb length was achieved, after which the gap thus produced was filled with autogenous bone graft and the bone internally fixed with a plate.

De Bastiani at the University of Verona in Italy was concerned by the incidence of complications experienced with the Wagner apparatus and, having designed the Orthofix monolateral external fixator to address many of the criticisms of currently available external fixation devices, developed the technique of *callotasis* – gradual, symmetrical distraction of the developing callus following a corticotomy.[2] The biological response provoked by this technique is very similar to that described by Ilizarov[3] in association with circular frames, or that observed many years previously by several groups of workers.[4,5,6,7] What De Bastiani showed, however, was that a circular fixator was not a prerequisite for excellent bone formation during lengthening procedures and in 1987 he published a series of 100 lengthenings in children and adults[2] which attested to the success of the technique.

Biological reconstruction of the skeleton is linked to the unique ability of bone to heal without scar formation.[8] The regenerative capacity of bone can be harnessed by an external fixator to acquire length, to correct deformity and to fill dead space. A deliberately produced transection of the bone produces an inflammatory response with the recruitment of osteoprogenitor cells. The latter give rise to osteoblasts that produce callus.[9] If a force, which can be longitudinal, angular or rotary, is applied to the developing callus, the reparative response can be maintained until a desired length is obtained, or a chosen degree of correction achieved. The woven scaffold is then gradually replaced by more mature bone which remodels in response to the stresses to which it is subjected.

The De Bastiani Technique for Callotasis

This combines a simple operative technique with a sophisticated fixator and well designed screws. The essential features are summarised in Table 42.1.

The fixator is mounted parallel to the long axis of the bone, to which it is attached by screws inserted at right angles to it. A metaphyseal or immediately submetaphyseal interruption in the bone is recommended, since this is a wider and more vascular region and has been shown to have better osteogenic potential than the diaphysis (De Bastiani et al 1987)[10]. A corticotomy is performed in order to try and preserve the medullary blood supply. Care is taken to preserve the periosteum since this layer has been shown to be the most important site of osteogenesis (Kojimoto et al 1988)[11]. De Bastiani recommended a vertical incision in the periosteum under direct vision prior to bone division and repair of the periosteum once the procedure is complete. Where the tibia was undergoing lengthening, a 1–2cm segment of the fibula was excised with no distal fixation of this bone.

Fixator parallel to the axis
Metaphyseal corticotomy
Respect for periosteum
Respect for medulla
Closed osteoclasis
Resection of fibula with periosteum
Immediate weightbearing
Delay before lengthening
Slow distraction
Neutralization period
Dynamization
Fixator removal

Table 42.1 The Essential Features of De Bastiani Callotasis

Distraction at a rate of 1mm per day is commenced when evidence of early callus formation is visible on X-ray. Once the planned increase in length has been achieved, the fixator column is locked and the neutralization period commenced. Well-formed callus is encouraged to consolidate by what De Bastiani labelled "dynamization". This involves unlocking the fixator's telescopic body and permitting it to slide freely or up to a silastic collar to allow transfer of load from the fixator to the newly formed segment. Once corticalization is evident on X-ray and the new bone clinically sound, the fixator is removed.

The Current Sheffield Callotasis Technique

While the principles described below are generally applicable to both monolateral and circular frames, specific details refer to the use of a monolateral frame, in most instances the Limb Reconstruction System (LRS). The femur, tibia and humerus are the most commonly lengthened bones, but with smaller devices now available, even bones as small as the metacarpals and phalanges can be treated.

A carefully performed osteotomy is mandatory for good callus formation. Preservation of the medulla and its blood supply was previously thought to be important (Ilizarov 1989a)[12]. There is considerable evidence, however, of rapid recovery of the medullary blood supply after reaming. In their rabbit study, Kojimoto et al (1988)[11] saw no reduction of the callus response after scraping away the endosteum. Delloye et al (1990)[13] sectioned the bone in mongrel dogs by corticotomy, osteotomy and osteotomy with a medullary plug and found no difference in callus response. Evidence that medullary division is unimportant is of value because of the technical difficulties in achieving a true "corticotomy". It is important, however, to treat the periosteum with respect and to avoid thermal necrosis of the bone.

The current technique in Sheffield for lengthening of the tibia involves tensioning the bone by 2 or 3mm with a distractor unit (Fig. 42.1a). Using the most direct surgical approach, the periosteum is divided longitudinally between two stay sutures to ensure subsequent correct coaptation. Bone levers are then passed around the bone so that their tips meet, thus protecting the periosteum from damage. A series of

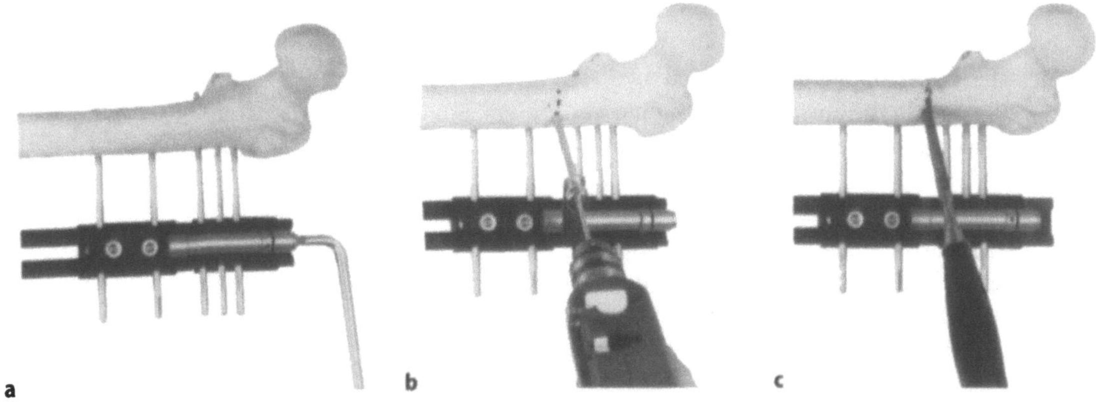

Fig. 42.1 The tension osteotomy. **a** The bone is tensioned using the compression-distraction unit. **b** A series of drill holes is made across the bone. **c** The bone is divided with an osteotome.

controlled drill holes is then made across the bone using a sharp 3.2mm drill at low speed (Fig. 42.1b). An osteotome is then used to divide the bone by connecting the drill holes together and finally dividing the posteromedial and posterolateral angles in the tibia (Fig. 42.1c). Since the bone has been pre-tensioned the bone ends will gently drift apart once the osteotomy has been completed. The latter is confirmed with a "triple test": exploration of the gap using a probe, assessment of the ease of distraction, and the appearance under image intensification. The osteotomy is then gently compressed, the periosteum reconstituted and the wound closed without a drain.

Prior to tibial osteotomy a fibular osteotomy is performed at the junction of its middle and distal thirds. More distal procedures may cause ankle instability. Premature consolidation of the osteotomy can be avoided by the removal of a small segment of fibula. This may, however, lead to a painful gap non-union.

The distal fragment is secured to the tibia with a 3.5mm unlagged cortical syndesmotic screw. This is because there is a tendency during lengthening for this distal fragment to migrate proximally, a situation which can lead to lateral subluxation of the ankle.

In longer lengthenings it is desirable to fix the head of the fibula to the tibia with a K-wire. In cases where both ends of the fibula are secured, a simple osteotomy may be sufficient.

Extended Callotasis

For longer lengthenings and where joint instability may be a problem, judicious use of soft tissue releases and joint stabilization as described by Vilarrubias[14] may be appropriate. In the tibia, for example, a percutaneous release of the Achilles tendon may be performed. This may, however, lead to loss of the active muscle stimulation induced by exercise and should not be undertaken lightly. In femoral lengthenings the knee should be supported in the extended position and in the tibia, the ankle should be supported in a plantigrade position in Plaster of Paris.

During the process of lengthening using the callotasis technique, considerable tension is generated in the soft tissues surrounding the limb and suitable precautions must be taken to protect adjacent joints. If joints at risk are splinted in the closed packed position and regularly stretched, the development of contractures is minimised. In certain situations, however, where, for example, there are associated burns and the soft tissues are poorly pliable, there is a greater tendency to develop joint contractures. In other cases there may be an underlying joint instability or cartilaginous disorder and the increased tension may produce subluxation or articular damage. In situations such as these, a modified monolateral fixator should be used to hold the joint at risk in a stable and slightly distracted position during the lengthening procedure. This will usually involve the use of constructs that hinge across the ankle and foot for tibial lengthening, or across the knee in femoral lengthening. The Sheffield Hybrid Fixator may be used for this purpose, enabling the joint in question to be mobilized after the soft tissue tension has been dissipated in the consolidation phase.

Bifocal lengthening is indicated where acquisition of more than 6cm is required, and is described in Ch. 44.

The choice of technique depends on both the risk factors and the surgical aims (Table 42.2; Saleh and Hamer 1993).[15] In Type 1 situations the original callotasis technique is adequate; for Type 2 and 3 problems, extended callotasis is recommended, and for Type 3 and 4 problems, acute correction template in conjunction with the LRS, or the circular fixator technique using the Sheffield Hybrid Fixator.

Type 1	Low-risk linear correction: Straight lengthening <20 per cent of starting length, with stable joints and no other "at risk" features.
Type 2	High-risk linear correction: Straight lengthening with joint instability, obesity, joint stiffness, or previous surgery, and/or other "at risk" features such as lengthening >20 per cent of starting length.
Type 3	Low-risk complex correction: Lengthening <20 per cent of starting length, with no other "at risk" features, but with soft tissue or bony angular correction.
Type 4	High-risk complex correction: Lengthening >20 per cent of starting length or other "at risk" features, with soft tissue or bony angular correction.

Table 42.2 Classification of the Degree of Risk in Lengthening Procedures

The Circular Frame Technique

Ilizarov Technique

The principles governing this method are similar to and predate those of the callotasis method. Instead of using screws and a single-sided fixator, tensioned Kirschner-wires and a circular frame may be used. The principles of surgery are similar to those described for callotasis. The advantage lies in the fact that pre-existing deformity and axial deviation occurring during lengthening may be corrected progressively by appropriate hinge and threaded rod placement. The fine wires provide better purchase in soft and cancellous bone and the technique may be used to correct concurrent soft tissue deformities such as equinus of the foot (Hardy et al 1991;[16] Saleh 1992;[17] Jackson and Saleh 1994[18]). Circular frames with transfixion wires are less well tolerated and carry an increased risk of nerve or vessel injury. It seems more appropriate, therefore, to reserve their use for complicated lengthenings or high risk situations. It is an unnecessary burden both for the patient and surgeon in more simple cases where a predictable result can be achieved with a monolateral frame (Saleh 1992;[17] Saleh and Scott 1992[19]). Problems of diaphyseal fixation exist because of the limited safe anatomical corridors, and screws are commonly used in this area. These circular frame techniques are used particularly for Type 4 problems: lengthening with angular or translational corrections; lengthening with multiapical deformities; lengthening in the presence of unstable joints.

The Sheffield Hybrid System

The Sheffield Hybrid Fixator is a new design which affords better stability while retaining elastic stiffness, circumferential beam support and strong fixation (Saleh et al 1997).[20] Metaphyseal fixation is achieved by attaching four wires at two levels off the ring, while diaphyseal fixation is secured with a strong clamp and screw system. Since the design of this clamp is similar to those of the Limb Reconstruction System, the two systems may be coupled together. For tibial lengthening, the use of two rings, one attached to each metaphysis with wires, enables the fibula to be transfixed both proximally and distally. The fibula-tibia relationship is thus constant, and a simple fibular osteotomy only, is required (Fig. 42.2). In addition, because the two rings are widely separated, soft tissue relaxation during lengthening is optimised.

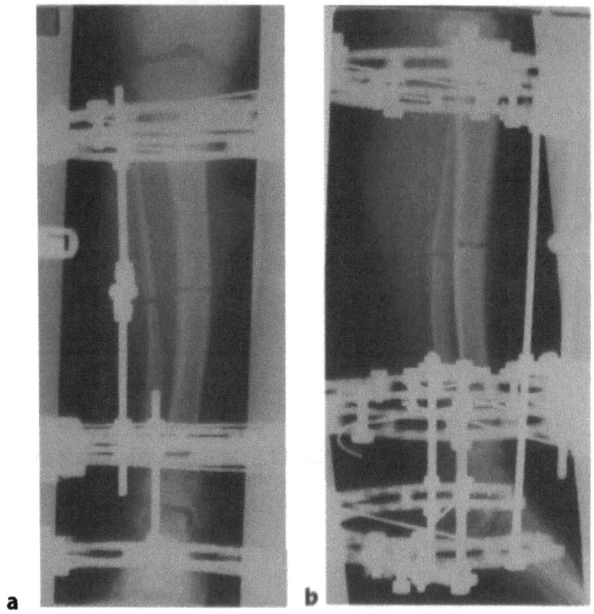

Fig. 42.2 Monofocal lengthening with correction of valgus using the Sheffield Hybrid Fixator. In this all-wire construct the fibula has been transfixed both proximally and distally and a simple fibula osteotomy only has been performed. **a** AP view with fixator in situ. **b** Lateral view, showing fixation extended on to the foot to protect the ankle and prevent equinus.

Post-Operative Management

High quality, frequent physiotherapy is the cornerstone of good post-operative management, with the object of acquiring and preserving a full range of joint movement and encouraging the patient to walk. Exercises normally commence immediately following operation and may be supplemented with continuous passive motion.

Distraction of the osteotomy site normally begins at about day 7 and the patient is discharged quite soon after this in most cases. Slow distraction appears to be uncontroversial. Both De Bastiani and Ilizarov recommend a rate of 1mm per day. Faster rates produce ischaemia and necrosis of bone, and slower rates may result in premature consolidation. The rate may be increased in rapid bone formers such as patients with Ollier's Disease, and reduced in poor bone formers such as the older patient. Rate titration is usually recommended according to the density and width of callus seen on carefully exposed X-ray plates. The rate may also be increased at the beginning of lengthening to prevent premature fusion and subsequently slowed down if soft tissue contractures occur. The frequency

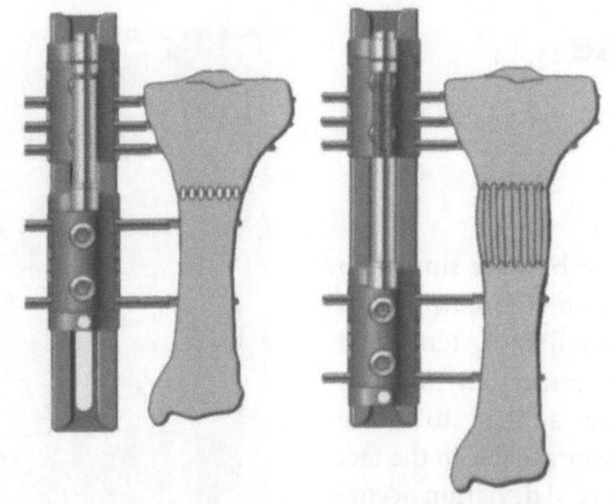

Fig. 42.3 Monofocal lengthening with the Limb Reconstruction System.

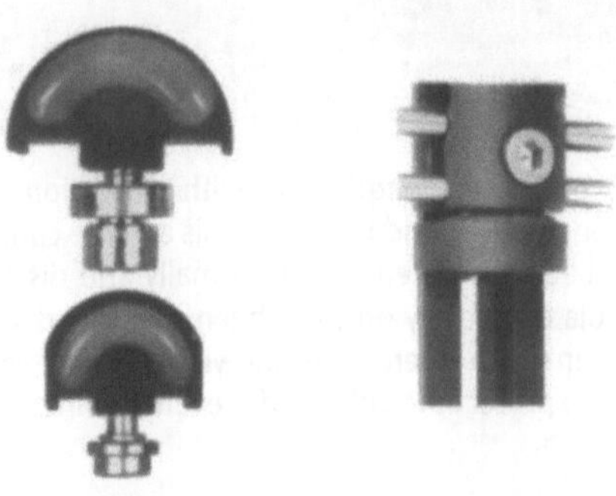

Fig. 42.4 The Dyna-Ring attachment.

of distraction is normally four increments daily, but dramatic osteogenesis has been seen with gradual continuous automated distraction (Ilizarov 1989b).[21] The optimal environment for bone may be very different from that of the soft tissues since the latter display viscoelastic characteristics and require long periods of recovery (Matsushita 1999).[22]

Where the Limb Reconstruction System is used (Fig. 42.3), the clamp locking screw of one of the clamps to which the distractor unit (compression-distraction unit) is connected is loosened each time distraction is performed, and tightened again at the end of the procedure. Distraction is effected by turning the screw in the end of the distractor unit one quarter turn in the appropriate direction. Patients are generally seen every two weeks during the lengthening or correction phase and once a month during the consolidation phase. An initial full segment radiograph is obtained to check the alignment in two planes and to ensure that the osteotomy site is opening satisfactorily. Bone quality at the distraction site can usually be assessed at four weeks following the commencement of distraction when a calcific front has moved from both bone ends into the distraction gap. Intermittent segment radiographs are recommended to assess

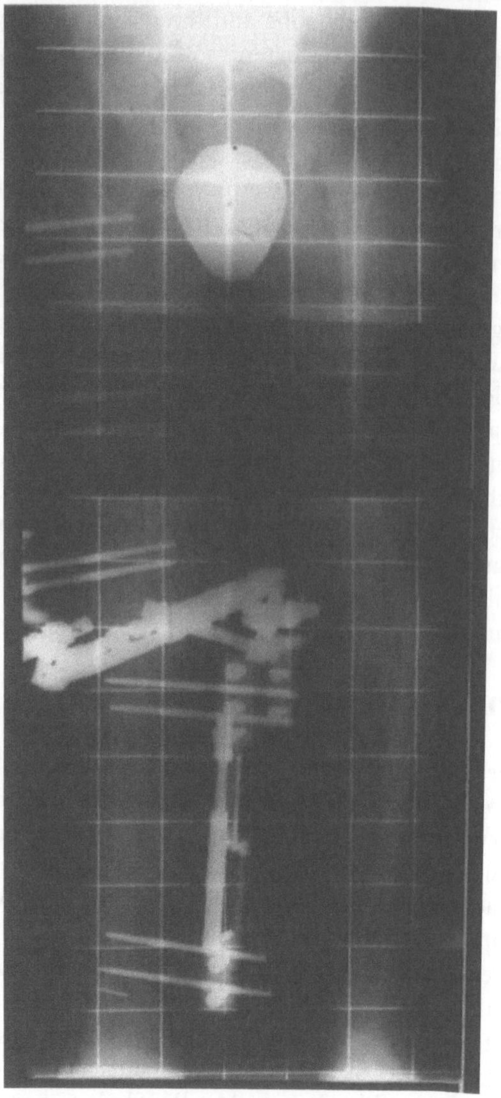

Fig. 42.5 Simultaneous monofocal lengthening in the tibia and bifocal lengthening in the femur. The knee is stabilized by the addition of a ring attached to the distal femoral and proximal tibial screw groups.

corrections and identify any unwanted angular deviation. At the conclusion of the lengthening or correction phase the fixator column is locked, and the phase of consolidation begins.

The point at which the regenerate is stable enough to be stressed is determined by evidence of obliteration of the radiolucent interzone and early corticalization. At this point, progressive transfer of weight to the newly formed bone will stimulate remodelling and reduce the time for which the fixator remains in place. This process of dynamization is achieved by loosening one of the clamps on the rail. If the femur has been lengthened, for example, the clamp proximal to the newly formed segment is loosened. In order to minimise any risk of collapse of the regenerate when dynamization is first instituted, a special module, the Dyna-Ring, may be used (Fig. 42.4). This incorporates a silicone cushion and is attached to the rail beneath the loosened clamp, with its silicone cushion facing the clamp and just in contact with it. The cushion permits limited micromovement of up to 2mm on weightbearing, thus preventing collapse, and allowing earlier conversion to the dynamic mode, if desired.

Once three cortices are visible on the AP and lateral radiographs, the fixator can be removed and a walking cast applied for 4–6 weeks. In the case of the femur, the fixator is removed for increasing periods during the daytime over a 4–6 week period. The patient is then followed up at appropriate intervals in the outpatient department until the pre-operative range of motion is obtained, full weightbearing achieved and remodelling complete. Fig. 42.5 shows an example of lengthening with joint protection.

Correction of Angular Deformity Developing During Monofocal Limb Lengthening by Callotasis

Monofocal lengthening with the Limb Reconstruction System (LRS) is often, but not invariably, associated with some degree of angular deviation due to the very considerable tension developed in the soft tissues. Where lengthening is carried out in the femur, the fixator is applied to the lateral aspect of the limb, and as a consequence, there will be a tendency for varus deviation to occur as lengthening proceeds. Conversely, in the tibia, where the fixator is applied to the anteromedial or medial aspect of the bone, the tendency is for valgus deviation to develop. The magnitude of such deviation is of the order of 1° per centimetre of lengthened bone. It is normal practice to correct such deformity at, or towards the end of the lengthening period, and accurate titration of the amount of correction can be achieved by incorporating a progressive correction clamp in the system.

There will also be situations where lengthening is required in a limb which also exhibits an angular deformity which will need to be corrected. In some of these, immediate angular correction prior to lengthening may be performed, and these techniques are described in Ch. 36. In other cases, progressive correction, often involving use of the Sheffield Hybrid Fixator Assembly may be appropriate (see Ch. 40). The present chapter, however, will consider the correction of deformity occurring during lengthening. Acute correction under anaesthesia may be performed by replacement of one of the straight clamps on the LRS with an adaptor unit and ball joint (see Ch. 36). Progressive corrections may be performed by replacing the straight clamp with either the Micrometric Swivelling Clamp or the Multiplanar Clamp. In cases where the OF-Garches System has been used, varus or valgus deformity occurring during lengthening may be corrected by unlocking the hinge mechanism.

The Micrometric Swivelling Clamp

An adult version only of this clamp is available (Fig. 42.6). For the correction of a deformity developing during lengthening it is used to replace a straight clamp which may be positioned anywhere along the rail. This can only be achieved if the rail and clamps are temporarily removed. To do this, the segment is first stabilized by means of a parallel fixator applied to the screw shafts externally to the Limb Reconstruction System. The original rail and clamps are removed and the Micrometric Swivelling Clamp is placed on the original rail in exchange for the appropriate straight clamp

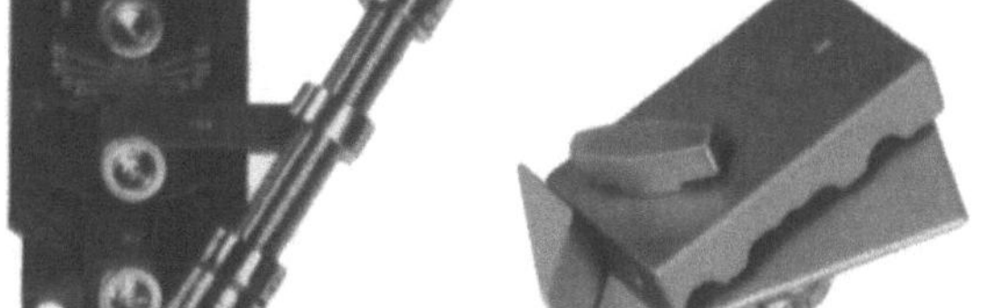

Fig. 42.6 The Micrometric Swivelling Clamp and its template.

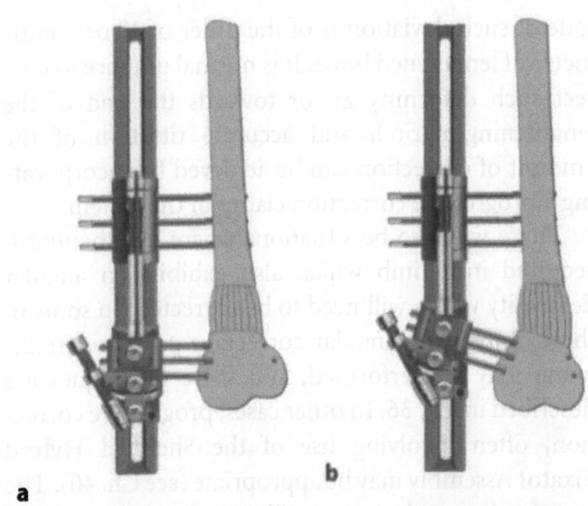

Fig. 42.7 Correction of a deformity developing during lengthening using the Micrometric Swivelling Clamp. **a** Varus deformity in the distal femur prior to correction. **b** Correction by callus manipulation. It should be noted from the relative positions of the clamps on the rail that the callus has initially been shortened to reduce tension in the soft tissues prior to correction of the deformity.

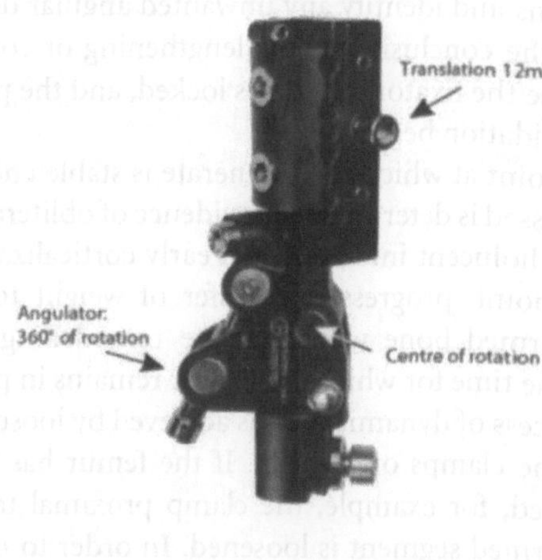

Fig. 42.8 The Multiplanar Clamp.

at the level of the deformity. The rail is then replaced on the bone screws and all the clamps and locking screws tightened firmly, as before. The temporary rail and clamps can then be removed. On the assumption that there is still some soft callus present, progressive correction of the deformity can now take place. Consideration of the geometry of the frame is important at this stage: if the rail is on the *concave* side of the deformity, correction can begin immediately, by turning the screw in the distractor unit, because correction will also involve shortening, and the soft tissue tension will not be increased. Note that after correction further lengthening may be required. However, if the frame is on the *convex* side of the deformity, correction would lengthen further at the same time, and the soft tissue tensions might be too great for the distractor on the clamp. In this situation, therefore, it is very important that the new callus is first shortened to reduce tension before the correction is made (Fig. 42.7). Pre-operative planning will reveal, and enable the surgeon to anticipate, the amount of shortening or lengthening that correction will cause. If the callus has matured to the point where it can no longer be manipulated in this way, an osteotomy would be required. In either case, it is important that correction is carried out under very careful radiological control.

The Multiplanar Clamp

This clamp (Fig. 42.8)can be attached to either end of the LRS rail and used to correct angular deformities in any plane, and up to 12mm of translation. Its use is described fully in Ch. 36 in association with the acute correction of deformity. The central part of the clamp,

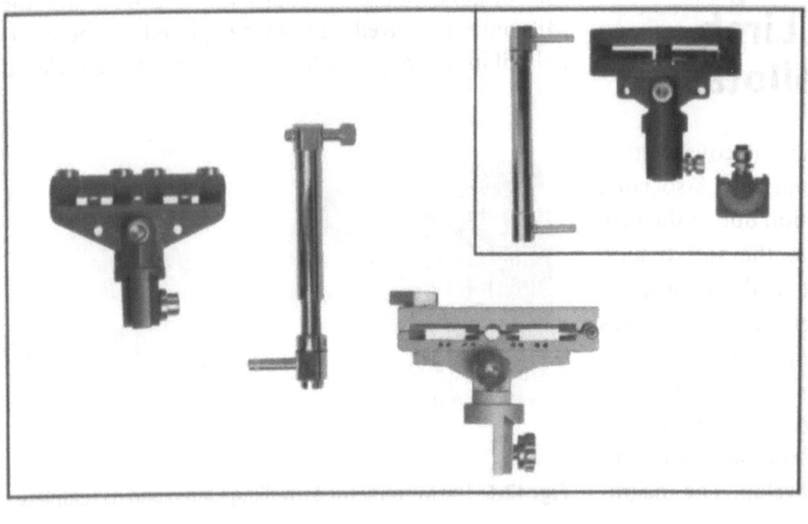

Fig. 42.9 The OF-Garches T-Clamp and template; the paediatric version is shown as an inset. Because the axis of rotation of the T-clamp passes through the centre of the osteotomy or lengthened segment translation should not occur during its use.

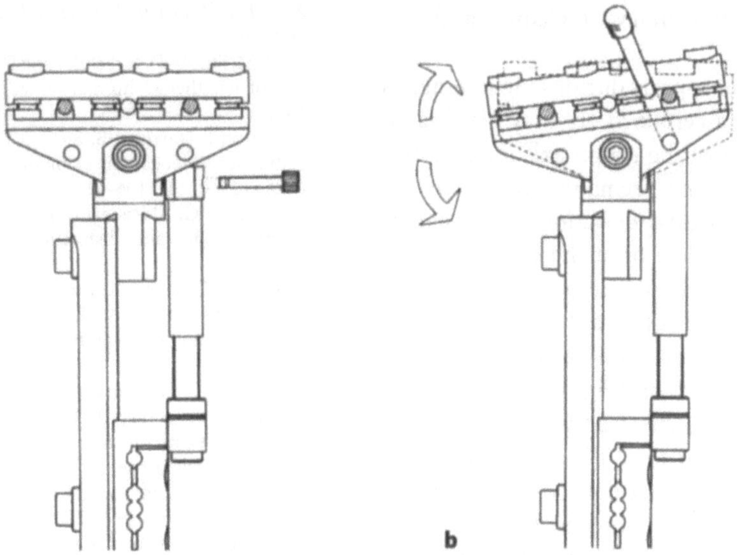

Fig. 42.10 The OF-Garches Clamp. Position of the removable locking pin **a** for lengthening **b** for angular correction.

the "angulator" can rotate through 360°, and can be locked in any desired position to determine the plane of correction independently of the bone screw positions. It is applied with a dedicated template. Its mode of use once again depends on the geometry of the frame, as described above.

The OF-Garches T-Clamp

This module (Fig. 42.9) attaches to one end of the Limb Reconstruction System rail. Its main use is for tibial lengthening in the upper metaphyseal region, to allow better control of valgus or varus deviation, although it can also be used for the acute correction of angular deviation (see Ch. 36). It has its own dedicated template. The OF-Garches T-Clamp can move in one plane only, and has swivelling screw seats which allow convergent siting of the upper screws. Its compression–distraction unit can be attached in one of two ways, depending upon whether lengthening or angular correction is desired (Fig. 42.10). A paediatric version is also available.

The application of the OF-Garches T-Clamp to the anterior aspect of the tibia is described in detail in Ch. 36. When used to lengthen the tibia at an upper tibial metaphyseal osteotomy, the compression–distraction unit is attached by inserting the removable locking pin into a cavity in the base of the clamp, as shown in Fig. 42.10a, and the clamp axis locking nut is firmly tightened. Extension of the compression-distraction unit by turning its screw clockwise once callus has started to form, will now lengthen the bone in its longitudinal

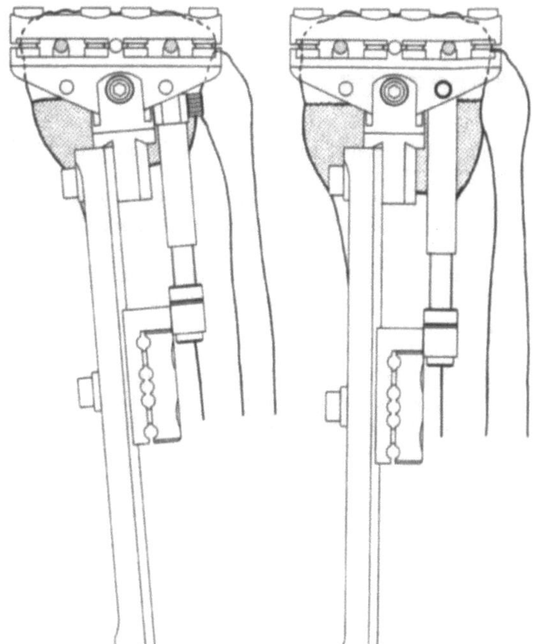

Fig. 42.11 Use of the OF-Garches T-Clamp to correct valgus deviation of the tibia occurring during lengthening. **a** Angular deviation has appeared during lengthening; note that the removable locking pin is connected to the base of the clamp. **b** Correction of angular deviation; note that removable locking pin is now connected to the wing of the OF-Garches clamp. The clamp axis locking nut is loosened and the straight clamp locking screw tightened.

axis between the OF-Garches T-Clamp and the straight clamp.

If a valgus deviation appears during lengthening, its cause must first be ascertained. It may be due to incomplete tightening of the clamp axis locking nut, bending of the screws, or premature fusion of the fibular osteotomy. If angular deviation occurs before the lengthening is complete or at the end of lengthening (Fig. 42.11a), correction can be performed at a rate of a quarter turn four times a day (0.25mm four times a day) with the compression–distraction unit on the same side as the deviation (Fig. 42.11b), with the removable locking pin inserted from anterior to posterior through the wing of the "T" as shown in Fig. 42.10b, the clamp axis locking nut loosened, and the straight clamp locking screw tightened. Once the deviation has been corrected, the position of the removable locking pin can be returned to that shown in Fig. 42.10a, the straight clamp locking screw loosened again, and lengthening resumed, if necessary.

References

1. Wagner H. 'Operative lengthening of the femur.' *Clin Orthop* 1978; 136: 125–42.
2. Aldegheri R, De Bastiani G, Renzi Brivio L. 'Allungamento diafisario dell'arto inferiore (studio di 78 casi).' *Chir Organi Mov* 1985; 70: 111–9.
3. Ilizarov GA. 'Clinical application of the tension-stress effect for limb lengthening.' *Clin Orthop* 1990; 250: 8–26.
4. Abbott LC. 'The operative lengthening of the tibia and fibula.' *J Bone Joint Surg* 1927; 9: 128.
5. Haboush EJ, Finkelstein H. 'Leg lengthening with a new stabilizing apparatus.' *J Bone Joint Surg* 1932; 14: 194.
6. Bosworth DM. 'Skeletal distraction of the tibia.' *Surg Gynecol Obstet* 1938; 66: 912.
7. Allan FG. 'Bone lengthening.' *J Bone Joint Surg* [Br] 1948; 30-B: 490-505.
8. Saleh M, Stubbs D, Street R, Lang D, Harris S. Histological analysis of lengthened human bone.' *J Paediatr Orthop* 1993; 2: 16–21.
9. Aaronson J, Harrison B, Stewart C, Harp J. 'The histology of distraction osteogenesis using different external fixators.' *Clin Orthop* 1988; 241: 106–116.
10. De Bastiani G, Aldegheri R, Renzi Brivio L, Trivella G. 'Limb lengthening by callus distraction (callotasis).' *J Paediatr Orthop* 1987; 7: 129–34.
11. Kojimoto H, Yasui N, Goto T, Matsuda S, Shimomura Y. 'Bone lengthening in rabbits by callus distraction. The role of periosteum and endosteum.' *J Bone Joint Surg* [Br] 1988; 70B: 543–9.
12. Ilizarov GA.' The tension-stress effect on the genesis and growth of tissues. Part 1: The influence of stability of fixation and soft tissue preservation.' *Clin Orthop* 1989; 238: 249–81.
13. Delloye C, Delefortrie G, Coutelier L, Vincent A. 'Bone regenerate formation in cortical bone during distraction lengthening.' *Clin Orthop* 1990; 250: 34–42.
14. Villarubias JM, Ginebreda I, Jimeno E. 'Lengthening of the lower limbs and correction of lumbar hyperlordosis in achondroplasia.' *Clin Orthop* 1990; 250: 143.
15. Saleh M, Hamer AJ. 'Bifocal Limb Lengthening: A Preliminary Report. *J Pediatr Orthop* 1993; Part B 2: 42–8.
16. Hardy JM, Tadlaoui A, Wirotius JM, Saleh M. 'The Sequoia circular fixator for limb lengthening.' *Orthop Clin N Am* 1991; 22: 663–75.
17. Saleh M. 'Technique selection in leg lengthening: the Sheffield Practice.' *Seminars in Orthopaedics* 1992; 7: 137–51.
18. Jackson A, Saleh M. 'The Ilizarov Technique' in: *Children's Orthopaedics and Fractures* Eds: Benson M, Fixsen J, MacNicol M. Churchill Livingstone: Edinburgh 1994, pp 502–11.
19. Saleh M, Scott BW. 'Pitfalls and complications of leg lengthening: The Sheffield experience.' *Seminars in Orthopaedics* 1992; 7: 207–22.
20. Saleh M, Yang L, Nayagam S. 'Can a Hybrid Fixator perform as well as the Ilizarov Fixator?' *J Bone Joint Surg* [Br] 1997; suppl IV p. 462.
21. Ilizarov GA. 'The tension–stress effect on the genesis and growth of tissues. Part 2: The influence of the rate and frequency of distraction.' *Clin Orthop* 1989; 239: 263–85.
22. Matsushita T, Nakamura K, Kurokawa T. 'Tensile forces in limb lengthening; histiogenesis or only mechanical elongation.' *Orthopedics* 1999; 22: 61–3.

Upper Metaphyseal Lengthening of the Tibia Using the OF-Garches

43

J.C. Pouliquen, C. Glorion and J. Langlais

Introduction

The incidence of valgus deviation and the problems with consolidation reported in various series of leg lengthenings in the literature, have focused the attention of this Unit, since 1985, on ways in which these two principal complications might be avoided. The technique of callotasis as described by De Bastiani et al[7] was used in an attempt to improve consolidation. A new distractor was designed, which could be applied very securely to the upper tibial metaphysis. This enabled a high metaphyseal osteotomy to be performed, which would encourage rapid consolidation, leaving scope for axial correction, if required, with a more easily mounted and less cumbersome implant than the circular Ilizarov fixator.

An initial report[16] evaluated the results of the first 47 tibial lengthenings by this method using Judet's lengthener in 15 cases, and the OF-Garches in 32. The present chapter describes the results obtained in 47 tibial lengthenings performed exclusively with the Orthofix device (OF-Garches).

Materials and Methods

We performed 69 upper metaphyseal lengthenings of the tibia between 1986 and 1993. To ensure that the series would be homogeneous, 22 patients were excluded. In 7 patients, valgus or varus deviations had been corrected by upper tibial callotasis in conjunction with a lengthening of less than 3cm. The treatment in these patients, therefore, was primarily axial correction, with lengthening as a secondary objective. In the initial group of 15 patients, the lengthener used was the Judet.[16,17]

In the present study 47 leg lengthenings performed using the callotasis technique and the OF-Garches lengthener in 40 children and adolescents (mean age 12.6 years; range 4–18 years) were reviewed. Five lengthenings were bilateral, 4 were performed twice on the same tibia, and one was performed three times. In six instances, lengthenings had previously been performed using other techniques. The causes of the limb discrepancy are shown in Table 43.1. In most cases, the aetiology was congenital or neurological. The 5 bilateral lengthenings were performed in patients of short stature: 2 patients with achondroplasia; 1 with Turner's syndrome, 1 with endocrine dwarfism and one with Leri and Weil's dyschondrosteosis. Thirty-five tibiae were straight before the treatment began, 6 had a valgus deviation and 6, a varus.

Lengthener

The lengthener used in this series was an Orthofix distractor, in which the orientation of the horizontal section can be adjusted in relation to the vertical section in the frontal plane. This model is of interest in that it permits total control of the diaphyseal axis in relation to the epiphysis, in a compact design which allows the patient to walk with minimal interference (Figs. 43.1, 43.2, 43.3).

Technique

The technique in all cases involved a subperiosteal tibial osteotomy and closure of the periosteum without drainage. Lengthening was commenced between the 9th and the 17th post-operative day, at a rate of 1mm per day in two equal stages (morning and afternoon). Patients

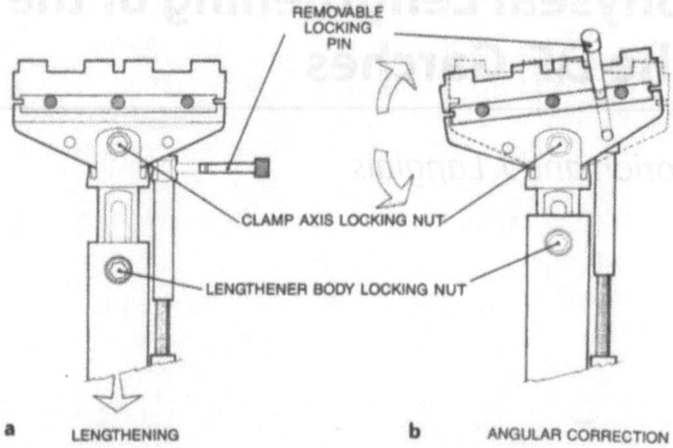

Fig. 43.1 **a** The position of the removable locking pin of the compression-distraction unit of the OF-Garches for lengthening along the axis of the bone. **b** For angular correction.

were encouraged to walk under conditions of normal weightbearing with a posterior splint to maintain the knee extended and the foot at a right angle to the tibial diaphysis. Lengthening was 5mm in excess of the final desired result to compensate for compaction of the callus during dynamization. When the callus was considered to have consolidated, the patient was readmitted to the hospital for removal of the lengthening device. This was accomplished in three stages: removal of the body of the lengthener; 3 days of walking with radiological assessment during this period, and finally removal of the implant screws and the syndesmosis screw(s).

The tibial osteotomy was performed in the upper metaphysis immediately below the anterior tibial tubercle in 42 cases, and in the metaphyseo-diaphyseal region in 5 cases. In all cases the tibia was sectioned by complete osteotomy without attempting to preserve the medullary canal. The approach to the fibula varied greatly. Except for 11 lengthenings in patients with complete fibular aplasia (with removal of a vestigial fibula in two cases), fibular osteotomy was performed in the supramalleolar region on 31 occasions, on 3 occasions it was performed below the neck of the fibula, and on 2 occasions at both sites. Tibio-fibular fixation was performed distally by means of a screw in 31 patients (one with tibio-fibular synostosis), proximally and

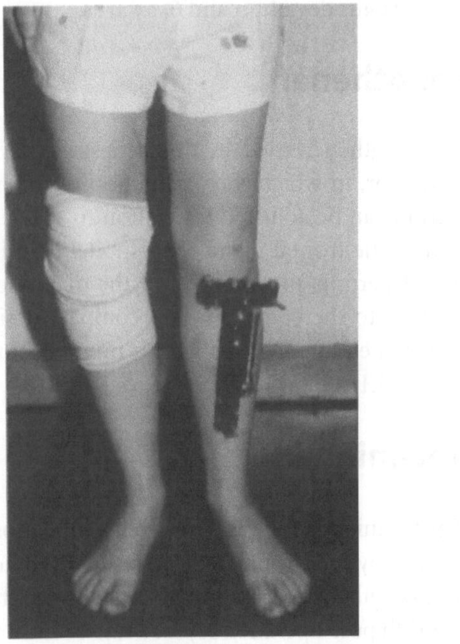

Fig. 43.2 The adult version of the OF-Garches used here in conjunction with an Orthofix telescopic lengthener.

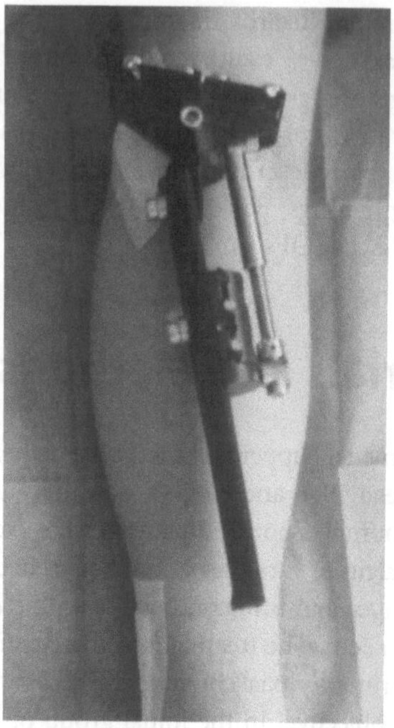

Fig. 43.3 The paediatric version of the OF-Garches used in conjunction with the Orthofix Limb Reconstruction System.

Aetiology	(n)	Age y/m	Discrepancy mm	Lengthening mm	Lengthening %	Dynamization C1	Dynamization C2
Non Acquired:							
Congenital	20	10.8	78	59	28	8	12
Syndrome	10	14.8	–	70	27.6	0	10
Dystrophic	1	12.0	45	45	16	0	1
Acquired:							
Neurological	13	13.3	47	41	14	8	5
Traumatological	2	16.6	50	45	14	0	2
Infectious	1	13.6	45	45	14	0	1
Total* or Mean	47*	12.9	63.5	55.2	22.7	16*	31*

Table 43.1 Aetiology of Discrepancy in Leg Length, Amount of Lengthening and Type of Dynamization in 47 Lengthenings in 40 Patients (19 Males, 21 Females). C1: Classical Dynamization; C2: using a Dyna-Ring.

distally in 3, and proximally only in 2. In 16 lengthenings, dynamization followed the protocol of De Bastiani and Aldegheri,[1,7] with loosening of the central body locking nut after one month of neutralization.

In the final 31 lengthenings, a Dyna-Ring dynamization collar was applied after one month of neutralization. This attaches to the male portion of the lengthener. It incorporates a silicone cushion and permits limited micromovement of up to 2mm on weightbearing. The newly formed callus may thus be dynamized during walking without fear that it will collapse. The Dyna-Ring was removed when the callus appeared solid enough for full dynamization to begin.

Complications were divided into four groups according to their severity, as proposed by Caton:[5] no complications; benign complications necessitating treatment without anaesthesia or a second operation; serious complications necessitating a second operation under anaesthesia, and severe complications resulting in permanent sequelae or discontinuation of lengthening. All complications encountered are shown in Table 43.7. It is imperative to detail complications in this way when reporting on a series of lengthenings as it is the only way in which different series of patients or different techniques can be reliably compared.

Results

Intra-operative Complications

Four complications in 3 patients were related to the operative technique. In case 18, there was malpositioning of the lengthener in the metaphysis, with valgus deviation and segmental translation. The device was re-sited, but the result was a consolidated valgus deformity requiring further operative correction. In case 52, one of the upper screws was too close to the patellar tendon and required re-siting 3 days after the first operation. In cases 60 and 61 (in the same patient), palsy of the peroneal nerve was discovered on the day after operation; it was due to compression from a plaster splint, and recovered without sequel.

Infections

Infection-related complications were mostly pin track infections, which responded to local treatment. The number of infections cited is probably an underestimate because some minor infections were not documented. A more serious infection (case 16) in the form of arthritis of the ankle, resulted from a pin used to stabilize the foot during lengthening in a patient with agenesis of the fibula; this infection resolved without sequelae after removal of the pin and drainage.

Screw-related Complications

Two screw-related complications were noted: one proximal screw was forced further into the bone than intended as a result of a fall (case 2), and one proximal screw fractured after a lengthening of 45mm (case 16). The screws in question were replaced.

Neurological Complications

Three patients (cases 10, 11, and 16), had parasthesia of the peroneal nerve during the lengthening period. After decreasing the daily amount of lengthening in these patients, the symptoms resolved.

Aetiology	Classical dynamization (n)	mm	Days	HI	Dyna Ring dynamization (n)	mm	Days	HI
Congenital	8	66.6	250	39.1	12	54.3	180.6	34.5
Syndrome	0	-	-	-	10	69.7	226	33.7
Dystrophic	0	-	-	-	1	45	218	49
Neurological	8	41.0	216	52.3	5	41.2	168	41.2
Traumatological	0	-	-	-	2	45	178	39
Infection	0	-	-	-	1	45	126	28
Total* or Mean	16*	53.8	233	45.7	31*	55.8	192.8	34.6

Table 43.2 Comparison of length of treatment (days) and healing index (HI) according to aetiology and type of dynamization used.

Complications		Benign (n)	Serious (n)	Severe (n)
Intraoperative				
	Screws	0	2	0
	Neurological(*)	2	0	0
Elongation period				
	Screws	4	2	0
	Sepsis from foot pin	0	1	0
	Distractor	0	0	0
	Neurological	3	0	0
	Vascular	0	0	0
	Knee (Flexion)	3	4	0
	Foot (Equinus)	0	2	0
	Deviation	2	5**	0
	Premature fusion of fibula	1	8	0
	Mental	2***	0	0
Consolidation period				
	Delayed fusion	0	1*	0
	Non-union	0	0	0
	Deviation at the callus site	0	2	0
	Fracture of the callus	0	1	0
Delayed complications				
	Fracture	0	1	0
Total complications		17	29	0

Table 43.3 Complications in 47 lengthenings.

(*) In the same patient , a posterior splint applied immediately after the procedure led to a peroneal nerve compression; this recovered without sequel.

(**) Two were due to premature fusion of fibula.

(***) In the same patient undergoing a bilateral lengthening.

Knee and Foot Contractures

Flexion deformity of the knee occurred in 7 instances during lengthening, despite daily application of a posterior splint. Three of these were readily reduced conservatively. In 2, a low level fracture of the femur occurred when reduction was attempted (cases 12 and 26). In cases 37 and 38, surgical release of the gastrocnemius muscle resolved the problem. In one patient equinus deformity of both feet was corrected by lengthening the Achilles tendon (cases 35, 36). Other equinus deformities of the foot responded to manipulation and support.

Errors of Deviation

Deviation is important and is the most frequent complication associated with leg lengthening. We had no cases of anterior or posterior bowing, or of varus deviation of the tibia, even when treatment went on for a long time. Seven cases of valgus deviation occurred during lengthening. Six patients had some degree of valgus deviation initially, which was made worse by lengthening, and in one patient the valgus deviation resulted from poor positioning of the implant (case 18).

Three patients (6 lengthenings) had severe varus deviation before lengthening (cases 25, 26, 37, 38, 46, 47). Lengthening was commenced on the tenth day following osteotomy, maintaining the initial deviation; correction of varus was then achieved by a medial elongation, of at least the predicted amount of lengthening. In 4 cases premature fusion of the fibula led to an overcorrection into valgus: in cases 37, 38, 61 a re-osteotomy of the fibula was performed; in case 60, a spontaneous chondrodiatasis of the upper fibular growth plate resulted in progressive correction of the

	Cases	None		Benign		Serious		Severe	
Aetiology	(n)	(n)	(%)	(n)	(%)	(n)	(%)	(n)	(%)
Congenital	20	10	50	5	25	5	25	0	0
Syndrome	10	1	10	2	20	7	70	0	0
Dystrophic	1	1	100	0	0	0	0	0	0
Neurological	13	5	40	3	23	5	37	0	0
Traumatological	2	0	0	0	0	2	100	0	0
Infectious	1	1	100	0	0	0	0	0	0
Total* or mean %	47*	18*	38	10*	21	19*	41	0*	0

Table 43.4 Number of patients (%) exhibiting complications of varying severity during the operative stage or during the elongation period, according to the aetiology of their condition.

	Cases	None		Benign		Serious		Severe	
Aetiology	(n)	(n)	(%)	(n)	(%)	(n)	(%)	(n)	(%)
Congenital	20	18	90	0	0	2	10	0	0
Syndrome	10	9	90	0	0	1	10	0	0
Dystrophic	1	1	100	0	0	0	0	0	0
Neurological	13	11	85	0	0	2	15	0	0
Traumatological	2	2	100	0	0	0	0	0	0
Infectious	1	1	100	0	0	0	0	0	0
Total	47	42	89	0	0	5	11	0	0

Table 43.5 Number of patients exhibiting complications of varying severity during the consolidation period or after the completion of programmme according to the aetiology of their condition.

valgus. In all cases, the initial deviation was completely corrected and the predicted lengthening achieved.

Seven valgus deviations occurred during lengthening. These were corrected using the angular correction facility on 4 occasions (with repeated fibular sectioning in cases 19 and 27). Three were only partially corrected and later required osteotomy (cases 3, 10 and 18).

Problems with Consolidation

In one case the callus fractured when the lengthener was removed; this was in a girl with fibular agenesis (case 44) who was undergoing a fourth lengthening of the same tibia. Application of a new device without exposing the fracture site was followed by consolidation within 3 months. In case 39, delayed union required bone grafting. In cases 36 and 42, we observed a valgus deviation at the callus site during the months following removal of the lengthener; these patients required re-operation.

Healing Time

The mean healing time, from application of the lengthener until its removal, or until treatment of a complication was completed, was 206 days (i.e., nearly 7 months). The Healing Index, as described by De Bastiani et al[7] was 39 days per cm. lengthened. This varied, however, according to whether classic dynamization or the Dyna-Ring was used.

With classic dynamization (16 cases), the healing index was 45.7 days per cm. lengthened, while in cases treated with the Dyna-Ring it was 34.6 days (treatment time 193 days for a mean lengthening of 55.8mm) (Table 43.2).

The healing index is clearly better with the Dyna-Ring method than with the classical method and the difference is significant ($P = 0.0036$).

Total Complications

Complications were frequent; 46 occurred in 47 lengthenings, (Table 43.3). Often, however, multiple interrelated complications occurred in the same patient (see Table 43.7).

In 18 cases there were no complications and in 10 there was only one benign complication. In 19, there was at least one serious complication necessitating a further operation under general anesthesia (Tables 43.4, 43.5).

In this series, 26 of 47 lengthenings (55 per cent) required little or no variation in the treatment schedule previously outlined to the parents, but 45 per cent of the lengthenings were accompanied by a complication that required a second unscheduled operation.

Lengthening of a tibia in which the growth plate was still open did not result in persistent deviation, and to date no accidental damage to the growth cartilage has been identified as a result of longstanding genu recurvatum.

Discussion

Consolidation of a progressively lengthened tibia has often been the dominant theme in studies of this kind, with fractures and non-unions generally considered to be the major complications. Anderson[2] suggested using a rigid frame; Wagner[20] advocates grafting, and Judet and Euvrard[8] used decortication in lengthening procedures. Merle d'Aubigné and Dubousset[10] recommended delayed lengthening in a "decortication sheath" whereas Ilizarov, as described by Sollogoub[19] stressed the importance of respecting the medullary vascularization and of conferring elasticity by a circular, semirigid frame. De Bastiani et al[7] base their approach on callotasis with delayed lengthening and dynamization.

Is the high metaphyseal callotasis of the tibia used in this series associated with fewer problems than the techniques previously used? To answer this question, we compared our complications with those reported in the major published studies (Table 43.6), and particularly with Damsin's multicentre series[5] of 57 lengthenings using the Ilizarov technique.

The incidence of neurological complications varied from 3 per cent in the series reported by Rigault et al,[18] to 46 per cent in that reported by Carlioz et al using the Wagner technique.[4] These variations probably result from differences in clinical assessment of the paralysis. The incidence of nervous complications (12 per cent) in Damsin's Ilizarov series[5] was the same as that in our own, but there were three persistent sequelae in Damsin's series, whereas there were none in ours.

The incidence of vascular complications in the literature is also extremely variable, ranging from 2 to 15 per cent.[9,12,15] As we stressed in a pilot study[14] and subsequently in our series of 108 tibial lengthenings by the Judet method,[13] vascular complications are not readily identified unless they are serious, with immediate onset. In Damsin's series,[5] as in our previous series,[16,17] an ischaemic syndrome leading to permanent paralysis was reported. The technique we used then involved scraping the upper tibial metaphysis, with the risk of damage to the tibio-fibular vascular

Authors	Kawamura	Coleman	Bijan	Carlioz	Rigault	Pouliquen	Aldegheri	Damsin	Pouliquen
Reference	9	6	3	4	18	13	1	5	this series
Technique	Anderson	Anderson Wagner	Anderson Wagner	Wagner	Judet Wagner	Judet	Orthofix*	Ilizarov	T Orthofix
Cases (n)	74	78	141	13	48	108	121	57	47
Neurological c.	32	7	?	46	3	22	?	12	12
Vascular c.	?	15	?	8	?	8	?	2	0
Benign cutaneous c.	?	26	20	23	?	58	?	14	9
Serious cutaneous c.	?	4	?	0	10	7	?	2	4.5
Serious deep infect.	?	0	?	0	3	2	?	0	0
Knee flexion	?	12	4	15	18	9	?	2	14
Equinus foot	32	21	16	77	42	70	?	21	4.5
Deviation	?	44	4	38	35	24	?	10	10
Fracture	15	23	4	8	11	7	?	10	2
Non-union	13	22	16	?	17	4	?	3	6
Healing index (days/cm)	?	?	?	?	?	48	42	42	39

c. = complications
Except cases and healing index all numbers are per cent.
* This series did not separate femoral and tibial lengthenings.

Table 43.6 Review of literature

bifurcation, but in our present series, there were no vascular complications.

Cutaneous complications are all pin-related. Minor complications are frequent in all series, but serious cutaneous complications are less common, peaking at below 10 per cent in the series of Rigault et al , in which both Judet and Wagner fixators were used.[18] True osteotomy site infections are non-existent with the Ilizarov technique, as stressed by Monte and Donzelli.[11] The same is true of the technique of callotasis used in our series.

Flexion deformity of the knee and equinus deformity of the foot are reported in all studies, with rates varying according to the assessment criteria used. The relative frequency of these two complications in the Ilizarov series[5] (genu flexum 2 per cent, equinus 21 per cent) was the reverse of that in our own series (genu flexum 14 per cent, equinus 4.5 per cent). The level of the tibial osteotomy, and thus the site of lengthening, is the probable cause of this difference. The more distal osteotomy of the Ilizarov technique has a greater effect on the soleus muscle, with more tendency to equinus and restriction of ankle movement. The higher osteotomy used in our technique affects mainly the gastrocnemius muscle, with a greater tendency to flexion deformity of the knee. The severity of these complications is not the same in the two series: 13 serious and two severe complications (23 per cent) in the Ilizarov series as compared with 6 serious and no severe complications in our own (8.5 per cent). These differences must, however, be viewed in the context of the substantial mean lengthening achieved (67mm) in the Ilizarov series versus 55.8mm in ours.

Valgus deviation of the tibia was a common complication in the series reported by Coleman and Stevens,[6] Carlioz et al,[4] and Rigault et al,[18] as well as in our earlier series of lengthenings by the Judet technique.[13] Our new techniques, with modular implants capable of correcting the deviation, reduced the incidence of this complication to 10 per cent at the end of the program in our present series. The cause of the 7 valgus deviations in our series was prior valgus deformity in 6 cases, one of them worsened by an initial error in technique and 6 worsened due to lengthening and/or as a result of fibular consolidation (2 cases). We need to prevent worsening of a pre-existing valgus and, when premature fusion occurs, to achieve

	Case	2	4	6	7	8	12	14	17	19	23	24	25	28	30	31	32	33	40	43	44	29	34
	Sex	F	F	M	F	F	M	M	M	M	M	M	M	F	F	M	F	M	M	M	F	F	F
	Age/years	9	4	15	8	14	15	7	10	6	10	14	12	15	7	6	11	10	16	13	14	12	14
	Aetiology	C	C	C	C	C	C	C	C	C	C	C	C	C	C	C	C	C	C	C	C	D	I
	Number of lengthenings	1	1	3	2	3	1	1	1	1	1	1	2	1	2	2	3	2	2	1	4	1	1
	Predicted discrepancy	70	120	50	80	60	75	70	190	50	40	40	120	45	100	150	80	45	35	60	70	45	45
	Predicted lengthening	50	70	50	60	60	75	65	60	50	45	40	75	45	65	75	50	45	35	55	50	45	40
Technique	Device	TG	TG	TG	TG	TG	TG	TG	TG	TG	TG	TG	TG	TG	TG	TG	TG	TG	TG	TG	TG	TG	TG
	Dynamization	C1	C1	C1	C1	C1	C1	C1	C1	C2	C2	C2	C2	C2	C2	C2	C2	C2	C2	C2	C2	C2	C2
Intra-operative Complications	Fixator-Screws																						
	Bone																						
	Soft tissues																						
Elongation period	Screws	dark grey (3)							grey										grey				
	Fixator																						
	Neurological																						
	Vascular																						
	Knee		grey	grey			dark grey												grey				
	Foot																						
	Deviation				grey													dark grey					
	Others							dark grey (1)															
	Fibular fusion									dark grey								dark grey					
Consolidation period	Delayed fusion																						
	Non-Union																						
	Refracture																				dark grey		
	Compl + deviation																						
	Others																						
Delayed complications																	dark grey (2)						
General	Mental																						
	No benefit																						
Data	Lengthening/mm	50	108	60	65	53	72	65	60	50	45	40	72	45	65	90	55	45	35	55	55	45	45
	Lengthening/ %	25	40	18	38	17	23	41	60	31	18	12	34	13	50	42	24	18	9	19	20	16	14
	Healing index (cm/day)	42	26	48	26	49	43	34	44	33.6	35	24	25	30	42.3	20	40.5	33	51	30	48	48.5	28
	Waiting (days)	17	14	10	17	9	15	15	12	11	11	10	10	11	12	10	13	10	10	10	13	10	10
	Elongation (days)	63	126	72	69	59	77	72	69	56	51	43	82	49	75	118	62	53	42	63	62	51	52
	Fusion (days)	130	141	206	83	192	218	134	183	101	95.5	43	88	75	188	52	148	85.5	127	90	188	157	64
	Total for treatment (days)	210	281	288	169	260	310	221	264	168	158	96	180	135	275	180	223	149	179	163	263	218	126

Table 43.7a Schematic summary of cases. Part A

White square = no complication; grey square = benign complication; dark grey square = serious complication; black square = severe complication. F = Female, M = Male. C = congenital, D = dystrophic, I = infection, N = neurological, S = short stature, T = traumatic; TG = OF-Garches. C1 = Classic Dynamization, C2 = Dyna-Ring used.

Number of lengthenings: 1 = first lengthening, 2 = second lengthening, etc.

(1) septic arthritis of ankle by a pin. (2) Tibial fracture 3 months later at the site of a half-pin track. (3) Due to a fall.

Case	1	3	5	9	10	11	13	15	18	22	39	42	45	20	21	26	27	35	36	37	38	46	47	16	41
Sex	M	F	F	F	F	M	M	F	F	F	F	F	F	F	F	F	F	M	M	M	M	F	F	M	M
Age/years	15	12	11	16	13	12	12	15	12	10	16	14	15	16	16	13	13	18	18	14	14	13	13	17	16
Aetiology	N	N	N	N	N	N	N	N	N	N	N	N	N	S	S	S	S	S	S	S	S	S	S	T	T
Number of lengthenings	2	1	1	1	1	1	1	1	1	1	1	1	1	1	1	1	1	1	1	1	1	1	1	1	1
Predicted discrepancy	50	40	50	40	30	60	60	45	50	45	45	45	50	-	-	-	-	-	-	-	-	-	-	50	50
Predicted lengthening	40	35	40	35	35	50	50	45	40	45	40	40	50	-	-	-	-	-	-	-	-	-	-	40	50
Device	TG	TG	TG	TG	TG	TG	TG	TG	TG	TG	TG	TG	TG	TG	TG	TG	TG	TG	TG	TG	TG	TG	TG	TG	TG
Dynamization	C1	C1	C1	C1	C1	C1	C1	C1	C2	C2	C2	C2	C2	C2	C2	C2	C2	C2	C2	C2	C2	C2	C2	C2	C2
Fixator-Screws																									
Bone																									
Soft tissues																									
Screws																									
Fixator																									
Neurological																									
Vascular																									
Knee																									
Foot																									
Deviation																									
Others																									
Fibular fusion																									
Delayed fusion																									
Non-Union																									
Refracture																									
Compl + deviation																									
Others																									
Delayed complications																									
Mental																									
No benefit																									
Lengthening/mm	45	35	38	35	35	50	50	40	40	45	40	45	35	70	70	60	60	85	85	90	90	30	55	40	50
Lengthening/ %	13	12	15	9	11	19	19	12	14	18	11	14	14	21	21	23	23	30	30	48	48	16	16	14	14
Healing index (cm/day)	37	48	55	44	54	82	38	61	43	40	45	37	41	37	37	30	30	31	31	27	27	62	34	32	45.8
Waiting (days)	15	15	15	10	15	14	17	10	10	11	10	10	10	10	10	10	10	10	10	11	11	10	10	10	10
Elongation (days)	51	41	40	40	39	56	55	48	42	49	47	51	41	82	82	72	72	99	99	111	111	35	65	46	57
Fusion (days)	101	112	154	104	135	340	118	185	120	120	123	106	94	167	167	98	98	155	155	121	121	142	112	72	162
Total for treatment (days)	167	168	209	154	189	410	190	243	172	180	180	167	145	259	259	180	180	264	264	243	243	187	187	128	229

Table 43.7b Schematic summary of cases. Part B.

See legends, table 7a

In case 46, healing index is 62 days/cm versus 34 in the other side (47) as lengtheners were both removed at the same time.

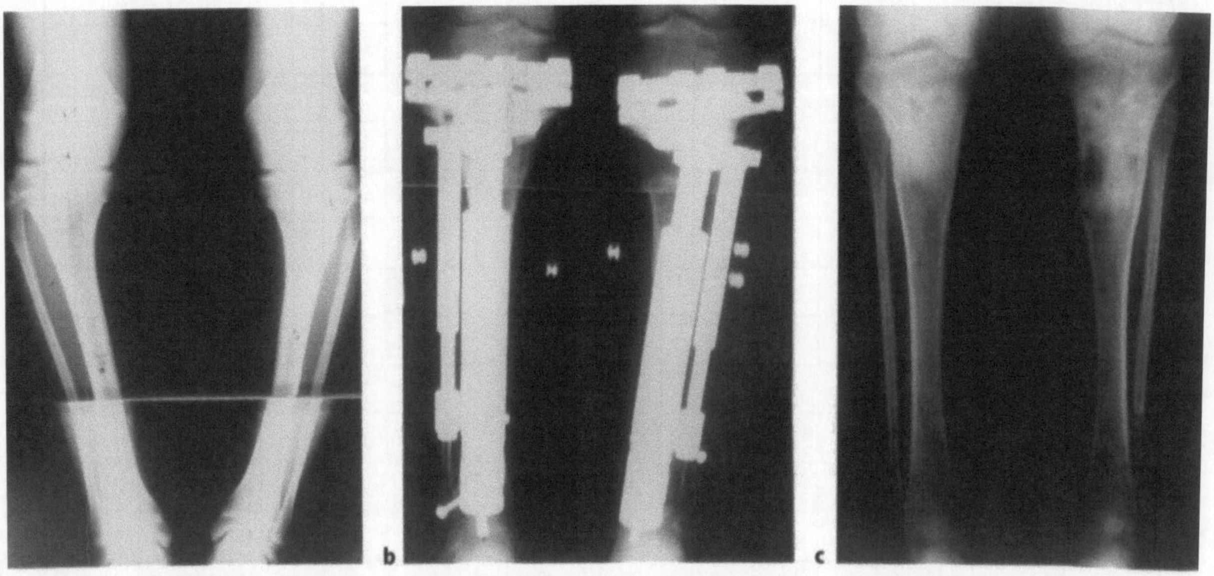

Fig. 43.4 Bilateral tibial lengthening in a 13-year-old girl with dyschondrosteosis. a Pre-operative varus deviation, short tibiae, unequal in length. b During treatment; correction of varus deviation in progress. c Final result: The amount of lengthening achieved was 30mm on the right side (Case 46) and 55mm on the left side (Case 47).

correction possibly by means of repeated fibular osteotomy, as advocated by Aldegheri et al.[1]

Use of the Orthofix OF-Garches allowed simple correction of valgus in 12 of 15 cases, limiting the need for subsequent tibial osteotomy. A high metaphyseal osteotomy rather than a diaphyseal osteotomy allows straightforward correction during the lengthening procedure (Fig. 43.3). This site has additional advantages if a second operation is needed since consolidation occurs more rapidly in the metaphysis than in the diaphysis. All six varus deformities were realigned and led to a straight tibia.

Consolidation of the lengthening site resulted in complications in only four cases: 1 fracture, 1 non-union and 2 with plastic callus (8.5 per cent). We attribute this highly satisfactory result partly to callotasis in conjunction with dynamization, and partly to the width and rapid organization of the callus at the high metaphyseal site used (Fig. 43.4). The improvement in outcome is striking when these results are compared with those of earlier series, even those of Damsin, who reported 13 per cent of complications associated with consolidation. When our overall results are pooled, the Healing Index is approximately the same as that obtained by Aldegheri et al[1] with high diaphyseal callotasis and by Damsin[5] with the Ilizarov technique.

Dynamization with the Dyna-Ring, in contrast, resulted in an improvement of 22 per cent in the healing index. The relatively small proportion of lengthening without complications is similar to that of other series and comparable to that reported by Caton[5] in a multicenter Wagner study. The proportion of lengthenings with slight or no variation in the preset treatment schedule was 55 per cent in our series and 54 per cent in Damsin's Ilizarov series.[5] These figure demonstrate clearly that even with a good technique and an experienced surgeon, tibial lengthening is a difficult undertaking.

The various series in the literature are not homogeneous. Earlier series included many lengthenings for the sequelae of poliomyelitis, whereas the more recent studies included many congenital or short stature cases. Moreover, several studies include femoral and tibial lengthenings in the same article. Comparison is therefore difficult. Rigault et al[18] stress the need to assess results according to aetiology. Our series makes it possible to compare the incidence of benign and serious complications in patients with differing aetiologies of disease (Tables 43.4 and 43.5). Forty per cent of patients were lengthened without any complications; 35 per cent of patients with a congenital discrepancy, 50 per cent of patients with neurological disease and 80 per cent of the patients with short stature had a serious complication either in the lengthening phase or in the consolidation phase. Our experience, therefore, does not suggest that tibial lengthening is easier in cases of neurological origin than in congenital cases.

Conclusions

Complications occurring during lengthening or after its completion have decreased with the advent of the newer techniques introduced by Ilizarov and De Bastiani and with the use of a modular implant allowing satisfactory control of axial deviation as well as callus maturation and mineralization.

The application of callotasis to tibial lengthening, with the facility for axial correction in the frontal plane, and a very high osteotomy, produced better results than those described in previously published series. The ease of application, good tolerance of the device, and minimal inconvenience to the patient, together with the axial micromovement permitted by the Dyna-Ring attachment, represent major improvements over other approaches. The method and the device can be used for most tibial lengthenings, and we believe, therefore, that the Ilizarov circular frame is appropriate in very few situations.

References

1. Aldegheri R, Renzi Brivio L, Agostini S. 'The callotasis method of limb lengthening.' *Clin Orthop* 1989; 241: 137–45.
2. Anderson M. 'Leg lengthening.' *J Bone Joint Surg* [Am] 1952; 34A: 150.
3. Bijan A, Akbarnia BA, Ghobadi F, Ganjavian M-S, Nasseri D. 'Experience of 141 tibial lengthenings and comparison of three methods.' *Clin Orthop* 1979; 145: 150-3.
4. Carlioz H, Pichon F, Barthelemy A, Lebard J P, Filipe G. 'Allongements progressifs selon la technique de Wagner. Résultats des 30 premiers cas.' *Rev Chir Orthop* 1980; 66: 473–83.
5. Caton J. Symposium, 65th SOFCOT Meeting, Paris. 'Traitement des inégalités de longueur des membres inférieurs et des sujets de petite taille chez l'enfant et l'adolescent.' *Rev Chir Orthop* 1991 ;77 (suppl 1): 32–80.
6. Coleman S, Stevens PM. 'Leg lengthening.' *Clin Orthop* 1978; 136: 92–104.
7. De Bastiani G, Aldegheri R, Renzi Brivio L, Trivella GP. 'Limb lengthening by callus distraction (callotasis).' *J Pediatr Orthop* 1987; 7: 129–34.
8. Judet R, Euvrard J. 'Inégalités de longueur des membres inférieurs.' *Act Orthop Hopital R Poincare* 1969; vol VII: 10–35.
9. Kawamura B. 'Limb lengthening. Experimental and clinical studies.' *J Bone Joint Surg* [Am] 1968; 50A: 851–77.
10. Merle D'Aubigné, R, Dubousset J. 'Correction des grandes inégalités des membres inférieurs avec ou sans correction simultanée des déviations latérales.' *Rev Chir Orthop* 1968; 54: 561–93.
11. Monte A D, Donzelli O. 'Comparison of differents methods of leg lengthening.' *J Pediatr Orthop* 1988; 8: 62–4.
12. Pouliquen J C. 'Allongement de membres.' *Ann Chir* 1989; 43: 329–33.
13. Pouliquen J C, Beneux J, Verneret C, Hardy J, Mener G. 'Allongement du tibia selon la methode de Judet. A propos de 108 cas chez l'enfant.' *Rev Chir Orthop* 1984; 70: 29–39.
14. Pouliquen J C, Chaboche P, Penneìot GF, Bergue A. 'Etude expérimentale du retentissement sur le cartilage de croissance et des parties molles de l'allongement progressif du fémur chez le lapin en période de croissance.' *Chir Pediatr* 1980; 21: 363–7.
15. Pouliquen J C, Gorodischer S, Verneret C, Richard L. 'Femoral lengthening in children and adolescents. A comparative study of 82 cases.' *Fr J Orthop Surg* 1989; 3: 162–73.
16. Pouliquen J C, Céolin J L, Langlais J, Pauthier F. 'Upper metaphyseal lengthening of the tibia by callotasis. Forty-seven cases in children and adolescents.' *J Pediatr Orthop* Part B, 1993; 2: 49–56.
17. Pouliquen J C, Glorion C., Céolin J L, Langlais J, and Pauthier F. 'Allongement métaphysaire supérieur du tibia. 57 cas effectués par la méthode du callotasis chez l'enfant et l'adolescent.' *Rev Chir Orthop* (in press)
18. Rigault P, Dolz G, Padovani J P, Touzet P, Mallet J F, Finidori G, Raux P. 'L'allongement progressif du tibia chez l'enfant. A propos de quarante-huit cas.' *Rev Chir Orthop* 1981; 67: 461–72.
19. Sollogoub I. *La méthode d'Ilizarov appliquée aux allongements des membres inférieurs chez l'enfant.* Thèse Medecine: Tours, 1986.
20. Wagner H. 'Operative Beinverlangerung.' *Chirurg* 1971; 42: 260–6.

Bifocal Lengthening

44

N. Yasui

Lengthening a single bone segment at two separate sites (bifocal lengthening) was first described by Ilizarov.[1] Three bony fragments produced by two metaphyseal corticotomies were held by a circular external fixator with a transfixing cross-tension wire system.[2] Although this frame was rather bulky, it was appreciated that bifocal lengthening procedures could offer a number of advantages over monofocal procedures; each lengthened segment is smaller, consolidation is faster and less tension is generated in the soft tissues.

Recently, more sophisticated external fixation devices have been developed to enable bifocal lengthening procedures to be carried out more conveniently.[3,4] The Orthofix Limb Reconstruction System (LRS) is a rigid monolateral fixator originally designed for segmental bone transport. The device can carry three separate clamps and is perfectly suitable for bifocal lengthening of the tibia and the femur. It is less bulky and more stable than the circular system and is well tolerated by the patient.

There is a knack, however, in using the monolateral device for limb lengthening. One should appreciate that the bone has a gradual tendency to deviate during lengthening.[3,5] The direction of deviation depends on the bone involved and the level of the osteotomy. When the proximal tibia is lengthened, for example, the bone tends to go into valgus and procurvatum as a result of opposing forces engendered by the lengthener antero-medially and the bulk of the calf musculature postero-laterally (Fig. 44.1). This valgus deviation of the tibia may be prevented by pre-setting the bone in slight varus at operation.[3,6]

The present author has been using bifocal lengthening primarily in patients with achondroplasia who have redundant soft tissues. This chapter describes the operative techniques of bifocal tibial lengthening using the Orthofix LRS. The principle of the method is based on the "callotasis" technique described by De Bastiani et al,[2,7] but the practical aspects have been modified by the current author.

Pre-operative Planning

Prior to surgery, the size of the bone to be lengthened is estimated radiographically using the slit scanogram[8] or by subtracting the 10–15 per cent magnification factor from the normal X-ray measurement. The Standard LRS is suitable for bones more than 20cm in length. For smaller bones in patients less than 12 years of age, a

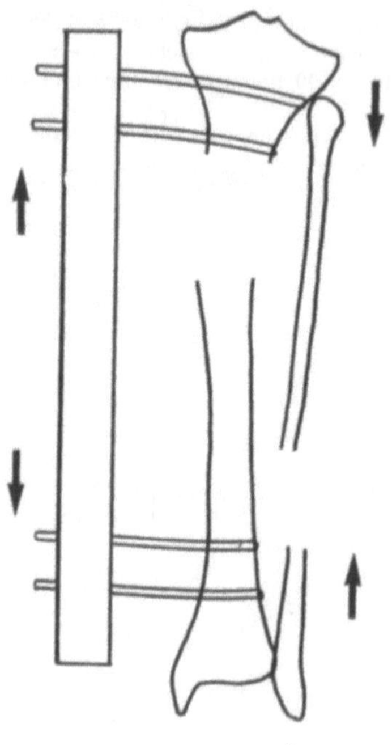

Fig. 44.1 The tibia has a tendency to go into valgus during lengthening.

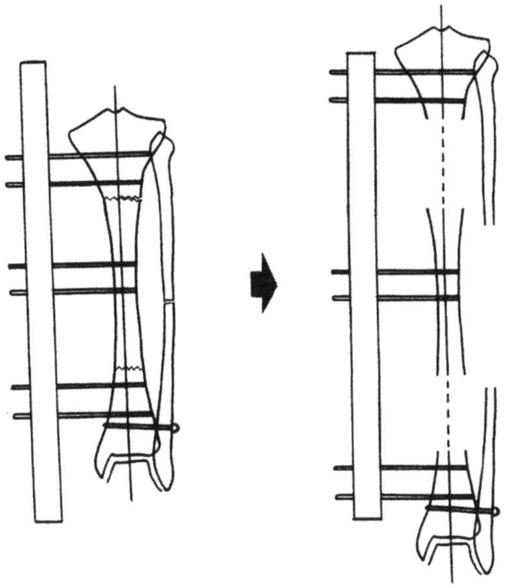

Fig. 44.2 The pre-operative plan is traced on the radiograph. Note that the bone is lengthened parallel to the body of the device.

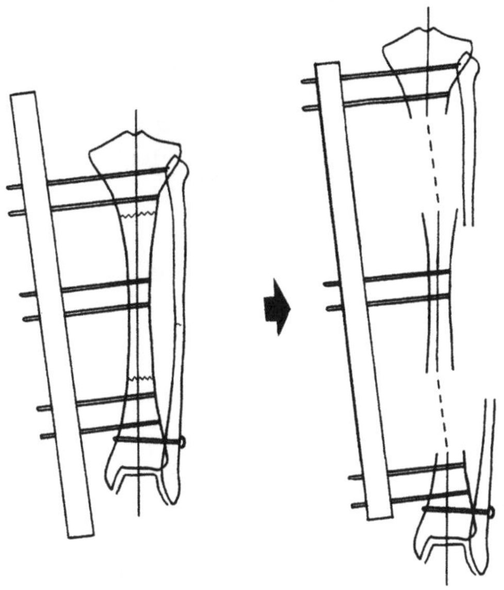

Fig. 44.3 Oblique application of the device causes oblique lengthening.

Paediatric Limb Reconstruction System is available.

The levels of screw insertion and the position of the osteotomy are traced on the radiograph pre-operatively. For a simple axial lengthening, the body of the monolateral lengthener should be placed parallel to the mechanical axis of the bone, so that the alignment of the limb does not change during lengthening (Figs. 44.2, 44.3). The alignment of the lengthened segment is thus predicted on the figure.

Operative Technique

The operation is performed under general anaesthesia in the following sequence; (1) insertion of the screws, (2) osteotomy of the fibula, (3) fixation of the fibula to the tibia, (4) double-level osteotomy of the tibia, and (5) application of the lengthening device.

1. Insertion of the Screws

The LRS with three clamps is applied to the antero-medial aspect of the tibia with six self-tapping screws (two in each clamp). In the original De Bastiani technique for standard monofocal lengthening, a rigid template was used as a guide to insert the individual screws parallel to one another and in the same plane.[2] The author, however, found that the commercially available template for bifocal lengthening allows substantial play between the template and the screw guide, the screw guide and the drill guide, and the drill guide and the drill. As a result, screws may occasionally be placed incorrectly. The author therefore uses the actual lengthening device as a template for exact pre-drilling and screw insertion (Fig. 44.4). There is much less play in this system because the individual screw guides are held directly in the definitive clamp. A swivelling clamp is used to hold the proximal two screw guides at an angle of 5° to the others. This slight tilt of the proximal two guides causes the tibia to be pre-set in slight varus and prevents valgus deviation of the bone during lengthening.

Under image intensifier control, a 3.2mm drill is inserted through the most proximal drill guide which is sited 2cm inferior to the tibial plateau. Drilling is performed while the assistant keeps the body of the device parallel to the long axis of the tibia (Fig. 44.5). This drill bit is left in situ in the drill guide and a second drill (4.8mm) is inserted through the most distal drill guide, perpendicular to the tibial axis (Fig. 44.6). The second drill bit is also left in situ in the drill guide and the remainder of the holes drilled using a (4.8mm) drill bit (Fig. 44.7).

The proximal 3.2mm drill bit is then removed and replaced by a self-tapping cancellous screw. The self-tapping cortical screws are then inserted in order (Fig. 44.8). In this manner, individual screws are placed exactly in the same plane on the antero-medial aspect

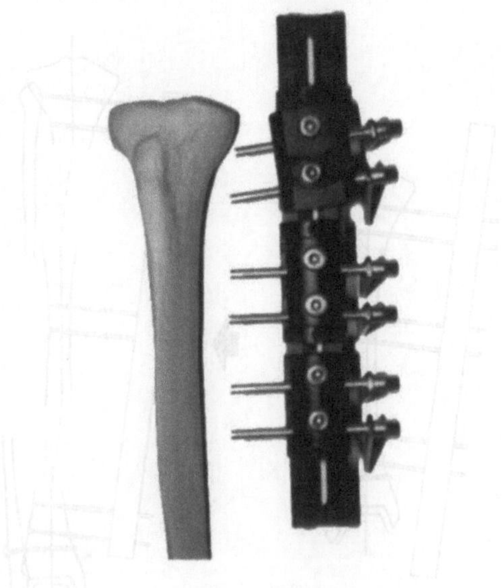

Fig. 44.4 Use of the lengthening device itself as a template.

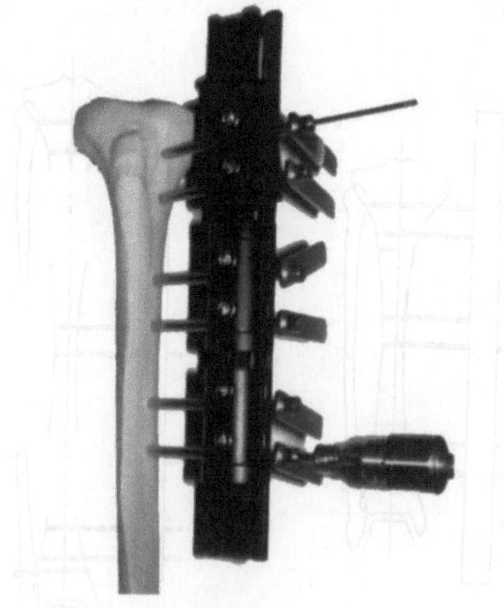

Fig. 44.6 With one drill bit still in situ in the most proximal hole, the most distal hole is now drilled.

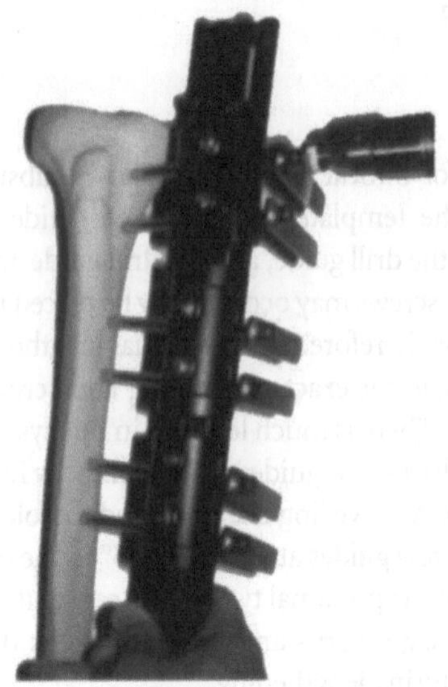

Fig. 44.5 Drilling the most proximal hole.

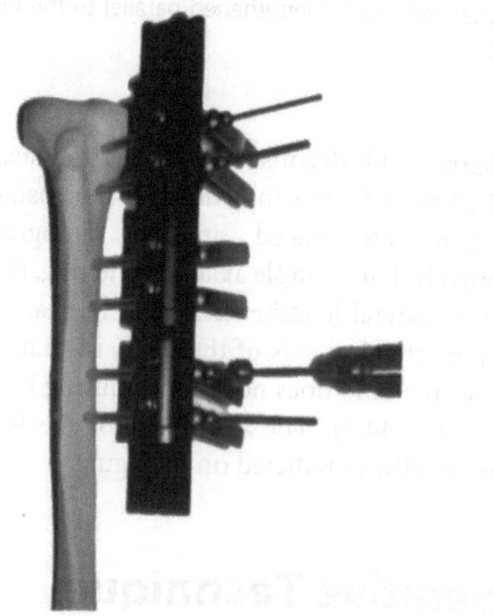

Fig. 44.7 The remaining holes are drilled.

of the tibia, and the proximal two screws have a tilt of 5° in relation the other screws (Fig. 44.8).

2. Osteotomy of the Fibula

The lengthening device is removed and osteotomy of the fibula performed in a bloodless field using a pneumatic tourniquet. In the original De Bastiani technique for monofocal tibial lengthening, a 2cm segment of the diaphysis in the distal third of the fibula was excised.[2,7] The object here is to avoid premature consolidation of the fibular osteotomy and to prevent proximal migration of the lateral malleolus during lengthening. The author prefers a simple osteotomy of the fibula in the mid-diaphysis using an oscillating saw with a thin blade. Instead of excising a segment of the bone, the distal fragment of the fibula is always fixed to the tibia with an AO screw (Fig. 44.11).

3. Fixation of the Fibula to the Tibia

With the ankle dorsiflexed 30°, a standard AO cortical screw with a diameter of 4.5mm is inserted through the fibula into the tibia percutaneously from a point 2cm above the lateral malleolus. The screw hole is pre-drilled with a 3.2mm drill and the thread is pre-cut

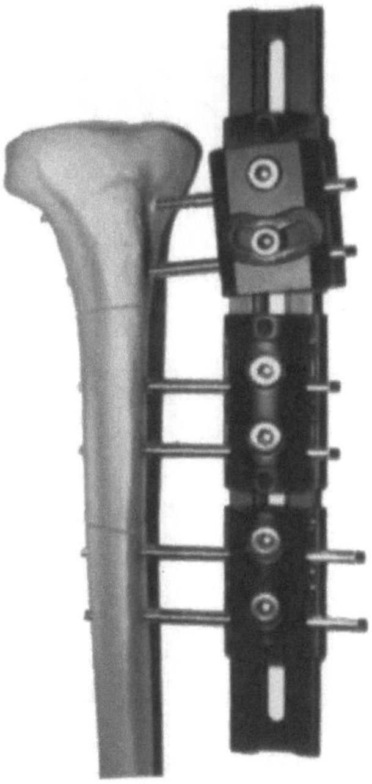

Fig. 44.8 All the screws in situ.

with a tapper. The tip of the screw reaches the medial cortex of the tibia (Fig. 44.11a).

When extensive lengthening of more than 10cm is planned, the proximal fibular fragment is also fixed to the tibia using a 2.4mm Steinmann pin (Fig. 44.11c). Under image intensifier control, the pin is inserted through the fibular head into the tibia. Great care should be taken to avoid damage to the common peroneal nerve which passes around the neck of the fibula. The prominent edge of the head of the fibula is the safe point for pin insertion. After the Steinmann pin has penetrated the medial cortex of the tibia and the skin, the tip of the pin is pulled forward until the blunt end reaches the fibular head and is buried under the skin.

4. Double Level Osteotomies of the Tibia

Two separate 2cm incisions are made on the anterior aspect of the tibia, one between the proximal and middle clamps and one between the distal and middle clamps. The periosteum is incised longitudinally, elevated and protected with thin retractors. Prior to osteotomy, the bone cortex is pre-drilled circumferentially to avoid the risk of crack formation. A 3.2mm drill is inserted into a short drill guide and placed on the anterior cortex. A series of holes is then drilled bicortically without any attempt to protect the intramedullary circulation. A drill stop is used, however, to prevent damage to the soft tissues beyond the posterior cortex. The osteotomy is accomplished by connecting the drill holes with a small chisel. Separation of the bone fragments is confirmed under image intensification, and the periosteum closed and sutured to cover the osteotomy.

5. Application of the Lengthening Device

Before the lengthening device is applied to the screws, the proximal swivelling clamp is removed and replaced by a straight clamp. All six screws are then clamped parallel to one another, thus pre-setting the proximal tibia in 5° of varus. (Fig. 44.9). The alignment of the bone and the body of the lengthener is checked radiologically. The separation of each osteotomy is confirmed during operation by gentle distraction using the compression-distraction units.

Post-operative Care

After a waiting period of eight days, distraction is commenced at a rate of 0.25mm/6 hours at each osteotomy site (Fig. 44.10). The separation of each tibial and fibular osteotomy is confirmed radiologically seven days from the start of distraction. The rate of distraction is gradually reduced as lengthening proceeds as shown in

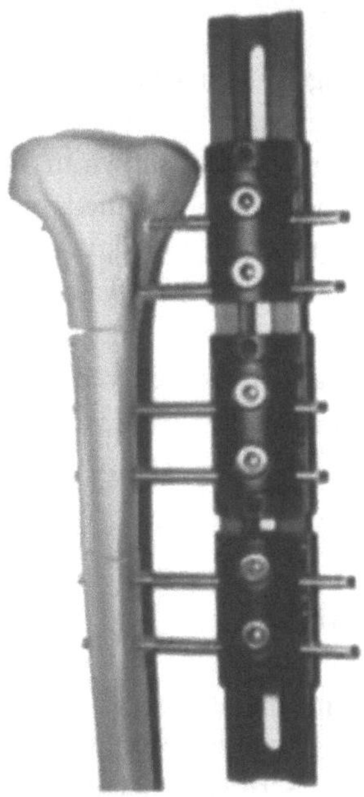

Fig. 44.9 All screws are clamped in parallel. Note that the proximal tibia is pre-set in 5° of varus.

Fig. 44.11. Thus, depending on the amount and quality of callus and the tension within the soft tissues, the rate of distraction will vary between 0.25mm/6 hours and 0.25mm/24 hours.[3] Early weightbearing is encouraged during the day and anti-equinovarus splints are applied at night (Fig. 44.12). Callus formation is monitored radiologically every three weeks. When the desired length has been achieved, the clamp locking screws on the proximal and distal clamps are locked, so that the lengthened segments are held in rigid fixation (neutralization) until signs of corticalization are evident. At this point the proximal and distal clamps are unlocked and dynamization of the lengthened segments begins. When solid union is confirmed, the screws are removed in a stepwise fashion (Fig. 44.11g).

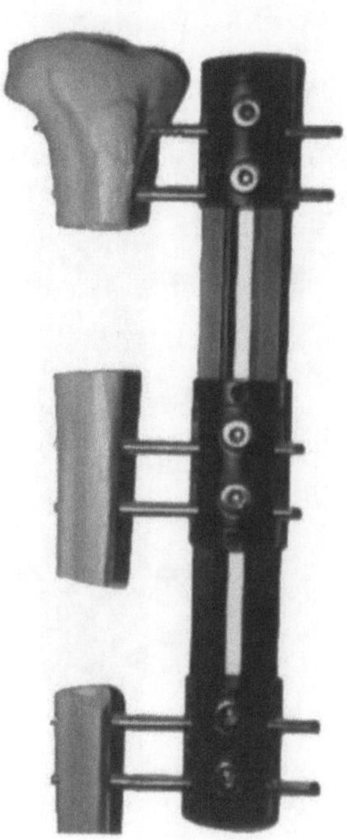

Fig. 44.10 Distraction at proximal and distal osteotomy sites.

Clinical Results

Since 1985, the present author has performed more than 250 limb lengthenings using monofocal procedures and various external fixators. In 1991, the Orthofix Limb Reconstruction System was introduced into Osaka Medical Centre and Research Institute for Maternal and Child Health. Since then, 27 limbs (23 tibiae and four femora) in 13 patients have been lengthened by bifocal procedures.

In eight patients with achondroplasia and two patients with hypochondroplasia, bilateral and bifocal tibial lengthening has been achieved. The mean age of these patients (eight male and two female) at operation was 13.1 years (range 10.5–16.0 years). The average increase in length achieved was 10.6cm (range 8–13cm). The average times for the various phases of the lengthening process are shown in Table 44.1. The Healing Index, which is obtained by dividing the overall treatment time (231 days) by the average increase in length (10.6cm) was 21.8. No major complications were encountered, although superficial pin-site inflammation was observed in most cases. The device and the procedures were well tolerated by the patients.

Discussion

In this chapter, the operative technique of bifocal tibial lengthening using the Orthofix Limb Reconstruction System has been described in detail. Based on the principle of "callotasis" described by De Bastiani et al,[2,7] various technical points have been modified: very precise drilling and screw insertion is performed using the actual lengthening device as a template; the tendency for the tibia to go into valgus during lengthening is prevented by pre-setting the bone in slight varus, and migration of the fibular fragments prevented by fixing them to the tibia. Instead of a corticotomy, which may or may not preserve intramedullary blood vessels, an osteotomy is performed, pre-drilling the cortex to avoid cracking the bone. A series of experimental studies by the author's group has demonstrated that the preservation of periosteum is more important than careful corticotomy if bone lengthening is to succeed.[9-11]

Post-operative management has also been modified. The rate of distraction is gradually reduced as lengthening proceeds. This is particularly important in bifocal procedures, since the overall rate of distraction

Phase	Days
Waiting period	8
Distraction period	130
Neutralization period	52
Dynamic loading period	41
Overall treatment time	231

Table 44.1 Average Time Course of Bifocal Tibial Lengthening

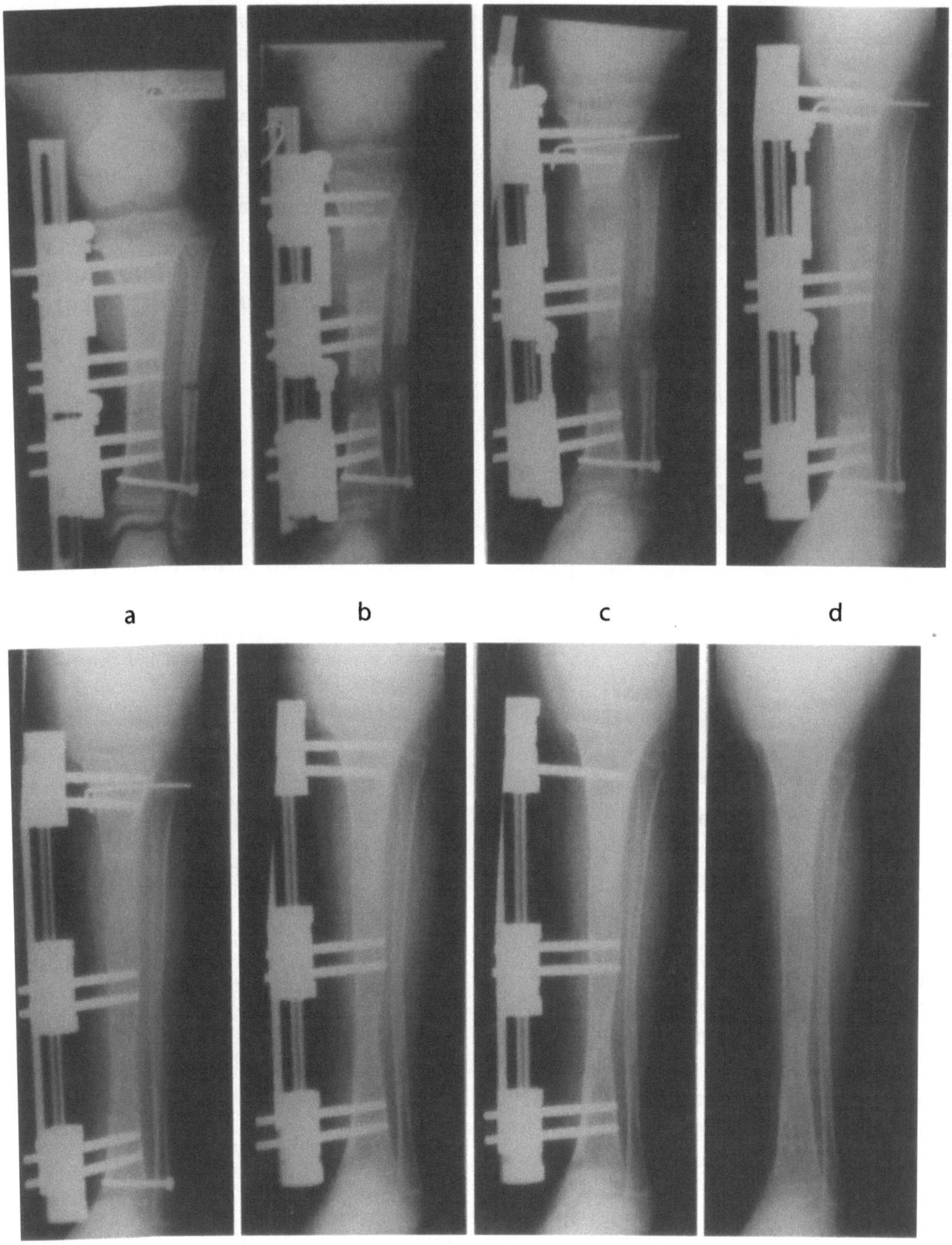

a b c d e f g h

Fig. 44.11 Bifocal tibial lengthening in a patient with achondroplasia (10-year-old girl). **a** Immediately following operation. The osteotomies of the tibia are poorly visible. **b** 32 days post-operation. Distraction had been carried out for 24 days at a rate of 0.25mm/6 hours at each osteotomy. The rate of distraction was thereafter reduced to 0.25mm/8 hours. Note that the proximal fibula had migrated downwards. **c** 50 days post-operation. The fibular head was fixed to the tibia with a Steinmann pin and the rate of distraction was further reduced to 0.25mm/12hours. **d** 109 days post-operation. The screws are slightly bent and the pre-setting of the proximal tibia in slight varus has led to spontaneous repositioning. **e** 136 days post-operation. A total of 12.5cm lengthening (7cm at the proximal and 5.5cm at the distal osteotomy, respectively) has been achieved. The clamp locking screws were tightened and the compression–distraction units removed (neutralization period). **f** 183 days post-operation. The clamp locking screws were unlocked and axial loading was encouraged (dynamization period). **g** 242 days post-operation. The most proximal pin has been removed. **h** 270 days post-operation. Solid union has been obtained. The tibia and fibula continued to grow after this stage, both in length and diameter.

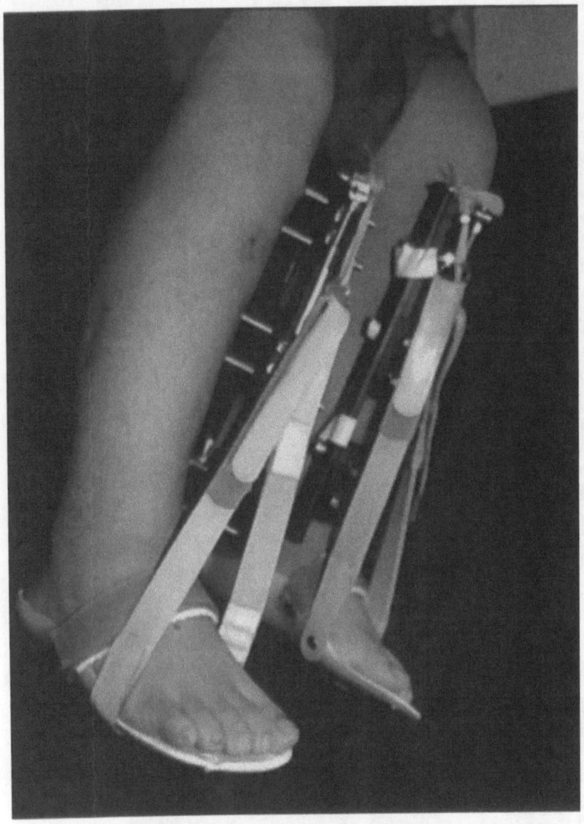

Fig. 44.12 Anti-equinovarus splint.

is still fast for the soft tissues. As long as premature consolidation is prevented, the more slowly the bone is lengthened, the better the soft tissues adapt. Stretching of the calf muscles is encouraged with physiotherapy, and anti-equinovarus splints are used at night. The author believes that continuous tension-stress is important to stimulate soft tissue growth.[12-14]

The Healing Index of 21.8 recorded in the current series of bifocal tibial lengthenings is significantly less than that reported in a previous study using monofocal procedures, where a Healing Index of 41.0[15] was recorded for patients with a similar background. Saleh and Hamer have also reported excellent results with bifocal limb lengthening using the Orthofix Limb Reconstruction System. They recorded a Healing Index of 21.5 for bifocal tibial lengthening in achondroplastic patients.[4]

Where extensive lengthening of more than 10cm is required, as in achondroplastics, bifocal limb lengthening has a number of advantages over monofocal procedures. It produces smaller lengthened segments, faster consolidation, and less tension in the soft tissues. The overall treatment time is significantly reduced so that the patient can return to normal life much earlier. More skilful surgical techniques and post-operative management, however, are required for bifocal procedures. Unskilful surgery can double the trouble.

References

1. Ilizarov G.A. 'Transosseous osteosynthesis.' in: Green S., ed. *Theoretical and clinical aspects of the regeneration and growth of tissue.* Springer-Verlag:Berlin, 1992.
2. Tachdjian M.O. 'Methods of limb lengthening.' in: Tachdjian M.O. ed. *Pediatric Orthopedics.* Saunders:Philadelphia, 1990.
3. Yasui N., Kawabata, H. and Nakanishi, H. 'Bilateral and bifocal lengthening in the tibia and the femur using a segmental slide lengthener.' *Int J Orthop Trauma* 1993; 3: 87.
4. Saleh M. and Hamer A.J. 'Bifocal limb lengthening: A preliminary report.' *J Pediatr Orthop* 1993; Part B 2: 42.
5. Paley D. 'Current techniques of limb lengthening.' *J Pediatr Orthop* 1988; 8: 73.
6. Price C.T. and Mann J.W. 'Experience with the Orthofix device for limb lengthening.' *Orthop Clin North Amer* 1991; 22: 651.
7. De Bastiani G., Aldegheri R., Renzi-Brivio L. and Trivella G. 'Limb lengthening by callus distraction (callotasis).' *J Pediatr Orthop* 1987; 7: 129.
8. Tachdjian M.O. 'Radiographic methods of measuring length of long bones.' in: Tachdjian M.O. ed. *Pediatric Orthopedics.* Saunders:Philadelphia, 1990.
9. Kojimoto H., Yasui N., Goto T., Matsuda S. and Shimomura Y. 'Bone lengthening in rabbits in callus distraction: The role of periosteum and endosteum.' *J Bone Joint Surg* [Br] 1988; 70-B: 543.
10. Yasui N., Kojimoto H., Shimizu H. and Shimomura Y. 'The effect of distraction upon bone, muscle, and periosteum.' *Orthop Clin North Amer* 1991; 22: 563.
11. Yasui N., Kojimoto H., Sasaki K., Kitada A., Shimizu H. and Shimomura Y. 'Factors affecting callus distraction in limb lengthening.' *Clin Orthop* 1993; 293: 55.
12. Ilizarov G.A. 'The tension-stress effect on the genesis and growth of tissues : Part I. The influence of stability of fixation and soft tissue preservation.' *Clin Orthop* 1989; 238: 249.
13. Ilizarov G.A. 'The tension-stress effect on the genesis and growth of tissues : Part II. The influence of the rate and frequency of distraction.' *Clin Orthop* 1989 239: 263.
14. Ilizarov GA. 'Clinical application of the tension-stress effect for limb lengthening.' *Clin Orthop* 1990; 250: 8.
15. Aldegheri R., Trivella G., Renzi-Brivio L., Tessari G., Agostini S. and Lavini F. 'Lengthening of the lower limbs in achondroplastic patients.' *J Bone Joint Surg* [Br]1988; 70-B: 69.

Limb Lengthening in High Risk Cases: The Importance of the Learning Curve

45

M.T. Dahl

Introduction

Complications of limb lengthening have long been a fundamental issue for surgeons performing bone lengthenings.[1,2,5,6,7,10,13] They occur so frequently that some authors use alternative words such as inconveniences,[4] problems,[14] and obstacles,[11] as descriptive terms for certain complications. The development of new technologies such as distraction osteogenesis or new devices such as the Orthofix Limb Reconstruction System (LRS) add new variations to the already difficult process of limb lengthening.

In this era of patient advocacy and informed consent, identifying, reporting and preventing errors in medicine has become increasingly important and therefore requires more interest and study.[3] This chapter demonstrates how complications occurring during limb lengthening can be predicted, and to some extent prevented, with planning and experience. A learning curve is used to display complication rates graphically, relative to experience. The analysis has four goals:

1. To identify limb deformities at high risk for lengthening complications and determine the relative complication risk.
2. To show how complication rates vary depending on the severity of the deformity.
3. To evaluate the effect surgical experience has on the complication rate in high risk cases.
4. To suggest strategies for the prevention of complications.

Materials and Methods

A customized database was created in 1989 to track the gradual limb length and deformity corrections performed by the author. Corrective surgeries entered into this database include: epiphysiodesis, bone lengthening, gradual deformity correction, non-union reconstruction, arthrodesis, contracture reconstruction, and osteosynthesis for acute fracture. The data presented in this chapter are taken from the database and are based on 327 consecutive bone lengthenings performed on 242 patients between 1985 and 1994. Only patients with lengthening as a component of their treatment were included in this review. Lengthenings involved the Wagner, De Bastiani, or Ilizarov techniques. The external fixators used were the Synthes (Wagner); Orthofix Dynamic Axial Fixator or LRS (De Bastiani); Ace (Fischer) or Richards (Ilizarov) (Table 45.1). The patient's age, gender, segment lengthened, length discrepancy, preoperative segment length, severity of deformity (relative complication risk), aetiology of deformity, duration of hospitalization, length of time the fixator was in place, amount of lengthening achieved, duration of follow-up, and complications, were recorded in the database. Measurements of length and angular defor-

Wagner	22
De Bastiani	104
Fischer	23
Ilizarov	178

Table 45.1 Methods of External Fixation

mity were made from scanograms and standing radiographs. Each case was retained in chronological order and was, in addition, categorized by technique. Data collection was prospective, beginning in 1989 and recorded at each clinic visit.

Complication rates were defined as the number of complications per lengthened segment. To simplify data presentation, these rates were averaged by year and plotted on a graph. Lines were drawn through consecutive points on the graph to produce the learning curves.

Classification of Complications

Any unwanted event was considered a complication (Table 45.2). The severity was assigned a grade of (I) minor, (II) serious, or (III) severe. Serious and severe complications were considered major in view of their associated morbidity. Minor complications (I) did not usually affect outcome or require extensive intervention, but might be linked to more severe complications. Complications that were either major and temporary, or minor and permanent, were considered to be serious (II). Severe complications (III) were those that required unplanned surgery or resulted in permanent sequelae. Major complications are the focus of this chapter.

Deformity Severity Scale (Relative Complication Risk)

A deformity severity scale was previously developed to correlate complication rates with the severity of the condition.[7] Length discrepancy is the primary factor used in the scale (Table 45.3). The presence of complication risk factors such as angulation, translation, rotation, contracture, non-union, infection, and congenital aetiology, increase the severity of the deformity. Lesser risk factors add to the complexity of treatment, but with proper planning, they do not usually compromise the end result. Greater risk factors significantly alter treatment plans and can seriously compromise the end result. The severity type increases one level if three lesser risk factors or two greater risk factors are present in addition to the length discrepancy.

	Minor	Major	
Complication	*Minor (I)*	*Serious (II)*	*Severe (III)*
Pin-site problems	Minor infections	Ring sequestrum	
Infection	Superficial wound	Deep wound	Osteomyelitis
Vascular			Vascular laceration or occlusion requiring repair
Neurologic	Hyperaesthesia	Neuropraxia	Permanent palsy
Medical		e.g. DVT, pneumonia	e.g. Cardiac arrest
Psychological			Requires change in treatment
Premature consolidation		Requires repeat corticotomy	
Delayed union/non-union		LI >2/adult or >1.5/child	Bone graft or retreatment necessary
Fracture		Repeat fixation	Osteotomy
Axis deviation >5°		6–10°	>10°
Subluxation		Temporary	Permanent
Contracture	<10°	11–20°	>20° and/or gait disturbance
Did not equalize	<2.5cm	2.5–5.0cm	>5.0cm

LI = Lengthening Index

Table 45.2 Complication Classification

Results

In Fig. 45.1 the number of lengthenings performed in the series in each severity type is shown. Of the 327 segments lengthened in 242 patients, 24 were in the upper extremities and 303 in the lower extremities. Primary lengthenings were performed in 223 segments, 70 were second lengthenings, 31 were third lengthenings, and 3 were fourth lengthenings. The average age of the patients was 13 years (range 2–56 years), and the average lengthening achieved was 4.7cm (range 2.2–18cm).

Minor Complications

Wire and pin-site complications (inflammation, infection, loosening, or metal failure) were poorly recorded before 1989, at which time a clinical grading system was initiated (Table 45.4). Wire and pin complications were rare in upper-extremity lengthenings. Most lower-extremity patients experienced wire or pin-site infections. However, the incidence of pin loosening and wire fracture dropped from 10 per cent in 1989 to a current rate of less than 3 per cent. A minor loss of joint motion (<10 per cent) occurred in 52 (16 per cent) of 327 lengthenings.

Major Complications (Grade Serious and Severe)

Major complication rates were particularly high and severe in the following instances: simultaneous lengthenings of congenital aetiology, congenitally short femurs, and large lengthenings (>15 per cent). Complications were most frequent in the following specific instances:

1. Simultaneous lengthening of the femur and tibia where the aetiology was congenital
2. Congenitally short femur
3. Type 3 fibular hemimelia
4. Congenital pseudarthrosis of the tibia
5. Infected segmental defects.

Both serious and severe complications are considered major, but the severe complications are more likely to result in re-operation or permanent sequelae. The current rate of major (serious and severe) complications in Type 1 deformities is 10 per cent. For Type 2 deformities, the major complication rate is 30 per cent. Type 3 deformities experience major complications 79 per cent of the time, while Type 4 deformities (the most severe deformities that this surgeon will treat with bone lengthening) sustained complications in 117 per cent (Fig. 45.2). This figure illustrates that the less severe the deformity, the lower the complication rate.

Deformity	Type 1	Type 2	Type 3	Type 4	Type 5
Length (%)	<15	16–25	26–35	>35	>50

Lesser Factors

- Angulation
- Translation
- Rotation
- Contracture
- Prior infection
- Anatomical location (femur, forearm or foot)
- Age (adult)
- Obesity
- Poor nutrition
- Neurological deficit

Greater Factors

- Congenital deformity
- Multi-site deformity
- Multiple surgeries
- Previous lengthening
- Non-union
- Bone loss
- Active infection
- Pre-operative instability

Table 45.3 Complication risk factors

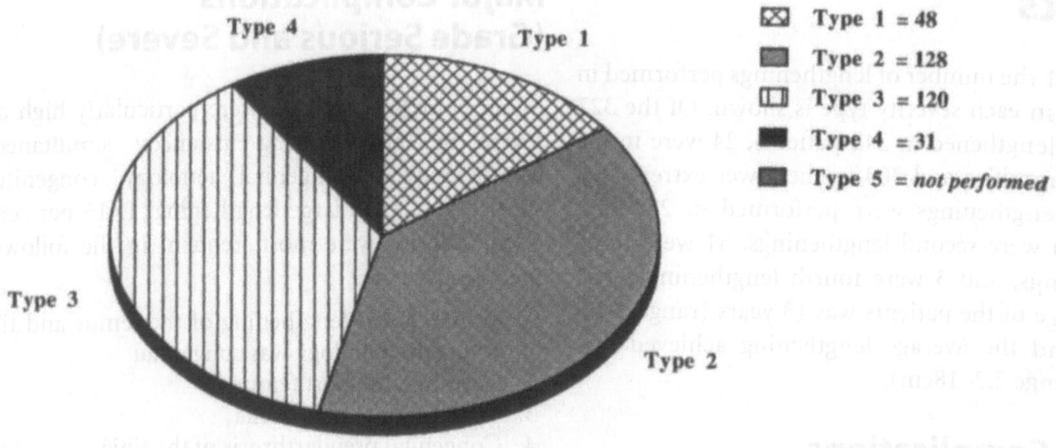

Fig. 45.1 The number of deformities corrected according to severity type.

Effect Of Experience on Major Complications (Grade Serious and Severe)

In lengthenings of lesser complexity (Type 1), complication rates diminish rapidly as experience is gained. Major complication rates do not diminish as rapidly with high risk lengthenings (Type 2, 3, and 4 deformities). Despite persistently high rates of major complications, however, it is notable that of these, fewer are severe as experience increases. A comparison of the percentage of serious (Grade II) and severe (Grade III) complications is shown in Fig. 45.3. From 1985 through 1994, a gradual decrease occurred in severe complications requiring unplanned surgeries.

Discussion

What accounts for the incidence of limb lengthening complications and what are the implications for their prevention? There are many reasons for the high frequency of complications during limb lengthening and these are illustrated in Fig. 45.4.

Learning Curves

A learning curve has the general form of a peak, followed by a downslope, levelling out to a plateau. The peak occurs initially, and reflects the high rate of complications associated with inexperience. The downslope represents the experience gained as the surgeon becomes more proficient. The plateau represents the

Grade	Appearance	Treatment
0	Normal	Weekly pin care
1	Inflamed	Daily pin care
2	Serous discharge	Topical antibiotics
3	Purulent discharge	Oral antibiotics
4	Osteolysis	Remove pin

Table 45.4 Wire and Pin Site Classification and Treatment

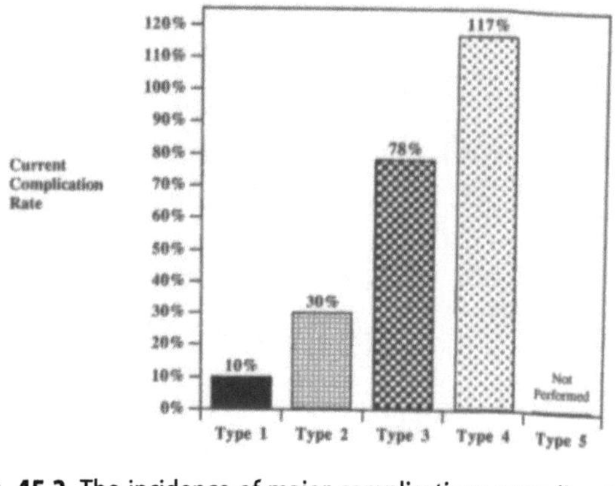

Fig. 45.2 The incidence of major complications according to severity type.

maintenance of a level of proficiency by continued practice.[9] A learning curve can be determined for any surgeon, device or biological principle in limb lengthening, and it is used to improve performance (Fig. 45.5).

Assessing Risk

Many deformity-associated features can affect the difficult process of limb lengthening. Some of these features are known to increase the risk of complications. The femur is considered to be more difficult to lengthen than the tibia. The presence of joint instability increases the chance of subluxation during lengthening. Simultaneous lengthening and treatment of a non-union increases the risk of complications. In an effort to correlate the author's complication rates with the features of deformities, a classification for severity of limb deformities (risk) was developed. The most easily measured feature, length discrepancy, is the basis of this scale (Table 45.3). The choice of risk factors was based on the experience of the author and of other orthopaedic surgeons reporting complications.[4,11,12] The validity of this classification is substantiated by trends in complication rates with further experience (Fig. 45.6).

Pre-operative Planning

The best method of treatment should offer an achievable outcome with the least risk. To attain this, a pre-operative plan and a problem list should be devised.[8] The list takes into consideration the deformity features (relative risk), underlying condition, treatment goals, patient and family expectations, and surgeon experience. Once complete, this list is manually written on an overlay tracing or computer digitization of the radiograph.

Designing Fixation

The overlay tracing is used as a worksheet to aid fixator design. Fixator clamps or rings are drawn orthogonal to the deformed bone segments. Hinges, connecting rods, and motor rods or fixator clamps are then drawn in place based on the apices of the deformity. The worksheet is cut with scissors at the proposed correction site and the segments are angulated into the desired position through the hinge sites, thereby testing the correction plan. Pin and/or wire locations are pre-operatively selected and illustrated on the worksheet (Fig. 45.7).

An additional pre-operative educational visit provides for surgeon re-evaluation and allows the patient and family to become familiar with the device. In the growing child, the plan is extended into maturity to be certain that expectations are reasonable and will be met.

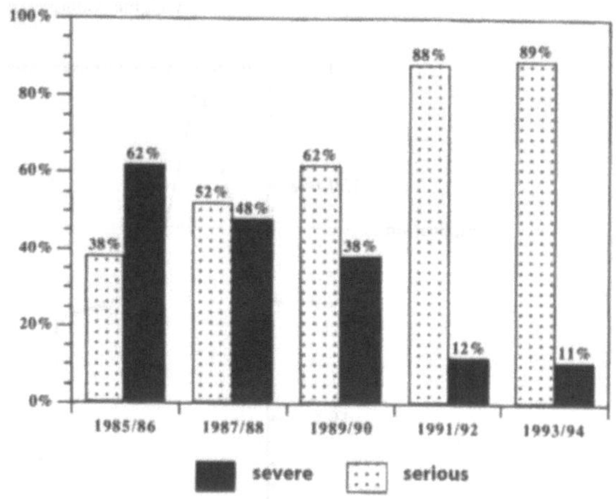

Fig. 45.3 Despite persistent major complications, the relative proportion of severe complications compared to serious, diminished with further experience.

Limb lengthening techniques consist of many evolving methods.

The limits of soft tissue tension and articular compression sequelae are not completely known.

Surgical principles in this changing field are incompletely documented, leading to repetition of mistakes.

Extensive planning is necessary with results dependent on the prediction of events before they occur.

Decisions made during even the simplest of lengthenings are often more complex than those made in other orthopedic conditions treated with an acute correction or conventional techniques.

Many events occurring in lengthening are not intuitively obvious, and may therefore come as a surprise on first encounter.

The process of limb lengthening requires a sustained level of attentiveness post-operatively, uncommon in other areas of orthopaedics.

Bad outcomes result from complex conditions (intrinsic), device failure (extrinsic), and judgement error (physician or patient).

There is no standard measurement of outcome.

Fig. 45.4 Possible causes of complications.

Post-operative Care

Many complications associated with limb lengthening are inter-related or linked. Identifying the links should diminish complications. For example, applying an unstable frame can result in axis deviation, which then subjects the regenerate bone to bending forces that

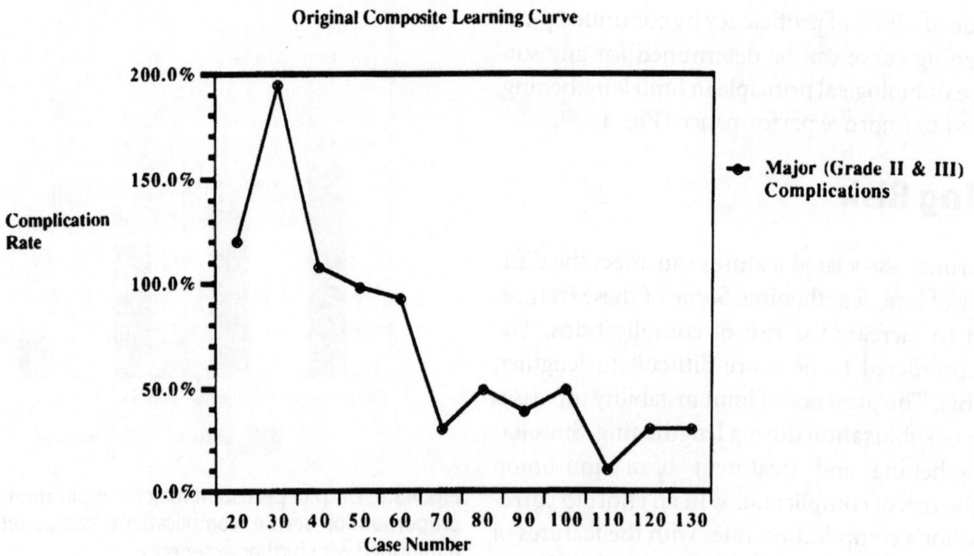

Fig. 45.5 The incidence of major (Grades II and III) complications as a function of the total number of lengthenings performed.

slow healing. The delay in consolidation results in prolonged external fixation and resultant disuse osteopenia. Pin loosening and sepsis may result in premature fixator removal with further bending of the regenerate or even fracture. These events are all linked to one another, as are the complications that result from their imperfect execution. Fig. 45.8 illustrates this linkage of complications.

Collection of Data: A Role for Computers

Computers can prove a useful tool for reducing the incidence and severity of complications; the use of computers has not, however, been well studied in medical settings. The difficulty of applying a computer program to limb lengthening becomes obvious when we consider the multitude of complex, integrated decisions that are made over a prolonged period of time. It is difficult to use computers as aids to decision making because the interpretation of events is not standardized, data gathering is individualized, and the results of treatment depend on a large number of decisions taken over a long period of time. Despite these shortcomings, the current generation of limb lengthening surgeons have an opportunity to contribute greatly to these methodologies through improved communication.

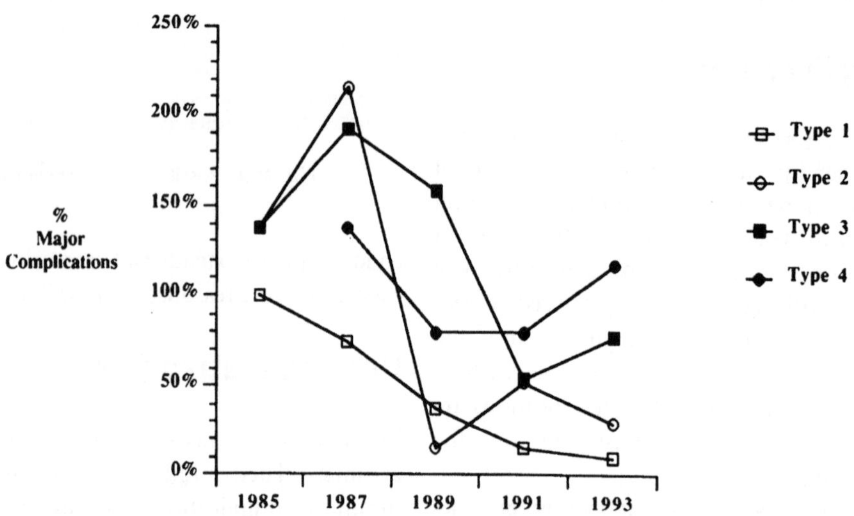

Fig. 45.6 The major complication rates are plotted by year for each severity of deformity. Note how steadily and rapidly rates diminish for the least severe deformities (Type 1), but persist at higher rates in more complex cases (Types 2, 3, and 4).

Outcome Measurements

The presence of serious or severe (major) complications can contribute to a bad result. These complications (i.e., fracture, axis deviation, subluxation, contracture) always impact upon the treatment plan, but if handled successfully, a good result may still be obtained. Major complications will certainly result in a higher cost and greater morbidity. Establishing methods to measure outcome or "limb quality" will help determine the best method of treatment (e.g. long leg shortening, short leg lengthening, prosthetic management, or combinations). The case illustrated in Fig. 45.9 demonstrates that a successful equalization of leg length does not necessarily mean a successful result.

Summary

How can limb length surgeons reduce the incidence and severity of complications in their practice?

1. After additional training specific to limb lengthening, the novice lengthening surgeon should gain proficiency with less complex lengthenings before proceeding to high risk cases.
2. The surgeon should establish a support team committed to the special needs of the patient undergoing lengthening.
3. A pre-operative plan or pathway must be established to predict the events that can occur, thereby minimizing or preventing complications.
4. Surgeons frequently performing limb lengthenings should agree on the definition and classification of complications occurring during and after limb lengthening.
5. These surgeons should construct a method of evaluating limb quality, assigning a rating for a given limb based on the patient's symptoms and satisfaction, as well as on measurements of static and dynamic function. These standards will help measure the success or failure of different limb lengthening procedures.
6. Finally, in conjunction with hospitals and clinics, data collection systems should be utilized to provide surgeons and staff with feedback. This evaluation of performance will produce the information required to track those who endeavour to perform this work. Analyses carried out by the systems installed must consider patients at high risk, the features of such patients' conditions, and the incidence of complications.

Avoiding Specific Complications

Pin and wire site inflammation and infection can be reduced but not eliminated. Location, insertion technique, biocompatability, hypersensitivity, stability and host medical factors must all be considered.

Fracture at the lengthening site is very distressing because it usually means the frame will need to be reapplied. Risk factors for fracture include: osteopenia, thin cross-sectional area, axis deviation, dysplastic bone, and adjacent joint stiffness. Training the regenerate before removing the frame, and protecting the regenerate after frame removal, are of value.

Premature consolidation can be anticipated in the young femur, the fibula, and at the convexity of the deformity. To avoid this complication, the latency period and lengthening rate should be individualized according to the quality and location of the regenerate, and the patient's age and health.

Delayed or non-union of lengthening sites can be avoided by stable, dynamic fixation. The latency period, lengthening rate, and rhythm must be individualized, with weekly radiographs.

Angulation can be avoided or corrected by precise hinge placement, frame stability, awareness of soft tissue tension, use of full length radiographs when completing the distraction phase, and maintenance of joint motion.

Stiffness usually occurs around the foot and ankle after bone transport in association with distal tibial non-unions. Prolonged joint immobilization prior to lengthening sets the stage for this insidious complication. Further immobilization with joint transfixion should be avoided, unless it is absolutely necessary to correct a contracture or to provide prophylaxis against subluxation. Lengthening of more than 15 per cent can overwhelm the joint or damage muscle fibres.

Knee subluxation is prevented by maintaining the joint in extension and avoiding ipsilateral femoral and tibial lengthening. Judicious use of pre-operative soft tissue releases (e.g. adductor, tenotomy, TAL) in congenital cases can be helpful.

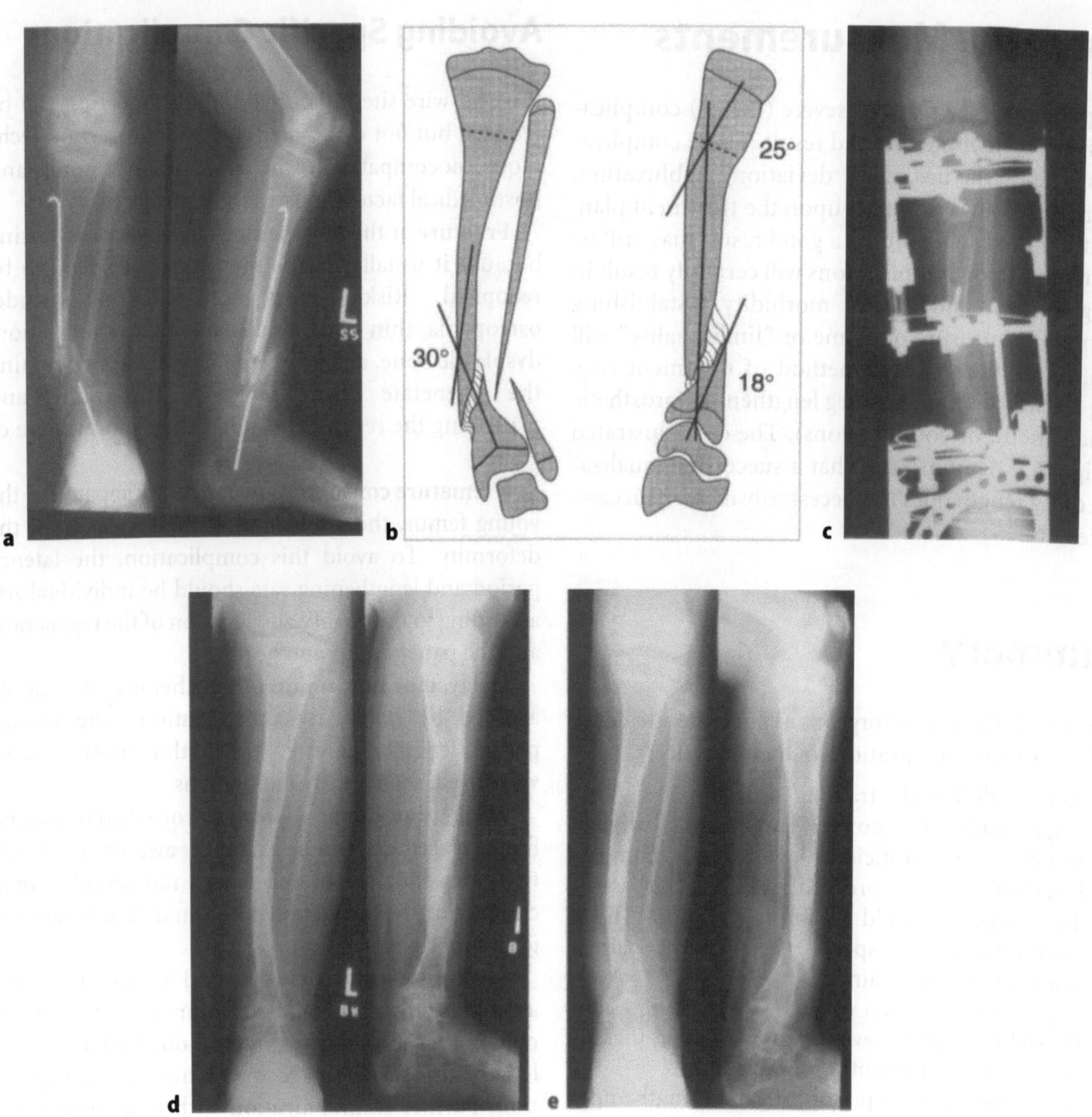

f

Problems:
1. Diagnosis - congenital pseudarthrosis of tibia
2. Ankle stiff
3. Leg length discrepancy 6.3 cm (30%)
4. Multiple surgeries
5. Broken rod
6. Non-union angulation 35° anteromedial
7. Proximal recurvatum 25°

Correction:
8. Closed distraction through non-union site
9. Proximal lengthening
10. Foot prophylaxis

Fig. 45.7 a This 6-year-old child with a multiply-operated congenital pseudarthrosis of the tibia and fractured internal fixation, presented with a flail non-union and a 6.3cm length discrepancy. This was considered a Type 4 deformity. **b** The pre-operative plan consisted in determining the apices of the deformities and their oblique plane, and designing and pre-assembling a circular fixator to match the existing deformity. **c** AP radiograph four weeks post-surgery demonstrates excellent bone formation in the closed distraction site distally, with atrophic lengthening proximally. The strategy was altered because of the atrophic new bone. Lengthening was discontinued. **d** AP and lateral radiographs 12 months post-correction demonstrate healing at both the lengthening and non-union sites with persistent translational and angular deformity through the dysplastic bone. **e** AP and lateral radiographs at 23 months post-lengthening show a refracture through dysplastic bone distally. This case illustrates the ability to correct severe deformities through pre-operative planning, precise execution and careful post-operative care; however, failure to achieve ideal alignment in dysplastic bone increased the chance of refracture. **f** Problem list.

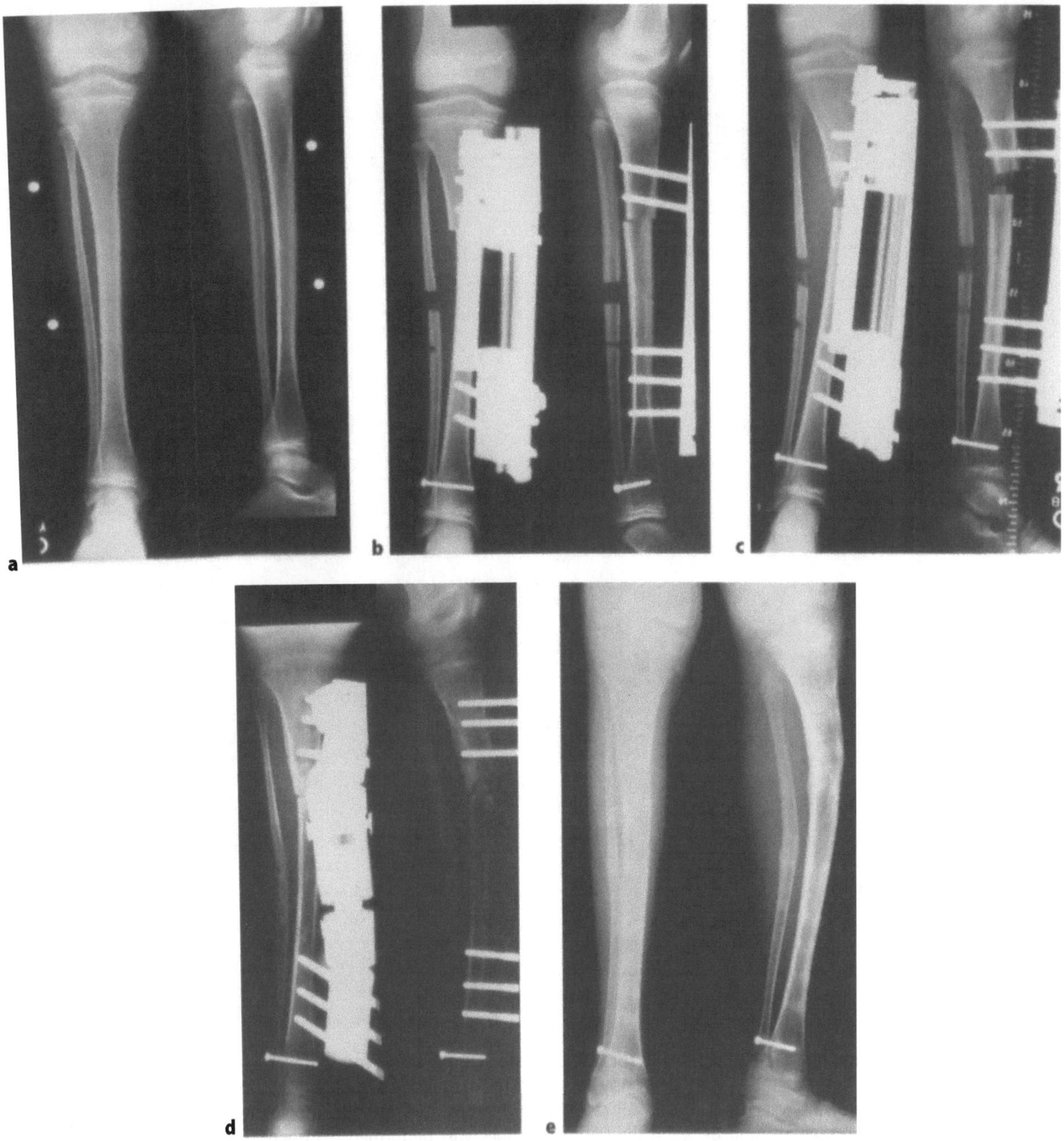

Fig. 45.8 **a** This fibular hemimelia with 17 per cent length discrepancy is considered a Type 2 deformity. **b** Post-operative AP and lateral radiographs show unstable monolateral external fixation. The construct has only two closely applied half pins proximally, which are not orthogonal to the mechanical axis of the bone. **c** Progressive pin osteolysis at the upper two pin sites with apex antero-medial deformity. Note the atrophic bone formation consistent with frame instability. **d** The surgeon recognized the frame instability, altered the fixator to a ball-joint construct and added an additional pin. **e** Post-lengthening AP and lateral radiographs show persistent angular deformity with only 1.5cm of length achieved.

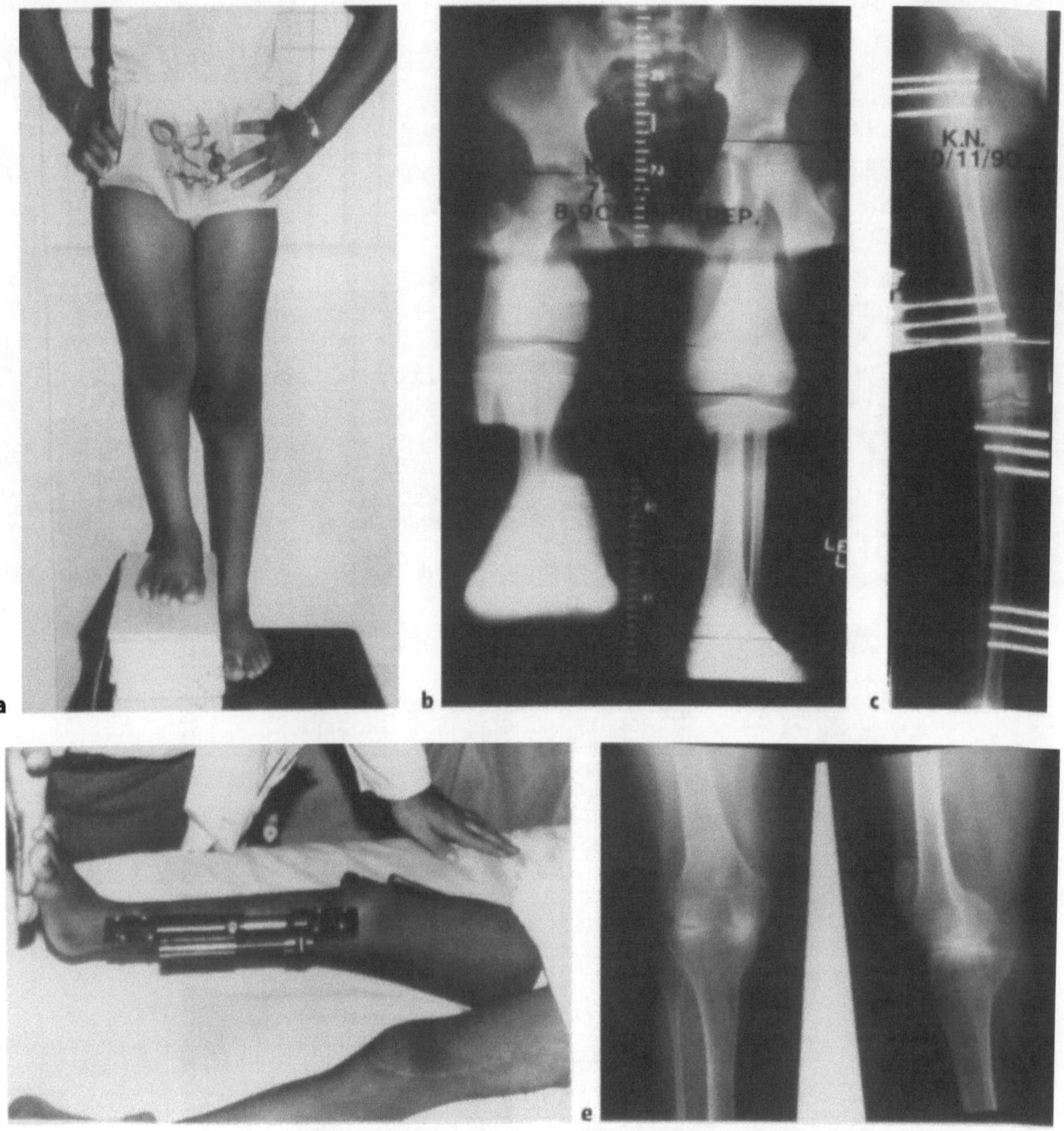

Fig. 45.9 a This 8-year-old girl had a congenitally short femur associated with a Type 1 fibular hemimelia with a projected discrepancy of 14cm. This is considered a Type 3 deformity because of the magnitude of the shortening, multiple levels, congenital aetiology, and instability of the knee joint. **b** The AP radiograph demonstrates a leg-length discrepancy of 8.9cm at initial presentation. **c** A 6cm lengthening, split between the femur and tibia, was performed with good healing. Three years post-lengthening, the child underwent a second procedure to lengthen the right femur and tibia again, 3cm each. **d** Knee joint and foot stiffness occurred. **e** The surgeon manipulated the knee shortly after fixator removal because of stiffness, resulting in severe fibrodesis of the knee joint. This knee contracture may have been prevented by lengthening one bone at a time, thereby avoiding severe compressive forces through the joint. Additionally, manipulation under anaesthesia shortly after lengthening is unsafe because of osteopenia and the potential for chondral damage.

Conclusion

The relative risk for limb lengthening complications can be determined pre-operatively on the basis of the features of the condition to be treated. Major complication rates increase relative to the severity of the deformity being treated. Upon review of the data, the occurrence of major complications in less complex cases (Types 1 and 2) was 10 per cent and 30 per cent respectively. For deformities of greater complexity (Types 3 and 4) the occurrence of major complications increased to 79 per cent, and 117 per cent. Complications persisted even with increased experience, but the severity of the complication was seen to diminish.

Orthopaedic surgeons will continue to be challenged by limb lengthening cases. In an attempt to diminish the incidence and severity of complications, the author recommends the following strategies:

1. The development of a pre-operative risk assessment;
2. Pre-operative planning;
3. Attentive and sustained post-operative care;
4. Data collection for continued assessment and improvement.

References

1. Abbott, L.C. 'The operative lengthening of the tibia and fibula.' *J Bone Joint Surg* 1927; 9:128–52.
2. Allan, F.G. 'Bone lengthening.' *J Bone Joint Surg* [Br] 1948; 30B:490.
3. Bates, D.W. et al 'Incidence of adverse drug events and potential adverse drug events: Implications for prevention.' *J Am Med Assn* 1995; 274: 29–34.
4. Codivilla, A. 'On the means of lengthening in the lower limbs, the muscles and tissues which are shortened through deformity.' *Am J Orthop Surg* 1905; 2: 353–69.
5. Coleman, S.S., Scott, S.M. 'The present attitude toward the biology and technology of limb lengthening. *Clin Orthop* 1991; 264: 76–83.
6. Compere, E. 'Indications for and against the leg lengthening operation.' *J Bone Joint Surg* 1936; 18: 692–705.
7. Dahl, M.T., Gulli, B., Berg, T. 'Complications of limb lengthening: A learning curve.' *Clin Orthop* 1994; 301: 10–8.
8. Dahl, M.T. 'The gradual correction of forearm deformities in multiple hereditary exostoses.' *Hand Clinics* 1993; 9: 707–18.
9. Glorion, Ch., Pouliquen, J.C., Langlais, J., Ceolin, J.L., Kassis, B. 'Allongement de femur par callotasis.' *Revue de Chirurgie Orthopedique* 1995; 81: 147–56.
10. Hughes, G.B. 'The learning curve in stapes surgery.' *Laryngoscope* 1991; 101: 1280.
11. Moseley, C., Mosca, V. 'Complications of Wagner leg lengthening.' in: *Behavior of the Growth Plate.* Edited by Hans K. Uhthoff and James J. Wiley. Raven Press: New York, 1988.
12. Paley, D. 'Problems, obstacles, and complications of limb lengthening by the Ilizarov technique.' *Clin Orthop* 1990; 250: 81.
13. Putti, V. 'The operative lengthening of the femur.' *J Am Med Assn* 1921; 77: 934.
14. Wagner, H. 'Operative lengthening of the femur.' *Clin Orthop* 1978; 136: 125.

The Complications of Leg Lengthening

46

M. Saleh and B.W. Scott

Surgical limb lengthening was first described in 1905[1] and successive surgeons have refined the technique.[2-8] However, acceptance of these techniques by the orthopaedic community has been slow and limited. Surgeons prefer instantaneous solutions to the problem of limb length discrepancy, such as shoe raises and orthoses, prostheses, amputation, and limb shortening. There are three main reasons for the lack of popularity of limb lengthening. First, complication rates have remained high. Second, surgery is only one step in a technique that is slow and time-consuming. Third, a large infrastructure is required because treatment is prolonged and considerable reliance is placed on patient compliance, family and community support, as well as hospital-based health care workers, such as nurses, physiotherapists, teachers, and social workers.

In the 1980s, the work of De Bastiani et al,[7,26] as well as that of Ilizarov,[5] did much to promote limb lengthening and built on the efforts of Heinz Wagner in the late 1960s and early 1970s. The most exciting concepts have evolved from Ilizarov's studies in distraction osteogenesis and, subsequently, soft tissue neogenesis. Each of these techniques had its origins in the mid-1950s and was not appreciated by Western doctors until the late 1970s.[9,10] Since that time, many surgeons in trauma and paediatric orthopaedics have developed special expertise in limb lengthening and reconstruction. Because leg lengthening is a relatively new, complex, and lengthy procedure, it is possible that mistakes will be made by surgeons, patients, and supporting staff. This is known as the "learning curve." This article discusses the pitfalls of such techniques, together with protocols for management and the reporting of complications. The common complications observed in limb lengthening are listed in Table 46.1.

Pre-operative Assessment

Anderson believed that good patient selection was the key to improved results.[4] The pre-operative period is used to assess the patient, to prepare the patient for surgery, and to develop a careful treatment plan (Table 46.2). The assessment may be undertaken on an outpatient basis and it is usually possible to develop an outline treatment plan. Medical, orthopaedic, and psychological risk factors should be established. Following this, patients with an unacceptably high degree of risk are offered alternative treatment and excluded from the programme. Preparation and training of the patient, however, is better performed on an inpatient basis. This period also provides an opportunity to develop a structured treatment plan well in advance of surgery. Documentation of the pre-operative condition clinically, photographically, and radiologically is vital.

Pre-operative Period: Outpatient Assessment

Aetiology

Lower limb lengthening may be required as a result of a number of congenital and acquired conditions, such as reduction deformities, hip dysplasia secondary to congenital dislocation of the hip, congenital pseudarthrosis of the tibia, poliomyelitis, spina bifida, Ollier's disease, post-irradiation shortening, and infection or trauma producing growth plate disturbance or angulations and malunion of fractures. Lengthening has also been performed in children with disproportionate short stature, e.g., achondroplasia, in which the limbs are short in relation to the trunk.[11,12] Patients with poor-quality tissues or unstable joints are a difficult, high-risk subgroup.

Bone	
	Premature consolidation
	Delayed consolidation and non-union
	Axial deviation angulation and translation
	Fracture
	Osteomyelitis
	Septic arthritis
Muscle and Joints	
	Muscle cramps
	Loss of range
	Contracture
	Subluxation
Nerve	
	Nerve injury - mixed or sensory
	Cord injury - paresis or paraplegia
Vessel	
	Bleeding and compartment syndrome
	Aneurysm
	Malignant hypertension
	Deep vein thrombosis/pulmonary embolus
Pin Sites	
	Pain
	Tethering
	Loosening
	Infection
Wound	
	Pain
	Haematoma
	Dehiscence
	Infection
Psychosocial	
	Crisis during or after lengthening
	Weight loss
	Withdrawal
	Depression
	Regression

Table 46.1 Complications of lengthening

Assessment	
	Aetiology
	Age
	Discrepancy
	Deformity
	Medical and surgical profile
	Psychological profile
Preparation	
	Educational needs
	Pin site care
	Physiotherapy (wheelchair)
Planning	
	Technique
	Timing

Table 46.2 Pre-operative assessment, preparation, and planning

Age

The majority of procedures are performed in children (a children-to-adults ratio of 4:1 in the author's practice), although an increasing number of adults with fracture-related shortening has been observed.[13,14] Lengthening may be performed on a patient of any age, but for practical and biological reasons it is more appropriate in younger patients and particularly before the development of fixed compensatory deformities. The optimum age group has found to be between 7 and 16 years of age. Younger children show remarkably rapid healing rates, but they tend to be less cooperative than older children. Children below the age of 5 years may need treatment because of major limb length discrepancy or progressive deformity. Deformity correction may be performed alone or in combination with a short unambitious lengthening. In these young children, pre-operative preparation and training for the patient, peer group, and family are vital.[15]

Discrepancy

The risks of lengthening relate to the duration and magnitude of the discrepancy, as well as other risk factors, such as age, aetiology and joint instability. In high-risk cases, repeated short lengthenings of less than 25 per cent of the segment length using the Vilarrubias or Ilizarov technique with joint protection are indicated. In low-risk cases, longer lengthenings up to 35 or 40 per cent may be considered. In achondroplasia, mesenchymal changes within connective tissue and redundant soft tissues enable lengthenings of 80 per cent and more to be achieved.[8,11,12] Measurement of the starting length and allowance for growth during treatment are vital to measure the success of surgery and estimate any growth acceleration caused by the procedure. Allowance for natural growth may be determined from growth prediction curves based on a series of anthropometric measurements and carpal bone age measurements.[16] Measurement of the discrepancy is difficult; of the clinical methods, standing on blocks of known thickness seems be more accurate and repeatable than direct measurement using a tape. Radiological methods such as conventional and computed tomography scanograms are also unreliable for a number of technical and observer-related reasons. We use the Friberg technique (Fig. 46.1)[17] to show the overall discrepancy and parallel beam scanograms to determine the segmental lengths and limb axis. Prediction of the measured discrepancy at maturity is difficult, although some impression may be gained from the straight line graph.[18] A method developed in Verona[19] is easier to use, but has not as yet been verified in longitudinal studies. The most reliable way to achieve symmetry is to perform the final lengthening at maturity.

Deformity

A bony or soft tissue deformity may lead to significant functional disability as well as a marked apparent length discrepancy. These deformities produce significant difficulties for any discrepancy measurement technique and it is easy to overestimate the effect of correction on limb equalization or underestimate it, which leads to extremely short lengthenings. In most cases, deformity should be corrected first because it is likely to be the major handicap to ambulation and will make lengthening more risky. The production of angular deformities is inherent in all lengthening techniques because of muscle imbalance. Femoral valgus and tibial varus will naturally tend to correct during lengthening, but femoral varus and tibial valgus should be addressed before starting lengthening because they will get worse. Joint ranges and muscle power should be carefully documented by the same person before and during lengthening. Specific radiographs may be taken; lateral bending radiographs of the thoracolumbar spine are useful to exclude fixed spinal deformity. Anteroposterior (AP) and lateral radiographs of the affected segment and standing mechanical axis films of the lower limbs also are useful. The mechanical axis is assessed using an AP radiograph of both legs from hip to ankle, with the patient standing on an appropriate block on the affected side to balance the pelvis; a 5cm grid is useful in this assessment (Fig. 46.2). In congenital cases or those with joint abnormalities, AP and lateral radiographs of the hip, laterals of the knee in extension and the tibia, ankle, and foot complex in the plantigrade position act as a useful baseline. Photographs should be taken of the whole patient, as well as AP, posteroanterior (PA), right, and left lateral views. These may be used to record preoperative deformities, such as genu valgus and femoral torsion and can be computerized for composite photography to show the effects of surgery on body proportions.[20,21]

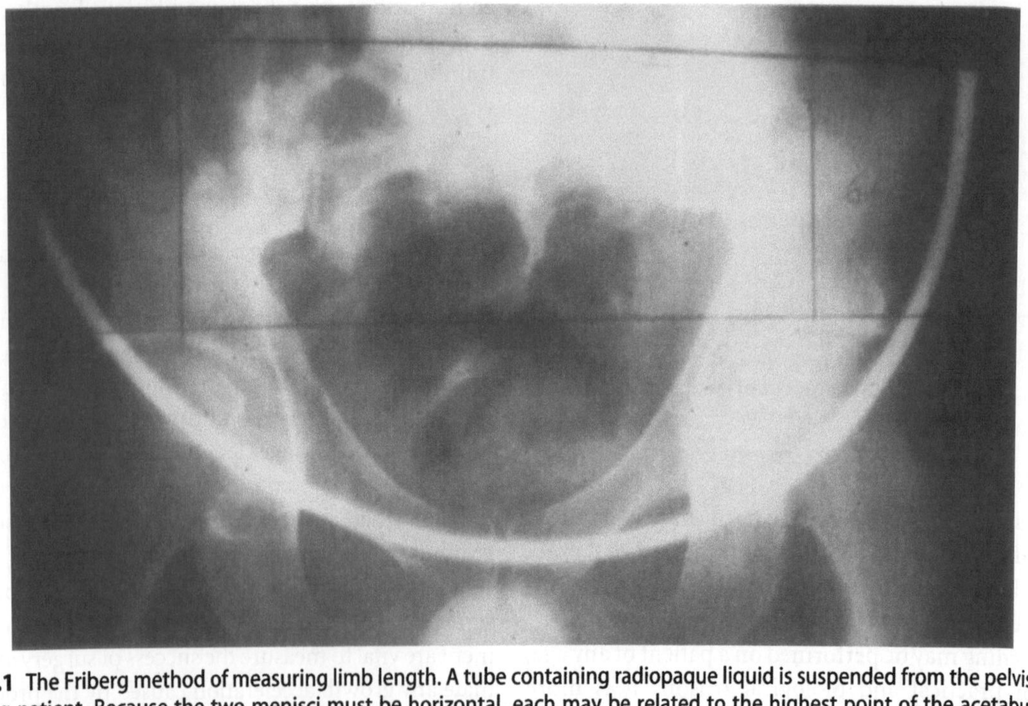

Fig. 46.1 The Friberg method of measuring limb length. A tube containing radiopaque liquid is suspended from the pelvis of the standing patient. Because the two menisci must be horizontal, each may be related to the highest point of the acetabulum to provide an accurate measurement of the discrepancy.

Medical and Surgical Profile

A full medical history should be taken to establish anaesthetic and surgical risk factors, e.g. cardiopulmonary compromise, blood dyscrasias (pin sites may be the source of a persistent diathesis), congenital cardiac anomalies (because bacteraemia may develop secondary to a pin site infection), and the presence of antibiotic allergies. Smoking should be discouraged because, apart from its general effects, it seems to have an adverse effect on callus formation.

Psychosocial Profile

Through several interviews with a patient and his or her family, it is possible to get a feel for psychosocial problems, but most orthopaedic surgeons have little knowledge in this area and it is better to work in conjunction with a social worker, clinical psychologist, counsellor, or teacher when lengthy procedures are planned. Discussion allows the patient and his or her family to understand the problems associated with the limb lengthening process. Through discussion, the doctor can make an assessment of how the patient and the family will cope, to determine the degree of preparation and support necessary. Studies performed in Sheffield Children's Hospital have identified a number of stressors, such as prolonged treatment times, wheelchair confinement leading to frustration and boredom, breakdown of routines within the family unit, and self-consciousness and embarrassment regarding dependency. These stressors may lead to psychological hazards, such as fear, anxiety, and panic before surgery, and depression, withdrawal, and regression after surgery. Psychological preparation may include modelling and role play in younger children and relaxation or self-hypnosis in older children. During treatment, open communication and normal family routines should be encouraged. The problems in adults are similar and considerable strain is placed on the spouse.

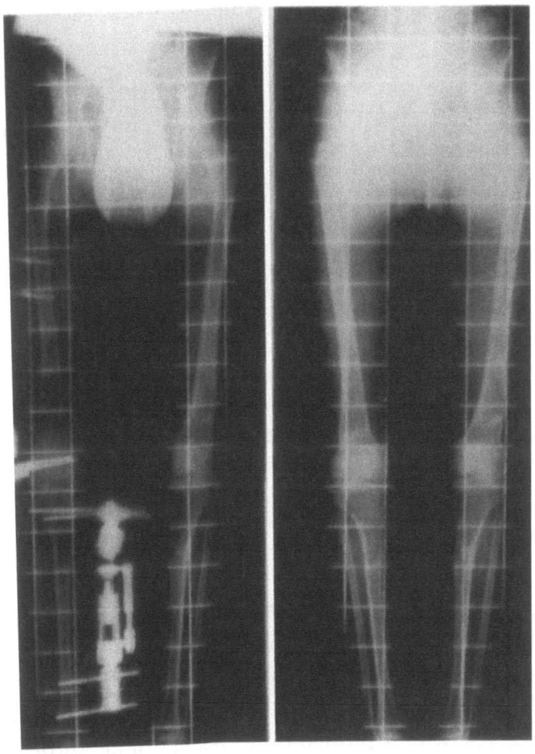

Fig. 46.2 Mechanical axis view. The 5 cm grid aids assessment.

Pre-operative Period: Inpatient Assessment

Preparation

During a 2-day in-patient admission, child patients and their families are able to familiarize themselves with the ward environment and routines and meet staff who will look after them in the peri-operative period. They are likely to be more receptive to information and training than in the highly stressful time immediately before surgery. Special educational requirements and home adaptations such as wheelchair access are evaluated. Child patients are encouraged to meet other children undergoing lengthening and to learn pin site care and physiotherapy regimes. General medical and anaesthetic assessments are carried out and epidural or patient-controlled analgesia is discussed. Some time is spent reassessing the patient clinically and radiologically until a complete operative plan is formulated and discussed with the health care team and patient. The type and extent of the fixation frame and stages of surgery are fully discussed. Finally, contact is made with community services and a date for surgery is planned.

Planning

Many lengthening techniques are available. Timing may depend on educational and sometimes social commitments, but surgery is usually indicated in anticipation of deteriorating mobility, developing deformity, or a discrepancy that is increasing at a rate beyond the corrective potential of surgery. The factors that must be assessed when planning a procedure or range of procedures up to maturity are listed in Table 46.3.

Torsion
Bony angulation
Osteoporosis
Joint instability
Scoliosis
Muscle weakness
Neurological lesion
Soft tissue contracture
Poor quality tissue
Infection
Poor cooperation

Table 46.3 Assessment

Peri-operative Period

Fixator Selection and Placement

Decisions regarding device selection depend on the clinical situation, device capability, and surgeon's skill and experience. The authors use a monolateral frame (Orthofix lengthener) for simple or bifocal lengthenings (Orthofix Limb Reconstruction System) and small single-axis corrections, but substitute a circular frame or use a hybrid construct if joint stabilization or substantial or multiplanar angular correction is required. Monolateral frames are usually applied antero-laterally on the femur to avoid discomfort as the foot flops into external rotation during sleep. Anterior mountings produce unacceptable muscle tethering. Some surgeons advocate postero-lateral placement to avoid tethering of fascia latae, but this position is awkward for the patient and tends to lead to internal rotation deformity at the hip and valgus at the knee. The fixator should be placed in the line of the mechanical axis to avoid varus and medial translation during lengthening. In proximal lengthening, muscle tethering may be reduced by avoiding distal placement of the distal screw cluster. Adequate skin releases should be performed to allow knee flexion to at least 90°. In the tibia, the medial position provides maximum stability but tends to rub the other leg and bunch up the posteromedial skin. Some surgeons believe that this position encourages valgus deformity and prefer an anterior position. The author's preference is for an anteromedial mounting, which provides good bony purchase without soft tissue impalement or interference with the other leg. The fixator should be placed parallel to the long axis of the bone. Distal screws may injure the saphenous nerve or long saphenous vein. Circular frames may be applied to all long bones, but safe corridors are limited in certain areas and frames are not generally well tolerated in the proximal humerus and proximal femur.

Screw Selection, Position, and Insertion

Screw shaft length should be selected according to the depth of soft tissues and position of the fixator. Templates are available to select the correct thread length. Cancellous screws should be used in wide metaphyseal zones and cortical screws in areas with a thick cortical buttress. There is an area within the metaphysis that the authors refer to as "no man's land". This area is not suitable for either type of screw because it is very narrow with thin cortical plates (Fig. 46.3). Screws should be placed high in the metaphysis but below the joint capsule or epiphysis to ensure a high submetaphyseal bone division. The insertion technique must be meticulous to avoid tissue necrosis and subsequent infection (Table 46.4).

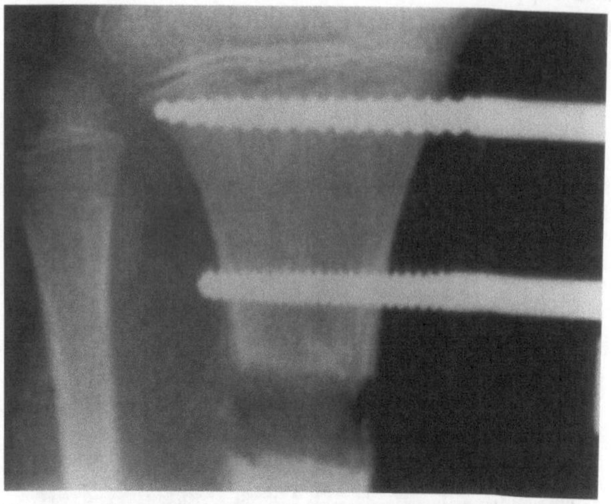

Fig. 46.3 "No man's land", an area with inadequate characteristics for satisfactory purchase of either cancellous or cortical screws.

Inserting Wires

Wires should be inserted from the side of maximum bulk or the side of important neurovascular structures. The skin is pushed towards the centre of the segment and the muscles are placed in their lengthened positions. The wire is pushed on to bone, drilling through bone only and then tapping through to the other side.

Create a soft tissue track
Push screw guide against the bone
Use a sharp clean drill
Use a slow drill speed 500 to 600 rpm
Drill with constant pressure
Avoid heating
Use a template to ensure correct screw seating in clamp
Clean drill between applications
Check joint range and release skin and fascia as necessary
Apply non-adherent absorbent dressings

Table 46.4 Avoiding pin site infection: surgical technique

Wires of 1.05mm diameter are used in young children and 1.5mm wires are used in older children and adults. Olive wires are used for pulling or counteracting angulation.

Bony Disruption

Ilizarov recommends a corticotomy that involves division of three-quarters of the cortical circumference with an osteotome and a closed osteoclasis of the remaining bone bridge. In practice, it is very difficult to avoid damaging the medulla and its blood supply. Many variations of this technique have been described, and certainly, better results are observed with this method than with high-energy bony divisions with powered saws. The periosteum should be repaired wherever possible. Having tried various methods, the most predictable procedure is observed to be an osteotomy under tension.[14,26] Confirmation of complete bone division is made by palpating a gap with a fine probe, radiological screening, and noting lack of resistance to fixator distraction. Incomplete osteotomy is often mistaken for premature fusion.

Fibula Resection and Stabilization

During tibial lengthening, the fibula may fuse prematurely or sublux proximally at the distal tibiofibular joint. A 1cm bone and periosteum resection should be performed and the distal tibiofibular joint temporarily secured with a Kirschner-wire or screw (Fig. 46.4).

Inpatient Post-operative Care

An indwelling epidural catheter or patient-controlled analgesia machine (Fig. 46.5) is set up in the recovery room. Providing a relatively pain-free environment is important to reduce pain memory in patients who will require a number of surgical procedures. The depth of analgesia must not prevent early active exercises. Bed exercises are started immediately and, in some cases in which joint stiffness is of particular concern, a continuous passive motion machine may also be used. Dressings are changed on day 2 before reduction of the analgesia schedule. The patient is encouraged to stand or perform wheelchair transfers early, to reaffirm self-respect, confidence and independence. Responsibility for pin site care is handed on to the patient and one aide after appropriate instruction and supervision (Table 46.5). Distraction is commenced on the 5th to the 10th post-operative day. Once begun, this is also the responsibility of the patient, who is instructed to complete a log book. Hospital discharge is goal orientated: satisfactory pin site care, good mobility and progress at physiotherapy, and usually, a post-operative radiograph showing satisfactory distraction. Community doctors, nurses, and physiotherapists are instructed on discharge so that continuity and confidence is maintained.

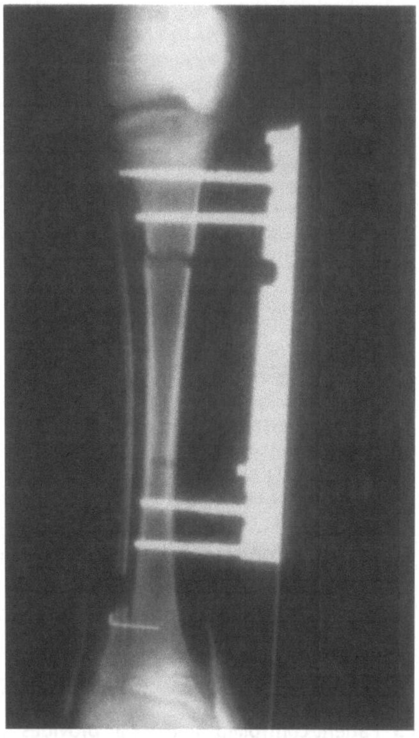

Fig. 46.4 A 1cm fibular resection and temporary fixation of the inferior tibiofibular joint to prevent premature fusion of the fibula and proximal migration.

Gauze dressings until bleeding and serous discharge stopped
Leave exposed
Clean once daily with saline
Massage skin around screws to avoid unwanted crusting and epithelialization
Avoid creams and powder sprays
Release tight skin
Encourage free drainage
Increase cleaning and massage if inflamed
Treat overt infection with antibiotics

Table 46.5 Avoiding pin site infection: post-operative care

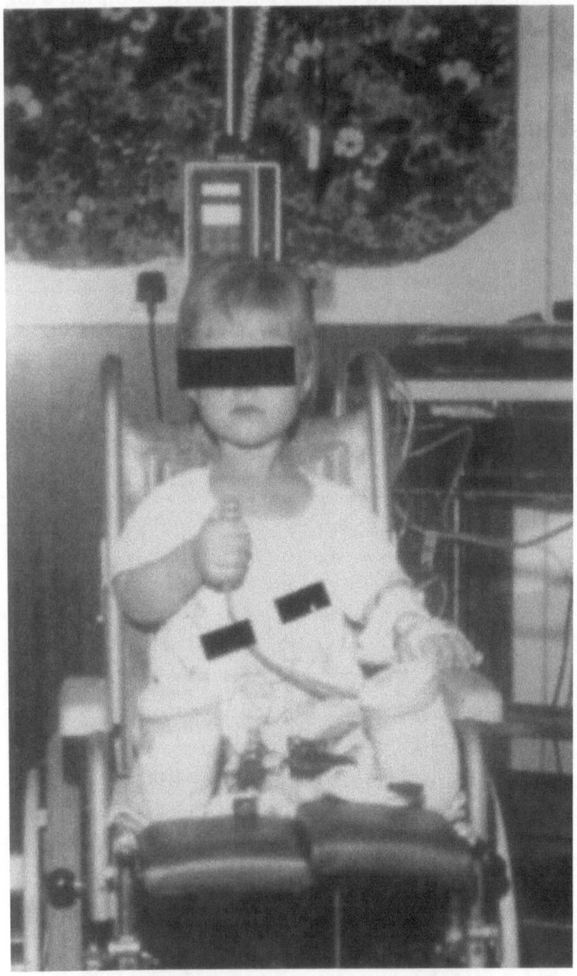

Fig. 46.5 Patient-controlled analgesia provides adequate comfort in the first and second post-operative days to allow exercising and pin site care.

Post-operative Care

Patients are generally reviewed weekly or bi-weekly during the early and middle parts of distraction and then monthly until 3 months after fixator removal. Each post-operative visit involves a review by the nurse (pin sites), physiotherapist (joint range, muscle tightness, or joint deformity), surgeon (unexplained pain, neurovascular integrity, length measurements, callus formation, angular deformity, and fixator maintenance), and, if necessary, the psychologist or social worker. Careful routines must be worked out, including limited use of radiographs to avoid large amounts of irradiation.

During distraction, routine monitoring is performed with AP radiographs centred on the area of interest (bone quality view) (Fig. 46.6). Radiographs of the whole segment (alignment views) (Fig. 46.7) are taken if there is any suspicion of angulation and to exclude osteolysis around the screws. Two orthogonal bone quality views are taken before dynamization and fixator removal. Alternative imaging methods, such as ultrasound and dual-emission X-ray absorptiometry, may be considered. The lengthening rate is usually 0.25mm four times per

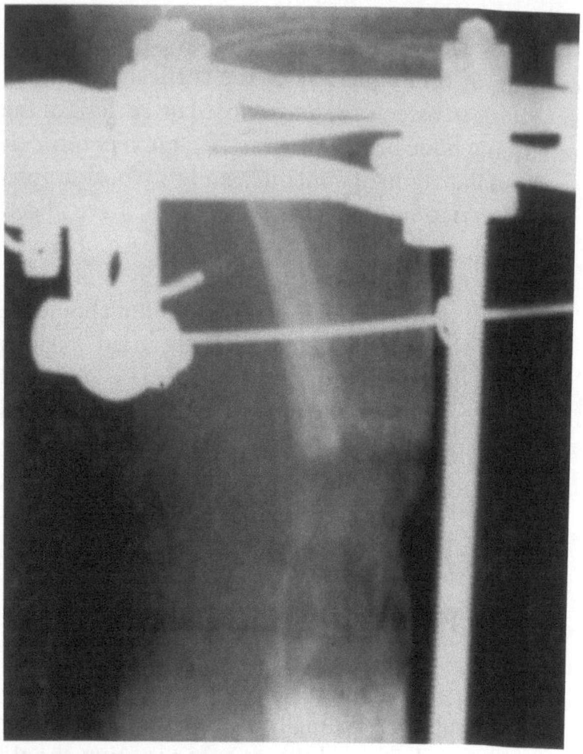

Fig. 46.6 Bone quality radiographs are taken in a predetermined orientation and localized to the area of interest. Exposures are recorded for repeatability and comparison purposes.

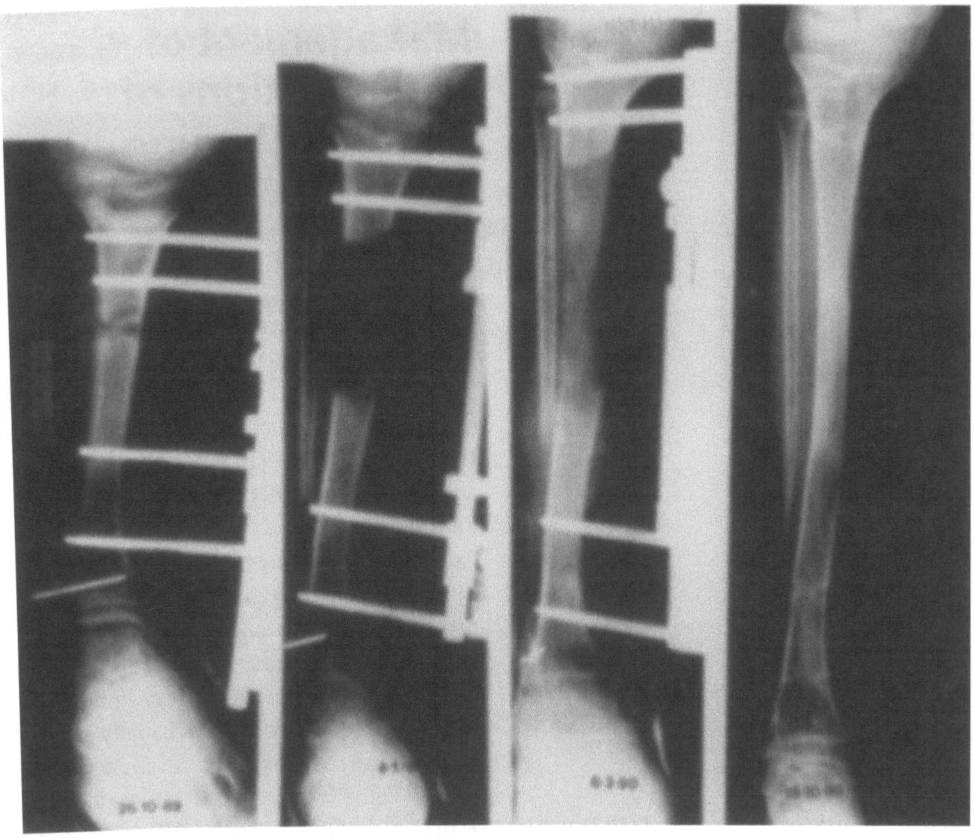

Fig. 46.7 Alignment views are taken to monitor overall progress of lengthening and to exclude angulation or osteolysis around the screws. (This series shows the evolution of callus during a 10cm lengthening.)

day. Poor callus formation may be limited by slowing down, stopping, or even reversing distraction.

Angular deviation should also be recognized early and corrected by manipulation of the callus, and, if necessary, changing the fixator configuration or adding additional screws. Slight overlengthening should be aimed for to allow for up to 5mm of collapse during the consolidation phase. If soft tissue tightness occurs, a further 10mm of length may be added and then slowly removed to relax the soft tissues. At the end of the lengthening phase, the fixator is locked. If physiotherapy parameters have been maintained, walking is encouraged, thus increasing bone loading. In the case of the Orthofix device, the frame may be made more elastic (dynamization), thus promoting bone loading in one of two ways. A Dyna-Ring may be applied, allowing 2mm of gradual compression of the callus column, or the body locking nut may be completely released, allowing free excursion of the telescoping body. The latter phase, known as dynamization, is usually initiated when at least three cortices are distinct on two orthogonal radiographs. Callus maturation should increase from this point up to the time of fixator removal. The treatment time is roughly divided into three equal parts: distraction, neutralization, and dynamization. An attempt should be made to standardize for both the positioning and exposure of radiographs to obtain truly comparable views on successive visits. It should be remembered, however, that radiographs are not quantitative, and variation in technique may mislead the surgeon regarding the progress of maturation. In a limb without significant angulation or joint stiffness, four complete cortices on two orthogonal radiographs are required before fixator removal. A stiff adjacent joint should be mobilized as much as possible and the bone protected by reducing the frame stiffness even further or removing the fixator and applying a protective orthosis to prevent fracture. In the case of circular frames, dynamization is a continuous process during distraction and consolidation owing to the inherent properties of the tensioned wires.

After fixator removal, follow-up should continue until all contractures have resolved or reached a plateau and there is radiological evidence of medullary recanalization. Screws may produce deep scars, particularly in the thigh, and appropriate patients may be offered scar revision surgery (Fig. 46.8).

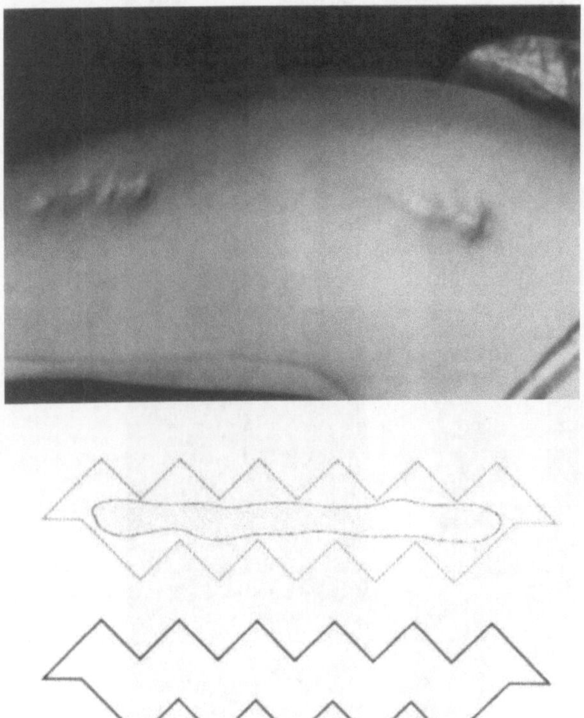

a b c

Fig. 46.8 **a** Deep pitted scarring at screw sites after a 6cm lengthening. **b** A W-plasty excision of epidermis is performed. The fat is undermined adjacent to the dermal island to the depth of the original depression and closed over the centre of the dermal island. Skin is closed using fine interrupted sutures. **c** With time the scar breaks up and fades.

Management of Complications of Leg Lengthening

Bone

Complications may occur early at the corticotomy or osteotomy site. If care is not taken with the osteotomy, lengthening may be prevented because of a small bony bridge and fractures may propagate into the adjacent screw hole. If the periosteum is not repaired carefully, there may be a delay in new bone formation, leading to a prolonged lengthening period and delayed consolidation.

Lengthening must obviously occur at a sufficient rate to prevent premature consolidation and also to produce well-mineralized new bone in the lengthening site. In most procedures, a rate of 0.25mm four times daily satisfies these criteria. If premature consolidation occurs, closed osteoclasis is usually sufficient to allow lengthening to continue. Premature fusion of the fibula (Fig. 46.9) may occur unless a generous (at least 1cm) resection is performed together with the surrounding periosteum. Premature consolidation is often observed in patients with Ollier's disease unless more rapid lengthening is performed.

Delayed consolidation is managed by slowing the lengthening rate in the earlier stages. If the growth zone in the centre of the distraction zone continues to widen or the column of bone becomes narrower, the distraction rate must be reduced (Fig. 46.10). Later, new bone formation may be accelerated by compressing the new bone and then redistracting. Bone formation may be poor in osteogenesis imperfecta, hypophosphataemic ricketts, Turner's syndrome and smokers. Plating and bone grafting should not be necessary. In the Sheffield Children's Hospital bone graft and plating have not been used and supplementary intramedullary fixation has been used in only 5 out of 150 cases, all except 2 in patients with osteogenesis imperfecta (Fig. 46.11).

Axial deviation during lengthening remains one of the most frequent complications requiring surgery and occurs more frequently where monolateral devices are used. It can still occur with a circular frame but can be more easily managed using differential distraction rates. The common deviations experienced are varus in the femur and valgus in the tibia.

Axial problems are caused by asymmetry of soft tissue tension; e.g., in the tibia, muscles may tend to lengthen more slowly than bone, producing valgus,

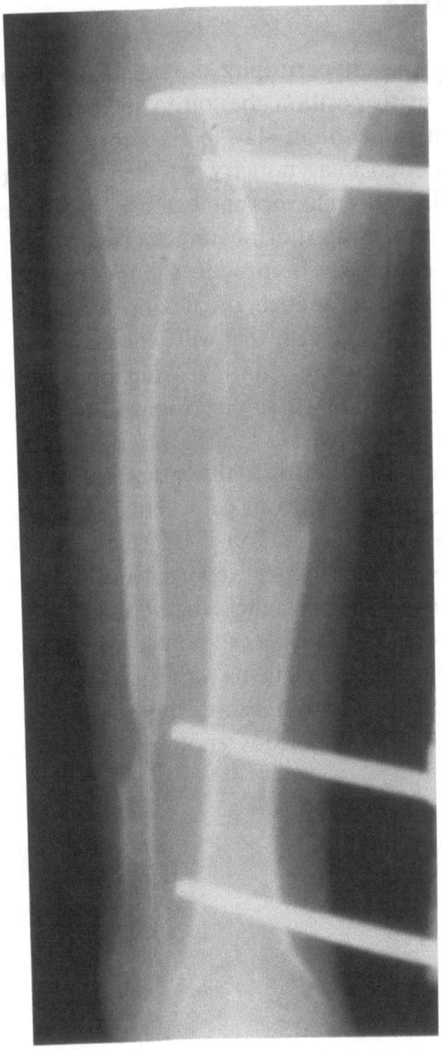

Fig. 46.9 Premature fusion of the fibula, if undiagnosed, will lead to progressive valgus deformity, proximal migration of the fibula, and screw loosening.

posterior angulation, and flexion contracture of the knee. Problems may also occur if the fixator is set away from the mechanical axis, which is valgus to the axis of the femur but along the axis of the tibia. The problem of angulation during lengthening is most elegantly solved by the substitution of a modular progressive correction clamp for an existing clamp (where the Limb Reconstruction System is used); by manipulation under anaesthesia and application of a ball jointed fixator or by removal of the device and immobilization in plaster. Correction by means of a modular progressive correction clamp is described in detail in Ch. 42, 'The Technique of Callotasis and its Application to Monofocal Limb Lengthening'. If recognized late, osteotomy may be required to correct both the angulation and its translational effect (Fig. 46.12).

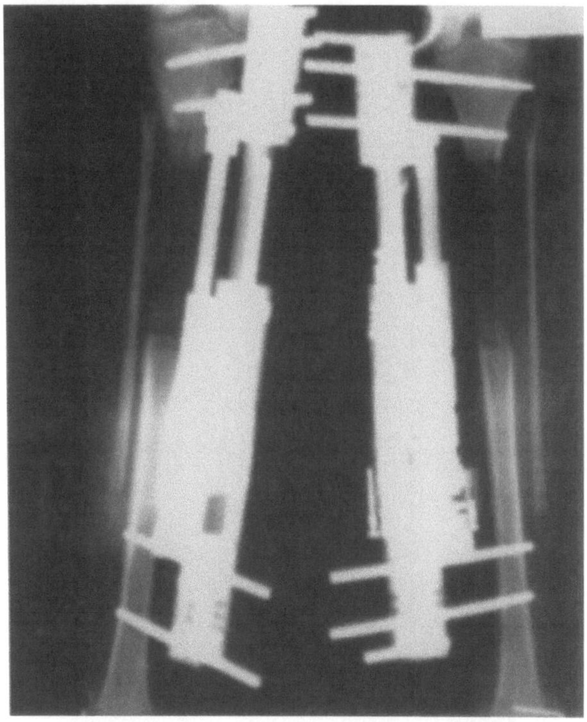

Fig. 46.10 Poor bone formation and a growth zone that is increasing in width are indicative of too rapid a distraction rate.

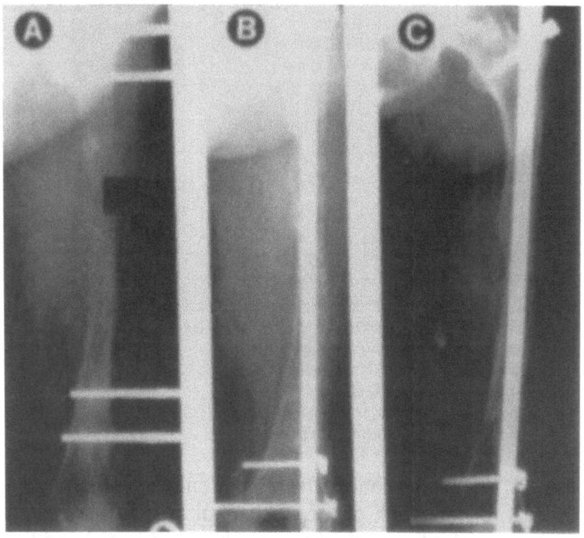

Fig. 46.11 Prophylactic nailing during the consolidation phase in osteogenesis imperfecta. **a** Appearance immediately before. **b** Early post-nailing. **c** Late post-nailing.

The rate of post-operative fracture varies with the method of lengthening. Luke et al[22] report a 37 per cent rate in Wagner lengthenings, whereas we have observed a 5 per cent refracture rate (using a modified Vilarrubias technique with callus distraction). The consequences of the fracture also vary significantly. Of Luke's cases 70 per cent required operative stabilization.

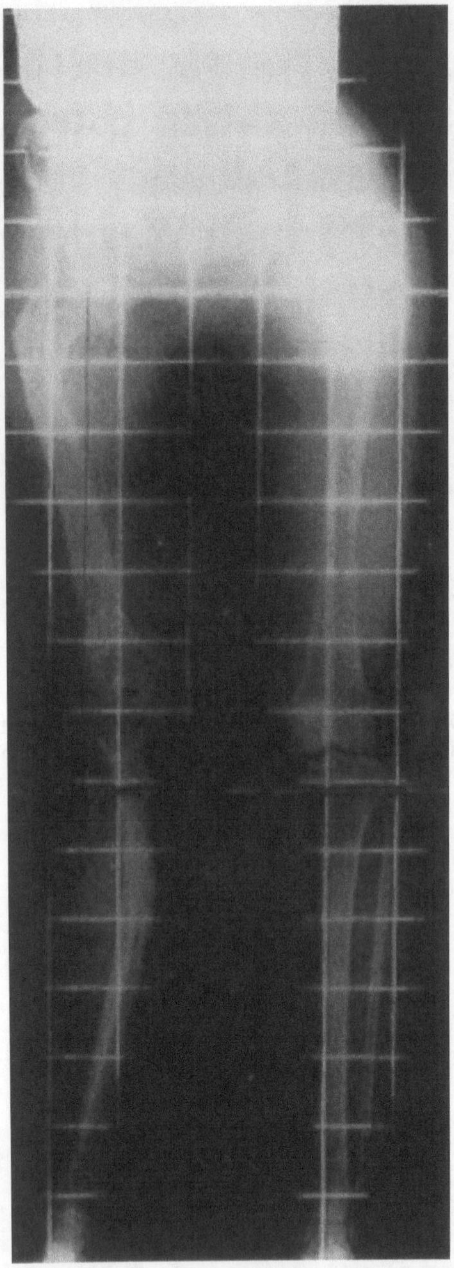

Fig. 46.12 Axial deviation after femoral and tibial lengthening leading to translation of the mechanical axis. To maintain a horizontal joint line to the knee, the hip is adducted and the ankle valgus.

Of five fractures in the Vilarrubias series, two femoral fractures in patients with congenitally short femora have required operative fixation with intramedullary rods, whereas the tibial fractures have been managed uneventfully with plaster techniques. Fractures in callotasis lengthening are usually of the stress pattern and have been noted to produce significant callus, which rapidly consolidates the lengthening site.

Muscles

Muscles may hypertrophy during distraction.[9] It is important to position the joints so that muscle will lengthen rather than stay in its shortened position. There is often an asymmetry between muscle strength and bulk between flexors and extensors with the larger muscle remaining short. Muscles crossing two joints are at special risk. This produces talipes equinus at the ankle, flexion at the knee, and flexion and adduction at the hip. If unchecked, this will worsen, producing a flexion contracture. As the flexion contracture increases, the joint will sublux (Fig. 46.13). At the knee, the tibia slides slowly backwards, often aided by associated cruciate deficiency. In the early stages, this is difficult to differentiate from contracture, but later may progress to full dislocation if treatment is not instituted. Jones and Moseley[23] reported a subluxation rate of 33 per cent in 21 Wagner lengthenings.

Appropriate strategies can reduce this rate substantially. Vilarrubias[8] lengthens with the ankle held in the plantigrade position in a cast. The Achilles tendon is elongated by percutaneous tenotomy. The knee is held

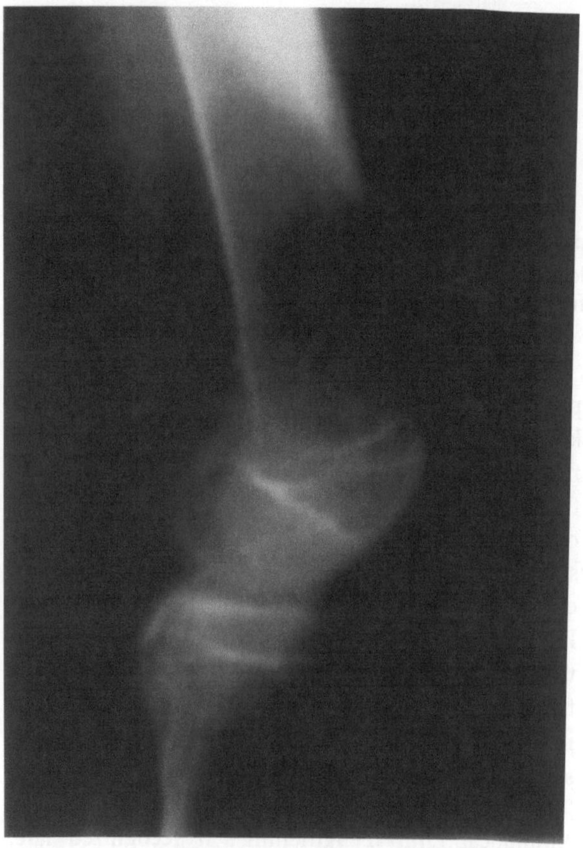

Fig. 46.13 Subluxation of the knee. Unlike simple flexion deformities, the tibia is displaced posteriorly on the femur.

in extension in a wheelchair with a leg platform while, to protect the hip, the patient is semi-recumbent. In femoral lengthenings, percutaneous release of the adductor longus, gracilis, rectus femoris straight head, sartorius, and fascia latae are performed. Physiotherapy is very important to maintain quadriceps strength. Flexion at the knee is discouraged. If a flexion contracture develops, the patient is admitted for more physiotherapy and continuous passive motion (CPM) is a useful adjunct. Dynamic splinting is of value both in prevention and treatment of knee subluxation.[27] Other techniques of value include the use of a stabilizer ring to prevent knee flexion (Fig. 46.14), reducing the rate of distraction, and compressing the lengthening site. Joint stiffness after lengthening is common in the short term but almost always resolves. The only longer-term problem in our series was persistent subtalar stiffness in a few patients.

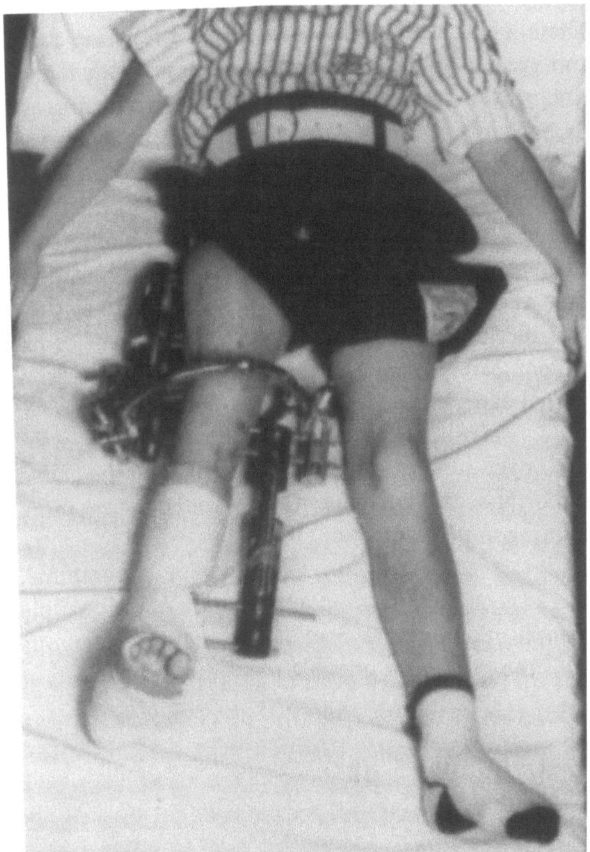

Fig. 46.14 A knee-stabilizing ring has been added to a monolateral fixator to protect the knee during the distraction phase. It may be disconnected for exercise.

Pin Sites

The aetiology of pin site infections has already been discussed. Infection around wires or screws is the most frequent problem encountered in lengthening. Pin site infections are classified by us according to their response to treatment as follows: grade I responds to local treatment including vigorous cleaning and massage; grade II responds to oral antibiotics; grade III responds to intravenous antibiotics or pin site release; grade IV responds to removal of pin; grade V responds to pin removal and surgery to control infection in bone; and grade VI is unresponsive to treatment (chronic osteomyelitis). In a thorough pin analysis of 65 lengthenings (274 pins) in Sheffield Children's Hospital, 29.6 per cent developed an infection (grade I to III), but only 1.1 per cent required curettage and/or pin removal. No cases of chronic osteomyelitis were recorded. No lengthenings failed to reach their goals because of pin problems.

It is important to involve patients in care of pin sites because of the need to clean and remove crusts daily. The area around the pin site should be massaged to prevent adhesions, and with early infection cleaning should occur two or three times per day. Skin release is rarely required with this regime. Pin site infections seem to be less of a problem when circular frames are used if appropriate tension is maintained, but wire breakage has been observed. In some cases, loose wires may be retensioned, but loose screws must be replaced.

Nerves

It is rare to produce neurological problems with lengthening. Problems may occur either with pin insertion or during distraction. The only nerve problem encountered with monolateral frames has been damage to the saphenous nerve. Application of a circular frame involves placing wires near nerves and a variety of nerve palsies has been observed, with the common peroneal frequently involved. Sensory nerve injury may be of considerable concern, as it may lead to permanent dysaesthesia.

Distraction may produce insidious paralysis. If toe movements are reduced and sensory loss occurs, the distraction must slow or stop. This usually produces a neurological improvement. Fortunately, this problem is rare. Paraplegia has been observed in one case where the bone of an achondroplastic patient with spinal stenosis was lengthened.

Vessels

Vascular problems are also unusual with modern techniques. Rapid distraction may cause malignant hypertension and cerebrovascular accident, but this is not a problem if the lengthening rate is kept to 1mm per day. Pins placed through or near arteries can cause bleeding with compartment syndrome, distal vascular insufficiency, or aneurysm. Deep vein thrombosis is rare in lengthening. Fortunately, none of these problems have been encountered in our series.

Pain

Leg lengthening is a procedure involving a prolonged period of fluctuating pain. Its management is split into stages. The post-operative pain may be severe in a patient whose bone has been lengthened at several sites and is best controlled either by indwelling epidural or by a patient-controlled analgesia pump. This can usually be discontinued by day 3 and treatment begun with dihydrocodeine or paracetamol. Aspirin derivatives and non-steroidal anti-inflammatory drugs may interfere with callus formation and their frequent use should be avoided.

Distraction is not usually painful, but if soft tissue tension increases, cramp-like pain may occur. Pin loosening will also produce discomfort. Control at the latter stages involves use of mild analgesics, occasionally transcutaneous electrical nerve stimulation, and, most usefully, involvement in diverting activities. Quiet music is useful at night to help with sleep.

Discussion

Careful planning and execution of leg lengthening procedures combined with a multidisciplinary approach will inevitably reduce complication rates. Nevertheless, lengthening remains high-risk surgery. Complication rates in all reports discussing lengthening have been high. In early reports these complications were often severe, producing long-term morbidity or even life threatening situations. At Sheffield Children's Hospital, a vigorous attempt has been made to reduce complications, but even so, patients entering the programme are told in detail of possible problems and that every patient is likely to experience at least one significant complication. It is equally important to tell the patients that very few of them will be left with any permanent sequelae. Some series stand out both because of the international standing of the authors and the remarkably low complication rates (Table 46.6).

The Wagner results have been included because the figure is low in relation to the complexity of the technique and other observed results with this technique. Several presentations and publications have reported complication rates of approximately 70 per cent.[12,24,27] These high rates may be caused by the learning curve and greater willingness to take on cases with higher risk. More realistically, meticulous reporting of perhaps less important events, such as pin site infections, may also be contributing to these high complication rates. As this type of surgery becomes more frequent, there is a need for standardized reporting. Many studies fail to report significant deformities, such as angulation, and results may be skewed by such variables as aetiology, patient selection, extent of in-patient care and support services, and prior unreported experience of lengthening. Such series also fail to consider the psychological trauma caused by prolonged surgery, patient satisfaction, and the added importance of permanent deformities over more minor complications.

Before embarking on a lengthening programme, the surgeon must have an appreciation of the possible complications and a plan for remedying situations with the minimum possible morbidity. Classification

Source	N	Segment/type	Complications (%)
Wagner[25]	58	Femur	44.8
De Bastiani[7]	100	Femur tibia achondroplasia	14.0
Ilizarov[3]	217	Tibia achondroplasia	8.8
Ilizarov[26]	237	Femur achondroplasia	5.6
Vilarrubias[28]	364	Femur tibia achondroplasia	12.9

Table 46.6 Complication rates in selected series

is difficult because complications differ markedly in their severity. Three attempts at classification are worthy of mention. Wagner[25] described a two-level system that included problems and complications. Problems were defined as "intrinsic, cannot be avoided and must be dealt with." A typical example would be a pin site infection. Complications were defined as "extrinsic and must be avoided," e.g., a serious bone infection.

In an excellent review, Paley[24] recommended a three-level system of problems, obstacles, and complications. Problems are defined by Paley as "difficulties being resolved during lengthening by non-operative methods" with obstacles defined as "difficulties being resolved by operative means." True complications were further classified into minor or major groups with major groups being subclassified into those that did not interfere with the original goals of treatment and those that did. At the Sheffield Children's Hospital, a similar three-level system has been in use for several years.[12] Complications were defined as mild, moderate, or severe. Following an analysis of 162 segments, the classification has been upgraded to meet the needs of outcome-related critical analysis.

Minor complications are those of no long-term functional or anatomical significance. They do not require anaesthesia or surgery (other than minor outpatient procedures under local anaesthesia) and do not affect the treatment plan. Examples include pin site infection of any grade, fixator problems, pin site releases, mild contractures, undisplaced and stress fractures, and behavioural disturbance. Moderate complications require a further general anaesthetic or operation for correction but are also of no long-term functional or anatomical significance. Examples include elongation of the Achilles tendon, manipulation of the callus under anaesthesia, insertion of a further screw or wire, scar revision, re-excision of the fibula, and osteosynthesis of a displaced or unstable fracture. Severe complications are of more concern because they constitute a significant functional or anatomical problem and are further divided into Type 1 (spontaneously improved or correctable by further surgery) and Type 2 (irremediable using present methods of treatment). Type 1 examples include failure of length gain, angulation, transient nerve injury, and reducible joint subluxations. Type 2 examples include osteomyelitis or septic arthritis, permanent joint stiffness, subluxation or dislocation, permanent nerve injury, and serious irreversible psychological disturbance. Axial deviations require further clarification and comment because they produce up to one-third of moderate and severe Type 1 complications, and site and orientation significantly affect their functional importance. It is suggested that up to 5° of tibial angulation in any plane is considered acceptable, i.e. not a complication, 6 to 10° a moderate complication, and greater than 10° a severe Type 1 complication. It is probable that more angulation may be accepted in the sagittal than in the frontal plane, but to introduce a more complex system would seem unnecessarily cumbersome. The situation in the femur is somewhat less clear because deformity is more easily tolerated. We have seen proximal femoral deformities of 45° in the sagittal plane with no apparent functional deficit and deformities of greater than 20° in the frontal plane that show as obvious cosmetic deformities, but again, with no functional deficit. These may be exceptional cases and the long-term effects are not clearly understood. We recommend the following description: less than 10° should be classified as normal, 11 to 15° should be classified as moderate, and greater than 15° classified as severe Type 1. Follow-up should be at least 1 year and, in the case of joint stiffness, the final functional outcome may not be known for at least 2 years after final corrective surgery.

Summary

The techniques of callus and soft tissue distraction have widened the surgeon's scope in the field of corrective and reconstructive surgery. Procedures are complex and lengthy and considerable time must be spent in pre-operative planning and patient preparation. Because treatment times are protracted, patients may have non-surgical problems, such as social, domestic, educational, and psychological problems, as well as problems that may be cared for by the nursing and physiotherapy staff. A multidisciplinary team approach is the first and most useful step in reducing complication rates. Concentrating this type of surgery in units with a relatively high throughput will improve results simply because of familiarity with the pitfalls of the technique. Complications are, however, inevitable but should be managed appropriately and minimized. The variety of the patients and their family units means that "cookbook" decisions cannot be applied. Nevertheless, more detailed recording of complications, together with analyses of patient satisfaction and functional outcome, may aid appropriate patient selection and improve operative planning. Functional outcome-related reporting of results at perhaps 2, 5, and 10 years after completion of treatment would be extremely valuable. Most lengthening series are too heterogeneous to make meaningful appraisals of subgroups of patients and operative techniques. Standardized complication reporting is integral, both to the grouping of disorders and treatments, and for meaningful comparisons between centres and methods.

Acknowledgments

The authors would like to thank Siobhan Shaw, assistant psychologist, and the charitable organization that supports our clinical work, the Sheffield Children's Hospital Limb Inequality Service.

References

1. Codivilla A: 'On the means of lengthening, in the lower limbs, the muscles and tissues which are shortened through deformity.' *Am J Orthop Surg* 1905, 2: 353-69.
2. Putti V: 'The operative lengthening of the femur.' *JAMA* 1921, 77:934.
3. Abbott LC: 'The operative lengthening of the tibia and fibula.' *J Bone Joint Surg* 1927, 9; 128-52.
4. Anderson WV: 'Lengthening of the lower limb: Its place in the problem of limb length discrepancy' in Graham WD (ed): *Modern Trends in Orthopaedic Surgery.* Butterworth: London, 1967, pp 1-22.
5. Ilizarov GA, Deviatov AA: 'Operative elongation of the leg.' *Ortop Travrmtol Protez* 1971, 32: 20-5.
6. Wagner H: 'Operative Beinverlangerung.' *Chirurg* 1971, 42: 260-6.
7. De Bastiani G, Aldegberi R, Renzi Brivio L et al: 'Limb lengthening by callus distraction (callotasis).' *J Pediatr Orthop* 1987, 7: 129-34.
8. Vilarrubias JM, Ginebreda 1, Jimeno E: 'Lengthening of the lower limbs and correction of lumbar hyperlordosis in achondroplasia.' *Clin Orthop* 1990; 250: 143-9.
9. Ilizarov GA: 'The tension-stress effect on the genesis and growth of tissues, Part 1, The influence of stability of fixation and soft tissue preservation.' *Clin Orthop* 1989, 238: 249–81.
10. Ilizarov GA: 'The tension-stress effect on the genesis and growth of tissues, Part 2, The influence of the rate and frequency of distraction.' *Clin Orthop* 1989, 239: 263-85.
11. Aldegheri R, Trivella G, Renzi-Brivio, et al: 'Lengthening in the lower limbs in achrondroplastic patients.' *J Bone Joint Surg* [Br] 1988, 70: 69-73.
12. Saleh M, Burton M: 'Leg lengthening: Patient selection and management in achondroplasia.' *Orthop Clin North Am* 1991, 22: 589-99.
13. Saleh M: 'Non-union surgery, Part 1. Basic principles of management.' *Int J Orthop Trauma* 1992, 14-8.
14. Ribbans WJ, Stubbs DA, Saleh M: 'Non-union surgery, Part 2. The Sheffield experience - One hundred consecutive cases. Results and lessons.' *Int J Orthop Trauma* 1992, 2: 19-24.
15. Weber G, Bregani P, Premoli F, et al: 'Surgical lengthening of the limbs in achrondroplastic children: A medical and psychosocial programme to select and treat patients' in Nicoletti B, Kopits SE, Ascani E, et al (eds): *Human Achrondroplasia – A Multidisciplinary Approach,* Plenum Press: New York, 1988, pp 461-2.
16. Anderson M, Green WT, Messner MB: 'Growth and predictions of growth in the lower extremities.' *J Bone Joint Surg* [Am] 1963, 45: 1-14.
17. Friberg O: 'Clinical symptoms and biomechanics of lumbar spine and hip joint in leg length inequality.' *Spine* 1983, 8: 643-51.
18. Moseley CF: 'A straight line graph for leg length discrepancies.' *J Bone Joint Surg* [Am] 1977, 59: 174-9.
19. Agostini S, Aldegheri R: *Chart of Anthropometric Values.* Universita di Verona, Clinica Ortopedica e Traumatologica, Valeggio SM(VR)
20. Nicolls MJ, Saleh M: 'Composite photographs in leg lengthening.' *Audiovisual Media Med* 1988, 11: 96-9.
21. Nicolls MJ: 'Computer aided manipulation of photographs in leg lengthening.' *Audiovisual Media Med* 1988, 13: 13-6.
22. Luke DL, Schoenecker PL, Blair VP, et al: 'Fractures after Wagner limb lengthening' *J Paediatr Orthop* 1992, 12: 20-4.
23. Jones DC, Moseley CF: 'Subluxation of the knee as a complication of femoral lengthening by the Wagner technique.' *J Bone Joint Surg* [Br] 1985, 67B: 33-5.
24. Paley D: 'Problems, obstacles and complications of limb lengthening by the Ilizarov technique.' *Clin Orthop* 1990, 250: 81-104.
25. Wagner H: 'Operative lengthening in the femur.' *Clin Orthop* 1978, 136: 125-42.
26. Ilizarov GA, Trokhova VG: 'Operative elongation of the femur.' *Ortop Travmato Protez* 1973, 34: 51-5.

An Historical Background to the Treatment of Non-Union

47

R.B. Simonis

Introduction

In Great Britain, before World War I, fractures were treated by general surgeons and bone setters. In fact, very few general surgeons were interested in the treatment of fractures and injuries, which was regarded as a troublesome chore. Their treatment was usually delegated to junior staff doctors and no attention was paid to the patient's rehabilitation.

Bone setters practised the art of fracture reduction long before there were any orthopaedic surgeons and they were in competition with the local doctors. The secrets of the bone setters were handed down from father to son, and were unpublished. Patients came to them from far afield as they built up a reputation. Their livelihood would have suffered if their techniques had been disseminated by publication.[8]

In 1875, Sir James Paget warned his colleagues that bone setters could obtain better results by massage and manipulation than the surgeons could by their methods. He suggested that surgeons should learn their techniques. Even now, in underdeveloped countries, patients with fractures often prefer to visit their local bone setters (witch doctors), rather than attend the local qualified doctor.

It was really World War I which put orthopaedics on the map. Hospitals were created for treating the wounded soldiers, and some of the more chronic orthopaedic conditions such as tuberculosis, osteomyelitis, septic arthritis and polio. After the war some of these hospitals remained open, treating civilian injuries. An attempt was made to form the British Orthopaedic Society in 1894. However, lack of interest in the treatment of fresh fractures, and a shortage of orthopaedic surgeons, closed the society four years later. It was not renewed until the foundation of the British Orthopaedic Association in 1918, just after World War I.[8]

Even by World War II, the provision of orthopaedic services was patchy in Great Britain. Most of the country had no orthopaedic services at all and there was little demand for any form of orthopaedic surgery. There were a few specialized centres like Oswestry in North Wales, and the Wingfield Orthopaedic Hospital at Oxford. However, as far as patients were concerned, the orthopaedic map was largely blank until the introduction of the National Health Service in 1948. It was only after 1948 that every British hospital introduced a fracture clinic. Specialist centres would usually treat "cold" orthopaedic cases and occasionally cases of non-union of fractures would come to them. In most hospitals the orthopaedic surgeon only had a few beds, which were grudgingly allocated to him by the general surgeons.

If the treatment of fresh fractures in the early 1900s was primitive; the treatment of non-unions was virtually non-existent. It is possible to glean from publications that the treatment of non-unions during the 19th century progressed from the insertion of a seton (first performed in 1802), to irritants applied either externally or internally, to stimulate the formation of callus. Successful ambulatory treatment, wearing some form of external brace, began to come into use after 1850. More modern treatment, such as bone grafting at the fracture site, did not start until about 1900.

Dr Edward Hartshorne wrote a thesis on the cause and treatment of pseudarthrosis in 1841.[6] He described a wide variety of non-surgical methods of treatment, including irritative applications of caustic potash (potassium hydroxide) to the skin over the fracture site, as well as injections into the fracture site. Friction of the bone ends against each other, as well as external friction and local pressure applied by splints, were used. Different kinds of electrical stimulation were also applied and various surgical treatments, including the passage of a seton-needle, armed with a skein of silk. Several surgeons treated non-union by resection of the bone ends and fixation of these ends with silver wire. In many cases this produced osteomyelitis, leading to amputation, which itself was sometimes used as definitive treatment for long-standing non-unions. By 1850 a perforator was used with holes bored through the bone and the non-union (Fig. 47.1). External fixation was provided by means of a Malgaigne spike; a strap and spike held the tibia against a splint (Fig. 47.2).

Before 1840 no good method of external fixation was available other than crude splints, and a "fracture box". The use of plaster of Paris in fresh fractures probably began in the 1840s. Initially starch and glue bandages were applied to the leg, and these then progressed to bandages painted with liquid plaster of Paris, using a brush. Plaster of Paris was used to make splints or moulds applied to one side of the limb; the extremity was not completely enclosed in plaster, because serious complications from tight plaster bandages were described. By about 1880, plaster of Paris bandages were in common use.

McEwen from Scotland, and Nussbaum from Germany, started bone grafting non-unions about 1890. It was not until after 1900 that the treatment of non-union of fractures by bone grafting became widely accepted.[3]

The treatment involved wide exposure of the non-union, resection of both ends of the bone down to bleeding, viable bone, and fixation, carpenter-fashion. In addition, large autogenous bone grafts were applied, and fastened with screws or wires. The limb would then be immobilized for a long period of time in a plaster cast. Even then bony union did not always result! The main reason for failure was that the vascularization of the bone ends was damaged by the exposure and the stripping of the periosteum, and this took a long time to recover.

The operative treatment of non-union has changed radically in recent years. The main reason for this lies in the recognition that the mesenchymal tissue in the non-union (scar, connective tissue and cartilage) is not inferior tissue which must be removed before surgery, but is a valuable matrix for callus formation. The "scar" tissue between the bone ends still possesses the power to differentiate into new bone. In 1920, Elmslie (St Bartholomew's and Royal National Orthopaedic Hospital, London) thought that it was unnecessary to remove this intervening tissue when bone grafting a pseudarthrosis.[5] Phemister (University of Chicago) rediscovered this fact in 1947.[10] He treated non-unions with sub-periosteal onlay grafts, without immobilization or resection of the non-union. His results were so good, and his operation so simple, that many surgeons still use this method today.

In 1949, Danis[4] (Brussels) proved that a pseudarthrosis of the forearm could heal under compression, provided by a plate, without excision of scar tissue, and without bone grafting. In 1953, Kuntscher showed that a pseudarthrosis in a long bone rapidly disappeared when it was fixed with an intramedullary nail.[7] Intramedullary reaming destroys the blood supply from the medullary cavity and, if the nailing is combined with an open operation, then the periosteal blood supply is also interrupted; so the non-union may persist.

It was Bohler (1963) who advocated the advantages of closed medullary nailing, which did not denude the

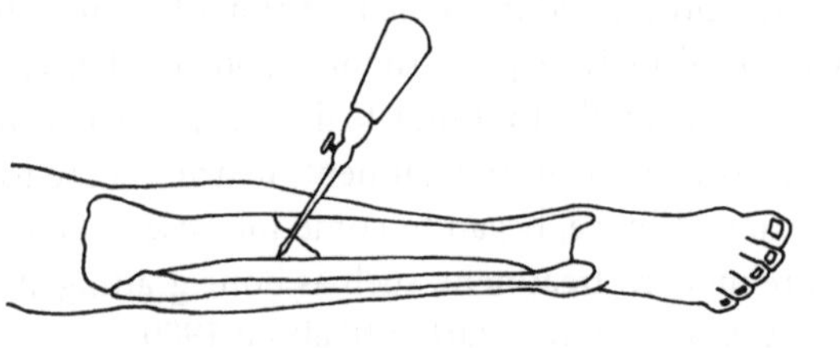

Fig. 47.1 Perforator (gimlet) passing through non-union.

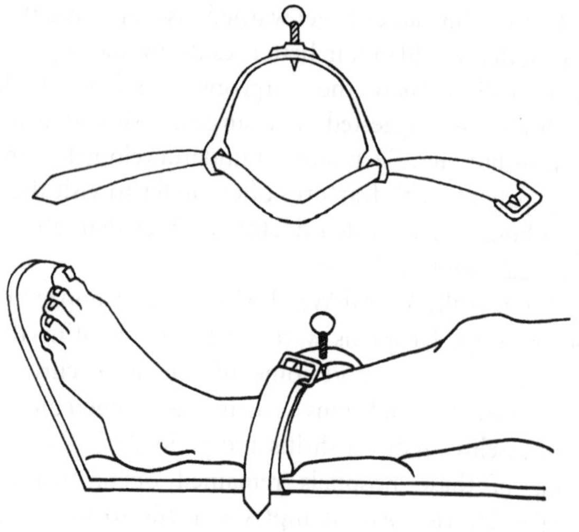

Fig. 47.2 Malgaigne's spike to fix a fractured tibia (1840).

periosteum of its blood supply. This was only really possible after the development of the image intensifier.

It was not until the late 1970s that external fixators were well enough designed to be able to provide rigid fixation and compression, both necessary to heal a non-union.

Thus, to heal a non-union, it is necessary rigidly to immobilize the bone ends, to create the local stimuli for the transposition of the mesenchymal tissue into bony callus. This can be obtained by three methods: compression plating, intramedullary nailing, or external fixation. All three have their definite indications, and all three can be combined with a bone graft. The vascularization of the non-union should be disturbed as little as possible.

Plating for Non-Union of Fractures

The use of metal to control the position of fractures was probably first attempted in the late 18th century. We can assume with virtual certainty that these attempts, before anaesthesia, antisepsis and antibiotics, were uniformly disastrous. It was not surprising, therefore, that until the end of the 19th century, open reduction and internal fixation was only used when all conservative treatment had failed. Delayed and non-unions were fixed in desperation, with the surgeon aware that there was a very high rate of complications.

At any given period of time, the status of orthopaedic implants has to be considered in the light of contemporary technology. Three developments were important in the gradual acceptance of internal fixation: (i) antisepsis, (ii) the advent of X-rays, and (iii) metallurgy.

It was not until Lister developed antisepsis, during the years 1860–70, that the complications of infection and gangrene became controllable and metallic internal fixation really started. It still required the "no-touch" technique devised by Sir William Arbuthnot Lane (1856–1938), to keep the rate of infection down to reasonable proportions.

The use of plates and screws was rare until the advent of X-rays in 1895. For the first time we could see what the surgery had achieved!

In the early days of internal fixation, one of the main problems was a tendency for metal implants to corrode; tissue reactions to material were not fully understood and there was no adequate science of biomechanics. Over the last 100 years this science has gradually improved; animal experiments detected that iron and carbon steels dissolved. The year 1926 saw the introduction of stainless steel with 18 per cent chromium and 8 per cent nickel, but this was still liable to disintegrate.

In 1936 vitallium started to be used for orthopaedic implants. This is a non-ferrous alloy of cobalt with chromium and molybdenum, and its inertness made it very suitable for orthopaedic implants. Titanium and its alloy appeared around 1947; as a pure metal it proved inert and corrosion resistant. Specifications for the various metals and alloys were laid down by the American Committee on Fractures in 1947. Since then there have been only minor changes in the composition of the metals used for implants.

Plate Design

The first bone plate was probably used by Hansmann in 1886. He fixed fractures with strips of unhardened nickel-plated sheet steel. One end of the plate was bent at right angles to protrude through the skin to facilitate retrieval of the plate about eight weeks after fixation. Lambotte, Lane, Sherman, Townsend and Gilfillan and Eggers, all played prominent roles in the development of the early bone plates (Figs. 47.3–47.7). The design of these plates continued to improve, providing greater strength and better conformity to the bone surface. As these designs were developed, new alloys became available, providing improved strength and acceptability by the body. These early plates all "fixed" the fracture fragments, representing an extension of the old principle of splintage. They substituted internal metal splints for the splints and plaster casts of closed treatment. So all these early plates did was to co-apt the fracture fragments. There was no mention of compression, which we now consider crucial both in the treatment of fresh fractures and non-unions.

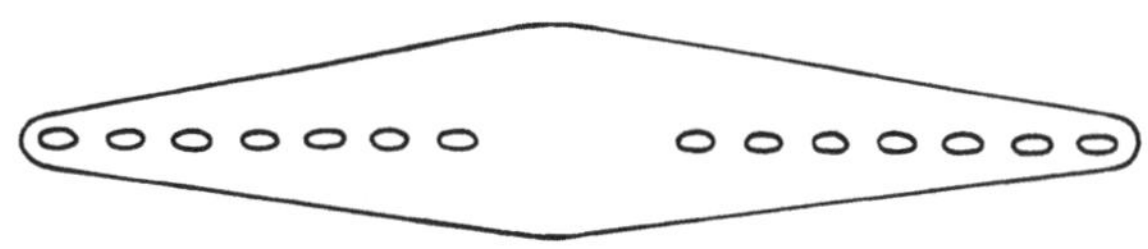

Fig. 47.3 Lambotte (1909).

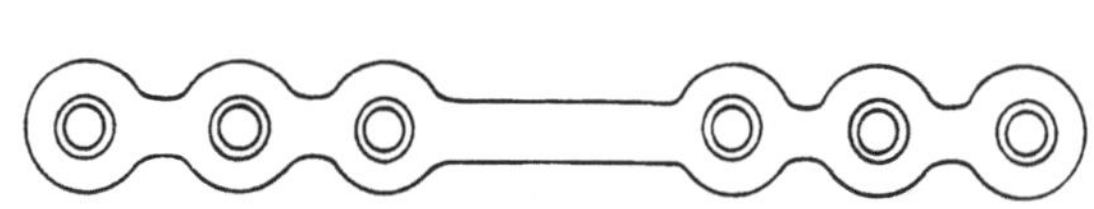

Fig. 47.4 Lane (1914).

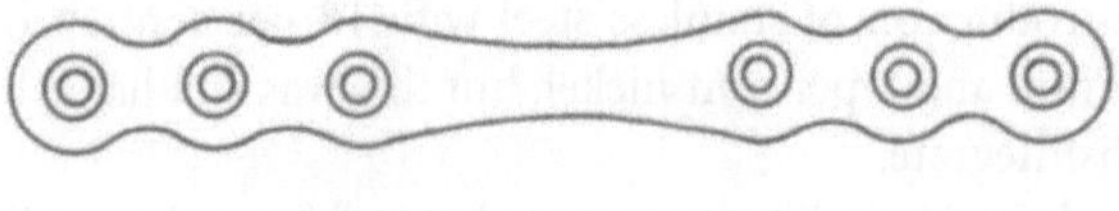

Fig. 47.5 Sherman (1912).

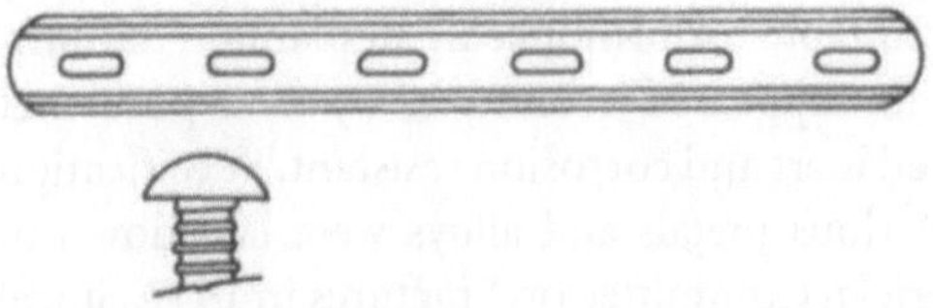

Fig. 47.6 Townsend and Gilfillan (1943).

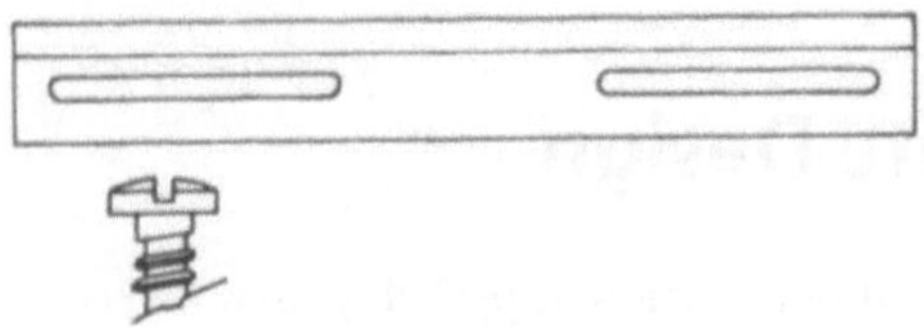

Fig. 47.7 Eggers (1948).

Compression

Fracture treatment initially sought to immobilize the bone fragments. Those who applied splints assumed that contractions of the muscle adjacent to the fracture would compress the fracture. Key introduced compression in 1932, for arthrodesis of the knee. He transfixed the femur and tibia with two pins in each bone. After removing the articular cartilage, he applied compression across the joint with two clamps secured to the pins. This technique was then used by Roger Anderson in 1934 for the treatment of fresh fractures. It eventually led to the development of the Charnley clamp, which again was used mainly for arthrodesis. Eggers in 1946 was the first to demonstrate that compression forces applied to healing bone fragments could speed up the rate of healing. However, his slotted plate (Fig. 47.7) was designed to allow the fracture fragments to slide together. "Sliding" was considered important because it narrowed the gap to be healed, not necessarily because it caused compression. The narrowing of the gap between the fragments was accomplished intra-operatively by manipulation of the fragments. Eggers considered that the most important pressure force was the action produced by the patient's muscles. It was not possible for the surgeon to adjust the amount of compression applied with his slotted plate.

Robert Danis[4] (1880–1962) of Brussels was the first surgeon to use a true compression plate in the treatment of acute fractures (Fig. 47.8). He wrote a treatise on the internal fixation of fractures, describing his plate, originally designed for the forearm. He provided data on 34 patients with fractures of radius and ulna. All 68 fractures healed satisfactorily following application of his plate. Three of these 34 patients had delayed union because of infection. He had less encouraging results with fractures of the humerus, tibia and femur. Other surgeons did not appear to obtain such good results with the plate, probably because of the difficulty of applying compression with the screw, which was very close to the bone.

Danis wrote that with rigid internal fixation, callus did not form. He stated that callus was not essential to fracture healing, and he devised the term "primary cortical healing". In 1948, Danis also showed that a pseudarthosis of the forearm could heal under compression, without excision of the scar tissue, and without bone grafting. It was this work that provided the stimulus for our contemporary treatment of both fresh fractures and non-union.

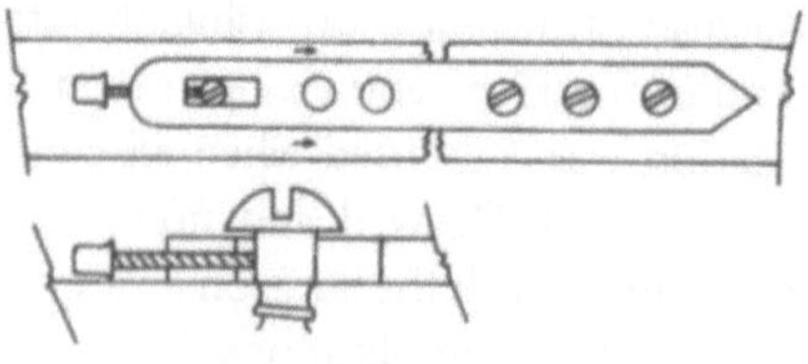

Fig. 47.8 Danis (1949).

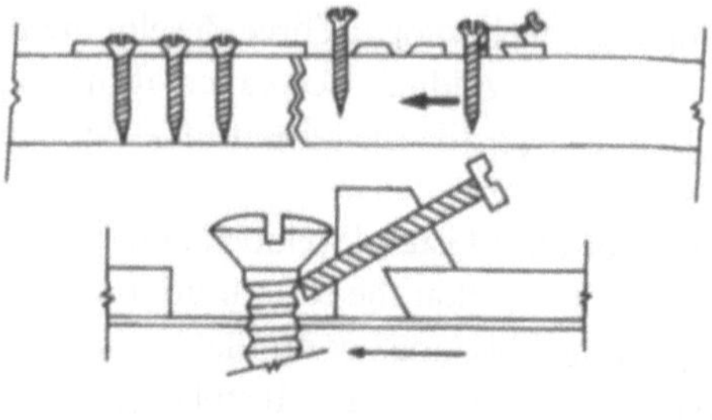

Fig. 47.9 Venable (1951).

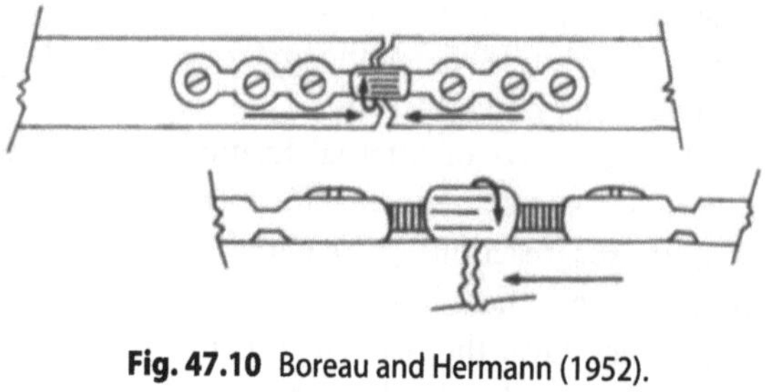

Fig. 47.10 Boreau and Hermann (1952).

Various other plates were devised to produce compression. In Venable's plate (Fig. 47.9), the compression screw was orientated obliquely to make it more accessible. Boreau and Hermann (Fig. 47.10) produced a compression plate, with a central turnbuckle, which actually weakened the device.

The Müller plate (Fig. 47.11) was an improvement on the Danis plate. It had a more sophisticated compression mechanism, secured to one end of the plate and to the bone.

In 1956, Bagby[1] described the first self-compressing bone plate; it had bevelled screw holes (Fig. 47.12). His concept was that the screws holding the plate to the bone could also compress the bone fragments, and that no additional device was necessary.

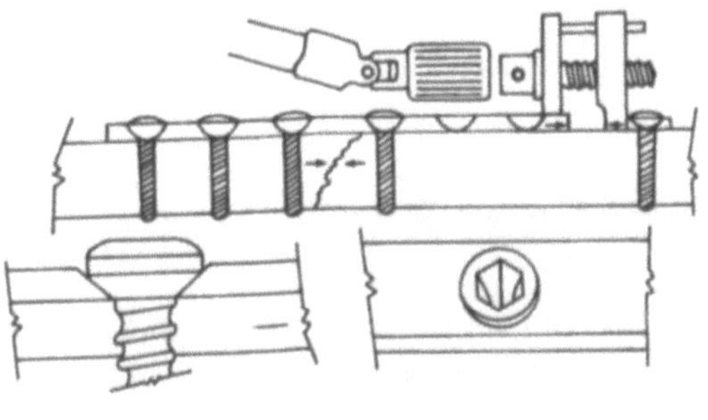

Fig. 47.11 Müller (1961).

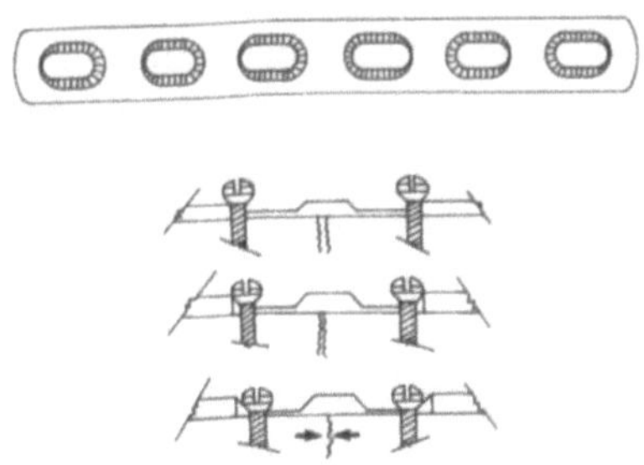

Fig. 47.12 Bagby plate (1956).

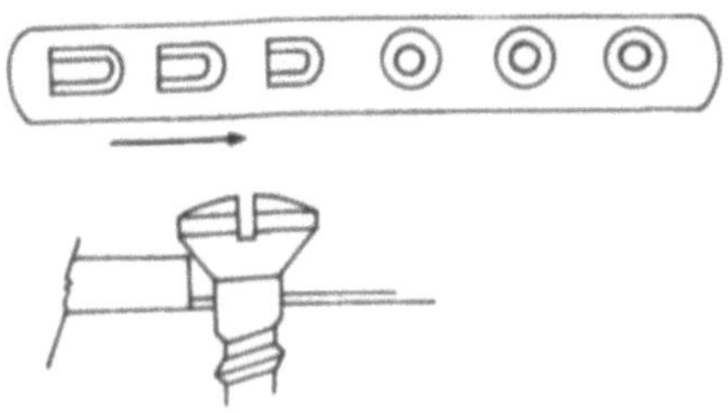

Fig. 47.13 Denham (England).

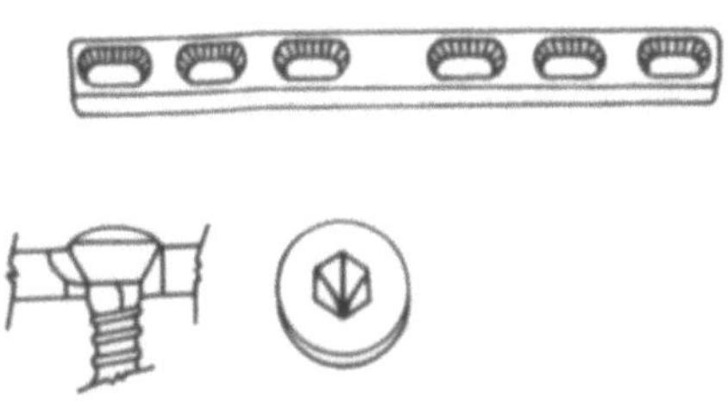

Fig. 47.14 Dynamic compression plate (ASIF).

The concept of the Bagby plate, using self-compressing holes, was subsequently incorporated in various other plates designed by Denham (Fig. 47.13), and other commercially available plates such as the dynamic compression plate (ASIF, Fig. 47.14).

In the early 1950s three Swiss workers, M E Müller, M Allgöwer and H Willenegger, began to study compression systems and founded the now famous *Arbeitsgemeinschaft Für Osteosynthesefragen* or "working party" on problems of internal fixation, generally known as AO[9]. They had shouldered screw holes in the plate. This resembled Bagby's plate (providing compression when the screws were tightened). They further suggested that by pre-bending the plate, compression could be applied across the surface as the plate was tightened down against the surface of the bone. They also developed lag screws, tension-band wires, and powered equipment with special tools for their insertion. Standardization of implants, and the AO instrument pack advanced the use of internal fixation.

History of Bone Grafting

Over 200 years ago, John Hunter demonstrated that separated fragments of bone could both survive and grow. He forecast the possibility of bone grafting in the future. The first successful bone transplantation was reported in 1879 by Sir William MacEwen (1848–1924) from Glasgow. He removed the whole shaft of the right humerus from a four-year-old boy who was suffering from osteomyelitis. Fifteen months later, MacEwen inserted small fragments of bone wedges removed from other children who had had corrective wedge osteotomies for bow legs. The new antiseptic surgery devised by Lister enabled him to do this without major complication. Further grafts were inserted a few months later, and sixteen months after the first procedure the humeral shaft had consolidated from end to end, and was only half an inch shorter than the other side. MacEwen saw this patient again 30 years later, in 1909. He had worked all his life as a carpenter and subsequently served in World War I. This famous case proved that bone grafting was a possibility. After 1900, most publications on the treatment of non-union usually included the use of bone grafts to promote union.

Fred Albee from New York put bone grafting on the map as a practicality in 1911. He adopted a carpenter's technique, fitting a cortical graft from the opposite tibia as a inlay into a cancellous bed at the new site. It was an exact fit, periosteum to periosteum, cortex to cortex, medulla to medulla. He used an electric saw with two blades. This technique caught on because of the ease of removing the tibial graft with the power saw, and because it was effective.

Various methods of grafting cortical bone were developed over the following years. These methods incorporated two important treatment principles, namely fixation and osteogenesis, in the management of non-union. Cortical bone is selected when there is bone loss and when stability is required. However, cortical bone is first resorbed by osteoclasts before significant osteoblastic activity can take place (creeping substitution). Thus cortical bone goes through a porous phase and is structurally less strong several months after its implantation. Some surgeons therefore supplement the graft with a plate. Cortical bone is less osteogenic than iliac cancellous bone. It has only been during the last 50 years that the special advantage of grafting with cancellous bone has been recognized.

Following Albee's paper on bone grafting, many modifications followed. Campbell used onlay grafts fixed with bone pegs, Henderson screwed his onlay grafts, and Tyerson used the fibula as an intramedullary graft. Nicoll[11] fixed blocks of iliac cortico-cancellous graft into defects in the shafts of long bones, using a metal plate, with good results.

Autogenous bone was obviously the ideal solution, but often the patient could not supply enough bone to fill a large defect. For this reason various methods of allograft were devised; even xenografts were used. Unfortunately, immunological rejection of the implant material and fracture of the graft precluded wide utilization of these grafts. In 1931, Svante Orell from Sweden deproteinised cadaveric human and animal bone by treating it with caustic potash and acetone to eliminate all soft tissues, in an attempt to remove antigenicity. All this did was to provide a scaffold, which was not particularly osteogenic. This technique did not last. Later, preserved beef bone had its vogue; deproteinised calf bone called "Kiel bone" could be cut to any shape and thickness for filling massive bone defects. Its incorporation was better if the bone was mixed with autogenous graft, or marrow cells aspirated from the patient's own ilium.

Bone Banks

Most orthopaedic surgeons occasionally have to remove healthy bone from their patients, and it is useful to preserve it. Inclan was the first to conceive of a bone bank in 1942. He stored the bone in blood or saline, just above 0° centigrade. Others have kept the bone in sealed glass containers at –24° centigrade, and others have boiled or autoclaved cadaveric bone. Once boiled, the bone is not antigenic but it is inert and replaced very slowly; incorporation takes a long time. Bone banks have gained more acceptance in recent years. Very strict screening of the donor must be used to avoid the passage of any infection.

Cancellous Bone Grafting

Cancellous bone revascularises more quickly, and has greater osteogenic properties than cortical grafts. As a result, massive cortical grafting is used less often in surgical practice today.

In 1947, Phemister, from Chicago, described a method of onlay bone grafting in non-unions without breaking down the fibrous ankylosis[10]. Until that time, the usual treatment for un-united fractures involved resection of the fibrous union and separation of the fracture surfaces. The fragments were aligned and then an onlay of thick cortical bone was fixed to the fragments with screws. The extremity was then immobilized in plaster. Phemister established that the "callus" associated with a non-union would ossify spontaneously when an adequate cancellous bone graft was applied, and that disturbance of the fibrous tissue between the fracture ends was unnecessary. Phemister bone grafting is still used today in the treatment of non-union, and has about a 90 per cent success rate.

Cancellous bone grafting became popular during World War II as a method of dealing with non– and delayed unions. It was also used in the treatment of the more difficult fresh fractures, particularly when there was an associated bony defect.

Free Vascularized Bone Grafts

Improvements in microsurgical techniques have made it possible to utilize vascularized bone transfer for the reconstruction of major bone defects. Iliac crest, posterior ribs, or fibula can be taken with their own vasculature and are therefore less dependent on the recipient bed for survival. Vascularised bone grafts are able to survive in irradiated beds and also in congenital pseudarthrosis of the tibia; two of the most difficult orthopaedic problems. Successful anastomosis of the nutrient vessels is accompanied by viability of both the bone and the marrow. One advantage of this technique lies in the ability to transfer bone with its overlying muscle and skin to cover major defects of bone and soft tissue (Fig. 47.15). The bone unites in a few weeks, and hypertrophies to the same size as the recipient bone within a few months. These grafts require time-consuming microsurgical techniques, but they have allowed many severely injured limbs to be salvaged.

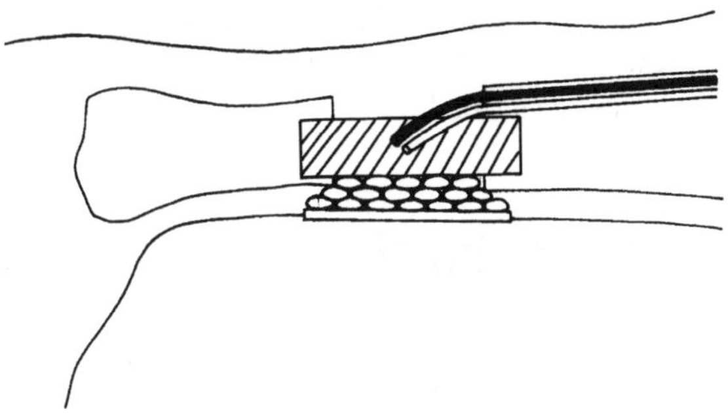

Fig. 47.15 Vascularised bone graft.

Intramedullary Nailing

The first reference to intramedullary fixation of fractures comes from 16th century writings suggesting that the Incas and Aztecs used sticks of wood pushed into the intramedullary canal for the treatment of non-union of long bones.[8] During the second half of the 19th century, the use of implants became more widespread. Dieffenback (Germany) in 1841 inserted ivory pegs through perforations which he had made at the fracture ends in cases of non-union.

Between 1870 and 1886 there were several reported cases of implants made of various materials. Malgaigne (France) used metal implants, and Ferraud (France) pushed ivory pegs down the medullary canal. By 1880, surgeons in Europe and the United States were experimenting with nails made of ivory, bone and iron for the treatment of pseudarthrosis. Various other implants were used for intramedullary fixation around this time; aluminium rods, ductile silver pins, and even knitting needles were used to treat femoral neck fractures. Hey-Groves, of Bristol, performed animal experiments with absorbable and non-absorbable intramedullary implants, finding metal pegs the most satisfactory. In 1918 he reported the use of steel rods in three cases of compound femoral fractures from gunshot injuries.

In the United States in the 1930s, the name of Rush became synonymous with fracture fixation. Rush Sr. and his two sons reported the treatment of Monteggia fractures by axial fixation using Steinmann pins, introduced through the olecranon. They later (1956) designed their own pins which they used for treating many different types of fracture and pseudarthrosis.

By the end of the 1930s, the concepts and techniques of intramedullary fixation took off with the work of Gerhard Kuntscher (1900–1972) from Germany. In 1939 he treated a sub-trochanteric fracture using an open section V-shaped steel nail. In 1940, he presented nailings of the femur, hip, tibia and humerus, at a meeting of the German Surgical Society. Whilst many surgeons involved in trauma at that time were sceptical of his techniques, he was supported by other colleagues from the University of Kiel, namely Maatz and Fischer, who helped him design other nails – conical, split and later the slotted clover leaf nails. In 1943, Kuntscher became commander of an army hospital in Finland, where he continued his pioneering work. The rest of Europe and North America learnt of his work by taking X-rays of returning prisoners of war.

In Vienna, Lorenz Bohler, a renowned trauma surgeon, was a keen advocate of Kuntscher's nailing techniques. Between 1941 and 1948 he performed closed nailings on 58 closed femoral fractures. By 1948 he recommended nailing for both upper femoral shaft fractures and non-unions of the femur. Bohler's life exhibited a remarkable change from that of a country doctor, to being in charge of a military hospital in World War I. In 1925, he was invited to Vienna to take charge of an accident hospital. Between the wars, he wrote a popular textbook on fracture treatment, and his acceptance of Kuntscher's nailing system gave it credibility. The first American intramedullary nailing was probably performed in 1945 by Macausland from Boston, using a tantalum nail, similar in design to one that he had removed from a returned American pilot.

Kuntscher continued developing his ideas after the war, and in 1952 introduced flexible guided reamers. Over the next 30 years, advances in instrumentation and techniques led to the development of interlocking screws to control both rotation and shortening.

Kuntscher continued to use intramedullary nailing for the treatment of non-union. He stated that to heal a non-union it was necessary to immobilize the ends of the bone at the fracture site and allow the fibrous tissue to change into bone; the vascularization should be disturbed as little as possible. Closed intramedullary nailing, preserving the periosteal blood supply, fulfilled these criteria. Between 1956 and 1961 Bohler treated 40 cases of non-union of the tibia, with closed or semi-closed intramedullary nailing, and all 40 cases healed by bony union.

Electricity

The first report of electricity being used in the treatment of non-union was by Mr Birch,[2] surgeon to St Thomas' Hospital, London, who:

> In 1812 treated an unconsolidated fracture of the tibia, below the middle, of 13 months' standing. The leg below the fracture could be moved easily in any direction, without exciting much pain. Shocks of electric fluid were passed through the space between the ends of the bone, both in the direction of the length of the limb and that of its thickness... After the limb was electricized, the ordinary apparatus for fractures of the leg was applied. The limb became less flexible in the situation of the fracture, and after continuation of the same treatment for six weeks, the man was able to walk and left the hospital cured.

This was only 13 years after Alessandro Volta (1745–1827), invented the battery in Italy.

Following this extraordinary report, many other anecdotal papers were published in medical journals, claiming great success! Electricity appeared to be an accepted technique in the treatment of delayed unions, until all sorts of wild claims were made of its effectiveness in treating a multiplicity of other complaints such as backache, migraine and pneumonia. Very quickly electricity fell into disrepute. The great German surgeon Dieffenback said in a public lecture in 1840[8]:

> No matter how perverse an idea may be in science, once it is thought of, someone or other will actually put it into practice... I need only remind you of how such a one has claimed to restore a sluggish fracture by applying one galvanic plate in the mouth and the opposite one in the anus.

The recent work on electricity started in Japan. In 1953, Yasuda published two important papers in an obscure Japanese journal. The first demonstrated the piezoelectric effect of bone, showing that when a bone is stressed or deformed a potential difference is created and a current passes along the bone. The other showed that a small amount of current applied to a bone stimulated osteogenesis at the cathode. A further paper in 1957 by Fukada and Yasuda confirmed that a voltage is passed when a bone is deformed. This was considered to be the physical mediator of Wolff's Law. Later, Andrew Bassett took on this work at Columbia University in New York. He confirmed that with a direct current, bone could be produced at the cathode and resorbed at the anode. Bassett went on to develop a machine capable of producing pulsed electromagnetic fields (PEMFs) which were applied to the limb through two external coils. These fields "induced" an electric current in the affected limb. This induced current accelerated soft tissue repair in nerve and tendon, as well as in healing bone. Exactly how electricity works has remained obscure, but because it works on all tissues, it is thought to create an effect at the cellular level.

The association of electricity with quackery still lingers on, but so many papers have been produced demonstrating the beneficial effects of both direct and induced currents, that it should be examined in greater detail. Carefully controlled double blind trials must be performed so that the place of electricity in fracture healing can be clarified.

External Fixation

Hippocrates (460–370 BC) described a method of external fixation (Fig. 47.16) as a means of immobilizing fractures. He was 2000 years ahead of his time. The development of the more modern external fixator is attributed to Malgaigne from Paris. His device was uncomfortable and often associated with infection, so it did not survive (Fig. 47.2).

Clayton Parkhill, who graduated in 1883, and became Professor of Surgery at the University of Colo-

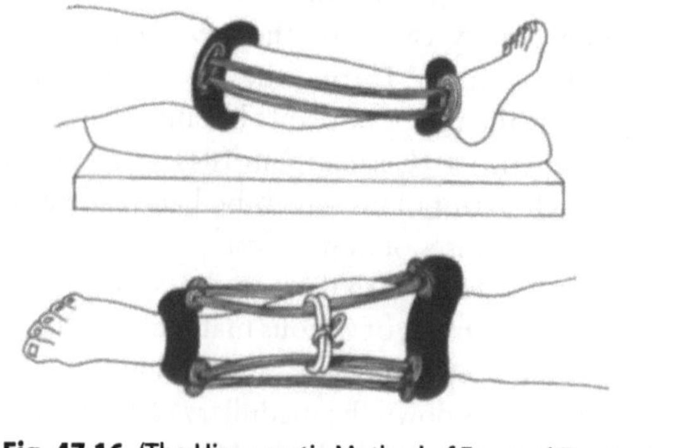

Fig. 47.16 'The Hippocratic Method of External Fixation'.

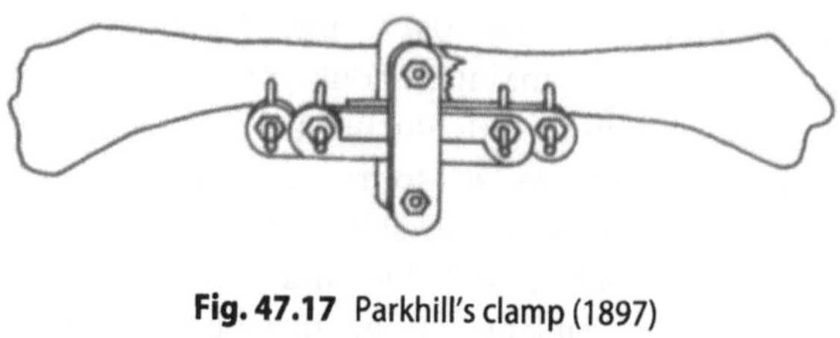

Fig. 47.17 Parkhill's clamp (1897)

rado, was an ingenious surgeon. Seeing the often catastrophic results of operating on fractures, he developed a new device with threaded half pins, screwed into the bone above and below the fracture, and connected by a metal clamp. The clamp consisted of two halves which could be fixed together once reduction had been obtained (Fig. 47.17).

External fixation continued to be developed because of the need to treat serious war injuries. In 1902 Albin Lambotte, from Belgium, working independently of Parkhill, developed his "fixateur" (Fig. 47.18). This was similar to Parkhill's, and could be used for fractures of the femur, tibia, forearm, humerus, clavicle and metacarpals. It was simple and rigid. He commented that use of the device had avoided the need for amputations where these had previously seemed inevitable.

The Parkhill and the Lambotte were the first two fixators widely available, and formed the basis of many which followed. Due to problems of infection, lack of stability and difficulty with alignment, fixators did not initially gain popularity.

Pin Development

Most modifications to the basic design of the external fixator in the early years relate to the pins themselves. Lambotte designed the first self-drilling, self-tapping pins. Codivilla, in a paper describing the first use of external fixation for leg lengthening (1905), recommended transfixion of the tibia to improve anchorage of the pins. Henri Judet in 1934 was the first to advocate insertion of half pins through both cortices. He showed the importance of pin track debridement to prevent necrosis and infection. It was not until 1973 that transfixing pins were threaded in the middle, to improve cortical hold.

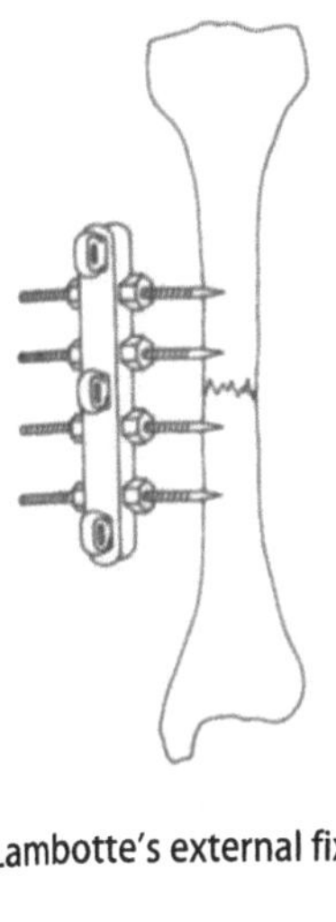

Fig. 47.18 Lambotte's external fixator (1902).

Adaptability of the External Fixator

One of the main drawbacks of systems based on the Lambotte or Parkhill fixator was the inability to change the position of the fragments in more than one plane. Articulations were introduced in the early 1930s permitting the possibility of altering position. Roger Anderson of Seattle in 1934 devised a way of fixing pins to moveable metal yokes, which were imbedded in plaster. Further modifications allowed them to be connected to a bar, thereby removing the need for plaster; multi-planar adjustment was now possible. The Anderson fixator was used during World War II. However, the problems of sepsis around the transfixion pins continued, and the technique had to be abandoned.

Otto Stader, a veterinary surgeon working towards the end of the 1930s, brought into common use a fixator originally designed for use on dogs. It was this system that prompted Raoul Hoffmann to develop his external fixator, which incorporated a universal ball joint, connecting external bars to strong pin clamps. The universal ball joint permitted three-dimensional fracture reduction, both at the time of application and subsequently. In addition, both compression and distraction could be applied. The Hoffmann frame was originally devised in 1938. It was later modified from a unilateral fixator to a quadrilateral frame by Vidal and Ardrey (Fig. 47.19). The Hoffmann and its modified versions gave, for the first time, reproducibly good results in the treatment of difficult fractures and non-unions.

Biology of External Fixation

Better understanding of the physiology of fracture healing has resulted in a change in the way the external fixator has been utilized. It has been known for some time that compression encourages the healing of

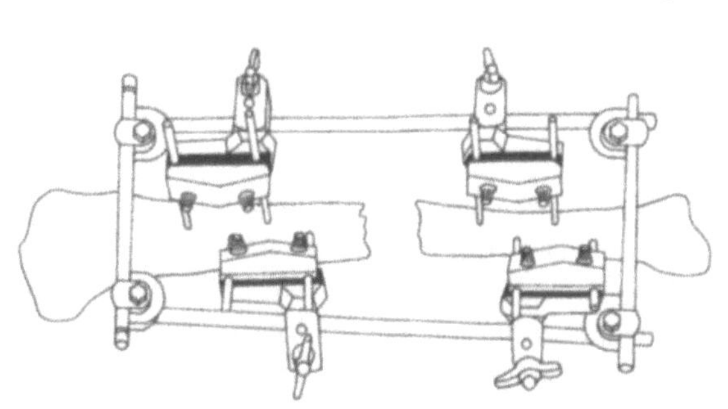

Fig. 47.19 Hoffmann–Vidal Frame.

arthrodeses and non-unions of fractures. Concepts of elastic fixation have been developed and micromovement has been shown to promote bony union at fresh fracture sites.

Dynamization, towards the end of fracture healing, strengthens the callus, speeds up consolidation and allows early removal of the fixator.

External fixators may be applied to function in one of three ways:

1. **Neutralization** Holding the limb out to length; protecting the fracture site from loading (i.e. neutralizing the loads).
2. **Compression** Compressing the fracture fragments together in an effort to increase stability and facilitate the healing of fresh fractures and non-unions.
3. **Distraction** Pulling the fracture fragments apart in order to form regenerate bone, and thus lengthen the limb.

Dynamic Axial Fixation

The first paper on the Dynamic Axial Fixator (Orthofix) was presented in 1984 by Professor G De Bastiani, from the University of Verona in Italy. He explained how, at that time, most surgeons tended to reserve external skeletal fixation for the more severe fractures with extensive soft tissue damage. The devices used then provided rigid fixation. Rigidity would prevent optimal primary bone healing, and the degree of stiffness provided by the frame would provoke only minimal stimulation of periosteal callus. This combination of poor primary healing with depressed secondary healing, resulted in an overall prolongation of healing time with possible refractures.

Professor F Burny, from Belgium, thought of external fixation as an alternative to other forms of fracture stabilization, and used it much more widely in simple closed fractures, as well as in the more complicated injuries. His method differed from those of Hoffmann and Vidal, in that he used a system which introduced a degree of elasticity into the fixator, producing stronger callus and faster healing. Working at the same time as Burny, De Bastiani developed the Dynamic Axial Fixator (DAF). This provides rigidity in the early phases of fracture healing, following which the system can be rapidly converted to a dynamic mode to provide micromovement and thus produce better callus formation and quicker bone healing. The Dynamic Axial Fixator has extended the range of indications for external fixation.

Initially, in 1984, the Dynamic Axial Fixator was used for the treatment of fresh fractures. Now, its ability to compress makes it, in addition, a useful tool for the treatment of non-union. Distraction at a corticotomy site in the shaft, can also produce bone lengthening. Development of the DAF has expanded the indications of external fixation to limb-lengthening and limb reconstruction, following bone loss after severe fractures.

Ilizarov External Fixation

Professor Gavriil Ilizarov working in Kurgan, in Western Siberia, developed his system of external fixation independently of De Bastiani. He was the son of a shepherd and was illiterate until the age of 12. His family could not afford to buy him shoes to walk to school. Being a quick learner, he progressed rapidly, graduating from medical school in 1943. He was then sent by the Government to the city of Kurgan, where conditions were primitive. Ilizarov was the only doctor for miles around, operating in a primitive log cabin, heated with a wood stove. He had to treat a lot of veterans returning from World War II. In this role he was forced to use his own ingenuity to treat the many non-unions and infected fractures he saw.

By 1951, Ilizarov had developed a system of external rings, attached to the limb by thin wires (bicycle spokes) driven through the bone (Fig. 47.20). These rings were connected by long threaded rods allowing compression of fractures and non-unions, expediting union. He also found that distraction could produce bony lengthening. Gradually Ilizarov's technique became accepted in the Soviet Union, and eventually he obtained funding for an 800-bedded hospital, the largest orthopaedic hospital in the world.

In 1978, Ilizarov successfully treated the famous Italian explorer, Carlo Mauri, who had an infected non-union following a climbing accident in the Alps. Mauri persuaded several Italian surgeons to visit Kurgan in the early 1980s, and they then started using the Ilizarov technique in Italy. Its use then spread through Europe to the United States.

The basic premise of Ilizarov's technique is that slow, constant tension on living tissues creates stresses which can stimulate and regenerate certain structures; specifically, bone, skin, muscle, nerves and blood vessels. By distracting a corticotomy in a long bone at the rate of 1mm per day, the bone can regenerate and lengthen. His circular frame allows axial regeneration (lengthening), as well as angular and rotational corrections. The indications for external fixation have now been widened further, to include the correction of deformities such as congenital dislocation of the hip and club foot.

Conclusion

With improved methods of management of fractures, one would expect fewer non-unions. This does not appear to be the case, however, for three main reasons. First, high speed transportation causes high velocity injuries and this produces a greater number of grossly comminuted and compound fractures. Second, there is an increase in mechanization, both in the industrial world and in the building trade, which also increases the number of complicated fractures. Finally, surgeons now have the ability to save legs that would previously have been amputated. Stabilization with external fixation, followed by arterial and soft tissue repair performed by plastic surgeons, allows the limb to be salvaged. It also produces cases for limb reconstruction, which may involve many orthopaedic operations over a long period of time.

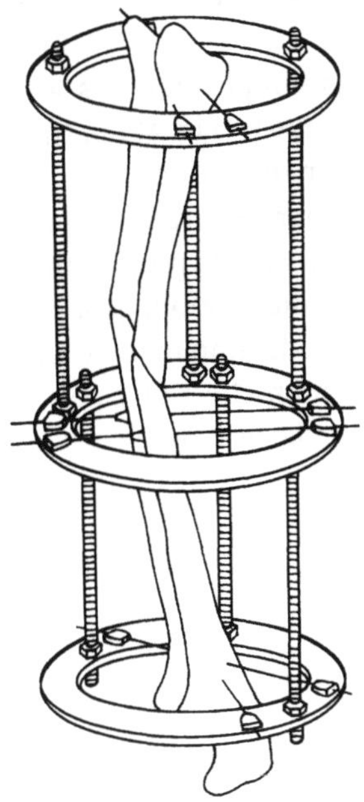

Fig. 47.20 Ilizarov Frame.

Nowadays tibial fractures constitute the majority of healing problems, but it is interesting to note that in 1935 Sever stated that non-union of the humerus produced more trouble than that experienced with any other bone. The reason that problems with tibial fractures are increasing is the fact that better initial management allows these legs to be salvaged. This may not necessarily be in the patient's best interest!

Acknowledgement

I would like to thank Miss Victoria Burden, from the photographic department of St Peter's Hospital, Chertsey, for the illustrations.

References

1. Bagby G. W., Washington. 'Compression Bone-Plating.' *J Bone Joint Surg* [Am] 1977; 59A: 625–31.
2. Bayer A (1816). *Traite des maladies chircurgicales.* Translated by Stevens A. H., as: *A Treatise in Surgical Diseases and the Operations Suited to Them.* New York.
3. Crawford R.R. 'History of the Treatment of Non-Union of Fractures in the 19th Century in the United States.' *J Bone Joint Surg* [Am] 1973; 55-A: 1685–1697.
4. Danis R. *Theorie et pratique de l'osteosynthese,* Masson: Paris, 1949.
5. Elmslie see Burrows H. J. 'Treatment of ununited fractures by bone grafting without resection of the bone ends.' *Proc Roy Soc Med* 1940; 33 : 157.
6. Hartshorne E. 'On the causes and treatment of pseudarthrosis and especially of that form of it sometimes called supernumary joint.' *Am J Med Sci* 1841; 1: 121–156.
7. Kuntscher G. *Praxis der Mark Nagelung,* Schatauer: Stuttgart, 1962.
8. Le Vay D. *The History of Orthopaedics.* The Parthenon Publishing Group, 1990.
9. Müller M. 'Internal fixation for fresh fractures and for non-union.' *Proc Roy Soc Med* 1963; 56: 455.
10. Phemister D. B. 'Treatment of ununited fractures by onlay bone grafts without screw or tie fixation and without breaking down of fibrous union.' *J Bone Joint Surg* 1947; 29: 946.
11. Nicoll E. A. 'The treatment of gaps in long bones by cancellous insert grafts.' J Bone Joint Surg [Br] 1956; 38B: 70–82.

The Principles of Non-Union Management 48

M. Saleh

Introduction

A "non-union" is a fracture of a bone induced either by trauma or surgery which fails to progress to union within a reasonable time span. Defining healing times is difficult. A diaphyseal tibial fracture, for example, may heal in 10 weeks or twelve months depending on endogenous and exogenous factors which in turn are modulated by the effects of surgery.

The "At Risk Fracture"

The fracture healing response in long bones should be well established by about six weeks and failure to initiate such a response may be indicative of delayed union. Delayed union, although a confusing term, is of practical value since it is the first manifestation of potential non-union. Bassett[1] considered this stage to appear between four and nine months after fracture. Healing is multifactorial, being dependant not only on the energy of injury but also on local and general host factors such as nutrition, site and quality of bone etc. Some fractures may be considered to be at risk of delayed healing, such as comminuted, displaced or open types.[2] Unstable fractures require surgical stabilization to prevent malunion and shortening, but inappropriate surgery may lead to non-union. Attempts have been made to define the state of non-union as a fixed period in time after fracture, for example: six months,[3] eight months[4] or 1 year.[5] The natural history of healing in a "high risk" fracture is not well understood, however, and may in fact exceed these stated times. Non-union may also be defined as a clinical or radiological state. Brighton[6] described it as "that condition existing in a fractured bone in which all reparative processes have ceased and yet bony continuity has not been restored". It seems more likely, however, that the reparative processes are in fact present but inadequate. This distinction is paramount to the proposed approach to treatment and is supported by Nicoll[2] who defined non-union as "a condition in which, in the opinion of the surgeon, the fragments would not have united with further conservative treatment".

The Fracture Environment

Fracture healing simply stated is a balance between repair and breakdown (Fig. 48.1). In a persistent non-union, breakdown may be occurring at a rate perhaps 1 per cent or so faster than repair, thus propagating the non-union effect. Factors propagating the non-union include: fracture site motion, gap, poor blood supply and infection. A reduction in these effects will alter the balance and even an effect of 2 per cent in favour of healing will produce healing, albeit slowly.

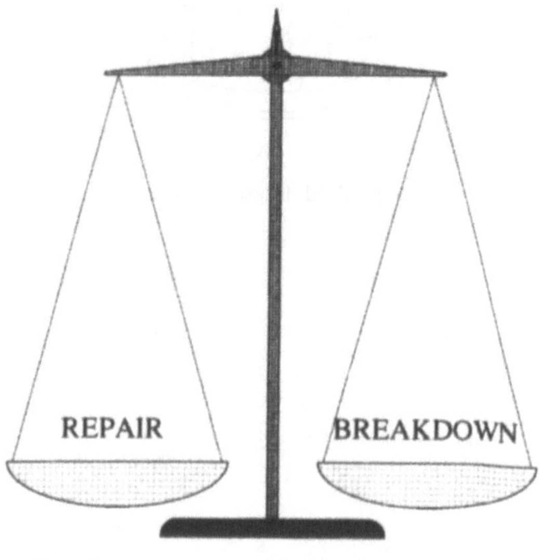

Fig. 48.1 There is a fine balance between repair and breakdown in normal bone.

The Classification of Non-Unions

There are three important categories of acquired non-union: hypertrophic, atrophic and infected. Acquired non-unions (Fig. 48.2) may be classified as hypertrophic (vascular) or atrophic (avascular) according to the radiological appearance or isotope uptake on bone scanning[7] (Fig. 48.3). Infected non-unions may be hypertrophic or atrophic. The diagnosis of infection is a clinical one, but positive culture of biopsy specimens is confirmatory. Two other types of non-union should be distinguished since they merit a different treatment approach. A highly mobile non-union with a large fracture gap on plain radiographs may be indicative of a true synovial pseudarthrosis. This may be confirmed on a bone scan showing a cold cleft between two hot ends[8] or at surgical exploration. A pseudarthrosis in infancy may be "congenital" and occurs mainly in the tibia, proximal femur or clavicle.[5] It usually presents with progressive deformity and some shortening followed by pain related to fracture. The radiological appearance may vary from a complete radiolucent gap to mild disruption of the bony architecture.

Diagnosis

Having established that a non-union exists, the reason why breakdown is proceeding faster than repair must be determined. Essentially, non-unions fit into two groups: simple failure of initial management of an "at-risk fracture" which usually presents early, and those difficult, resistant non-unions in disillusioned and often depressed patients who have undergone a downward spiral of unsuccessful operations. The success rate in treating the former group will inevitably be much higher.

History

The precise nature of the initial injury (including the magnitude, direction and duration of force) will indicate the degree of tissue disruption and therefore the "fracture at risk". Ideally, clinical information allowing appropriate grading according to Tscherne[9] or Gustilo[10] should be available. The type of primary management will provide more information about the fracture environment; for example, soft tissue damage and contami-

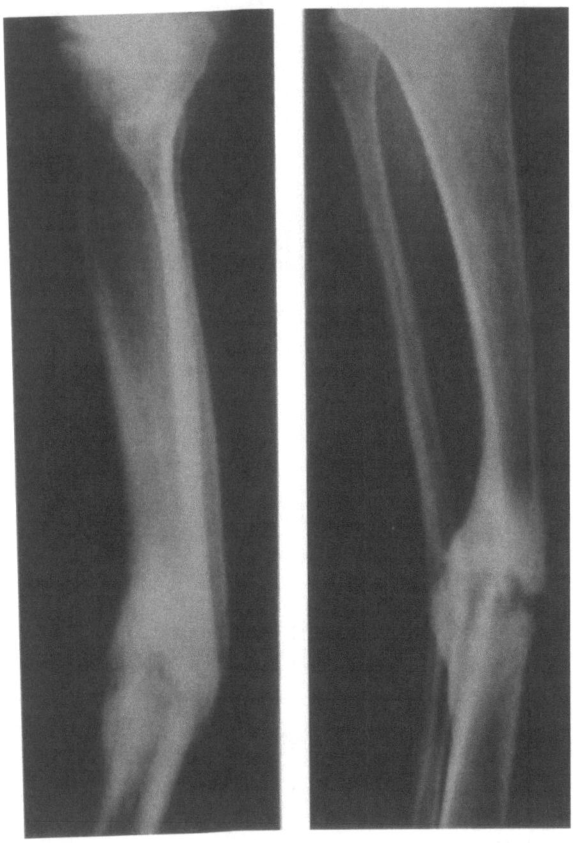

Fig. 48.2 Lateral and AP radiographs of an angulated non-union.

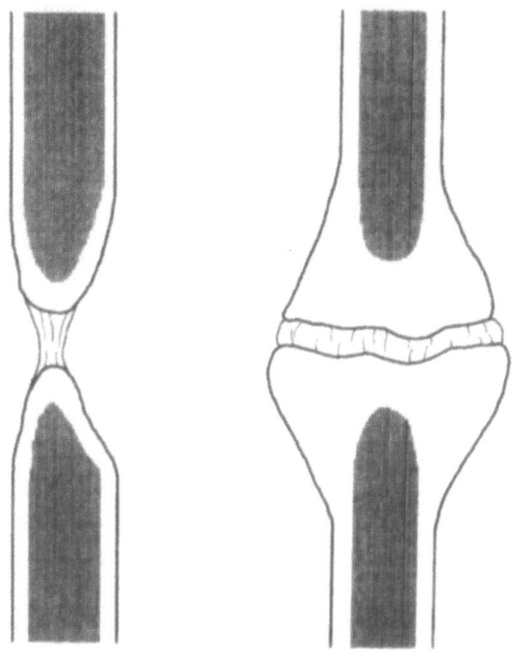

Fig. 48.3 A line drawing depicting the main differences between hypertrophic and atrophic non-union. Note the small amount of callus and resorption of the bone ends in the atrophic non-union. Compare that with the higher callus activity and larger surface area of contact in the hypertrophic non-union tending to make these non-unions "stiff" on clinical examination.

nation in the wound. Secondary, or later management, provides information on subsequent operative procedures which influence the fracture environment; for example, in rigid plate fixation soft tissues are stripped off the bone[11] and the callus response eliminated[12]. Any past evidence of sepsis, whether superficial or deep, must be ascertained by direct questioning. The patient's specific complaints (pain, loss of function, deformity), present level of activity and expectations, will influence the operative plan.

Examination

The examination should include an assessment of the general mental and physical state of the patient. The patient must be prepared to accept what is often a protracted treatment programme and convalescence. An assessment must be made of the quality of the soft tissues, including the position of wounds and incisions. Fracture site tenderness or movement (fracture stiffness) and neurovascular integrity in the limb are evaluated. The range of movements at every joint in the limb must be measured to identify contractures, angular and rotational deformities at the fracture site and the body's capacity to cope with a bony deformity. For example, if there is a 15 degree varus deformity of the hindfoot in a tibial non-union and only 15 degrees of valgus available at the subtalar joint on the normal side, the subtalar joint is working at the limit of its range in walking, thus limiting function and feeding the non-union effect. Any limb length discrepancy must be noted because pelvic tilt will produce shear forces at the fracture site and lead to back pain and a limp.[13]

Investigations

It is helpful to review the progress of the fracture radiologically, from the initial degree of comminution and displacement through to the type and position of fixation devices. Subsequent investigations must be comprehensive but need not be complex. Radiographs coned on the area of interest will normally provide sufficient information regarding the quality of the bone at the fracture site (Fig. 48.4). These films provide baseline and monitoring information; up to four views should be taken, and the position and exposure information recorded for reproducibility. Radiographs should also be taken for alignment and include the joint above and below. The degree of angular deformity and, to a lesser extent, rotational and translational malalignment, will produce shear stresses on the fracture site and impair healing. In lower limb fractures the mechanical axis of the limb should be assessed using full length radiographs against a 5cm grid (Fig. 48.5). Limb segment length may be measured precisely using conventional or CT scanograms (Fig. 48.6). Overall limb length measurements may be made using the Friberg technique.[13] A loop of tubing containing radio-opaque dye is placed around the waist of a standing patient. An antero-posterior radiograph of the pelvis is taken (Fig. 48.7). The limb length discrepancy is represented by the differential between the level of the meniscus and femoral head on each side. Tomograms are useful when looking for sequestra and assessing juxta-articular fractures. Technetium bone scans are rarely indicated; indium labelled white cell scans[14] may, however, be useful to assess infection. If a sinus is present, a sinogram may aid identification of septic foci.

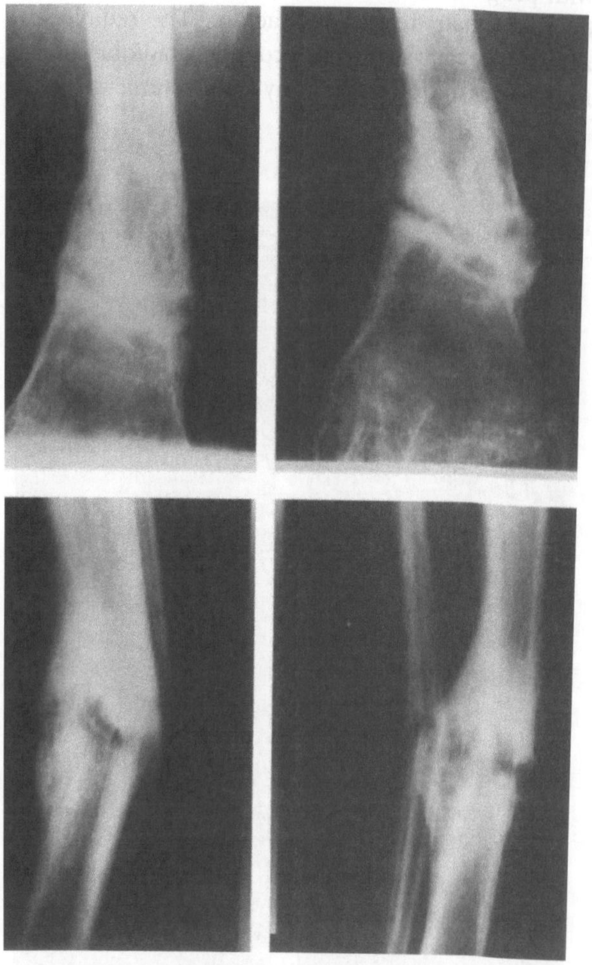

Fig. 48.4 Radiographs coned down on to the fracture/lengthening site to assess bone quality. The dose of radiation used is recorded for repeatability and to allow more accurate comparison between films.

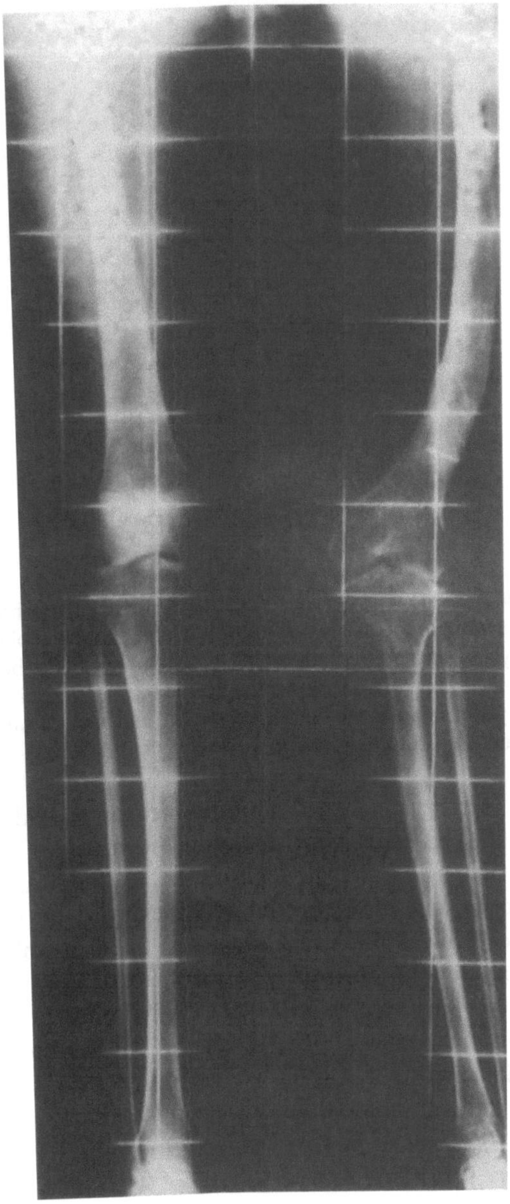

Fig. 48.5 AP Mechanical axis view radiograph. Taken standing, with a 5cm grid in front of the X-ray plate.

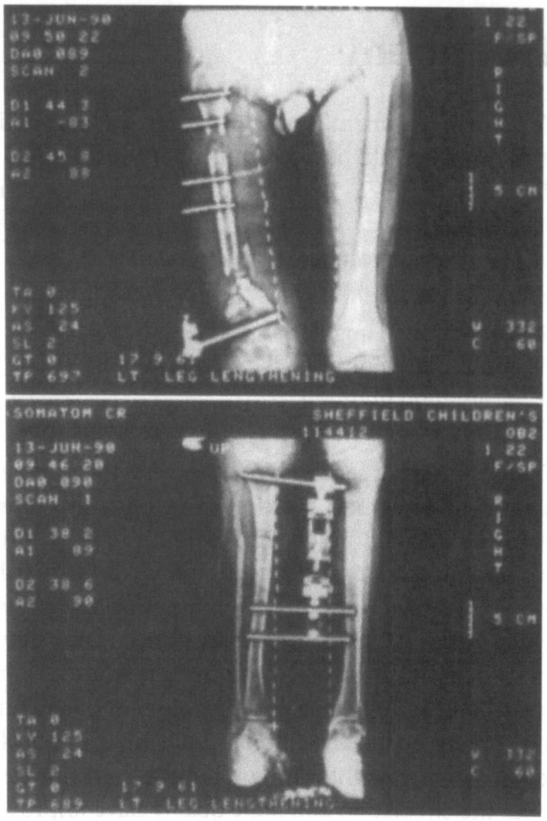

Fig. 48.6 CT scanogram taken during a bone transport. A cursor can be positioned on the video screen by the operator allowing measurement of bone lengths. The degree of accuracy is limited by the screen resolution and the consistent positioning of the cursor.

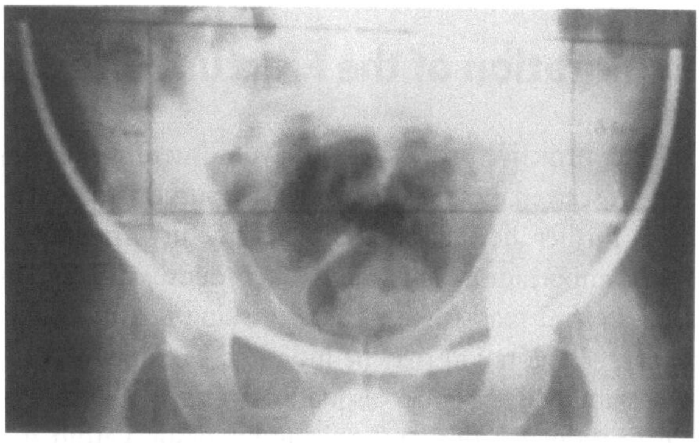

Fig. 48.7 The Friberg method of measuring limb length. On a standard standing AP pelvic radiograph, a tube containing radiopaque liquid is hung in front of the pelvis and allowed to settle. Since the two menisci must be horizontal, the difference in distance from this line to an equivalent point on each side (e.g. the highest point of the acetabulum), will be an accurate estimate of the difference in overall leg length.

Other investigations should assess previous and present infections with bacteriology reports for culture and antibiotic sensitivities. Where the organism is unknown, or infection is suspected but not proven, suspicious areas of the bone may be biopsied in clean air facilities and subjected to aerobic and anaerobic culture.[15,16] The laboratory analysis should also take place in clean air facilities to reduce the risk of contamination.[15] Prior to open surgery, it may be useful to discuss antibiotic treatment with a clinical bacteriologist. Arteriograms or Doppler studies may be indicated to evaluate the arterial state of the limb and are helpful if free vascularised grafts are required. In areas with unstable scarring, there may be difficulty in closing the wound or a risk of wound necrosis if exploration is performed. This is particularly common over the tibia and a plastic surgery opinion should be sought prior to surgery.

Treatment

The aim of treatment is not only to recover continuity at the fracture site but also to produce restoration of the mechanical axis and thereby maximize the functional result.

Treatment objectives include:

1. improvement in bone and soft tissue quality
2. correction of angulation and length
3. mobilization of stiff adjacent joints
4. promotion of union
5. eradication of infection.

There is no strict sequence for these treatment objectives; each issue may, however, contribute in varying degrees to the non-union effect. For example, if a limb has been in plaster for a long period the bone may be osteoporotic and the adjacent joints stiff. An orthosis which blocks movement at the fracture site but allows movement at the adjacent joints may improve bone quality and act as a valuable preparatory step to definitive surgery. In the lower limb, a built-up shoe may be required and weightbearing should be encouraged. Once the circulation and bone quality have improved and joints are more mobile, definitive surgery may be considered. The mobile adjacent joints will act as torque converters and relieve stress that would otherwise be transmitted to the fracture site as a shear stress, producing fracture breakdown.

Exploration of the Fracture Site

It is an attractive proposition to avoid fracture site surgery in scarred areas. At the very least, surgery may produce further devitalisation of the fracture fragments. More important, scar tissue is often dense, difficult to separate and masks tissue planes, risking neurovascular injury.[17] Exploration may be indicated to improve fracture stability using either a square osteotomy[18,19] or internal fixation. Fibrous or cartilaginous tissue within the non-union may, however, have osteogenic potential[20,21] For this reason, local surgery should be avoided unless there is necrotic tissue, infection, muscle interposition or a true synovial pseudarthrosis. In hypertrophic non-unions, healing may be encouraged by appropriate stabilization combined with either compression or distraction, whereas atrophic non-unions may require exposure and preparation for bone grafting. Bone regeneration may be encouraged by local revascularizing measures such as osteoperiosteal decortication (Fig. 48.8),[19] osseous and soft tissue scarifications[22] or centromedullary perforations as advocated by Trueta.

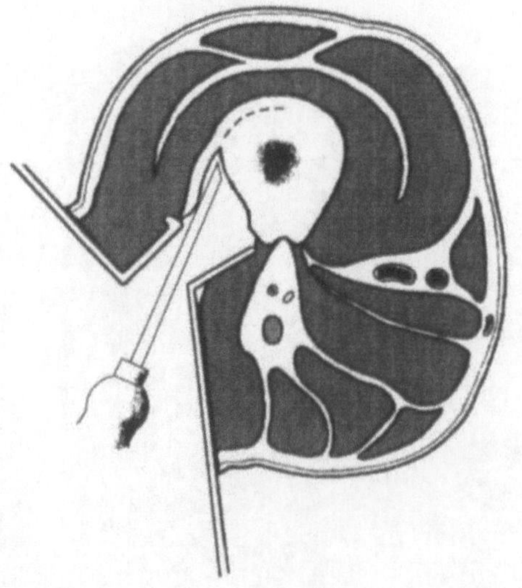

Fig. 48.8 Osteoperiosteal decortication. Chips of cortical bone still attached to the overlying periosteum and peripheral blood supply are elevated from the whole circumference of the bone using a chisel. When the underlying bone has been stabilized this layer of vascularized bone graft can be held in place with a few periosteal sutures.

If surgery is indicated, a utility incision should be used and reused to avoid “tram line” scarring and soft tissue damage. A tourniquet is used to aid the surgical approach and the bone should be exposed on one surface only. Bone levers should be avoided unless circumferential exposure of the fracture ends is required; for example, in a square osteotomy. If it is important to assess bone vascularity, the tourniquet should be released early or avoided altogether.

Treatment should follow three principles:

1. REALIGNMENT
2. STABILIZATION
3. STIMULATION

Realignment

The importance of realignment and the adverse effects of shear stresses were recognised by Bohler,[18]: “it must be emphasized that in the extremities, weightbearing on the callus should be in the proper axis and should not produce a bending or a rubbing”.

An angulated fracture may be realigned immediately in a closed fashion by passing an intramedullary nail across the fracture. If performed as a closed procedure, reaming will distribute bone graft to the endosteal surface of the fracture. Often, however, fracture reduction requires a limited open reduction, and in these cases the wound should be closed before reaming, to preserve the graft. If the fracture is stiff, a

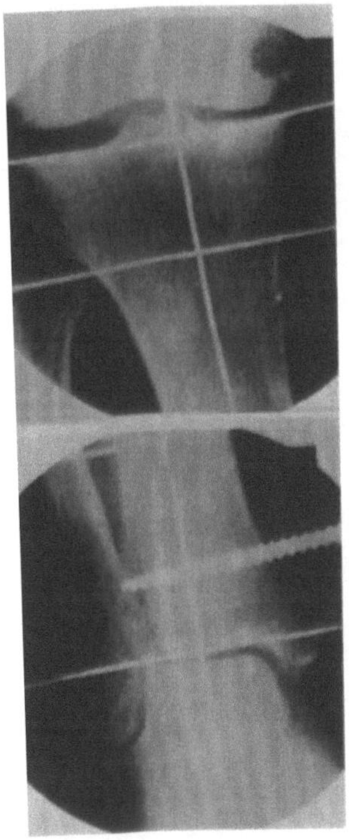

Fig. 48.9 Alignment grid. Per-operative AP views taken using an image intensifier. With the longitudinal line aligned to the mid-points of both the ankle and knee joints the joint surfaces can be seen to be parallel to the perpendicular lines. The long axis can be checked by panning along the bone.

percutaneous osteotomy under radiological control combined with a closed gentle osteoclasis may aid initial realignment. Neurological sequelae may occur with sudden corrections; for example, the common peroneal nerve in correction of the valgus tibia. Angular correction may be checked per-operatively using an image intensifier and alignment grid. The alignment grid consists of a Perspex sheet in which is embedded a grid of lead wires with a central longitudinal reference line and horizontal lines at equidistant intervals. The grid is enclosed in a sterile bag and placed under the limb being aligned thus allowing accurate positioning of the bone ends and joints on the operating table[23] (Fig. 48.9).

Realignment may also be performed progressively after surgery using a circular external fixator. In Fig. 48.10, a supracondylar femoral non-union is angulated in anterior and lateral angulation with half a diameter of lateral translation. Correction was achieved progressively after applying a circular frame and distracting the non-union (Fig. 48.11).

In hypertrophic non-unions correction of deformity and length may be achieved with circular frames or monolateral frames by gradual corrective callus distraction (Fig. 48.12). If the bone ends are atrophic re-alignment may require a square osteotomy for

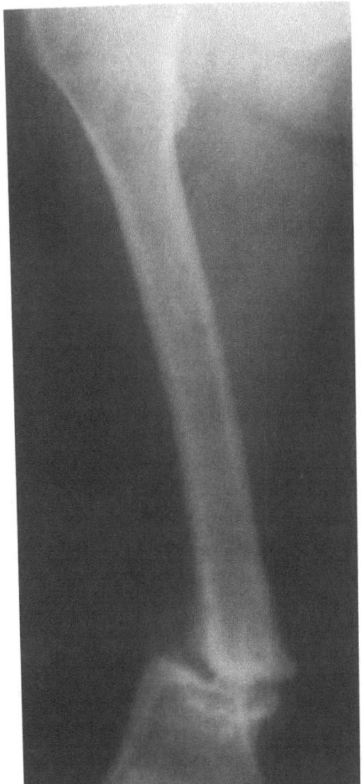

Fig. 48.10 Radiograph of an angulated, displaced non-union. The angulation is in more than one plane.

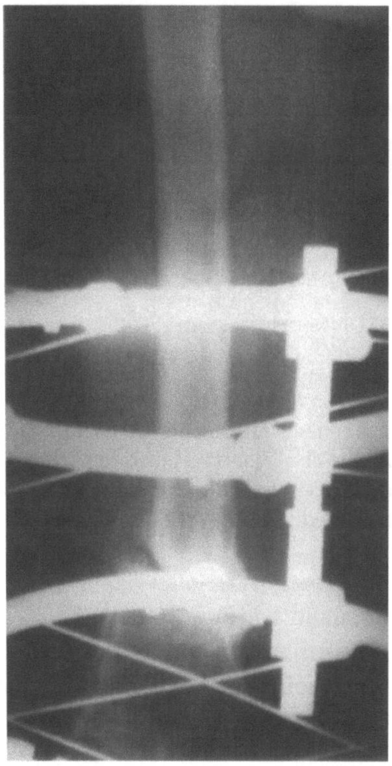

Fig. 48.11 The same bone as in Fig. 48.10 after gradual correction in several planes using a circular frame.

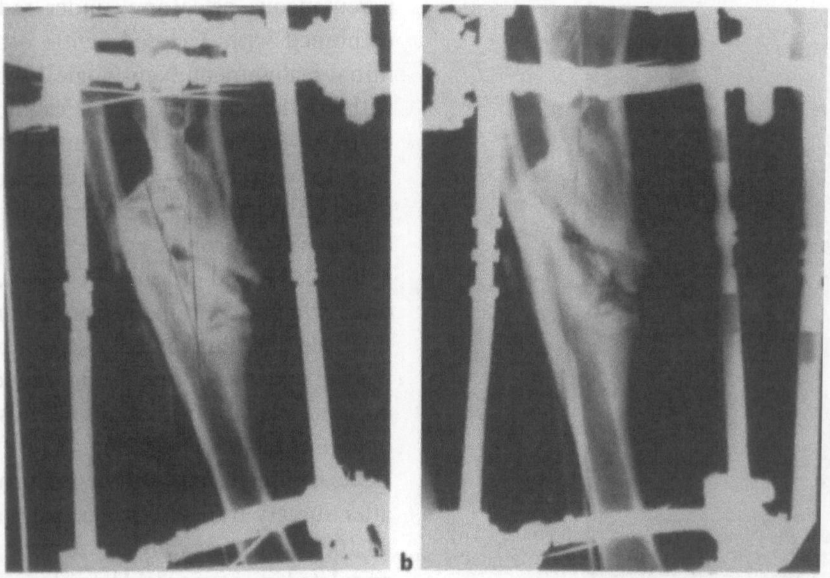

Fig. 48.12 AP radiograph of a hypertrophic non-union in which lengthening was achieved by gradual callus distraction. **a** Before distraction, **b** after distraction.

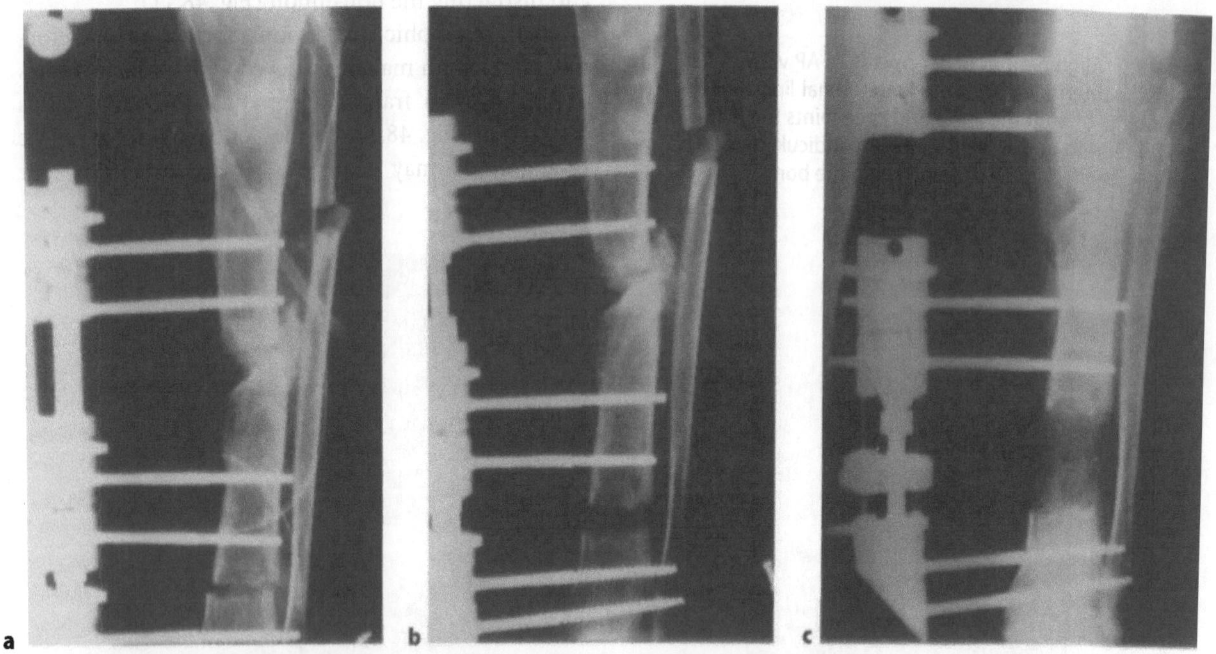

Fig. 48.13 A series of radiographs of an infected pseudarthrosis of the tibia. The pseudarthrosis was excised and the bone ends squared off. The tibial defect was then compressed for 3 weeks. **a** A further two pins were then added distally and a corticotomy performed between middle and distal pin-sites. **b** As compression continued at the proximal site, the distal osteotomy was distracted. **c** The distal site was then lengthened further to restore leg length. Note the presence of a 1cm fibular resection osteotomy.

improved stability and bone contact. This will result in shortening which may be corrected in the same procedure by lengthening the bone in the metaphysis, the simultaneous compression–distraction technique[24] (Fig. 48.13).

In the lower leg, if the fibula is intact, an osteotomy must be performed to allow tibial realignment and fracture apposition (Fig. 48.13). In the forearm, limb length is not so critical and parallel bone shortening may be more appropriate to realign the radio-ulnar articulations (Fig. 48.14). Conversely, the shortened ununited bone may be lengthened by inserting an interposition graft[25] (Fig. 48.15) or by callus lengthening (Fig. 48.16).

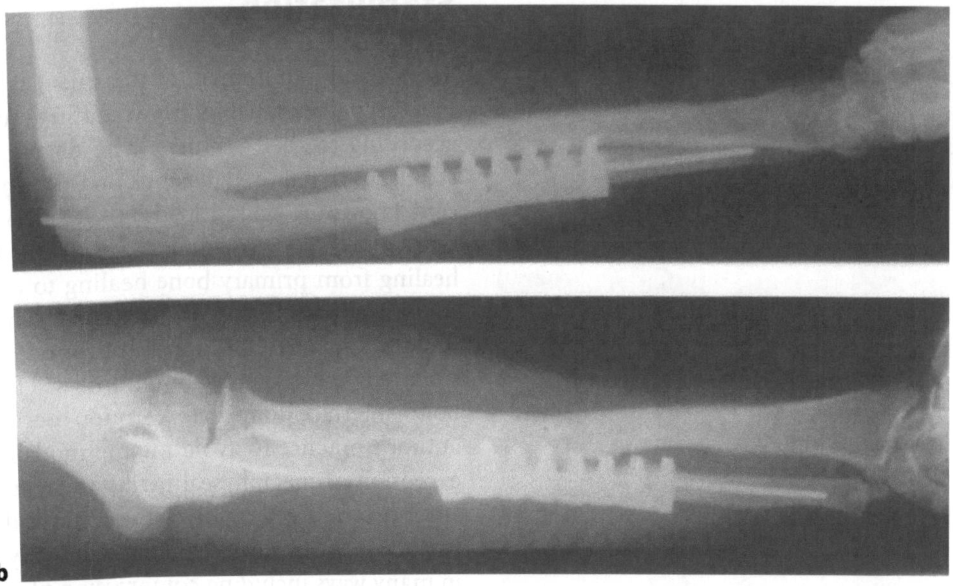

a

b

Fig. 48.14 **a** AP radiograph of a non-union of the ulna with shortening; **b** the alignment of the distal radio-ulnar joint was restored by shortening of the radius.

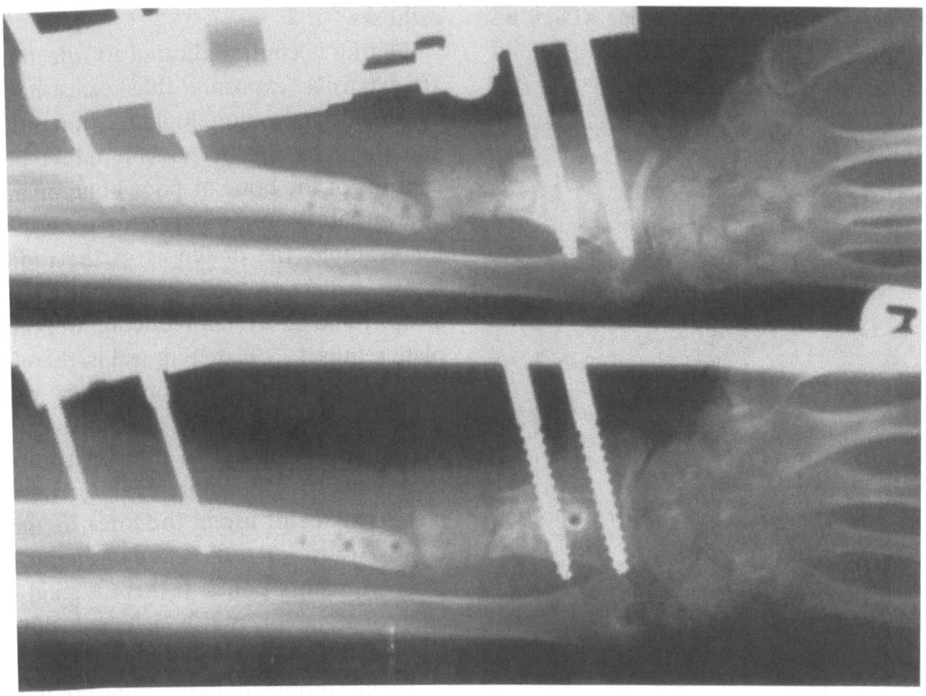

Fig. 48.15 AP radiograph of a shortened ununited radius in which the radio-ulnar joint was realigned by lengthening the radius using an interposition graft.

Re-alignment should include correction of soft tissue deformities; for example, correction of an equinus foot or flexion contracture of the knee. These procedures may be carried out using conventional open soft tissue releases and tendon lengthening or by closed distraction methods using circular frames.[24] In Fig. 48.17, an example of tibial non-union, simultaneous correction of valgus angulation and equinus was performed, the latter using hindfoot and forefoot wires. Note that a hinge is used to position the fulcrum of movement accurately.

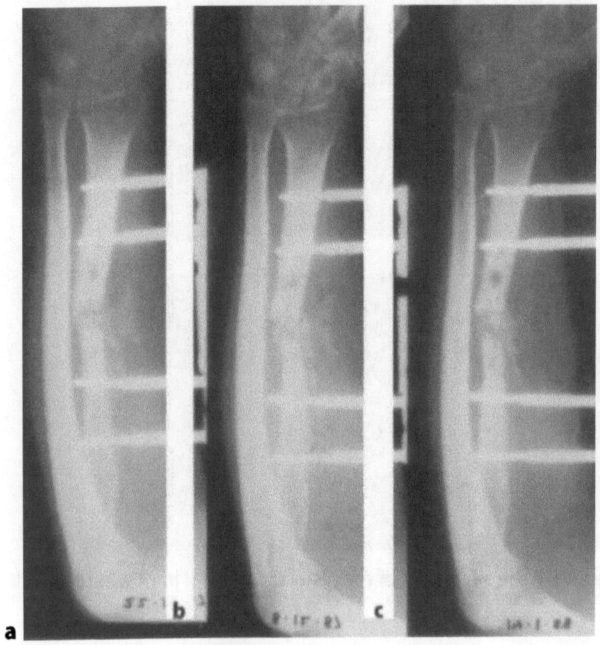

Fig. 48.16 AP radiographs of another shortened ununited radius, this time lengthened by callus distraction. **a** Day 0. **b** Six weeks. **c** Eleven weeks.

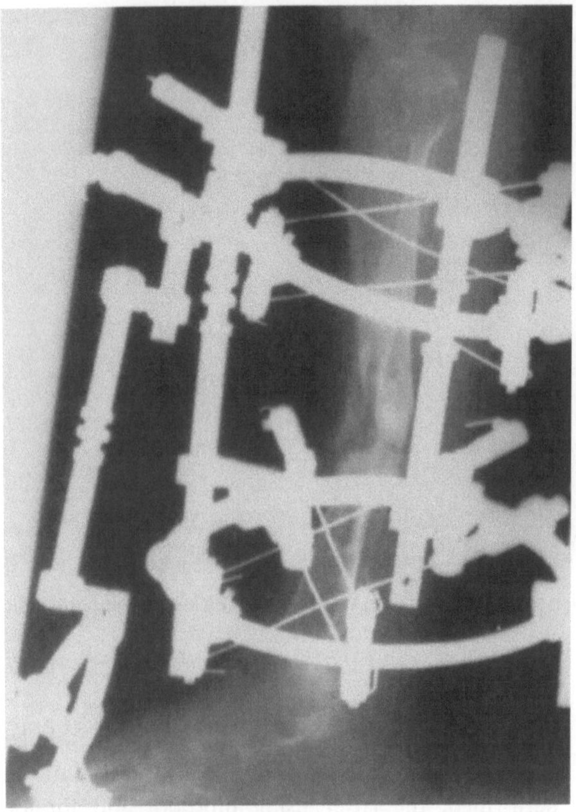

Fig. 48.17 Lateral radiograph of a tibial non-union treated with a circular frame for correction of valgus angulation of the bone with simultaneous correction of equinus deformity of the foot using a forefoot wire.

Stabilization

The second requirement of treatment is stabilization. Fractures are capable of accepting some loading according to their stiffness. The degree of accessory stabilization required depends on this property, a concept known as shared loading. Stabilization may be rigid or elastic, providing a spectrum of biological healing from primary bone healing to callus repair.[26] Rigid fixation relies on primary cortical healing which is slow[12] and therefore most appropriate to implants since a rigid external fixation frame will fail at the pin-bone interface long before union occurs. It is the author's practice to avoid mixing modalities with the exception of metaphyseal periarticular fractures. The latter may be fixed rigidly with screws and neutralized by a more elastic device. Stabilization may be achieved in many ways including compression plating,[27,28] flexible plating with paraskeletal clamps,[29] flexible stacked nails,[30,31] close fitting intramedullary nails,[32] external fixators capable of an elastic mode[33,24,34] or plasters and orthoses.[35]

Plating is contraindicated in infection. It requires an extensive exposure thus exacerbating the pre-existing devitalization. Rigid fixation must be achieved and this may not be possible either because of the contour of the bone or poor bone quality. It may be appropriate in some hypertrophic non-unions only, for example, the diaphysis of the radius and ulna. Stress protection occurs, leading to cortical bone atrophy and an overall reduction in bony stiffness on plate removal.[12,36] Plate removal is, therefore, theoretically required; but revision surgery carries its own risks. Stress protection and its sequelae may be prevented by the use of more elastic plates such as those made of carbon fibre reinforced resins.[37] Mennen plates may be of use in the forearm and fibula; they claim to cause less soft tissue damage and may be left in place in mature bones. If there is good bony contact additional stability may be achieved with tension band wiring.[38]

Locked intramedullary nailing produces fixation by control of the medullary cavity. It is particularly useful in osteoporosis but should be avoided where there is a history of infection or active infection. Reaming in association with tight fitting intramedullary devices has been shown to impair the endosteal circulation temporarily and, therefore, repair mechanisms.[39] In practice, however, closed nailing produces elastic fixation and is associated with an exuberant callus response. Healing will be rapid if the procedure is closed but closed techniques are demanding and

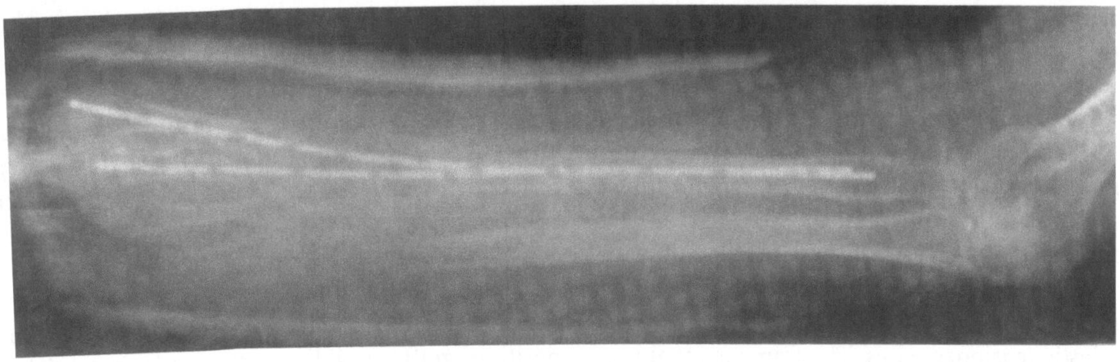

Fig. 48.18 AP radiograph of the forearm showing bundle nailing of a non-union of the distal radius. The distal ends of the flexible nails are placed in the metacarpals, the proximal ends in the radius.

closed osteotomies difficult.[40] Open nailing is performed as a last resort but risks violating both the periosteal and endosteal surfaces of the bone. Some surgeons use a Kuntscher nail in association with a derotation plate. This combination is inappropriate both biologically and biomechanically. In femoral non-unions the nail should always be statically locked. In the tibia, however, this is often unnecessary because of the shape of the bone and the lower mechanical stresses involved. Bundle stacked nailing is useful in the upper limb and relies on local multiple point fixation as pre-bent nails are used to fill the medullary canal. They may be inserted closed and provide elastic fixation with surprisingly good rotational stability (Fig. 48.18).

External fixation is perhaps the most useful technique overall. There are obvious advantages; the metal is away from the fracture site so the technique is indicated in infected cases. The fracture may be controlled by compression, neutralization or distraction (ligamentotaxis).[41] Monolateral frames with 6mm pins such as the Dynamic Axial Fixator (Orthofix srl, Verona, Italy) designed by Professor De Bastiani are ideal for most applications and allow conversion from rigid to dynamic or elastic fixation.[42] The application technique must be meticulous, the pins being placed at right angles to the axis of the bone and the fixator parallel to the axis of the limb to enable dynamization to occur (Fig. 48.19). The hospital and community staff must be capable of dealing with pin sites adequately to avoid infection. A practical solution with reliable patients is to encourage self-care. Large pins, however, do not provide good purchase in osteoporotic bone. Despite their dynamization capability there is some risk of delayed healing, and stress protection may occur with fixators that are too stiff. There may be inhibition of joint movement, particularly where fixation pins transfix muscles around the femur and humerus.

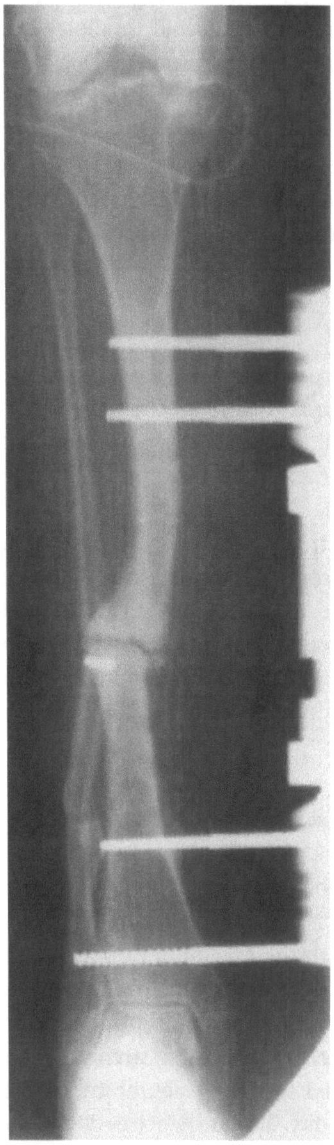

Fig. 48.19 Radiograph showing good positioning of an Orthofix unilateral external fixator with the pins at right angles to the bone surface and the body of the fixator parallel to the long axis of the bone.

Circular external fixation frames of the Ilizarov pattern, represented in this context by the Sheffield Hybrid Fixator, are also valuable.[24] They produce better fixation in osteoporotic bone than monolateral frames and have the theoretical advantage of circumferential control of the fracture environment. Stiffness is built into the frame by the ring diameter, number, position, separation and tension of wires inserted. Axial movement at the fracture site is effected by weightbearing and muscle contraction on the relatively elastic tensioned wires. The frame is capable of adaptation for progressive reduction of a fracture as well as lengthening and multilevel surgery.[43]

In some situations stabilization may be achieved with plaster and other casting materials. Radiolucent materials should be selected to allow accurate monitoring of the fracture response. The selective use of hinges will allow joint mobilization at a time when some loss of external fracture support may be accepted, i.e. as a preliminary event to definitive fracture stabilization or as a late event prior to removal of the stabilizing device.

Stimulation

The final pre-requisite of treatment is to stimulate healing. Three basic mechanisms underlie bone regeneration: osteogenesis, osteoinduction and osteoconduction.[44] Osteogenesis is carried out by pre-existing differentiated bone forming cells. Osteoinduction involves differentiation of uncommitted connective tissue cells into bone forming cells in the presence of an inductive stimulus. Osteoconductive grafts behave as a nonviable scaffolding for the ingrowth of vessels and new bone by creeping substitution. Most of the methods described involve one or more of these mechanisms.

Bone Grafting

Autogenous bone grafting is the mainstay of non-union treatment. It is contraindicated in the presence of active infection, with the exception of open grafting used in the Papineau technique which will be described below. Cancellous bone is used for its osteogenic potential and cortical bone for structural strength. The iliac crest donor site is a source of significant and often understated morbidity. The incidence of donor site complications in one series was 9.4 per cent and included: chronic wound pain and hypersensitivity, buttock anaesthesia, muscle herniation, meralgia paraesthetica and even subluxation of the hip.[45] Meralgia paraesthetica is also described by Weikel and Habal.[46] In another series, chronic donor site pain was reported in 25 per cent of patients but associated particularly with tricortical grafts.[47] A limited percutaneous approach for harvesting graft using a trefine is preferred to open techniques.[48] Bone should be gently packed into prepared cavities within the non-union site after a limited (Fig. 48.20) or percutaneous (Fig. 48.21) approach. Larger defects may be prepared and keyed to accept a precisely measured bicortical interposition graft providing osteogenic potential and structural support. In more homogeneous non-unions, onlay grafting may be performed using thin cortico-cancellous strips. Medullary canal reaming is another potent source of cancellous graft.

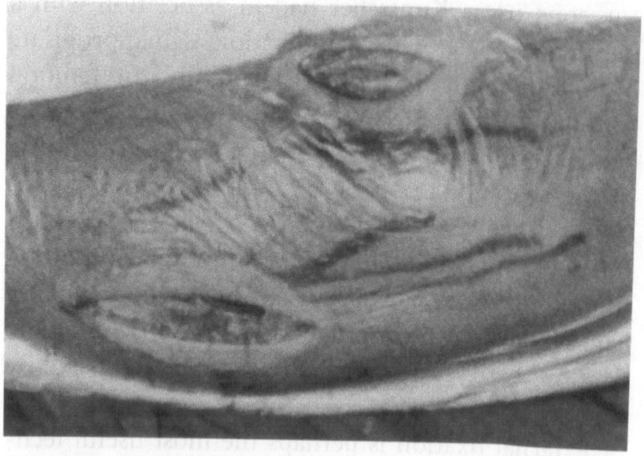

Fig. 48.20 Photograph of the incisions used to perform limited open bone grafting to the forearm.

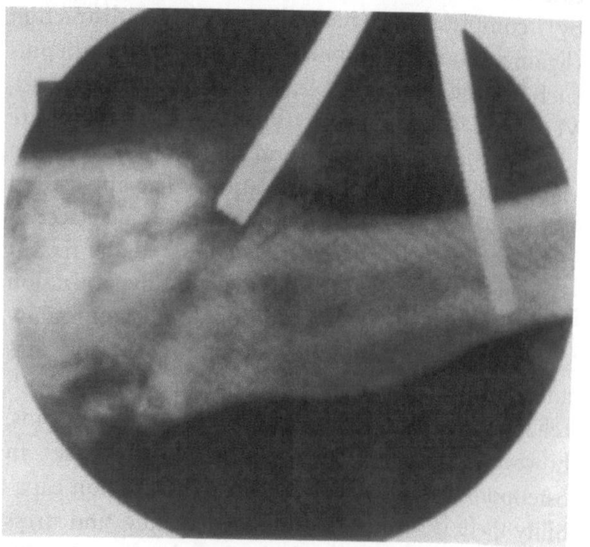

Fig. 48.21 Radiograph showing percutaneous bone grafting. Here a trephine is being used to remove a core of tissue into which a cancellous or cortico-cancellous bone graft obtained in a similar manner from the iliac crest, can be inserted.

Mechanical Stimulation

Wolff[49] proposed two laws of bone remodelling; first, skeletal elements are strategically placed to resist imposed forces and second, the total mass of bone is adjusted according to the magnitude of prevailing mechanical loads. In order to increase bone loading the patient must be encouraged to exercise the limb[18,24] and the external stabilizing mechanisms should be progressively reduced. Where external fixation has been used, the frame may be made more elastic by removing some of the pins or in the case of the Dynamic Axial Fixator, by releasing the body locking nut and allowing some axial movement. Controlled micromovement is also considered to be a potent stimulus.[50,51] Statically locked intramedullary nails may be unlocked, providing a more elastic fracture environment.

Electrical Stimulation

Methods using electrical signals to stimulate bone formation have been used in clinical practice since the early seventies. There are three main types in use today.

1. Direct current stimulation by either semi-invasive methods[52] or implantable devices.[53]
2. Inductive stimulation with pulsed electromagnetic fields (PEMFs) using external coils and low frequency asymmetrical waveforms.[1] More recently, coils have become available with vascular specific signals which have proven efficacy for soft tissue problems such as venous ulceration[54] and these may be of value in the incorporation of large structural grafts.
3. Capacitively coupled signals using stainless steel plates in contact with the skin over the non-union site, typically using a 60kHz sinusoidal five volt peak-to-peak signal powered by a portable battery pack.[55] These non-invasive systems are particularly useful in infected non-unions where bone grafting or other invasive techniques would be inappropriate.

Vascular Stimulation

Stimulation may include walking,[18] the use of the muscle pump[56,57], use of the A-V Impulse System (Orthofix Vascular Division)[58,59] and fascio-cutaneous or muscle flaps.[60,61] Osteotomies within the same segment will also increase the local circulation.[62] Stabilization of the non-union and the PEMF vascular signal may promote vessel ingrowth.

Infected Non-Unions

Infection is a common sequela after open fractures and after internal fixation.[63] Burri stated that "although the technique of (plate) osteosynthesis is steadily improving, due to the increasing volume of operative procedures, the absolute number of infections secondary to the open reduction of fractures will increase".[64] This has been borne out in practice and infection following rigid plate osteosynthesis represents "the worst non-union scenario" with motion, a gap, poor blood supply and infection. Infected atrophic non-union is the single most important reason why plating of open fractures should be deprecated and plating of tibial fractures by inexperienced surgeons should be banned altogether.

Infection increases the local circulation by 5–10 times and wherever possible surgical exploration should be performed under tourniquet. Methylene blue may be injected into draining sinuses in an attempt to identify septic foci. Exploration aims to control infection by excision of necrotic tissue including bone, and removal of metalwork. Parenteral antibiotics should not be given until bacteriological specimens have been taken. Antibiotic-loaded bone cement[65] may be inserted into the cavity. Stabilization should be achieved by means of external fixation, although some authors have successfully used internal fixation with plates[20,66] or intramedullary nails.[67] Lesser degrees of infection may respond to improved vascularity secondary to closed measures with appropriate external fixation.[24] Secondary procedures aim to provide bony continuity and include bone grafting away from the infected plane, for example posterolaterally in the tibia,[40] open grafting of partial defects[68] and bone transport[24] after complete diaphysectomy.

Management of Bone Gaps

Bone defects may be due to the initial trauma or to diaphysectomy for infection, congenital pseudarthrosis or tumour. Until recently, bone gaps were managed by autogenous cancellous bone grafting, interposition grafts or in the tibia, fibula pro tibia transfer.[69] Recent advances include the use of massive allografts,[70] replacement by metal implants, free vascularized bone grafts and bone transport. Vascularized bone grafts[60] require specialist surgical techniques and long operation times. They are associated with significant donor site morbidity and require long periods to hypertrophy. Bone gaps are most satis-

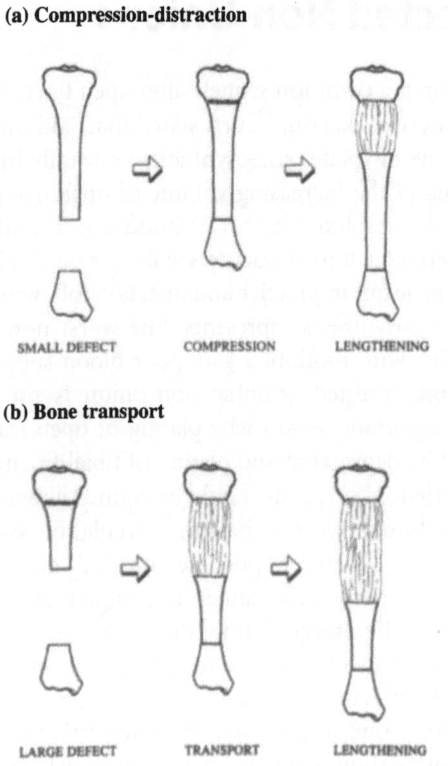

Fig. 48.22 **a** For small bone defects, compression of the defect is followed by osteotomy and lengthening at the other end of the bone. **b** In larger defects, lengthening and compression occur simultaneously so the middle segment of bone is transported to fill the defect. Once the defect has been closed, further lengthening can be carried out as required.

factorily closed by simultaneous compression and distraction for small defects (less than 3cm in the tibia or 5cm in the femur) or transport for longer defects (Fig. 48.22). Limb lengthening techniques with spontaneous callus formation are utilized either to restore length, or to transport a middle fragment to fill a bone gap. The new osteotomy and effort of distraction will produce a general hyperaemic effect in the limb segment beneficial to the non-union. A major attraction is the restriction of surgery to the involved limb segment. In Fig. 48.23 a segmental fracture of the femur with bone loss has been realigned and the defect closed by transport. Further lengthening was performed to produce limb length equality.

Post-operative Care

Follow-up should be on a monthly basis or if necessary more frequently. The patient should also see the same members of staff to provide continuity of care and appropriate emotional support. The mental welfare of the patient is very important as patient cooperation is vital to much of the treatment described. Clinic staff should therefore be on a constant lookout for signs of stress or depression resulting from the long periods of immobility or hospital treatment. Routine evaluation should include a clinical soft tissue assessment and radiological assessment of the bone. A bank of X-ray

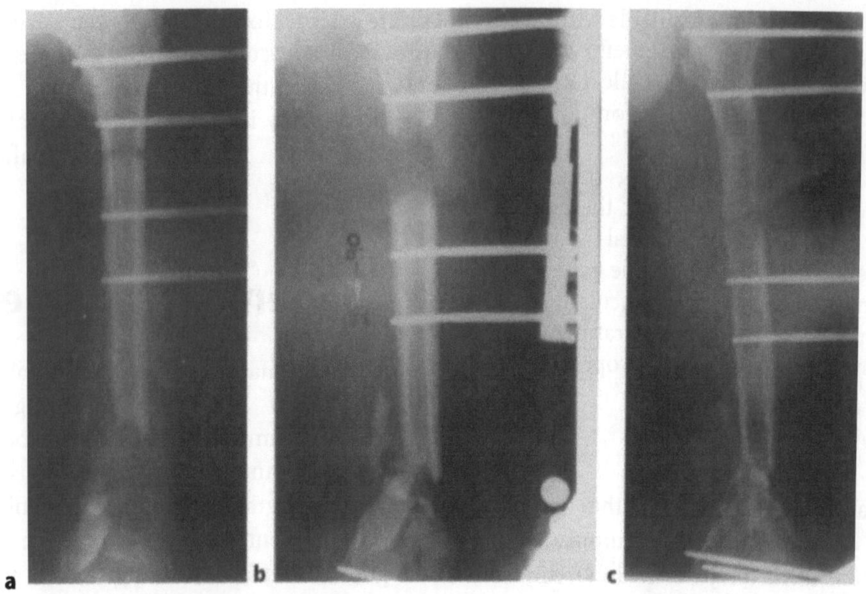

Fig. 48.23 Radiographs showing a large defect of the lower end of the femur following segmental fracture, being closed by bone transport. The limb was then lengthened by further callus distraction. **a** Day 0: the fixator is applied with screws to the proximal end, shaft and what remains of the distal end of the femur. A corticotomy has been performed just below the lesser trochanter. **b** Day 50: the middle segment of bone is pulled down through the thigh tissues which remain static. **c** 1 year: transport is now complete and the bone is uniting at the distal end. Plenty of new bone can be seen forming in the lengthening site.

viewing boxes is required to follow the progress of a fracture. Physiotherapy and progressive reduction in fracture support should be provided until the joints are mobile and the fracture clinically and radiologically united. A polypropylene or block leather orthosis is then provided until the fracture has remodelled or the patient is capable of a full range of activities without symptoms. Insoles, shoe raises and other orthoses may be required pending secondary surgical procedures such as toe surgery, limb lengthening, and soft tissue releases such as quadricepsplasty.

Conclusions

The basic principles of non-union management have been described, namely, realignment, stabilization and stimulation. Future improvements in non-union surgery will include objective methods of measuring fracture stiffness, as well as bony and soft tissue recovery. Dexa scanning, CT reconstruction and NMR scans require evaluation. There may be valuable chemical and hormonal mediators of bone regeneration. Some non-unions are incurable either in practical terms, because the patient is unable, physically or mentally, to cope with the operative programme, or because there is no viable therapeutic option. Amputation is a good solution if approached with a positive mental attitude and appropriate patient preparation. The most suitable cases for amputation are those with irretrievable infected non-unions and those with significant neurological deficits.

References

1. Bassett C, Mitchell B, Gastan S. 'Treatment of Ununited Tibial Diaphyseal Fractures With Pulsing Electromagnetic Field.' *J Bone Joint Surg* [Am] 1981, 63A: 511–23.
2. Nicoll E. 'Fractures of the Tibial Shaft. A Survey of 705 Cases.' *J Bone Joint Surg.* [Br] 1964, 46B:373–87.
3. Crenshaw A. 'Delayed Union and Nou-union of Fractures' Ch 7 in *Campbell's Operative Orthopaedics.* 6th Edition. Eds. Edmonson A, Crenshaw A, the CV Mosby Company, 1980.
4. Muller M. 'Reconstructive Bone Surgery. Supplement.' in *Manual of Internal Fixation, Techniques Recommended By the AO-Group.* 2nd Edition. Eds. Muller M, Allgower M, Schneider R, Willenegger H. Springer-Verlag:Berlin Heidelberg New York, 1979.
5. Sharrard W. 'Bone and Joint.' Ch 14 in *Wound Healing For Surgeons.* Eds; Bucknell T, Harold Ellis. Balliere Tindel, 1984
6. Brighton C. 'Use of Constant DC In the Treatment of Non-Union.' AAOS Instructional Course Lectures 31: 94–103, 1982.
7. Weber B, Cech O. *Pseudoarthrosis.* Eds, Bern-Stuttgar-Wein, Huber, 1976
8. Esterhai J, Brighton C, Heppenstall R et al, 'Detection of Synovial Pseudarthrosis by TC Scintigraphy – Application To Treatment of Traumatic Non-Union With Constant Direct Current.' *Clin Orthop* 1981, 161: 15.
9. Tscherne H, Gotzen L. (Eds) *Fractures With Soft Tissue Injuries.* Springer-Verlag, 1984.
10. Gustilo R, Mendoza R, Williams D. 'Problems In the Management of Type III (Severe) Open Fractures: A New Classification of Type III Open Fractures.' *J Trauma* 1984, 24: 742–6.
11. Trueta J *Studies of the Development And Decay of the Human Frame.* William Heinemann Ltd: London, 1968.
12. McKibbin B. 'The Biology of Fracture Healing In Long Bones.' *J Bone Joint Surg.* [Br] 1978, 60b: 150.
13. Friberg O. 'Clinical Symptoms and Biomechanics of Lumbar Spine and Hip Joint In Leg Length Inequality.' *Spine* 1983, 8:643–51.
14. Lavender J, Peters A, Ring D, Henderson R, 'Radionuclide Scintigraphy' Ch 8 in *Infection In the Orthopaedic Patient.* Eds; Coombs R, Fitzgerald R. Butterworths: London, 1989.
15. Elson R. 'Revision Arthroplasty.' Ch 15 in *Complications of Total Hip Replacement.* Ed. Ling R, Churchill Livingstone: Edinburgh, 1984.
16. Coombs R, Jessop J. 'Biopsy In Orthopaedic Infection.' Ch 10 in *Infection In the Orthopaedic Patient.* Eds; Coombs R, Fitzgerald R. Butterworths: London, 1989.
17. Ratliff A. 'Vascular And Neurological Complications.' in *Complications of Total Hip Replacement.* Ed, Ling R, Churchill Livingstone: Edinburgh, 1984.
18. Bohler L. 'The Treatment of Pseudarthrosis.' in *The Treatment of Fractures.* Wilhelm Maudrich: Vienna, 1929.
19. Judet R, Patel A. 'Muscle Pedicle Bone Grafting of Long Bones By Osteoperiosteal Decortication.' *Clin Orthop.* 1972, 87: 74–80.
20. Nicoll E. 'Closed And Open Management of Tibial Fractures.' *Clin Orthop.* 1974, 105: 144–53.
21. Phemister D. 'Treatment of Ununited Fractures By Onlay Bone Grafts Without Screw Or Fixation And Without Breakdown of the Fibrous Union.' *J Bone Joint Surg.* 1947, 29: 946–60.
22. Colchero F, Orst G, Vidal J. 'La Scarification Son Interet Dans Le Traitement de L'Infection Osteo-Articulaire Chronique Fistulisee A Pyogenes.' *Int Orthop* 1982, 6(4): 263–71.
23. Saleh M, Harriman P, Edwards D. 'A Radiological Method For Producing Precise Limb Alignment.' *J Bone Joint Surg* [Br] 1991, 73-B No.3: 515–6.
24. Ilizarov G. 'Clinical Application of the Tension-Stress Effect For Limb Lengthening.' *Clin Orthop.* 1990, 250: 8–6.
25. Hagen K, Bunkle H. 'Treatment of Congenital Pseudarthrosis of the Tibia With Free Vascularised Bone Graft.' *Clin Orthop.* 1982, 166: 34–44.
26. Chao Eys, Aro H 'Biomechanics And Biology of External Fixation.' Chapter 11 in *External Fixation And Functional Bracing* Ed. Coombs R, Green S Sarmiento A. Orthotext: London, 1989.
27. Muller M. 'Treatment of Non-Union In Fractures of Long Bones.' *Clin Orthop.* 1979, 138:141–53.
28. Rosen H. 'Compression Treatment of Long Bone Pseudarthrosis.' *Clin Orthop.*1979, 138: 154–66.
29. Mennen V. 'A New Bone Holding Clamp For General Use During Internal Fixation of Fractures.' *S Afr Med J* 1981, 60: 580.
30. Hackethal K. *Die Bundelnagelung.* Springer: Berlin-Gottingen-Heidelberg, 1961.
31. Barranowski D, Brug E. 'Current Indications For Intramedullary Bundle Nailing.' *Unfallchirurg.* 1989, 92(10): 486–94.
32. Kempf I, Grosse A, Abalo C. 'Locked Intramedullary Nailing.' *Clin Orthop.* 1986, 212: 165–73.
33. De Bastiani G, Aldegheri R, Brivio L. 'The Treatment of Fractures With A Dynamic Axial Fixator.' *J Bone Joint Surg* [Br]1984, 66-B No.4, 538–45.
34. Borrione F, Hardy J. *Le Fixateur Externe Circulaire Sequoia, Technique Applications.* Springer-Verlag: Paris, 1990.
35. Sarmiento A. 'Functional Bracing of Tibial Fractures.' *Clin Orthop.* 1974, 105: 202.

36. Woo S L-Y, Akeson W, Coutts R, et al 'A Comparison of Cortical Bone Atrophy Secondary To Fixation With Plates With Large Differences In Bending Stiffness.' *J Bone Joint Surg* [Am] 1976, 58-A: 190–5.
37. Tayton K, Johnson-Nurse C, McKibbin B, et al 'The Use of Semi-Rigid Carbon-Fibre-Reinforced Plastic Plates For Fixation of Human Fractures. Results of Preliminary Trials.' *J Bone Joint Surg* [Br] 1982, 64-B: 105–11.
38. Schatzker J, Alho A, Sheehan J. 'Screws And Plates And their Application.' Chapter 3 in *Manual of Internal Fixation, Techniques Recommended By The AO-ASIF Group*. 3rd Edition. Eds. Muller M, Allgower M, Schneider R, Willenegger H. Springer-Verlag, 1991.
39. Rheinlander F. 'Tibial Blood Supply In Relation To Fracture Healing.' *Clin Orthop.* 1974, 105: 34–81.
40. Johnson K. 'Management of Malunion And Non-Union of the Tibia.' *Orth Clin N Am* 1987, Vol. 18 No. 1: 157–71.
41. Vidal J, Buscayret C, Connes H, et al 'Guidelines For Treatment of Open Fractures And Infected Pseudarthroses By External Fixation.' *Clin Orthop.* 1983, 180: 83–95.
42. Aro H, Kelly P, Lewallen D, et al 'Comparison of the Effects of Dynamisation And Constant Rigid Fixation On Rate And Quantity of Bone Osteotomy Union In External Fixation.' From Transactions of 34th Annual Meeting of Orthopaedic Research Society, Atlanta, Georgia. Vol 13: P 303, Feb 1988.
43. Paley D, Chaudray M, Pirore A, et al 'Treatment of Malunions And Mal-Non-Unions of the Femur And Tibia By Detailed Preoperative Planning And the Ilizarov Techniques.' *Orth Clin N Am* 1990, Vol 21, No 4, 667–91.
44. Glowacki J, Mulliken J. 'Demineralised Bone Implants.' *Clin Plast Surg* 1985, 12: 233.
45. Cockin J. 'Autologous Bone Grafting: Complications At the Donor Site.' *J Bone Joint Surg* [Br] 1971, 53-B: 153.
46. Weikal A, Habal M. 'Meralgia Paraesthetica: A Complication of Iliac Bone Procurement.' *Plast Reconstr Surg* 1977, 60: 572–4.
47. Summers B, Eisenstein S. 'Donor Site Pain From the Ileum.' *J Bone Joint Surg* [Br] 1989, 71-B: No.4, 677–80.
48. Saleh M. 'Bone Graft Harvesting. A Percutaneous Technique.' *J Bone Joint Surg* [Br] 1991, 73-B: No.5, 867–8.
49. Wolff J. *The Law of Bone Remodelling*. Translated by Maquet P and Furlong R. Springer-Verlag, 1986.
50. Goodship A, Kenwright J. 'The Influence of Induced Microenvironment Upon the Healing of Experimental Fractures.' *J Bone Joint Surg* [Br] 1985, 67-B: 650–5.
51. Kenwright J, Goodship A. 'Controlled Mechanical Stimulation In the Treatment of Tibial Fractures.' *Clin Orth* 1989, 241: 36–47.
52. Brighton C. 'The Semi-Invasive Method of Treating Non-Union With Direct Current.' *Orth Clin North Am* 1984, 15(1): 33–45.
53. Paterson Sir Dennis. 'Treatment of Non-Union With A Constant Direct Current: A Totally Implantable System.' *Orth Clin North Am* 1984, 15(1): 47-59.
54. Ieran M, Zaffuto S, Bagnacani M, et al 'Effect of Low Frequency Pulsing Electromagnetic Fields on Skin Ulcers of Venous Origin In Humans: A Double Blind Study.' *J Orthop Res* 1990, Vol. 8, No. 2, 276–82.
55. Brighton C, Pollack S. 'Treatment of Recalcitrant Non-Union With A Capacitively Coupled Electrical Field. A Preliminary Report.' *J Bone Joint Surg* [Am] 1985, 67(A): 577–85.
56. Trueta J. 'Muscle Contraction And Interosseous Circulation.' *J Bone Joint Surg* [Br] 1965, 47-B: 186.
57. Trueta J. 'Blood Supply And the Rate of Healing of Tibial Fractures.' *Clin Orth* 1974, 105: 11–25.
58. Andrews B, Somerville K, Austin S, Wilson N, Browse NL. 'Effect of foot compression on the velocity and volume of blood flow in the deep veins.' *Brit J Surg* 1993, 80: 198–200.
59. Morgan R, Cardan G, Psaila J, Gardner A, Fox R, Woodcock J. 'Arterial flow enhancement by impulse compression.' *Vasc Surg* 1991, 8–16.
60. Weiland A, Moore J, Hotchkiss R. 'Soft Tissue Procedures For Reconstruction of Tibial Shaft Fractures.' *Clin Orth* 1983, 178: 42–53.
61. Vasconez L, Bostwick J, Mcgraw J. 'Coverage of Exposed Bone By Muscle Transposition And Skin Grafting.' *Plast Reconstr Surg* 1974, 53: 526.
62. Svesnikov A, Barabash A, Cheplenko T,et al 'Radionuclide Studies of Osteogenesis and Circulation in Substitution of Large Defects of the Leg Bones In Experiment.' *Ortop Travmotol Protez* 1984, 11: 33.
63. Clifford R, Beauchamp C, Kellum J, et al 'Plate Fixation of Open Fractures of the Tibia.' *J Bone Joint Surg* 1988, 70-B: 644–8.
64. Burri C, Passler H, Henkemeyer H. 'Treatment of Post-Traumatic Osteomyelitis With Bone, Soft Tissue And Skin Defects.' *J Trauma* 1973, Vol 13, No 9 799-810.
65. Klemm K. 'Clinical Applications of Gentamicin-PMMA Beads.' Chapter 26 in *Infection In the Orthopaedic Patient*. Eds. Coombs R, Fitzgerald R. Butterworths, 1989.
66. Weber B, Brunner C. 'The Treatment of Non-Unions Without Electrical Stimulation.' *Clin Orth* 1981, 161: 24–32.
67. Klemm K. 'Treatment of Infected Pseudarthrosis of the Femur And Tibia With An Interlocking Nail.' *Clin Orth* 1986, 212: 174-81.
68. Papineau L, Alfageme A, Dalcourt J, et al 'Chronic Osteomyelitis; Excision And Open Cancellous Bone Grafting After Extensive Saucerisation.' *Int Orthop* 1979, 3: 165–76.
69. Blauth W, Vontorne O. 'Die Fibula-pro-Tibia-Fusion (Hahn-Brandes-Plastik) in Der Behandlung Von Knochendefeklen Der Tibia.' *Z Orthop* 1978, 116: 20–6.
70. Mankin H, Gebhardt M. 'The Use of Frozen Cadaveric Allografts In the Management of Patients With Bone Tumours of the Extremities.' *Orth Clin N Amer* April 1987, 275–91

A Review of the Management of Non-Unions Using Orthofix External Fixation Systems

49

M. Saleh

In Sheffield a large tertiary referral service was developed by Professor John Sharrard in 1979 for the treatment of difficult non-unions. The Dynamic Axial Fixator (DAF) was introduced in 1982 to deal with severe, intractable cases, many of which were infected. A review of this early experience is presented in order to analyze the appropriate role and use of the DAF. The first 22 segments treated with the DAF were reviewed[1] at the First Riva Congress in 1986 on recent advances in external fixation. Fractures were held in neutralization but post-operative compression was employed in some instances, using the fixator's compression–distraction device. The overall healing rate was 62.5 per cent and although fractures treated by progressive compression healed, undesirable angulation occurred.

By 1990, 52 cases had completed treatment and these were reviewed for an International Conference in Montpellier.[2] The technique of application was far more meticulous, and emphasis was placed on the use of short-bodied fixators and supplementary screws to keep the distance from the fracture site to the inner screws at 6cm or less (Fig. 49.1). Careful attention was paid to the restoration of alignment and lengthening procedures were offered if required. Fractures were held in neutralization or compression, but progressive compression was not used. The healing rate improved to 69 per cent, with the majority of failures being femoral applications. Only 44 per cent of femoral fractures united and it was concluded that in such cases, with long fixator-to-bone distances, bone loss at the fracture site and, in many cases, osteoporosis, the fixators were working beyond their realistic mechanical limits. The Limb Reconstruction System, although designed for bifocal treatments, offers greater stability than the DAF due to the absence of ball joints. and the facility to provide screw support close to the fracture site and along the whole length of the limb segment. The use of these devices in the femur, together with bone grafts or square resection osteotomies to permit the bone to take more load, led to improved results (Fig. 49.2).

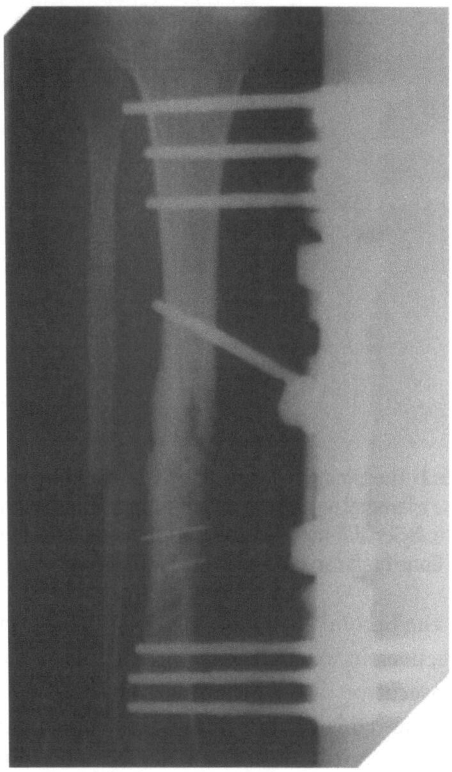

Fig. 49.1 Short body fixator plus supplementary screw to stabilize a tibial non-union.

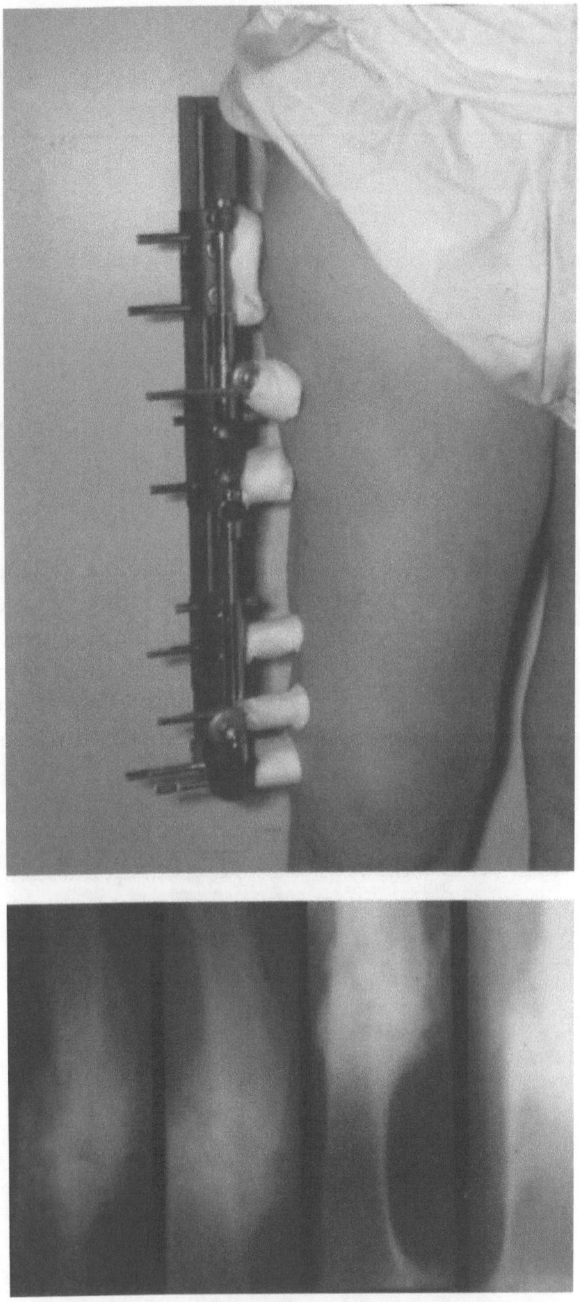

Fig. 49.2 The Limb Reconstruction System and bone graft to stabilise a femoral non-union. **a** Clinical appearance with fixator in place. **b** Serial X-rays (left to right) showing healing of non-union. Bone graft can be seen in the initial view.

At the Second Riva Congress in 1992, on current perspectives in external and intramedullary fixation, 91 consecutive cases, including the initial 52 cases, were reviewed.[3] All non-union foci were treated in neutralization or distraction (Saleh and Royston 1995);[4] compression was not used. If further length was required, a metaphyseal osteotomy and bifocal treatment was performed (Saleh and Rees 1995).[5] Despite the failures in the initial cohort an overall healing rate of 80.7 per cent was achieved.

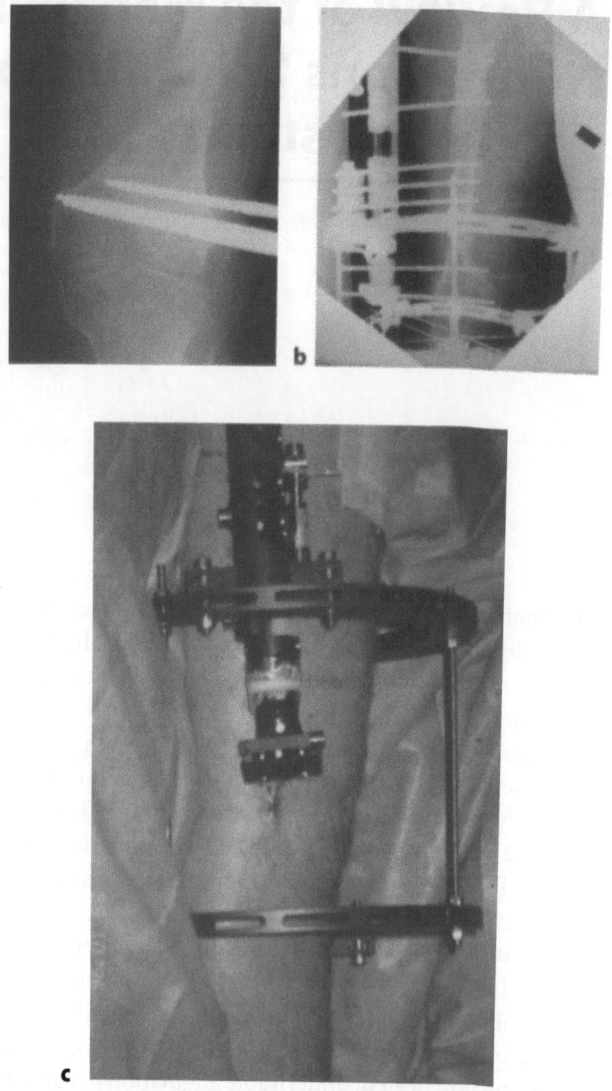

Fig. 49.3 Distal femoral non-union stabilized with the Limb Reconstruction System with a metaphyseal clamp for the distal femur, and coupled to a Sheffield Hybrid Fixator to take fixation across the knee for added stability. **a** Non-union prior to stabilization. **b** X-ray showing assembly in situ. **c** Clinical view of assembly.

Distal femoral non-unions remained a problem, however, because of the limited purchase for bone screws in the intercondylar region, and knee stiffness. The overall effect of the lower leg lever arm and stiff knee is to produce loosening of the distal femoral fixation. In these cases, a metaphyseal clamp is used to ensure optimal purchase in the distal femur and the fixation is taken across the knee by coupling a Sheffield Hybrid Fixator (SHF) from the mid-femoral diaphyseal screws to the proximal tibial diaphysis. Using this technique the stress on the distal femoral fixation is reduced (Fig. 49.3).

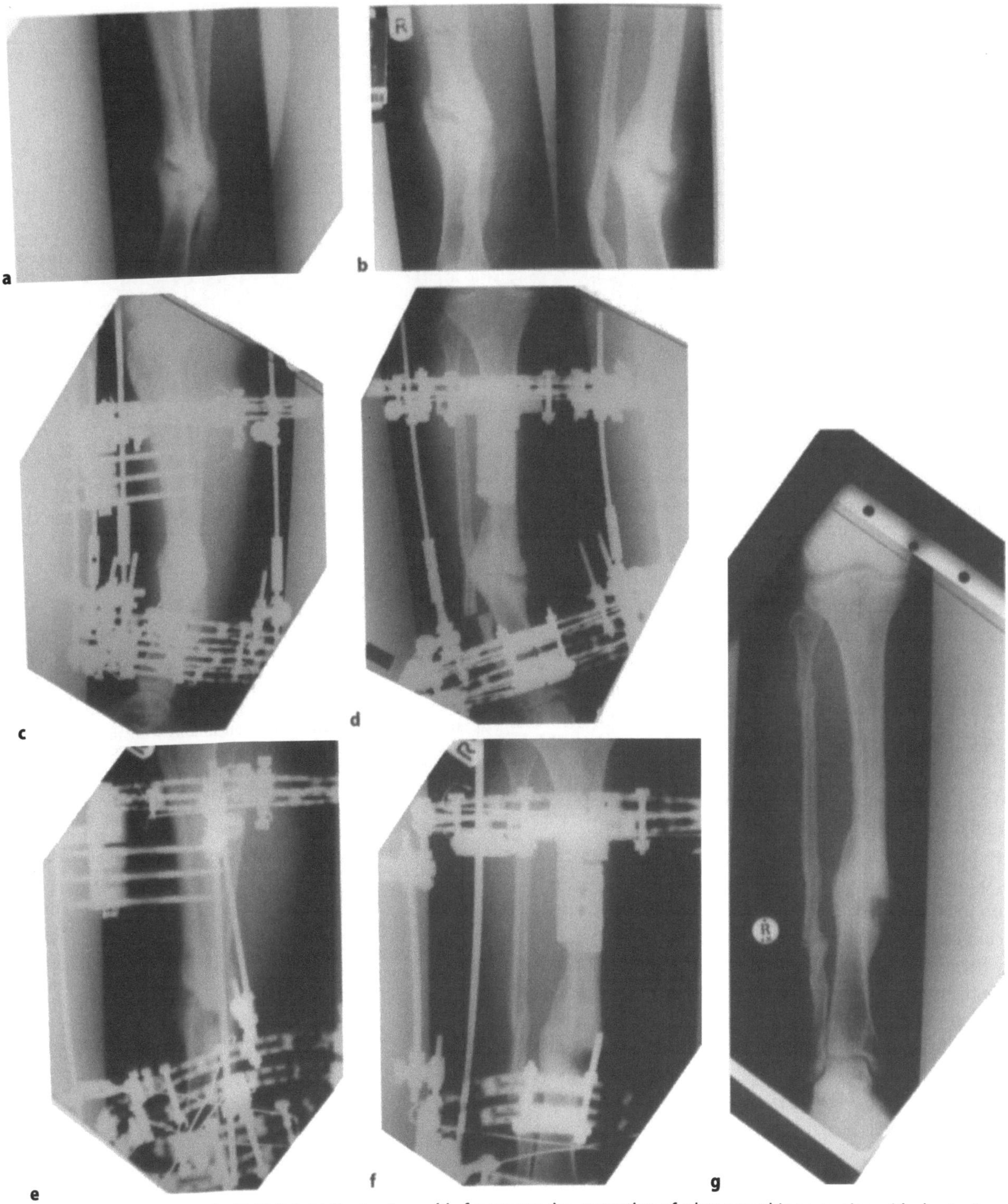

Fig. 49.4 Use of the Sheffield Hybrid Fixator Assembly for progressive correction of a hypertrophic non-union with shortening, anterior angulation and varus deformity. This 35-year-old male HGV Driver was involved in a road traffic accident, sustaining a grade III-B open tibial fracture. He was treated initially with K-wires and external fixation. The wound became infected and he had debridement and soleal flap. The fracture remained ununited and a bone graft was performed. When the fracture was considered to be united and he returned to work. He was never comfortable and later developed bowing of his leg for which he was treated in a cast. He was then referred to Author's unit where he was diagnosed as having a hypertrophic non-union with shortening, anterior angulation and varus deformity. **a, b** X-rays prior to treatment. **c, d** The Sheffield Hybrid Fixator was applied and an osteotomy performed through the non-union; immediate post-operative X-rays. **e, f** Progressive oblique plane correction was carried out. **g** Full correction was achieved and firm bony healing followed.

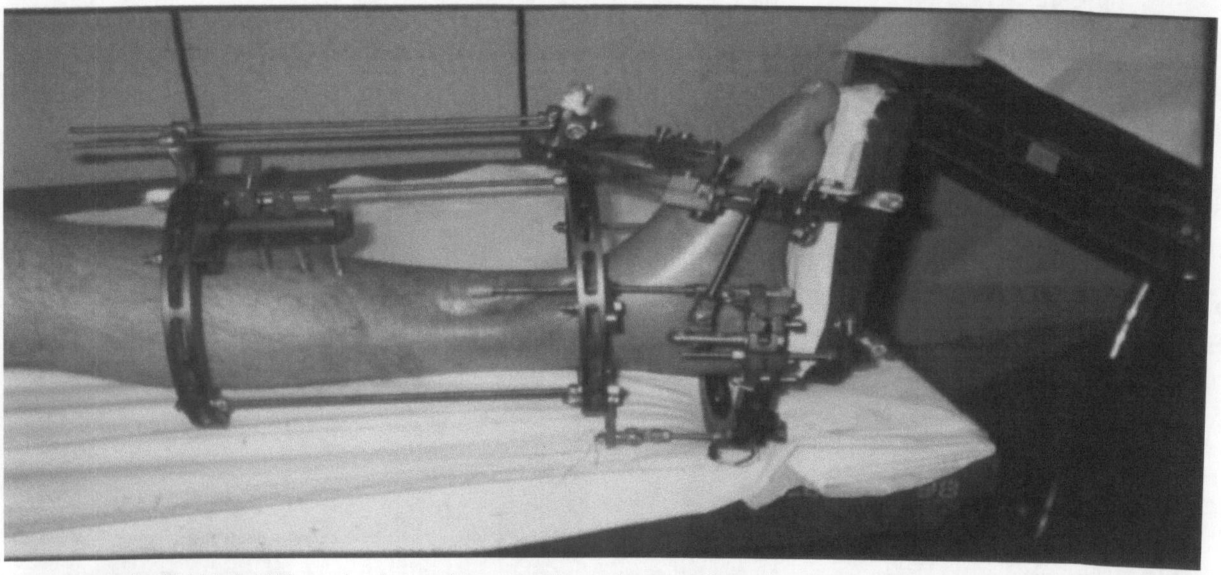

Fig. 49.5 A Sheffield Hybrid Fixator has been taken across the ankle to stabilize a distal tibial infected non-union. Note the sandal to permit weightbearing.

Following the use of sound principles for management as outlined in Ch. 48, a review of 100 consecutive non-unions was carried out, revealing an 87 per cent healing rate (Ribbans et al 1992).[6] Monolateral external fixation remains one of the most important techniques of stabilization for non-unions. Between 1987 and 1995, 251 non-unions were treated in this unit using various methods of stabilization (Table 49.1). In a recent review of 113 monolateral cases, 102 had healed without recourse to any other stabilization technique, representing a 90 per cent success rate. Following further fixation 7 more healed and 4 went on to amputation. Interestingly, all but one of the revision cases and all the amputations occurred in patients who smoked. Since its introduction in 1995, the Sheffield Hybrid System is now used to treat those cases which were previously treated using an Ilizarov frame. Hybrid fixation has particular advantages in tibial non-unions because of the ability to perform progressive correction (Fig. 49.4) and to cross the ankle to stabilize distal tibial non-unions or to correct contractures in the ankle and foot (Fig. 49.5).

Monolateral External Fixation	34%
Circular/Hybrid External Fixation	27%
Locked Intramedullary Nailing	20%
Plating	12%
Miscellaneous	7%

Table 49.1 Techniques of stabilization used in the treatment of 251 cases of non-union in Sheffield 1987–1995 (breakdown by percentage)

References

1. Sharrard WJW, Saleh M. 'The Dynamic Axial Fixator in the Treatment of Non-union and Pseudarthrosis.' First Riva Congress: Recent Advances in External Fixation. Riva del Garda, Italy, 28–30 September 1986; Abstract Book, p. 92–3.
2. Saleh M. 'The Treatment of Non-unions with the Dynamic Axial Fixator.' Conference: Evolution of External Fixation and Orthofix: From Static to Dynamic. University of Montpellier, Montpellier, France, 28–30 June 1990; Abstract Book, p.177.
3. Saleh M. 'Treatment of non-union of fractures with the DAF.' Second Riva Congress: Current Perspectives in External and Intramedullary Fixation. Riva del Garda, Italy, 27–31 May 1992; Abstract Book, p. 140.
4. Saleh M, Royston S. 'Management of non-union of fractures by distraction with correction of angulation and shortening.' *J Bone Joint Surg* [Br] 1996; 78-B: 105–9.
5. Saleh M, Rees AR. 'Bifocal surgery for deformity and bone loss – bone transport and compression–distraction compared.' *J Bone Joint Surg* [Br] 1995; 77-B: 429–34.
6. Ribbans WJ, Stubbs DA, Saleh M; 'Non-union surgery Part II. The Sheffield experience – 100 consecutive cases Results and lessons.' *Int J Orthop Trauma* 1992; 2: 19–24.

Bifocal Techniques for Non-Union and Deformity

50

M. Saleh and A. Rees

Introduction

Patients with limb shortening and diaphyseal bone loss or deformity (angulation and/or non-union) secondary to trauma have caused a considerable challenge to orthopaedic surgeons. Deformity correction alone using modern techniques such as nailing and external fixation may leave residual shortening, resulting in concomitant disability. Segmental skeletal defects due to trauma or resection of bone for infection have conventionally been treated with massive autogenous cancellous bone grafts (Christian et al 1989), or vascularized bone grafts (Weiland et al 1983a, 1983b). In the case of infection, sequestration of the graft is a problem. In such situations resection of the bone, granulation of the bed and Papineau type open grafting (Papineau et al 1979) have been used. These methods may not be capable of allowing realignment or restoration of limb length and may be associated with significant donor site morbidity. In our practice we have used the Papineau technique for partial defects but where infection involves the whole diaphysis or a bone defect exists secondary to trauma, newer techniques of callus distraction which allow mobilization of joints and address the leg length discrepancy are preferred (Saleh 1992a, Ribbans et al 1992).

In the 1950s and 1960s in Kurgan, in the former USSR, Ilizarov developed a radically different method of treating these defects using external fixation, compression of the defect and limb lengthening with spontaneous callus formation. In 1969 he described this technique and called it bifocal distraction compression osteosynthesis (Ilizarov and Ledyaev 1992). The bone segment is fixed proximally and distally by the external fixation frame. A corticotomy (bone division sparing the medulla) is performed in the metaphysis of the bone furthest from the defect and this is gradually distracted after a delay of five to seven days. The bone is thus lengthened by callus distraction. The defect is gradually closed at the same rate by the segment of bone between the corticotomy and the defect moving down to meet the opposite end rather like a lift in a lift shaft. When the defect is closed, the distraction may be continued further to address any residual limb length discrepancy. This method applies to larger defects and is known as bone transport; smaller defects may be closed at the time of surgery and then compressed, length being gradually restored in the metaphysis; this is termed compression–distraction. Both these techniques have significant advantages over conventional methods. First, surgery is confined to the affected segment. Second, using technetium uptake studies, the metaphyseal osteotomy has been shown to increase the blood supply to the bone by 2.2 times (Sveshnikov et al 1984). This has important implications when the healing of a non-union of the tibia is considered. Paley et al (1989) demonstrated the value of this clinically, and believed that adding a corticotomy improved union rates in atrophic non-unions. Human studies have also demonstrated that the bone formed by callus distraction – which in this case is used to replace the defect – remodels to a quality similar to that of normal bone (Saleh et al 1993a).

In Sheffield three bifocal strategies are used in the management of deformity and bone defects associated with shortening. Large bone defects are treated by bone transport, and smaller defects are treated by compression–distraction (Fig. 50.1a). Diaphyseal deformities are treated by compression–distraction

Compression–distraction										
Patient no.	Age	Diagnosis	Infection	Segment	Defect cm	Short cm	Angulation	Time from injury	Prev. ops	Frame type*
1	19	non-union	yes	tibia	0	6	yes	36 mos	5	LRS
2	41	non-union	no	femur	0	6.5	yes	60 mos	5	CIRC
3	25	open fracture	no	femur	2	7	yes	4 mos	1	LRS
4	36	non-union	no	tibia	1	2.5	yes	84 mos	4	LRS
5	30	non-union	no	tibia	0	3	yes	24 mos	2	CIRC
6	22	non-union	no	tibia	1	2	yes	28 mos	4	LRS
7	24	malunion	no	femur	0	7	yes	25 mos	3	LRS
8	42	non-union	yes	tibia	0	3.5	yes	17 mos	4	LRS
Bone Transport										
Patient no.	Age	Diagnosis	Infection	Segment	Defect cm	Short cm	Angulation	Time from injury	Prev. ops	Frame type*
9	33	non-union	no	tibia	3	3.5	yes	120 mos	3	LRS
10	22	non-union	yes	tibia	4	4	yes	11 mos	2	CIRC
11	29	open fracture	no	femur	7	2	no	0.25mos	1	LRS
12	20	open fracture	no	femur	6	2	no	2 mos	1	LRS
13	39	non-union	no	tibia	3	1.5	no	17 mos	3	CIRC
14	32	non-union	yes	tibia	6	1	no	7 mos	3	CIRC
15	34	non-union	yes	tibia	5	3	no	72 mos	10	LRS
16	52	non-union	yes	tibia	3	2	yes	8 mos	4	CIRC

Table 50.1 Details of the 16 patients who had either compression-distraction or bone transport. *LRS = Limb Reconstruction System, CIRC = Circular Frame

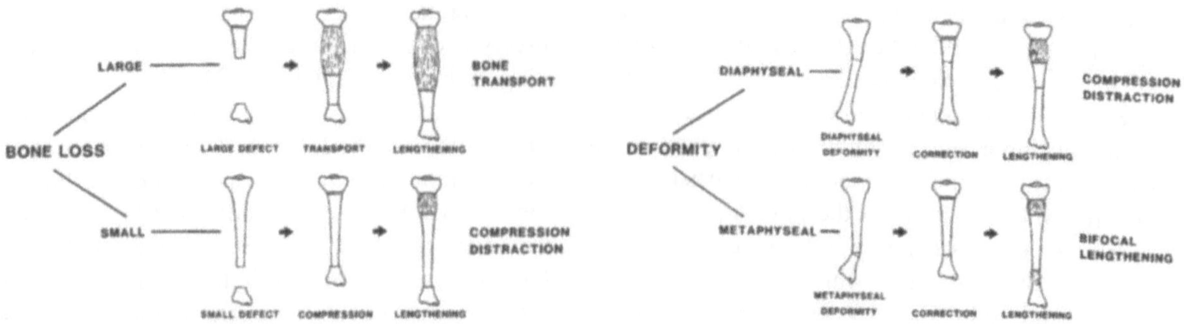

a b

Fig. 50.1 **a** Management of bone loss. **b** Management of shortening with deformity.

and metaphyseal deformities and some diaphyseal hypertrophic non-unions by bifocal lengthening (Saleh and Hamer 1993b) (Fig. 50.1b).

This chapter presents the results of the first sixteen patients treated bifocally in Sheffield. There were no cases of bifocal lengthening. A comparison between gradual (bone transport) and immediate (compression–distraction) closure of the defect is made.

Patients and Methods

Sixteen consecutive male patients with bone loss and deformity have undergone reconstruction, with an average follow-up of 24 months (range 8–66 months) from completion of treatment. The patients were aged between 19 and 52 years (mean 31.5 years). There were

5 femoral fractures and 11 tibial fractures. There were 12 cases of non-union, six having active infection, one malunion with shortening and three cases of open fracture with initial bone loss.

Shortening ranged between 1cm and 7cm (mean 4.8cm) and bone defects ranged between 1cm and 7cm (mean 3.7cm).

There were three acute cases with bone loss, all in the femur. These presented between one and 16 weeks from injury (mean 7.6 weeks) and all had only one previous operative procedure. The remaining 13 cases were salvage procedures in patients on average 39 months from injury (range 7 months to 10 years) who had had on average 3.8 previous procedures (range 2–10). Further details of the patient group are shown in Table 50.1.

Treatment in all cases included a metaphyseal osteotomy under tension for lengthening (Saleh

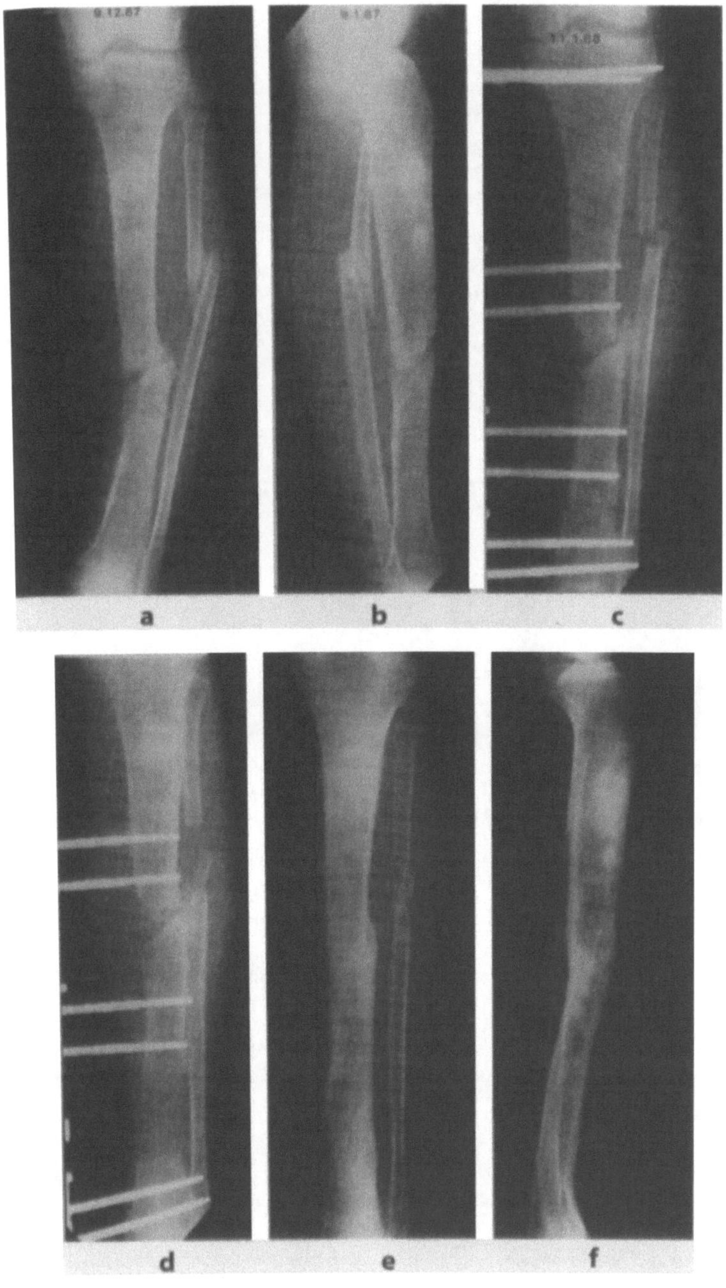

Fig. 50.2 Compression–distraction of an infected, non-united tibia. **a, b** Pre-operative radiographs show sclerosis proximally from previously infected pin sites which contraindicated proximal metaphyseal osteotomy. **c** Distal osteotomy, square osteotomy of the non-union site and compression. **d** Distal lengthening. **e,f** End result.

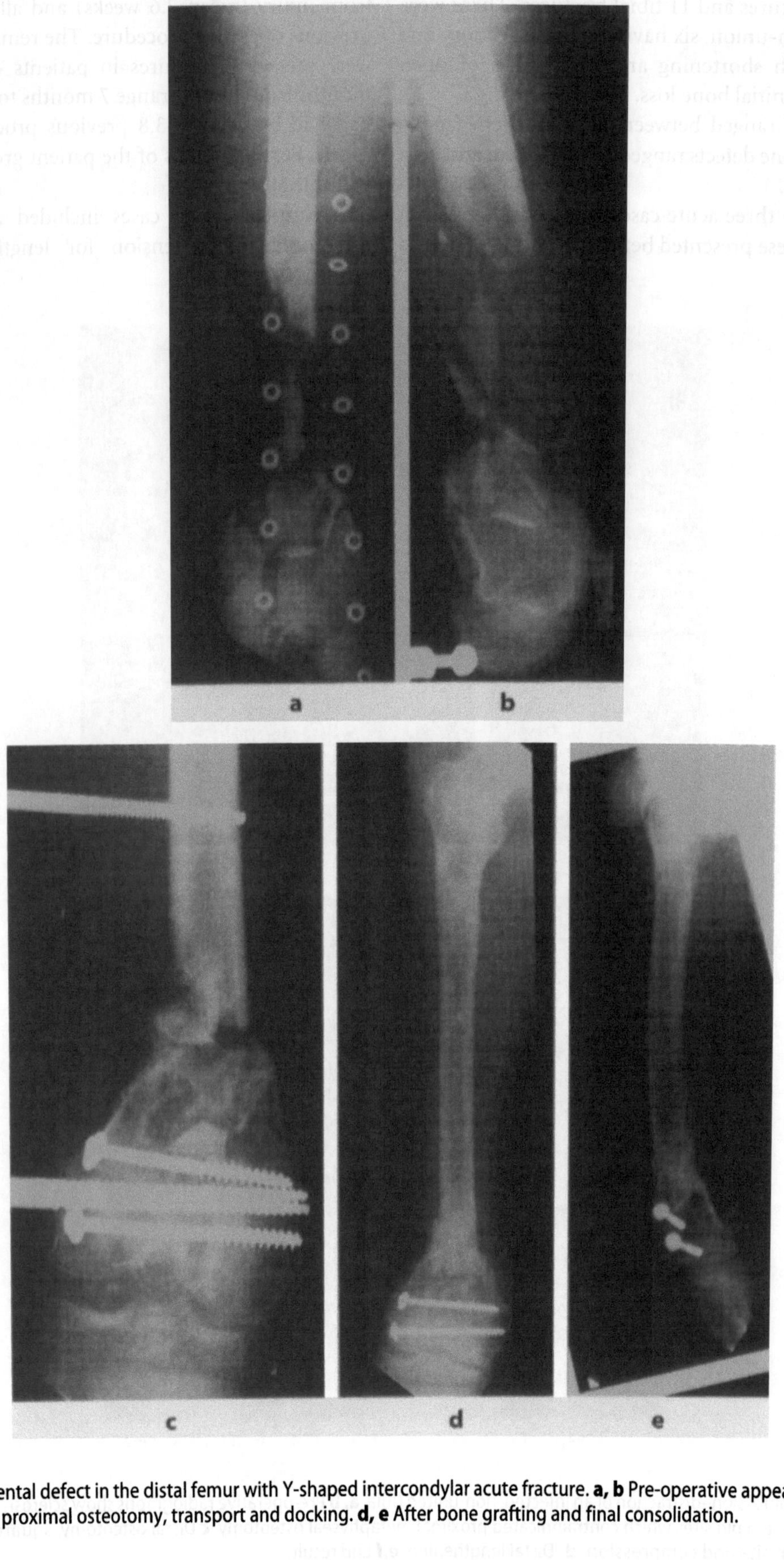

Fig. 50.3 Segmental defect in the distal femur with Y-shaped intercondylar acute fracture. **a, b** Pre-operative appearance. **c** After internal fixation, proximal osteotomy, transport and docking. **d, e** After bone grafting and final consolidation.

1992b). Diaphyseal deformity was treated by either a closing wedge or opening osteotomy and compression (Fig. 50.2). Bone defects from trauma or resection of abnormal or infected bone were treated by initial compression when less than 3cm in the tibia and less than 5cm in the femur. Larger defects were treated by bone transport (Fig. 50.3). In this series eight patients were treated with compression–distraction and eight with bone transport.

Fixation was achieved by means of the Orthofix unilateral Limb Reconstruction System (LRS) in 10 cases, and a circular frame (Sequoia, ATS, Paris) in 6 cases. In general a unilateral frame was used unless the defect was close to a joint, the bone was osteoporotic or gradual correction of angulation was necessary. Intra-operative alignment was ensured by the use of fluoroscopy and an alignment grid (Saleh et al 1991).

Since the majority of these cases were salvage procedures where amputation may have been the only reliable alternative treatment option, it is difficult to assess the results using conventional functional scores. Results were determined according to whether the treatment had achieved the goals of union, equalization of leg length, correction of the deformity and eradication of infection. The results were categorized as follows:

Excellent: all goals achieved; no major complication;

Good: most goals achieved; no major complication;

Fair: some goals achieved; no major complication;

Poor: failure of goals, or major complication.

A major complication was defined as one which persisted following the end of treatment.

Results

At a mean follow up of 24 months (range 8–66 months) following removal of fixation all the patients had excellent or good results. Twelve patients had an excellent bony result with equalization of leg length, union and correction of deformity with no major complications. There were four good results in femoral cases where limb length equality was not achieved. In one case (number 3) screw loosening in osteoporotic bone precluded further lengthening; in another case (number 2) the patient was over 2 metres tall and there was not sufficient frame stability to lengthen further. In a further case (number 12) lengthening was deliberately stopped short of equalization to prevent knee stiffness in a patient whose fracture involved the femoral condyles, requiring simultaneous internal fixation (Fig. 50.3). After removal of the frame, knee movement returned and the patient has since undergone and completed a further lengthening. In another patient (number 7) discomfort in the leg led to cessation of lengthening 2cm from equality, and premature removal of the frame for domestic reasons lead to a fracture requiring treatment with a further fixator, resulting in good alignment and function but a 3cm limb length discrepancy.

In the cases of bone transport, the average time to union was 16 months (range 11–24 months) whereas with compression–distraction the average time to union was 9.8 months (range 5–12 months). This difference is partly explained by the fact that in bone transport the defect is closed gradually, thus prolonging the time before healing can commence at the non-union (docking) site. Another important factor is that the bone transport group underwent more lengthening (mean 6.5cm compared with a mean of 4.7cm for compression–distraction). However, the healing index, which is the time to consolidation per cm lengthened, was similar at 2.4 months for bone transport and 2.65 months for compression–distraction. In the case of bone transport, the limiting factor was usually union at the fracture site, whereas with compression–distraction, the limiting factor was consolidation at the lengthening site.

Bone grafting was necessary at the docking site in 7 cases to promote consolidation. Of these, 5 were cases of bone transport and 2 were compression–distraction. Two cases required bone grafting at the lengthening site, one compression–distraction and one bone transport.

Minor complications were common. Most of these were pin site infections which resolved satisfactorily with antibiotic treatment. In two cases, poor bone quality resulted in intractable pin site infection with loosening of the frame, one in the case of a unilateral frame and one with a circular frame. In both cases this was fortunately close to the time of consolidation of the fracture site and plaster protection following removal of the frame was sufficient to achieve union. In a further case, loosening of the wires of one ring led to frame instability requiring further pin fixation.

Frame adjustment was necessary in 5 cases. There were 2 fractures during treatment, one above an Orthofix screw and one through lengthening callus. The latter required further external fixation and both united satisfactorily without adversely affecting the result. In one bone transport, the docking site eventually healed following frame removal and further frame application with bone grafting.

Infection was eradicated in the six infected cases.

A mean of 2.2 additional operative procedures were required in the bone transport patients compared to one additional procedure in the cases treated by compression–distraction. Five patients required no additional procedures; 4 from the compression–distraction group and only one from the bone transport group. Although circular frames took longer to apply, there appeared to be no difference between the results with circular compared to monolateral frames.

Discussion

The bifocal techniques of diaphyseal correction, compression or transport and metaphyseal lengthening produced excellent results in 12 cases. In the other four cases, all femoral, good results were achieved. In thirteen of the cases prior conventional treatment had failed. The treatment times with these bifocal techniques were long and in some cases may have been prolonged by our inexperience. In view of these intrinsically long treatment times careful patient selection is necessary.

These results represent the early experience in Sheffield with these techniques, and as time has progressed, the technique has been refined and results have become more reliable. Bone transport is inherently more complicated than compression–distraction with correspondingly longer treatment times and further operative procedures being necessary. There are several inherent problems. Because the defect is closed gradually, there is a time delay before bony contact and compression occurs at the docking site, thus prolonging the treatment time. The transported segment of bone can be deviated as it passes through the soft tissues, leading to translation at the docking site. We did not experience blocking of the transported segment by dense scar tissue but on one occasion (case 14) a bony block occurred requiring a further operation to insert an olive wire to deviate medially the transported bone temporarily. If the contact area at the docking site is small, limited bone grafting will be necessary. Bone grafting at this site was required in 5 out of the 8 cases of bone transport. Occasionally, the leading edge of the transported segment is relatively avascular (Green et al 1992) and this also can delay union unless trimming of the sclerotic end is performed. This procedure has been performed in our unit, but was not required in any of the cases presented. Unlike conventional limb lengthening and compression–distraction, the screws or wires move with the bone, cutting their way through the soft tissues, resulting in the need for soft tissue releases under local anaesthetic. Occasionally, a long necrotic skin track trailing the wire or screw occurs, which heals progressively and spontaneously. In a more recent case where both wires and screws were used, no difference was seen in the size or depth of this necrotic track.

Compression–distraction is a much simpler procedure. Since the defect is closed on the table there should be no problem of translation. Good bony apposition is obtained on day one and healing can commence then, without delay. These differences are reflected in our results. Bone transport patients had much longer non-union site consolidation times and, although the time to consolidation per centimetre lengthened (healing index) was similar in the two groups, it was union at the docking site that limited removal of the frame in these patients. In the compression–distraction group on the other hand, the limiting factor was time to consolidation of the lengthening site. A more significant difference in healing index may have been seen if longer lengthenings had been performed in the compression–distraction group. In this series the mean length gain was 3.7cm (range 2–6cm) in the compression–distraction group and 6.5 cm (range 4–8cm) in the bone transport group. When the femur is compared to the tibia there is a trend for the femur to consolidate faster (a healing index of 2.1 months per cm for the femur as compared with 2.85 months per cm for the tibia).

In the 4 cases of prolonged treatment (greater than 15 months) delay of consolidation at the docking site occurred. Three of these cases had no bone grafting, two had had no resection of the bone ends and three were the three earliest cases performed. In the fourth case there was a problem with docking, and translation of the transported segment had occurred.

Although Ilizarov originally described the procedure without bone graft or resection and in some series this has been adhered to (Paley et al 1989, Morandi et al 1989, Dagher and Roukoz 1991), other authors have recommended resecting bone to achieve a satisfactory docking configuration (Cattaneo et al 1992, Green et al 1992). Green also found bone grafting necessary on occasion, and on biopsy at the time of grafting found empty lacunae at the forward end of the transported segment indicating avascular bone. While routine bone grafting does not seem to be necessary, we feel that it is indicated when the contact area is small. We use percutaneous harvesting of bone from the iliac crest (Saleh 1991) which is associated with less morbidity than conventional open harvesting (Kreibich et al 1994).

Many authors have reported high complication rates and the need for further procedures with bone transport (Green et al 1992, Paley et al 1989, Cattaneo et al 1992, Marsh et al 1994). In our series further operations were necessary at a rate consistent with the intrinsic complexity of the procedure and, although minor complications occurred, none were serious or persisted following the end of treatment. In part this may be due to careful patient selection and preparation prior to surgery.

Criteria for deciding whether to opt for initial closure of the defect (compression–distraction) or to employ bone transport have not been widely reported. In our series, compression–distraction was performed when the defect was less than 3cm in the tibia and less than 5cm in the femur. Bone transport was performed for larger defects. These recommendations may include a significant safety margin and it remains to be seen as to whether the acute closure of larger defects as reported by Giebel (1991, and in this book, Ch. 52) is safe enough to allow bone transport to be performed less frequently.

What is evident from this series is that treatment times are prolonged and that more additional procedures are necessary with bone transport. In part, the additional time to consolidation of the non-union site is accounted for by the time taken for the transported segment to cross the defect in the bone before the process of healing can commence. For example, with a gap of 6cm closing at 1mm per day, this is an additional 60 days of treatment (in our series this adds a mean of 1.5 months to the treatment time) but even where this is taken into account, treatment times are prolonged. Treatment times may be shortened by bifocal transport in longer defects and these strategies may be important since it is our impression that complications increase when treatment times are in excess of 15–18 months. Treatment times may also be reduced by effecting an initial shortening of part of the defect followed by a shorter transport (Catagni 1992) or longer immediate shortenings (Giebel 1991). These procedures have the advantage of producing shared stability between the bone ends and the fixator earlier in the treatment period thus offloading the fixator and reducing the likelihood of fixation failure. Another strategy recommended by some authors (Raschke et al 1992) is bone transport over a nail, which enables the fixation frame to be removed prior to consolidation.

The choice of fixator may remain one of personal preference, but most other series have used either circular frames (Paley et al 1989, Morandi et al 1992, Cattaneo et al 1992) or unilateral fixators (Marsh et al 1994). We have used both and find the Orthofix unilateral fixator (LRS) a simple system with excellent rigidity. We prefer it to the circular frame as it is less cumbersome, quicker to apply and better tolerated by the patient, but where the fracture was near a joint, where the bone was osteoporotic, or where gradual correction of angulation was necessary, we used a circular frame. Where previous microvascular free flaps have been performed it may not be safe to use transfixion wires in the transported segment because of the risk of pedicle transection.

In conclusion, this early experience of bone transport and compression–distraction in fracture management has shown that the technique produces union of the fracture and, in the majority of cases, restoration of leg length with few complications. It has the advantage over more conventional methods of restricting major surgery to the affected segment, and addresses both alignment and length with a single treatment. The technique, however, is complicated, requires careful monitoring and good patient compliance. Preoperative preparation of patients is mandatory in all elective procedures and surgery should be performed in a centre with routine experience of callus distraction (Saleh 1992b, Saleh and Scott 1992). The treatment strategy should be matched to the patient's requirements, and one should aim to complete treatment within 18 months. Compression–distraction is simpler (requiring less additional procedures) than bone transport, and should be undertaken in preference when it is possible to close the defect directly. We do not know at present how large a defect can be closed acutely although we have subsequently had some experience of partial immediate closure with subsequent slow progressive closure of larger defects. When it is necessary to perform bone transport we believe that to optimise conditions for healing, the necrotic or infected bone ends should be resected and fashioned in such a way as to enhance docking. The frame should be carefully mounted so as to be parallel in both planes to prevent translation, and bone grafting of the docking site, if necessary, should be performed early.

References

Cattaneo A., Catagni M., Johnson E.E. 'The treatment of infected non-unions and segmental defects of the tibia by the methods of Ilizarov.' *Clin Orthop* 1992; 280: 143–52.

Catagni M. Personal communication 1992.

Christian E.P., Bosse M.J., Robb G. 'Reconstruction of large diaphyseal defects, without free fibular transfer, in grade IIIB tibial fractures.' *J Bone Joint Surg* [Am] 1989; 71A: 994–1004.

Dagher F., Roukoz S. 'Compound tibial fractures with bone loss treated by the Ilizarov technique.' *J Bone Joint Surg* [Br]1991; 73B: 316–21.

Giebel G. 'Resektionsdebridement mit kompensatorischer Kallusdistraktion.' *Unfallchirurg* 1991; 94: 401–8.

Green S.A., Jackson J.M., Wall D.M., Marinow H., Ishkanian J. 'Management of segmental defects by the Ilizarov intercalary bone transport method.' *Clin Orthop* 1992; 280:136–42.

Ilizarov G.A., Ledyaev V.I. 'The replacement of long tubular bone defects by lengthening by distraction osteotomy of one of the fragments'. in *Clin Orthop* 1992; 280: 7–10.(Original in Russian *Vestn Khir* 1969; 102: 77)

Kreibich N., Scott I., Wells J., Saleh M. 'Donor site morbidity after conventional and percutaneous bone graft harvesting.' Accepted *J Bone Joint Surg* [Br] 1994; 76B: 847–8.

Marsh J.L., Prokuski L.J., Biermann J.S. 'Comparison of conventional treatment vs bone transport for the treatment of chronic infected non-union of the tibia. *Clin Orthop* 1994; 301:139–49.

Morandi M., Zembo M.M., Ciotti M. 'Infected tibial pseudarthrosis – a 2-year follow-up on patients treated by the Ilizarov Technique.' *Orthopaedics* 1989; 12: 497–508.

Paley D., Catagni M.A., Argnani F., Villa A., Benedetti G.B., Cattaneo R. 'Ilizarov treatment of tibial non-unions with bone loss.' *Clin Orthop* 1989; 241: 146–65.

Papineau L.J., Alfageme A., Dalcourt J.P., Pilon L. 'Chronic osteomyelitis; excision and open cancellous bone grafting after extensive saucerisation.' *Int Orthop* 1979; 3 :165–76.

Raschke M.J., Mann J.W., Oedekoven G., Claudi B.F. 'Segmental transport after unreamed intramedullary nailing.' *Clin Orthop* 1992; 282: 233–40.

Ribbans W.J., Stubbs D.A., Saleh M. 'Non-union Surgery Part II. The Sheffield Experience – 100 consecutive cases, results and lessons.' *Int J Orthop Trauma* 1992; 2: 19–24.

Saleh M., Harriman P., Edwards D.J. 'A radiological method for producing precise limb alignment.' *J Bone Joint Surg* [Br]1991; 73B: 515–6.

Saleh M. 'Non-union Surgery Part I. Basic Principles of Management.' *Int J Orthop Trauma* 1992a; 2: 4–18.

Saleh M. 'Technique selection in limb lengthening: The Sheffield Practice.' *Seminars in Orthop* 1992b; 7: 137–51.

Saleh M., Scott B.W. 'Pitfalls and Complications of Leg Lengthening: The Sheffield Experience.' *Seminars in Orthop* 1992; 7: 207–222.

Saleh M. 'Bone Grafting Harvesting: a percutaneous technique.' *J Bone Joint Surg* [Br]1991; 73B: 867–8.

Saleh M., Stubbs D.A., Street R.J., Lang D.M., Harris S.C. 'Histologic Analysis of human lengthened bone. *J Paed Orthop* 1993; 2[B]: 16–21.

Saleh M., Hamer A. 'Bifocal lengthening – preliminary results' *J Paed Orthop* 1993; 2[B]: 42–8.

Sveshnikov A.A., Barabash A.P., Chepelenko T.A., Smotrova L.A., Larionov A.A. 'Radionuclide studies of osteogenisis and circulation in substitution of large defects of the leg bones' in *Experiment Ortop Travmatol Protex* 1984; 11: 33–7.

Weiland A.J., Moore J.R., Daniel R.K. 'Vascularised bone grafts. Experience with 41 cases.' *Clin Orthop* 1983a;174: 87–95.

Weiland A.J., Moore J.R., Hotchkiss R.N. 'Soft tissue procedures for reconstruction of tibial shaft fractures.' *Clin Orthop* 1983b; 178: 42–53.

The Treatment of Chronic Infected Non-Unions

51

S. Meletiou and J.L. Marsh

The diagnosis and treatment of chronic infected non-union is one of the most complex and challenging problems in orthopaedics. The clinician needs a comprehensive understanding of the pathophysiology in order to develop a clinical approach. This requires the use of available diagnostic modalities and familiarity with a full range of treatment options. Each patient has a unique set of clinical variables; some broad classification of infected non-unions is helpful, however, in planning treatment. The principles of treatment consist of adequate surgical debridement, appropriate cultures to guide specific antimicrobial therapy, fracture stabilization, and reconstruction of both the soft tissues and the bone. The relative indications for amputation versus limb salvage need to be considered by the physician and patient.

Classification

Cierny has classified osteomyelitis based on both local disease and host factors, which together determine appropriate management and prognosis.[8] There are four anatomical types of local disease: medullary, superficial, localized, and diffuse (labelled I–IV respectively). Diffuse osteomyelitis (Type IV) is through and through involvement of an entire intercalary segment with soft tissue involvement. This type is most characteristic of chronic infected non-unions.[8]

The second part of Cierny's clinical staging is the physiological classification of the patient. The class A patient has a normal response to trauma and infection and a normal capacity to heal. The class B patient has either local factors (B^L), systemic factors (B^S), or a combination ($B^{L/S}$) which impede the ability to respond to treatment. For the class C patient, potential morbidity and/or mortality of treatment outweighs the possible benefits and thus, only palliative measures are advised. The anatomical and physiological classifications are combined to form a clinical stage (i.e. IIA, $IIIB^{L/S}$). In this manner the interaction between local disease and host factors are present in the staging and considered when forming a treatment plan. The focus of the rest of this chapter will be on chronic infected non-unions, which are staged as IVA–IVC.[8]

A classification of post-traumatic osteomyelitis proposed by May et al[31] is focused on the tibia and delineates expected time frames of treatment for differing levels of involvement. The classification is based on the osseous defect after initial skeletal and soft tissue debridement. Type I osteomyelitis has an intact tibia and fibula capable of functional support. Treatment consists of debridement, antibiotics, and soft tissue coverage. The average rehabilitation period until walking without support or upper extremity aids is from six to twelve weeks. Type II osteomyelitis has a metaphyseal or a diaphyseal defect of greater than 30 per cent width without a complete disruption in tibial continuity. Treatment is similar to Type I with the additional need for bone grafting. The expected rehabilitation time is longer, usually three to six months. Type III and IV injuries have tibial defects of 6cm or less and greater than 6cm respectively. Type III defects can be bridged by autogenous bone graft, but Type IV require more extensive osseous reconstruction, such as vascularized bone grafts. The rehabilitation period averages from twelve to eighteen months, compared to six to twelve for Type III. Type V defects are similar to Type IV without an intact fibula. Posterolateral and fibula-pro-tibia graft procedures are not an option and the rehabilitation time is likely to be greater than eighteen months.[31]

This system delineates differences in non-union types which may affect surgical options and provides the surgeon and patient with information that can help define the length of the treatment and rehabilitation periods. This can assist the patient in making an informed decision prior to committing to limb reconstruction or choosing amputation.

We have found that chronic infected non-unions present with two levels of severity requiring two different treatment strategies. A Type 1 chronic infected non-union usually has a history of infection or an open wound but is not draining at the time of entering treatment. The radiograph has a hypertrophic appearance. The diagnosis of infection is made by clinical suspicion combined with a positive radiographic study (indium white cell scan) and culture. This type is frequently the result of failed external fixation and the infecting organisms are often low grade. Skeletal stabilization by external fixation, axis correction, and limited debridement will often produce union.

The Type 2 chronic infected non-union is overtly infected and the radiograph has an atrophic appearance. Polymicrobial infection is common and there is usually considerable dead bone. It commonly results from failure to obtain soft tissue coverage or following failed plating. Segmental skeletal resection is required to cure the infection. Fig. 51.1 summarizes these three classifications of chronic infected non-union.

Diagnosis

Radiology

When the radiograph demonstrates cortical destruction, periosteal reaction, mixed bone destruction and formation as well as sequestrum, the diagnosis of infection is clear. In these cases, the clinical diagnosis of infection is also obvious (draining wound, etc.). In some cases, tomograms or computed tomograms (CT) enhance the clinician's ability to appreciate cortical destruction or a sequestrum not detected on plain films. In other cases, however, despite these studies, the clinical and radiological diagnosis of infection may be uncertain. When the history raises a suspicion of infection, further investigations are indicated prior to treatment.

Magnetic resonance imaging (MRI) is very sensitive for detecting changes within the marrow. Early

	Classification System	Basis of System	Description
Cierny	Stage IVA Stage IVB Stage IVC	General anatomical description Host physiological status	Through and through medullary involvement A. normal immune response B. local and/or systemic compromising factors, i.e. diabetes, malignancy, tobacco abuse, venous stasis, radiation fibrosis C. potential morbidity of limb salvage in excess of benefits
May	Type III Type IV Type V	Size of post-debridement defect Expected length of treatment course	III. tibial defect <6 cm, rehab 6-12 months IV. tibial defect >6 cm, rehab 12-18 months V. type IV without usable intact fibula, rehab > 18 months
Meletiou and Marsh	Type 1 Type2	Anatomical and radiographic appearance Microbiology Delineation of treatment strategies	1.Hypertrophic non-union with low-grade infection. Commonly monomicrobial 2. Atrophic non-union, with drainage, cellulitis, exposed bone or hardware. Usually polymicrobial

Fig. 51.1 Three classification systems for chronic infected non-unions.

osteomyelitis, with inflammatory infiltrate and marrow oedema, produces a low intensity signal on the T1 image and increased signal intensity on STIR and T2 weighted images. Surrounding soft tissue planes are poorly defined due to oedema. There is a wide zone of transition between normal marrow and diseased marrow. In chronic osteomyelitis, the tissue planes are more distinct, there is cortical thickening, and the zone of transition within the marrow is more distinct.[50]

Unger et al compared MRI to technetium-99m methylene diphosphonate (Tc-99m-MDP) scintigraphy in acute osteomyelitis and noted sensitivities of 92 per cent and 82 per cent and specificities of 96 per cent and 65 per cent respectively. MRI was more accurate than Tc-99m-MDP at differentiating cellulitis from osteomyelitis. In fact, the bone marrow was noted to have a normal signal in the absence of osteomyelitis even in cases of cellulitis extending to the periosteum.[52] These authors also noted an increase in T1 signal in cases of healed osteomyelitis.[52]

Unfortunately, there are limitations to MRI that decrease its usefulness for the evaluation of chronic infected non-unions. In this setting, it is rather non-specific. Other non-infectious causes of inflammation such as previous surgery, neoplastic processes, healing fracture, bone contusions, and infarcts can simulate the signal changes found in osteomyelitis. In addition, the presence of any hardware limits the utility of MRI.

Tc-99m-MDP scintigraphy alone is highly sensitive but not specific, and it cannot differentiate non-union from infected non-union. Esterhai et al noted 100 per cent uptake at 24 non-union sites, but only 13 had biopsy evidence of osteomyelitis.[14] Sequential Tc-99m-MDP and gallium-67 (Ga67) scans have been evaluated to detect infection associated with a non-union; however, the false-negative rate has been reported to be as high as 82 per cent.[13,45]

Tc-99m-MDP/Indium-111-labelled leukocytes (In-111-WBC) scanning is more accurate for the detection of osteomyelitis in the presence of fracture

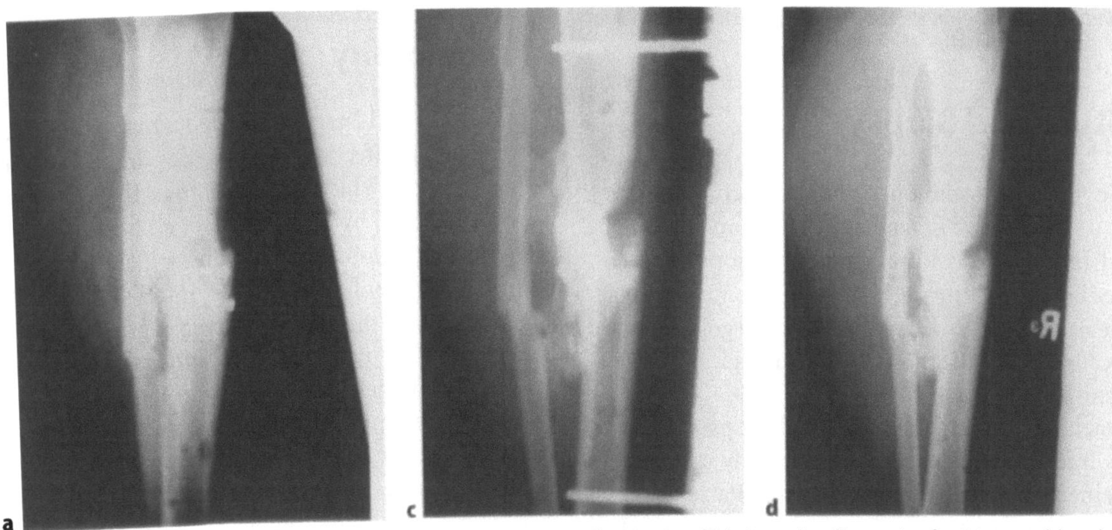

a c d

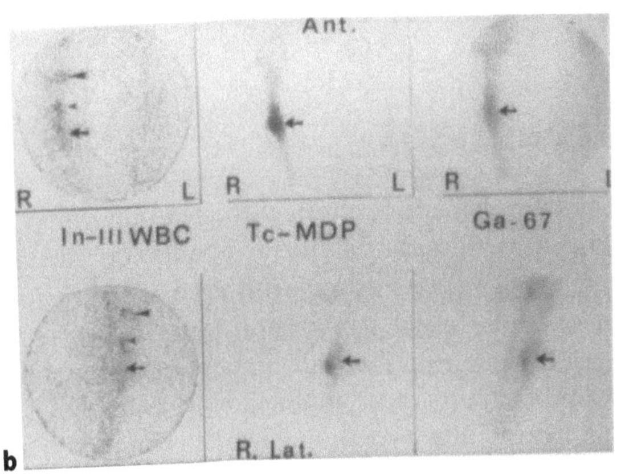

b

Fig. 51.2 **a** This lateral radiograph of a 34 year-old male one year after a Type III tibia and fibula fracture treated initially with external fixation, demonstrates a possible sequestrum at a proximal pin site without clear radiographic evidence of infection at the fracture site. The previously open wound was healed but a pin site continued to drain. **b** There was increased uptake at the fracture site on the sequential Tc-99m-MDP/In-111-WBC Scan. White cells localized at both the fracture site and at the pin sites (arrows). He was treated with hardware removal, limited irrigation and debridement of the non-union site, overdrilling of the pin sites, application of an Orthofix ball joint external fixator, antibiotics, and posterolateral bone graft. Intra-operative cultures grew *S. aureus*. **c** A lateral radiograph demonstrates the fixator and a maturing graft 3months after surgery. **d** There was solid union on the lateral radiograph taken 8 months post-operatively, and there was no clinical evidence of infection.

non-union (Fig. 51.2). The criteria used for a positive study is In-111-WBC localization which corresponds to a region of increased Tc-99m-MDP uptake and is greater than that of non-adjacent or contralateral bone marrow. Sequential scans are thought to be advantageous over In-111-WBC scintigraphy alone for bony localization and for determining the extent of the infection.[47] Nepola et al reported a sensitivity of 86 per cent and a specificity of 84 per cent for sequential Tc-99m-MDP/In-111-WBC.[35] There is an increased false-positive rate for Tc-99m-MDP/In-111-WBC scans at sites of failed arthrodesis, non-union of intra-articular fractures, and metaphyseal non-unions adjacent to joints where there is active traumatic arthropathy.[46]

With these caveats in mind, our current recommended use of scintigraphy is combined Tc-99m-MDP/In-111-WBC scans for screening patients with delayed diaphyseal union or non-union and a history of an open fracture, wound complication, drainage, infection or other radiographic findings suggestive of infection.[35] The radioisotope scans in Fig. 51.2 demonstrate occult infection in a case that might otherwise have been treated with an intramedullary nail.

Culture and Biopsy

While imaging techniques can be useful screening tools, the definitive diagnosis of infection is made by direct biopsy and culture. Operative biopsy and culture of bone, sequestrum, loculated pus, and orthopaedic devices within an infected field is the gold standard for accurate identification of all pathological microorganisms.

Mackowiak et al evaluated the diagnostic value of sinus track cultures and found that only 44 per cent contained the operative pathogen.[27] Patzakis et al reported similar results (57 per cent).[38] Perry et al found superficial swabs were as accurate as needle biopsy, but both were inaccurate when compared to operative culture. The authors postulate that there are numerous microenvironments within an infected area and there is a high probability that a needle biopsy will miss some of these, thus failing to identify a pathogen. In cases where there is a pathogen, the usefulness of swabs and needle biopsy rises.[39] This is supported by other authors.[38]

When analyzing intra-operative cultures, it is important to be aware of the incidence and type of clinically unimportant positive cultures at the institution. Dietz et al reported a 58 per cent incidence of positive cultures from clean elective orthopaedic procedures. In this study, none of the common pathogens such as *Staphylococcus aureus* or *Pseudomonas aeruginosa* were found, and colony counts were five or less for all but one species. Broth cultures, in particular, were noted to have high false-positive rates. These findings suggest that clinically unimportant bacteria can frequently be grown and that there may be a critical number of colony counts, below which there is no pathological significance.[12] Results are likely to differ between hospitals and a similar study at each might prove useful.

Our current recommendations for definitive diagnosis of chronic osteomyelitis include multiple intra-operative aerobic, anaerobic and (when indicated) fungal cultures from the deep tissues. This provides the best opportunity for isolating pathogens from all microenvironments within the wound. We do not recommend superficial swabs or needle biopsies as these results are, at best, difficult to interpret. Finally, the common intra-operative contaminants present at each institution should be known in order to aid interpretation of culture results.

Microbiology

Patzakis et al and Perry et al noted a high incidence of polymicrobial infection (58 per cent and 32 per cent respectively).[38,39] This was higher than the 13 per cent previously noted by Mackowiak et al, possibly due to an important emphasis on obtaining material from all microenvironments within the infected area.[27] For similar reasons, they also observed a greater number and variety of pathogens. *S. aureus* is the most common pathogen, reportedly present in roughly 60 per cent of patients. *P. aeruginosa* is second, present in 20–30 per cent of cases. Other organisms commonly present include Bacteriodes species, Enterobacteriaceae, Streptococcus, Peptostreptococcus, and *S. epidermidis.*[27,38,39]

Treatment

The management of chronic infected non-union has four arms: surgical debridement, antibiotic therapy, soft tissue reconstruction with dead space management, and skeletal stabilization with osseous repair. Each of these arms is equally important and treatment within each proceeds simultaneously. We feel that the subdivision into Type 1 and Type 2 is important as it affects treatment strategies. This will be addressed within each of the following sections.

Surgical Debridement

Initial surgical debridement takes place at the same time as biopsy and culture. All infected, necrotic, and avascular tissue as well as all foreign bodies/hardware must be excised, leaving a viable yet contaminated tissue bed. Pre-operative planning is important. The surgeon should use the plain films, scintigraphy, and possibly CT scans to help determine the three-dimensional extent of the infection and the surgical debridement. Incisions should be planned to take advantage of old scars and to include excision of sinus tracks, if possible. The approach must give excellent exposure of the infected bone.

The most challenging aspect of debridement is in determining how much is adequate. Currently, the most useful criterion for adequate debridement is the achievement of uniform punctate bleeding from the debrided surface, the so-called "paprika" sign. Swiontkowski used laser Doppler flowmetry as an adjunct to surgical debridement in osteomyelitis. In twelve of thirteen cases, debridement to depths where the bone recorded "blood cell flux" signals of at least 75mv resulted in control of the infection.[48] This technique may hold promise in assisting the surgeon to determine the viability of bone fragments and, thus, their need for resection.

Curettage will remove much of the obviously infected or necrotic bone and the use of a pneumatic burr may be helpful. It is also important to irrigate while burring to avoid heat necrosis. After burring, uniform haversian bleeding from the bone surface should be obtained. Loose bone fragments should be resected, as they will not remain viable without soft tissue attachments. An important aspect of the debridement is hardware removal, as its continued presence may perpetuate the infection. Soft tissue stripping should be minimized as it creates more necrotic bone, a haven for the bacteria. Pulsatile lavage (with or without antibiotics) should be liberally used throughout the procedure. All sinus tracks should be excised; those with suspicious changes in appearance, drainage, etc. require wide excision and evaluation for epidermoid carcinoma. Necrotic and infected soft tissues should also be excised.

Adhering to these general principles, somewhat different strategies can be developed for Type 1 and Type 2 chronic infected non-unions. Debridement of the Type 1 will usually be limited. It is not normally necessary to resect much cortical bone and the remaining defect is generally small and not segmental. These non-unions are hypertrophic with viable non-infected bone attempting to repair. This bone does not need to be resected. Infection will be localized at the non-union site and will respond well to limited debridement.

The Type 2 infected non-unions generally will require segmental resection. The resection should be done radically to a clean level. Removal of all infected or sequestered material is accomplished with this one resection. The remaining bone ends are checked for viability and cultured. If the extent of infection is less clear, a gradual proximal and distal resection may be required.

Antibiotic Therapy

Antibiotic selection and use is a crucial aspect of treatment and both systemic and local methods of drug delivery can be employed.

All antibiotics should be stopped at least one week prior to the initial debridement in order to improve the yield of intra-operative cultures. After debridement, broad spectrum intravenous antibiotics should be started since there is a high incidence of polymicrobial infections.

When culture results return, antibiotics should be selected to treat all of the pathogens. It is important to choose antibiotics with a high predicted blood level/mean inhibitory capacity (MIC) ratio. One study has demonstrated a direct relationship between the maximal peak blood level of aminoglycosides/MIC ratio and the rate of clinical response.[33] The increase in the rate of response occurred up to a point where peak blood levels were eight times that of the MIC.

The use of steady-state serum bactericidal tests in cases of chronic osteomyelitis has also been shown to be predictive of therapeutic efficacy in a prospective study. Peak titres of 1:16 or greater had a 91 per cent predictive value for cure, whereas titres less than 1:16 had a predictive value for failure of 71 per cent. Trough titres of 1:4 or greater were predictive of cure in 100 per cent while trough titres less than 1:2 had a predictive value for failure of 100 per cent.[55] This study employed six weeks of combination parenteral and oral antibiotics.

Antibiotic-impregnated PMMA bead chains are an effective local delivery system for antibiotics and may decrease the need for prolonged systemic antibiotics. The beads are placed in the dead-space created by the surgical debridement. The wound is closed with a tissue graft or a watertight dressing. For chronic infected non-union, Calhoun demonstrated in a controlled, randomized clinical trial that gentamycin-impregnated beads plus peri-operative antibiotics were as efficacious and cost-effective as four weeks of intravenous antibiotics. Beads place a high concentration of antibiotics at the site of infection producing bactericidal seroma levels for weeks to months.[2] Furthermore, the serum-to-haematoma ratio is between 1:40 and 1:70, which avoids many of the potential systemic side-effects of antibiotics.[3].For maximum effectiveness, the technical aspects of bead construction, cement selection and antibiotic dosage/selection should be closely followed.[2,3,23]

Duration of antibiotic therapy has never been well established. Six weeks of treatment, however, is considered by most to be appropriate. Due to the greater likelihood of cure in Type 1 cases, we feel that one week of parenteral antibiotics followed by five weeks of oral antibiotics is sufficient. This avoids the potential complications of long-term intravenous therapy. Mader has demonstrated equivalent efficacy between oral ciprofloxacin and parenteral antibiotics for the treatment of chronic osteomyelitis in a prospective randomized study.[28] For Type 2 infected non-unions we use four to six weeks of intravenous antibiotics as recommended by others.[53]

Soft Tissues

In Type 1 infected non-unions, primary wound closure is usually possible. Where soft tissue debridement is more extensive, rotational flaps are often sufficient. The medial gastrocnemius can be used for wounds over the proximal third of the tibia, and the soleus for wounds over the middle third. This is followed by split-thickness skin grafting.

Type 2 chronic infected non-unions involve greater soft tissue loss, and rotational flap coverage may be inadequate. Several authors have described free tissue transfer to provide wound coverage.[7,18,54] Latissimus dorsi and rectus abdominis free muscle flaps are the most commonly used transfers. Pre-operative arteriograms are required to determine the adequacy of the blood supply to the extremity and to plan the anastomosis. Weiland reported a 79 per cent success rate in 33 patients with chronic osteomyelitis treated by free tissue transfer. The most common cause of failure was an inability to obtain adequate arterial flow into the transferred tissue despite normal-looking vessels on the pre-operative arteriogram.[54] Early flap coverage has been shown to be advantageous, as it provides a vascular envelope around the non-union site. This may aid in the progression to union.[1,5,9] There is also evidence, at least in acute open fractures, that early soft tissue coverage results in a lower incidence of infection, due to the ability of a well-vascularized wound to clear a larger inoculum of bacteria and prevent subsequent colonization.[9,15,30]

A new method, which we prefer for handling the soft tissue defect in Type 2 chronic infected non-unions, involves the use of bone transport and the allied technique of compression–distraction. This has decreased the need for free tissue transfer in our hands. Simultaneous transport of bone and the overlying soft tissues into the defect results in secondary wound closure without the need for surgery on remote sections of the body.

Skeletal Stabilization Methods

After the initial debridement has been completed, skeletal stabilization is required. The options are casting, plate fixation, intramedullary nailing, and external fixation.

Plaster casts can be used as an adjunct to compression plating, after removal of an external fixator, or as an isolated method of skeletal stabilization. Freeland described a 100 per cent union rate in 23 infected non-unions treated with posterior bone-grafting, long leg casting, and early weightbearing. The average time to union was 5.5 months.[16]

Compression plating of infected non-unions has been advocated, particularly in cases where there is adequate wound coverage.[22,26,43] Rosen evaluated 24 cases, and recorded an 83 per cent union rate. Of the 16 cases without drainage pre-operatively, 7 developed drainage post-operatively, and 6 out of 8 cases that were draining pre-operatively persisted post-operatively. Persistent infection post-operatively was clearly a problem with this technique. The author emphasised union as the first goal, followed by control of the infection.[43]

Intramedullary (IM) nailing has been employed for infected non-unions of the femur and tibia. Klemm combined IM nailing with closed suction irrigation and intravenous antibiotics, followed by nail removal and re-reaming to remove potential endosteal sequestrum after healing. Fracture union was obtained in 89.5 per cent of femoral infected non-unions and in 62.5 per cent of tibial. Tibial infected non-unions initially treated by plate fixation had particularly poor results (0 per cent union); this was thought to be due to compromising both the periosteal and endosteal blood supply to the non-union site.[24] This author now uses external fixation for the treatment of chronic infected non-unions. Miller treated 19 stage IV infected tibial non-unions with reamed IM nailing followed by open wound management with occlusive saline dressings. Fracture union occurred in 18. He believed that reaming helped to reestablish the medullary blood supply to the non-union. His use of open wound management techniques was felt to be a potentially important difference from the technique described by Klemm.[32]

A drawback of internal fixation, whether it be compression plating or IM nailing, is the placement of a biomaterial within an infected bed of tissue. Gristina et al, and others, have demonstrated the adherence of bacteria to the surface of biomaterials via a glycocalyx enclosed biofilm. This biofilm acts as a protective barrier to host defences as well as to antimicrobial therapy. Furthermore, the biofilm makes accurate microbiological sampling difficult, leading to an underestimation of the number of polymicrobial infections, which potentially prevents adequate antimicrobial therapy.[21] The use of internal implants for infected non-union will therefore inevitably lead to a significant rate of persistent infection and we do not advocate it.

External fixation is the most popular method of skeletal stabilization in infected non-unions and has several advantages over internal fixation. These include minimal soft tissue stripping and devascularization of the bone, and the lack of biomaterials within an infected wound. External fixators do not require another surgical procedure for removal.

The Orthofix system in particular has the additional advantage of easy frame dynamization. Using this monolateral external fixation system for the treatment of chronic infected non-union, Marsh et al reported an 87 per cent union rate with 87 per cent free from infection.[29]

The Orthofix Limb Reconstruction System (LRS) offers additional possibilities for osseous and soft tissue reconstruction which are used in the treatment of Type 2 infected non-unions. This system consists of a monolateral external fixation frame with clamps which slide along a rail. The skeletal defect is reconstructed by bone transport or compression–distraction (Fig. 51.3). Bone transport involves the production of an osteotomy at a site proximal or distal to the segmental defect, creating a free fragment which, along with the overlying soft tissues, is transported into the defect, gradually closing it. Once contact occurs, union is stimulated by autogenous cancellous bone grafting and/or compression across the contact site. Compression–distraction (sometimes referred to as shortening–lengthening in this context) acutely shortens the limb to close the segmental osseous and soft tissue defect. (See Ch. 52.) A remote osteotomy and distraction is then used to regain limb length.

Marsh et al employed bone transport and compression–distraction in the treatment of chronic infected non-unions. When compared to conventional treatment (external fixation, bone grafting, and soft tissue covering), the transport group had better resolution of limb length discrepancy. There was no difference in union rate, eradication of infection, treatment length, or incidence of complications.[29] However, extensive bone grafting or free tissue transfers were not required, and limb lengths were accurately restored.

Methods To Stimulate Osseous Repair

Hypertrophic infected non-unions without a segmental defect (i.e. Type 1 chronic infected non-unions) may only require skeletal stabilization. This has been

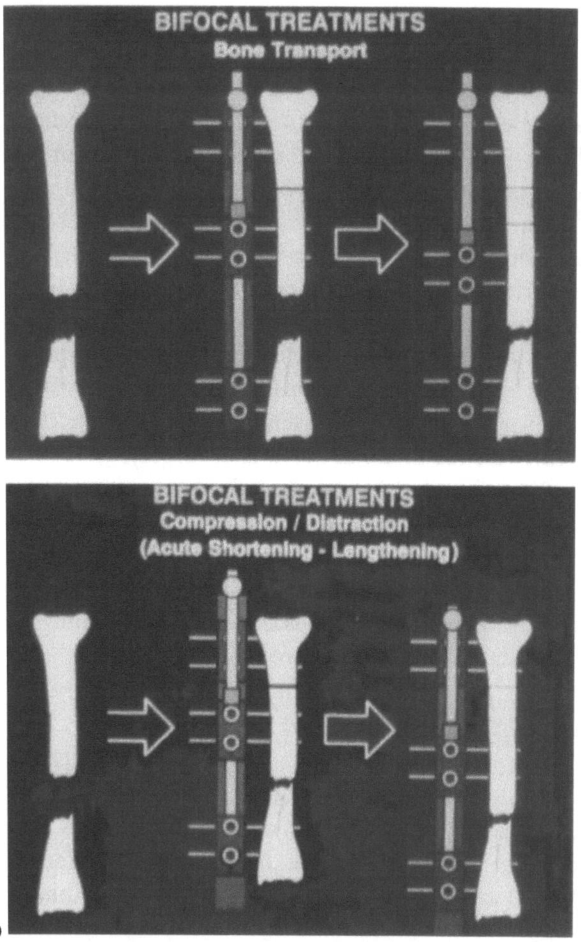

a

b

Fig. 51.3 The two Bifocal Treatment Strategies utilizing the Limb Reconstruction System. **a** Bone transport. **b** Compression–distraction (shortening–lengthening).

successful in selected cases employing IM nailing, compression plating, and external fixation.[24,29,34]

Atrophic non-union and cases with a segmental defect (Type 2) require osseous reconstruction. The simplest method is an open or Papineau cancellous bone grafting. This requires good vascularity to be successful. The bony bed is treated with whirlpool baths and wet-to-dry dressings until pink granulation tissue forms. The wound is then superficially redebrided and filled with cancellous ribbons. Once the graft is covered with granulation tissue (crowned), skin coverage can be obtained through marginal healing or split thickness grafting. If the defect is large, it may require filling in several layers. The graft is incorporated and heals via creeping substitution.[8] One shortcoming is the fact that the skin coverage is tenuous and may suffer recurrent ulceration. As a result, we prefer soft tissue coverage rather than this open bone graft technique.

Posterolateral bone grafting of infected tibial non-unions has been employed successfully and has the advantage of not requiring direct reconstruction of the infected non-union site, even in cases of segmental defect. Through a posterolateral approach, the interosseous membrane is exposed between 5 and 8cm above and below the fracture site. Corticocancellous bone graft is laid along the posterior aspect of the interosseous membrane between the tibia and the fibula above and below the fracture. Post-operative immobilization is with a long leg cast. Freeland reported union in all 23 cases and cessation of drainage in 21 of the 23.[16] Others have reported similar results in cases of non-infected non-union.[40,42] The complications associated with this procedure include persistent angular deformity, shortening, and the risk of neurovascular injury at the time of surgery.

Transfer of the ipsilateral fibula on a peroneal vascular pedicle has been described as a means of osseous reconstruction.[6,31] This method requires an intact ipsilateral fibula and cannot be used in cases where the peroneal vessel is the only artery supplying the distal limb. The fibula responds to weightbearing by hypertrophy. Until union is achieved, however, the limb is somewhat destabilized by this procedure.

The transfer of free vascularized fibular grafts can reconstruct large osseous defects without the shortcomings noted above. An osteomyocutaneous flap can be obtained if there is a soft tissue defect. Vascularized grafting, due to its intrinsic blood supply, results in earlier establishment of bony union and, at least theoretically, greater resistance to infection compared to free or cancellous bone. Yajima reported survival in 30 of 33 free vacularized fibular transfers for cases of infected non-union. Recurrence of infection was noted in four, three of which responded to saucerization.[56] Free vascularized transfers have been described using the ilium, scapula, and rib as donor material.[49,51]

Distraction osteogenesis (see Skeletal Stabilization Methods) offers a technique for osseous repair performed on the same limb without extensive bone grafting. Good results have been reported with both ring and monolateral fixators.[4,11,19,36,37] The technique using the LRS has become the preferred technique for the treatment of Type 2 chronic infected non-unions in our hands. The only disadvantage of these techniques is the long treatment time, requiring prolonged periods of external fixation.

Future directions in the area of osseous reconstruction for infected non-unions may involve the use of recombinant proteins. Recombinant human bone morphogenetic protein (rhBMP-2) has been shown to induce bone and cartilage formation in an orthotopic site in rats.[57] Recombinant human osteogenic protein-1 has been demonstrated to elicit healing of large segmental bone defects in primates.[10] This research holds promise and may augment or circumvent the methods primarily used today.

Limb Salvage Versus Amputation

For many chronic infected non-unions, amputation should be considered as an alternative to limb reconstruction. Unfortunately, there is little information available to guide the clinician in deciding which patient would be best served by amputation. In addition, there are few studies to evaluate the quality of life in patients treated with limb salvage compared to those treated with amputation for infected non-union. Lerner et al did a quality-of-life comparison between patients with post-traumatic non-union, lower extremity amputation, and chronic refractory osteomyelitis. Using the Arthritis Impact Measurement Scale (AIMS) and the Psychosocial Adjustment to Illness Scale (PAIS), they found that the presence of pain had a significantly negative effect on outcomes in patients with non-union and osteomyelitis. This study demonstrated poorer functional and psychological results in patients with chronic osteomyelitis than in those with non-union or amputation. The study did not, however, compare patients with successful reconstruction to those treated with amputation.[25]

Georgiadis has compared limb salvage with amputation for acute open tibial fractures with soft tissue loss. Patients with successful limb salvage were noted to have more complications, necessitating more operations and a longer hospital stay than those treated with amputation. Hospital cost for limb salvage was approximately double that for the amputation patients. Quality-of-life evaluation was similar between the two groups, but a larger percentage of those who underwent limb salvage considered themselves severely disabled, and significantly fewer were working.[17]

For each individual patient with chronic infected non-union, it is important to weigh the risks and benefits of limb salvage versus amputation. Some investigators have noted that 10–15 per cent of their patients (Cierny stage IVC) were functionally better served by an amputation.[8] Whether this is the appropriate percentage is unknown, and depends on the patient profile being treated. It is a challenge for the future to determine which patients would be best served by amputation, and to determine guidelines that will work to the patient's benefit.

Authors' Preferred Method

For chronic infected non-union, we use external fixation exclusively for skeletal stabilization. In the vast majority of cases, this has been monolateral external fixation, although there are indications for tensioned wire fixation. We classify infected non-unions into two broad categories, which is somewhat artificial since infected non-unions exist on a spectrum. The two categories do, however, have differences in aetiology, microbiology, radiographic appearance and, as will be discussed here, management. This has therefore been a useful distinction.

Type 1

These non-unions usually have a history of infection or were previously open fractures. On examination, however, there is usually little evidence of active infection. The soft tissue envelope is sealed or there is minimal evidence of drainage. On clinical examination, these non-unions are frequently stiff, and plain radiographs show a hypertrophic appearance. There is not usually any hardware in place, since these non-unions are most commonly the result of failed external fixation or failed conservative treatment.

Microbiologically, these are monomicrobial infections, primarily with gram positive organisms, often coagulase negative Staphylococcus. A high index of clinical suspicion based on a history of previous infection or severe open fracture will suggest a diagnosis of infected non-union in these cases. Sequential Tc-99m-MDP/In-111 scanning will often confirm the diagnosis of occult infection. This investigation is especially helpful in those cases otherwise well suited for intramedullary nailing; that is, diaphyseal fractures that are well aligned. If the indium scan is positive, we would not stabilize the non-union with an intramedullary nail, but would choose external fixation instead.

Surgical management of Type 1 infected non-unions begins with open biopsy and debridement. Debridement is often limited to clearly dead and infected bone. A skeletal defect is not created. Old external fixation screw sites that show evidence of infection are over-drilled. Pre-operative investigation with plain films, tomograms, or CT scans will direct the surgeon to suspicious areas for sequestration. The soft tissues are amenable to primary closure over the non-union site.

Stabilization is by monolateral external fixation. Ring fixation with tensioned wires would be used only for periarticular non-unions where it was considered that this method of fixation would be better than monolateral screws. Axis correction is critical for optimal results, as well as for stimulating repair. For this reason, a device such as the Orthofix Monolateral Fixator, which permits intra-operative adjustment of alignment, is preferred. Accurate correction of the limb axis is facilitated by the use of fluoroscopy, and if the opposite leg is placed in the lithotomy position, this facilitates biplanar radiographs of the affected limb. The Orthofix Limb Alignment Grid[44] aids in fluoroscopic assessment and adjustment of limb alignment. In the case of the tibia, fibular osteotomy, and in some cases, a limited osteoclasis is necessary to obtain alignment. In general, we prefer immediate correction with one of these techniques, rather than gradual correction with hinged fixators.

At the present time, it is uncertain which mechanical forces will optimally stimulate repair when applied to a non-union. Type 1 infected non-unions have traditionally been treated with compression. It is now clear, however, that in certain situations, distraction is an excellent stimulus for osteogenesis. We currently choose that mechanical force which will best stabilize the non-union site. In many cases this will be compression, but non-unions with an oblique shear plane and shortening are best stabilized in slight distraction.

Post-operatively, organism-specific intravenous antibiotics are administered until the wounds are healed. We recommend a short course (7–10 days) of intravenous antibiotics followed by appropriate oral antibiotics to complete a 4–6 week course. The fixator is locked either in distraction or compression, according to that originally chosen. Progressive forces are not used. At 4–6 weeks, the fixator is dynamized and loading increased progressively to full weightbearing. The fixator is removed when the non-union is fully healed.

Using these techniques, the surgeon should expect satisfactory results, with union and resolution of infection in the majority of cases of Type 1 infected non-union. In our hands, the healing rate has been around 90 per cent. Fig. 51.4 demonstrates the work-up and treatment of a Type 1 non-union using these techniques.

Type 2

In these non-unions, the diagnosis of infection by history, examination, and plain radiographs is obvious. There is a history of chronic drainage, often associated with failure of soft tissue coverage and exposed bone. Examination confirms active infection, drainage, and cellulitis indicating diffuse soft tissue involvement. Radiographs typically have an atrophic appearance with sequestered bone and involucrum present at and near the non-union site. Failed plate fixation, failure of soft tissue coverage, or severe infection after intramedullary nailing will give this clinical picture. These non-unions frequently have polymicrobial infections, most often involving gram negative organisms.

The surgeon and the patient must make a decision between limb salvage and amputation. In each case, multiple factors must be considered. These include patient-related factors such as age, associated medical problems, smoking history, occupation, expectations, psychological profile, and duration of the infected non-union. Local factors in the limb to be considered include the condition of the distal part of the extremity, sensation on the bottom of the foot, vascularity, extent of bone involvement, and type of infecting organisms.

If a decision is made to salvage the limb, extensive debridement of bone and soft tissues is required as the first step. This will usually create a soft tissue and skeletal defect. Multiple cultures should be obtained to identify all micro-organisms involved. In contrast to Type 1 infected non-unions, the debridement for Type 2 should be aggressive. If there is any suggestion of infection or avascularity, the suspected area, be it bone or soft tissue, should be excised. Motorized instruments can assist with bony debridement. The criteria for adequate debridement that we have used is healthy, bleeding bone and soft tissues. This debridement is done as an initial staging procedure. Post-operatively, organism-specific intravenous antibiotics are given for six weeks. If the soft tissue defect is amenable to suture closure, this is done over tobramycin polymethylmethacrylate antibiotic bead chains. This debridement in conjunction with subsequent antibiotics should be planned to cure the infectious process.

In most cases, after debridement there will be a segmental defect in the bone, and a large soft tissue wound, both of which require reconstruction. Conventional treatment has been to reconstruct the soft tissue defect by muscle transfer. This frequently requires free tissue transfer using, for instance, the latissimus dorsi muscle. This is followed by bone grafting for the osseous defect. In recent years, we have preferred to use a combined strategy where the soft tissues and bone are reconstructed simultaneously without free tissue transfer or extensive grafting. This requires the use of bone transport techniques.

The limb is stabilized with the LRS, a monolateral rail with multiple sliding pin clamps. The defect is stabilized by two of these pin clusters. A low energy osteotomy is then created at a different level with a third pin cluster stabilizing across this osteotomy. A section of bone and overlying soft tissues is then gradually transferred into the defect beginning 7–10 days after creation of the osteotomy, at a rate of 1mm per day. Until closure, the wound is managed with routine open wound management techniques with once or twice daily dressing changes. Since bone is not exposed, there is no drying or desiccation, and the open bed rapidly granulates. With this technique, the majority of the reconstruction is performed on the injured limb segment without extensive grafting or tissue transfers from other body parts. Fig. 51.5 demonstrates the use of open wound techniques to treat a Type 2 infected non-union of the femur.

In acute injuries, the healing process is expedited by partial or complete closure of the bony defect immediately, followed by limb lengthening at the remote osteotomy site. This compression–distraction (shortening–lengthening) technique is less applicable to chronic infected non-unions because the chronic nature of the problem leads to stiffening of the surrounding soft tissues. In addition, an intact fibula should not be sacrificed solely to obtain limb shortening. The fibula provides valuable stability to the limb and, in addition, might be required later for grafting or reconstruction. Nevertheless, we advocate as much primary closure of the defect as is easily obtainable.

When contact between the transported segment and the segment on the other side of the defect is achieved, a routine procedure to stimulate union at the docking site is recommended. Our preference has been limited decortication through a small incision and

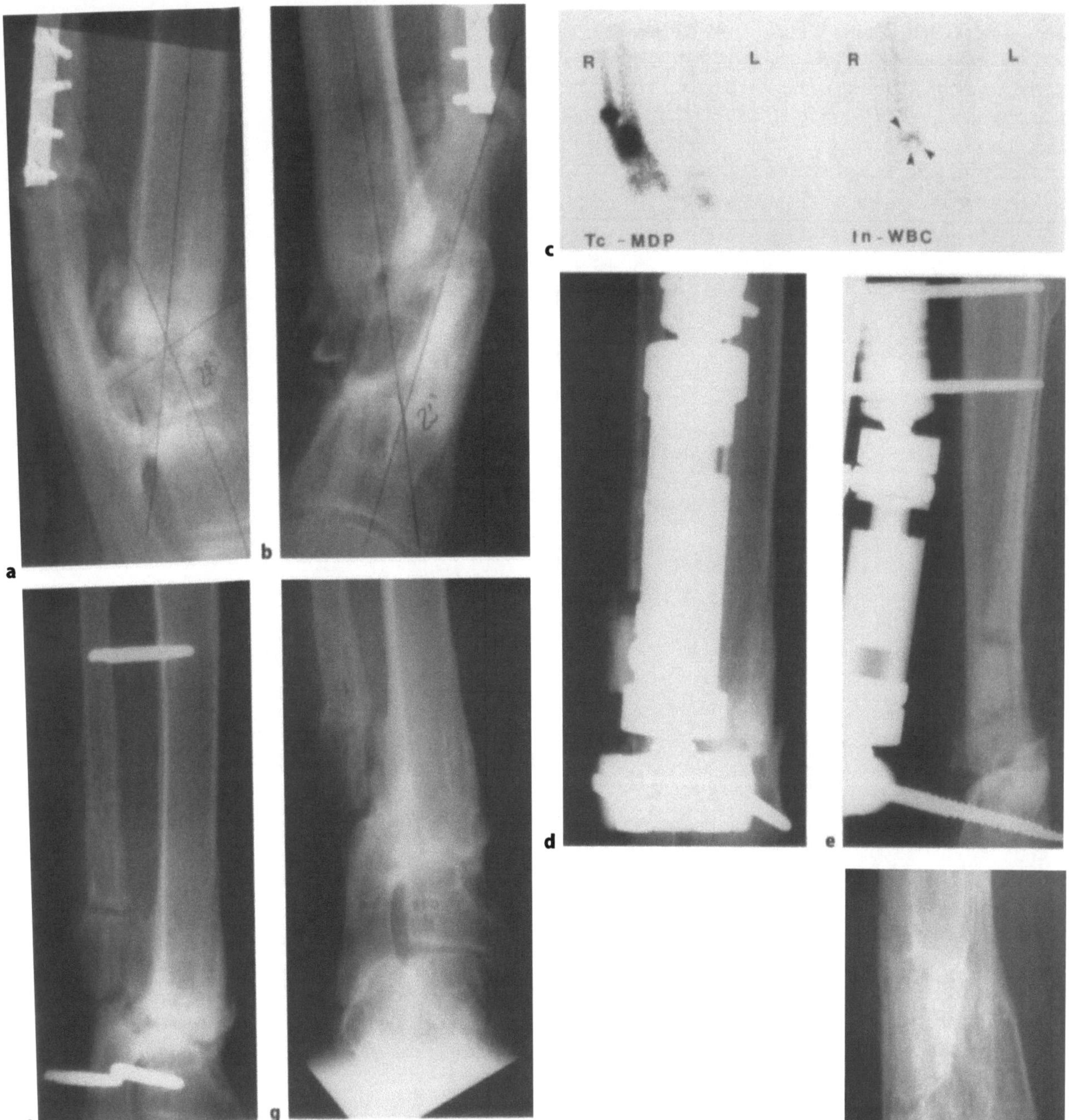

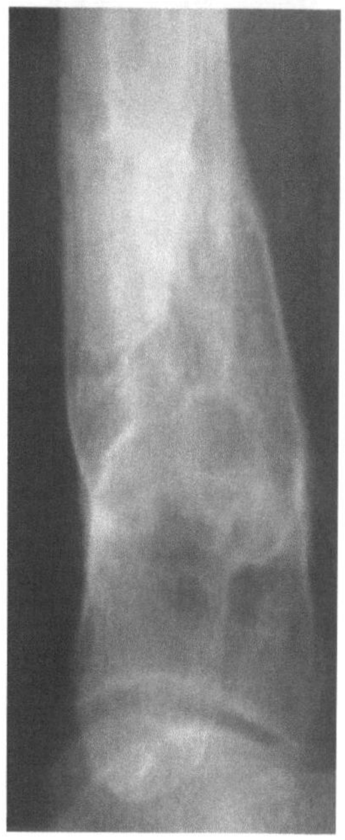

Fig. 51.4 **a** Anteroposterior; **b** Lateral radiographs of a 60-year-old female after failed closed treatment and a secondary failed plating for a distal third tibia and fibula fracture, show a hypertrophic angulated non-union. The plating was complicated by wound breakdown and infection, necessitating plate removal and prolonged antibiotic therapy. At the time of presentation she had been off antibiotics for three months, had pain on ambulation and increasing varus deformity and had a 1×1cm medial ulcer with minimal drainage. Because of the low grade clinical appearance and hypertrophic radiograph, this was classified as a Type 1 infected non-union. **c** Her Tc-99m-MDP/In-111-WBC Scan demonstrates white cell uptake at the fracture site (arrows). **d** Anteroposterior and **e** lateral radiographs demonstrate the alignment after limited debridement, tibial osteoclasis and realignment, and fibular osteotomy. Cultures grew *S. aureus*, for which she received six weeks of intravenous antibiotics. A small anterolateral iliac crest bone graft was applied at the non-union site. Currently we would not choose to bone graft this Type 1 non-union. **f** An anteroposterior radiograph taken six months later at the time of fixator removal shows healing. **g** Anteroposterior and **h** lateral radiographs 18 months after beginning treatment, show sound union and maintained alignment. There was no clinical evidence of infection.

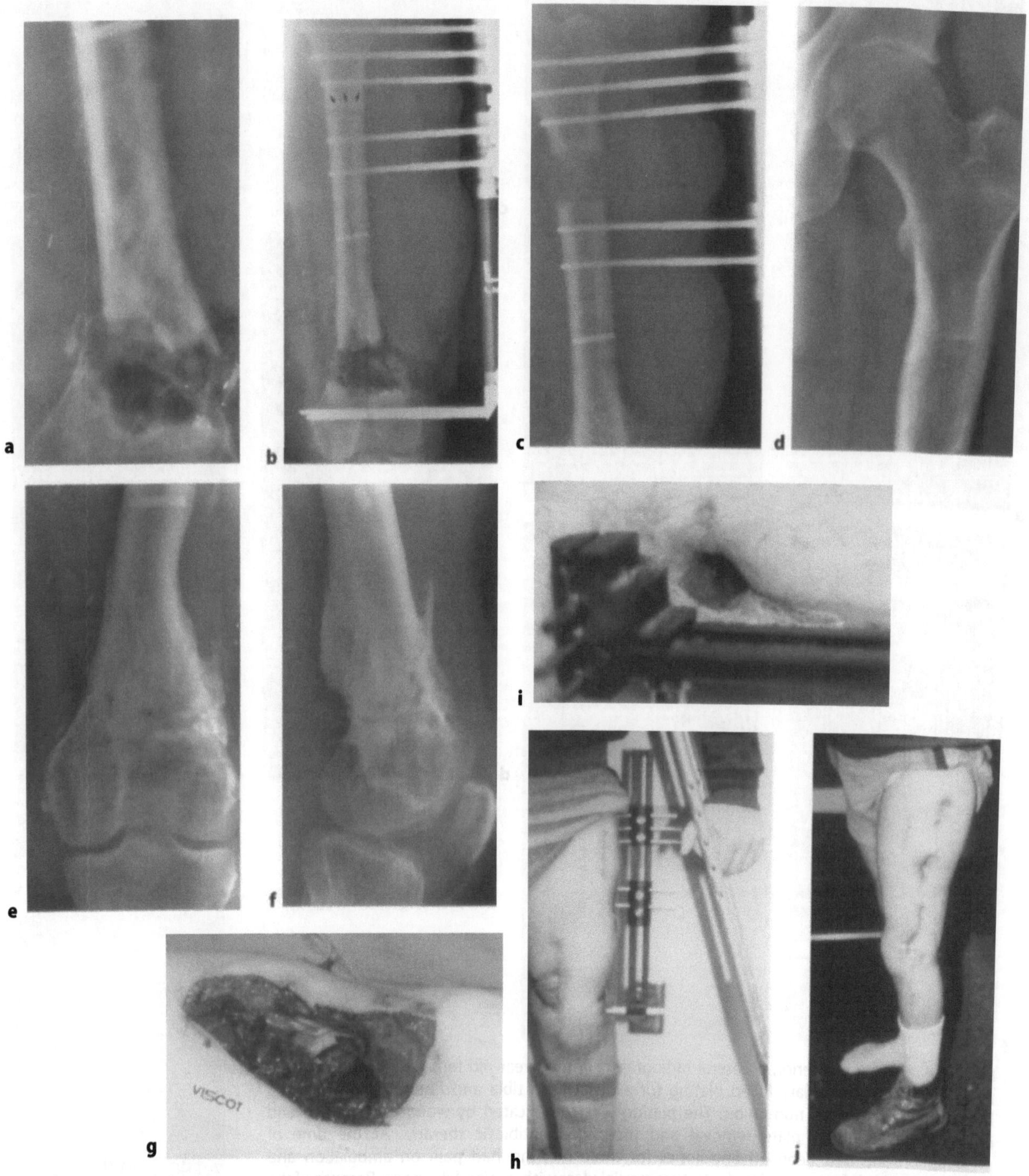

Fig. 51.5 **a** An anteroposterior radiograph of a 20-year-old male, 6 months after a high velocity gunshot wound of the distal femur, demonstrating a partial defect with residual dead bone. He had lateral purulent drainage. This infected non-union was classified as Type 2. After debridement there was a 5cm segmental defect. Cultures were positive for *S. aureus*. **b** Anteroposterior radiograph taken after application of the LRS, and a subtrochanteric osteotomy (arrows). His wound was packed open and he received two weeks of intravenous antibiotics. **c** Three months later there was radiographic contact, early healing of the defect and maturing proximal distraction osteogenesis. His wound was healed. A small lateral bone graft from the iliac crest had been applied at the contact site one month previously. **d** Two years later, a radiograph of the area of distraction osteogenesis showed nearly complete remodelling. The distal femur was solidly healed on both **e** anteroposterior and **f** lateral radiographs. **g** Demonstrates the appearance of the wound during the original debridement. The wound gradually closed during bone transport. **h, i** Two months after beginning treatment, the lateral wound was almost closed. **j** At the conclusion of treatment three months after frame removal, all wounds were healed.

cancellous grafting at this site. This stimulates repair, and speeds union at this critical level.

As is the case with Type 1 infected non-unions, the indications for tensioned wire fixators or hybrid fixators include small periarticular segments which require stabilization. In addition, these complex non-unions are often associated with cross-ankle equinus contractures, and simultaneous stabilization and correction of the foot deformity is possible with more complex ring fixators (see Ch. 49). When the defect is in the distal femur and the knee is stiff, the forces on the distal femoral site may be such that stabilization is required across the knee, and we have preferred to do this with ring fixation systems.

As for Type 1 infected non-unions, the fixator should be left in situ until the limb is fully healed. We have assessed this on serial radiographs, looking for bridging callus at the docking site, and restoration of cortical integrity on three out of four biplanar views at the distraction site. Recently, the Orthofix Orthometer has become available enabling serial monitoring of the bending stiffness of a limb. Fixator removal is considered to be safe when a stiffness of 15 Newton meters has been achieved in the tibia.[41] We have had no experience with the use of this device.

One of the problems with these treatment methods for Type 2 chronic infected non-unions is the long treatment time. Patients should be counselled preoperatively regarding the length of treatment required to reconstruct the limb, as unexpectedly long periods of external fixation can lead to patient dissatisfaction if inadequate information has been given. One of the causes of failure in our hands has been premature removal of the fixator. Currently available methods to speed treatment are two-level corticotomies for longer defects (see Ch. 50) and early grafting at the docking site to speed healing at this level. While transport over nails has been reported, we have not considered it applicable to the chronic infected non-unions in our practice. Methods which may be available in the future to speed both the distraction and the healing rate include stimulation by pulsed electromagnetic fields, ultrasound, and the use of newer osteoinductive agents to hasten osseous repair.

References

1. Byrd HS, Spicer TE, Cierney G III: 'Management of open tibial fractures.' *Plast and Reconstr Surg* 1985; 76: 719–28.
2. Calhoun JH, Henry SL, Anger DM, Cobos JA, Mader JT: 'The treatment of infected non-unions with Gentamicin-Polymethylmethacrylate antibiotic beads.' *Clin Orthop* 1993; 295: 23–7.
3. Calhoun JH, Mader JT: 'Antibiotic beads in the management of surgical infections.' *Am J Surg* 1989; 157: 443–49.
4. Cattaneo R, Catagni M, Johnson EE: 'The Treatment of Infected Non-unions and Segmental Defects of the Tibia by the Methods of Ilizarov.' *Clin Orthop* 1992; 280: 143–52.
5. Caudle RJ, Stern PJ: 'Severe open fractures of the tibia.' *J Bone Joint Surg* [Am] 1987; 69-A: 801–7.
6. Chacha PB, Ahmed M, Daruwalla JS: 'Vascular pedicle graft of the ipsilateral fibula for non-union of the tibia with a large defect.' *J Bone Joint Surg* [Br] 1981; 63-B: 244–53.
7. Christian EP, Bosse MJ, Robb G: 'Reconstruction of large diaphyseal defects, without free fibular transfer, in Grade-IIIB tibial fractures.' *J Bone Joint Surg* [Am] 1989; 71-A: 994–1004.
8. Cierny G III: 'Classification and treatment of adult osteomyelitis' in: *Surgery of the Musculoskeletal System* 1990, Churchill Livingstone Inc., pp.4337–79.
9. Cierny G III, Byrd S., Jones RE: 'Primary versus delayed soft tissue coverage for severe open tibial fractures: A comparison of results.' *Clin Orthop* 1983; 178: 54–62.
10. Cook SD, Wolfe MW, Salkeld SL, Rueger DC:'Effect of recombinant human osteogenic protein-1 on healing of segmental defects in non-human primates.' *J Bone Joint Surg* [Am] 1995; 77-A: 734–50.
11. Dendrinos GK, Kontos S, Lyritsis E: 'Use of the Ilizarov Technique for Treatment of Non-Union of the Tibia Associated with Infection.' *J Bone Joint Surg* [Am] 1995; 77-A: 835–46.
12. Dietz FR, Koontz FP, Found EM, Marsh JL: 'The importance of positive bacterial cultures of specimens obtained during clean orthopaedic operation.' *J Bone Joint Surg* [Am] 1991; 73-A: 1200–6.
13. Esterhai J, Alava A, Mandell GA, Brown J: 'Sequential technietium-99m/galluim-67 scintigraphic evaluation of subclinical osteomyelitis complication fracture non-union.' *J Orthop Res* 1985; 3: 219–25.
14. Esterhai JL, Brighton CT, Heppenstall RB, Alavi A, Mandell GA: 'Detection of synovial pseudarthrosis by 99mTc scintigraphy: Application of treatment of traumatic non-union with constant direct current.' *Clin Orthop* 1981; 161: 15–23.
15. Fischer MD, Gustilo RB, Varecka TF: 'The timing of flap coverage, bone grafting, and intramedullary nailing in patients who have a fracture of the tibial shaft with extensive soft tissue injury.' *J Bone Joint Surg* [Am] 1991; 73-A: 1316–22.
16. Freeland AE, Mutz SB: 'Posterior bone-grafting for infected ununited fracture of the tibia.' *J Bone Joint Surg* [Am] 1976; 58-A: 653–6.
17. Geordiadis GM, Behrens FF, Joyce MJ, Earle AS, Simmons AL: 'Open tibial fractures with severe soft-tissue loss: Limb salvage compared with below-the-knee amputation.' *J Bone Joint Surg* [Am] 1993; 75-A: 1431–40.
18. Gordon L, Chiu EJ: 'Treatment of infected non-unions and segmental defects of the tibia with staged microvascular muscle transplantation and bone grafting.' *J Bone Joint Surg* [Am] 1998; 70-A: 377–86.
19. Green SA: 'The Ilizarov method.' *Orthop Clin N America* 1991; 22: 677–87.
20. Green SA, Dlabal TA: 'The open bone graft for septic non-union.' *Clin Orthop* 1983; 180: 117.
21. Gristina AG, Costerton JW: 'Bacterial adherence to biomaterials and tissue.' *J Bone Joint Surg* [Am] 1985; 67-A: 264–73.
22. Gustilo RB: 'Management of Infected Non-union' in: *Orthopaedic Infection – Diagnosis and Treatment.* 1989 by WB Saunders Co., pp.139–54.
23. Klemm KW: 'Antibiotic bead chains.' *Clin Orthop* 1993; 295: 63–76.
24. Klemm KW: 'Treatment of infected pseudarthrosis of the femur and tibia with an interlocking nail.' *Clin Orthop* 1993; 295: 63–76.
25. Lerner RK, Esterhai JL Jr., Polomano RC, Cheatle MD, Heppenstall RB: 'Quality of life assessment of patients with posttraumatic fracture non-union, chronic refractory

osteomyelitis, and lower-extremity amputation.' *Clin Orthop* 1993; 295: 28–36.
26. Lifeso RM, Al-Saati F: 'The treatment of infected and uninfected non-union.' *J Bone Joint Surg* [Br] 1984; 66-B: 573–9.
27. Mackowiak PA, Jones SR, Smith JW: 'Diagnostic value of sinus-tract cultures in chronic osteomyelitis.' *JAMA* 1978; 239: 2772–5.
28. Mader JT, Cantrell JS, Calhoun J: 'Oral Ciprofloxacin compared with standard parenteral antibiotic therapy for chronic osteomyelitis in adults.' *J Bone Joint Surg* [Am] 1990; 72-A: 104–10.
29. Marsh JL, Prokuski L, Biermann JS: 'Chronic infected tibial non-unions with bone loss: Conventional techniques versus bone transport.' *Clin Orthop* 1994; 301: 139–46.
30. Mathes SJ, Alpert BS, Chang N: 'Use of the muscle flap in chronic osteomyelitis: Experimental and clinical correlation.' *Plast and Reconstr Surg* 1982; 69: 815–28.
31. May JW, Jr., Jupiter JB, Weiland AJ, Byrd HS: 'Current concepts review: Clinical classification of post-traumatic tibial osteomyelitis.' *J Bone Joint Surg* [Am] 1989; 71-A: 1422–28.
32. Miller ME, Ada JR, Webb LX: 'Treatment of infected non-union and delayed union of tibia fractures with locking intramedullary nails.' *Clin Orthop* 1989; 245: 234-8.
33. Moore RD, Lietman PS, Smith CR: 'Clinical response to aminoglycoside therapy: Importance of the ratio of peak concentration to minimal inhibitory concentration.' *Journal of Infectious Disease* 1987; 155: 93–9.
34. Muller ME, Thomas RJ: 'Treatment of non-union in fractures of long bones.' *Clin Orthop* 1979; 138: 141–53.
35. Nepola JV, Seabold JE, Marsh JL, Kirchner PT, El-Khoury G: 'Diagnosis of infection in ununited fractures.' *J Bone Joint Surg* [Am] 1993; 75-A: 1816–21.
36. Paley D: 'Current techniques of limb lengthening.' *J Pediatric Orthop* 1988; 8: 73–92.
37. Paley D, Catagni MA, Argnani F, Villa A, Benedetti GB, Cattaneo R: 'Ilizarov treatment of tibial non-unions with bone loss.' *Clin Orthop* 1989; 241: 146–65.
38. Patzakis MJ, Wilkins J, Kumar J, Holtom P, Greenbaum B, Ressler R: 'Comparison of the results of bacterial cultures from multiple sites in chronic osteomyelitis of long bones.' *J Bone Joint Surg* [Am] 1994; 76-A: 664–5.
39. Perry CR, Pearson RL, Miller GA: 'Accuracy of cultures of material from swabbing of the superficial aspect of the wound and needle biopsy in the preoperative assessment of osteomyelitis.' *J Bone Joint Surg* [Am] 1991; 73-A: 745–8.
40. Reckling FW, Waters CH III: 'Treatment of non-unions of fractures of the tibial diaphysis by posterolateral cortical cancellous bone-grafting.' *J Bone Joint Surg* [Am] 1980; 62-A: 936–41.
41. Richardson JB, Cunningham JL, Goodship AE, O'Connor BT, Kenwright J: 'Measuring stiffness can define healing of tibia fractures.' *J Bone Joint Surg* [Br] 1994; 76-B: 389–94.
42. Rijnberg WJ, vanLinge B: 'Central grafting for persistent non-union of the tibia: A lateral approach to the tibia, creating a central compartment.' *J Bone Joint Surg* [Br] 1993; 75-B: 926–31.
43. Rosen H: 'Compression treatment of long bone pseudarthroses.' *Clin Orthop* 1979; 138: 154–66.
44. Saleh M, Harriman P, Edwards DJ: 'A radiological method for producing precise limb alignment.' *J Bone Joint Surg* [Br] 1991; 73-B: 515–6.
45. Schauwecker DS, Park HM, Mock BH, et al: 'Evaluation of complicating osteomyelitis with Tc-99m MDP, In-111 granulocytes, and Ga-67 citrate.' *J Nucl Med* 1984; 25: 849–53.
46. Seabold JE, Ferlic RJ, Marsh JL, Nepola JV: 'Periarticular bone sites associated with traumatic injury: False-positive findings with In-111-labelled white blood cells and Tc-99m MDP scintigraphy.' *Radiology* 1993; 186: 845–49.
47. Seabold JE, Nepola JV, Conrad GR, Marsh JL, Montgomery WJ, Bricker JA, Kirchner PT: 'Detection of osteomyelitis at fracture non-union sites: Comparison of two scintigraphic methods.' *AJR* 1989; 152: 1021–7.
48. Swiontkowski MF: 'Criteria for bone debridement in massive lower limb trauma.' *Clin Orthop* 1989; 243: 41–7.
49. Taylor GI, Townsend P, Corlett R: 'Superiority of the deep circumflex iliac vessels as the supply for free groin flaps: Clinical work.' *Plast Reconstr Surg* 1979; 64: 745.
50. Tehranzadeh J, Wang M, Mesgarzadeh M: 'Magnetic resonance imaging of osteomyelitis.' *Clinical Reviews in Diagnostic Imaging* 1992; 33: 495–534.
51. Teot L, Bosse JP, Maufarrege R, Papillon J, Beauregard G: 'The scapular crest pedicled bone graft.' *Int J Microsurg* 1981; 3: 257.
52. Unger E, Moldofsky P, Gatenby R, Hartz W, Broder G: 'Diagnosis of osteomyelitis by MR imaging.' *AJR* 1988; 150: 605–10.
53. Wagner DK, Collier BD, Rytel MW: 'Long-term intravenous antibiotic therapy in chronic osteomyelitis.' *Arch Int Med* 1985; 145: 1073–8.
54. Weiland AJ, Moore JR, Daniel RK: 'The efficacy of free tissue transfer in the treatment of osteomyelitis.' *J Bone Joint Surg* [Am] 1984; 66–A: 181–93.
55. Weinstein MP, Stratton CW, Hawley HB, Ackley A, Reller LB: 'Multicenter collaborative evaluation of a standardized serum bactericidal test as a predictor of therapeutic efficacy in acute and chronic osteomyelitis.' *Am J Med* 1987; 83: 218–22.
56. Yajima H, Tamai S, Mizumoto S, Inada Y: 'Vascularized fibular grafts in the treatment of osteomyelitis and infected non-union.' *Clin Orthop* 1993; 293: 256–64.
57. Yasko AW, Lane JM, Fellinger EJ, Rosen V, Wozney JM, Wang EA: 'The healing of segmental bone defects, induced by recombinant human bone morphogenetic protein (rhBMP-2): A radiographic, histological, and biomechanical study in rats.' *J Bone Joint Surg* [Am] 1992; 74-A: 659–70.

Infected Non-Unions with Soft Tissue Loss: the Shortening–Lengthening Technique

52

G. Giebel

Bifocal procedures may be used to treat fractures associated with a major soft tissue defect and denuded bone, or delayed or non-unions with osteomyelitis and soft tissue necrosis. In such cases it is necessary to cover the bone rapidly with viable soft tissue or it will become necrotic after two or three days. This is accomplished by shortening the bone and subsequently lengthening it by callus distraction.

It is sometimes possible to cover the defect with locally imported musculo-cutaneous flaps, and in the distal third of the tibia particularly, the soft tissue defect can be covered with a free flap, usually derived from the latissimus dorsi. The disadvantages of such a technique are severalfold: the mutilation of a perfectly healthy, intact muscle from the back; a complex operative procedure, and a cosmetic result that will cause many patients to avoid public swimming pools or seaside holidays.

It was for this reason that we began, in 1987, to use the "shortening–lengthening technique" to cover these soft tissue defects with exposed bone (Giebel 1991). The first stage involves shortening the extremity by resection of a segment of bone within the defect such that the available soft tissues on either side of it can be brought together. When the defect has been covered in this way, subsequent corticotomy with callus distraction at a level distant from the lesion, restores the extremity to its former length (Fig. 52.1). In about 80 per cent of these cases, the shortening–lengthening technique as described below can be used. This technique can readily be performed using one Orthofix Limb Reconstruction System (LRS) or two Orthofix telescopic lengtheners at the same time.

Indications

This technique is indicated for soft tissue defects with denuded bone, which cannot be closed by the importation of local flaps and which require the resection of ideally, no more than five, or at maximum, seven centimetres of bone for soft tissue cover to be effected.

Technique

Initially, a relatively small segmental resection is performed to determine how much of the bone can be covered. This initial shortening is carried out in combination with a fasciocutaneous flap in order to limit the amount of shortening (Fig. 52.2).

If insufficient bone has been removed, an additional one or two centimetres are resected to shorten the extremity further, enabling the existing soft tissues, together with the fasciocutaneous flap, to cover the bone completely without tension. In open fractures the soft tissues are quite supple, and complete cover is usually achieved readily. In the presence of osteomyelitis, on the other hand, the soft tissues are very stiff, and it may not be possible to achieve the full amount of shortening required in a single operation. In these circumstances, therefore, the soft tissues should be gradually opposed at the bedside over the next two to three days, until the bone ends are in contact.

At the time of the first operation and segmental resection it usually possible to perform a corticotomy at a distant site where the condition of the overlying soft tissues is good. Lengthening at this site can then begin after a waiting period of six days. In a minority of

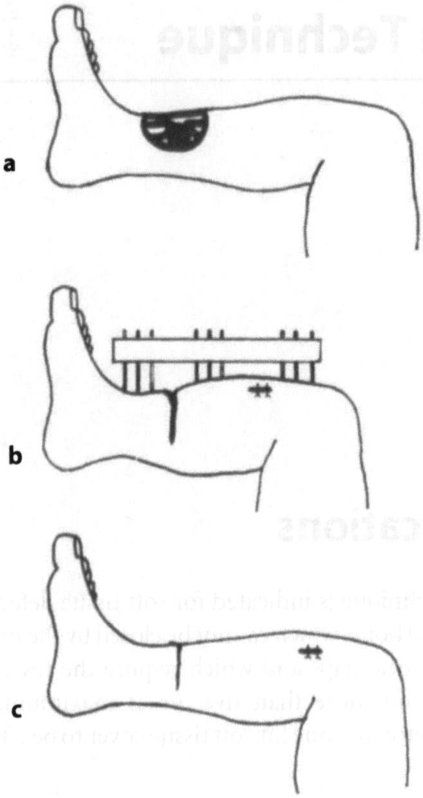

Fig. 52.1 The technique of shortening–lengthening to cover a soft tissue defect. **a** Open tibial fracture with soft tissue loss. **b** Shortening of the leg with segmental resection of bone. At the same operation proximal corticotomy is performed. Distraction will begin 6 days later. **c** The original length of the extremity is now restored through callus distraction.

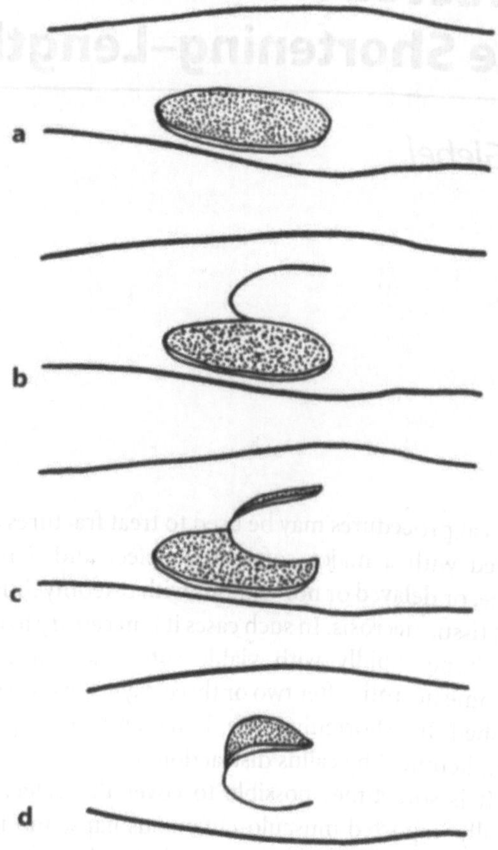

Fig. 52.2 The technique of shortening combined with a fasciocutaneous flap to cover a soft tissue defect with exposed bone. **a** The defect. **b** The incision. **c** Repositioning of the flap. **d** Shortening of the tibia now allows the defect to be covered.

cases only, it may be necessary to perform the corticotomy at a second operation. One such circumstance would be where the soft tissues over the region of sound bone have become infected or damaged for any reason.

The simplest way to perform a shortening–lengthening procedure is to use two separate fixators. In this way, fracture reduction, shortening and lengthening can be managed independently. In most cases it is better, however, to use one fixator with three clamps which can control the entire procedure (Fig. 52.3d). Where one fixator only is used, the technique can be performed as a one-stage or two-stage procedure. In the one-stage procedure, shortening and corticotomy are performed in a single operation (Fig. 52.3). In the two-stage procedure, these steps are carried out at separate operations (Fig. 52.4). The Orthofix Limb Reconstruction System (LRS) is a very useful device in this context. The two outer clamps stabilize the joint-bearing segments, while the middle clamp fixes the mobile central fragment.

Before the rail is applied it is particularly important to ensure good alignment. To achieve this, temporary use of an Orthofix paediatric fixator with small pins (e.g. 4.0/3.5 or 4.5/3.5mm) can be useful. Once reduction has been achieved, the LRS can be applied and after a waiting period of six days lengthening by callus distraction at the corticotomy site can begin.

In infected cases, debridement of the infected area is carried out during the first operation. The septic area is initially covered and the corticotomy performed under sterile conditions. Following this, the corticotomy incision is covered with sterile dressings and the septic wound exposed for debridement.

The corticotomy should be carried out with minimal exposure of the bone (Giebel 1987, Ilizarov 1992). Through a 1.5–2.0cm incision, the bone is divided using a chisel; Hohman retractors are not used. Callus distraction is performed with the Orthofix in the usual way (Aldegheri et al 1989, De Bastiani et al 1987). About 1cm of the fibula should be resected to avoid premature fusion of the bone ends.

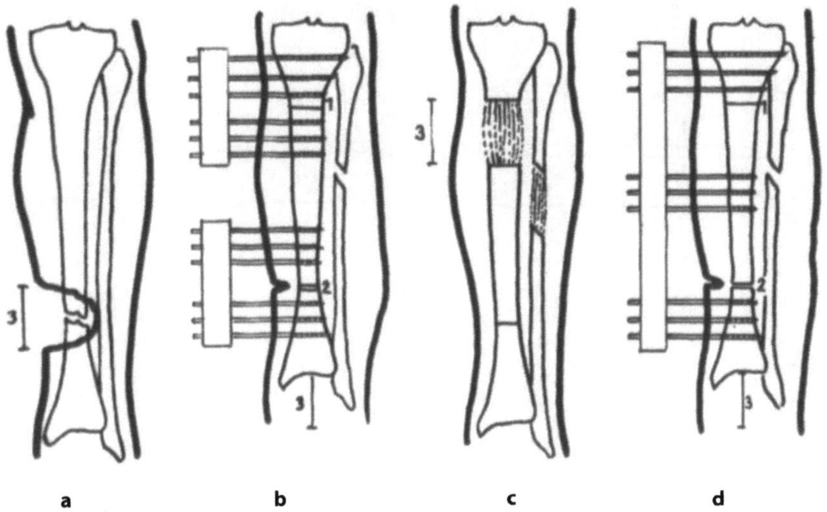

Fig. 52.3 Use of external fixation (Orthofix) for the shortening–lengthening technique (one-stage procedure). The one-stage procedure is used for an open fracture with a soft tissue defect and exposed bone in circumstances where the bone cannot be covered with a local flap. **a** Following the accident; major soft tissue defect with exposed bone. **b** Resection debridement (2) with shortening of the extremity at the site of the fracture until the available soft tissues can cover the defect. Corticotomy (1) and stabilization with external fixation at the same time. **c** The original length of the extremity is now restored through callus distraction. Distance 3 represents the extent of the shortening which is equivalent to the length regained by callus distraction. **d** The technique using a single lengthener (Limb Reconstruction System) with three clamps.

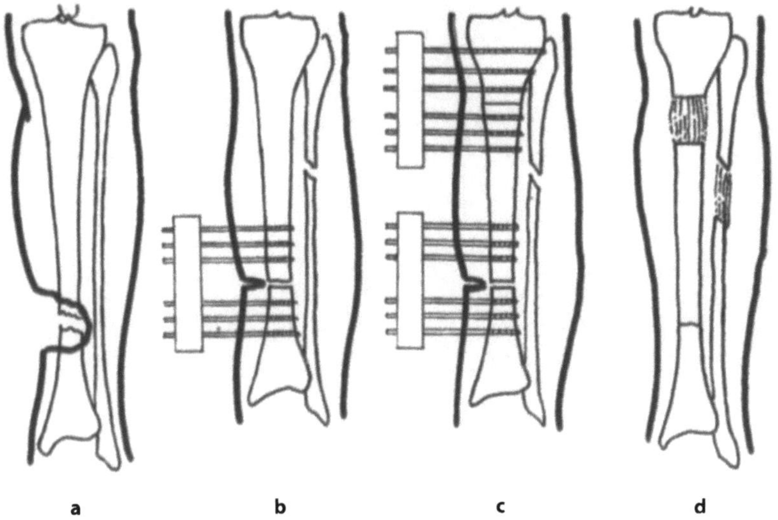

Fig. 52.4 The two-stage procedure using the same technique as that illustrated in Fig. 52.3. This would be employed where there is extensive soft tissue damage or where infection in the limb is widespread. **a** After the accident. **b** After resection, debridement and shortening, enabling closure of the soft tissue defect. **c** Corticotomy will follow at a second operation, when the condition of the soft tissues has improved. **d** Restoration of the original length by callus distration.

Post-Operative Management

Six days after the operation distraction is commenced at a rate of one millimetre per day. When the desired length has been reached, distraction is stopped and the neutralization period begins. X-rays are taken every two to four weeks during the distraction phase and every month during the neutralization period. The length of the leg can be monitored by measuring the extremity directly as well as on X-rays. This can be prove difficult where joint contractures are present. Physiotherapy is mandatory if pain is to be minimized and contractures avoided. Stretching exercises are most important, and are designed to lengthen both the muscles and the fascia. Fig. 52.5 is an illustrative case.

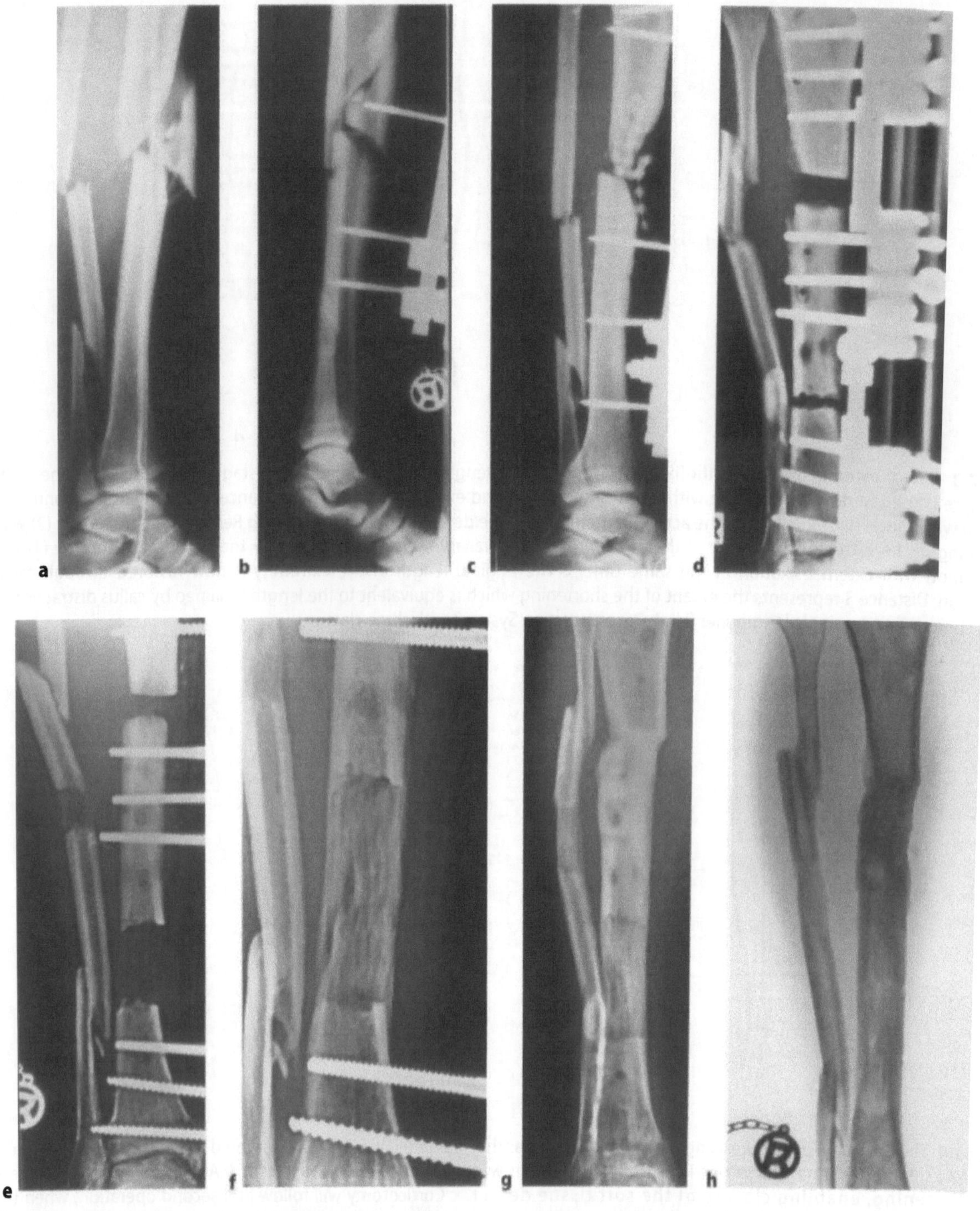

Fig.52.5 **a** After a motorcycle accident this 42-year-old man sustained a type III (Gustillo and Anderson) open fracture of the leg. **b** Atypical stabilization with an external fixator. **c** Pin track infection via the butterfly fragment screw was followed by acute osteitis and necrosis of this fragment, which was removed, and the defect filled with antibiotic beads. **d** Because of the soft tissue necrosis, segmental resection with shortening of the extremity was carried out to enable closure of the soft tissue defect; at the same operation distal corticotomy for segmental transport was performed; the proximal gap is the shortened area and the distal gap the corticotomy. **e** Increasing distraction of the corticotomy is visible. **f** Increasing callus formation in the gap with mineralization occurring. **g, h** Healing at the proximal docking side was achieved without the need for bone grafting.

Next page: **i** Clinical view showing soft tissue necrosis with an antibiotic chain over the anterior surface of the tibia. **j** This could not be covered with a muscle flap due to severe contusion of the triceps surae muscle. After resection-debridement with shortening of the extremity, closure of the soft tissue defect was possible. After this, the condition of the soft tissue improved considerably. Healing occured after the removal of the external fixator. **k, l** The leg regained its former length and the cosmetic result is better than would have been the case if local or free flaps had been used.

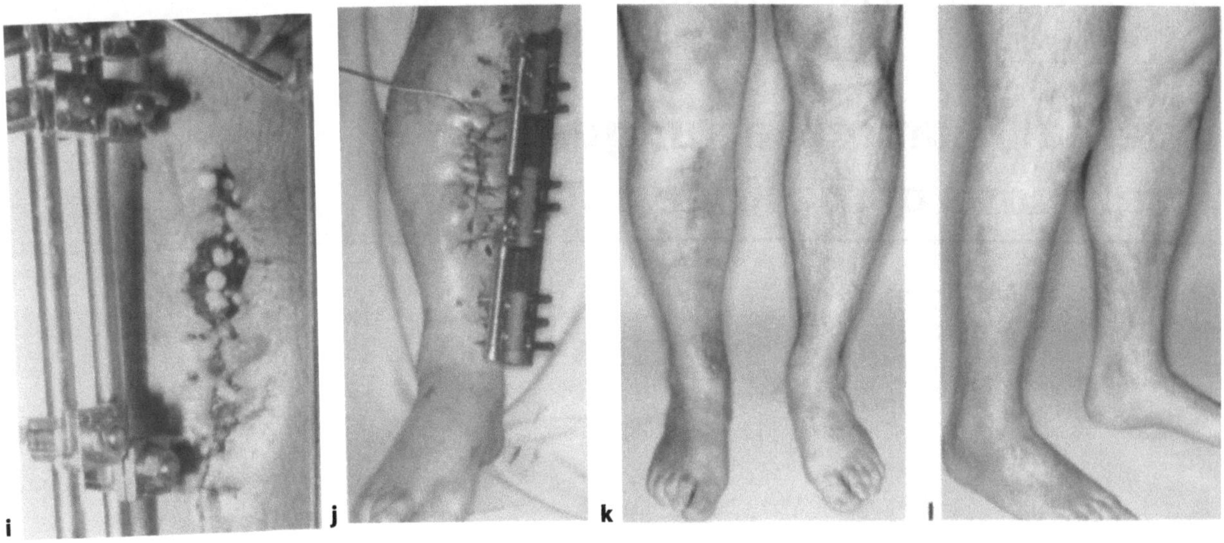
i j k l

Fig. 52.5 (continued)

Discussion

The shortening–lengthening technique is a safe procedure, and in comparison with free-flap procedures, is less demanding for both the patient and the surgeon. It is formulated on physiological principles, produces excellent cosmetic results, can be performed in virtually any hospital by a competent surgeon familiar with external fixation techniques, and does not demand special microsurgical training or knowledge. Using this technique we have been able to reduce the incidence of our free flap operations for covering denuded bone to 20 per cent of that prior to the introduction of the procedure.

The incidence of temporary complications is high, but permanent sequelae are rare, providing the surgeon who performes the procedure is personally involved in the aftercare of the patient. If severe pain is experienced, lengthening should be stopped for a few days and stretching exercises increased until the pain subsides. Pin track infections should be treated in the usual way. If contractures develop, physiotherapy should be intensified and splints used. If translation or axial malalignment are observed, these should be corrected before the bone heals. If premature consolidation should occur, a second corticotomy should be performed at the same level as the previous one.

From the outset, the patient treated with this technique should be closely monitored by the surgeon performing it. The amount of shortening needed can be reduced if it is combined with a fasciocutaneous flap. If more than 5–7cm of shortening would be necessary to enable the defect to be covered, a free flap may be better. In most cases a one-stage procedure is possible, thereby reducing the number of operations needed. Overall hospitalization time for the patient undergoing this procedure is relatively short.

References

Aldegheri, R., L. Renzi-Brivio, S. Agostini: 'The Callotasis method of limb lengthening.' *Clin Orthop* 1989; 241: 137–145.

De Bastiani, G., R. Aldegheri, L. Renzi-Brivio, G. Trivella: 'Limb Lengthening by callus distraction (Callotasis).' *J Pediatr Orthop* 1987; 7: 129–134.

Giebel, G.: 'Extremitätenverlängerung und die Behandlung von Segment-Defekten durch Kallusdistraktion.' *Chirurg* 1987; 58: 601–606.

Giebel, G.: 'Resektions-Débridement mit kompensatorischer Kallusdistraktion.' *Unfallchirurg* 1991; 94: 401–408.

Ilizarov, G. A.: *Transosseous Osteosynthesis* (1992), Springer: Berlin, Heidelberg, London, 1st. Edition.

SECTION 4 ARTHRODESIS

External Fixation Techniques for Arthrodesis of the Knee and Ankle

53

M. Saleh and M. Rickman

Introduction

Arthrodesis, or fusion of the major joints, is an uncommon procedure and often the last procedure in a long line of attempts to salvage the joint. In joints such as the hip and knee, the results of primary arthroplasty are generally excellent, and even revision arthroplasties give satisfactory results in most cases. This explains why primary arthrodesis of these joints is unusual. In the case of the ankle, however, the results of ankle joint arthroplasty have been rather disappointing, and here, primary arthrodesis is a more acceptable procedure.

Arthrodesis of the Knee

Historically, knee arthrodesis was performed for painful knee conditions and for degenerative arthritis prior to the successful introduction of arthroplasty. Usually the bone was in good condition and square cut osteotomies excising the articular cartilage left large healthy bone surfaces which could be approximated in 15° of flexion and held efficiently in compression with a simple clamp device (Charnley 1951)[1]. This device consisted of two Steinmann pins one of which was inserted above and one below the arthrodesis level and connected by threaded rods to permit compression. Stability was dependent on having a large coapted bony surface and Charnley clamps were used routinely for primary arthrodesis. As an alternative to the Charnley clamps where bone quality is good, a single monolateral fixator mounted anteriorly may be used (Fig. 53.1).

Commonly today, arthrodesis is performed for major trauma with bone loss and following the removal of joint replacements. In the latter scenario, there is often significant bone and soft tissue loss and the bone may be of poor quality. In aseptic cases, satisfactory results have been reported with long radius Kuntscher intra-medullary nails (Fern et al 1989).[2] In infected cases and those that are not suitable for nailing, stability may be achieved with long term orthoses or external fixation. Where failure of arthrodesis occurs, this may be due to failure to eradicate infection, to bone loss at the joint surfaces, to inadequate stabilization, or any combination of these. In such situations, the use of external fixation as originally described by Charnley fails to provide adequate stability in the sagittal plane. Equally, an anteriorly mounted DAF may fail to provide adequate coronal plane support. The problem is exacerbated in cases where much of the distal femoral surface has been removed in order to fit a prosthesis. In these circumstancess, bi-planar fixation is needed (Fidler 1983).[3] Fidler described the use of Charnley clamps combined with an anteriorly mounted Wagner monolateral fixator. Where there is adequate metaphyseal bone stock stability may be provided by a circular or hybrid fixator with wires in metaphyseal bone. In most cases, however, the metaphyseal bone is poor, and adequate fixation may only be obtained using diaphyseal screws. Two techniques using the Orthofix system are capable of achieving biplanar fixa-

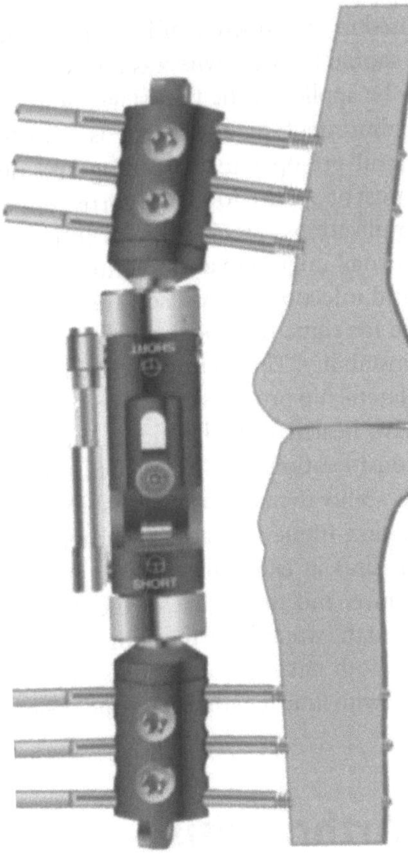

Fig. 53.1 Knee arthrodesis in a patient with good quality bone; anteriorly placed ProCallus fixator in situ, with three screws in each clamp.

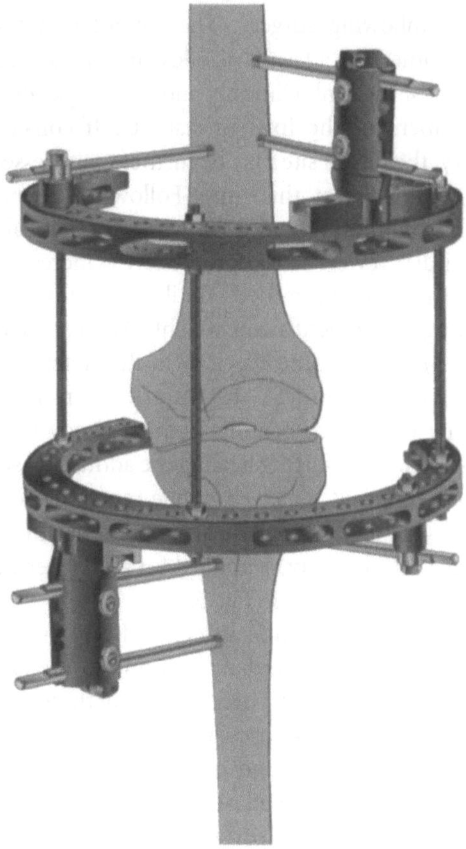

Fig. 53.2 Knee arthrodesis using the Sheffield Hybrid Fixator Assembly. Hinges may be used to facilitate the correct flexion angle.

tion; a Sheffield Hybrid Fixator with screws (Fig. 53.2) or the use of a combination of anterior and laterally placed dynamic axial fixators. The anterior fixator may use an Iowa body or the Link system; the lateral fixator is of straight design and may be either a ball-jointed fixator or a lengthener allowing for a 15° flexion angulation. A description of the operative technique follows.

Surgical Technique

The surgical approach to the knee is usually through the old wound anteriorly, and a similar approach may be used in cases of primary arthrodesis. Where present, the prosthesis is removed, together with any bone cement and non-viable tissue. The joint surfaces are resected and fashioned to give a good functional result, usually in slight flexion as described above. A minimal amount of bone is removed, the aim being to achieve as large a bone contact area as possible. Small areas of contact following prosthesis removal increase the chances of instability which can lead to failure of osteosynthesis. In infected cases, antibiotic beads may be inserted followed by parenteral antibiotics. A bone graft is normally required and this may be inserted primarily or, in the case of infection, at a second stage. Percutaneous autogenous bone graft harvested from the iliac crest may be used (Saleh 1992;[4] Kreibich et al 1994)[5] and in addition, any bone removed to aid alignment of the arthrodesis, as well as the patella, can also be used.

When the Sheffield Hybrid Fixator is used, two two-thirds rings of appropriate size are connected together using three threaded bars. Hinges may be inserted to achieve the correct flexion angle. Stable fixation may be achieved using two screws in the Sheffield clamp and an additional screw mounted in a single screw holder 60°–90° to the first group for each level, i.e. diaphysis of femur and diaphysis of tibia (Fig. 53.2). Partial weightbearing (30–40 per cent of body weight), with crutches, should commence on the day following operation, and increase progressively over the treatment period. Physiotherapy for the hip and ankle should begin as soon as possible, usually within the first one or two days following surgery. The patient is generally allowed home after a few days following a review of the alignment of the limb clinically and radiologically, and an assessment of the fixation stability. If considered necessary, the fusion site may be further compressed by a few millimetres at this time. Following discharge, patients should return every 3–4 weeks for clinical and radiological review. A progressive increase in weightbearing is permitted until the construct is supporting the patient's full weight. At this stage, in order to introduce some elasticity to the system as the arthrodesis starts to heal, the threaded bars may be exchanged for reduction units with the body locking nuts released. With further healing the additional single screws are removed, followed by the remainder of the screws and the fixator. If necessary, a plaster cylinder or removable orthosis may be applied for a final period. A case history is illustrated in Fig. 53.3.

As an alternative, two fixators may be applied, one in the anterior (sagittal) plane and one in the lateral (coronal) plane, in the normal way, using three screws in each clamp. A compression–distraction unit is applied to each fixator and compression exerted by turning the screw in the end of each until good contact is felt between the bone surfaces. Bony contact, and therefore stability, should be confirmed by image intensification and direct visualization. If the distances from the clamps to the level of the arthrodesis are large, supplementary screws may be added to the bodies of the fixators. This technique is usually stable and permits early weightbearing. Dynamization is not employed in this indication. The fixators will normally remain in place for between 3 and 6 months, and progressive de-stabilization may be introduced to load the bone gradually and encourage final healing. To do this, the supplementary screws are removed first, followed by the middle screws in each clamp, followed by one of the fixators, and finally by the second fixator. The order of fixator removal will depend on the progress to healing but the antero-posterior moment is normally the most important to counteract and it follows, therefore, that the lateral fixator would be removed before the anterior fixator. A case history is illustrated in Fig. 53.4.

The use of intramedullary nailing has three main drawbacks: it entails a long operation, and involves reaming of both femoral and tibial medullary cavities, resulting in major blood loss. This means that the patient needs to be able to withstand such a procedure both from a medical and an anaesthetic standpoint. This is not normally the case with external fixation, which, in comparison, can be applied much more rapidly and less traumatically. Furthermore, where nailing is used in the presence of infection, a two-stage procedure should be used, whereas an external fixator can usually be applied at the first stage. Since no post-operative adjustment of alignment is possible with nailing, careful pre-operative planning and operative technique must be applied to ensure correct alignment.

The complications associated with intramedullary nails include nail migration and fracture, trochanteric fractures, and infection. They also generally require a dorsal brace for some time post-operatively, to avoid rotational instability. They cannot be used in the presence of ipsilateral hip prostheses, or if previous femoral fractures have healed with significant malalignment. The main considerations with external fixation remain the patient's ability to manage and rehabilitate with an external fixation frame in place. Fractures can occur through pin sites in externally fixed cases, but deep infection is rare, and the nature of the device allows better access to the wound. Furthermore, external fixation permits both post-operative adjustment and the ability to deal with limb length discrepancy (Fig. 53.3).

Ankle Arthrodesis

Ankle arthrodesis is an accepted method of treatment for disabling arthritis from a variety of aetiologies. Some surgeons have turned to total ankle replacement, but the results of this have so far been disappointing. Many feel that the functional results achievable with primary ankle arthrodesis are good enough to question the need for ankle joint arthroplasty. Arthrodesis achieves pain relief and allows for correction of deformity and instability. Numerous series have been published, all with largely similar results and complication rates (Mazur et al 1979,[6] Barr and Record 1953,[7] Ratcliffe 1959,[8] Kennedy 1960,[9] Verhelst et al 1975,[10] Morrey and Weiderman 1980).[11] The fact that many different techniques are reported indicates that no single surgical method is universally accepted as being superior to any other. Compression arthrodesis may be achieved with internal or external fixation. Internal compression arthrodesis has been shown to be associated with non-union rates of up to 26 per cent (Holt et al 1991,[12] Kirkpatrick et al 1991,[13] Mears et al 1991).[14]

Non-union rates of up to 37.5 per cent have been reported for external compression techniques (Charnley 1951,[1] Hagen 1986,[15] Scranton et al 1980).[16]

External fixation may be achieved with Charnley clamps (Charnley 1951).[1] The technique relies upon good bone stock, a competent Achilles tendon and careful placement of the anterior talar Steinmann pin

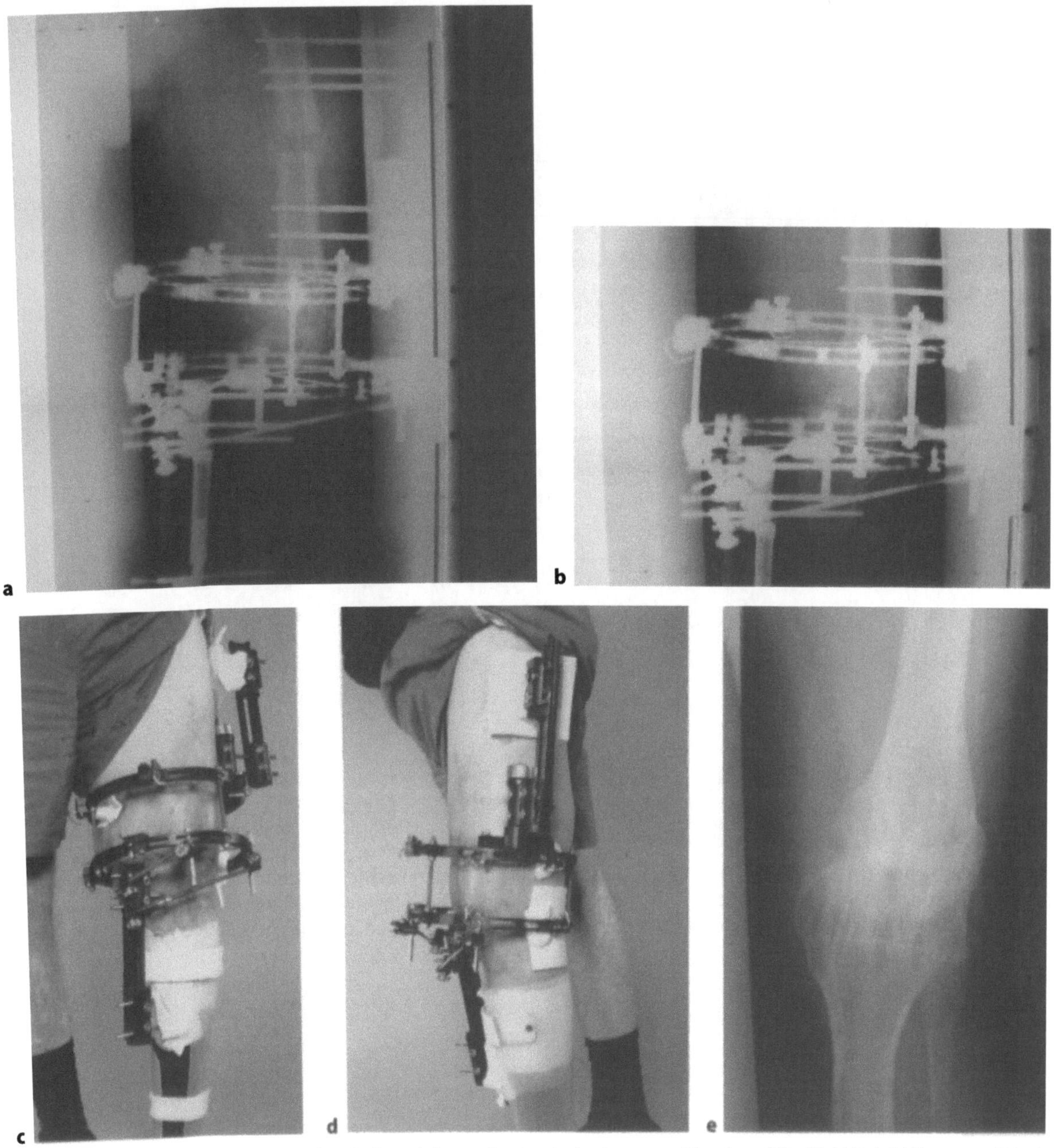

Fig. 53.3 Case Report 1: Failed knee arthrodesis and shortening treated using a combination of Sheffield Hybrid Fixator and Limb Reconstruction System. A 55-year-old male was involved in a severe road traffic accident in 1981, during which he sustained an open, comminuted, supracondylar fracture of the femur extending into the knee, a fracture of the clavicle, fractured ribs, a fracture of the little finger and a head injury. The femoral fracture was initially treated by traction, healing in malunion with 3cm shortening and a stiff knee. He was referred to another centre where a quadricepsplasty was performed but he continued to suffer from a stiff and painful knee. He ultimately underwent knee fusion in 1985. He managed well until he had another accident which resulted in a fracture through the arthrodesis. He was then treated first in a Thomas splint and subsequently in plaster. The fracture remained ununited and painful. At this stage he was referred to author's unit with a non-union, pain and deformity. On examination he had 9cm of shortening, 30° of external rotation, 35° of flexion and 25° of varus. He was treated by revision arthrodesis, correction of the deformity and lengthening by distraction osteosynthesis using a Sheffield Hybrid Fixator Assembly across the arthrodesis and 30cm LRS rails for femoral and tibial lengthening. **a,b** X-ray images with the fixator assembly in situ; bifocal lengthening in progress. **c, d** Clinical appearance. **e** The arthrodesis healed in good alignment; his limb length and axis were fully corrected and he returned to full ambulation and independence.

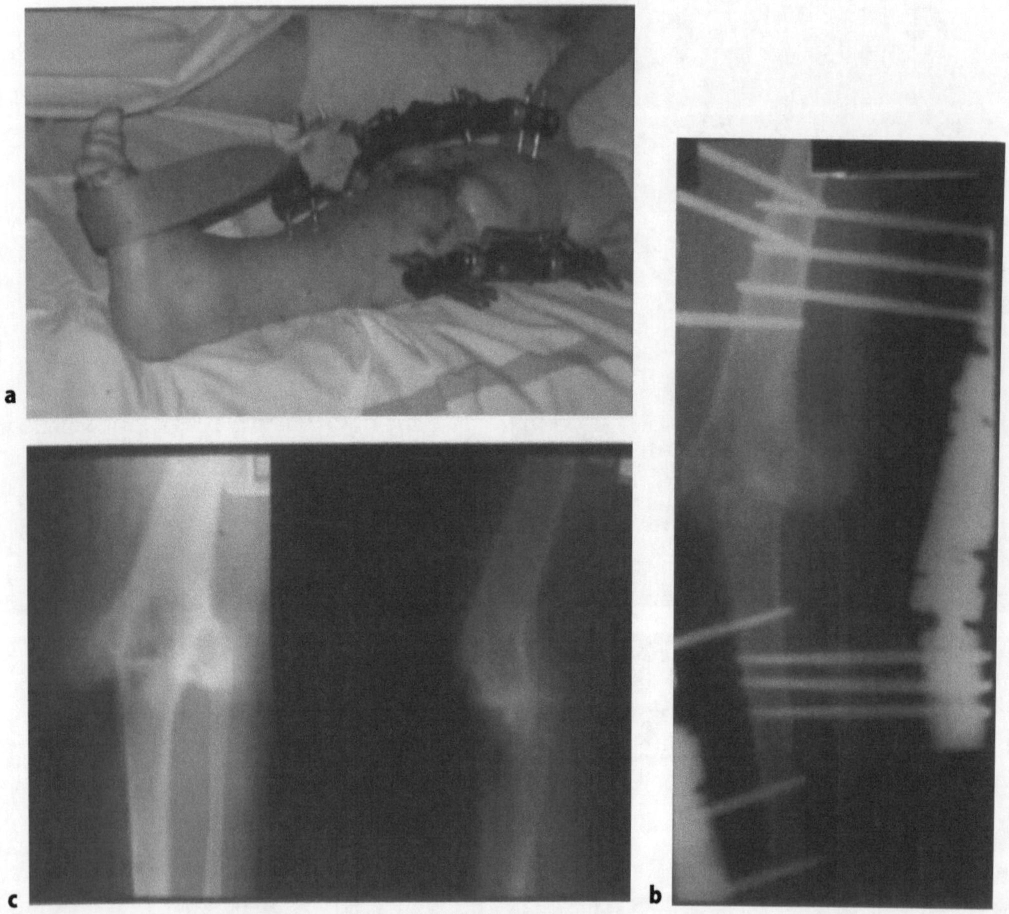

Fig. 53.4 Case report 2: A lady of 68 years underwent knee replacement. Deep infection occurred requiring extensive debridement followed by fasciocutaneous flap cover. Stability was achieved with an anteriorly mounted DAF with Iowa body and a lateral fixator applied. **a** Clinical appearance. **b** X-ray appearance. **c** Final X-ray; healed with a good functional result.

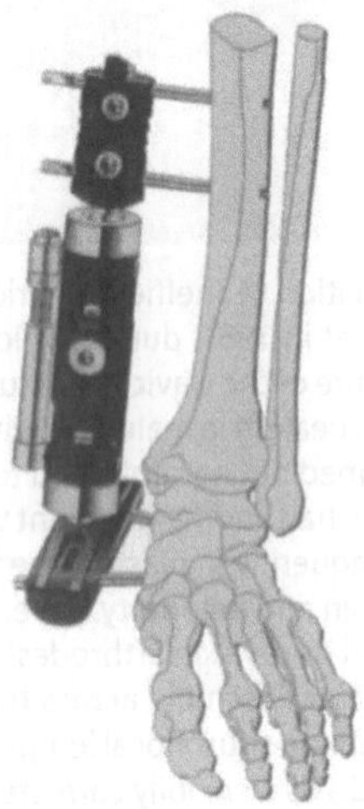

Fig. 53.5 Ankle arthrodesis using the ProCallus Fixator with a Torbay-Garches clamp distally.

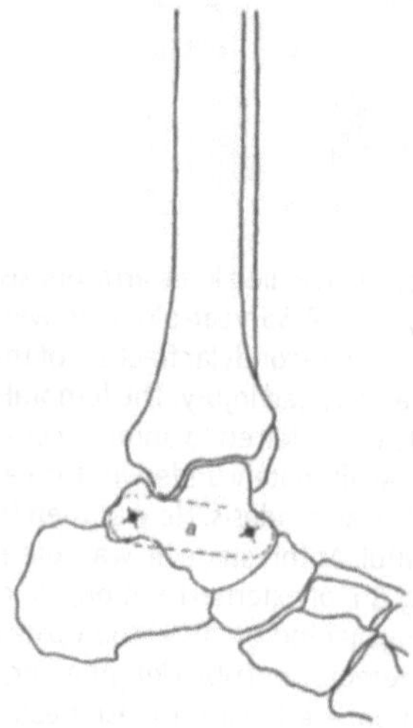

Fig. 53.6 Position of the distal screws in the talus for tibio-talar fusion.

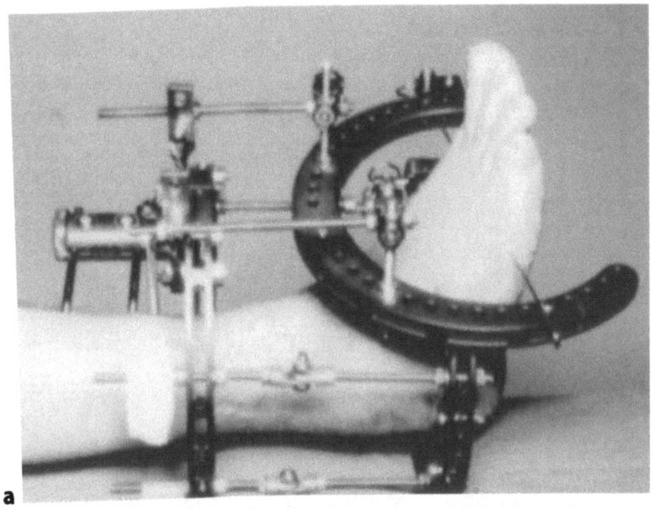

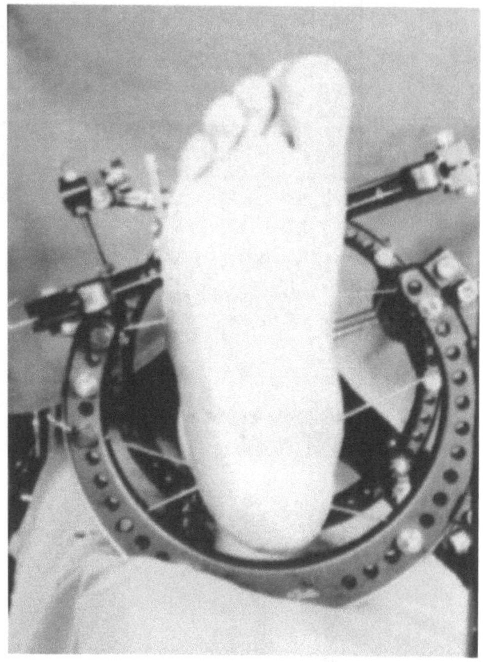

Fig. 53.7 The Sheffield Hybrid Fixator Assembly for ankle fusion. **a** lateral view. **b** view from beneath.

to achieve stable compression fixation. A medially applied Dynamic Axial Fixator with a Torbay-Garches or T-clamp distally may also produce stable compression fixation in the presence of good bone stock (Figs. 53.5 and 53.6). Compression is applied more effectively to the medial than the lateral side, making it less appropriate in revision or osteoporotic cases.

The presence of infection or inadequate soft tissue coverage precludes the use of internal fixation, while poor bone quality and altered anatomy render it more difficult, and less likely to be successful. Unfortunately, these problems often occur together, making salvage in these cases a formidable undertaking. In this situation, internal compression arthrodesis is often not feasible, or associated with generally poor results. Circular external fixation using the Sheffield Hybrid Fixator may be used successfully in such circumstances since the fixator provides even, long term support around the arthrodesis site (Fig. 53.7). Limited joint exposure and articular debridement is required and post-operative adjustment of alignment may be performed. In addition, extending the frame proximally together with an additional osteotomy of the tibia and fibula permits correction of length discrepancy. The results even in revision surgery have been good (O'Doherty et al 1992).[17] We have used two varieties of external fixation, monolateral fixation and hybrid fixation, and the use of each is discussed below.

Monolateral External Fixation

Fig. 53.5 shows the use of an Orthofix ProCallus fixator applied to the medial aspect of the tibia. A straight clamp is used for the proximal screws in the tibial diaphysis. Distally, either a Torbay-Garches clamp or T-clamp with two screws placed in the talus can be used, or a straight clamp, with screws in the talus and calcaneum respectively, for tibio-talar joint fusion. Where subtalar and tibio-talar double fusion is required, the T-Garches clamp with two pins in the calcaneum can be used.

Access to the ankle joint is generally by one of two methods. The most commonly used is the anterior approach, using a vertical incision between extensor hallucis longus and extensor digitorum. This affords good access to the joint centrally, with minimal dissection. If more extensive dissection is required, the lateral approach as described by Gatellier and Chatang (1924)[18] can be used, dividing the fibula and turning down the lower end on the calcaneo-fibular ligaments. The articulating surfaces are then debrided, removing all articular cartilage, and the bone surfaces modified to allow close apposition of the distal tibia and upper surface of the talus. Any large resections should be made on the tibial side of the joint. If local osteoporosis is marked, or there are other reasons why healing may be delayed, a bone graft can also be added.

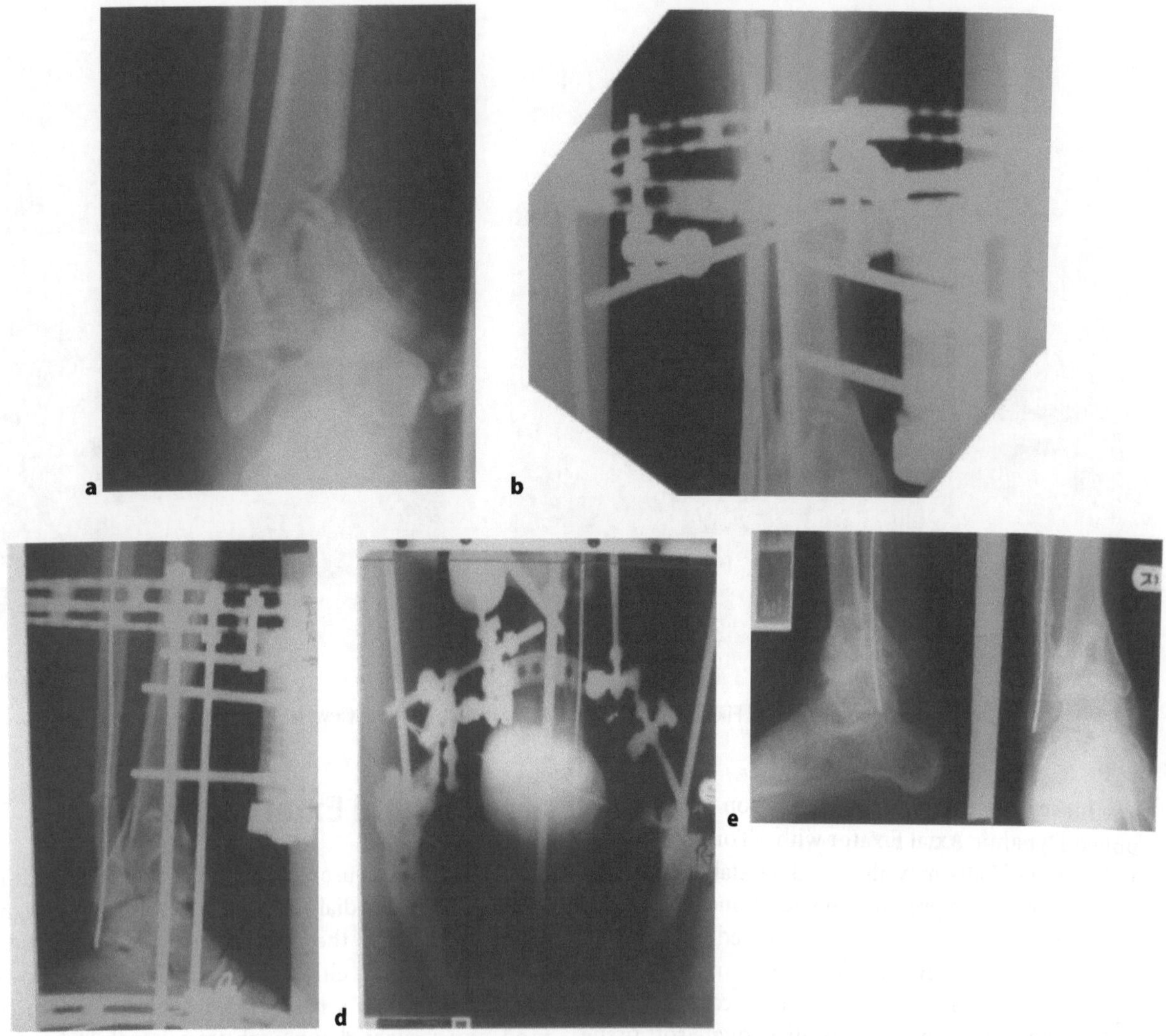

Fig. 53.8 Case Report: Acute ankle fusion using the Sheffield Hybrid Fixator. **a** A 26-year-old male was involved in a high energy road traffic accident sustaining an acetabular fracture and a right pilon fracture (Ruedi and Allgower Type III). When admitted to the author's unit he was noted to have poor quality skin over the ankle and considerable swelling. **b, c, d** A trans-articular Sheffield Hybrid Fixator Assembly was initially applied, followed by formal arthrodesis. **e** Sound union was achieved with good restoration of limb function.

The distal screws are inserted first. Where both are placed in the talus, the anterior screw passes through the neck of the talus and the second screw is sited posteriorly (Fig. 53.6). Both screws are inserted in a plane exactly parallel to the articular surface of the tibia. Two proximal screws are inserted into the medial face of the tibia such that when the fixator is mounted its telescopic body will be open by about 2cm, to allow the debrided bone surfaces to be subjected to symmetrical axial compression before the body locking nut of the fixator is tightened.

The application technique where a straight clamp is used distally is essentially similar, with the exception that the more proximal of the two distal screws passes through the body of the talus anterior to the medial malleolus, and the more distal passes through the calcaneum, a little posterior to the first screw, avoiding the neurovascular bundle.

A posterior splint may be used for the first two or three days. Physiotherapy for mobilization of the knee joint and exercises to strengthen the quadriceps and hamstring muscles are commenced as soon as the patient is comfortable, which is usually within one or two days of the operation.

Partial weightbearing (maximum 20–30kg) may commence on the first or second post-operative day, and may be gradually increased over the next four to six weeks to full weighbearing. Serial X-rays should be taken to confirm the maintenance of alignment and to follow the progress of fusion. Some slight loss of compression may occur during the initial days following operation. The degree of compression should therefore be checked, and adjusted, where indicated, after two or three days. Further checks and adjustments should be made at each follow-up visit, every three to four weeks.

Fusion has usually occurred after three months, at which time the fixator is removed.

Hybrid Fixation

Where hybrid fixation is used, the Sheffield Hybrid System extended to the foot (Fig. 53.7) is a highly stable construct. A full ring is secured to the lower third of the tibia with a Sheffield clamp and two screws and an offset supplementary screw. A two-thirds ring is secured to the os calcis with two, three, or occasionally four wires and this ring is connected by three threaded bars to the tibial ring. A third ring is attached to the forefoot using two wires inserted through the metatarsal necks. Foot wires should not be tensioned to more than 6–800N. The forefoot ring is connected to the hindfoot and tibial rings with threaded bars and hinges. Post-operatively, the foot position may be adjusted by compressing or distracting the threaded bars. A sandal may be used to permit touch or partial weightbearing. A case history is illustrated in Fig. 53.8.

The functional success of ankle arthrodesis will depend to a large extent on the position finally achieved. The mobility of the foot and subtalar joints (where the latter have not been fused) allow a surprisingly good functional result, with patients often able to walk without a limp. The optimal position of the arthrodesis has been reported as neutral flexion, slight valgus angulation of the hind foot and 5–10° of external rotation. This position has also been shown to place the least strain on the knee joint.

References

1. Charnley J. 'Compression arthrodesis of the ankle and shoulder.' *J Bone Joint Surg* [Br] 1951; 33-B: 180.
2. Fern ED, Stewart HD, Newton G. 'Curved Kuntscher nail arthrodesis after failure of knee replacement.' *J Bone Joint Surg* [Br] 1989; 71B: 588–90.
3. Fidler MW. 'Knee arthrodesis following prosthesis removal. Use of the Wagner apparatus.' *J Bone Joint Surg* [Br] 1983; 65B: 29–1.
4. Saleh M. 'Bone Graft Harvesting: a percutaneous technique.' *J Bone Joint Surg* [Br] 1991; 73B: 867–8.
5. Kreibich DN, Wells J, Scott IR, Saleh M. 'Donor site morbidity at the iliac crest: comparison of percutaneous and open methods.' *J Bone Joint Surg* [Br] 1994; 76B: 847–8.
6. Mazur JM et al 'Ankle Arthrodesis. Long term follow up with gait analysis.' *J Bone Joint Surg* [Am] 1979; 61-A: 964–75.
7. Barr JS, Record EE. 'Arthrodesis of the ankle – Indications, operative technique and clinical experience.' *New England J Med*; 1953: 248: 53–6.
8. Ratcliffe AHC. 'Compression arthrodesis of the ankle.' *J Bone Joint Surg* [Br] 1959; 41-B: 524–34.
9. Kennedy JC. 'Compression arthrodesis of the ankle.' *J Bone Joint Surg* [Am] 1960; 42-A: 1308–16.
10. Verhelst MP et al 'Arthrodesis of the ankle joint with complete removal of the distal part of the fibula.' *Clin Orthop* 1975; 118: 93–9.
11. Morrey BF and Weideman GP. 'Complications and long term results of ankle arthrodesis following ankle trauma.' *J Bone Joint Surg* [Am] 1980; 62-A: 777–84.
12. Holt ES, Hanson ST, Mayo KA, Sangeorzan BJ. 'Ankle arthrodesis using internal screw fixation.' *Clin Orthop* 1991; 268: 21–8.
13. Kirkpatrick JS, Goldner JL, Goldner RD. 'Revision arthrodesis for tibiotalar pseudarthrosis with fibula onlay-inlay graft and internal screw fixation.' *Clin Orthop* 1991; 268: 29–36.
14. Mears DC, Gordon RG, Kann SE, Kann JN. 'Ankle arthrodesis with an anterior tension plate.' *Clin Orthop* 1991; 268: 56–64.
15. Hagen RJ. 'Ankle arthrodesis. Problems and pitfalls.' *Clin Orthop* 1986; 202: 152–62.
16. Scranton PE, Fu FH, Brown TD. 'Ankle arthrodesis: a comparative clinical and biomechanical evaluation.' *Clin Orthop* 1980; 234: 151.
17. O'Doherty DP, Street R, Saleh M 'The use of circular external fixators in the management of complex disorders of the foot and ankle.' *The Foot*, 1992; 2:135–42.
18. Gatellier J, Chatang. 'Access to fractured malleolus with piece chipped off at back.' *J Chir* 1924; 24: 513.

SECTION 5 ARTICULATED DISTRACTION

Introduction

M. Saleh

Articulated distraction is a technique that is unique to external fixation. The external fixator is used to cross a joint and a hinge is placed within the fixation system to permit movement. Its use both in orthopaedic trauma and limb reconstruction is increasing. It is referred to in earlier chapters of this book in relation to injuries of the elbow (Ch. 14), wrist (Ch. 16), hand (Ch. 19), ankle (Ch. 27) and contractures of the knee and foot (Ch. 40). The two chapters in this section describe in detail the application of this technique in joint stiffness in the upper limb (Ch. 54) and in hip disease (Ch. 55).

Joint Stiffness in the Upper Limb: the Arthrodiatasis Technique

54

D. Pennig

Introduction

To allow adequate ambulation in mammals the development of sophisticated joints was necessary. Further evolution provided an upper extremity in primates which became indispensible for complex tasks. It allowed the use of tools, and in mankind the upper limb may be rated more important than the lower limb. This is reflected in the space allocated to the hand on the cerebral cortex. An impairment of joint function in the upper limb may create a significant disability.

The upper limb serves to position the hand in a way that allows it to execute its highly differentiated tasks. The elbow and shoulder joints play an important role in the free functioning of the hand and an impairment of their function may therefore only be compensated to a certain degree. The joints of the upper limb are highly sophisticated with the shoulder being very movable. The elbow allows flexion and extension and together with the distal radio-ulnar joint permits the radius to rotate around the humero-ulnar axis. This brings the hand into a position to execute its tasks; the mechanical properties of the carpal bones have yet to be fully understood The thumb in opposition to the fingers possesses the most versatile carpo-metacarpal joint. Carpo-metacarpal joints II, III and IV do not generally contribute to finger movement whereas carpo-metacarpal joint V allows the fifth finger some movement in the dorso-volar plane. Further distally, the MP, PIP and DIP joints resemble hinges with the MP joints developed in such a way that with increasing flexion the stability of the joint increases.

The restoration of function in joint impairment not only requires a full understanding of the patient's needs but also a sound understanding of the complex anatomy of the upper limb. Relevant details of the anatomy are provided in Ch. 12.

Prior to the development of surgical and orthopaedic techniques, joint impairment was a sad fate and there was little hope for improvement. Patients suffering from joint stiffness were crippled, and their place in society more or less determined. With a better understanding of joint design, joint function and biomechanical properties, surgical techniques were devised to improve function in disabling joint stiffness.

The History of Restoration of Joint Function

More than a hundred years ago an operative technique was described to treat complete stiffness or ankylosis of the mandibular joint (Helferich 1894) and one year later in elbow joint stiffness (Wolff 1895). It is remarkable that even then, the upper limb received such attention. The first, however, to treat a condition involving joint impairment was von Esmarch in 1860 and he again dealt with a condition that must have been an extremely serious and worrying disability for the patient, stiffness of the mandibular joint. Esmarch solved this problem by creating an extra-anatomical joint and did not attempt to restore the original joint.

In the lower limb, Reha Barton from Philadelphia performed an osteotomy in 1826 below the greater trochanter, to restore function in the leg. Again, an extra-anatomical position for the newly created joint was chosen. The technique aimed at improving the position of the leg and creating a mobile non-union.

The latter however did not happen reproducibly. Sayre in 1862 resected a semi-lunar piece of bone above the lesser trochanter in a stiff hip joint. Unfortunately, the patient died seven months later, but the post-mortem examination revealed an interesting nearthros (Fig. 54.1). Later in the nineteenth century the surgical technique was altered. Maunder in 1875 recommended a subcutaneous arthrolysis, and Julius Wolff in 1889 performed an open arthrolysis as the treatment of choice in joint stiffness. The first publications on this technique by Julius Wolff concentrated on the elbow joint. It was, however, evident that the loss of cartilage and damage to the articulating surfaces required some form of additional procedure, which Verneuil in 1863 had devised theoretically for ankylosis of the mandibular joint. He interposed a muscle flap and called it interposition arthroplasty. It took 30 years for Helferich to further develop interposition arthroplasty. After careful and minimal resection of the ankylosed joint, a pedicle flap from the temporalis muscle was interposed in the mandibular joint. Interposition arthroplasty quickly became popular in other joints. A brief episode involved the use of artificial materials (celluloid plates, pig bladder and wall of

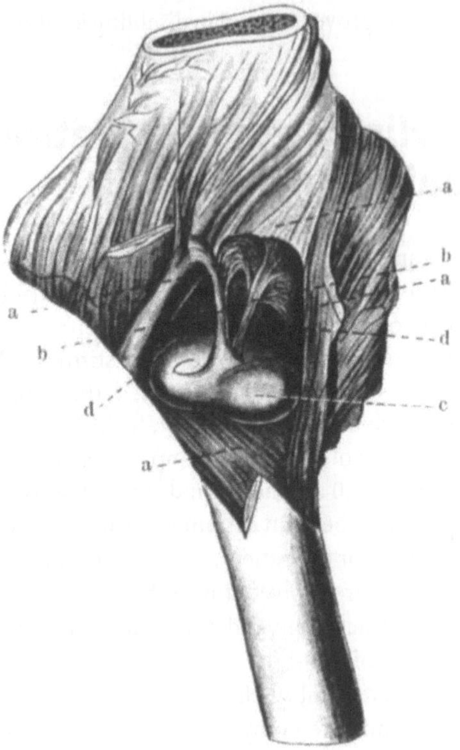

Fig. 54.1 Cadaver specimen 7 months after resection of a semi-lunar piece of bone above the lesser trochanter in a stiff hip joint (a) A pseudo-capsule had formed. (b) Neathros with ligament structures. (c) Cartilage covering the bone end. (d) Neo-acetabulum.

ovarian cysts) to be transplanted. There was, however, little success, and in 1934 Erwin Payr considered this to be a dead end.

Modern arthroplasty took off at beginning of the 20th century with vascularized flaps and a more sophisticated surgical technique together with an improvement in asepsis. Early contributions in the American, French and Italian literature indicate that joint surgery became an intensely discussed topic. In England as well as in Scandinavia the technique met with certain reservations, but in Germany von Esmarch, Payr and Lexer contributed significantly to the progress. Lexer in 1920 published material dealing with 439 arthroplasties and Payr in more than 800 pages described in 1934 his experience with in excess of 400 cases.

It was Payr who systematically studied the technique of interposition arthroplasty as well as the general pathophysiology of joint stiffness in animal experiments. Fascinating results were published in rabbits. Figs. 54.2 and 54.3 show cross-sections through joints treated by interposition arthroplasty.

In clinical practice, however, there were a fair number of failures. In some cases the stiffness recurred, while others developed an unstable joint. The underlying pathology in some cases such as haemophiliacs, was detrimental, and there was little success. To understand the failures, Payr studied in great detail the differences between species. In animals it is almost impossible to create an ankylosis or arthrodesis surgically without installing hardware permanently. Even long-term immobilization does not succeed. After the immobilizing device is removed the animal will start to move around and use the limb. The animal is well capable of tolerating pain since without movement its fate is sealed. Immediate use of the limb is the result and spontaneous development of a nearthros the consequence. Payr also described significant differences between wild animals and domesticated animals.

Payr understood that after an interposition arthroplasty post-operative treatment played an important role. He favoured extension to avoid undue pressure on the interposed tissue which most likely would have resulted in necrosis of the flap. He also used orthotic devices to overcome contractures. Devices allowing joint motion under distraction were not available to him.

In 1975, restoration of knee and elbow function with a hinge distractor apparatus was described (Volkov and Oganesian 1975). This apparatus not only allowed movement, it also permitted gradual reduction of a dislocated joint followed by restoration of function. Along the same lines, Robert Judet used a

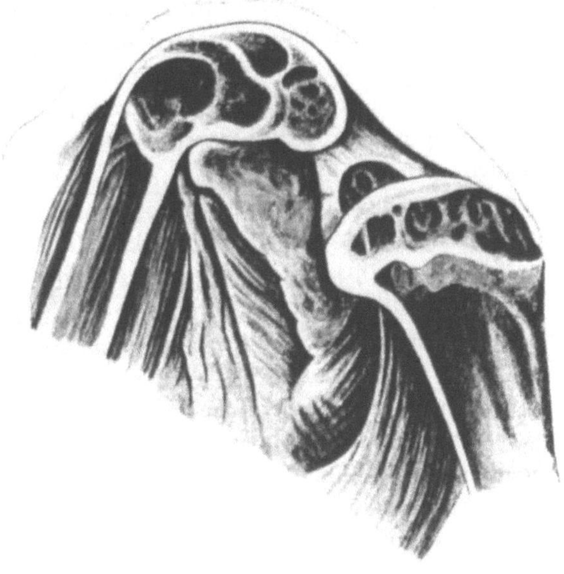

Fig. 54.2 Creation of a neathros after resection in a rabbit. Sagittal cross-section showing cartilage covering the bone ends (32 days after surgery).

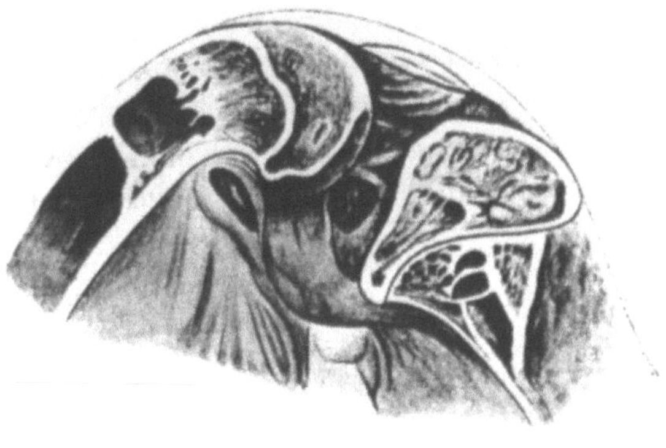

Fig. 54.3 70 days after surgery formation of synovial fluid in the pseudo-capsule was observed as well as cartilage formation on both new joint members.

unilateral and bilateral distractor on the elbow and ankle joints. This device did not allow reduction but it did permit distraction of the joint and movement around a functional axis. The technique was tested in dogs. The cartilage of the tibial pilon and the talus were excised until the subchondral cancellous bone was visible. The distractor allowed the creation of a permanent gap of 4–8mm. After 3–6 months the dogs showed an almost normal range of motion and in histological studies the interposed material resembled "normal cartilage". Based on these results the devices were tested in the elbow and the ankle joint with remarkable success.

Devices similar to the Volkov apparatus have been described recently but experience remains rather anecdotal (McKee et al 1998).

Our experience in the upper limb with fixator controlled distractional arthroplasty, described as arthrodiatasis, is based on 46 cases with most of the clinical cases involving the elbow and finger joints.

Pathophysiology of Joint Stiffness

The term stiffness implies that the normal active and/or passive range of motion is lost. There is variation in the normal range of motion of a joint depending on age, training, hereditary factors and environment. This is best illustrated in the available movement in the Japanese hip joint which is used to squat, compared to that in western civilizations. If the opposite limb is not affected, the range of motion of a given joint may be compared to the unaffected side to determine an individual's range of motion.

There is a difference between active and passive motion, and active motion may also be reduced by pain. If pain is eliminated there may be an increased range of movement in a joint.

Congenital Stiffness

Patients with primary dysplasia of upper limb joints may have a normal range of motion but may also have some impairment. Most commonly, impaired function is the late result of a brachial plexus injury affecting shoulder, elbow, wrist and hand. The shoulder is generally affected most frequently.

Transient Stiffness

Transient stiffness is encountered after periarticular and intra-articular injuries and in the case of the elbow, physiotherapy may be expected to resolve it within 3–4 months. More acute stiffness develops in cases where the joint locks due to a loose body in osteochondrosis dissecans. As soon as the loose body is removed or displaced from the articular surfaces the joint is unlocked and movement restored. Overuse of a joint may also lead to temporary loss of function.

Neurological Stiff Shoulder

Muscular action may be impaired in spasticity or because of nerve injuries; where a joint is not used throughout its appropriate range of motion a loss of motion will be observed.

Acquired Stiffness

The most common cause of stiffness is post-traumatic and this occurs after joint or periarticular injury and occasionally even after prolonged immobilization in diaphyseal fractures. The response is partly due to the intra-articular pathology but an inflammatory cause is also present.

The general causes of stiffness include:

- joint malalignment
- cartilage destruction
- shortening of ligaments and capsules
- intra-articular fibrosis with fibro-fatty tissue
- post-traumatic incongruence
- postinfection
- degenerative
- congenital
- iatrogenic

Extra-articular causes include:

- impaired gliding function of muscles and/or tendons after injury
- burn injuries
- muscular imbalance due to nerve damage or spasticity.

It is not unusual to find a combination of extra- and intra-articular causes and it is not sufficient to resolve the intra-articular pathology unless the muscle power will be capable of moving the joint later on. It is not the target of the operation to have a better radiological image of the joint, but to improve motion and function.

One of the main problems in joint stiffness is the development of fibro-fatty tissue leading to the clinical diagnosis of arthrofibrosis. The cascade of events leading to fibrosis and scar formation shows how the fibrotic healing of gliding surfaces is initiated (Fig. 54.4).

The healing pattern is influenced by several factors including joint stability and movement of the injured tissues. The effect of early controlled mobilization on periarticular structures is complex. The biological response to joint instability is an increased fibroblastic activity with formation of fibrosis in an attempt to generate stability. This, however, leads to non-directed and non-functional stabilization resulting in stiffness.

The concept of transarticular fixation with motion capacity allows controlled restitution of joint mobility. During the first weeks after injury the reparative process requires movement within the normal range to define the working length of ligaments, muscles and capsule. The ligament repair process with increased activity of fibroblasts causes the collagen fibres to line up parallel to the line of tension. A lack of tension would result in disorientation of the fibres, formation of scar tissue and arthrofibrosis. Haematoma formation and cellular debris cause obliteration of the joint with the formation of fibro-fatty tissue within it and are important factors in the development of joint impairment.

As a result of impact it is not uncommon for an articular defect to be associated with flake fractures and cartilage abrasions. The repair process in articular fractures starts with a fibrin clot filling the remaining gaps. The cell system available for repair will contain chondrocytes which after several days may create a surface of fibrocartilage. The fibrin clot repair and the early cellular response must be protected. Early excessive loading of the joint, however, may disrupt the repair process (Buckwalter 1992, 1995) and a fixator which allows a certain degree of distraction of the joint will support the repair. When moving the joint again the articular surfaces must be protected against excessive shear forces. Not only may inappropriate loading of articular components lead to a redisplacement of the fractures, it also may be detrimental to the repair process.

The role of early mobilization in joint injuries has been studied experimentally in dogs (Behrens et al 1989). Comparing rigid fixation with limited motion after articular injuries it was evident that the latter

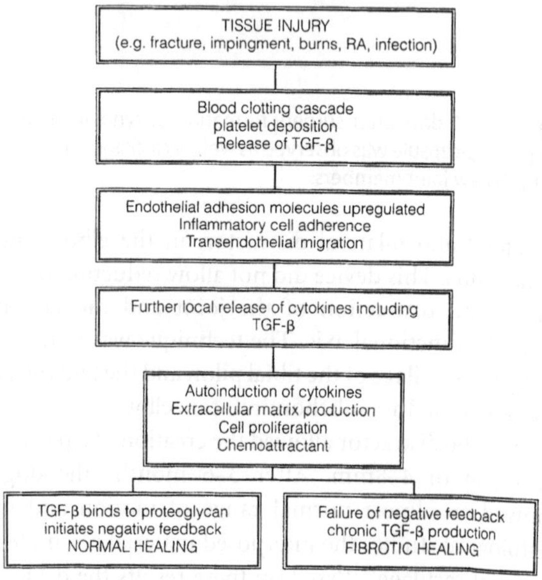

Fig. 54.4 Cascade of events leading to fibrosis and scar formation in the joint (from Crossan J, Meek D, Darmani H (1997) *Fibrosis and adhesion formation in: Joint Stiffness of the Upper Limb.* Copeland SA, Gschwend N, Landi A (Eds). Martin Dunitz: London).

group recovered the proteoglycan content of the cartilage whereas the rigidly fixed group showed further degeneration when functional loading occurred.

Pathophysiologically, in a stiff joint the water content of the cartilage increases while the proteoglycan content decreases. Radiographic narrowing of the joint line is the consequence.

The Principles of Arthrodiatasis

Joint Distraction and Mobilization With External Fixation

In joint stiffness the finely-tuned components of the joint do not allow normal motion. Whatever the intra- or periarticular pathology, joint capsules and ligaments will at some point have lost their normal elasticity and will be unable to stretch appropriately. This process develops rather slowly. In arthrodiatasis we attempt to reverse the process (Fig. 54.5) which may be complicated by joint subluxation. On the side to which one of the joint members is displaced there are shortened ligaments and capsule. One-stage reduction, if at all successful, will cause significant pressure on the cartilage which may deteriorate under excessive loading (Fig. 54.6). Arthrodiatasis, therefore, attempts in these cases to stretch ligaments beyond their normal length and the joint is subsequently reduced, held in this position and moved gradually.

The three phases of arthrodiatasis are:

Distraction	intra-operatively
Relaxation	6–10 days
Mobilization	5–8 weeks

It is a continuous process and not a one-stage procedure. Distraction is only possible with extension, which is best provided by an external apparatus with pins anchored in the bone. Distraction is performed during surgery and may be repeated several times, which takes 15–60 minutes. This serves to stretch the ligaments and to distract the joint capsule. The average amount of distraction depends on the degree of stiffness as well as the duration of the problem. Table 54.1 gives an idea of the amount of distraction effected with the fixators used in our department.

In the presence of subluxation or even complete dislocation, the rate of distraction may be higher to overcome the severe shortening of the ligaments and capsule. It may be necessary in these cases to use a sequential strategy and start with distraction intra-operatively. Post-operative distraction may be necessary at a rate of 1–4mm a day depending on the pain response of the patient and the joint treated. Shoulder, elbow and wrist joints may be treated in this way whereas MP and PIP joints may usually be reduced intra-operatively following distraction. After the distraction phase the relaxation phase lasts 6–10 days. In long-standing contractures it is closer to 10 days and in those of shorter duration, closer to 6. In the MP and PIP joints we do not immobilize for more than 6 days. The relaxation phase of ligaments and capsules and of muscles and tendons crossing the joint is followed by the mobilization phase. Mobilization is permitted with unilateral external fixators which are specifically designed for a particular joint. There are dedicated fixators for elbow, wrist, MP and PIP joints (Fig. 54.7) which serve not only to maintain distraction but also to allow mobilization around the rotational centre of the joint. The total treatment time is usually 6–8 weeks from surgery to removal of the device. It may be necessary to prolong this phase in patients responding slowly or in cases with interposition arthroplasty. In such cases a total treatment time of 9–12 weeks is advocated.

The external fixators used for the purpose of joint mobilization maintain alignment and distraction. They allow mobilization within the given range of motion of the joint. The patient needs to understand the mechanics of the device and it is therefore necessary to select patients for this treatment. Physiotherapy is performed two to three times per day and the fixator may be locked in a particular position overnight. When dealing with flexion contracture of the wrist, for example, it is most important to regain full extension, and the fixator is locked overnight in the position of maximum correction achieved during the last physiotherapy session of the day. This helps the volar liga-

Shoulder	15–25mm
Elbow	12–17mm
Wrist	5–10mm
MP joint	5–7mm
PIP joints	4–6mm

Due to elasticity of fixators and bone screws, not all of the distraction will be exercised on the joint.

Table 54.1 Amount of distraction in arthrodiatasis

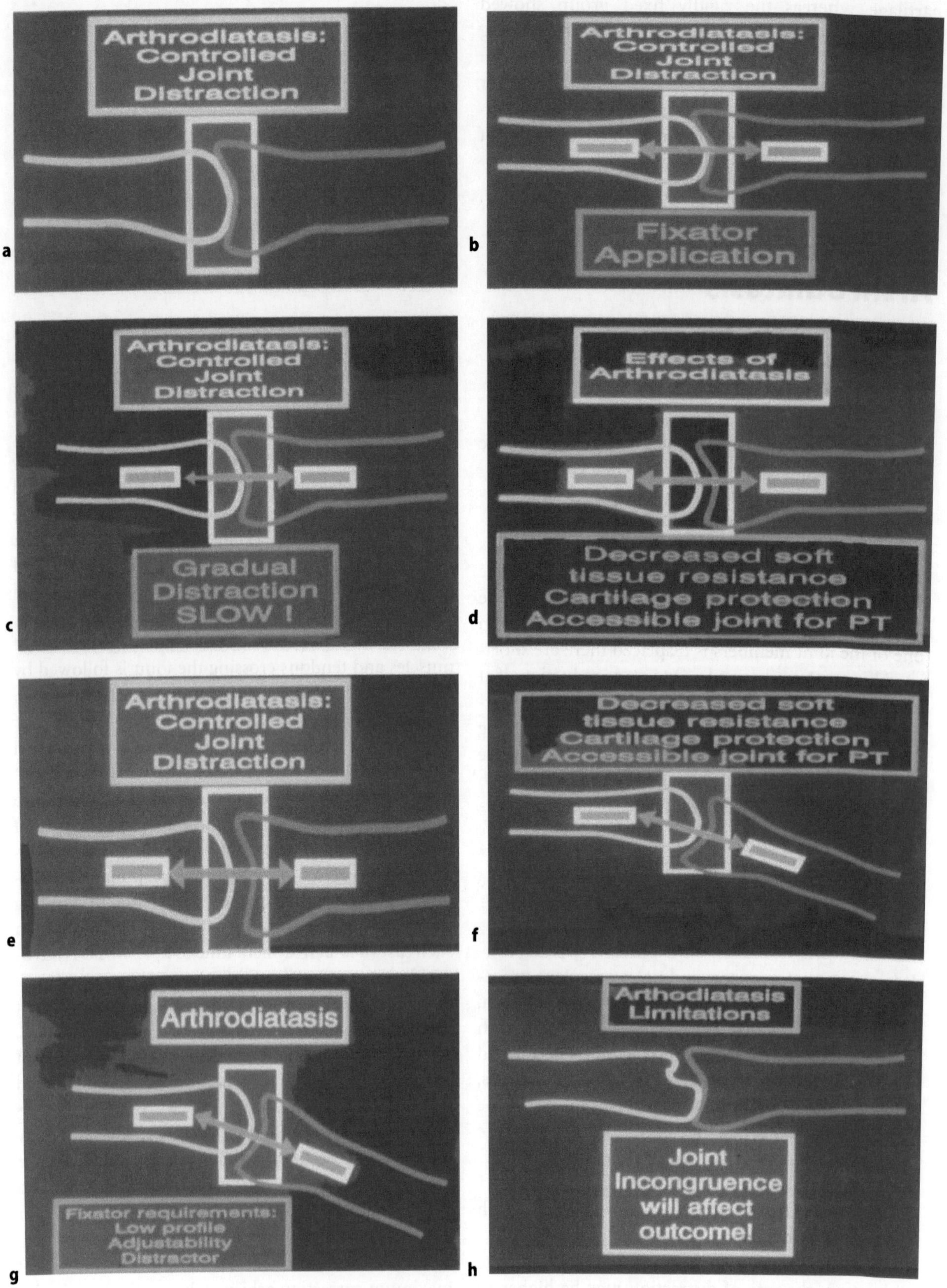

Fig. 54.5 a–h Principles of arthrodiatasis: Controlled joint distraction. (PT = physiotherapy)

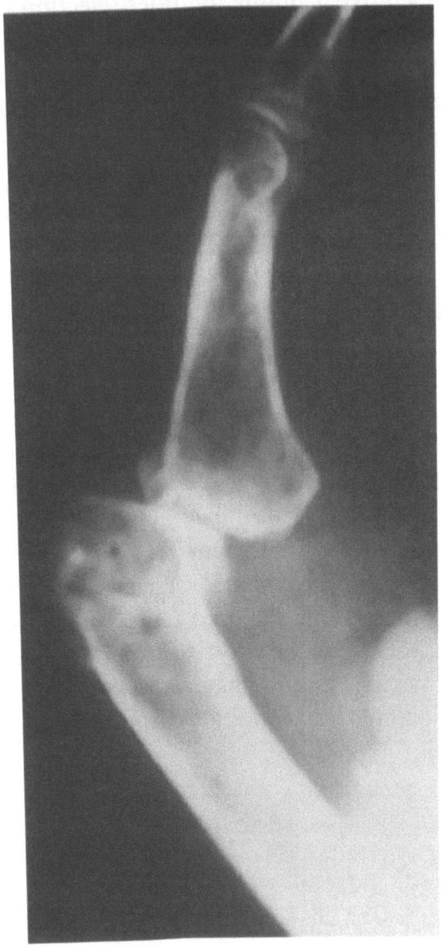

Fig. 54.6 Chronic subluxation in the metacarpo-phalangeal joint in the index finger. Note: narrow joint line in the remaining contact area as well as shortened ligaments on the dorsal side which are stretched, whereas the ligaments on the volar site are shortened.

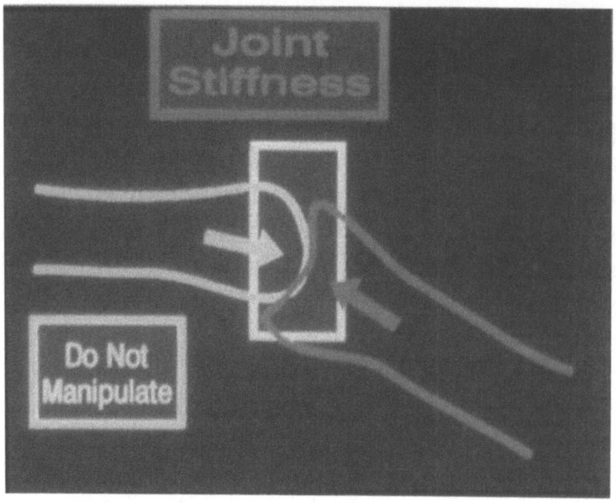

a

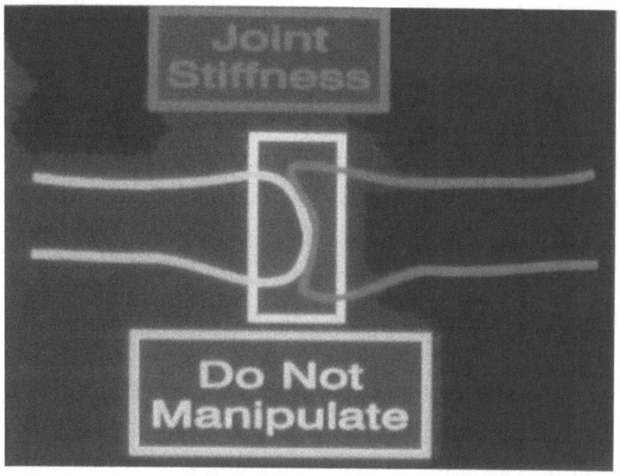

b

Fig. 54.8 a Manipulation under anaesthesia is not recommended in joint stiffness. **b** Forced manipulation will lead to undue stress on the cartilage surface and may damage the joint.

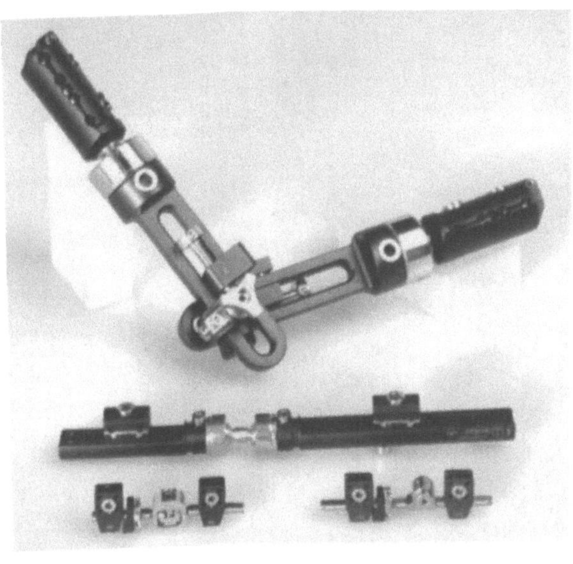

Fig. 54.7 Fixators used for arthrodiatasis: elbow fixator, wrist fixator, standard miniFixator, hinged miniFixator.

ments to relax and stretch overnight. Physiotherapy is continued from here during the next day. In a mixed flexion and extension contracture of the elbow we prefer to alternate, locking the fixator in maximum flexion on one night and in extension on the next.

We routinely administer indomethacin 50mg twice a day for 4–6 weeks provided there are no contraindications. Since nerve irritation is not uncommon at some stage, we also provide the vitamin B complex for the entire treatment period.

The fixator is usually removed 6–8 weeks after surgery but in slow responders or in cases with interposition arthroplasty and/or long standing problems, the fixator remains in situ for 9–12 weeks. During treatment the mechanical performance of the fixator is monitored, and lubrication of the device may be required.

The technique of arthrodiatasis is best employed in departments with ample experience in external fixation and joint reconstruction. It requires a team approach, careful evaluation and counselling of the patient and dedicated aftercare. The most important aspect, however, is to understand the patient's requirements and to analyze the particular reason why he or she is seeking an improved function of the joint. A sober approach when predicting the potential benefit will serve both the patient and the surgeon well. The patient will invariably have received prior physiotherapy and been through a variety of other conservative approaches before being seen in the department, with this as a last resort. A certain percentage of patients will have had mobilization under anaesthesia, which is never practised in our department. In arthrofibrosis with fibro-fatty tissue in the joint this may lead to avulsion of cartilage flakes as well as to undue loading of the articular surfaces in the presence of shortened ligaments (Fig. 54.8). There is no way to control these risks and we do not, therefore, advocate the use of mobilization under anaesthesia or physiotherapy under continuous brachial plexus anaesthesia.

Operative Technique

When using arthrodiatasis with external fixation a sound knowledge of the equipment used as well as the anatomical landmarks is mandatory. Without substantial experience in external fixation the learning curve will be frustrating for both patient and surgeon.

Pre-operative assessment will record the range of motion of all joints of both upper limbs. Measurement of grip strength may also be helpful. A full neurological examination including nerve conduction studies is mandatory, especially in the shoulder, the elbow and the wrist. Standard X-rays of both sides are taken to allow a comparison between affected and unaffected sides. In the shoulder and elbow CT-studies are carried out followed by an arthro-CT and an arthrogram (Fig. 54.9). The latter helps to assess the status of the joint capsule which in some cases may completely fail to extend when filled with a contrast medium. The CT-scan is used to identify an intra-articular malunion. Heterotopic bone formation is often present but will not necessarily be obstructing joint motion. If heterotopic ossification has led to bony bridges, these will need to be resected prior to joint distraction. Osteophytes, especially at the tip of the olecranon or on the coronoid process in the elbow joint, may be the mechanical reason for a loss of extension and/or flexion and again, the CT-scan will help to determine the need for their removal.

Pre-operative planning includes selection of screw sites as well as the positions of necessary incisions for removal of hardware or heterotopic bone. An open arthrolysis is not part of the technique but percutaneous lengthening of, for example, the triceps tendon may be required. An understanding of the underlying pathology is of the utmost importance for a successful operative approach in these cases.

Shoulder

Experience with arthrodiatasis in the shoulder is limited. Possible indications include acquired stiffness after trauma not responding to physiotherapy and arthroscopic debridement. Subluxation or displacement of the humeral head may be an indication. The true primary stiff shoulder may very well be an indication but its aetiology is controversial.

In addition to the standard radiographs described above, a Rockwood view to evaluate the subacromial space is necessary. MRI may also play a role in the study of pathological conditions around the shoulder.

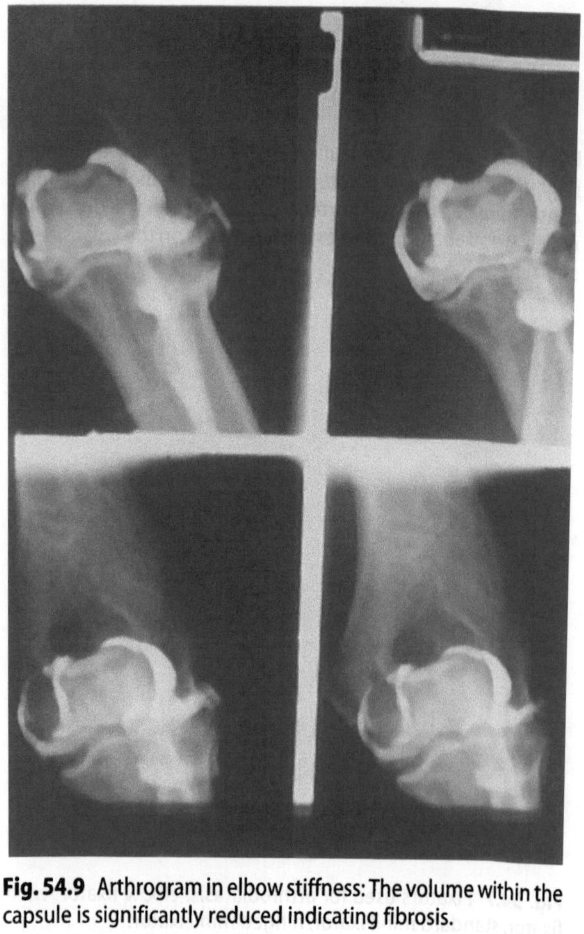

Fig. 54.9 Arthrogram in elbow stiffness: The volume within the capsule is significantly reduced indicating fibrosis.

Fixator application in the shoulder is anterior and an elbow fixator is used. The first screw is placed in an open fashion through the coracoid process (Fig. 54.10a). Good purchase can be expected provided the coracoid process is penetrated correctly by the screw. Predrilling with a 3.2mm drill and the use of a 4.5/3.5mm screw is advisable. If the coracoid process is large, a 6/5mm screw may be used after predrilling with a 4.8mm drill. The second screw, again inserted in a open fashion, is placed parallel to the glenoid articular surface at a safe distance from the capsule. The central connecting unit is placed as close to the shoulder joint as possible. A straight clamp or extended range clamp is employed and the elbow fixator attached to it. The screws for the distal clamp are placed at the insertion of the deltoid muscle, carefully avoiding transfixion of the muscle fibres. The arm is placed in 30° abduction but otherwise in a neutral position. Distraction starts during surgery and may be a repetitive process. The amount of fixator distraction is 15–25mm and widening of the joint space must be observed with the image intensifier (Fig. 54.10b) and documented post-operatively. It may be necessary to redistract in the post-operative phase. The relaxation phase will be closer to 10 than to 6 days in most cases. Shoulder mobility may be tested in the conscious patient after the relaxion phase is over and for this purpose the central connecting unit and the medial ball joint are unlocked. The fixator body may be removed during the second phase of mobilization to allow physiotherapy to gain more motion. In the shoulder application, total fixator time should not exceed 6 weeks (Fig. 54.10c).

Only a few cases have been treated in this way and the technique must therefore be used with caution. It is not suitable for the unstable shoulder, but may help to augment other procedures aiming at regaining stability of the joint. It may also help supplement a corrective osteotomy in order to regain joint alignment.

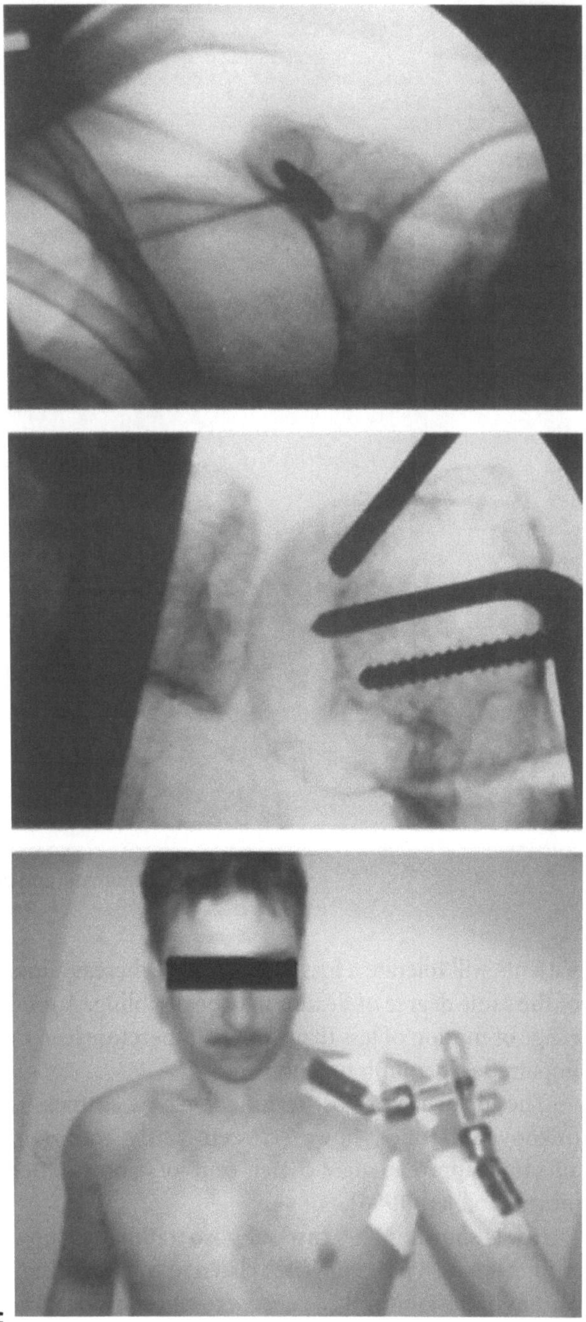

a

b

c

Fig. 54.10 **a** Insertion of a 4.5/3.5mm screw in the coracoid process of the scapula. **b** Joint distraction to facilitate derotational osteotomy in posterior subluxation of a shoulder joint. **c** Fixator application in a shoulder.

Elbow

To make use of the unique upper limb, elbow function requires a stable and pain-free joint with an adequate range of motion. Elbow motion has been investigated in healthy volunteers and 90 per cent of daily living activities could be carried out in an arc of motion between 30 and 130° of extension and flexion. Pro- and supination of 50° in each case was also required. The functions studied included sports and work activities (Morrey and Chao 1976). In elbow stiffness most

	Non-traumatic stiffness (with no progressive local trauma)		Post-traumatic stiffness (outcome of local trauma)
Extra-articular	Neuromuscular diseases	Extra-articular	Muscular retraction (Volkman's contracture)
	Spasticity (spastic palsy)		
	Muscle imbalance		Myotendinous adhesions
	(outcome of obstetric palsy)		sequel to humerus fractures
	Ossifications		iatrogenic
	Cranial trauma/long-term coma		Skin retraction
	Ossifying myositis		burns
	Skin retraction		retracted scars
	epidermolysis		Ossification of extra-capsular tissues
	bullous		Secondary degenerative arthritis
	Multifactorial causes		Capsular retraction
	arthrogryposis		sequel to dislocation
	dermatosclerosis		outcome of epiphyseal fracture
Articular	Primary degenerative arthritis	Articular	Articular incongruence
	Synovial chondromatosis		articular fractures
	Rheumatic proliferative synovitis		incongruity of articular surfaces
	Pigmented villonodular synovitis		sequel to long-term dislocation
	Haemophilic arthropathy		osteochrondral free bodies
	Infected arthritis or its outcome		Capsular ossification

Table 54.2 Non traumatic and post-traumatic stiffness in the elbow

patients will tolerate a loss of extension whereas a loss of the same degree of flexion may be disabling. A total range of motion of less than 100° will therefore lead to impaired upper limb function.

The incidence of post-traumatic elbow stiffness is unknown. It does, however, seem fairly common, affecting approximately 5 per cent of elbows after injury (Sojbjerg 1996).

It was shown in 200 cases of post-traumatic elbow stiffness that 38 per cent were related to fracture dislocations of the joint and 20 per cent to elbow dislocation (Mohan 1972). Radial head fractures accounted for 10 per cent of the cases. The injury pattern itself is only one aspect in the development of post-traumatic stiffness; prolonged immobilization also seems to be an important factor, and the elbow joint should not, in our opinion, be immobilized for longer than 6 days.

Post-traumatic elbow stiffness is best classified according to the position of the contracture as extension or flexion stiffness, and an assessment of the function of adjacent joints (shoulder and wrist) is also required. The causes of post-traumatic stiffness can be divided into articular and extra-articular. Mixed pathology is, however, often the reason for limitation of elbow function. Extra-articular causes include muscular and skin retraction, fibrosis of ligaments and capsule and heterotopic bone formation with bony bridging of the joint. Intra-articular causes include obliteration of the joint with fibro-fatty tissue and articular incongruence with secondary degenerative arthritis (Table 54.2).

Pre-operative evaluation includes a detailed history of the aetiology of the disability and a full clinical examination. When moving the elbow into maximal flexion and extension, gliding of the joint must be palpated. Plain radiographs are necessary and an arthrogram helps to evaluate the remaining joint space. A CT scan and an arthro-CT (Fig. 54.9) are also required. The CT helps to decide whether heterotopic bone formation is present and whether it limits function mechanically. MRI does not seem to be helpful. Diagnostic arthroscopy as a routine measure is not recommended since the joint is tight and iatrogenic injuries of the cartilage may result.

Ulnar, radial and median nerve function should be studied pre-operatively using nerve conduction tests. The ulnar nerve is especially vulnerable on increased flexion in cases where a lack of motion has persisted for a prolonged period, and decompression is recommended.

Before operative procedures are carried out on an elbow with limited motion conservative measures such as physiotherapy and dynamic splinting should be exhausted. We do not advocate manipulation under anaesthesia or a continuous brachial plexus block. This may cause intra-articular damage by avulsion of cartilage fragments when the fibro-fatty tissue which lines the joint ruptures.

While release operations have been described in the literature (Urbaniak et al 1985; Morrey 1990; Sojbjerg 1996) distraction arthroplasty has not been used routinely, and was first described some years ago (Volkov and Oganesian 1975). Since that time limited series have been published (Deland et al 1987; Judet and Judet 1978; Regan and Reilly 1990; Regan et al 1991; McKee et al 1998).

The key to application of the elbow fixator is proper identification of the rotational axis of the humero-ulnar joint. The patient is positioned supine and a hand table is used. A tourniquet is not applied. With the shoulder in internal rotation, the elbow is placed on its medial side. It should be supported by a rolled up towel so that a true lateral view of the elbow joint can be obtained with the image intensifier. The operation must not commence before the image shown in Fig. 54.11a is visible on the image intensifier screen. A 2mm × 150mm Kirschner-wire is used and its tip is placed on the proximal border of the circle (Fig. 54.11b). When distracting along the axis of the humerus the central connecting unit will move distally into the centre of rotation, and prior to distraction along the humeral link the 2mm Kirschner-wire must be removed. The K-wire is drilled through the lateral condyle in the direction of the X-ray beam. The power drill is disconnected and the position of the K-wire is checked. Provided that the point of entry is at the proximal point of the circle, the K-wire can now be bent until the part protruding from the skin is parallel to the rotational axis (Fig. 54.11.c and 54.12a, b). This avoids repeated placement of the wire. With the K-wire in the correct position, the fixator is now used as its own template (Fig. 54.13) and the humeral screws are inserted first.

Placement of the humeral screws and ulnar screws follows the procedure described in Ch. 14.

The main benefit of distraction arthroplasty is lengthening of the inevitably shortened ligaments and fibrotic capsule (Fig. 54.14a, b). At the same time the humero-ulnar and humero-radial joint surfaces will be separated and this helps to protect the cartilage. If the joint is stiff and tight, closed manipulation may lead to excessive loading of the remaining cartilage and further damage to the articular structures may be expected. Since shortening of the ligaments and capsule occurs over a period of time, the reversal of this process (arthrodiatasis) should also be slow. Simultaneous distraction along the humeral and ulnar links will result in symmetrical distraction of the joint and avoid impingement of either the olecranon or the coronoid process on the capitulum humeri (Fig. 54.15a–c).

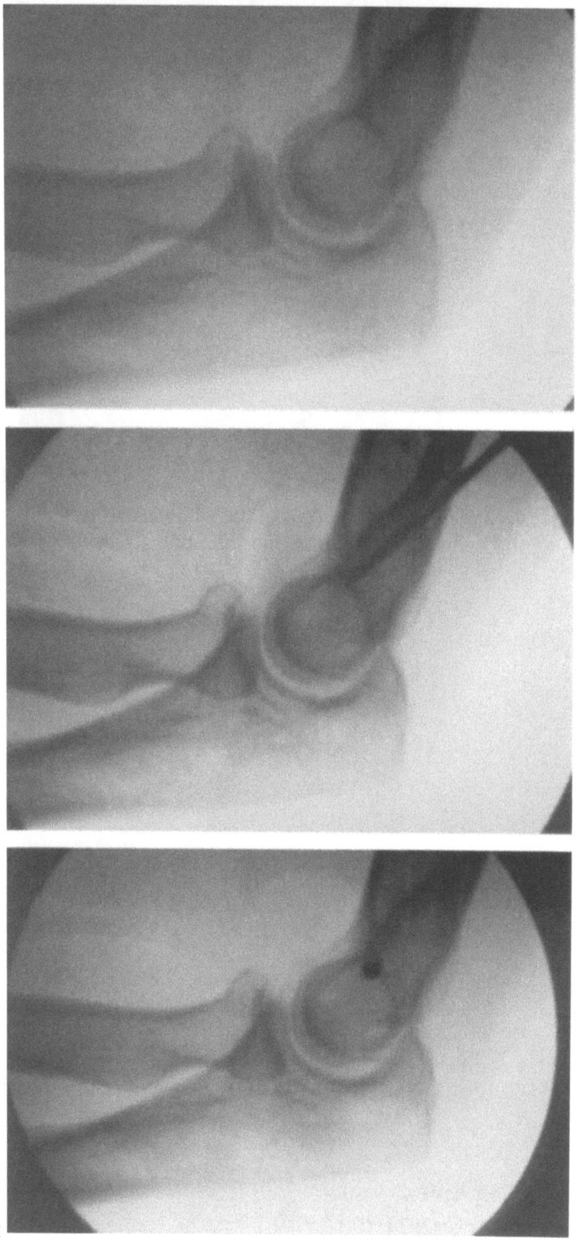

a b c

Fig. 54.11 **a** Ideal lateral image of the elbow prior to insertion of the 2mm K-wire. **b** The tip of the K-wire pointing at the proximal border of the circle. **c** Correct proximal positioning of the K-wire to allow joint distraction.

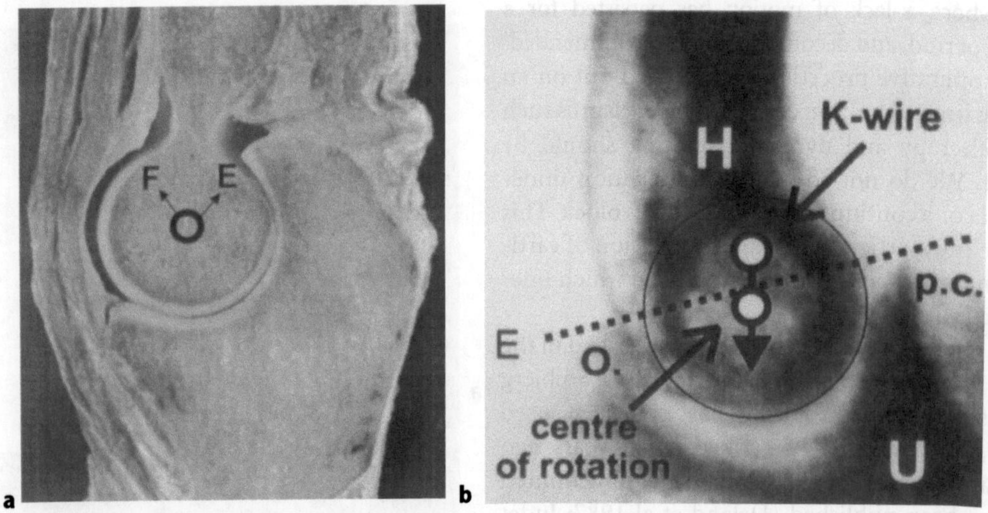

Fig. 54.12 **a** The rotational axis of the elbow illustrated in a sagittal cross-section, F = flexion, E = extension. **b** When using the humeral distractor the position of the K-wire will shift from the proximal border of the ring structure to the centre of

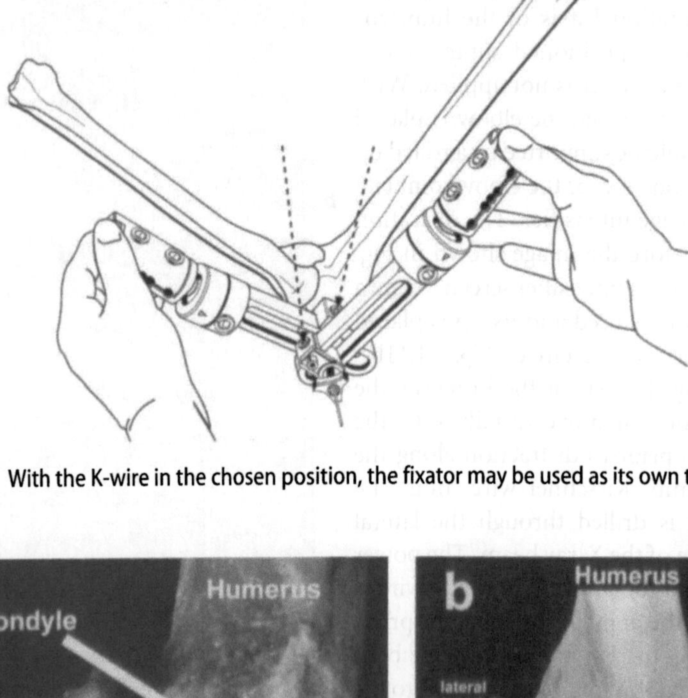

Fig. 54.13 With the K-wire in the chosen position, the fixator may be used as its own template.

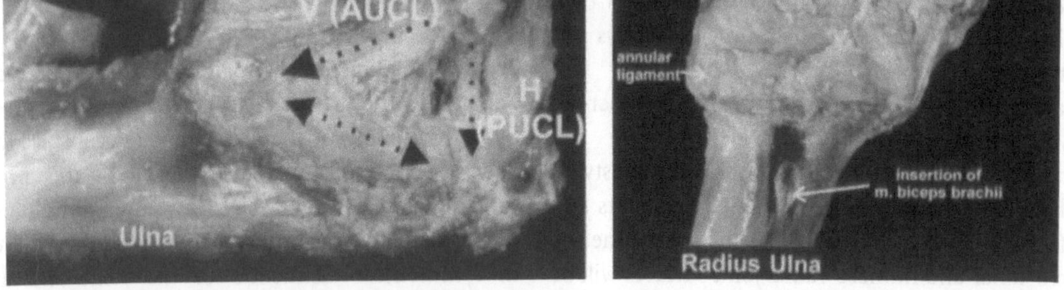

Fig. 54.14 **a** Ligament attachment on the medial side of the humerus. AUCL = anterior ulnar collateral ligament, PUCL = posterior ulnar collateral ligament. **b** Anterior aspect of joint capsule and annular ligament in the elbow.

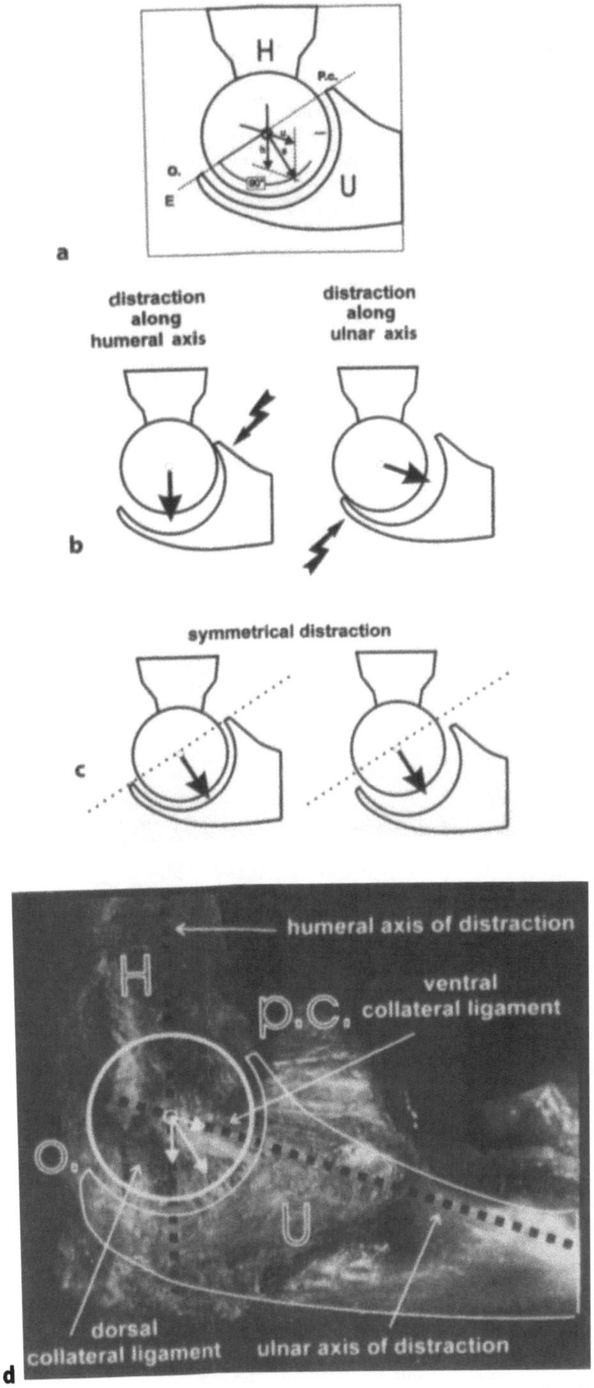

Fig. 54.15 a Simultaneous humeral and ulnar distraction leads to symmetrical distraction of the humero-ulnar joint (H-Humerus, U-Ulna, O-Olecranon, E-Plane of distraction, P.c. Coronoid process). **b** Distraction along the humeral axis alone leads to impingement of the coronoid process (left), distraction along the ulnar axis alone to impingement of the olecranon process (right). **c** Symmetrical distraction leads to widening of the joint without impingement. **d** Lateral view of the humero-ulnar joint. The dotted lines indicate the axis of the humerus (H) and the ulna (U). Distraction along the ulnar line lengthens the ventral ulnar collateral ligament; along the humeral link the dorsal ulnar collateral ligament is lengthened. (P.C.) coronoid process; (O) olecranon.

The total degree of distraction depends on the resistance of the soft tissues and the humeral distractor is turned a total of 10–12 times (= 10–12mm) (Fig. 54.16) while the ulnar distractor is turned 3–5 times (= 3–5mm) clockwise.

In most cases with significant stiffness the capacity of the elbow fixator to distract may not be sufficient. In these cases we insert the fixator pins as described above into the humerus and the ulna. A standard Orthofix fixator or a short Orthofix fixator placed on the humeral pins is used with two additional pins in a T-clamp inserted in the olecranon (Fig. 54.17a–d).

It is important to align the elbow fixator prior to applying the distraction fixator and to mark the fixator clamp positions on the humeral and ulnar screws. All components of the elbow fixator with the exception of the clamp cover screws must be left locked when temporarily removing the device to apply the distraction fixator. We prefer postero-lateral pin insertion into the olecranon for better purchase and better visualization of joint distraction in the lateral view. Standard compression–distraction units are used in these cases and we distract and redistract 10–15mm over a minimum of 30 minutes. The standard fixator is then removed and the elbow fixator applied. With the elbow fixator mounted, distraction along the humeral and the ulnar links is performed as described above. Radiographic control of joint distraction is mandatory prior to moving the elbow into flexion and extension (Fig. 54.17e–g). This movement is performed exerting gentle force, aiming for 100° of total motion. After

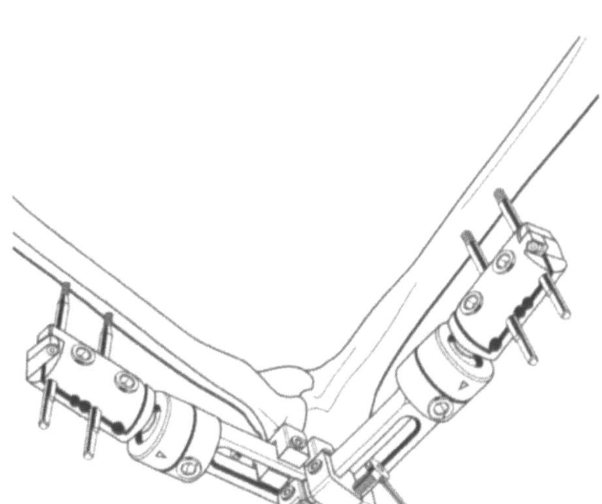

Fig. 54.16 A small distractor placed on the humeral link. This will shift the axis and requires the K-wire (and therefore the central connecting unit) to be placed approximately 7mm proximal to the ideal centre of rotation prior to distraction.

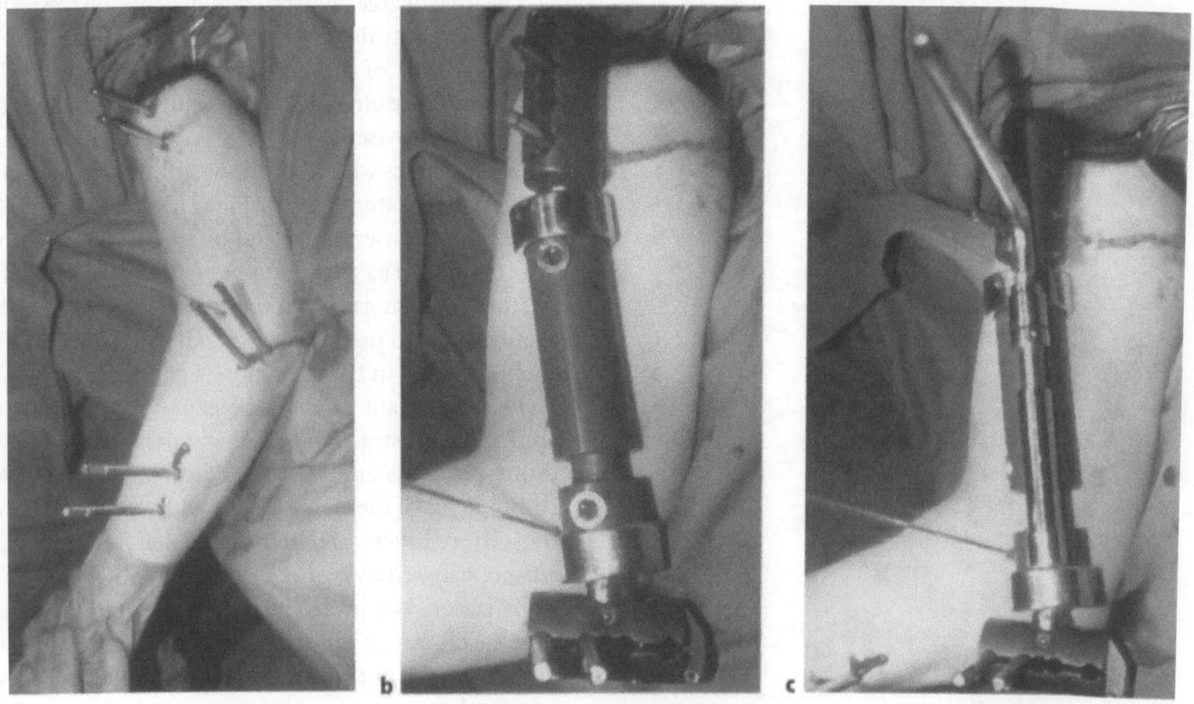

a b c

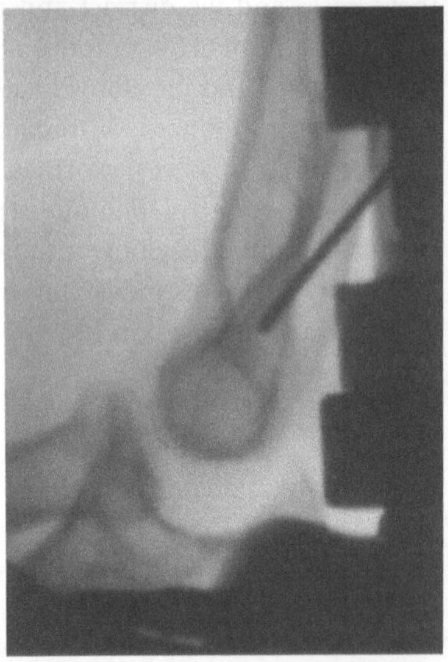

d

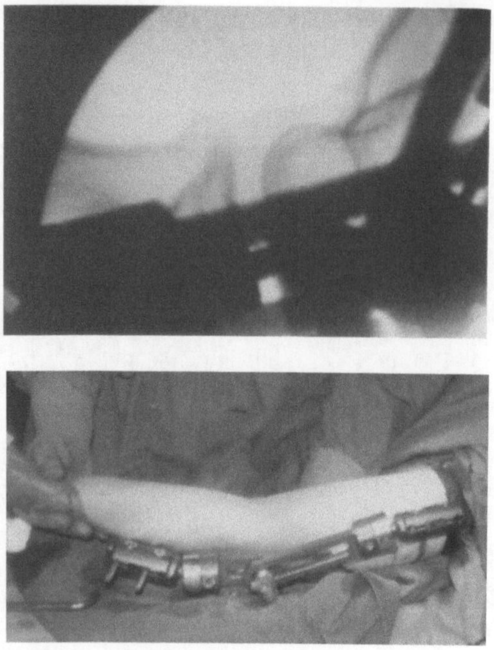

e g

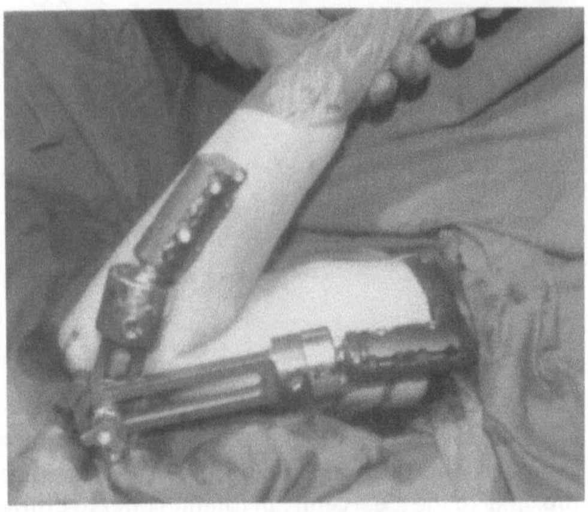

f

Fig. 54.17 **a** Use of a standard Orthofix fixator in a case of significant stiffness. The fixator is mounted proximally on the humeral screws used for the elbow fixator and distally on two 4.5/3.5mm screws placed in the olecranon slightly obliquely to allow visualization of the joint. **b** The fixator in place. **c** Use of a standard compression–distraction unit to widen the joint (12–15mm). **d** Effect of distraction on a humero-ulnar joint. **e** After reapplication of the elbow fixator distraction along the humeral and ulnar link is performed. This widens the space between the radial head and the capitulum humeri. **f** Flexion after distraction, small distractors removed. **g** Extension after distraction, small distractors removed.

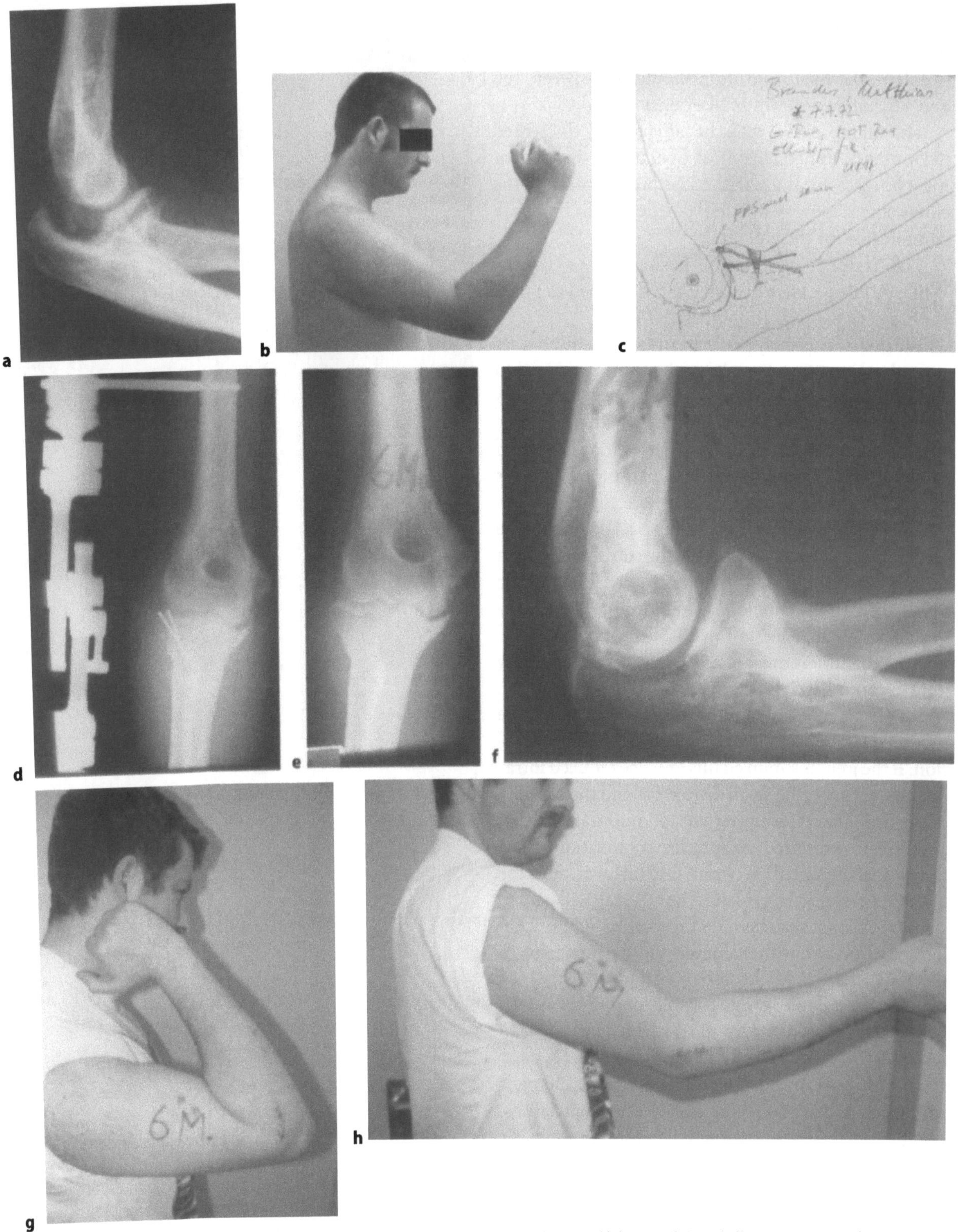

Fig. 54.18 **a** Chronic subluxation 9 months after trauma in a 25-year-old manual labourer. **b** Fixed elbow position in this patient. **c** Pre-operative planning for corrective osteotomy of the subcapital radial head with bone grafting and fixation. **d** Post-operative AP film. Notice the widening of the joint. **e** AP film 6 months post-operatively. **f** Lateral film 6 months after correction and removal of osteosynthetic material from the radial head. Correct alignment of the joint. **g** Flexion 6 months after operation. **h** Extension 6 months after operation.

intra-operative movement under anaesthesia the fixator is locked. If a lack of flexion was the main problem, the fixator position should be between 100 and 120° of flexion from full extension.

The ulnar nerve may be affected by increased flexion and immediately post-operatively the patient must be assessed. If dysaesthesia is present, placing the elbow in a more extended position will be more comfortable for the patient.

The fixator remains in this position for 6–10 days. While intra-operative distraction is described as phase 1, phase 2 is the relaxation phase.

We do not routinely perform any soft tissue releases since the distraction capacity of the fixator will lead to elongation of the shortened structures. CT studies including an arthro-CT will indicate whether the joint space is obliterated by bony fragments which have then to be removed through a limited arthrotomy. This is particularly important in cases where the olecranon fossa shows bony apposition. If this is not removed the olecranon will not glide into the olecranon fossa during extension. On the anterior side heterotopic bone formation should be removed when bony bridging is established in the CT-scan. Intra-articular fracture malunion must be evaluated. Since the elbow joint is a non-weightbearing joint only a malunion which affects movement of the olecranon process, the coronoid process and/or the radial head requires revision. If the joint is subluxed this must be reduced intra-operatively using the small distractors and the capacity of the ball joints. It is important to understand that in addition to posterior or anterior subluxation, rotational malalignment between the forearm and the humerus may also be present. The CT-scan will help to assess rotational malalignment. Posterior subluxation is often associated with malunion and/or shortening of the radial head and the proximal radius. This may require correction to create a stable joint (Fig. 54.18).

The relaxation phase for the distracted ligaments to respond to forces applied to them lasts 6–10 days. From post-operative day 1 indomethacin 2 × 50mg is administered provided there are no contraindications. This helps to avoid formation of heterotopic bone. We do not routinely use radiotherapy. Phase 3, the mobilization phase, commences on the completion of phase 2, with the central connecting unit unlocked.

The patient will require physiotherapy 2–3 times per day and cryotherapy is used prior to physiotherapy. Analgesics may also be required prior to the physiotherapy session, but we do not advocate the use of continuous brachial plexus anaesthesia. The elbow fixator central connecting unit is locked overnight and we alternate the position between the maximum

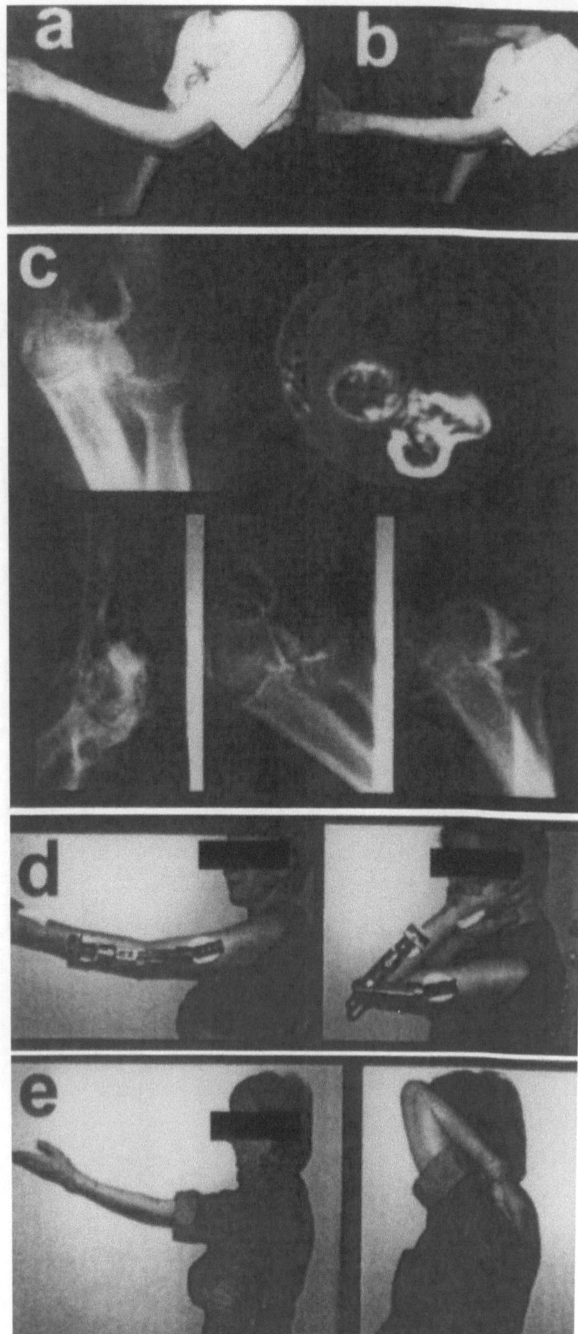

Fig. 54.19 a, b Maximal extension and maximal flexion in a 30-year-old woman having suffered a posterior radial dislocation. **c** The arthrogram indicates an abnormal joint space and arthrofibrosis. **d** Extension/flexion with the fixator in situ after two weeks. **e** Extension/flexion two weeks after fixator removal.

flexion achieved during physiotherapy and maximum extension. A protocol is helpful to make sure that the elbow will remain in maximum flexion one night and in maximum extension the next (Fig. 54.19). The ulnar nerve should be monitored carefully and any loss of motor function may need urgent intervention. We do not, however, suggest anterior transposition. Nerve conduction studies may be required to monitor the ulnar nerve during the mobilization phase.

To increase flexion and/or extension the standard compression–distraction unit is inserted into the cams of the fixator. By turning the compression–distraction screw clockwise at a rate of 1–4mm (1–4 full turns) per day the elbow will move into flexion (Fig. 54.20a). Counterclockwise turns with the compression–distraction unit will move the elbow into extension. To straighten the elbow fixator out fully, spacers are used to reach maximal extension (Fig. 54.20b).

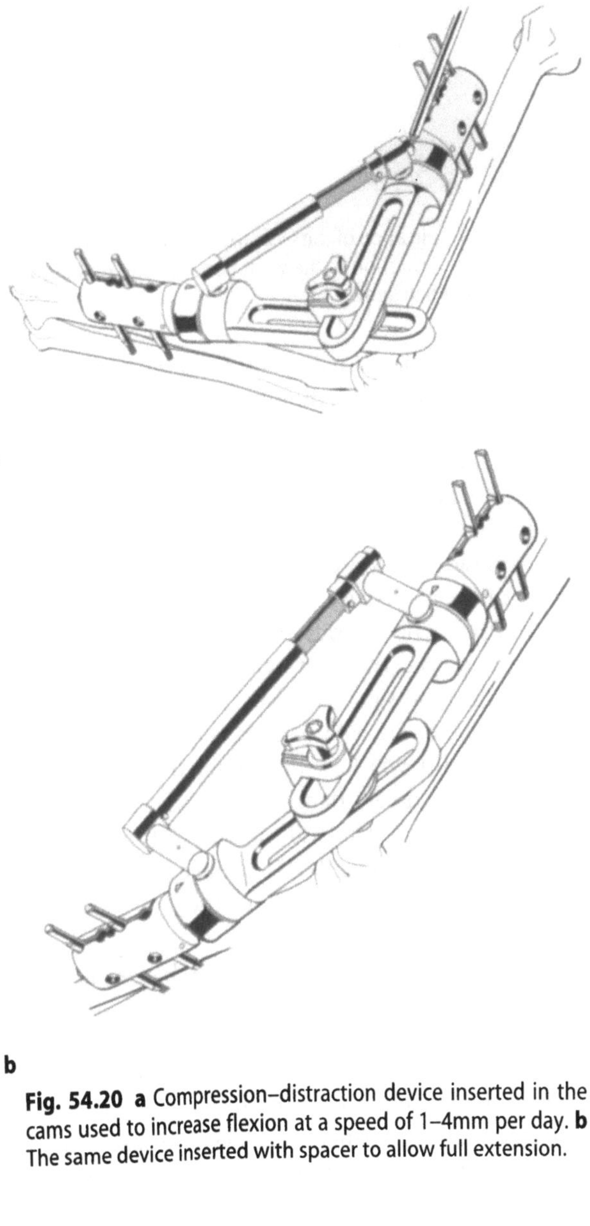
a
b

Fig. 54.20 a Compression–distraction device inserted in the cams used to increase flexion at a speed of 1–4mm per day. b The same device inserted with spacer to allow full extension.

The use of mechanical distraction or compression should never be too vigorous, and the patient's response should be carefully monitored. It must never be used alone but should be supplemented with active and passive physiotherapy.

X-ray control is carried out post-operatively and thereafter every other week. The fixator remains in situ for six weeks and a longer period may be required if the response is slow. The target is 100° of motion and flexion is more important than extension.

Pin site care is identical to the procedure described for acute cases. See Ch. 11.

The successful use of arthrodiatasis in elbow stiffness requires considerable clinical experience and is best performed in centres with an appropriate case load. The patient should be informed what to expect from the procedure. To achieve a satisfactory result, patient selection is important. Of equal importance is the post-operative management which ideally is carried out in the department performing the operation. The same holds true for pin site care and the department must be familiar with external fixation procedures in reconstructive cases.

Wrist

In the wrist, post-traumatic stiffness is not uncommon. Failure to respond to physiotherapy and loss of useful wrist motion are indications for intervention.

Extra-articular causes of stiffness include burns and tendon adhesions. Tendon problems may in addition require tenolysis, whereas contractures due to burns may respond to slow distraction with a fixator alone.

Extra-articular radial malunion should be corrected first if the degree of malunion merits an operative intervention. Corrective osteotomy of the distal radius is described in Ch. 16. The most common indication for arthrodiatasis is intra-articular joint stiffness with the wrist in normal alignment and not requiring any bony correction. This is not uncommonly encountered in cases of distal radius fractures with prolonged immobilization. Arthrodiatasis should not be used in cases with a history of algodystrophy or in patients who may develop this condition.

The Pennig II wrist fixator with a compression–distraction module on the metacarpal side and a gliding module on the radial side is used (Fig. 54.7). The fixator is applied strictly in the frontal (coronal) plane and the distal ball joint must be aligned with the so-called centre of rotation, the lunate-capitate joint line.

For the successful application of this technique, the individual characteristics of each case must be taken into account. Brachial plexus anaesthesia or general anaesthesia is recommended. A tourniquet may be used. Pre-operative preparation of the arm includes shaving of the skin surfaces and washing of both the forearm and the hand with a non-coloured disinfectant.

A hand table is used. The forearm is placed in neutral rotation. The fixator is applied to the second metacarpal and the middle/distal third of the radius in the frontal (coronal) place. The detailed application technique is described in Ch. 16.

An image intensifier should be used to verify the position of the screws and penetration of the far cortex by all four screws when they have been introduced. The screws should not be advanced too far; due to their tapered design, they will become loose if they are backed out.

The fixator should be fully assembled exactly as shown in Fig. 54.21. It is essential that the dot on the cam is facing the threaded neck before each security collar is tightened. Failure to follow this procedure exactly may result in loosening of the collars. The collars are now screwed home fully and, with all other screws loosened, the fixator is applied to the bone screws already in situ, positioning it at a distance of 15–20mm from the skin.

The distal ball joint is exactly aligned with the lunate-capitate joint line (Fig. 54.22).

If there is no joint subluxation, distraction is performed intra-operatively. The target is to achive a joint space twice the normal, intra-operatively (Fig.

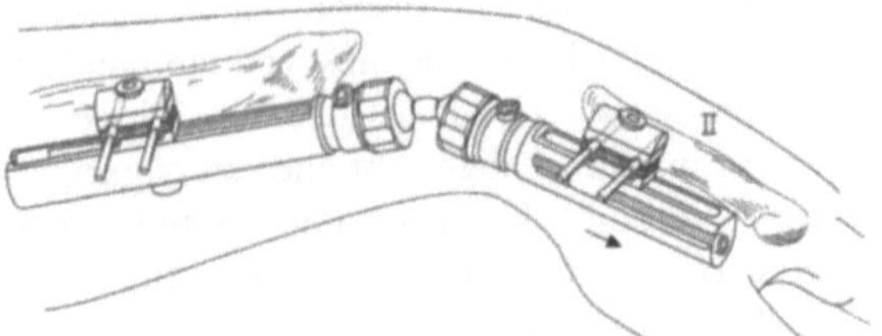

Fig. 54.21 Wrist fixator with long module (left) and compression–distraction module (right).

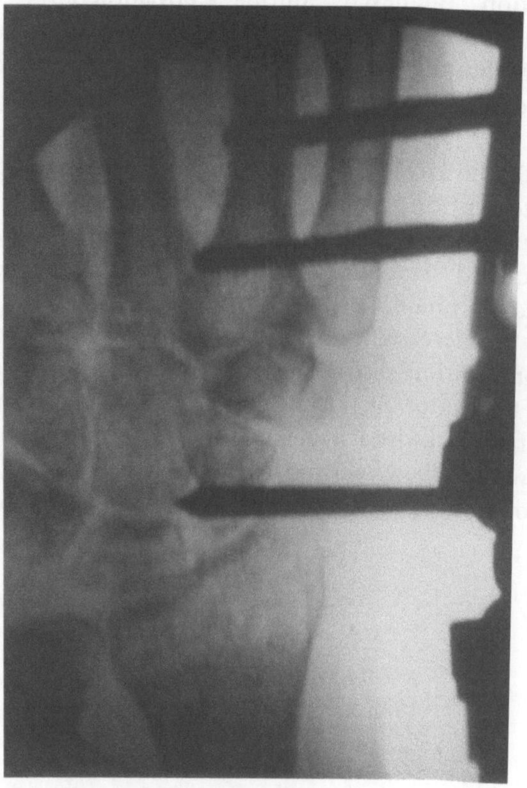

Fig. 54.22 Application of the wrist fixator. Alignment of the so-called centre of rotation of the wrist (lunate-capitate joint line) with the distal ball joint.

54.23). The patient's pain response after waking from anaesthesia is carefully monitored and if MP and PIP joint stiffness develop or significant swelling of the dorsum of the hand is visible, distraction must be reduced. One full turn of the compression–distraction module screw counterclockwise equals 1mm. After a few days redistraction may be performed, and the final width of the joint space should not exceed three times the normal. The relaxation phase lasts 10 days and mobilization is carried out by unlocking the distal ball joint. If the most significant loss of motion is extension (Fig. 54.24a, b; Fig. 5425a–h) as is often the case, the physiotherapist will lock the fixator overnight in the position of maximal extension achieved during the last session of the day. This will further assist in stretching the strong volar ligaments. If loss of flexion is the main problem the wrist will be maintained in flexion overnight.

We agree with Palmer and Nelson that extension is more important than flexion, whereas Ryu seems to feel that both extension and flexion are equally important (Table 54.3). In the second mobilization phase, during the last two weeks the fixator should remain unlocked and the patient instructed to take a more active role in mobilizing the wrist. Fixator application

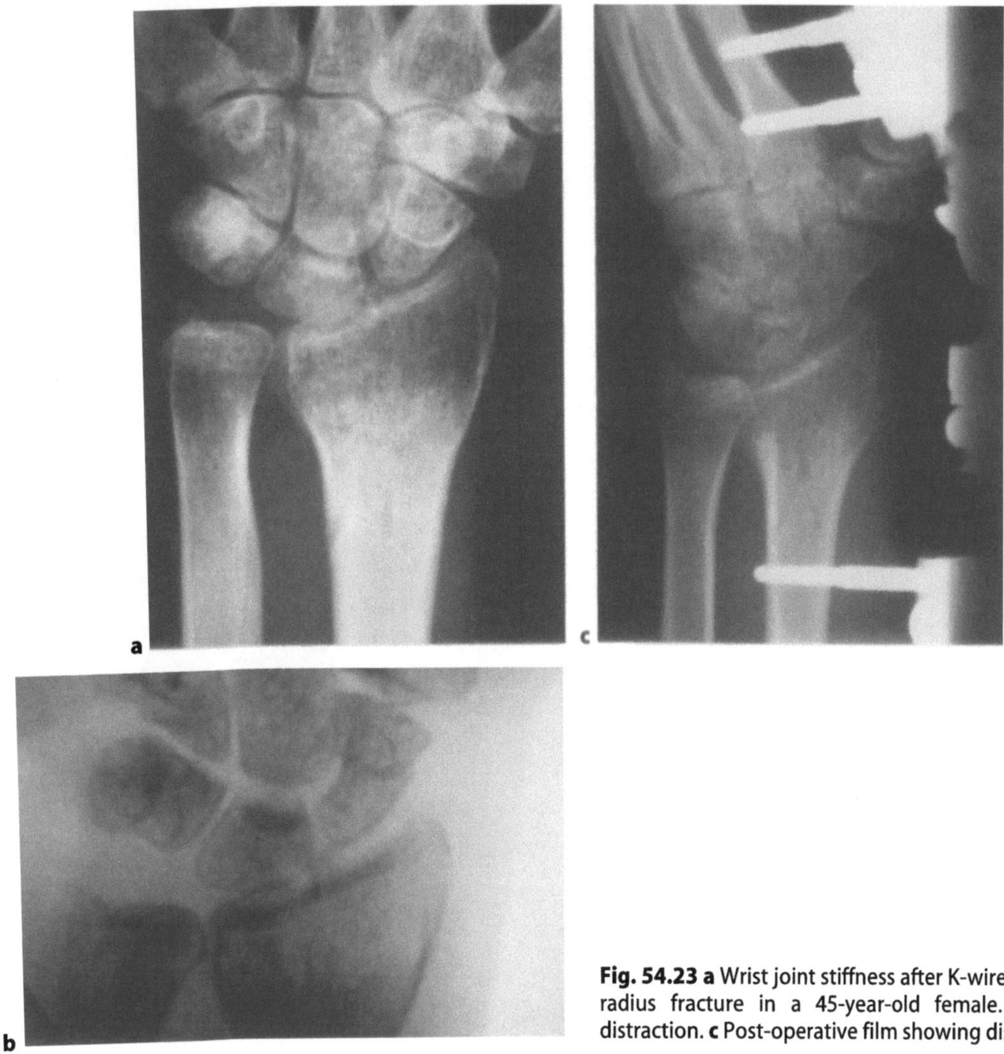

a

c

b

Fig. 54.23 **a** Wrist joint stiffness after K-wire fixation of a distal radius fracture in a 45-year-old female. **b** Intraoperative distraction. **c** Post-operative film showing distracted joint.

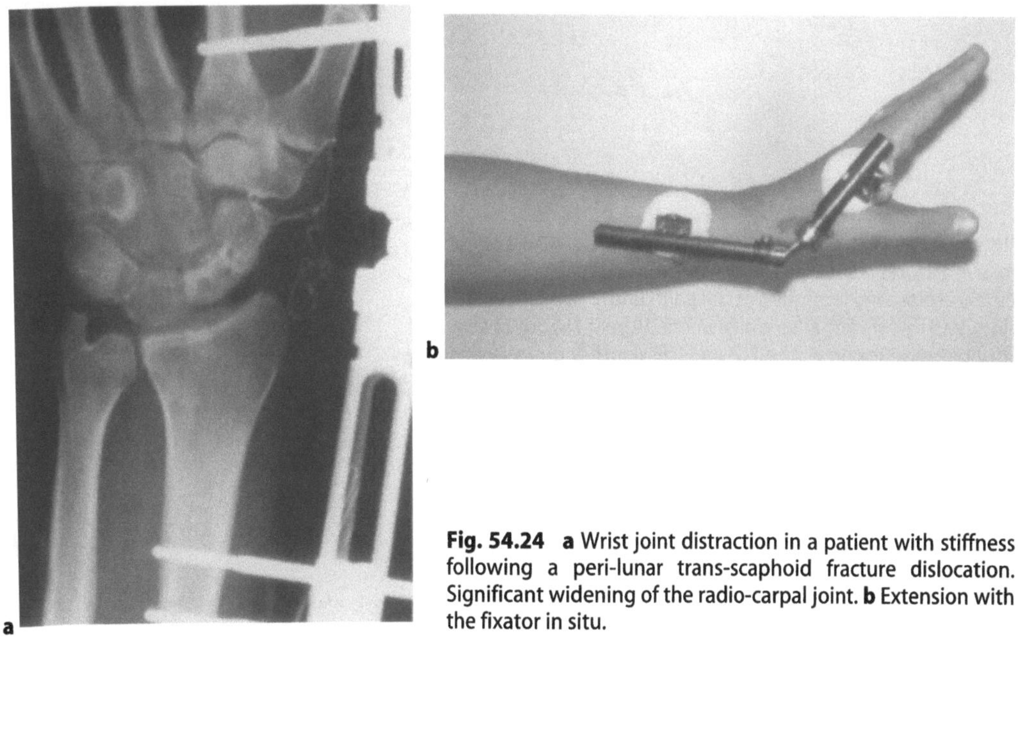

b

a

Fig. 54.24 **a** Wrist joint distraction in a patient with stiffness following a peri-lunar trans-scaphoid fracture dislocation. Significant widening of the radio-carpal joint. **b** Extension with the fixator in situ.

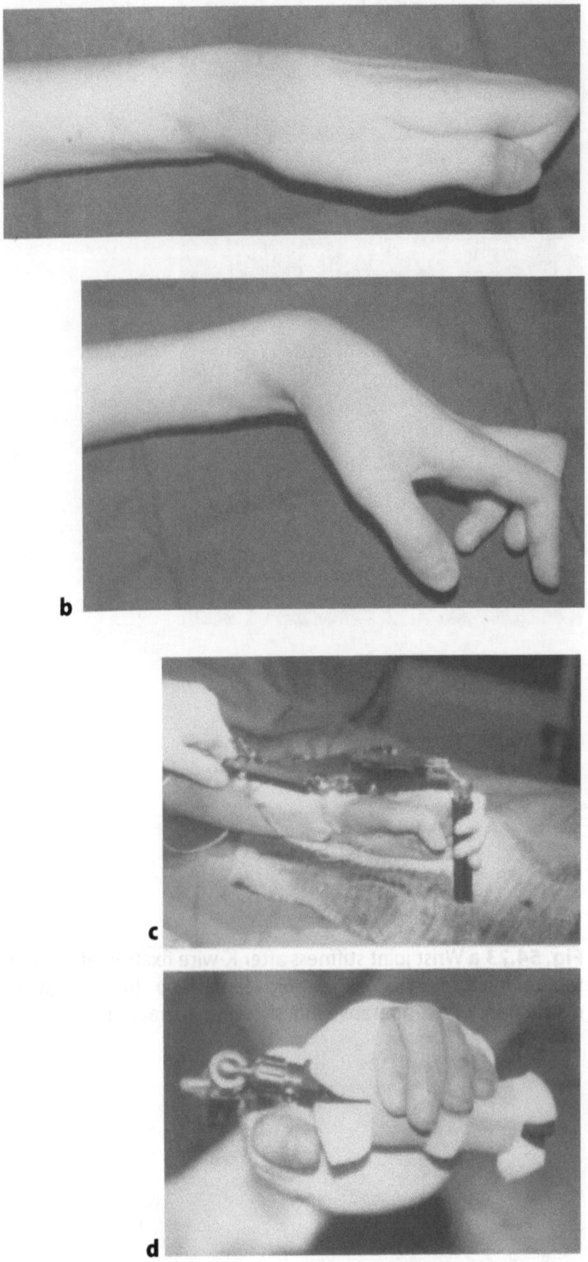

a b c d

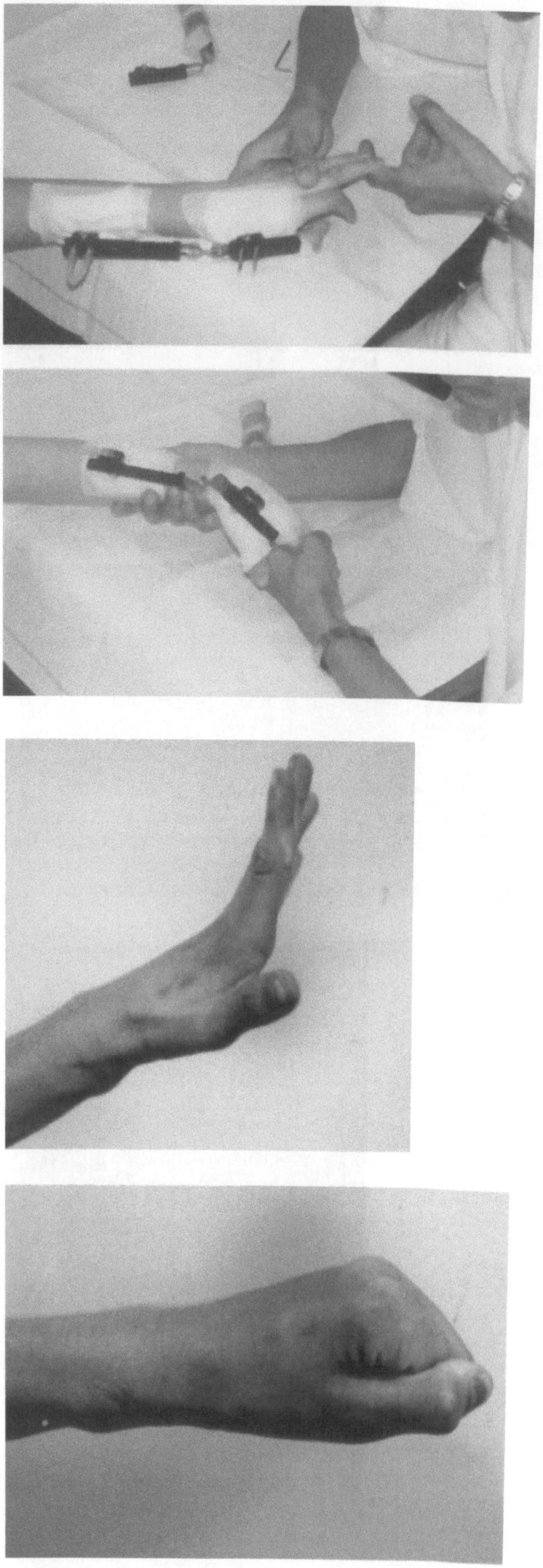

e f g h

Fig. 54.25 **a** One year after a complete laceration of the volar structures (tendons and nerves just proximal to the wrist joint and a second laceration in the palm of the hand involving index and middle finger tendons) in this 10 year old boy, a claw position with flexion of the PIP and DIP joints is observed on extension of the wrist. **b** When the wrist is flexed maximum extension in MP and PIP joints is shown. **c** The wrist joint was distracted and tenolysis and neurolysis performed at wrist and palm levels. A second fixator was attached to the metacarpal screws to support the fingers. **d** Padding of the second fixator to allow access to the fingers for physiotherapy. **e** Physiotherapy on the finger joints. Note that the second fixator is removed temporarily and will be re-applied at the end of the session to secure the movement gained during physiotherapy. **f** After unlocking the distal ball joint movement of the wrist joint with physiotherapy. **g** Extension and **h** flexion of the fingers one year after surgery.

times should not exceed six weeks in these cases.

In acute fractures, overdistraction of the wrist joint must be avoided since it may trigger algodystrophy. In the chronic situation described above this risk is much less, but careful supervision is required to detect early signs of algodystrophy.

Hand

In the MP and PIP joints, it is particularly important to establish the cause of finger stiffness. Arthrodiatasis will only solve intra-articular and periarticular (ligaments and capsule) problems, retractile scars and skin adhesions. It will not help to treat the sequelae of injuries of flexor or extensor tendons and pronounced arthritic changes not will respond favourably to the technique.

	Palmer (1985)	Nelson (1990)	Ryu (1991)
Flexion (Fl)	5°	28°	40°
Extension (Ex)	30°	37°	40°
RD	10°	12°	10°
UD	15°	27°	30°

RD: radial deviation. UD: ulnar deviation

A hypermobile patient may complain of wrist stiffness although his ROM is still within normal limits. A stiff wrist may be fixed in Fl, Ex, RD, UD: the most cumbersome position is a wrist in a flexed or radially-deviated position as the grip position is in extension and ulnar deviation.

Table 54.3 Useful wrist range of motion

Metacarpophalangeal and Interphalangeal Joints

A normal metacarpophalangeal joint will show increased joint space under manual distraction (Fig. 54.26a–c). If rotational malalignment is present in an MP or IP joint it must be detected pre-operatively (Fig. 54.27) since it is important in terms of placement of the threaded wires. Step one consists of application of a standard MiniFixator with 2mm threaded wires. In stiffness of metacarpophalangeal joint II the first fixator is applied from the dorso-ulnar side, whereas in cases involving the fifth finger this fixator is mounted

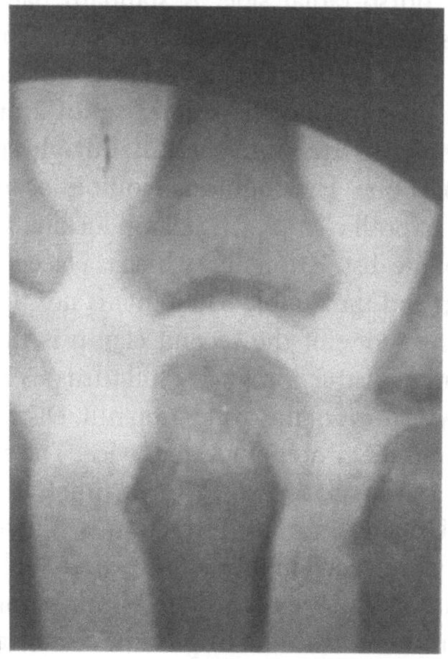

a

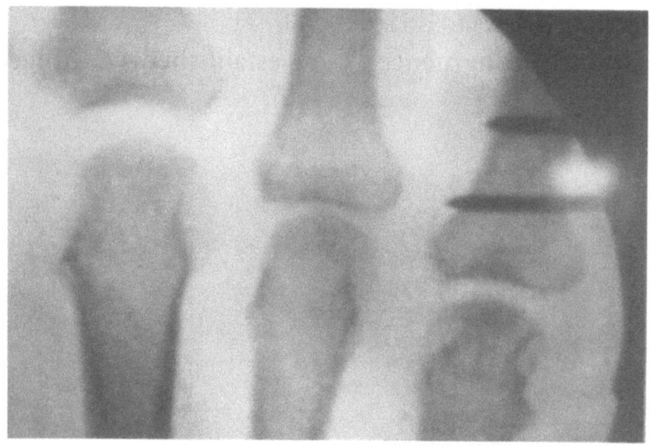

b

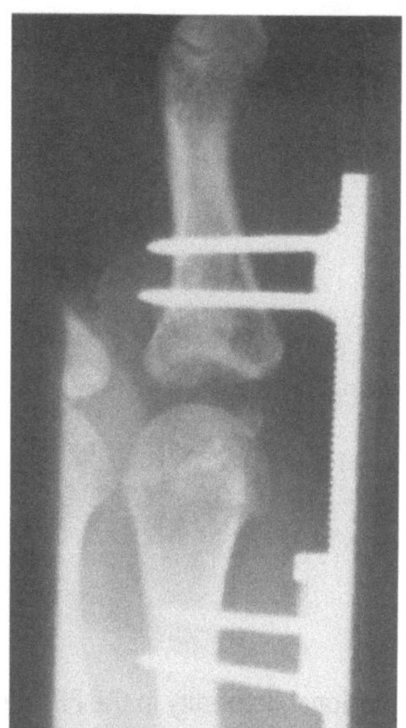

c

Fig. 54.26 **a** Manual distraction of MP joint III. The joint is now twice as wide as normal. **b** In comparison with the MP joint III the affected MP joint is distracted but still requires further distraction. **c** Maximum distraction in an MP joint.

from the dorso-radial side. A standard ball jointed fixator is used with a distraction nut. The 2mm threaded wires are inserted parallel into the shaft of the proximal phalanx and the second set of 2mm wires subsequently inserted into the distal diaphysis of the metacarpal bone. The double ball joint is locked as are the cams of both clamps. The clamp locking screw on the side of the distraction nut (which is placed between the clamp and the double ball joint) is not tightened; the locking screw of the second clamp is tightened. Now 5mm of distraction (= five full turns) is achieved by clockwise turns of the distraction nut. Distraction is released and the process repeated twice. The aim is to produce a joint space two to three times as wide as normal. Usually, 5mm of distraction is sufficient but more may be needed in those cases where subluxation is present. In these circumstances joint congruence must be restored with the help of the fixator and it is necessary to unlock the double ball joint and the clamp locking screws to do so.

Once congruence is re-established, a hinged MiniFixator is mounted. In the index finger this device is applied from the radial side and in the fifth finger from the ulnar side. The centre of rotation in the metacarpal head is targeted from the appropriate side with a 1.8/2mm Kirschner-wire under radiographic control. Correct placement is checked in both planes. The hinged MiniFixator is then slid over the Kirschner-wire with the distraction nut between the hinge and the distal clamp. Placing the distraction nut between the hinge and the proximal clamp would shift the centre of rotation which is not appropriate. Two 2mm threaded wires are inserted parallel into the proximal phalanx through the clamp seats closest to the bar, starting with the most distal wire. The same procedure is carried out in the proximal clamp. After locking the proximal clamp to the threaded bar, correct alignment of the K-wire marking the centre of rotation is reconfirmed. Simultaneous distraction of the initially applied MiniFixator and the hinged MiniFixator is now carried out. Distraction of 5–7 mm is performed

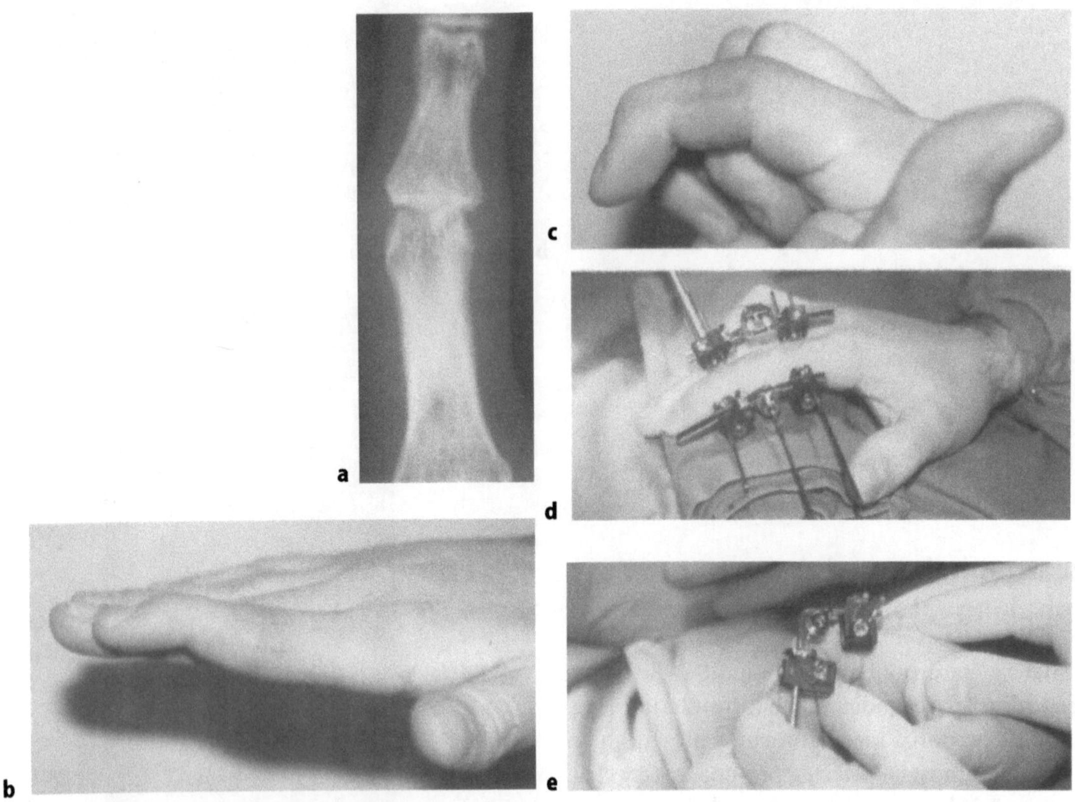

Fig. 54.27 **a** Rotational deformity in the PIP joint of the index finger in a 24-year-old male following intra-articular fracture. Note the rotational deformity. **b** Extension in the PIP joint. **c** 10° of flexion only in the PIP joint. **d** A standard miniFixator with a distraction nut is mounted from the dorso-ulnar side. After correction of the rotational deformity the hinged MiniFixator is applied from the radial side. Simultaneous distraction of the joint is performed and the standard MiniFixator removed. **e** Intra-operative movement of the PIP joint. **f** Reduction of the PIP joint. **g** Lateral film of the PIP joint. **h** Extension after 8 days; the fixator central unit was unlocked two days previously. **i** Full flexion present 8 days after surgery. **j** Extension in the PIP joint two weeks after fixator removal. **k** Flexion in the PIP joint two weeks after fixator removal.

alternately on either side. Correct opening of the MP joint must be verified using the image intensifier. After 5–10 minutes the distraction in the standard MiniFixator is released and again an image intensifier check is made to see if the hinged MiniFixator will allow the joint to remain distracted symmetrically. It may be necessary to repeat the process of distraction.

The standard MiniFixator is now removed and the joint moved with the hinged MiniFixator. The Kirschner-wire is removed. Most commonly, loss of flexion will be the problem and the hinged MiniFixator should be locked in flexion at the end of surgery. The vascularity of the skin on the extensor side must be carefully observed for adequate perfusion. If this is critical, a position of reduced flexion must be adopted. The fixator is left in this position for six days following which movement is commenced after unlocking the hinge. Again, physiotherapy will place the MP joint alternately in extension and flexion overnight. The patient is encouraged to perform physiotherapy alone in addition to working with the physiotherapist (Fig. 54.28a–e).

In metacarpophalangeal joints III and IV application of a hinged MiniFixator is not possible. For these joints two standard MiniFixators are used in a V-shape to distract the joint. One of the devices will be removed during the operation after distraction of the joint to three times its normal width has been achieved. Subluxation of the joint is now resolved and for this the procedure as described for MP joints II and V is followed. After correct joint alignment has been obtained redistraction of the joint is performed. After six days the double ball joint and one of the clamp locking screws is unlocked and physiotherapy commenced. This will not permit a full range of motion (Fig. 54.29a, b). Locking of the MiniFixator clamp locking screws after physiotherapy is carried out under distraction.

In PIP joints the same principles apply – a combination of a standard MiniFixator with a hinged

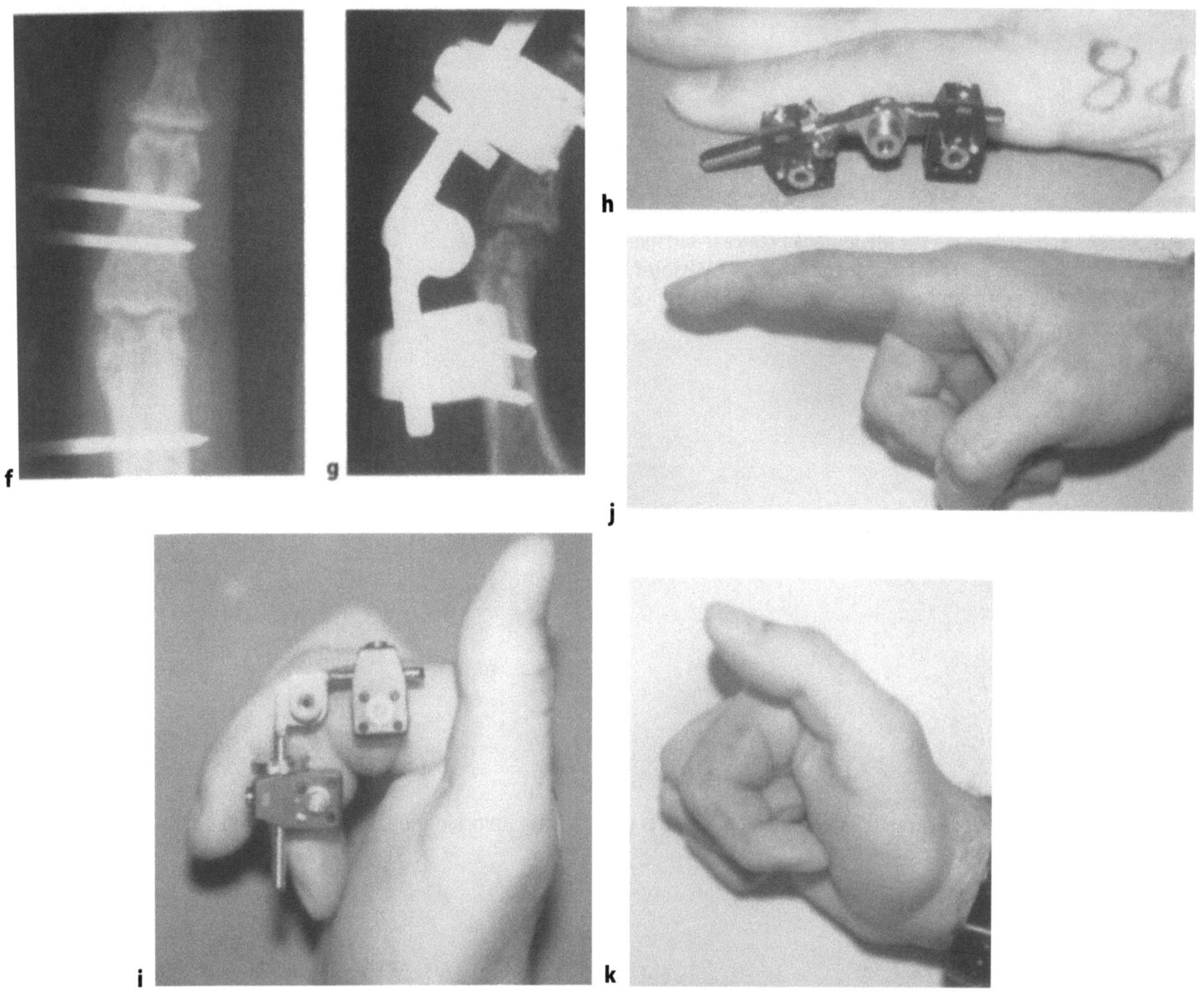

f g h j i k

Fig 54.27 (continued)

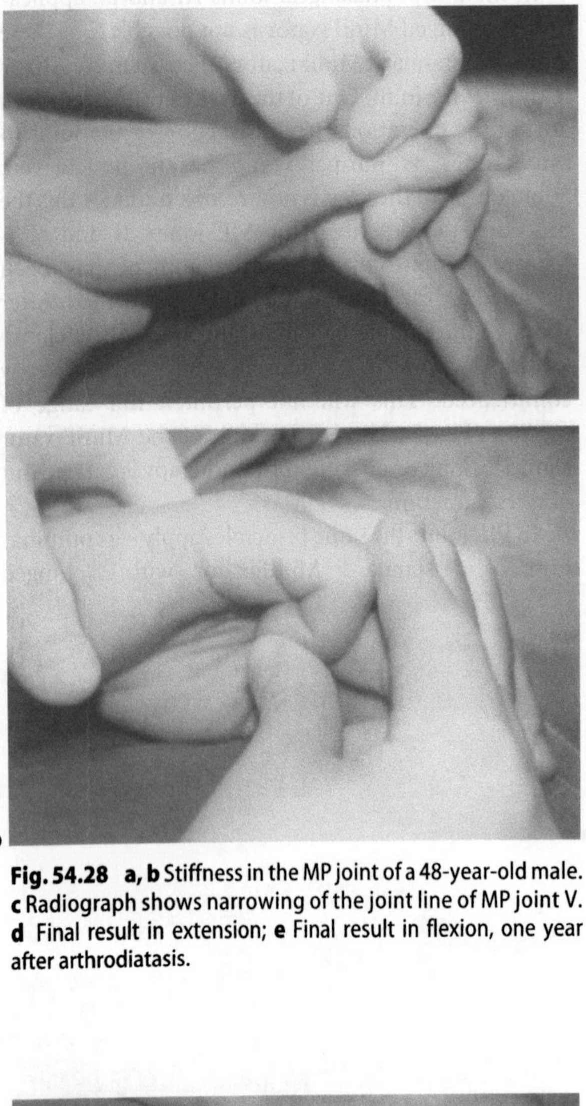

a

b

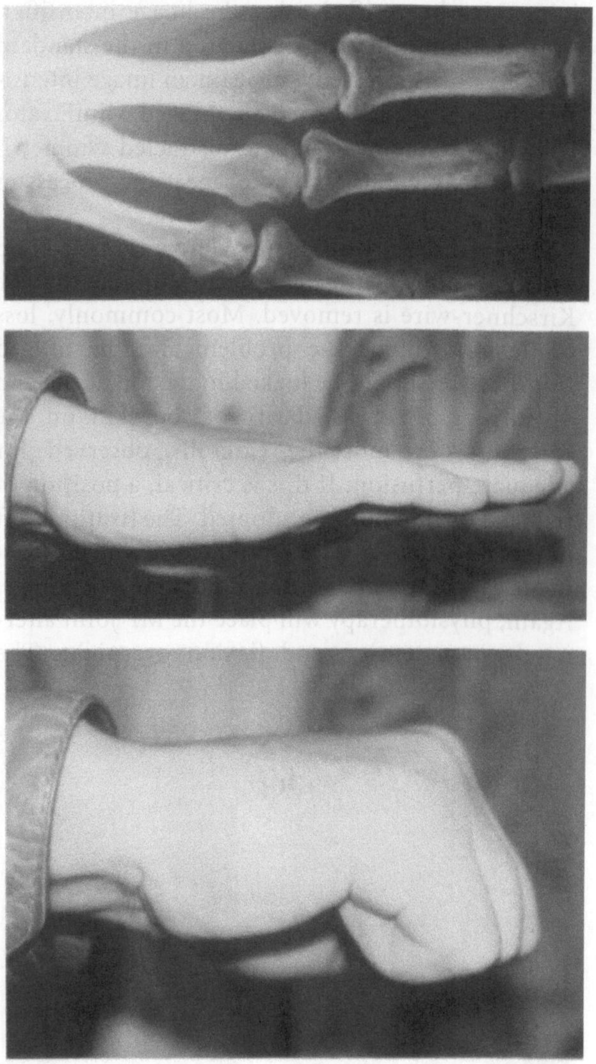

c

d

e

Fig. 54.28 **a, b** Stiffness in the MP joint of a 48-year-old male. **c** Radiograph shows narrowing of the joint line of MP joint V. **d** Final result in extension; **e** Final result in flexion, one year after arthrodiatasis.

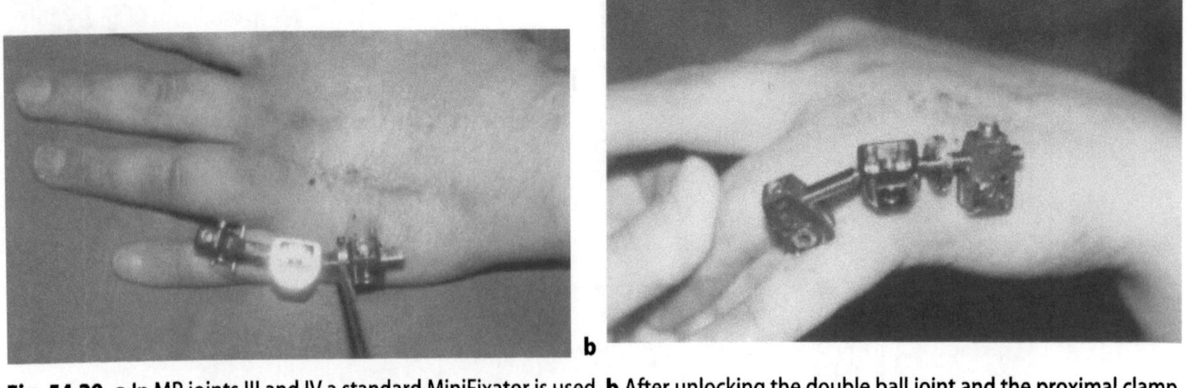

a

b

Fig. 54.29 **a** In MP joints III and IV a standard MiniFixator is used. **b** After unlocking the double ball joint and the proximal clamp locking screw physiotherapy is performed.

MiniFixator is again used (Fig. 54.7a–k). In the PIP joint of the index finger the standard fixator is applied from the dorso-ulnar side and the hinged MiniFixator from the radial side. In the middle finger the standard fixator is applied from the dorso-radial side and the hinged MiniFixator from the ulnar side. The same holds true for the ring and the fifth fingers. The amount of distraction is 4–6mm. Intra-operatively, distraction of the PIP joint will generate a joint space about twice that of normal. It is important to correct any subluxation and also any rotational malalignment (Fig. 54.30a–c). The post-operative treatment follows the guidelines set out for MP joint stiffness.

Interposition Arthroplasty

Interposition arthroplasty is a more important technique in the lower limb. It may, however, be necessary, especially in the elbow joint, to interpose tissue to regain some gliding surface where there is severe loss of cartilage. The techniques of interposition arthroplasty have been described elsewhere and we recommend the use of a flap raised from the triceps tendon. In the PIP joint there will invaribly be significant scarring especially after open or crush injuries. In these cases, where the cartilage has been destroyed, we raise a flap from the proximal phalanx and interpose it in the joint (Fig.

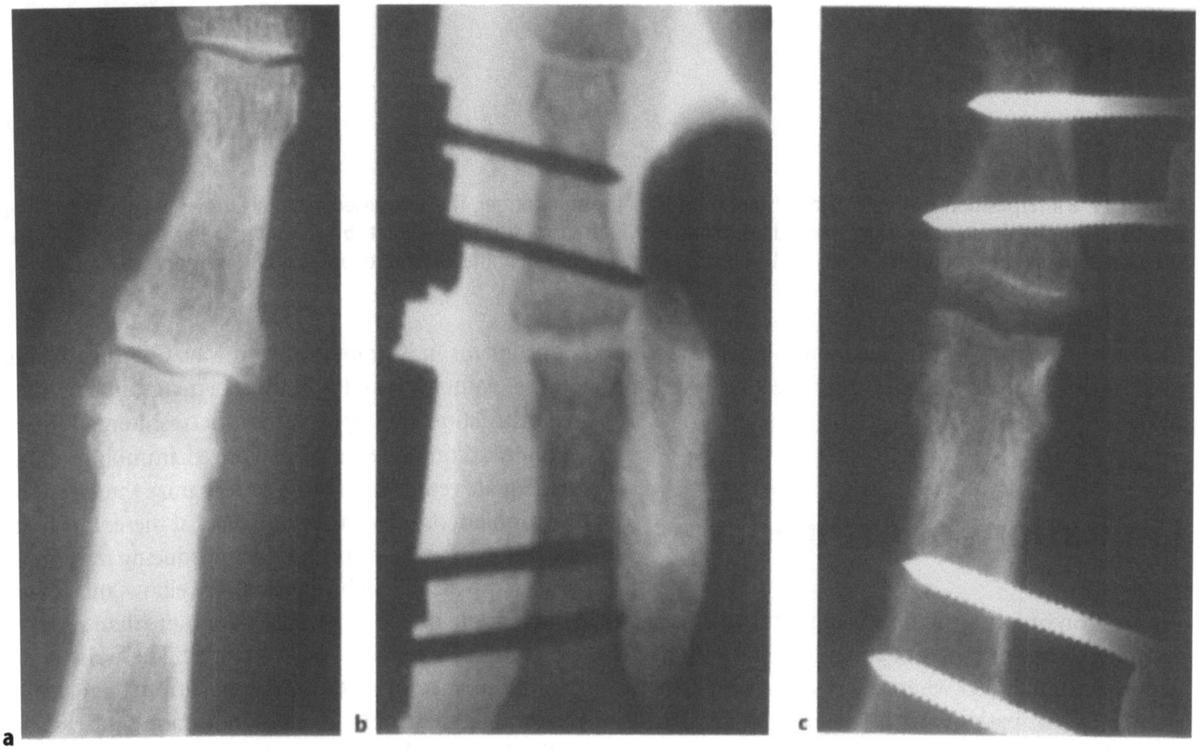

a b c

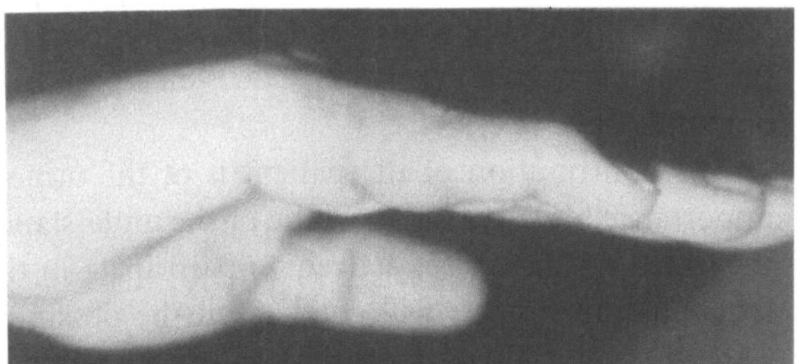

d

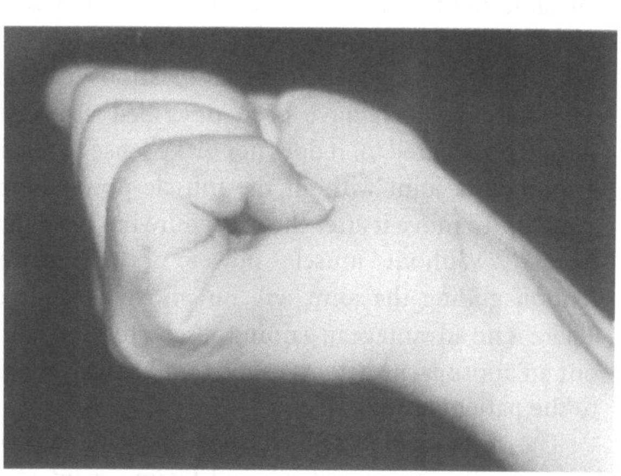

e

Fig. 54.30 **a** Stiffness in a PIP joint of a 30-year-old female. Note rotational subluxation as well as narrowing of the joint line. **b** Intra-operative distraction of the PIP joint. Note reduction of the joint with correct congruence. **c** Post-operative film showing significant distraction of the PIP joint. **d** Extension; **e** Flexion at the end of treatment (6 months).

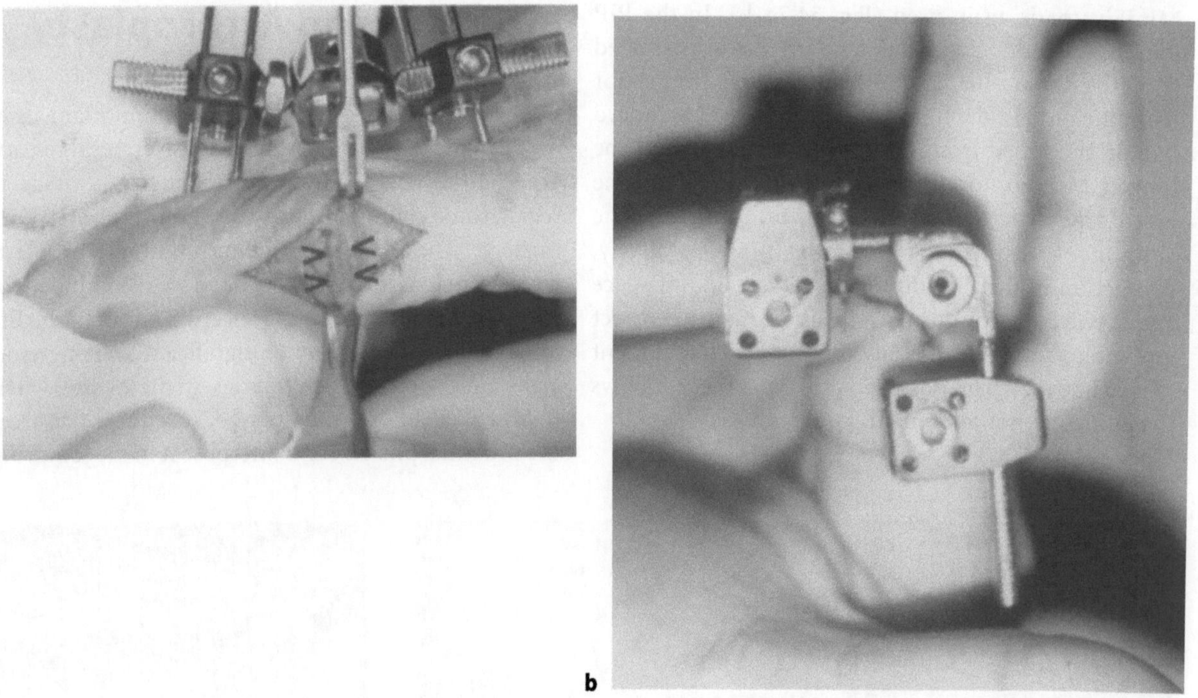

a b

Fig. 54.31 **a** Interposition arthroplasty in PIP joint stiffness of the index finger. The interposed material (arrows) is gained from the scar tissue on the dorso-radial side. A standard minifixator is used to distract the joint. **b** After interposing the flap a hinged minifixator was mounted and the standard MiniFixator removed. Flexion of the PIP joint two weeks after surgery.

54.31a, b). The fixator will remain in situ in distraction in these cases for 12 weeks both in the elbow and the PIP joint.

Limitations of Arthrodiatasis

Restoration of joint function using arthrodiatasis is a complex technique and not suitable for all patients. It is not recommended where there are severe arthritic changes, or in patients with rheumatoid arthritis or unstable joints. In these cases, however, it may be useful in association with other techniques to stabilize the joint. The general contraindications to external fixation which have been described elsewhere should be adhered to. It does not make sense to regain motion in a joint without the muscle power being available to move it after the procedure has been performed. Without muscle power or unimpaired tendon gliding the joint will not move as desired. There is no advantage in gaining passive motion without an appropriate active component being available to the patient as well.

The techniques described above may be supplemented with other procedures, and it is important never to be too dogmatic and believe that the fixator will solve all problems in a straightforward way. Careful analysis of the pathology and sound experience in articular reconstruction are important for success. Joint stiffness is often a consequence of prolonged immobilization, inadequate reduction, failure to recognize the extent of the problem or often, a combination of these. It is best, therefore, to prevent stiffness by introducing motion as soon as possible. We believe that the elbow and finger joints should not be immobilized for more than six days following soft tissue or bony trauma. The wrist is an exception since in distal radius fracture patients may develop algodystrophy if, after an intra-articular distal radius fracture, the joint is mobilized too early and pain occurs. While we allow pro- and supination from day one in these patients, flexion and extension is permitted only after three weeks.

The contribution of the patient is of the utmost importance for success. Only if he or she understands the principle and agrees actively to participate in the rehabilitation process will good results be obtained. Careful supervision of the patient within the unit and during the outpatient phase is another key factor. Ideally, the patient should be seen by the same surgeon in the outpatient department at each consecutive visit. Physiotherapy is prescribed twice daily for the entire period of fixator treatment and generally five times per week thereafter for an extended period.

Successful use of the technique of arthrodiatasis requires senior surgeon expertise and this must also be available in the post-operative phase.

References

Behrens F, Kraft EL, Oegema T (1989) 'Biomechanical Changes in Articular Cartilage after Joint Immobilization by Casting or External Fixation.' *Orthop Res* 7 (3):335–43.

Buckwalter JA (1992) 'Mechanical Injuries of Articular Cartilage.' *The Iowa Orthopaedic Journal* Vol 12: 50–7.

Buckwalter JA (1995) 'Should Bone, Soft Tissue and Joint Injuries be Treated with Rest or Activity?' *Orth Res* 13:155–6.

Deland JT, Walter PS, Sledge CB et al (1987) 'Biomechanical basis for elbow hinge-distractor design.' *Clin Orthop* 215: 303–12.

Esmarch von (1860) 'Die Behandlung der narbigen Kieferklemme durch Bildung eines künstlichen Gelenkes im Unterkiefer.' *Beitr prakt Chir* H 2.

Helferich (1894) 'Ein neues Operationsverfahren zur Heilung der knöchernen Kiefergelenkankylose.' *Verh dtsch Ges Chir.* 504.

Judet R, Judet T (1978) 'Arthrolyse et arthroplastie sous distracteur articulaire.' *Revue de Chirurgie orthop,*dique 64: 353–65.

Lexer (1920) *Wiederherstellungschirurgie.* Johann Ambrosius Barth:(Leipzig) 2. Auflage.

McKee MD, Bowden SH, King GJ et al (1998) 'Management of recurrent, complex instability of the elbow with a hinged external fixator.' *J Bone Joint Surg* [Br] 80-B. No. 6: 1031–6.

Mohan K (1972) 'Myositis ossificans of the elbow.' *Int Surg* 57(6): 475–80.

Maunder (1875) *Brit Med J*: 586–7.

Morrey BF (1990) 'Posttraumatic contracture of the elbow.' *J Bone Joint Surg* [Am] 72A: 601–18.

Morrey BF, Chao EY (1976) 'Passive motion of the elbow joint.' *J Bone Joint Surg* [Am] 58A: 501–8.

Nelson DL (1990) 'The functional range of motion of the wrist.' American Society for Surgery of the Hand, 45th Annual Meeting, Toronto.

Palmer AK, Werner FW, Murphy D et al (1985) 'Functional wrist motion: a biomechanical study.' *J Hand Surg* 10A: 39–46.

Payr E (1934) *Gelenksteifen und Gelenkplastik.* Erster Teil. Springer: Berlin.

Regan WD, Reilly CD (1993) 'Distraction arthroplasty of the elbow.' *Hand Clin* 9: 719–28.

Regan WD, Korinek SL, Morray BF et al (1991) 'Biomechanical study of ligaments around the elbow joint.' *Clin Orthop* 271: 170–9.

Ryu J, Cooney WP III, Askew IJ et al (1991) 'Functional ranges of motion of the wrist joint.' *J Hand Surg* 9A: 409–19.

Sayre (1898) 'Remarkable repair after excision of hip.' *N.Y. Med Rec* 13: 355.

Söjbjerg JO (1996) 'The stiff elbow.' *Acta Orthop Scand* 67(6): 626–31.

Urbaniak JR, Hansen PE, Beissinger SF et al (1985) 'Correction of posttraumatic flexion contracture of the elbow by anterior capsulotomy.' *J Bone Joint Surg* [Am] 67A: 1160.

Verneuil (1863) *Gaz d et Chir.* 97–101.

Volkov MV, Oganesian OV (1975) 'Restoration of Function in the Knee and Elbow with a Hinge-Distractor Apparatus.' *J Bone Joint Surg.*[Am] Vol 57-A: 591–600.

Wolff J (1895) Über die Operation der Ellenbogengelenkankylose. *Berliner klinische Wochenschrift* 43: 44.

Wolff J (1897) 'Zur Arthrolysis cubiti.' *Berliner klinische Wochenschrft* 46: 1017–8.

Supplementary Bibliography

Bennighoff A, Goerttler K. (1980) 'Lehrbuch der Anatomie des Menschen.' in: Ferner H. Staubesand J (eds.) *Allgemein Anatomie, Cytologie und Bewegungsapparat,* Bd.1 Urban 38; Schwarzenberg: München Wien Baltimore.

Bhattacharyya S. (1974) 'Arthrolysis: a new approach to surgery of posttaumatic stiff elbow.' *J Bone Joint Surg* [Br] 56B: 567.

Breen TF, Gelbermann RH, Ackermann GN (1988) 'Elbow flexion contractures: Treatmant by anterior release and continous passive motion.' *J Hand Surg* [Br] 13: 286.

Bryan RS, Bickel WHT (1971) 'Condylar fractures of the distal humerus.' *J Trauma* 11: 830.

Cobb TK, Linscheid RL (1994) 'Late correction of malunited intercondylar humeral fractures. Intraarticular osteotomy and tricortical bone grafting.' *J Bone Joint Surg* [Br] 76B: 622–6.

Copeland SA, Gschwend N, Landi A, Saffar P (Eds) (1997) 'Joint Stiffness of the Upper Limb.' Martin Dunitz Ltd.: London.

Costa P, Giancecchi F, Cavazzuti A, et al (1991) 'Internal and external fixation in complex diaphyseal and metaphyseal fractures of the humerus.' *J Orthop Trauma* 17 (1): 87–94.

Ewald FC (1986) 'Reconstruction of complex elbow problem' Ch. 13. in: Tullos HS (ed.) *Instructional course lectures,* vol. XXXV, 108–15.

Fuss FK (1991) 'The ulnar collateral ligament of the human elbow joint. Anatomy, function and biomechanics.' *J Anat* 175: 203–12.

Gausepohl T, Koebke J, Pennig D et al (1997a) 'Anatomische Grundlagen zur Anwendung der unilateralen externen Fixation an Oberarm, Unterarm und Hand.' *Osteosyn Int* 5: 76–88.

Gausepohl T, Pennig D, Mader K (1997b) 'Der transartikuläre Bewegungsfixateur bei Luxationen und Luxationsfrakturen des Ellenbogengelenkes.' *Osteosyn Int* 5: 102–10.

Gausepohl D, Pennig D (1998) 'Luxationen und Luxationsfrakturen des Ellenbogens - Einsatz des Bewegungsfixateurs.' in: *Ellenbogenchirurgie in der Praxis* (Meyer RP, Kappeler U, eds) Springer: Berlin-Heidelberg-New York: 161–82.

Glynn JJ, Niebauer J (1976) 'Flexion and extension contracture of the elbow: surgical management.' *Clin Orthop* 117: 289–91.

Green DP, McCoy H (1979) 'Turnbuckle orthotic correction of elbow-flexion contractures after acute injuries.' *J Bone Joint Surg* [Am] 61A: 1092.

Gutierrez LS (1964) 'A contribution to the study of the limiting factors of elbow extension.' *Acta Anat* (Basel) 56: 146–56.

Husband JB, Hastings H (1990) 'The lateral approach for operative release of posttraumatic contracture of the elbow.' *J Bone Joint Surg* [Am] 72A: 1353.

Johannsson H, Olerud S (1971) 'Operative Treatment of intercondylar fractures of the humerus.' *Trauma* 11(10: 836–43.

Kapandji IA (1970) *The physiology of joints. Annotaded diagrams of the mechanics of the human joints,* vol.1,2. Livingstone: Edinburgh London: 78–101, 102–21.

McKee M, Jupiter J, Toh CL et al (1994) 'Reconstruction after malunion and non-union of intra-articular fractures of the distal humerus.' *J Bone Joint Surg* [Br] 76(B): 614–21.

Mingione A, Barca F (1991) 'Anatomophysiopathology.' in: Celli J (ed) *The elbow traumatic lesions.* Springer: Berlin-Heidelberg-New York-Tokyo.

Morrey BF (1985) 'Functional anatomy of the ligaments of the elbow.' *Clin Orthop* 201: 84–90.

Morrey BF (1994a) 'Distraction arthroplasty', Ch. 17. in: Morrey BF (ed) *The Elbow.* Raven: New York, 307–27.

Morrey BF (1994b) 'Limited extensile triceps reflecting exposures of the elbow', Ch. 1. in: Morrey BF (ed) *The Elbow.* Raven: New York, 3–19.

Morrey BF (1994c) 'Posttraumatic stiffness: distraction arthroplastry', Ch. 29, 2nd edn. in: Morrey BF (ed) *The elbow and its disorders.* Saunders: Philadelphia, 476–91.

Morrey BF, Askew LJ, An KN (1988) 'Strength function after elbow arthroplasty' *Clin Orthop* 234: 43–50.

Morrey BF, Tanaka S, An KN (1991) 'Valgus stability of the elbow.' *Clin Orthop* 265: 187–95.
Pennig D: *Treatment of fracture and deformities in small bones. The Pennig Minifixator. Operative Technique.* Orthofix Srl., Bussolengo, Italy.
Pennig D: *The Pennig dynamic wrist fixator. Operative Technique.* Orthofix Srl., Bussolengo, Italy.
Pennig D, Gausepohl T (1997) *The elbow fixator. Operative Technique.* Orthofix Srl., Bussolengo, Italy
Pennig D, Gausepohl D (1998) 'Die posttraumatische Ellenbogensteife – Gelenkdistraktion mit Fixateur externe als Behandlungskonzept.' in: *Ellenbogenchirurgie in der Praxis* (Meyer RP, Kappeler U eds) Springer: Berlin-Heidelberg-New York: 183–205.
Pennig D, Gausepohl D, Mader K (1999) 'Transarticular fixation with motion capacity in fracture dislocations of the elbow.' *Injury* Suppl (in press).
Reha-Barton (1828) Reference see Payr E.
Rydholm U, Tjörnstrand B, Petterson H et al (1984) 'Surface replacement of the elbow in rheumatoid arthritis.' *J Bone Joint Surg* [Br] 66B: 737–41.
Shahriaree H, Sjadi K, Silver CM et al (1979) 'Excisional arthroplasty of the elbow.' *J Bone Joint Surg* [Am] 81A: 922–927.
Walker N, Jacob HAC (1981) 'Biomechanische Untersuchungen am Ellenbogengelenk.' *Orthopade* 10: 253–255.
Weizenbluth M, Eichenblat M, Lipskeir E et al (1989) 'Arthrolysis of the elbow: 13 cases of posttraumatic stiffness.' *Acta Orthop Scand* 60: 642.
Willner P (1948) 'Anterior capsulectomy for relief of flexion contractures of the elbow following fracture.' *J Bone Joint Surg* 26: 71–86.

Articulated Distraction of the Hip

55

R. Aldegheri, G. Trivella and M. Saleh

Conservative surgery for osteoarthrosis has waned in popularity since the advent of total hip arthroplasty.[6,7,10,14,17] The long-term implications of failure and repeated revision arthroplasty in young patients, however, support the need for surgery aimed at joint conservation. This study was set up in the hope of finding a procedure that would arrest or even reverse the degenerative process and delay the need for joint arthroplasty.

Articular cartilage defects are capable of repair and replacement; the long-term durability of the newly formed tissue is, however, unknown.[5,11] Salter et al[13] demonstrated the value of continuous passive motion in the repair of articular cartilage defects in adolescent and adult rabbits. Intra-articular adhesion formation was also reduced in those animals treated with intermittent active motion or continuous passive motion compared with those that were immobilized. Improved healing of articular cartilage has been observed in the animal model with continuous passive motion and intermittent movement using an external fixator (articulated distraction). Judet and Judet[9] excised the cartilage layer from the surfaces of the tibiotarsal joints of dogs. A hinged external fixator was placed across the joint for 30 days, maintaining a joint space of 4 to 8mm. After the dogs were killed at one year, they found "callus whose macroscopic and microscopic appearance was close to that of normal articular cartilage."

Articulated distraction using a circular fixator has been used with success to mobilize joint contractures and reduce old dislocations of the elbow and knee.[15] Satisfactory results were obtained in 31 knees and 28 elbows after one to six years of follow-up. Judet and Judet[9] used monolateral hinged distractors to stabilize and mobilize the elbow, knee, and ankle joints in patients with post-traumatic arthritis and other joint pathologies. Thirteen of 16 arthritic ankles were considered to have a good result after a mean follow-up time of 16 months. In both series, articulated distraction was used in combination with limited arthroplasty. Recently, the biomechanical basis[4] and clinical application[12] of such techniques in the elbow have been described.

The term arthrodiatasis was coined to describe a regime of articulated distraction and open surgery of the hip employed in Verona since 1979.[1,2] Arthrodiatasis is derived from the Greek *arthro* (joint), *dia* (through), and *tasis* (to stretch out).

Articulated distraction of the hip provides off-loading of muscle and body forces and distraction of the joint space by means of an external fixator[3] that crosses the hip joint. Sagittal plane hip movement is encouraged by the addition of a hinge. Creating a space between the bony surfaces, reducing mechanical stress, and providing movement are initiated in an attempt to restore the synovial circulation and encourage fibrous repair of the articular cartilage without the formation of adhesions. Open surgery to release soft-tissue contractures or to improve joint congruence (by limited arthroplasty or screw fixation of loose fragments) may be required to facilitate movement.

Materials and Methods

An independent observer reviewed the medical records and radiographs of 80 patients treated at the Institute of Clinical Orthopaedics and Traumatology at the University of Verona in Verona, Italy. The 56 male and 24 female patients had an average age of 34 years (range 9–69 years).

Diagnoses varied, with avascular necrosis in 35 patients, osteoarthrosis in 20 patients, chondrolysis in 15 patients, and miscellaneous conditions in 10 patients (Tables 55.1).The indications for surgery included at least two of the following: (1) continuous pain, (2) severe restriction of movement, or (3) walking limited to less than 15 minutes with or without crutches or canes.

Specific treatment was dictated by the condition and its severity. If hip motion was satisfactory and the joint was radiographically congruent, articulated distraction alone could be used. If motion was reduced, soft-tissue releases as described by Voss,[16] and extra-articular perforations as described by Forbes-Mackenzie,[8] were added. If joint incongruence existed, limited joint arthroplasty or screw fixation of large osteochondral defects was also used.

Sixteen patients had articulated distraction alone using the standard dynamic axial fixator developed by De Bastiani, with a single axis articulating unit (Fig. 55.1). The other 64 patients underwent additional surgery.

Surgical Technique

The range of hip motion is assessed under general anaesthesia. Significant limitation of joint motion under anaesthesia necessitates soft-tissue release during surgery. Any further arthroplasty, such as capsulorrhaphy, bone contouring, or fixation of osteochondral fragments, is carried out at that time.

Accurate alignment of the external fixator with its rotating axis in line with the hip-joint flexion-extension arc is critical. With the hip held in 10° to 15° of abduction, the cortical screws are placed in the pelvis, engaging the outer and inner tables. The proximal or pelvic fixation can be accomplished either axially with a straight clamp or transversely with a T-clamp attachment. The distal two cortical screws are placed in the femoral diaphysis using the template. The template is then removed and the actual fixator applied to the four screws. A third screw can be added to one or both clamps to improve fixation (Fig. 55.2).

The fixator is left in place for as long as tolerated, usually between 6 and 10 weeks. Removal of the fixator is usually precipitated by loosening of the pelvic screws. Partial weightbearing is allowed for limited periods each day to avoid premature loosening of the screws. The hip should be moved frequently. Continuous passive motion was not used in this series but may be valuable.

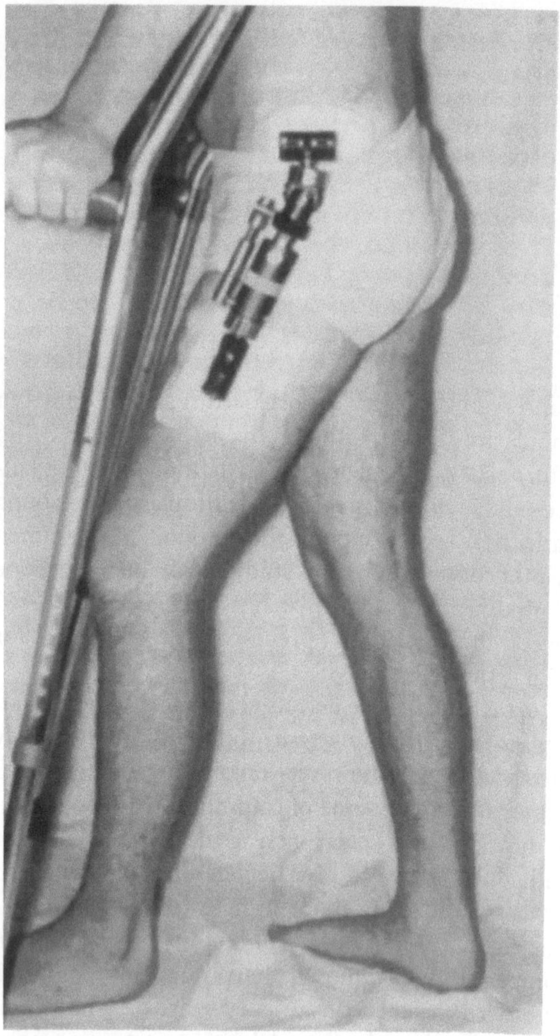

Fig. 55.1 Patient with hinged, articulated fixator in place (with T-clamp proximally).

Results

A good clinical result was defined as (1) a resumption of normal activities with no pain or mild pain only after a prolonged exercise, (2) greater than 150° total arc of motion with 90° flexion and 20° in abduction, adduction, and internal and external rotation, and (3) independent ambulation for at least 30 minutes.

Since the surgical operations were carried out during a four-year period and the initial study period was seven years, there were some patients who had not completed five years of follow-up evaluation. Questionnaires were sent to these patients and clinical examination was arranged. Forty-six good results were achieved (Table 55.2). Table 55.3 shows the results at a minimum follow-up period of five years. Radiographic improvement did not always parallel clinical improvement (Fig. 55.3).

A statistical analysis using logistic regression showed no correlation between cause, operation variant, or gender; however, there was a strong correla-

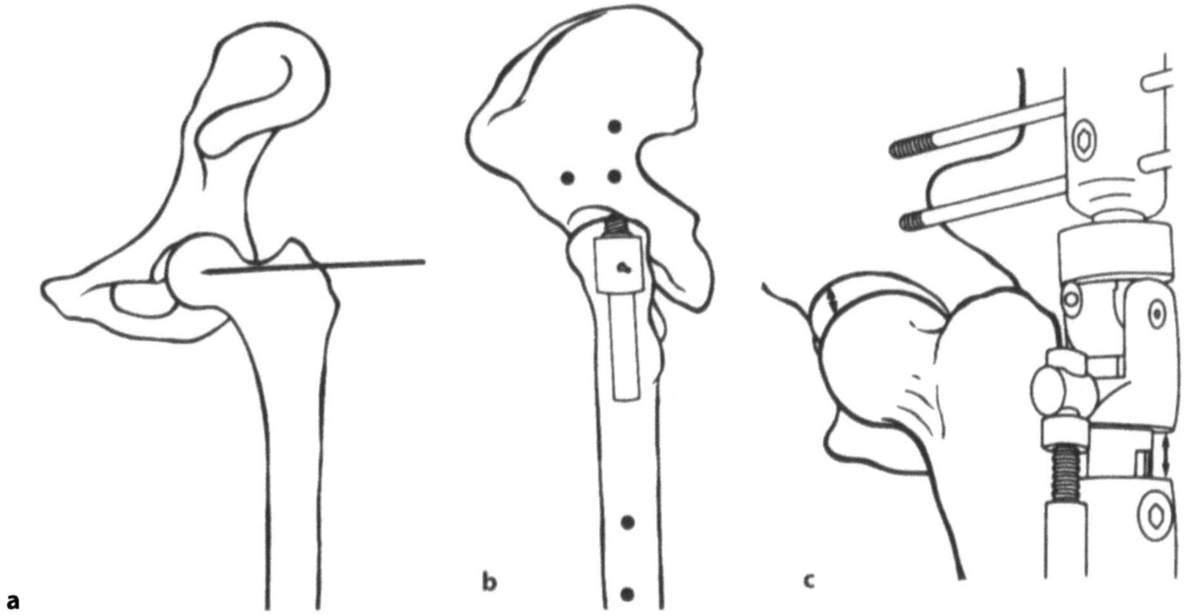

Fig. 55.2 a An image intensifier is used to place a guide wire into the centre of rotation of the hip. **b** The template guide for the articulated body is then inserted over the guide wire noting the relationship of pelvic and femoral screw fixation. **c** The compression–distraction unit is distracted until a 5mm joint space is seen on image intensification.

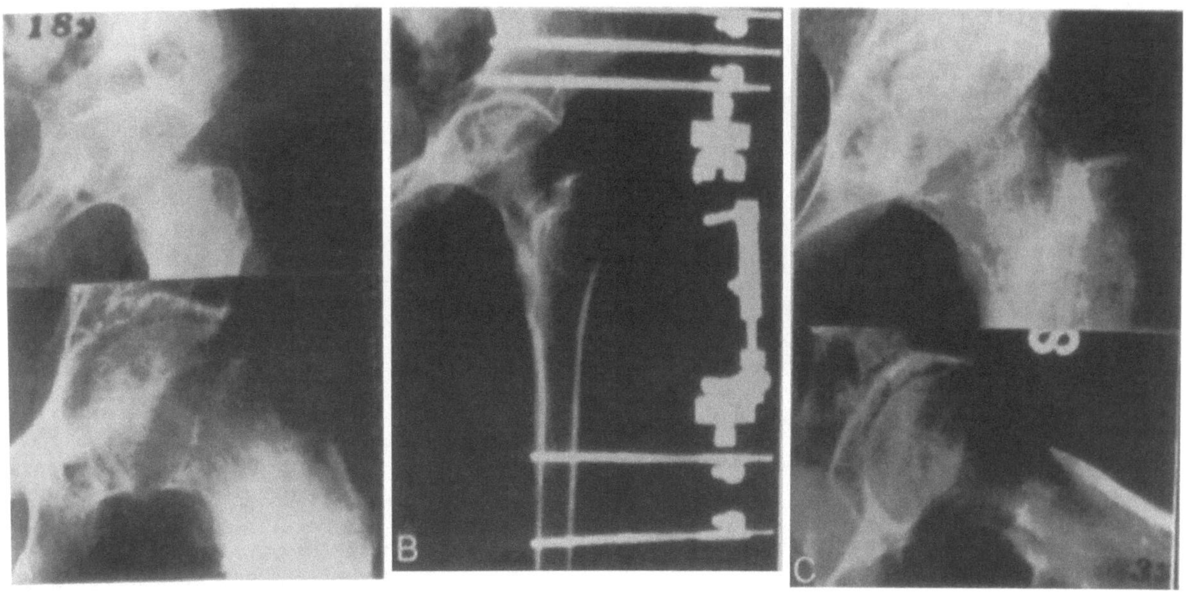

Fig. 55.3 Articulated distraction with extra- and intra-articular soft-tissue release was performed in this 18-year-old man with chondrolysis secondary to slipped upper femoral epiphysis. Ankylosis was present in flexion, abduction, and external rotation. The composite radiographs show the minimal motion. **a** Before operation, after soft-tissue release. **b** During distraction. **c** Three years post-operatively A good clinical result was achieved and still remained at the 7-year follow-up evaluation.

tion with age ($p < 0.05$). Only four good results were achieved in patients over the age of 45 years, three with primary osteoarthrosis and one with traumatic avascular necrosis.

In the early part of the study, four patients with inflammatory arthropathy were operated on with uniformly disappointing results. If patients with inflammatory arthropathy and patients older than the age of 45 years are excluded, there were 42 good results in 59 patients, representing a 71.2 per cent success rate.

Aetiology	Surgery AD	STR	LA	PER	SF	Total
Avascular necrosis						
Idiopathic II*	4					4
Idiopathic III*					1	1
Idiopathic IV*		7	2	5		14
Fracture	2	4	2			8
Fracture dislocation		2	2	1		5
Hodgkins					1	1
Thalassemia		1				1
Seq septic arthritis			1			1
Osteoarthrosis						
Primary		12		2		14
Dysplasia		6				6
Chondrolysis						
SUFE	6	8	1			15
Miscellaneous						
Seq CDH	2	1				3
Ankylosing spondylolisthesis.		2				2
Rheumatoid arthritis		2				2
Coxa profunda	2					2
Seq septic arthritis		1				1
Total	16	46	8	8	2	80

AD, articulated distraction alone; STR, soft-tissue release; PER, perforations; LA, limited arthroplasty; SF, screw fixation; CDH, congenital dysplasia of the hip; Seq, sequela; SUFE, slipped upper femoral epiphysis.

* Staging after Ficat and Arlet (1980).

Table 55.1 Diagnosis and Treatment Regimens

For patients younger than 45 years of age, good clinical results were achieved in the six cases of osteoarthrosis, the three cases of hip dysplasia, 14 of 15 cases of chondrolysis (93.3 per cent), five of nine cases of traumatic avascular necrosis (55.5 per cent), ten of 19 cases of idiopathic avascular necrosis (52.6 per cent),[6,7] two cases of post-septic arthritis, and one case each of avascular necrosis after Hodgkin's disease and thalassemia. Good results were achieved in the two cases of screw fixation, 12 of 13 cases of articulated distraction alone (92.3 per cent), six of eight arthroplasties (75 per cent), and 22 of 31 soft tissue releases (71 per cent). Capsular perforations did not improve any results.

Aetiology	Surgery AD	STR	LA	PER	SF	Total
Avascular necrosis						
Idiopathic II*	4					4
Idiopathic III*					1	1
Idiopathic IV*		4	1			5
Fracture	1	2	1			4
Fracture dislocation			2			2
Hodgkins					1	1
Thalassemia		1				1
Seq Septic arthritis			1			1
Osteoarthrosis						
Primary		7				7
Dysplasia		2				2
Chondrolysis						
SUFE	5	8	1			14
Miscellaneous						
Seq CDH	2	1				3
Seq Septic arthritis		1				1
Total	12	26	6	0	2	46

AD, articulated distraction alone; STR, soft-tissue release; PER, perforations; LA, limited arthroplasty; SF, screw fixation; CDH, congenital dysplasia of the hip; Seq, sequela; SUFE, slipped upper femoral epiphysis.

* Staging after Ficat and Arlet (1980).

Table 55.2 Successful Results At a Minimum Follow-Up Time of Five Years

There were no serious complications, although three patients developed pain related to the pelvic screws. In one patient, this led to premature removal of the device.

Discussion

With time-limited success of prosthetic hip arthroplasty in younger patients, a minimally invasive procedure to relieve pain and restore function can temporize before larger operations such as osteotomy or prosthetic arthroplasty. Even at rest, the hip is loaded because of significant muscle forces. Any operation must address mechanical and biological objectives. Arthrodiatasis neutralizes muscle and weightbearing forces and creates a potential space where cartilage repair may occur.

Movement encourages a synovial circulation and allows nutrition and, therefore, fibrous repair of articular cartilage without adhesion formation. Prior reports of soft-tissue release or other lesser arthroplasties have indicated less than satisfactory results. The authors believe that the addition of articulated distraction significantly improved results for at least five years.

Avascular Necrosis					Pre-operative			Post-operative		
Patient	Gender	Age	Subset	Op	Pain	ROM	WD	Pain	ROM	WD
1	m	36	1 IV	STR	2	1	2	1	0	0
2	f	50	#	STR	2	1	2	0	0	0
3	m	21	#	LA	2	2	3	1	0	1
4	m	16	Th	STR	2	2	2	0	0	1
5	m	40	I II	AD	2	2	2	0	0	0
7	m	44	I IV	STR	2	1	3	0	0	0
10	m	35	#	AD	2	2	3	0	0	0
11	m	29	I II	AD	2	1	3	0	0	1
14	f	34	I IV	STR	2	2	2	0	0	1
16	m	40	#	STR	2	1	2	0	0	0
21	m	44	#D	LA	2	2	3	1	0	1
22	m	36	I III	SF	2	1	2	0	0	1
24	m	28	#D	LA	2	1	2	0	0	1
26	m	9	Sep	LA	2	1	2	0	0	0
29	m	40	I II	AD	2	1	3	0	0	0
30	f	39	I IV	STR	2	1	2	0	0	0
32	m	35	Hod	SF	2	1	3	1	0	1
33	m	45	I IV	LA	2	1	3	1	0	0
35	f	43	I II	AD	2	1	2	0	0	0

Pain: 0 = no pain; 1 = pain after pro1onged exercise (two hours standing or active work); 2 = continuous pain day and night.

ROM: 0 = at least 90° flexion and 20° abduction, adduction, and internal and external rotation; 1 = severe restriction of movement less than 40° flexion and 0° to 5° movement in abduction, adduction, internal, and external rotation; 2 = no movement.

WD: 0 = walking without sticks or crutches for two to three hours in any environment; 1 = walking without sticks or crutches for 30 to 60 minutes in any environment; 2 = walking without sticks or crutches less than 15 minutes duration within the home and work environment; 3 = walking with sticks or crutches less than 15 minutes duration within the home and work environment.

STR, soft-tissue release; LA, limited arthroplasty; AD, articulated distraction alone; SF, screw fixation; OP, operation.

Table 55.3 Comparison of pre- and post-operative clinical state for patients with successful results

		Osteoarthrosis			Pre-operative			Post-operative		
Patient	Gender	Age	Subset	op	Pain	ROM	WD	Pain	ROM	WD
39	m	45	P	STR	2	1	3	1	0	1
45	m	55	P	STR	2	1	2	0	0	0
47	m	41	D	STR	2	1	2	1	0	1
49	f	45	P	STR	2	1	2	1	0	1
50	f	41	P	STR	2	1	3	1	0	0
51	m	42	D	STR	2	1	2	1	0	1
52	f	45	P	STR	2	1	2	0	0	0
53	f	52	P	STR	2	1	2	0	0	0
55	m	49	P	STR	2	1	3	1	0	1
		Chondrolysis			Pre-operative			Post-operative		
56	m	17		STR	2	2	3	1	0	1
57	m	18		AD	2	2	2	0	0	0
58	f	13		AD	2	2	3	1	0	1
59	f	14		AD	2	2	2	1	0	1
60	f	10		AD	2	1	2	0	0	0
61	m	18		STR	2	1	2	0	0	0
62	m	19		STR	2	2	2	0	0	0
63	f	14		AD	2	1	2	0	0	0
64	m	20		LA	2	1	2	0	0	0
65	m	17		STR	2	1	2	0	0	0
66	m	16		STR	2	1	2	1	0	0
68	m	20		STR	2	2	2	1	0	1
69	m	14		STR	2	1	2	0	0	0
70	m	18		STR	2	1	2	0	0	0
		Miscellaneous			Pre-operative			Post-operative		
72	f	14	CDH	AD	2	2	3	1	0	1
73	m	23	CDH	STR	2	2	3	0	0	1
75	f	15	CDH	AD	2	1	1	1	0	0
80	f	23	Sep	STR	2	1	2	1	0	0

Pain: 0 = no pain; 1 = pain after prolonged exercise (two hours standing or active work); 2 = continuous pain day and night.

ROM: 0 = at least 90° flexion and 20° abduction, adduction, and internal and external rotation; 1 = severe restriction of movement less than 40° flexion and 0° to 5° movement in abduction, adduction, internal, and external rotation; 2 = no movement.

WD: 0 = walking without sticks or crutches for two to three hours in any environment; 1 = walking without sticks or crutches for 30 to 60 minutes in any environment; 2 = walking without sticks or crutches less than 15 minutes duration within the home and work environment; 3 = walking with sticks or crutches less than 15 minutes duration within the home and work environment.

STR, soft-tissue release; AD, articulated distraction alone; LA, limited arthroplasty; OP, operation. P, primary; D, dysplasia.

Table 55.3 (continued)

Satisfactory results were achieved in more than 70 per cent of patients aged 45 and younger. The procedure was ineffective in patients older than 45 years or in those with inflammatory arthropathy. Extra-articular perforation as a supplementary procedure was uniformly unsuccessful. Articulated distraction alone is a minimally invasive procedure and is associated with a high success rate in those patients with a good range of movement under anaesthesia. Correct application of the device and closely supervised rehabilitation are major determinants of the outcome. The pelvic screws must gain secure fixation. The transverse axis of the mechanical joint must be aligned with the centre of the femoral head. Flexion of the hip with a minimum radiographic separation of the joint space of 5mm, corresponding to about 10mm on the dynamic axial fixator, must be possible without resistance.

Often a good clinical outcome was associated with poor radiological appearances, including an irregular joint space and bony incongruence. A discrete joint space was always observed, however. This discrepancy between a pain-free, mobile hip and its radiological appearance is difficult to explain but may be interpreted as a functional adaptation of the femoral head to loading stress.

A cautionary note must be raised since pin tracks are a theoretical site of bacterial colonization and, therefore, for potential contamination of the operative field of a subsequent replacement arthroplasty.

Acknowledgments

The authors thank Miss Elena Henley and Mr. David Robson of the Department of Probability and Statistics, University of Sheffield, England.

References

1. Aldegheri, R.: 'Arthodiatasi d'anca.' *Ortopedia E Traumatologia Oggi.* 1981; 1: 103.
2. Aldegheri, R., and Trivella, G.: 'L'artrodiatasi nel trattamento dell'anca rigida dopo epifisiolisi.' *Revista Italiana di Ortopedia e Traumatologia Pediatrica* 1985; 1:137.
3. De Bastiani, G., Aldegheri, R., and Brivio, L. R.: 'The treatment of fractures with a dynamic axial fixator.' *J Bone Joint Surg* [Br] 1984; 66B: 538.
4. Deland, J. T., Garg, A., and Walker, P. S.: 'Biomechanical basis for elbow hinge-distractor design.' *Clin Orthop* 1987; 215: 303.
5. Eisenstein, A., and Rothschild, S.: 'Biochemical abnormalities in patients with slipped capital femoral epiphysis; and chondrolysis. *J Bone Joint Surg* [Am] 1976; 58A:459.
6. Ficat, R. P., and Arlet, J.: *Ischaemia and necrosis of bone.* Williams and Wilkins: London, 1980, p. 196.
7. Ficat, R. P.: 'Idiopathic bone necrosis of the femoral head. Early diagnosis and treatment.' *J Bone Joint Surg* [Br] 1985; 67B:3.
8. Forbes-Mackenzie, J.: 'Osteoarthritis of hip and knee. Description of a surgical treatment.' *Br Med J* 1936; 306: 8.
9. Judet, R., and Judet, T.: 'Arthrolyse et arthroplastie sous distracteur articulaire.' *Rev de Chirurgie Orthopedique* 1978; 64: 353.
10. Maistrelli, G., Fusco, U., Avai, A., and Bombelli, R.: 'Osteonecrosis of the hip treated by intertrochanteric osteotomy – a four-to-15-year follow-up. *J Bone Joint Surg* [Br] 1988, 70B: 761.
11. Mankin, H. L: 'Response of articular cartilage to mechanical injury.' *J Bone Joint Surg* [Am] 1982; 64A:460.
12. Morrey, B. R: 'Post-traumatic contracture of the elbow.' *J Bone Joint Surg* [Am] 1997; 2A: 601.
13. Salter, R. B., Simmonds, D. R, Malcolm, B. W., Rumble, E. L, Macmichael, D., and Clements, N. D.: 'The biological effect of continuous passive motion on the healing of full thickness defects in articular cartilage.' *J Bone Joint Surg* [Am] 1980; 62A: 1232.
14. Salvati, E. A., Robinson, H. L, and O'Dowd, T. D.. 'Southwick osteotomy for severe chronic slipped capital femoral epiphysis: results and complications.' *J Bone Joint Surg* [Am] 1980; 62A: 561.
15. Volkov, M. V., and Oganesian, O. V.: 'Restoration of function in the knee and elbow with a hinge-distractor apparatus.' *J Bone Joint Surg* [Am] 1975; 57A: 591.
16. Voss, C. L: 'Uber die methode der muskularen dekompression (temporare hangehufte).' *Int Chi. Orthop*, Paris, 1966.
17. Wilson, P. D., Jacobs, B., and Schecter, L: 'Slipped capital femoral epiphysis: An end-result study.' *J Bone Joint Surg* [Am] 1965; 47A: 1128.

Index

A

B

C

G

H

I

R

S

MIX
Papier aus verantwortungsvollen Quellen
Paper from responsible sources
FSC® C105338

If you have any concerns about our products,
you can contact us on
ProductSafety@springernature.com

In case Publisher is established outside the EU,
the EU authorized representative is:
Springer Nature Customer Service Center GmbH
Europaplatz 3, 69115 Heidelberg, Germany

Printed by Libri Plureos GmbH
in Hamburg, Germany